Granulocyte Responses to Cytokines

IMMUNOLOGY SERIES

Editor-in-chief

NOEL R. ROSE

Professor and Chairman
Department of Immunology and Infectious Diseases
The Johns Hopkins University
School of Hygiene and Public Health
Baltimore, Maryland

European Editor

ZDENEK TRNKA

Basel Institute for Immunology
Basel, Switzerland

1. Mechanisms in Allergy: Reagin-Mediated Hypersensitivity, *edited by Lawrence Goodfriend, Alec Sehon and Robert P. Orange*
2. Immuopathology: Methods and Techniques, *edited by Theodore P. Zacharia and Sidney S. Breese, Jr.*
3. Immunity and Cancer in Man: An Introduction, *edited by Arnold E. Reif*
4. *Bordetella pertussis*: Immunological and Other Biological Activities, *J. J. Munoz and R. K. Bergman*
5. The Lymphocyte: Structure and Function (in two parts), *edited by John J. Marchalonis*
6. Immunology of Receptors, *edited by B. Cinader*
7. Immediate Hypersensitivity: Modern Concepts and Development, *edited by Michael K. Bach*
8. Theoretical Immunology, *edited by George I. Bell, Alan S. Perelson, and George H. Pimbley, Jr.*
9. Immunodiagnosis of Cancer (in two parts), *edited by Ronald B. Herberman and K. Robert McIntire*
10. Immunologically Mediated Renal Diseases: Criteria for Diagnosis and Treatment, *edited by Robert T. McCluskey and Guiseppe A. Andres*
11. Clinical Immunotherapy, *edited by Albert F. LoBuglio*
12. Mechanisms of Immunity to Virus-Induced Tumors, *edited by John W. Blasecki*
13. Manual of Macrophage Methodology: Collection, Characterization, and Function, *edited by Herbert B. Herscowitz, Howard T. Holden, Joseph A. Bellanti, and Abdul Ghaffar*
14. Supressor Cells in Human Disease, *edited by James S. Goodwin*
15. Immunological Aspects of Aging, *edited by Diego Segre and Lester Smith*
16. Cellular and Molecular Mechanisms of Immunologic Tolerance, *edited by Tomáš Hraba and Milan Hašek*
17. Immune Regulation: Evolution and Biological Significance, *edited by Laurens N. Ruben and M. Eric Gershwin*
18. Tumor Immunity in Prognosis: The Role of Mononuclear Cell Infiltration, *edited by Stephen Haskill*
19. Immunopharmacology and the Regulation of Leukocyte Function, *edited by David R. Webb*

20. Pathogenesis and Immunology of Treponemal Infection, *edited by Ronald F. Schell and Daniel M. Musher*
21. Macrophage-Mediated Antibody-Dependent Cellular Cytotoxicity, *edited by Hillel S. Koren*
22. Molecular Immunology: A Textbook, *edited by M. Zouhair Atassi, Carel J. van Oss, and Darryl R. Absolom*
23. Monoclonal Antibodies and Cancer, *edited by George L. Wright, Jr.*
24. Stress, Immunity, and Aging, *edited by Edwin L. Cooper*
25. Immune Modulation Agents and Their Mechanisms, *edited by Richard L. Fenichel and Michael A. Chirigos*
26. Mononuclear Phagocyte Biology, *edited by Alvin Volkman*
27. The Lactoperoxidase System: Chemistry and Biological Significance, *edited by Kenneth M. Pruitt and Jorma O. Tenovuo*
28. Introduction to Medical Immunology, *edited by Gabriel Virella, Jean-Michel Goust, H. Hugh Fudenberg, and Christian C. Patrick*
29. Handbook of Food Allergies, *edited by James C. Breneman*
30. Human Hybridomas: Diagnostic and Therapeutic Applications, *edited by Anthony J. Strelkauskas*
31. Aging and the Immune Response: Cellular and Humoral Aspects, *edited by Edmond A. Goidl*
32. Complications of Organ Transplantation, *edited by Luis H. Toledo-Pereyra*
33. Monoclonal Antibody Production Techniques and Applications, *edited by Lawrence B. Schook*
34. Fundamentals of Receptor Molecular Biology, *Donald F. H. Wallach*
35. Recombinant Lymphokines and Their Receptors, *edited by Steven Gillis*
36. Immunology of the Male Reproductive Organs, *edited by Pierluigi E. Bigazzi*
37. The Lymphocyte: Structure and Function, *edited by John J. Marchalonis*
38. Differentiation Antigens in Lymphohemopoietic Tissues, *edited by Masayuki Miyasaka and Zdenek Trnka*
39. Cancer Diagnosis In Vitro Using Monoclonal Antibodies, *edited by Herbert Z. Kupchick*
40. Biological Response Modifiers and Cancer Therapy, *edited by J. W. Chiao*
41. Cellular Oncogene Activation, *edited by George Klein*
42. Interferon and Nonviral Pathogens, *edited by Gerald I. Byrne and Jenifer Turco*
43. Human Immunogenetics: Basic Principles and Clinical Relevance, *edited by Stephen D. Litwin, with David W. Scott, Lorraine Flaherty, Ralph A. Reisfeld, and Donald M. Marcus*
44. AIDS: Pathogenesis and Treatment, *edited by Jay A. Levy*
45. Cell Surface Antigen Thy-1: Immunology, Neurology, and Therapeutic Applications, *edited by Arnold E. Reif and Michael Schlesinger*
46. Immune Mechanisms in Cutaneous Disease, *edited by David A. Norris*
47. Immunology of Fungal Diseases, *edited by Edouard Kurstak*
48. Adoptive Cellular Immunotherapy of Cancer, *edited by Henry C. Stevenson*
49. Colony-Stimulating Factors: Molecular and Cellular Biology, *edited by T. Michael Dexter, John M. Garland, and Nydia G. Testa*
50. Introduction to Medical Immunology: Second Edition, *edited by Gabriel Virella, Jean-Michel Goust, and H. Hugh Fudenberg*
51. Tumor Suppressor Genes, *edited by George Klein*
52. Organ-Specific Autoimmunity, *edited by Pierluigi E. Bigazzi, Georg Wick, and Konrad Wicher*
53. Immunodiagnosis of Cancer: Second Edition, *edited by Ronald B. Herberman and Donald W. Mercer*

54. Systemic Autoimmunity, *edited by Pierluigi E. Bigazzi and Morris Reichlin*
55. Molecular Immunobiology of Self-Reactivity, *edited by Constantin A. Bona and Azad K. Kaushik*
56. Tumor Necrosis Factors: Structure, Function, and Mechanism of Action, *edited by Bharat B. Aggarwal and Jan Vilček*
57. Granulocyte Responses to Cytokines: Basic and Clinical Research, *edited by Ronald G. Coffey*

ADDITIONAL VOLUMES IN PREPARATION

Introduction to Medical Immunology, Third Edition, *edited by Gabriel Virella*

Granulocyte Responses to Cytokines

Basic and Clinical Research

edited by

Ronald G. Coffey

University of South Florida College of Medicine
Tampa, Florida

Marcel Dekker, Inc. New York • Basel • Hong Kong

Library of Congress Cataloging-in-Publication Data

Granulocyte responses to cytokines : basic and clinical research /
edited by Ronald G. Coffey.
p. cm.
ISBN 0-8247-8655-6 (alk. paper)
1. Granulocytes. 2. Mast cells. 3. Colony-stimulating factors
(Physiology) 4. Cytokines. I. Coffey, Ronald G.
[DNLM: 1. Cytokines--metabolism. 2. Granulocytes--drug effects.
W1 IM53K v. 57 / WH 200 G7643]
QR185.8.G73G73 1992
616.07'9--dc20
DNLM/DLC
for Library of Congress 92-18487
CIP

This book is printed on acid-free paper.

MARCEL DEKKER, INC.
270 Madison Avenue, New York, New York 10016

Current printing (last digit):
10 9 8 7 6 5 4 3 2 1

PRINTED IN THE UNITED STATES OF AMERICA

Series Introduction

At the dawn of experimental immunology, Elie Metchnikoff described phagocytosis as the fundamental process by which cells ingest foreign particles. The phenomenon not only links all animals from amoeba to man, but also accounts for the most pervasive mechanism of resistance to infection. That such a mechanism has endured through so many eons of evolution is the best evidence of its value for survival of the species.

Despite their historical and phylogenetic priority, phagocytes are too often overlooked as a critical element in protective immunity. Yet every child with chronic granulomatous disease, a metabolic defect in granulocyte function, is dramatic testimony to the role of phagocytosis in day-to-day protection against potentially pathogenic infectious agents. The disease emphasizes the importance of phagocyte metabolism in destroying ingested pathogens.

The new tools provided by modern immunology and molecular biology now permit us to analyze the processes of phagocytosis—mobilization, accumulation and activation. In the present volume, Dr. Coffey and his co-authors give an account of the critical role played by cytokines in regulating granulocytic phagocytes. It is a book that would have fascinated Metchnikoff. Contemporary readers will find it no less informative.

Noel R. Rose

Preface

Granulocytes are the first line of defense against several pathogens, parasites, and certain tumor cells. Unfortunately, granulocytes also contribute in a major way to the symptoms of inflammation, allergy, cardiovascular disease, and shock. Cytokines are polypeptides secreted by cells of the immune system and by a few other cells that provide accessory cell functions for the immune system. Cytokines are, in a sense, hormones, but usually are produced transiently and act locally. They are extremely potent, acting at picomolar concentrations (about a thousandth of the effective concentrations of most endocrine hormones).

In the mid-1980s, reports began to appear concerning the regulation by cytokines of mature granulocyte functions. Although this information has been virtually explosive, we are just beginning to understand the complex cytokine language of communication among leukocytes and other tissues. Recombinant methods for producing large quantities of cytokines have permitted, in the last few years, extensive clinical trials for a host of disorders. Granulocyte colony-stimulating factor (G-CSF) and granulocyte-macrophage colony-stimulating factor (GM-CSF) were recently licensed for clinical use in the United States (Nightingale SL, JAMA 1991; 265:2315). It therefore seemed timely to collect, under one cover, information about the basic physiological functions of granulocytes, the modification of these functions by cytokines, and the clinical experience with cytokines relevant to granulocytes.

The cell types included for discussion are neutrophils or polymorphonuclear leukocytes (PMNs), eosinophils, and both basophils and their fixed tissue counterparts, the mast cells. This book would be considerably larger if all clinically tested cytokines were to be considered, but in keeping with the focus on granulocytes, only the relevant colony-stimulating factors (CSFs) having predominant (but not exclusive) effects on these cells were selected for clinical discussion. Clinical applications of interleukins (ILs), interferons (IFNs), and other cytokines are therefore not considered.

The first part consists of nine chapters that outline the roles of neutrophils, eosinophils, basophils, and mast cells in health and disease. The basic information on the development and metabolic functions of each cell type is followed by detailed descriptions of the intracellular signaling systems invoked by a variety of stimuli. Part A concludes with a discussion of cyclic nucleotide regulation in granulocytes. This information is essential for understanding the mechanisms by which cytokines affect cellular functions. Important observations on the effects of cytokines on certain functions can be found in some of these chapters as well as the next section (see table).

The 16 chapters in Part B describe basic research on the effects of cytokines on granulocytes. The first effect to be discovered, the promotion of cell development and maturation within the bone marrow, is presented in Chapter 10, and is followed by a discussion in Chapter 11 of effects on emigration of granulocytes. This activity is a prerequisite for most of the inflammatory effects of granulocytes, also discussed in Chapters 1 and 18. Effects of specific cytokines on mature neutrophils constitute the subjects for Chapters 12–19. Rapidly developing information on eosinophil stimulation by cytokines is presented in Chapters 20 and 21, and effects on basophil and mast cell function and viability are discussed in Chapters 22 and 23. Chapter 24 describes cytokine effects on the growth of malignant cells, effects that would indicate caution in the use of cytokine therapy for certain leukemias. This part concludes with a description of effects of cytokines on granulocyte adhesion, an important process in the development of the inflammatory phase of asthma.

Part C contains four chapters that outline preclinical and clinical studies with the CSFs. Trials have been conducted for a variety of conditions ranging from genetic to drug- or virus-induced granulocytopenias and immunodeficiencies. Although the focus has been on reconstitution or expansion of blood cell numbers, the in-vitro and in-vivo studies described in the second and third parts indicate that enhanced functions as well as numbers may result from therapies involving granulocyte-stimulating CSFs. It is apparent that caution should be exercised to avoid possible effects that promote growth of certain cancers (see Chapter 24) and that exacerbate inflammatory or allergic conditions because of the use of the cytokines (Chapter 25).

The synthesis of cytokines by granulocytes is not expressly discussed in this book. However, neutrophils have recently been found to produce interleukin-1 and tumor necrosis factor, albeit in much smaller quantities than monocytes and macrophages. Mast cells produce a host of cytokines, as discussed in Chapter 7 (see Table 8). Since many of the factors produced by the cells also have actions on the cells of origin, they may be considered as autocrine regulators.

Several useful tables summarizing cytokines and their actions can be found in Chapters 5 (Table 2), 7 (Table 7), 10 (Table 1), 11 (Table 1), 18 (Table 1), 22 (Tables 1, 2), and 24 (Table 1). Hematopoiesis is illustrated in Chapters 1 (Figure 2), 10 (Figures 1 and 2 and Table 1), and 25 (Figure 1).

Our knowledge about cytokines and their actions on granulocytes is still rapidly expanding. The proliferation of basic mechanistic studies in this area is absolutely dazzling. The adoption of new therapeutic modalities based on these discoveries will surely provide some of the most exciting medical advances of the next century. This book will, we hope, provide a strong theoretical background as well as sufficient clinical information to spur these efforts.

Ronald G. Coffey

Table Cytokines and Chapters[a] in Which They Are Discussed

IL-1	5, 6, 7, 8, 10, **11, 14,** 18, **22,** 24, 25
IL-2	6, 10, **14,** 18, 25
IL-3	6, 7, 8, 10, **21, 22, 23,** 24, 25, **26**
IL-4	7, 10, 18, **20,** 24, 25
IL-5	6, 7, 10, 18, **21, 23,** 25
IL-6	10, 18
IL-7	10
IL-8	10, **11, 13,** 18, **22,** 25
IL-9	10
G-CSF	5, 10, 11, 24, **26, 27, 29**
GM-CSF	5, 6, 7, 9, 10, 11, 14, **16, 17,** 18, **21, 22, 23,** 24, **26, 28, 29**
HRA[b]	7, 22
HRF[c]	7, 22
IFN-α	5, 10, 22
IFN-β	10, **20**
IFN-r	5, 6, 7, 8, 10, 11, 14, **15, 20,** 22, 25
LIF[d]	**12**
M-CSF	10, **25, 26**
MIF[f]	7
TGF-β[g]	10, 24
TNF-$_\alpha$	5, 10, **11, 14, 18, 19,** 25
TNF-$_\beta$	10, 11, **14, 18**

[a] Numbers in boldface indicate chapters in which the cytokine is a focus for discussion.

[b] Histamine-releasing activity.

[c] Histamine-releasing factor.

[d] Leukocyte-inhibitory factor.

[e] Leukemia-inhibitory factor.

[f] Macrophage-inhibitory factor.

[g] Transforming growth factor-β.

Contents

Series Introduction (*Noel R. Rose*) iii
Preface v
Contributors xiii

Part A Functions of Granulocytes

1. Neutrophil Activation and Function in Health and Disease 1
Kent J. Johnson, James Varani, and James E. Smolen

2. The Neutrophil Respiratory Burst Mechanism 47
Linda C. McPhail, Susan L. Strum, Peter A. Leone, and Silvano Sozzani

3. Regulation of Lipoxygenase Enzymes in Leukocytes 77
Jack Y. Vanderhoek

4. Activation of Leukotriene Production in Granulocytes: Effects on Cell Activation 87
Anthony W. Ford-Hutchinson

5. G-Proteins and the Role of Second Messengers in the Regulation of the Human Neutrophil 107
Pramod M. Lad, John S. Kaptein, Ching-Kow E. Lin, Cosmas I. Kalunta, Stephen J. Scott, and David Guoqing Gu

6. Eosinophil Activation and Function in Health and Disease 137
Randa I. Abu-Ghazaleh, Hirohito Kita, and Gerald J. Gleich

7. Basophils and Mast Cells: Piecemeal Degranulation in Situ and ex Vivo: A Possible Mechanism for Cytokine-Induced Function in Disease 169
Ann M. Dvorak

8. Signal Mechanisms in the Activation of Basophils and Mast Cells 273
Donald MacGlashan, Jr.

9. Effects of Cyclic Nucleotides on Granulocytes 301
Ronald G. Coffey

Part B Effects of Cytokines: Basic Research

10. Regulatory Effects of Cytokines on Myelopoiesis 339
F. Herrmann and R. Mertelsmann

11. Cytokine-Stimulated Emigration of Granulocytes in Vivo 351
Dennis E. Van Epps

12. Physiological Studies with Human Leukocyte Inhibitory Factor 373
Larry Borish and Ross Rocklin

13. The Biology of NAP-1/IL-8, a Neutrophil-Activating Cytokine 387
Jens-M. Schröder and Enno Christophers

14. Activation of Neutrophils by Interleukins-1 and -2 and Tumor Necrosis Factors 417
Antonio Ferrante

15. Modulation of Neutrophil Functions by γ-Interferon 437
Giorgio Berton and Marco A. Cassatella

16. Activation of Neutrophils by Granulocyte-Macrophage Colony-Stimulating Factor 457
John F. DiPersio and Camille N. Abboud

17. Biochemical Effects of Human Granulocyte-Macrophage Colony-Stimulating Factor (GM-CSF) on the Human Neutrophil 485
Richard Sullivan

18. Mechanisms of Host Tissue Damage by Cytokine-Activated Neutrophils 499
Antonio Ferrante, Inge C. Kowanko, and Edna J. Bates

19. Tumor Necrosis Factor Stimulation of Neutrophils for Antitumor Activity 523
Hungyi Shau and Robert L. Roberts

20. Interferon Activation of Eosinophils 535
C. De Simone, S. Tzantzoglou, G. Santini, F. Sorice, E. Jirillo, and C. Rumi

21. Regulation of Human Eosinophil Production and Function by Interleukin-5 549
Angel F. Lopez, M. Frances Shannon, Mon-Ming Chia, Linda Park, and Mathew A. Vadas

22. Cytokine Stimulation of Human Basophil Histamine Release 573
Mary Haak-Frendscho and Allen P. Kaplan

23. Hemopoietic Growth Factors Regulate Basophil Function and Viability 587
Koichi Hirai, Yutaka Morita, and Terumasa Miyamoto

24. Effects of Hematopoietic Growth Factors on Nonhematopoietic Cells 601
Shoukat Dedhar and Connie Eaves

25. Effects of Cytokines on the Expression of Adhesion Molecules in Allergic Diseases 615
Eduardo Calderón

Part C Effects of Cytokines: Clinical Research

26. Granulocyte Colony-Stimulating Factors as Therapeutic Agents 637
Robert E. Donahue and Steven C. Clark

27. G-CSF and M-CSF: Preclinical and Clinical Results 651
F. Herrmann, A. Lindemann, and R. Mertelsmann

28. Clinical Trials of Granulocyte-Macrophage Colony-Stimulating Factor for the Treatment of Aplastic Anemia 661
Saroj Vadhan-Raj

29. Clinical Trials of Granulocyte Colony-Stimulating Factors for Treatment of Bone Marrow Depression Associated with Cancer Chemotherapy 671
Graham J. Lieschke and George Morstyn

Abbreviations 695

Index 699

Contributors

Camille N. Abboud, M.D. Hematology Unit, Department of Medicine, University of Rochester School of Medicine and Dentistry, Rochester, New York

Randa I. Abu-Ghazaleh, M.D., Ph.D. Mayo Clinic and Mayo Foundation, Rochester, Minnesota

Edna J. Bates, Ph.D. Department of Immunology, University of Adelaide and Adelaide Children's Hospital, Adelaide, South Australia

Giorgio Berton, M.D. Institute of General Pathology, University of Verona, Verona, Italy

Larry Borish, M.D. Department of Medicine, National Jewish Center for Immunology and Respiratory Diseases, University of Colorado Health Sciences Center, Denver, Colorado

Eduardo Calderón, M.D. Division of Allergy and Clinical Immunology, Department of Internal Medicine, James A. Haley V.A. Hospital and University of South Florida, Tampa, Florida

Marco A. Cassatella, M.D. Institute of General Pathology, University of Verona, Verona, Italy

Mon-Ming Chia Institute of Medical and Veterinary Science, Adelaide, South Australia

Enno Christophers, M.D. Department of Dermatology, University of Kiel, Kiel, Germany

Steven C. Clark, Ph.D. Genetics Institute, Inc., Cambridge, Massachusetts

Ronald G. Coffey, Ph.D. Department of Pharmacology and Therapeutics, University of South Florida College of Medicine, Tampa, Florida

Shoukat Dedhar, Ph.D. Department of Cancer Research, British Columbia Cancer Agency, Vancouver, British Columbia, Canada

C. De Simone, M.D. Università di L'Aquila, L'Aquila, Italy

John F. DiPersio, M.D., Ph.D. Hematology Unit, Department of Medicine, University of Rochester School of Medicine and Dentistry, Rochester, New York

Robert E. Donahue, V.M.D., S.M. Clinical Hematology Branch, National Heart, Lung, and Blood Institute, Bethesda, Maryland

Ann M. Dvorak, M.D. Departments of Pathology, Beth Israel Hospital and Harvard Medical School, Boston, Massachusetts

Connie Eaves, Ph.D. Terry Fox Research Laboratory, British Columbia Cancer Agency, Vancouver, British Columbia, Canada

Antonio Ferrante, Ph.D., M.R.C.Path. Department of Immunology, University of Adelaide and Adelaide Children's Hospital, Adelaide, South Australia

Anthony W. Ford-Hutchinson, Ph.D. Department of Pharmacology, Merck Frosst Centre for Therapeutic Research, Pointe Claire-Dorval, Quebec, Canada

Gerald J. Gleich, M.D. Department of Immunology and Division of Allergic Diseases and Internal Medicine, Mayo Clinic and Mayo Foundation, Rochester, Minnesota

David Guoqing Gu, M.S. Regional Research Laboratory, Kaiser Foundation Hospitals, Los Angeles, California

Mary Haak-Frendscho, Ph.D. Department of Cell Biology, Genentech, Inc., South San Francisco, California

F. Herrmann, M.D., Ph.D. Department of Internal Medicine I, University of Freiburg, Freiburg, Germany

Koichi Hirai, M.D., Ph.D. Department of Medicine and Physical Therapy, University of Tokyo School of Medicine, Tokyo, Japan

E. Jirillo, M.D. Università di Bari, Bari, Italy

Kent J. Johnson, M.D. Departments of Pathology and Pediatrics, The University of Michigan Medical School, Ann Arbor, Michigan

Cosmas I. Kalunta, MT (ASCP) Regional Research Laboratory, Kaiser Foundation Hospitals, Los Angeles, California

Allen P. Kaplan, M.D. Department of Medicine, State University of New York at Stony Brook, Stony Brook, New York

John S. Kaptein, Ph.D. Regional Research Laboratory, Kaiser Foundation Hospitals, Los Angeles, California

Hirohito Kita, M.D. Mayo Clinic and Mayo Foundation, Rochester, Minnesota

Inge C. Kowanko, Ph.D. Department of Immunology and University Department of Pediatrics, University of Adelaide and Adelaide Children's Hospital, Adelaide, South Australia

Pramod M. Lad, Ph.D. Regional Research Laboratory, Kaiser Foundation Hospitals, Los Angeles, California

Peter A. Leone, M.D. Section of Infectious Diseases, Department of Medicine, Wake Forest University, Bowman Gray School of Medicine, Winston-Salem, North Carolina

Graham J. Lieschke, M.B.B.S., B.Med.Sc., F.R.A.C.P. Ludwig Institute for Cancer Research, The Royal Melbourne Hospital, Victoria, Australia

Ching-Kow E. Lin, Ph.D. Regional Research Laboratory, Kaiser Foundation Hospitals, Los Angeles, California

A. Lindemann Department of Internal Medicine I, University of Freiburg, Freiburg, Germany

Angel F. Lopez, M.D., Ph.D. Institute of Medical and Veterinary Science, Adelaide, South Australia

Donald MacGlashan, Jr., M.D., Ph.D. Division of Clinical Immunology, Johns Hopkins University School of Medicine, Baltimore, Maryland

Linda C. McPhail, Ph.D. Section of Infectious Diseases, Department of Medicine, Wake Forest University, Bowman Gray School of Medicine, Winston-Salem, North Carolina

R. Mertelsmann Department of Internal Medicine I, University of Freiburg, Freiburg, Germany

Terumasa Miyamoto Department of Medicine and Physical Therapy, University of Tokyo School of Medicine, Tokyo, Japan

Yutaka Morita, M.D., Ph.D. Department of Medicine and Physical Therapy, University of Tokyo School of Medicine, Tokyo, Japan

George Morstyn, Ph.D., F.R.A.C.P. Department of Medical and Clinical Affairs, Ludwig Institute for Cancer Research, The Royal Melbourne Hospital, Victoria, Australia

Linda Park Immunex Corporation, Seattle, Washington

Robert L. Roberts, M.D.,Ph.D. Department of Pediatrics, Division of Immunology/Allergy, UCLA School of Medicine, Los Angeles, California

Ross Rocklin, M.D. Department of Clinical Research, Boehringer Ingelheim Pharma, Inc., Ridgefield, Connecticut

C. Rumi, M.D. Policlinico "A. Gemelli," Rome, Italy

G. Santini Università " La Sapienza," Rome, Italy

Jens-M. Schröder, Ph.D. Department of Dermatology, University of Kiel, Kiel, Germany

Stephen J. Scott, B.Sc. Regional Research Laboratory, Kaiser Foundation Hospitals, Los Angeles, California

M. Frances Shannon Institute of Medical and Veterinary Science, Adelaide, South Australia

Hungyi Shau, Ph.D. Department of Surgical Oncology, UCLA School of Medicine, Los Angeles, California

James E. Smolen, Ph.D. Departments of Pathology and Pediatrics, The University of Michigan Medical School, Ann Arbor, Michigan

F. Sorice, M.D. Università "La Sapienza," Rome, Italy

Silvano Sozzani, Ph.D. Istituto di Richerche Farmacologiche Mario Negri, Milan, Italy

Susan L. Strum, M.S. Section of Infectious Diseases, Department of Medicine, Wake Forest University, Bowman Gray School of Medicine, Winston-Salem, North Carolina

Richard Sullivan, M.D. Department of Medicine, Baylor College of Medicine, Houston, Texas

S. Tzantzoglou, Ph.D. Università "La Sapienza," Rome, Italy

Mathew A. Vadas, M.D., Ph.D. Institute of Medical and Veterinary Science, Adelaide, South Australia

Saroj Vadhan-Raj, M.D. Department of Clinical Immunology and Biological Therapy, University of Texas, M.D. Anderson Cancer Center, Houston, Texas

Dennis E. Van Epps, Ph.D. Applied Cellular Biology Center, Applied Sciences Division, Baxter Healthcare Corporation, Round Lake, Illinois

Jack Y. Vanderhoek, Ph.D. Department of Biochemistry and Molecular Biology, The George Washington University School of Medicine and Health Sciences, Washington, D.C.

James Varani, Ph.D. Departments of Pathology and Pediatrics, The University of Michigan Medical School, Ann Arbor, Michigan

A

Functions of Granulocytes

1

Neutrophil Activation and Function in Health and Disease

KENT J. JOHNSON, JAMES VARANI, and JAMES E. SMOLEN
The University of Michigan Medical School, Ann Arbor, Michigan

I. INTRODUCTION

The neutrophil is a highly specialized type of white blood cell or leukocyte whose function in its mature form is the ingestion and killing of invading bacteria and other microorganisms. Because of this specialized function, the neutrophil acts as the first line of defense against invading pathogens and since the time of Metchnikoff it has been appreciated that the neutrophil is the primary infiltrating cell present in the cellular phase of the acute inflammatory response. Of interest is the fact that even during the time of Metchnikoff there were disagreements on whether the neutrophil was harmful as well as protective to the host (1). The neutrophil is the most numerous of leukocytes in the blood and normally constitutes 50–70% of the total. However, during pathologic conditions such as bacterial infections, their number in the circulation can increase dramatically. This increased number of circulating neutrophils is called leukocytosis (1,2).

The nomenclature of neutrophils is somewhat confusing, with many different names having been used to describe this cell. The neutrophil is one of a group of cells in the blood called white blood cells or leukocytes because they do not contain hemoglobin (3). Leukocytes can be further divided into two groups based on whether or not cytoplasmic granules are present. As shown in Figure 1, the neutrophil has distinct cytoplasmic granules which has led to another term for the neutrophil: i.e., the granulocytes, with the cells differentiated by the staining characteristics of the cell granules. The neutrophil granules characteristically do not stain with the Wright stain, hence the name neutrophil. In some species, such as the rabbit, the neutrophil granules will stain. Hence the term heterophil is also used occasionally (4,5).

Neutrophils are also characterized by their distinctive nucleus. As illustrated in Figure 1, the nucleus is polymorphous and usually consists of three to five sausage-shaped masses of chromatin connected by fine threads. This variable or polymorphous shape of

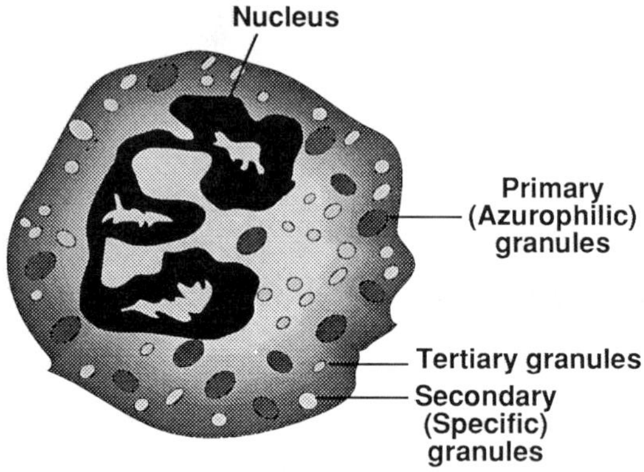

Figure 1 Drawing of a mature human neutrophil to illustrate the characteristic polymorphous nucleus and cytoplasmic granules.

the nucleus has led to the neutrophil also being called a polymorphonuclear leukocyte, PMN, or poly for short (6). Finally, since the neutrophil is capable of phagocytosis, it has also been called a phagocyte. For the purposes of this chapter, the term neutrophil will be used except where indicated.

II. NEUTROPHIL DIFFERENTIATION AND MATURATION

Most mature blood cells in the blood, including neutrophils, are very short lived and thus need to be constantly replaced. For example, studies have suggested that 4×10^8 cells/h are replaced (7).

Neutrophils, like other cells of the hematopoietic system, are derived from the bone marrow. As shown in Figure 2, there are three major steps in the neutrophil differentiation process leading to the formation of a mature neutrophil, which are described in several recent reviews (7–12). The initial differentiation process involves the proliferation of the pleuripotential stem cell, which is felt to be the common precursor for all blood cells. The concept that a single stem cell can give rise to myeloid and erythroid cells is supported by the use of chromosomal markers, marrow transplants in mice, and the clonality of cells in leukemia (11,12). The second stage consists of progenitor cells, which at this point are committed to a given hematopoietic linkage. These cells proliferate clonally but may be derived from more than one cell and require several growth factors as described below (11–14). The third and final stage of maturation consists of precursor cells which can be identified morphologically and cytochemically as to cell lineage—in this case, granulocytic (8,9). During this last neutrophil stage, proliferation and maturation result in the successive production of morphologically distinct cells called myeloblasts. Further maturation occurs without cell division. Subsequent maturation leads to the band cell or juvenile neutrophil with its segmented nucleus (Figure 2). This final maturation sequence from the myeloblast to the mature neutrophil is thought to take around 14 days. Mature neutrophils are then released into the blood, where their circulating half-life is only around 7 h. At that time they then enter tissues for 1–4 days and their ultimate fate is unknown, although it is felt that many are excreted into the gastrointestinal tract as well as being destroyed by the

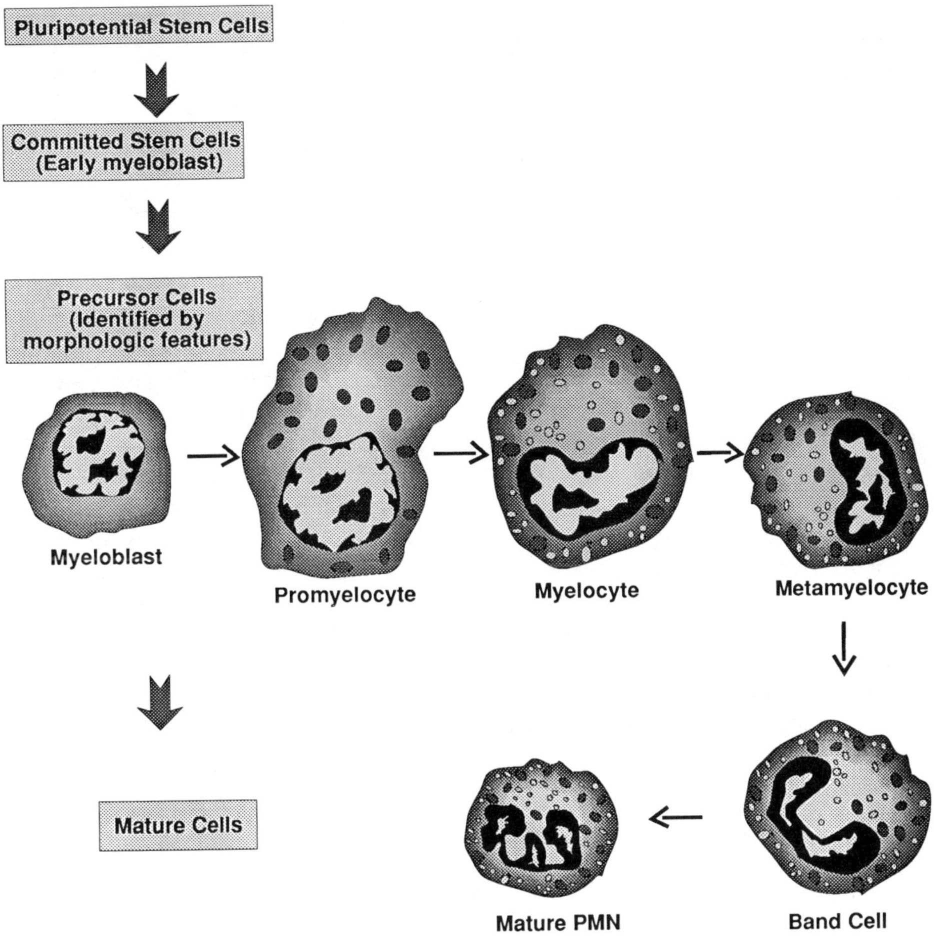

Figure 2 Differentiation and maturation of the neutrophil in the bone marrow. Hematopoiesis occurs as a result of the successive clonal proliferation of three classes of cell. The final class consists of precursor cells which can be identified morphologically.

spleen (15). The number of neutrophils formed by the marrow is very high due to their short life in the circulation, with as many as 10 billion neutrophils being released from the bone marrow daily.

The differentiation and maturation of hematopoietic cells in the bone marrow is controlled by several glycoproteins and peptide growth factors (7,16). There are several of these growth factors involved in the differentiation and maturation of neutrophils and macrophages. These growth factors are called colony-stimulating factors (CSFs) because of their ability to stimulate colony formation of maturing hematopoietic cells in tissue culture. As described by Metcalf (16), five colony-stimulating growth factors have been identified which regulate neutrophil and macrophage hemopoiesis (Table 1).

These growth factors act primarily to induce proliferation of the neutrophil/or macrophage-committed progenitor cells. Granulocyte-macrophage colony-stimulating

Table 1 Growth Factors Implicated in Granulocyte Differentiation and Maturation

1. Granulocyte colony-stimulating factor (G-CSF)
2. Granulocyte-macrophage colony-stimulating factor (GM-CSF)
3. Macrophage colony-stimulating factor (M-CSF)
4. Multipotential colony-stimulating factor (multi-CSF) (IL-3)
5. Interleukin-6 (IL-6)

Source: From Ref. 16.

factor (GM-CSF) and multipotential colony-stimulating factor (multi-CSF or IL-3) induce the proliferation of granulocytes and macrophages, whereas granulocyte colony-stimulating factor (G-CSF) and interleukin-6 (IL-6) affect primarily granulocyte proliferation. Macrophage colony-stimulating factor (M-CSF) induces primarily macrophage proliferation (16–18). These CSFs have multiple biological effects on these cells rather than just proliferation. They also enhance survival of the cells by stabilizing the cell membrane, inducing cellular differentiation and maturation, as well as stimulating the functional activity of mature cells (16). These growth factors are produced by a wide variety of cells, including monocytes and macrophages, lymphocytes, fibroblasts, and endothelial cells, and GM-CSF has been identified in biological fluids and tissues (7,19,20). The exception to this is multi-CSF or IL-3, which is produced only by the T-lymphocyte. In addition to the localized production of CSFs in the bone marrow by macrophages and fibroblasts, the monocyte/macrophage-derived cytokines TNF and IL-1 stimulate endothelial cell, fibroblast, and lymphocyte production of these factors (21,22).

There are a number of factors which inhibit or modulate hemopoiesis. These factors includes those agents which can inhibit the proliferation of progenitor cells directly, such as prostaglandins, interferons, chemotactic peptides, TNF, and transforming growth factor B. Other modulatory or inhibitory agents such as lactoferrin inhibit the release of GM-CSF from monocytes (23–25). Thus the regulation of the proliferation and differentiation of neutrophils in the bone marrow depends on a complex interrelationship among various stimulatory and inhibitory factors produced locally in the marrow as well as systemically by several different types of cells. Central to this process is the stimulation of monocytes and macrophages by agents such as bacteria or viruses which release cytokines (IL-1, TNF), which in turn induce the release of the colony-stimulating factors from the other cell types (26).

III. CONSTITUENTS OF THE NEUTROPHIL AND THEIR BIOLOGICAL ACTIVITY

Since neutrophils are designed to function as the first line of defense against invading microorganisms, it is only logical that they have developed potent toxins that are capable of destroying these invading pathogens. In fact, the neutrophil has developed two primary ways to accomplish this task. The first involves the release of granule constituents and the second involves the generation of reactive oxygen products produced by a cell membrane-associated enzyme system unique to phagocyte cells. In the following discussion we will describe the biologically active constituents of both of these systems and their postulated roles in the destruction of invading pathogens, as well as their role in the development of neutrophil-mediated tissue injury.

A. Neutrophil Granules

As described above, cytoplasmic granules as well as the distinctive polymorphous nucleus characterize the neutrophil, and the granules contain several potent proteolytic enzymes as well as other agents which function to aid in the killing of ingested organisms. Three major types of granules have been described, with over 20 granule constituents having been identified.

1. Primary (Azurophilic) Granules

As illustrated in Table 2, primary or azurophilic granules are so named because they are the first to appear during hemopoiesis. This granule is correctly called a primary lysosome in that it contains acid hydolytic enzymes which when fused with the phagocytic vacuole becomes a secondary lysosome.

Several types of hydrolases as well as other active biologic agents are present in the primary granule. The first group of hydrolytic enzymes are the acidic hydrolases. As the name implies, these are hydrolytic enzymes which have optimal activity at acidic pH. In this group are a series of acidic proteases—specifically, cathepsin B and D. These proteases, which are differentiated by their specificity for certain synthetic substrates, have been described as capable of degrading fibronectin and other extracellular matrix glycoproteins including basement membranes. In addition, they are capable of activating leukokinin involved in kinin production, and cathepsin D has also been described as being bactericidal (27–29). Because of their optimal activity at acidic pH, their role in tissue injury has been questioned (29).

A number of other acid hydolases are present in the primary granule which have specific enzymatic glycosidase functions as well as generalized hydrolytic properties. Thus, for example, β-glucuronidase catalyses the hydrolysis of β-D-glucuronide to D-glucuronic acid, β-glucosaminidase catalyzes the hydrolysis of D-glucosamine to D-glucose, and β-galactosidase catalyzes the hydrolysis of β-D-galactoside to D-galactose (30,31). These enzymes have proven to be useful markers of primary granule release during such events as phagocytosis and chemotaxis (32,33).

The main proteinase activity in the primary granule is the result of serine proteinases, which have optimal activity at neutral pH and are therefore called neutral proteinases. The most significant is elastase, but cathepsin G is also in this category. Cathepsin G is highly cationic, and this is thought to be responsible for its ability to act as a bactericidal agent (34). It does degrade extracellular matrix proteins such as elastin and collagen, but much less efficiently than elastase (35). Finally, cathepsin G can cleave proteins, including complement and immunoglobulins, and it has also been described as being capable of cleaving angiotensin (36).

The main neutrophil proteinase activity present in the human neutrophil is elastase, which is present in concentrations as high as 3 pg/cell (37). The name elastase refers to enzymes which can degrade elastin, and in the human neutrophil it refers to a series of five isozymes present in the primary granule (38). In terms of biological activity, elastase has been described as having a multiplicity of effects (37–43). In addition to degrading elastin, it degrades virtually all other extracellular matrix proteins. For example, it actively degrades collagens, both fibrillar as well as nonfibrillar (40). It also cleaves a wide variety of plasma proteins, including immunoglobulins and complement proteins (42), and has been described as being directly cytotoxic to some types of eukaryotic cells (43). Interestingly enough, it does not appear to be particularly bactericidal by itself, but rather potentiates myeloperoxidase-dependent killing of bacteria

Table 2 Neutrophil Granule Constituents and Their Biologic Activity

Granules	Biological activity
Primary (azurophilic) granules	
Acid hydrolases	
Cathepsins B and D	Activate leukokinins, hydrolyze proteoglycans Hydrolyze basement membrane, bactericidal (cathepsin D)
β-Glucosaminidase N-acetyl-glucuronidase β-Glucuronidase α-Mannosidases	Hydrolyze several biochemicals
Neutral proteinases	
Cathepsin G	Bactericidal, highly cationic ? Degrades connective tissue Inactivates bradykinin Activates angiotensin Cleaves proteins (complement and immunoglobulins)
Elastase	Degrades collagen, elastin, and proteoglycans (extracellular matrix) Cleaves plasma proteins (I, complement, etc.) Not bactericidal (potentiates MPO killing of bacteria) Cytotoxic
Myeloperoxidase (MPO)	Oxidative bactericidal effects
Cationic proteins	
Defensins Bactericidal/permeability increasing protein (BPI)	Destroys bacteria and other microorganisms
Lysozyme	Bactericidal—hydrolyses bacterial cell wall proteoglycans
Secondary (specific) granules	
Lysozyme	Bactericidal—hydrolyzes cell wall proteoglycan
Collagenase	Metalloproteinase activated by oxidants Hydrolyzes collagens type I, II, and III
Lactoferrin	Iron chelator—prevents iron-dependent oxidant formation (·OH) Cell adhesion
Vitamin B_{12} binding protein	Binds B_{12}—function unknown
C5a-cleaving enzyme	Produces chemotactic peptide C5a
Plasminogen activator	Neutral protease that activates plasminogen to form plasmin
Cytochrome b_{558}	Associated with the respiratory burst
Membrane receptors	
FMLP receptor	Chemotactic peptide
C3b1 receptor	Modulates cell motility
Laminin receptor	Cell adhesion
Alkaline phosphatase	Hydrolyzes phosphoric acid esters at alkaline pH (9–10); increased levels in acute infections; decrease levels in chronic myelogenous leukemia
Tertiary Granules	
Gelatinase	Metalloproteinase activated by oxidants—hydrolyzes denatured collagen (gelatin); degrades mature collagen (types IV, V, and XI)
Membrane receptors	
Laminin C3b1	Cell motility and adhesiveness

(44). As will be described later, elastase is felt to play an important role in tissue inflammation by virtue of its ability to degrade most types of extracellular matrix.

Myeloperoxidase (MPO) refers to the neutrophilic peroxidase enzyme which, like other peroxidase enzymes in the body, catalyzes the conversion of hydrogen peroxide to various products. Myeloperoxidase is present in very high concentrations in the azurophilic granule, with studies suggesting that this enzyme makes up as much as 5% of the dry weight of the cell (44). The purified enzyme is an intense green color, and the greenish color of pus is due to this enzyme (45). Myeloperoxidase is detected by the peroxidase stain, and this has proved useful in the diagnosis of granulocytic leukemias (46).

The presence of large amounts of myeloperoxidase certainly suggests that this enzyme is important in neutrophil function. In fact, myeloperoxidase does appear to be important in the killing of ingested bacteria by the neutrophil. By itself, myeloperoxidase has little effect. However, when combined with H_2O_2 and a halide such as chloride, potent oxidant bactericidal activity is generated (47–49). As shown in Figure 3, organisms ingested by the neutrophil activate the cells respiratory burst with the formation H_2O_2. This H_2O_2 combines with myeloperoxidase to form an H_2O_2-halide-generated oxidant which is toxic to bacteria, virus, fungi, and protozoans (47–49). Most of the myeloperoxidase interaction occurs in the phagolysosome, but significant myeloperoxidase is released into extracellular fluids and outside the cell. Not only is myeloperoxidase involved in killing of pathogens, it has also been implicated in tissue injury, as will be described later. The importance of myeloperoxidase as a bactericidal agent is

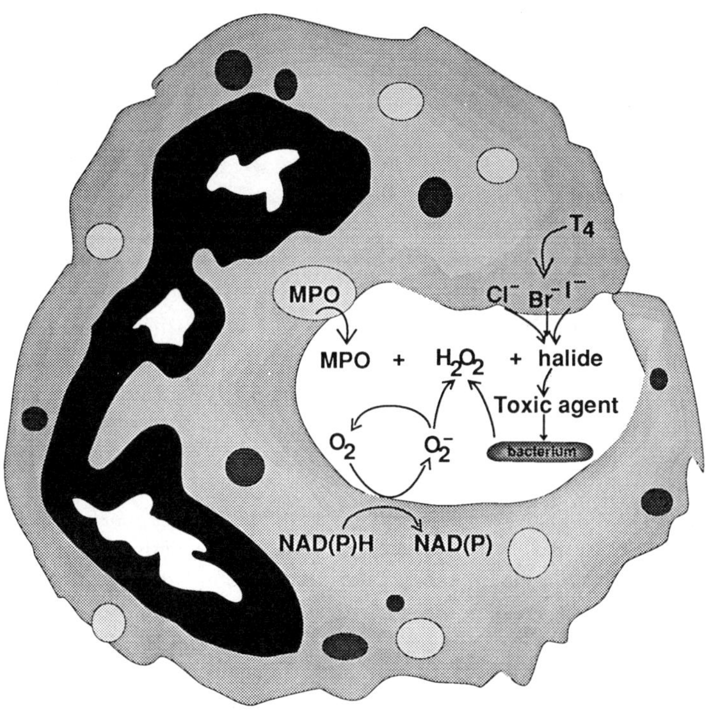

Figure 3 Myeloperoxidase-oxidant bactericidal effects in the neutrophil phagolysosome.

illustrated by individuals who have a genetic deficiency of the enzyme. These patients have impaired killing of some types of bacteria and fungi (50,51).

Lysozyme (muramidase) is a small (around 14,500 MW), very cationic enzyme which is widely distributed in the body, including in the azurophilic and especially the secondary granules of neutrophils (52). It is bactericidal for some types of bacteria such as Gram-positive organisms by virtue of its ability to hydrolyze bacterial cell walls. However, many bacteria, including most of the Gram-negative organisms, are resistant to this enzyme (53). Since most pathogenic bacteria are resistant to the effects of lysozyme, it has been suggested that it serves in vivo to clear up cellular debris (54).

Finally, the primary granule contains a series of five to seven cationic proteins in addition to those previously described, all of which have potent bactericidal activity. The best described of these proteins include the defensins, as well as a single protein called bactericidal/permeability-increasing protein or BPI (55–59). These proteins bind to electrostatically negatively charged surface sites of Gram-negative bacteria with a subsequent breakdown of the permeability barrier of the bacteria (59).

2. *Secondary (Specific) Granules*

Secondary or specific granules are synthesized later than azurophilic granules, during the myelocyte stage of neutrophil development; as the name implies, they are unique for the neutrophil (60). In the mature neutrophil they are twice as numerous as the azurophilic granules and can be distinguished morphologically as well as histochemically by virtue of the fact that they are peroxidase negative (60,61). They are also different from the azurophilic granules in that they are not lysosomes, and the contents of these granules are designed primarily for secretion rather than internal use, even though significant release of azurophilic granule contents occurs as well (36,37,62). The contents of the secondary granules are given in Table 2. Lysozyme, described previously as a component of the azurophilic granule, is also present in much higher levels in the secondary granule (54).

Lactoferrin is an 80,000-MW glycoprotein which functions to avidly bind iron. It is present only in the specific granules of neutrophils although, like other granule contents, it is released extracellularly during cell activation (63,64). Its precise role has yet to be determined. However, in nonsaturated or apo form it has bactericidal as well as bacteriostatic effects on some types of bacteria, presumably by removing iron from use by the bacteria (65). Depending on the degree of iron saturation of the lactoferrin, it has been described as either enhancing or inhibiting the formation of the iron-dependent hydroxyl radical (66). In fact, studies from our laboratory have shown a protective effect of apolactoferrin on tissue injury, suggesting that the protein can also potentially act as an important protective screen against oxygen radical-induced cell injury (67). It has also been implicated as being an important adhesion protein for neutrophils (68).

The secondary granule also contains a neutrophil collagenase. Collagenase, like gelatinase, which is located in the tertiary granule, is a metalloproteinase and is present and secreted in a latent, inactive form (41,69,70). Recent studies suggest that these metalloenzymes are activated by chlorinated oxidants such as hypochlorous acid (41), and once activated, these enzymes can cleave many of the different types of collagen. For example, collagenase can cleave types I, II, and III collagens, whereas gelatinase can degrade types II, V, and XI collagens (69,70). This oxidant-dependent activation of proteases is potentially of great significance in the pathogenesis of neutrophil-induced tissue injury. This will be addressed in greater detail later.

Other enzymes present in the secondary granules include a plasminogen activator and an enzyme that cleaves the complement component C5 to form C5a, which is a potent neutrophil chemoattractant (71,72).

The secondary granules also appear to be involved in cell adhesion, motility, and cell activation. For example, the granule contents not only have the ability to form C5a, but their plasma membranes possess complement receptors for C5a and the formal peptide (f-Met-Leu-Phe) chemotactic factors as well as laminin receptors (73–75). In addition, the specific granules contain cytochrome b_{558} and an FAD flavoprotein (75). These granule components appear to translocate to the cell membrane and are involved in cell motility (complement receptors) and activation of the respiratory burst (75,76). In support of this hypothesis, patients whose neutrophils lack specific granules have defective neutrophil chemotaxis and cell adherence and are less efficient at killing of bacteria (75).

3. *Tertiary Granules*

As shown in Table 2, there are granules which are not well characterized that have the secretory characteristics of secondary granules (77). These granules are called tertiary, and the primary constituent of these granules is gelatinase, which, as described above along with collagenase, is a metalloenzyme activated by oxidants (41). It is capable of cleaving some types of intact collagen, as well as denatured collagen or gelatin (77,78). The membranes of the tertiary granules also contain factors which are involved in neutrophil function, in this case complement C3bi receptors, which may be important in neutrophil adherence to target cells (79).

B. Neutrophil Oxidant Formation

In addition to granule constituents, neutrophils are capable of producing another group of powerful bactericidal agents: reactive oxygen products; these agents are powerful oxidizing species (oxidants) which are formed as intermediate products in the reduction of molecular oxygen to water. All cells produce oxidants in small amounts, and oxidant formation occurs during many normal biological functions of the cell, including mitochondrial electron transport and during the formation of cyclooxygenase products (80–82). However, neutrophils and other phagocytic cells possess an additional enzyme system to generate high levels of oxidants; the respiratory burst NADP/NADPH oxidase enzyme that is located in the plasma membrane and is activated when the cell is stimulated (83,84). The details of the activation of this enzyme system will be covered in detail in Chapter 2. For our purposes, in terms of neutrophil function, this oxidase system produces several highly reactive oxidant species which have potent biological effects. As shown in Figure 4, the primary oxidants formed include the superoxide anion (O_2^-), hydrogen peroxide (H_2O_2), as well as metabolic products of H_2O_2. As shown in Figure 5, the first of these involves the reaction of O_2^- with H_2O_2 in the presence of iron, which results in the formation of the hydroxyl radical (·OH) via the chemical reaction called the modified Haber Weiss or Fenton reaction. Lactoferrin, the iron-binding protein from the secondary granule, can either enhance or inhibit the formation of the hydroxyl radical, depending on the degree of iron saturation (85,86). The other main way that H_2O_2 is metabolized occurs when a peroxidase enzyme such as myeloperoxidase reacts with H_2O_2 in the presence of a halide to form a hypohalous acid, of which hypochlorous acid (HOCl) is the most common (87) (Figure 5).

The primary function of these oxidants is to kill organisms phagocytized by the neutrophil, with the formation of these oxidants presumably being responsible for most of

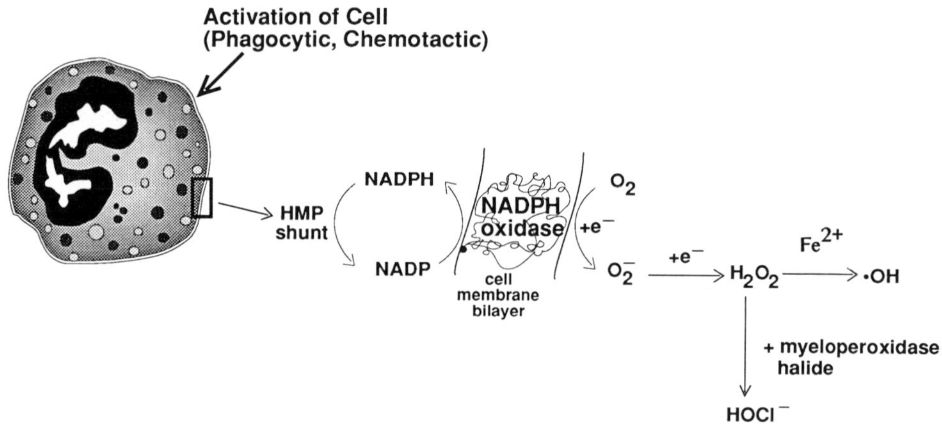

Figure 4 Membrane-associated NADP/NADPH oxidase enzyme system and its production of reactive oxygen products.

the killing of bacteria by these cells. The oxidants most responsible for the bactericidal effects include H_2O_2 and/or its metabolic products HOCI or ·OH (88,89). The importance of these oxidants in the killing of bacteria by neutrophils is illustrated by patients who have chronic granulomatous disease of childhood (CGD). The neutrophils from these patients lack the NADPH oxidase system, and these patients are highly susceptible to bacterial infections. Their neutrophils in vitro show a markedly decreased ability to kill bacteria (90,91).

The production of oxidants by neutrophils and other phagocytic cells is not without risk in that the extreme reactivity of these oxidants, particularly the hydroxyl radical, is capable of damaging host eukaryotic cells as well as prokaryotic bacteria (92–94). The

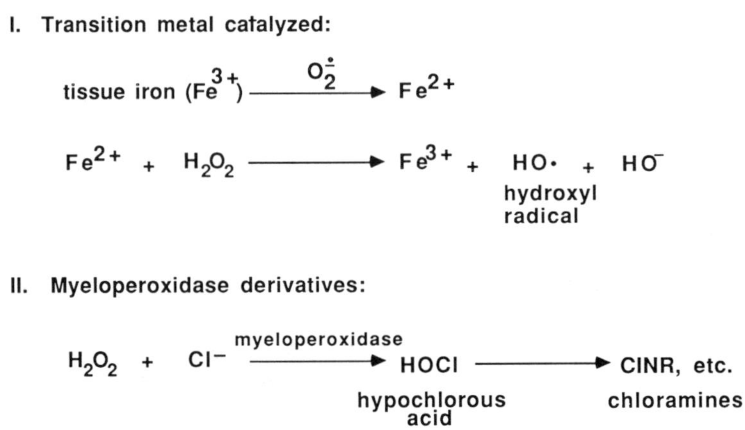

Figure 5 Metabolic reduction products of H_2O_2.

exact way in which the oxidants exert their cytotoxic effects has not been clarified, but several intracellular targets have been identified. Perhaps the most important are the toxic effects of oxidants on nucleic acids. It has long been known that radiation cytotoxicity is oxidant mediated—specifically, ·OH—and the primary target appears to be DNA, with nucleic acid-base modifications and strand breaks identified (80,95,96). Damage by other agents, such as hydroxide and some types of drug-induced injury, are felt to be mediated by similar mechanisms (80).

Other primary intracellular targets include membrane lipids as well as many proteins. Oxidants react with the cholesterol and fatty acids of cell membranes and form lipid peroxides (97,98). The significance of this lipid peroxidation in terms of cytotoxicity is unclear (99). However, some studies report that lipid peroxidation results in an alteration in the structural integrity of the cell membrane with a loss of normal ionic gradients and an influx of Na^+ and Ca^{2+}. The Na^+ influx leads to cell swelling because of increased intracellular H_2O, and the Ca^{2+} influx induces the formation of Ca^{2+}-dependent phospholipases and kinases which augment the injury (100,101). Finally, proteins are susceptible to oxidant attack, and protein polymerization can result from oxidation of amino acid residues and cross-linking of peptides (102,103). Even though oxidants are not felt to cleave peptide bonds, they alter the biological activity of some proteins as well as rendering the protein more susceptible to proteolysis (104).

Since oxidants are capable of causing injury to cells, several antioxidants are normally present to protect the cells from injury, as shown in Table 3. Vitamins E and C have been identified as antioxidants, and both are present in the cell. Vitamin E, in particular, is highly lipophilic and is present in cell membranes in high concentrations, where it acts to prevent lipid peroxidation (105).

The major way that a cell protects itself from oxidant injury is by the use of antioxidant enzyme systems. The primary way that O_2^- is removed from cells is by the

Table 3 Cellular Defenses Against Oxidant Injury

I. Vitamins
  A. Vitamin E (a-tocopherol)
  B. Vitamin C

II. Enzymes
  A. Superoxide dismutase (SOD)
  B. Catalase
  C. Glutathione (GSH) peroxidases

III. Iron chelators
  A. Lactoferrin
  B. Transferrin

IV. Scavengers
  A. Ceruloplasmin
  B. Other cell components
    1. Amino acids
    2. Unsaturated fatty acids
    3. Sugars

enzyme superoxide dismutase (SOD). SOD, first described by McCord and Fridovich, is actually a group of three metalloenzymes that catalyze the conversion of O_2^- to H_2O_2 and O_2 (106). Two enzyme systems appear to be primarily responsible for metabolizing H_2O_2. The first is catalase, a heme enzyme present in the cytosol and organelles: and the second is glutathione peroxidase, which is a cytosolic enzyme. Both function to convert H_2O_2 to H_2O and O_2. Of the two enzymes, glutathione peroxidase appears to play a more important role in protecting the cell against H_2O_2-mediated injury (107–109). Other agents which have been shown to have antioxidant activity include ceruloplasmin, which is responsible for the majority of antioxidant activity in the blood, and materials classified as "scavengers" of oxidants because of their ability to transfer electrons between themselves and oxidant species such as ·OH. Examples include mannitol, ethanol, dimethylthioureau (DMTU), and dimethyl sulfoxide (DMSO). Finally, iron chelators such as lactoferrin and transferrin have been found to be protection against oxidant-induced cell injury, presumably by their binding of iron and thus preventing the formation of ·OH via the iron-dependent Fenton reaction. Generally, the naturally occurring enzymes SOD, catalase, and iron chelators such as desferoxamine are more effective at protecting cells from oxidant injury (110). In this regard, there is also evidence that increasing the levels of antioxidant enzymes in the cell such as glutathione peroxidase renders the cell more resistant to killing.

In summary, neutrophils as well as other phagocytic cells generate high levels of reactive oxygen products when stimulated. These oxidants have potent bactericidal effects, but they are also toxic to the cells of the host, with many potential targets in the cells have been identified. Protective mechanisms have evolved to protect cells from free radical injury, but under certain conditions such as inflammation these defense mechanisms can be overwhelmed and tissue injury occurs.

IV. NEUTROPHIL ACTIVATION

The way in which a neutrophil is activated by diverse stimuli to release its granule contents or generate reactive oxygen products is referred to as stimulus-response coupling. The current model for the stimulus-response coupling pathway in the neutrophil is thought to involve the sequence of intracellular events shown in Figure 6. Evidence for each event in the stimulus-response coupling pathway will be considered separately.

A. Receptors and Stimuli

Neutrophil responses can be evoked by a variety of particulate and soluble stimuli. Opsonized particles, immune complexes, and chemotactic factors produced during the inflammatory process activate neutrophils by binding to specific cell surface receptors. Of the neutrophil chemotactic receptors, the N-formyl peptide receptor is the best characterized. N-formyl peptides, the synthetic analogs of bacterial products, induce a variety of neutrophil responses and have been extensively employed as activating stimuli. Specific receptors for the chemotactic peptide, N-formyl-methionyl-leucyl-phenylalanine (fMet-Leu-Phe), have been identified on the neutrophil surface (111–113), and binding of the formyl peptide to its receptor correlates with its ability to induce chemotaxis and degranulation (114). The fMet-Leu-Phe receptor is stereospecific (114), appears to have both high- and low-affinity binding sites (115–117), and has an apparent molecular weight of 50–70 kDa (118–121). An intracellular

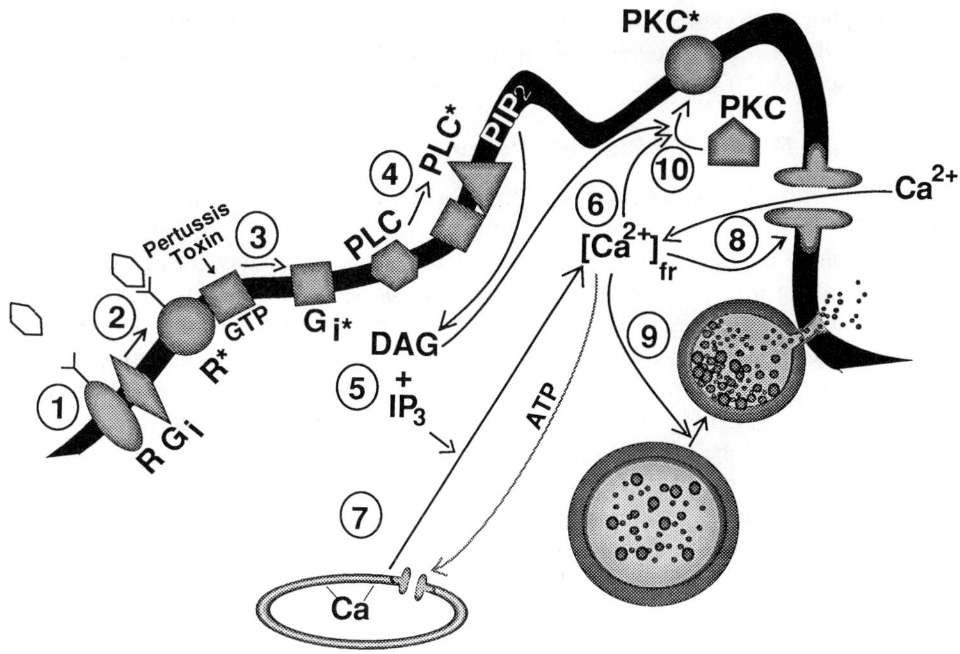

Figure 6 Model of stimulus response coupling in the neutrophil leading to degranulation. The signal transduction mechanisms alluded to in the text are illustrated schematically in this figure. The resting state of the cell is represented in the lower left side (1) by an unoccupied cell surface receptor [R] coupled with an inactive G_i-like guanine nucleotide binding protein [G_i]. Binding of a specific ligand to this receptor (2) leads to conformation changes in this protein [R*] and activation of the accompanying G-protein [square figure]. Activation of this G-protein is blocked by pertussis toxin and involves the binding of GTP, leading to an activated G-protein [G_i^*]. This G-protein (3) then interacts with a polyphosphatidylinositol-specific phospholipase C [PLC, hexagon] leading to the activation of this enzyme [PLC*, triangle] (4). PLC* cleaves an endogenous lipid, namely, phosphatidylinositol bisphosphate [PIP_2], yielding diacylglycerol [DAG] and inositol trisphosphate [IP_3] (5). IP_3 is known to liberate calcium from bound intracellular stores (7), leading to a rise in intracellular free calcium $[Ca^{2+}]_{fr}$ (6). This increase in intracellular Ca_{fr}^{2+} is augmented by an influx from the extracellular space [right side of figure] (8). DAG, in consort with elevated Ca_{fr}^{2+}, activates protein kinase C [PKC, hexagon] (10), leading to translocation of this enzyme to membranous sites [PKC*]. Elevations in intracellular free calcium alone are known to induce the secretion of granule constituents to the extracellular space [lower right side] by fusion of granule membranes with the plasma membranes (9). This process is augmented by the presence of GTP. These transduction mechanisms are discussed in greater detail in the text.

location has also been suggested for the fMet-Leu-Phe receptor, since neutrophil activation results in enhanced fMet-Leu-Phe binding in normal cells (122), but not in egranulated neutrophil cytoplasts (123). These receptors have been identified on the membranes of specific granules (124) and are biochemically similar to those on the plasma membrane (125,126), suggesting that they are mobilized to the cell surface following stimulation and may thus serve a modulatory role. The receptor occurs in several forms, associated with guanine nucleotide-binding proteins (G-proteins) (127–131) and the cytoskeleton (127,132) [see (133,134) for reviews].

Neutrophils also express receptors for a wide variety of other agonists. However, the N-formylated peptide receptor is archetypal, and space limitations preclude a more detailed discussion of the other varieties.

B. Guanine Nucleotide Binding Proteins

Recent data strongly suggest that receptors for the chemotactic stimuli fMet-Leu-Phe, C5a, LTB_4, and PAF are coupled to cellular responses through a guanine nucleotide-binding protein similar to the inhibitory protein, G_i, of the adenylate cyclase system. Evidence linking a G-protein to these receptors has been provided by studies demonstrating that guanine nucleotides can regulate the affinity of the fMet-Leu-Phe, PAF, and LTB_4 receptors (135–140). A high-affinity GTPase located in neutrophil plasma membranes is stimulated by these same receptor-mediated stimuli, but not by the phorbol ester, PMA (141–144). This enzymatic activity is likely to be involved in terminating the activation of the guanine nucleotide-binding protein.

Studies using pertussis toxin have proven instrumental in the understanding of G-protein involvement in the proposed stimulus-response coupling pathway. Pertussis toxin ADP-ribosylates the alpha-subunit of G_i of the adenylate cyclase system and also a 40,000 to 41,000-Da protein in neutrophil plasma membranes (145–152). Initial studies demonstrated a strong correlation between the ability of the toxin to catalyze the ADP-ribosylation of the membrane protein and to affect cellular responses initiated by surface receptors. However, pertussis toxin did not alter intracellular cyclic AMP levels, suggesting that the G-protein involved was distinct from G_i of the adenylate cyclase system (145,150). More recently, purification and characterization of a guanine nucleotide-binding protein in neutrophils have shown that this protein differs both structurally and immunochemically from previously reported guanine nucleotide-binding proteins (148,149,151–158).

Not only can neutrophil responses be abolished by pertussis toxin, but stable guanine nucleotides can induce secretion in their own right as well as enhance Ca^{2+}-induced secretion in permeabilized neutrophils (159,160). While pertussis toxin inhibits fMet-Leu-Phe-induced secretion from intact cells, secretion in response to guanine nucleotides, PMA, and Ca^{2+} is not inhibited in the permeabilized cell system, suggesting that a second G-protein may be involved at more distal sites in secretion (160).

C. Phospholipases

A membrane-associated phosphoinositide-specific (161) phospholipase is activated upon stimulation with chemotactic stimuli. In particular, phospholipase C hydrolyzes phosphatidylinositol-4,5-bisphosphate (PIP_2) and phosphatidyl inositol-4-monophosphate (PIP_1) (162–166) to the putative second messenger products inositol 1,4,5-trisphosphate (IP_3) and 1,2-diacylglycerol (DAG) (162–164). In permeabilized neutrophils, IP_3 has been shown to interact with a specific intracellular receptor (167) and stimulate the release of Ca^{2+} (168,169).

It is believed that guanine nucleotide-binding proteins are involved in the receptor-mediated activation of phospholipase C (170). Chemotactic factors stimulate reductions in PIP_2 levels and increase inositol phosphate levels (171,172). These changes are not observed if cells are pretreated with pertussis toxin (172,173). Fluoride treatment, which stimulates G-proteins, also directly stimulates the accumulation of inositol lipids

(174), while stimuli which do not interact with cell surface receptors, such as PMA and A23187, do not induce IP_3 formation (163,164). It has been suggested that G-proteins regulate phospholipase C activity by lowering the Ca^{2+} requirement necessary for activation to resting Ca^{2+} levels (175,176). Guanine nucleotides have been shown to stimulate IP_3 production in permeabilized neutrophils (175,177). This effect is enhanced by fMet-Leu-Phe and inhibited by pertussis toxin.

More recently, it has been proposed that phospholipase D, which preferentially uses phosphatidylcholine to produce phosphatidic acid (PA) (178,179), is involved in neutrophil activation. The evidence is growing that PA accumulation by this enzyme is critical in cellular responses (179–188).

D. Calcium

The importance of Ca^{2+} as an effector of cellular function has received widespread attention in recent years. Like other cell types, the intracellular Ca^{2+} concentration in resting neutrophils is maintained at submicromolar levels by a plasma membrane-bound Ca^{2+}-ATPase pump (189–191). There is substantial evidence that intracellular Ca^{2+} levels rise in stimulated neutrophils and that these increments may directly or indirectly bring about cell responses. Studies employing the fluorescent probes quin-2 and fura-2 as the Ca^{2+} probe indicate that, following stimulation with fMet-Leu-Phe, intracellular Ca^{2+} rises almost immediately from a resting level of 0.1 μM to 1 μM (192–201). There appear to be two separate pools involved in regulating the stimulus-induced rise in intracellular Ca^{2+} levels: There is an initial IP_3-mediated mobilization of Ca^{2+} from intracellular depots followed by an influx of extracellular Ca^{2+}. The initial mobilization of intracellular Ca^{2+} liberated in response to IP_3 appears to regulate directly the permeability changes to Ca^{2+} across the plasma membrane. Indeed, these calcium channels are insensitive to both fMet-Leu-Phe and IP_3, but are opened if intracellular Ca^{2+} is raised above 10^{-7} M Ca^{2+} (202).

In an effort to demonstrate Ca^{2+}-dependent secretion directly, neutrophils have been permeabilized by a variety of means, including the cholesterol-complexing agents saponin (203), digitonin (138,168,204–206), and streptolysin O (207), Sendai virus, (160,208,209), and high-voltage electrical fields (210,211), and then exposed to Ca^{2+} in EGTA-containing media. With some exceptions (203), these studies have shown that micromolar levels of Ca^{2+} alone are sufficient to induce the release of both specific and azurophil granule constituents (160,201,207–209,211), although specific granule secretion requires lower Ca^{2+} concentrations. The implications that azurophil and specific granule exocytosis differ in this Ca^{2+} requirements is supported by intact cell studies using quin-2 and ionomycin to establish the desired intracellular Ca^{2+} concentrations (212). While secretion can be modulated by both guanine and adenine nucleotides and by PKC activation, it appears that the primary intracellular trigger for exocytosis is Ca^{2+}.

How might this divalent cation mediate degranulation? At the most primitive level, Ca^{2+} may promote membrane fusion intracellularly through its interactions with negatively charged head groups of membrane phospholipids (213,214). Furthermore, polylysine and other metal cations have been shown to induce aggregation and fusion of phospholipid vesicles in a pH-dependent fashion (213,214). The pH dependence of fusion may be related to the ability of hydrogen ions to provide a charge-neutralizing effect (215). Thus, Ca^{2+} may change the physical properties of granules and membranes in such a way as to allow them to come into close apposition (216).

Ca^{2+} may play a role in the fusion process by regulating proteins that participate in the fusion process. For instance, phospholipase A_2, the enzyme responsible for the liberation of arachidonic acid, is present in both granule and neutrophil membranes (217–222). The membrane-bound enzyme is activated during stimulation (223,224) and is Ca^{2+} dependent (225). Phospholipase A_2-treated plasma membranes have been shown to induce the release of chromaffin granule contents, suggesting that arachidonic acid or one of its metabolites may participate in membrane fusion processes (226).

Ca^{2+} may likewise interact with other proteins to regulate fusion. Synexins belong to a class of Ca^{2+}-binding proteins originally found in adrenal chromaffin cells (227). Recently, three synexin-like proteins have been isolated from human neutrophils with properties similar to the synexins found in adrenal chromaffin cells (228). These proteins not only demonstrate the ability to aggregate specific granules in the presence of Ca^{2+}, they also induce the rapid fusion of granules with liposomes. Rapid fusion is highly dependent on the presence of Ca^{2+} and arachidonic acid. Other Ca^{2+}-binding proteins called lipocortins have been detected in neutrophils (229–233), and some of these lipocortins have aggregating and fusion-promoting activity (234). Finally, it has been reported that neutrophil plasma membranes, but not granule membranes, are particularly prone to Ca^{2+}-induced fusion with liposomes (235). It should be apparent that a detailed understanding of membrane fusion is not yet in place.

E. Protein Kinase C

The phorbol ester, phorbol 12-myristate 13-acetate (PMA), has been used extensively as an activating stimulus to investigate the stimulus-response coupling pathways that are operative in neutrophils. The phosphorylation state of a wide variety of intracellular proteins changes upon stimulation with PMA (236–239). These changes occur in parallel with the induction of neutrophil functional responses and have also been observed with chemotactic peptide stimulation (239,240), suggesting the involvement of a protein kinase in the activation pathway. The ability of PMA to elicit neutrophil responses has been attributed to the activation of a Ca^{2+}-sensitive, phospholipid-dependent protein kinase (protein kinase C or PKC). High levels of PKC have been detected in neutrophils (241,242). In other cell types, it has been demonstrated that the intracellular receptor for PMA is PKC (243,244). In neutrophils, both receptors for PMA and PKC activity are located in the cytoplasm of resting cells and redistributed to the plasma membrane following cell activation (245). Immunocytochemical data suggest that this shift in activity represents translocation from the cytosol to the membrane in both neutrophils (246) and HL60 cells (247).

It is generally believed that activation of the kinase is achieved physiologically by 1,2-diacylglycerol which is derived from the hydrolysis of phosphatidylinositols following receptor activation (162–165). Consistent with this notion is the observation that synthetic diacylglycerols also activate neutrophils by interacting with the same intracellular receptor as PMA (248). The mobilization of diacylglycerol following receptor activation may activate PKC by sensitizing the enzyme to resting levels of intracellular Ca^{2+}, because PMA reduces the K_m for the putative Ca^{2+} receptor, PKC, into the submicromolar range (243).

The close correlation between the activation of PKC and neutrophil functions (236,245,248–251) and the synergy between the activation of PKC agonists and other stimuli (249,250,252,253) has suggested a role for this enzyme in stimulus-response coupling. While PKC has been implicated in the phosphorylation changes occurring following cell activation (236–238,241,242), neutrophils also contain other kinases in addition to PKC which may also be involved in cell activation (254–258). The inability of the PKC inhibitors H-7 and H-9 (259,260) to block neutrophil activation in response to several stimuli supports this possibility and suggests that PKC activation is not a necessary requirement for cell activation by all activating agents.

V. THE ROLE OF THE NEUTROPHIL IN ACUTE INFLAMMATION

Neutrophils have long been recognized as being the principal cell type present in the second or cellular phase of the acute inflammatory response. Usually within the first 24 h after the initiation of the tissue injury, neutrophils accumulate at the site of injury (261,262). As illustrated in Figure 7, neutrophils are attracted into the site by a sequence of events beginning with the elaboration of chemical mediators which attract the neutrophils from the circulation by events involving margination and adhesion of the neutrophils to the endothelium followed by diapedesis or migration of the neutrophils through the blood vessels into the injury site. These chemical mediators are called chemotactic factors and include such inflammatory mediators as products of complement activation (C5a), lipoxygenase pathway products (LTB_4), the generation and release of cytokines from lymphocytes and macrophages (IL-I, TNF, IL-8), and bacterial chemotactic products (263–266). These chemotactic factors diffuse away from the site of injury, creating a concentration gradient which attracts circulating neutrophils into the area. After attraction of the neutrophils by the chemotactic factors, margination and adherence of the neutrophils to the vascular endothelial cells occurs. This adherence to vascular endothelium requires glycoproteins on the surface of the neutrophils and endothelial cells. These "adhesive glycoproteins" include fibronectin and laminin as well as those present on the surface of the neutrophil and endothelial cell. The neutrophil adhesive glycoproteins are designated as MO-1, LFA-1, and P150-95. The adhesive glycoproteins present on the surface of endothelial cells include ICAM-1, which serves as a receptor for the LFA-1 neutrophil glycoprotein and ELAM-1 (267–269). In the case of the leukocyte adhesive glycoproteins, inflammatory mediators such as chemotactic factors increase the adherence of leukocytes to target cells in vitro. Endothelial cell expression of ICAM-I and ELAM-I can also be increased by inflammatory mediators such as endotoxin and cytokines such as tumor necrosis factor and interleukin-I (268). The importance of these adhesive glycoproteins in neutrophil function in vivo is illustrated by individuals who genetically lack the leukocyte adhesive proteins MO-1 and P150-95. These individuals are susceptible to increased bacterial infections (270).

The adherence of the leukocyte to the endothelium is a necessary prerequisite for their subsequent emigration or diapedesis into the tissues and subsequent activation. Historically, this adherence was not felt to cause enough neutrophil activation to harm the endothelial cell. However, it is now apparent that under certain circumstances the endothelium is injured or destroyed by the neutrophil. In fact, in some types of acute inflammation, such as adult respiratory distress syndrome (ARDS), the pulmonary microvascular endothelial cell appears to be the primary target. Whether the endothelial cell or other cells or matrices are the primary target, neutrophil adherence to the target is a critical event in the activation and release of potent inflammatory mediators by the leukocyte, with adherence causing enhanced oxygen radical generation and granule release (271).

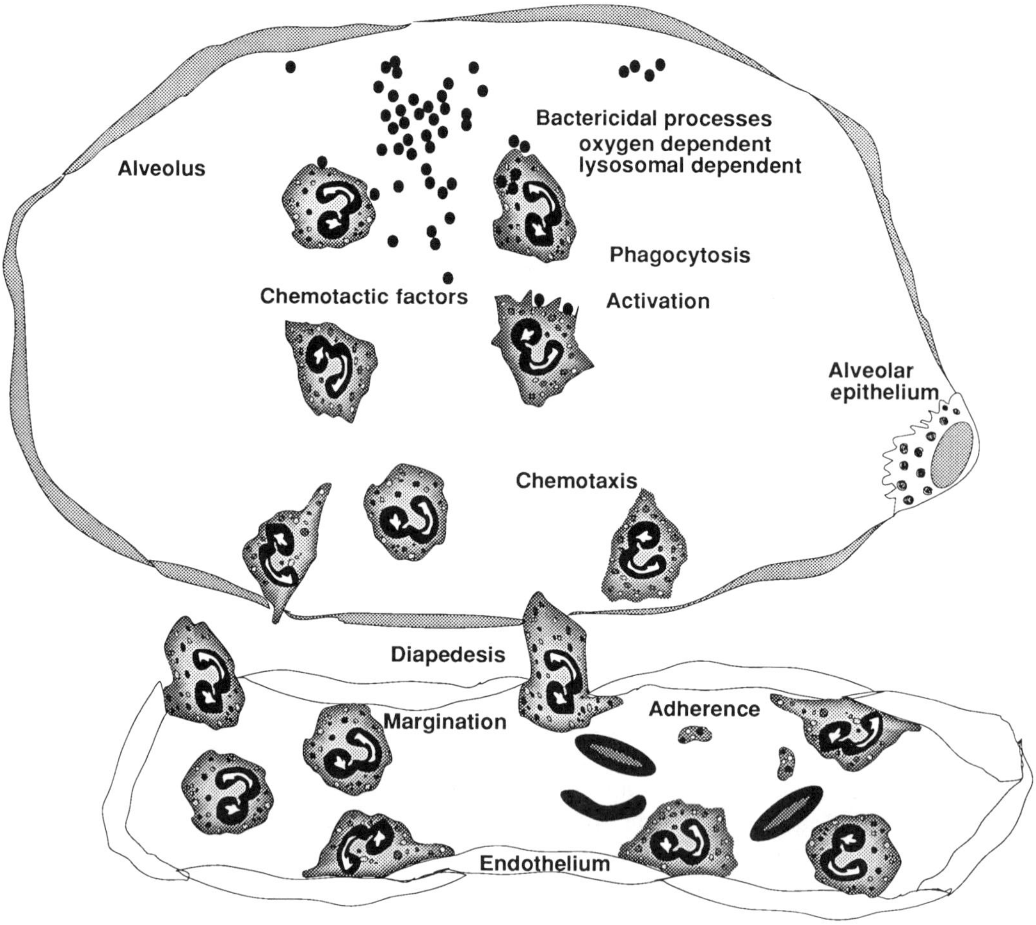

Figure 7 A drawing of acute bacterial pneumonia to illustrate the sequence of events leading to neutrophil recruitment and activation in sites of acute inflammation. Chemotactic factors derived from bacteria and complement attract neutrophils from the circulation via a concentration gradient. The neutrophils attach to the pulmonary capillary endothelial cells via neutrophil and endothelial cell adhesive glycoproteins such as ICAM-1 and LFA-1. The neutrophils then migrate (diapedesis) through the vessel wall and once in the tissues are activated by various soluble and particulate stimuli—in this case, bacteria. Once activated, the neutrophils phagocytize and destroys the bacteria. However, potent neutrophil proteases and oxidants which destroy the bacteria are also released into the extracellular space, where they induce tissue injury by altering intracellular matrix as well as destroying parenchymal cells.

VI. TISSUE INJURY BY NEUTROPHILS

Once the neutrophil is present at the site and activated, it provides the most important first line of defense against injurious agents such as pathogenic bacteria or fungi. In addition, neutrophils perform an important debridement function by removing dead cells and other cellular debris. However, it is clear that activated neutrophils are a two-edged sword, with the ability to harm as well as protect the host. Much of the tissue injury seen in inflammatory diseases such as ARDS, rheumatoid arthritis, or bacterial infection is linked to neutrophil activation and release of potent inflammatory mediators (272–274).

The products released from the neutrophil that cause tissue injury have been the subject of intensive study, with most attention focusing either on the release of the granule proteases or on the activation of the plasma membrane-associated respiratory burst NADPH oxidase enzyme with the generation and release of toxic oxygen products. In the following discussion we will first look at the evidence implicating reactive oxygen products as mediators of acute tissue injury. Next we will examine the evidence that proteases are involved. Finally, we will summarize studies that suggests that neutrophil protease/oxidant interactions are critical in the development of the tissue injury.

A. Neutrophil Oxidants and Tissue Injury

In many human diseases, neutrophil-derived oxygen radicals have been implicated in the pathogenesis of the acute tissue injury. In adult respiratory distress syndrome (ARDS) or infant RDS, neutrophils are predominant early on and the injury is associated with H_2O_2 generation in lavage fluid and expired breath of these patients as well as evidence of oxidative inactivation of the main antiprotease screen alpha-1-antiproteinase (α1pi) (275–277). Other human diseases where neutrophil oxidants are implicated include ischemic reperfusion injury of organs such as the heart, CNS, or GI tract, and glomerulonephritis (278,279).

Experimentally, as mentioned previously, oxidants are clearly cytotoxic (80,92–96), and oxidants have clearly been shown to cause tissue injury directly in in vivo animal models and in isolated perfused organs. For example, in models of acute lung injury, enzymes and enzyme substrates that directly produce O_2^- or H_2O_2 cause lung injury that can be inhibited by SOD, catalase, and hydroxyl radical scavengers or ion chelators (280,281). Using stimulated neutrophils or macrophages as the source of the oxidants results in the same spectrum of injury. In whole animals, acute lung injury induced by immune complexes, systemic complement activation, endotoxin, and thermal injury also appears to be largely mediated by the formation of oxidants by neutrophils and macrophages (282–287). In the majority of these systems the addition of the antioxidant enzymes and/or iron chelators at the time of the initiation of the injury is very protective, with the bulk of the evidence favoring the concept that the hydroxyl radical is primarily responsible for the initiation of the tissue injury. Thus, in humans as well as in animal models of human disease, neutrophil oxidants are increasingly implicated in the evolution of tissue injury.

B. Neutrophil Proteases and Tissue Injury

Even though oxidants are highly reactive and have potent cytotoxic effects, their actions are not specific, rather, they react with the first available target such as a plasma membrane. This relative nonspecificity and short half-life of oxidants, as well as the fact that certain types of acute tissue injury are not oxidant dependent, has led to renewed interest in the potential role of neutrophil granule constituents in the induction of acute tissue injury. Of all the granule constituents present as described earlier, the proteolytic enzymes appear to have the greatest potential to act as mediators of acute tissue injury. Historically, proteases have long been suspected as being important pro-inflammatory agents, with most studies suggesting that proteases primarily target extracellular matrix components such as collagens and elastin, leading to disordered repair of damaged organs and fibrosis (288–292). Neutrophil proteolytic enzymes that have been primarily implicated in this regard include the serine-neutral proteases elastase and cathepsin G and the metalloproteinases collagenase and gelatinase. Most of the evidence implicating proteases as pro-inflammatory agents involves elastase. Very little work has been done on the other three enzymes in terms of their pro-inflammatory effects. Elastase is present at high levels in the primary granule, and during cell activation and degranulation some of the granule contacts including elastase are released into the extracellular milieu. In vitro, elastase has the ability to degrade almost all components of the extracellular matrix, including fibrillar collagen, proteoglycans, fibronectin, and type IV collagen as well as elastin. In addition, elastase cleaves a variety of proteins, including some associated with the inflammatory response such as immunoglobulins, complement proteases, and fibrinogen (293,294). Some studies also suggest that elastase is directly cytotoxic to endothelial cells (295).

In vivo studies on the role of neutrophil elastase in tissue injury have focused largely on emphysema and other types of chronic obstructive pulmonary disease (COPD). In humans the association was first made in patients who developed panacinar emphysema secondary to a deficiency of the main circulating protease inhibitor alpha-1-antitrypsin (alpha-1-antiprotease). Subsequently, evidence has accumulated that emphysema induced by cigarette smoking is also associated with elastase, with the free protease detected in the lung tissues (296–298). Free elastase activity has also been identified in lavage fluid of cystic fibrosis patients (299). Other diseases where free elastase activity in tissues has been detected as well as elastase bound to alpha-1-proteinase inhibitors include ARDS, pancreatitis, and rheumatoid arthritis (300–303). Experimental in vivo studies have demonstrated that proteases such as papain or, more specifically, free elastase produce emphysema (304–306). The role that proteases such as elastase may play in the induction of acute tissue injury is unclear. Some studies suggest an important role in experimental acute glomerular injury (307,308).

The second major group of proteinases released by the activated neutrophil is the metalloproteinases. This includes a collagenase as well as a gelatinase. As mentioned previously, these proteases are present at high levels in specific granules and tertiary granules and are felt to play an important role in bactericidal effects. Like other granule constituents, they are released to a certain extent into the extracellular space during neutrophil activation, and these proteinases can cleave several types of intact as well as denatured collagen or gelatin (309). These enzymes are released in a latent, inactive form, so whether or not these enzymes play a role in the induction of acute tissue injury is unclear. However, recent evidence suggests that these latent enzymes can be activated by the generation of the myeloperoxidase-dependent oxidant HOCI (310). Thus, there is renewed interest in the possible proinflammatory role of these enzymes.

In summary, activated neutrophil serine and metalloproteinases are present during inflammatory disease in vivo, and in vitro they have potent effects on extracellular matrix and may even be directly cytotoxic. However, proof that these proteinases are involved directly in acute tissue injury in vivo is lacking. Instead, there is accumulating evidence that neutrophil oxidants and proteases act synergistically to produce acute tissue injury as outlined below.

VII. MECHANISMS OF NEUTROPHIL-MEDIATED ENDOTHELIAL CELL INJURY

As indicated above, there is ample evidence that activated neutrophils are capable of producing tissue injury. In some human disease processes such as ARDS, evidence suggests that the endothelium of the pulmonary vascular bed is the primary target. Because of this, our laboratory as well as several other laboratories have invested considerable effort in understanding the mechanisms by which vascular endothelial cells can be injured by activated neutrophils. The final sections of this review will briefly summarize what has been learned as a result of these studies. Although most of the work has focused on endothelial cells as the target, one needs to keep in mind that injury to other types of cells present in paranchymal organs may involve similar mechanisms.

A. Intracellular Events in Neutrophil-Mediated Endothelial Cell Injury

Studies conducted in the late 1970s and early 1980s with human umbilical vein endothelial cells and with large vessel arteries convincingly demonstrated a central role for H_2O_2 in neutrophil-mediated injury. Studies by Sacks et al. (311), Weiss et al. (312), and Martin (313) each demonstrated that the endothelial cell injury resulting from activated human neutrophils could be largely prevented by catalase but not superoxide dismutase. Injury was not unique to endothelial cells, because other studies with bacteria, fibroblasts, red blood cells, and a variety of tumor cells also demonstrated the critical involvement of H_2O_2 in cytotoxicity (314,315). The mechanism of H_2O_2-induced injury has not been fully elucidated in any of these studies. A role for the peroxidase-halide generation of HOCI has been identified in certain of these models, but a role for ferrous iron-catalyzed hydroxyl radical formation has also been implicated.

A series of studies were therefore carried out in our laboratory to investigate the mechanism by which human neutrophils injured endothelial cells from bovine pulmonary artery (316). The data from these studies (Table 4) showed that lethal injury could be induced by activation of the neutrophils with either immune complexes, zymosan, or phorbol esters, but not with formyl peptide-treated or platelet-activating factor-treated neutrophils. The degree of injury was most closely correlated with the amount of hydrogen peroxide produced ($r = 0.995$) but also correlated well with superoxide anion (O_2^-) generation ($r = 0.904$). There was no correlation with proteolytic enzyme release.

Not surprisingly in light of these findings, inhibitor studies (Table 5) showed no protection with soybean trypsin inhibitor, slight protection with superoxide dismutase, and good protection with catalase. Inhibitor studies showed further that sodium azide, a myeloperoxidase inhibitor, did not protect, but that HO· scavengers such as mannitol and dimethythiourea (DMTU) and the iron chelator deferoxamine did protect (Table 5). Taken together, these data strongly suggest that human neutrophil killing of bovine pulmonary artery endothelial cells involves the generation of H_2O_2 and its conversion to the highly toxic HO· radical. In subsequent studies it was shown with rat pulmonary artery endothelial cells that the same spectrum of inhibitors would also protect these cells from the lethal injury mediated by activated human neutrophils (Table 5).

Table 4 Activation of Human Neutrophils for Endothelial Cell Killing: Correlation with Oxidant Production but Not Protease Release[a]

Stimulating agent	O_2^- production (nmol 5×10^6 cells/h)	H_2O_2 production (nmol 5×10^6 cells/h)	Protease release (mg protein hydrolyzed) (nmol 5×10^6 cells/18 h)	Cytoxicity (% specific ^{51}Cr release)
None	10 ± 1	<1	20 ± 1	3 ± 1
Phorbol ester	37 ± 0	20 ± 1	51 ± 10	40 ± 7
Immune complex	46 ± 1	14 ± 1	59 ± 2	32 ± 8
Zymosan	16 ± 1	8 ± 0	32 ± 1	10 ± 2
FMLP	19 ± 1	1 ± 0	63 ± 5	0
Platelet-activity factor	16 ± 2	1 ± 0	45 ± 2	3 ± 1

[a] See Ref. 316 for details.

Table 5 Killing of Bovine and Rat Pulmonary Artery Endothelial Cells by Neutrophils in the Presence of Various Inhibitors[a]

	Cytotoxicity (% specific ^{51}Cr release)	
Inhibitor[b]	bovine	rat
None	27 ± 3	36 ± 4
SBTI	24 ± 4	41 ± 4
SOD	20 ± 7	47 ± 3
Catalase	9 ± 1	18 ± 3
Deferoxamine	5 ± 2	14 ± 3
DMTU	8 ± 3	Not done
Mannitol	13 ± 2	Not done
Sodium azide	30 ± 4	54 ± 2

[a] See Ref. 316 for details.

[b] SBTI = soybean trypsin inhibitor; SOD = superoxide dismutase; DMTU = dimethylthiourea.

Efforts to follow up on these observations have led us to examine the events which occur within the target endothelial cell under attack by neutrophils (317). As shown in Table 6, pretreatment of either rat or bovine pulmonary artery endothelial cells with deferoxamine following by washing confers a high degree of protection on these cells against subsequent injury by activated neutrophils. In contrast, pretreatment of the neutrophils with the same agent followed by washing does not inhibit their ability to subsequently injure the target cells. These observations suggest that the iron which is critical for interaction with H_2O_2 is derived from sources within the target cells. In additional studies, we were able to demonstrate that deferoxamine penetrates the endothelial cells and forms a complex with target cell iron. In the presence of deferoxamine, iron is slowly released from the cells. However, the rate at which this occurs is too slow to account for the observed protection. We favor the hypothesis, therefore, that the complexing of iron with deferoxamine protects by either preventing iron reduction from the Fe^{3+} form to the Fe^{2+} form or by removing it from close proximity to critical intracellular target molecules.

Table 6 Protection of Bovine and Rat Pulmonary Artery Endothelial Cells Against Neutrophil-Mediated Killing with Deferoxamine

	Percent protection	
Conditions of treatment[a]	Bovine	Rat
Endothelial cells treated	88 ± 3	94 ± 2
Neutrophils treated	−3 ± 1	Not done

[a] Endothelial cells were treated for 4 h with 5 mM deferoxamine and then washed two times prior to addition of neutrophils. Neutrophils were treated for 30 min and then washed two times prior to addition to endothelial cell monolayers and activation. See Ref. 317 for details.

Iron must be present as the reduced form (Fe^{2+}) to participate in HO· generation from H_2O_2. Yet nearly all of the iron within cells is in the Fe^{3+} form. It can be assumed, therefore, that a source of reducing equivalents must be present within susceptible cells to reduce iron from the Fe^{3+} form to the Fe^{2+} form. The enzyme xanthine oxidase is a good candidate for such a source in the rat pulmonary artery endothelial cells, since rat tissues are rich in this enzyme. This enzyme can exist in two functional forms. In the dehydrogenase form it uses NAD^+ as the electron acceptor, but in the oxidase form it uses O_2 as the electron acceptor, generating O_2^- in the process. That the xanthine oxidase-generated O_2^- may be involved in the cytotoxicity process is suggested by the finding that exposure of the endothelial cells to factors that result in cytotoxicity causes a conversion of the enzyme from the dehydrogenase form to the oxidase form and by the finding that inhibitors of xanthine oxidase protect the endothelial cells against killing by activated neutrophils or reagent H_2O_2. These data, which have been described in recent reports (318,319), are summarized in Table 7. A role for xanthine oxidase in killing of bovine pulmonary artery endothelial cells by activated neutrophils has not yet been examined by us. However, Rodell et al. (320) reported that inhibitors of bovine pulmonary artery endothelial cell xanthine oxidase would also protect these cells.

As part of our effort to delineate the role of endothelial cell xanthine oxidase in the cytotoxicity process, we examined the cells for the presence of substrate (xanthine and hypoxanthine) for this enzyme (319). Cells were labeled for 45 min with ^{14}C-adenosine. Following this, they were washed two times to remove unincorporated label and then incubated for varying periods of time in control buffer or in the presence of H_2O_2. At the end of the incubation period, extracts were prepared and analyzed by HPLC for ^{14}C-labeled metabolites of adenosine. In control cells we observed that approximately 75% of the incorporated radioactivity was found in a fraction co-migrating with ATP (Figure 8). Figure 8 also shows that within 15 min of exposure to H_2O_2 there was a precipitous fall in intracellular radioactivity with a concomitant increase in extracellular radioactivity. The fall in intracellular radioactivity was reflective of a loss of ATP. However, there was no concomitant buildup of ATP in the extracellular fluid (Figure 8). In order to identify the metabolites present in both intracellular and extracellular pools, samples were obtained from cells and from extracellular fluid 30 min after exposure to buffer alone or to H_2O_2. The samples were separated by HPLC and compared to authentic standards. Table 8 shows the profile of metabo-

Table 7 Protection of Rat Pulmonary Artery Endothelial Cells Against Neutrophil-Mediated Killing and H_2-Mediated Killing with Xanthine Oxidase Inhibitors

	Percent protection against killing by	
Inhibitor	Activated neutrophils	H_2O_2
Allopurinol	64 ± 4	65 ± 10
Oxypurinol	28 ± 2	59 ± 2
Lodoxamide	13 ± 1	Not done

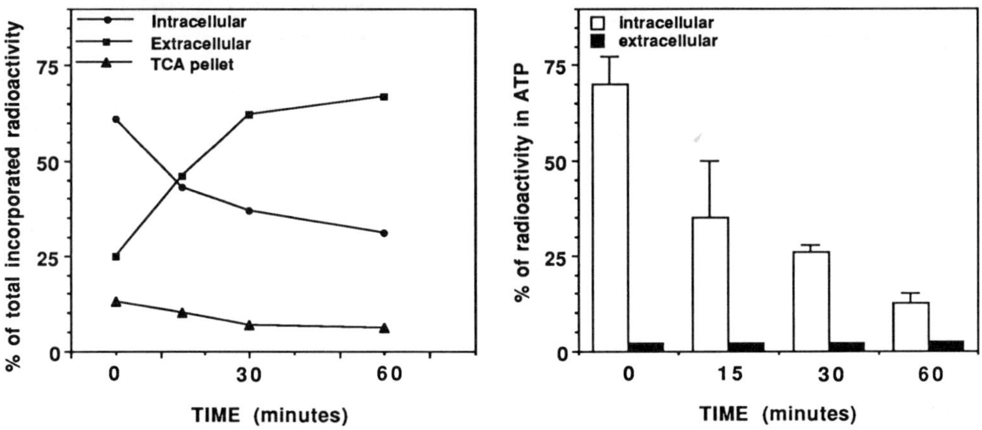

Figure 8 Time course of total radioactivity and ATP loss from rat pulmonary artery endothelial cells after exposure to H_2O_2. Cells were labeled with ^{14}C-adenosine and exposed to 500 nmol/ml H_2O_2 for varying periods of time. Intracellular and extracellular radioactivity and ATP levels were then determined. The data represent the average radioactivity (A) and percentage of radioactivity (B) co-migrating with authentic ATP. See Ref. 319 for details.

lites obtained. The major finding was that the drop in ATP levels following H_2O_2 exposure was accompanied by a buildup of xanthine and hypoxanthine. By 30 min of exposure to H_2O_2, up to 20% of the originally incorporated radioactivity was found in these fractions. It is of interest that although ATP levels fell rapidly after H_2O_2 exposure, this was, of itself, not indicative of cytotoxicity. The addition of catalase to the buffer 30–60 min after treatment with H_2O_2 resulted in substantial protection from killing, even though the greatest changes in ATP levels had already taken place. In addition, agents which provided significant protection against killing, including deferoxamine and allopurinol, did not inhibit the loss of ATP from the H_2O_2-exposed cells or the buildup of xanthine and hypoxanthine. These data are therefore consistent with the suggestion that the loss of ATP per se is not responsible for oxidant injury but may participate by providing substrate for the generation of oxidant species within the target cell.

The model of endothelial cell injury developed on the basis of these findings is illustrated in Figure 9 and can be summarized as follows: It suggests that neutrophil-mediated killing of rat pulmonary artery endothlelial cells requires activation of surface NADPH oxidase, resulting in the generation of O_2^- and subsequently, H_2O_2, requires availability of ferrous iron and an oxidant (presumably derived from xanthine oxidase activity) within the target cell and ultimately involves the generation within the target cell of $HO\cdot$ by ferrous-iron reduction of H_2O_2.

It should not be implied that the scenario described above is the only way in which activated neutrophils can injure the vascular endothelium. It has been shown by Harlan et al. (321,322) that activated neutrophils can cause disruption of intact endothelial cell monolayers by an oxygen radical-independent, protease-dependent mechanism. While this is not associated with lethal injury to the endothelial cells, disruption of the vascu-

Table 8 Distribution of Radioactivity Following Incorporation of ^{14}C-Adenosine into Rat Pulmonary Artery Endothelial Cells and Exposure of the Cells to H_2O_2[a]

	Metabolite (percent of total radioactivity)						
Source	ATP	ADP	AMP	NAD/IMP	ADO	INO	X/HX
Cell associated							
Buffer alone	60 ± 13	12 ± 4	3 ± 3	5 ± 1	<1	<1	<1
H_2O_2	17 ± 7	9 ± 1	4 ± 1	8 ± 3	1 ± 1	1 ± 1	3 ± 1
Extracellular							
Buffer alone	<1	<1	<1	<1	<1	<1	1 ± 1
H_2O_2	<1	<1	<1	<1	<1	6 ± 5	15 ± 7

[a] ADO = adenosine; INO = inosine; X/HX = xanthine/hypoxanthine. Values shown are averages ± standard deviations. See Ref. 319 for details.

lar lining could have important consequences for the establishment or amplification of inflammatory processes. In addition to this model of nonlethal endothelial cell injury, studies by other investigators have shown that microvascular endothelial cells can be lethally injured by neutrophil-derived proteolytic enzymes (323). Neutrophil elastase and a membrane-bound neutrophil protease have been implicated as potential effector

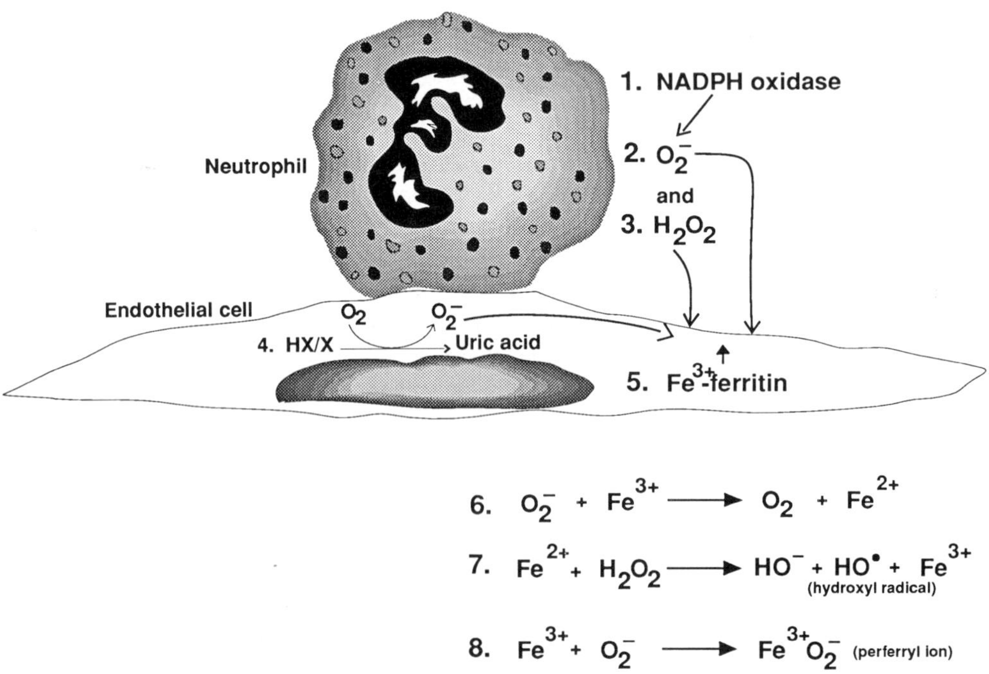

Figure 9 Model of endothelial cell killing by activated neutrophils.

moieties responsible for the injury in these models (323,324). Perhaps the most interesting model, in light of the findings presented in this review, is one described by Rodell et al. (320) showing that inhibitors of xanthine oxidase protect bovine pulmonary artery endothelial cells from elastase-mediated injury. The implication of this is that even in protease-mediated endothelial cell injury, there is a role for events which occur within the target cell and these events may depend on the generation of an oxidant.

B. Synergistic Interaction of Leukocyte Products in Endothelial Cell Injury

Although oxidants play a critical role in inflammatory injury to the vascular endothelium, recent studies suggest that the extent of injury can be magnified through the interaction of other inflammatory mediators with neutrophil oxidants. These include cytokines such as interleukin-1 (IL-1) and tumor necrosis factor-α (TNF-α), neutrophil proteases and other hydrolytic enzymes, cationic proteins, which are present in large amounts in the neutrophil granule, as well as various phospholipids which may be present at sites of inflammation as a result of cell death or microbial accumulation.

Studies by Ginsburg et al. (325) have demonstrated that a variety of disparate substances (having only their highly cationic nature in common) can bind to the surface of endothelial cells. In concentrations at which these cationic substances are nontoxic, they render the endothelial cell much more sensitive to oxidant injury. Substances which can function in this manner include cationic proteins of neutrophil granules, nuclear histone proteins, polyamino acids such as polylysine and polyhistidine, polyamines, and cationic antibiotics such as polymyxin B. Figure 10 depicts the effects of such interactions on the endothelium. It can be seen that histone and H_2O_2 synergize in the killing of endothelial cells. This effect is apparently due to an irreversible binding of the histone to the endothelial cell surface. Washing the cells prior to addition of oxidant does not eliminate the synergistic effect. Neutralization of the cationic charge with polyanethole sulfonate, a strongly anionic substance, however, does completely block the synergistic killing (Figure 10).

Oxidant injury to endothelial cells can also be potentiated with other agents capable of altering the endothelial cell surface. Table 9 shows that exposure of the target cells to lysophosphatidylcholine at subtoxic concentrations increases the sensitivity of the cells to injury. Lysophosphatidyl compounds are generated by the action of phospholipase A_2 and may be present in large amounts at sites of inflammation. Some of these phospholipid moieties intercalate readily into cell membranes. Presumably it is binding to the endothelial cell membrane that is critical because, as was observed with histone, the lysophosphatides cannot be easily removed by washing after they have become bound to the target cell. In the presence of an excess of phosphatidycholine, however, synergistic injury is prevented (Table 9). Not surprisingly, polyanathole sulfonate, which prevents the interaction of histone with the target cells, has no effect on the interaction of lysophophatidylcholine with the same cells.

The direct effects of cationic substances and lysophosphatides on endothelial cells provides one mechanism for the magnification of vascular damage at sites of inflammation. The same agents may also potentiate damage by a direct effect on neutrophils present at the inflammatory sites. Ginsburg and his associates (326,327) have

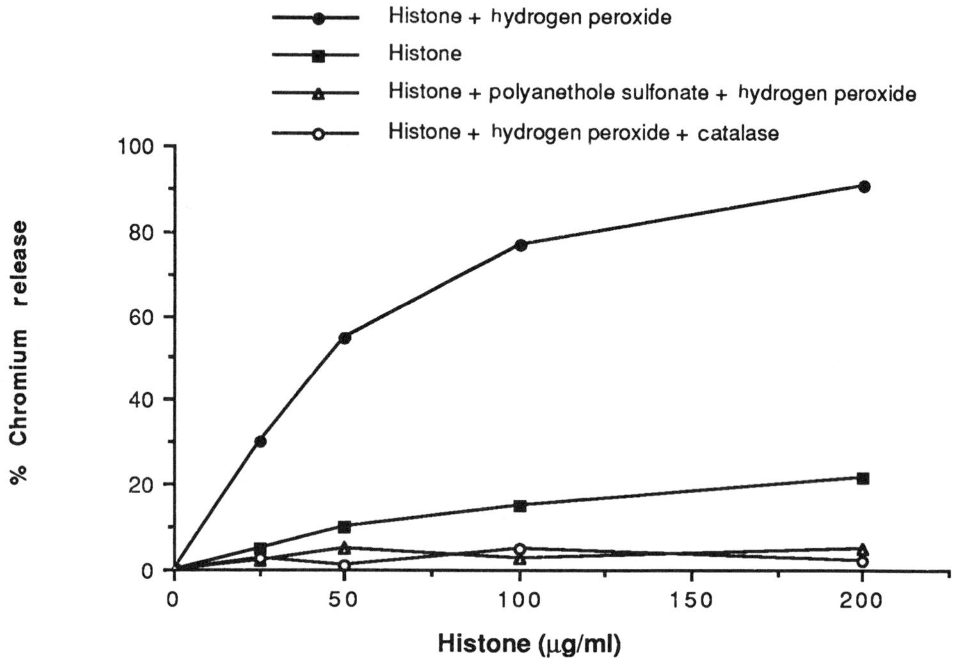

Figure 10 Synergistic killing of rat pulmonary artery endothelial cells by H_2O_2 and histone. Cells were treated with sufficient glucose oxidase (0.128U) in the presence of glucose to generate a sublytic amount of H_2O_2. In the presence of increasing amounts of histone, this amount of H_2O_2 produced increasing amounts of endothelial cell killing. Neutralization of either H_2O_2 with catalase or histone with polyanethole sulfonate inhibited killing.

shown in a series of studies that both cationic proteins and lysophosphatides can bind to the neutrophil surface to enhance the respiratory response to soluble stimuli. The end result is a greater production of reactive oxygen metabolites, includes H_2O_2. Thus the same agents that increase endothelial cell sensitivity to oxygen radicals concomitantly increase levels of these same reactive metabolites.

Given the observations cited above, it is not surprising that various hydrolytic enzymes can also potentiate endothelial cell injury by neutrophils. Studies from our laboratory (328) have shown that a number of different proteolytic enzymes do not induce lethal injury to endothelial cells unless present in high quantity over an extended period of time (8h or more). In much lower quantities, however, these same enzymes can dramatically increase sensitivity to oxidant injury. Enzymes that alter the phospholipid structure of cell membranes potentiate sensitivity to oxidant injury in a similar manner. Whether these invitro observations can be related to invivo events is not known at present. However, since inflammatory sites, particularly sites of microbial infection, may contain a rich mixture of cationic substances, proteolytic enzymes, phospholipases, and phospholipid breakdown products, these substances may contribute to the tissue damage observed at sites of inflammation by enhancing endothelial cell sensitivity to neutrophil-generated H_2O_2 as well as by augmenting the generation of H_2O_2 by neutrophils.

Table 9 Synergistic Killing of Endothelial Cells by H_2O_2 and Lysophosphatidylcholine

Treatment	Percent ^{51}Cr release
H_2O_2 (100 nmol)	1 ± 1
Lysophosphatidylcholine (1 μg)	8 ± 6
H_2O_2 + lysophosphatidylcholine	56 ± 11
H_2O_2 + lysophosphatidylcholine + 50 μg phosphatidylcholine	23 ± 10
H_2O_2 + lypophosphatidylcholine + 50 μg polyanethole sulfonate	62 ± 8
histone (75 μg)	12 ± 1
H_2O_2 + histone	66 ± 5
H_2O_2 + histone + 50 μg phosphatidylcholine	66 ± 6

In addition to the products of neutrophils themselves, metabolites generated by other cells at the site of the inflammatory lesion or systemically may modulate leukocyte interaction with the endothelium. Monocyte-derived cytokines, in particular, have been shown to influence the interaction of neutrophils with the endothelium. Interleukin-1 (IL-1) and especially tumor necrosis factor-α (TNF-α) have a variety of effects that can potentiate endothelial cell injury. Some of these effects are directed toward the neutrophil, while others involve the endothelial cells directly. A major effect seen at the level of the neutrophil is an activation of the respiratory burst (329,330). At the endothelial cell level, IL-1 and TNF-α act to increase expression of leukocyte adhesion molecules (331,332). These include intercellular adhesion molecule (ICAM), endothelial-leukocyte adhesion molecule (ELAM), and vascular cell adhesion molecule (VCAM). Up-regulation of these moieties is thought to promote neutrophil binding to the endothelium at sites of inflammation. In addition to activating neutrophils and promoting their adhesive interaction with the endothelium, these same cytokines also alter endothelial cell behavior in ways that could enhance their sensitivity to injury or be directly injurious. Although most studies have indicated that normal vascular endothelial cells are resistant to direct cytotoxicity by TNF-α, recent studies have shown that killing may occur under appropriate conditions (333). In addition, studies from our laboratory have shown that pretreatment of rat pulmonary artery endothelial cells with TNF-α renders these cells more sensitive to killing by activated neutrophils (334). The in vivo significance of this is unknown. We have speculated that endothelial cells near inflammatory foci may, by virtue of their exposure to high levels of TNF-α, be rendered sensitive to subsequent injurious stimuli. The recent finding by Rothstein and Schreiber (335) that TNF-α synergizes with bacterial products and leukocyte factors to bring about hemorrhagic necrosis and shock in experimental animals is consistent with this.

C. Summary

Neutrophil damage to the vascular endothelium is a complex, multifaceted event. Two points need to be made in summarizing the information that is available at present.

First, neutrophils have multiple mechanisms capable of injuring the endothelium independently, but the injury seen at sites of inflammation is probably a result of synergistic interaction among the various effector mechanisms. Second, the target endothelial cells are not passive bystanders but rather participate actively in their own injury. Thus, understanding the molecular events that occur during inflammatory vascular disease requires understanding the biochemical processes that occur in the target cell as well as the biochemical processes of the effector cell.

VIII. CONCLUSION

As this chapter illustrates, the neutrophil is a marvelously complex cell that contains a large array of potent biological mediators designed to maximize its ability to kill invading microorganisms. The evolutionary development of these potent microbicidal agents is a two-edged sword in that many of these same neutrophil products such as oxidants and proteases that destroy microorganisms also clearly are capable of killing host cells and altering connective tissue matrix. Based on studies outlined in this chapter, neutrophil oxidants and proteases acting individually as well as in concert appear to be responsible for much of the tissue injury. Given this information, it should be possible to develop selective strategies for inhibition of neutrophil-mediated tissue injury without interfering with the cells' ability to kill invading microorganisms.

REFERENCES

1. Palmblad J. The role of granulocytes in inflammation. Scand J Rheum 1984; 13:163–72.
2. Ryan G, Majna G. Acute inflammation: a review. Am J Pathol 1977; 86:185.
3. Diggs LW, Sturm D, Bell BA. The morphology of human blood cells. Philadelphia: WB Saunders, 1956.
4. Cline MJ. The white cell. Cambridge, MA: Harvard University Press, 1975.
5. Baggiolini M, Hirsch JG, DeDuve C. Resolution of granules from rabbit heterophil leukocytes into distinct populations by zonal sedimentation. J Cell Biol 1969; 10:529–41.
6. Cooke WE, Ponder E. The polynuclear count. Philadelphia: JB Lippincott, 1927.
7. Metcalf D. The molecular control of normal and leukemia granulocytes and macrophages. Proc R Soc Lond B 1987; 230:389–423.
8. Bainton DF. Morphology of neutrophils and neutrophil precursors. In: Williams WF, Beutler E, Ersliv AJ, Lichtman MA, eds. Hematology, 4th ed. New York: McGraw-Hill, 1990:761–8.
9. Ackerman GA. Ultrastructure and cytochemistry of the developing neutrophil. Lab Invest 1968; 19:290–302.
10. Golde DW, Cline MJ. Regulation of granulopoiesis. N Engl J Med 1974; 291:1388–95.
11. Quesenberry, P. The hematopoietic stem cell. In: Williams WJ, Beutler E, Erslev NJ, Lichtman MA, eds. Hematology, 4th ed. New York: McGraw-Hill, 1990:129–147.
12. Quesenberry P, Levitt L. Hematopoietic stem cells. N Engl J Med 1979; 301:755, Part II 301:819, Part III 301:868.
13. Iscave NN, Till JE, McCulloch EA. The proliferative states of mouse granulopoietic progenitor cells. Proc Soc Exp Biol Med 1970; 134:33.
14. Moore MAS and Williams N 1974. Functional morphologic and kinetic analysis of the granulocyte-macrophage progenitor cell. In: Robinson WA, ed. Hemapoiesis in culture: Second International Workshop. (DHEW publication no. 74–205).
15. Klebanoff SJ, Clark RA, eds, The neutrophil: function and clinical disorders. New York: North-Holland, 1978:74–5.

16. Metcalf D. The molecular control of cell division, differentiation, commitment and maturation in haemopoietic cells. Nature 1989; 339:27–30.
17. Metcalf D. The molecular control of normal and leukaemic granulocyte and macrophages. Proc R Soc Lond B 1987; 230:389–423.
18. Ikebachi K, Wong G, Clark SC. Interleukin 6 enhancement of Interleukin-3 dependent proliferation of multipotential hemopoietic progenitors. Proc Natl Acad Sci USA 1987; 84:9035–9.
19. Johnson GR, Metcalf D. Sources and nature of granulocyte-macrophage colony stimulating factor in fetal mice. Exp Hematol 1978; 6:327–35.
20. Kaury MJ, Prognell IB. Retroviruses induce granulocyte-macrophage colony stimulating activity in fibroblasts. Nature 1982; 299:638–640.
21. Zucali JR, Dinarello CA, Oblon DJ. Interleukin I stimulates fibroblasts to produce granulocyte-macrophase colony-stimulating factor (GM-CSF). Proc Natl Acad Sci USA 1986; 83:8669.
22. Munker R, Gasson J, Ogawa M, Koeffler HP. Recombinant human tumor necrosis factor induces proliferation of granulocyte-monocyte colony stimulating factor mRNA and protein from lung fibroblasts and vascular endothelial cells in vitro. Nature 1986; 323:79.
23. Broxmeyer HE, Williams DE, Lu L. Biomolecules associated with suppression of myelopoiesis in normal conditions and during myeloid leukemia and other related disorders. In: Najman A, Guign M, Corin NC, Mary JY, eds. Inhibitory factors in the regulation of hematopoiesis. Paris, France: John Wiley Eurotext, 1987.
24. Pelus LM, Broxmeyer HE, Kurland JI, Moore MAS. Regulation of macrophage and granulocyte proliferation: specificities of prostaglandin E and lactoferrin. J Exp Med 1979; 150:277.
25. Peetre C, Gulberg U, Nilsson E, Olsen I. Effects of recombinant tumor necrosis factor on proliferation and differentiation of leukemia and normal hemopoietic cells in vitro. Relationship to cell surface receptor. J Clin Invest 1986; 78:1644.
26. Golde DW, Gasson JC. Gytokines: myeloid growth factors. In: Gallen JI, Goldstein IM, Synderman R, eds. Inflammation: basic principles and clinical correlates. New York: Raven Press, 1988:253.
27. Hakomori S, Fukuda M, Sekiguchi K, Carter WB: Fibronectin laminin and other extracellular glycoproteins. In: Piez KA, Ruddi AH, eds. Extracellular matrix biochemistry. New York: Elsevier, 1984:229–75.
28. Cochrane CG, Aiken BS. Polymorphonuclear leukocytes in immunologic reactions. The destruction of vascular basement membrane in vivo and in vitro. J Exp. Med 1966; 124:733–52.
29. Thorne KJI, Oliver RC, Barrett AJ. Lysis and killing of bacteria by lysosomal proteinases. Infect Immun 1976; 14:555–63.
30. Tomasic J, Keglevic D. The kinetics of hydrolysis of synthetic glucuronic esters and glucuronic esters by bovine liver and *Escherichia coli* β-glucuronidase. Biochem J 1983; 133:789–95.
31. Wallenfels K, Weil R. The enzymes, vol. VII, 3d ed., Boyer PD, ed. New York: Academic Press, 1972.
32. Pruzansky JJ, Patterson R. Subcellular distribution of histamine in human leukocytes. Proc Soc Exp Biol 1967; 124:56–9.
33. Becker EL, Showell HJ. The ability of chemotactic factors to induce lysosomal enzyme release II. The mechanisms of release. J Immunol 1974; 112:2055–62.
34. Odeberg H, Olsson I. Antibacterial activity of cationic proteins from human granulocytes. J Clin Invest 1975; 56:1118–24.
35. Travis J. Structure, function and control of neutrophil proteinases. Am J Med 1988; 84(6A):37–42.
36. Havermann K, Janoff A, eds. Neutral proteases of human polymorphonuclear leukocytes. Baltimore: Urban and Schuartzenberg, 1978.

37. Ohlsson K, Olsson I. The neutral proteases of human granulocytes. Isolation and partial characterization of granulocytic elastases. Eur J Biochem 1974; 42:519–27.
38. Baugh R, Travis J. Translation of collagen messenger RNA in a cell-free system derived from wheat germ. Biochemistry 1976; 15:836–41.
39. Starkey PM, Barratt AJ, Burleigh MC. The degradation of articular collagen by neutral proteinases. Biochim Biophys Acta 1977; 483:386–97.
40. Gosline JM, Rosenblood J. Elastin. In: Piez KA, Reddi AH, eds. Extracellular matrix biochemistry. New York: Elsevier, 1984:191–227.
41. Weiss S. Tissue destruction by neutrophils. N Engl J Med 1989; 320(6):365–76.
42. Henson PM, Henson JE, Fitlschen C, Kimani G, Bralton DL, Riches DWH. Phagocytic cells: degranulation and secretion. In: Gallin JI, Goldstein IM, Synderman R, eds. Inflammation: basic principles and clinical correlates. New York: Raven Press, 1988:363–80.
43. Janoff A. Elastase in tissue injury. Ann Rev Med 1985; 36:207–16.
44. Schultz J, Kaminker K. Myeloperoxidase of the leukocyte of normal human blood. I. Content and localization. Arch Biochem Biophys 1962; 96:465–7.
45. Agner K. Verdoperoxidase. Adv Enzymol 1943; 3:137–48.
46. Hayhoe FGJ, Cowley JC. Acute leukemia: cellular morphology, cytochemistry and fine structure. Clin Haematol 1972; 1:49.
47. Klebanoff SJ. Phagocytic cells: products of oxygen metabolism. In: Gallin JI, Goldstein IM, Snyderman R, eds. Inflammation, basic principles and clinical correlates. New York: Raven Press, 1988:391–333.
48. Belding ME, Lebanoff SJ, Roy CG. Peroxidase mediated virucidal systems. Science 1970; 167:195–6.
49. Wright CD, Bowie JU, Gray GR, Nelson RD. Candidacidal activity of myeloperoxidase: mechanisms of inhibitory influence of soluble cell wall mannan. Infect Immunol 1983; 42:76–80.
50. Lehrer RI, Cline MJ. Leukocyte myeloperoxidase deficiency and disseminated candediasis: the role of myeloperoxidase in resistance to candida infection. J Clin Invest 1969; 48:1478–88.
51. Klebanoff SJ. Myeloperoxidase: contribution to the microbicidal activity of intact leukocytes. Science 1970; 169:1095–7.
52. Stryer L. Biochemistry, 2d ed. San Francisco: WH Freeman, 1981.
53. Spitznagel JK. Non-exidative antimicrobial reactions of leukocytes. In: Synderman R, ed. Contemporary topics in immunobiology, vol. 14, chap. 10: Regulation of leukocyte function. New York: Plenum Press, 1984.
54. Chipman DM, Sharon N. Mechanism of lysozyme action. Lysozyme is the first enzyme for which the relation between structure and function has become clear. Science 1989; 165:454–65.
55. Lehrer RI, Ganz T, Selsted ME, Phagocytic defects I. Abnormalities outside of the respiratory burst. Oxygen-independent bactericidal systems. Mechanisms and disorders. Hematol Oncol Clin N Am 1988; 2:159.
56. Selsted ME, Szklorek D, Lehrer RI. Purification and antimicrobial activity of antimicrobial peptides of rabbit granulocytes. Infect Immun 1984, 45:150.
57. Ganz T. Extracellular release of antimicrobial defenses by human polymorphonuclear leukocytes. Infect Immun 1987; 56:568.
58. Weiss J, Victor M, Elsbach P. Role of charge and hydrophobic interactions in the action of bactericidal permeability increasing protein of neutrophils on gram negative bacteria. J Clin Invest 1983; 71:540.
59. Elsbach P, Weiss J. Phagocytic cells: oxygen independent antimicrobial systems. In: Gallin JT, Goldstein Im, Synderman R. Inflammation: basic principles and clinical correlates. New York: Raven Press, 1988:449–53.

60. Bainton DF, Ullyat JL, Farquhar MG. The development of neutrophilic polymorphonuclear leukocytes in human bone marrow. Origin and content of azurophil and specific granules. J Exp Med 1971; 134:907–34.
61. Klebanoff SJ, Clark RA. The neutrophil: function and clinical disorders. New York: North Holland, 1978:23–5.
62. Leffell MS and Spitznagel I. Intracellular and extracellular degranulation of human polymorphonuclear azuorphil and specific granules induced by immune complexes. Infect Immun 1974; 10:1241–9.
63. Masson PL, Heremans JF, Schonne E. Lactoferrin, an iron binding protein in neutrophilic leukocytes. J Exp Med 1969; 130:643–58.
64. Bennett RM, Kakocinsky T. Lactoferrin content of peripheral blood cells. Br J Haematol 1978; 39:509.
65. Bullen JJ, Roger HJ, Griffiths E. Role of iron in bacterial infection. Curr Top Microbol Immunol 1978; 35:792.
66. Ambruso DR, Johnson RB. Lactoferrin enhances hydroxyl radical production by human neutrophils, neutrophil particulate fractions, and an enzymatic generating system. J Clin Invest 1981; 67:352.
67. Ward PA, Till GO, Kunkel R, Beauchamp C. Evidence for role of hydroxyl radical in complement and neutrophil dependent tissue injury. J Clin Invest 1983; 72:780–801.
68. Oseas R, Yang HH, Baehner RL. Lactoferrin: a promoter of polymorphonuclear leuckotye adhesiveness. Blood 1981; 57:939.
69. Weiss SJ, Peppin GJ. Collagenolytic metalloenzymes of the human neutrophil: characteristics, regulation and potential function in vivo. Biochem Pharmacol 1986; 35:2189–97.
70. Hay ED. Cell biology of the extracellular matrix. New York: Plenum Press, 1981.
71. Wright DG, Gallin JL. Modulation of the inflammatory responses by products released from human polymorphonuclear leukocytes during phagocytosis. Generation and inactivation of the chemotactic factor C5a. Inflammation 1975; 1:23.
72. Granelli-Pepirnon A, Vassalli JD, Reich E. Secretion of plasminogen activator by human polymorphonuclear leukocytes. Modulation by glucocorticoids and other effectors. J Exp Med 1977; 146:1693.
73. Fletcher MP, Gallin JI. Human neutrophils contain an intracellular pool of putative receptors for the chemoattractant N-formyl-methionyl-leucyl-phenylalinine. Blood 1983; 62:792.
74. O'Shea JJ, Brown EJ, Seligmann M. Evidence for distinct intracellular peak of receptors for C3b and C3bi in human neutrophils. J Immunol 1985; 134:2580.
75. Smolen JE, Bower LA: Function of neutrophils. In: Williams WJ, Beutler E, eds. Hematology, 4th ed. New York: McGraw-Hill, 1990:782.
76. Barregaard N. The respiratory burst of phagocytosis: biochemistry and subcellular localization. Immunol Lett 1985; 11:165.
77. Murphy G, Britz U, Baggiolini M, Reynolds JJ. The latent collagenase and gelatinase of human polymorphonuclear leukocyte. Biochem J 1980; 192:517.
78. Dewald B, Bretz V, Baggiolini M. Release of gelatinase from a novel secretory compartment of human neutrophils. J Clin Invest 1982; 70:518.
79. Harlan JM, Killen PD, Senecal FM. The role of neutrophil membrane glycoprotein GP-150 in neutrophil adherence to endothelium in vitro. Blood 1985; 66:165.
80. Freeman BA, Crapo JD. Biology of disease. Free radicals and tissue injury. Lab Invest 1982; 47(5):412–26.
81. Dionisi D, Galeotti T, Terranova T, Azzi A. Superoxide radicals and hydrogen peroxide formation in normal and neoplastic tissues. Biochem Biophys Acta 1975; 403:292.
82. Mason RP, Kalyanaraman B, Trainer BE, Eling TE. A carbon centered free radical intermediate in the prostaglandin synthetase oxidation of arachidonic acid: spin trapping and oxygen uptake studies. J Biol Chem 1980; 256:5019.

83. Weiss SJ, LoBuglio AF. Phagocyte-generated oxygen metabolites and cellular injury. Lab Invest 1982; 47:5.
84. Babior BM. Oxygen-dependent microbial killing by phagocytes. N Engl J Med 1978; 298:659–68; 721–5.
85. Winterbaum CC. Lactoferrin-catalysed hydroxyl radical production: additional requirement for a chelating agent. Biochem J 1983; 210:15–9.
86. Aruma OI, Halliwell B. Superoxide-dependent and ascorbate-dependent formation of hydroxyl radicals in the presence of iron. Are lactoferrin and transferrin promoters of hydroxyl radical generation? Biochem J 1987; 241:273–8.
87. Weiss SJ, Klein R, Slivka A, Wei M. Chlorination of taurine by human neutrophils: evidence for hypochlorous acid generation. J Clin Invest 1982; 70:598–607.
88. Klebanoff SJ. Myeloperoxidase-halide-hydrogen peroxide antibacterial system. J Bacterial 1968; 95:2131–8.
89. Fantone JC, Ward PA. Polymorphonuclear leukocyte-mediated cell and tissue injury. Oxygen metabolites and their relation to human disease. Human Pathol 1985; 16(10):973–7.
90. Baehner RL, Boxer LA, Davis J. The biochemical basis of nitroblue tetrazolium reduction in normal human and chronic granulomatous disease polymorphonuclear leukocytes. Blood 1976; 48:309.
91. Curnutte JT, Babior BM. Chronic granulomatous disease. In: Harris H, Hirschhorn K, eds. Advances in human genetics, vol. 16. New York: Plenum Press, 1987:229–97.
92. Fantone JC, Ward PA. Role of oxygen-derived free radicals and metabolites in leukocyte-dependent inflammatory reactions. Am J Pathol 1979; 107:397–417.
93. Weiss SJ. Neutrophil (PMN) generated hydroxyl radicals (OH·) destroy RBC targets. Clin Res 1979; 27:466A.
94. Warren JS, Johnson KJ, Ward PA. Oxygen radicals in cell injury and cell death. Pathol Immunopathol Res 1987; 6:301–15.
95. Myers LS. Free radical damage of nucleic acids and their components. In: Pryer WA, ed. Free radicals in biology, vol. 4. New York: Academic Press, 1980:95.
96. Zeloc RE, Cromroy HL, Bolch WE, et al. Inhalid ozone as a mutagen I. Chromosome aberrations induced in Chinese hamster lymphocytes. Environ Res 1971; 4:262.
97. Mead JF. Free radical mechanisms of lipid damage and consequences for cellular membranes. In: Pryor WA, ed. Free radicals in biology, vol. 1. New York: Academic Press 1976:51–68.
98. Tappel AL, Dillard CJ. In vivo lipid peroxidation measurement via inhaled pentane and protection by vitamin E. Fed Proc 1981; 40:174.
99. Gutteridge JMC. Lipid peroxidation. In: Halliwell I, ed. Oxygen radicals and tissue injury. Bethesda: FASEB Publication, 1988:9–19.
100. Farber JL. Biology of Disease. Membrane injury and calcium hemostasis in the pathogenesis of coagulative necrosis. Lab Invest 1982; 47:114.
101. Maridenneaw I, Broquet P, Garay RR. Na^+ and K^+ transport damage induced by oxygen free radicals in human red cell membrane. J Biol Chem 1983; 258:3107.
102. Raubul WT, Tappel AL. Damage to protein, enzymes and amino acids by peroxidizing lipids. Arch Biochem Biophys 1966; 113:5–8.
103. Raubul WT, Tappel AL. Polymerization of protein induced by free radical lipid peroxidation. Arch Biochem Biophys 1966; 173:150–5.
104. Fligiel SEG, Lee EC, McCoy JP, Johnson KJ, Ward PA. Protein degradation following treatment with hydrogen peroxide. Am J Pathol 1984; 115:418–25.
105. Lucy JA. Functional and structural aspects of biological membranes: a suggested structural role of vitamin E in the control for membrane permeability and stability. Ann NY Acad Sci 1972; 203:4–11.
106. Michelson AM, McCord JM, Fridovich I. (eds). Superoxide and superoxide dismutases. New York: Academic Press, 1977.

107. Roos D, Weenig RS, Wyss SR, Aebi HE. Protection of human neutrophils by endogenous catalase: studies with catalase deficient individuals. J Clin Invest 1980; 65:1515–22.
108. Laurence RA, Burk RK. Glutathione peroxidase activity in selenium deficient rat liver. Biochem Biophys Res Commun 1976; 71:952–8.
109. Orrenius S, McConkey DJ, Nicotera P. Mechanisms of oxidant-induced cell damage. In: Cerutti PA, Fridovich I, McCord JM, eds. Oxy-radicals in molecular biology and pathology. New York: Alan R. Liss, 1988:327–39.
110. Fantone JC, Ward PA. Role of oxygen derived free radicals and metabolites in leukocyte-dependent inflammatory reactions. Am J Pathol 1982; 107(3):396–418.
111. Williams LT, Snyderman R, Pike MC, LEfkowitz RJ. Specific receptor sites for chemotactic peptides on human polymorphonuclear leukocytes. Proc Natl Acad Sci (USA) 1977; 74:1204–8.
112. Aswanikumar S, Corcoran B, Schiffmann E, Day AR, Freer RJ, Showell HJ, Becker EL, Pert CB. Demonstration of a receptor on rabbit neutrophils for chemotactic peptides. Biochem Biophys Res Comm 1977; 74:810–7.
113. Niedel J, Wilkinson S, Cuatrecaseas P. Receptor-mediated uptake of ^{125}l-chemotactic peptide by human neutrophils. J Biol Chem 1979; 254:10700-6.
114. Schiffmann E, Aswanikumar S, Venkatasubramanian K, Corcoran BA, Pert CB, Brown J, Gross E, Day AR, Freer RJ, Showell AH, Becker EL. Some characteristics of the neutrophil receptor for chemotactic peptides. FEBS Lett 1980; 117:1–7.
115. Walter RJ, Marasco WA. Direct visualization of formylpeptide receptor binding on rounded and polarized human neutrophils: cellular and receptor heterogeneity. J Leuk Biol 1987; 41:377–91.
116. Mackin WM, Huang CK, Becker EL. The formylpeptide chemotactic receptor on rabbit peritoneal neutrophils. I. Evidence for two binding sites with different affinities. J Immunol 1982; 129:1608–11.
117. Sklar LA, Mueller H, Omann G, Oades Z. Three states for the formyl peptide receptor on intact cells. J Biol Chem 1989; 264:8483–6.
118. Niedel J, David J, Cuatrecasas P. Covalent affinity labelling of the formyl peptide chemotactic receptor. J Biol Chem 1980; 255:7063–6.
119. Schmitt M, Painter RG, Jesaitis AJ, Preissner K, Sklar LA, Cochrane CG. Photoaffinity labeling of the N-formyl peptide receptor binding site of intact human polymorphonuclear leukocytes. A label suitable for following the fate of the receptor-ligand complex. J Biol Chem 1983; 258:649–54.
120. Huang CK. Partial purification and characterization of formylpeptide receptor from rabbit peritoneal neutrophils. J. Leukocyte Biol 1987; 41:63–69.
121. Allen RA, Jesaitis AJ, Sklar LA, Cochrane CG, Painter RG. Physicochemical properties of the N-formyl peptide receptor on human neutrophils. J Biol Chem 1986; 261:1854–7.
122. Gallin JI, Wright DG, Schiffmann E. Role of secretory events in modulating human neutrophil chemotaxis. J Clin Invest 1978; 62:1364–74.
123. Gallin JI, Metcalf JA, Roos D, Seligmann B, Friedman MM. Organelle-depleted human neutrophil cytoplasts used to study f Met-Leu-Phe receptor modulation and cell function. J Immunol 1984; 133:415–21.
124. Allen RA, Erickson RW, Jesaitis AJ. Identification of a human neutrophil protein of Mr 24000 that binds N-formyl peptides: co-sedimentation with specific granules. Biochim Biophys Acta 1989; 991:123–33.
125. Gardner JP, Melnick DA, Malech HL. Characterization of the formyl peptide chemotactic receptor appearing at the phagocytic cell surface after exposure to phorbol myristate acetate. J Immunol 1986; 136:1400–5.
126. Fletcher MP, Gallin JI. Human neutrophils contain an intracellular pool of putative receptors for the chemoattractant N-formyl-methionyl-leucyl-phenylalanine. Blood 1983; 62:792–9.
127. Painter RG, Zahler Bentz K, Dukes RE. Regulation of the affinity state of the N-

formylated peptide receptor of neutrophils: role of guanine nucleotide-binding proteins and the cytoskeleton. J Cell Biol 1987; 105:2959–71.

128. Polakis PG, Uhing RJ, Snyderman R. The formylpeptide chemoattractant receptor copurifies with a GTP-binding protein containing a distinct 40-kDa pertussis toxin substrate. J Biol Chem 1988; 263:4969–76.

129. Williamson K, Dickey BF, Pyun HY, Navarro J. Solubilization and reconstitution of the formylmethionylleucylphenylalanine receptor coupled to guanine nucleotide regulatory protein. Biochemistry 1988; 27:5371–7.

130. Polakis PG, Evans T, Snyderman R. Multiple chromatographic forms of the formylpeptide chemoattractant receptor and their relationship to GTP-binding proteins. Biochem Biophys Res Commun 1989; 161:276–83.

131. Cupo JF, Allen RA, Jesaitis AJ, Bokoch GM. Reconstitution and characterization of the human neutrophil N-formyl peptide receptor and GTP binding proteins in phospholipid vesicles. Biochim Biophys Acta 1989; 982:31–40.

132. Jesaitis AJ, Bokoch GM, Tolley JO, Allen RA. Lateral segregation of neutrophil chemotactic receptors into actin- and fodrin-rich plasma membrane microdomains depleted in guanyl nucleotide regulatory proteins. J Cell Biol 1988; 107:921–8.

133. Allen RA, Traynor AE, Omann GM, Jesaitis AJ. The chemotactic peptide receptor. A model for future understanding of chemotactic disorders. Hematol Oncol Clin N Am 1988; 2:33–59.

134. Jesaitis AJ, Allen RA. Activation of the neutrophil respiratory burst by chemoattractants: regulation of the N-formyl peptide receptor in the plasma membrane. J Bioenerg Biomembr 1988; 20:679–707.

135. Snyderman R, Pike MC, Edge S, Lane B. A chemoattractant receptor on macrophages exists in two affinity states regulated by guanine nucleotides. J Biol Chem 1984; 98:444–8.

136. Sklar LA, Bokoch GM, Button D, Smolen JE. Regulation of ligand-receptor dynamics by guanyl nucleotides: rapidly interconverting states for the neutrophil formyl peptide receptor. Fed Proc 1986; 45:5705a (abstr).

137. Goldman DW, Chang FH, Gifford LA, Goetzl EJ, Bourne HR. Pertussis toxin inhibition of chemotactic factor-induced calcium mobilization and function in human polymorphonuclear leukocytes. J Exp Med 1985; 162:145–56.

138. Sklar LA, Bokoch GM, Button D, Smolen JE. Regulation of ligand-receptor dynamics by guanine nucleotides. Real-time analysis of interconverting states for the neutrophil formyl peptide receptor. J Biol Chem 1987; 262:135–9.

139. Ng DS, Wong K. GTP regulation of platelet-activating factor binding to human neutrophil membranes. Biochem Biophys Res Comm 1986; 141:353–9.

140. Sherman JW, Goetzl EJ, Koo CH. Selective modulation by guanine nucleotides of the high affinity subset of plasma membrane receptors for leukotriene B4 on human polymorphonuclear leukocytes. J Immunol 1988; 140:3900–4.

141. Hyslop PA, Oades ZG, Jesaitis AJ, Painter RG, Cochrane CG, Sklar LA. Evidence for N-formyl chemotactic peptide-stimulated GTPase activity in human neutrophil homogenates. FEBS Lett 1984; 166:165–9.

142. Feltner DE, Smith RH, Marasco WA. Characterization of the plasma membrane bound GTPase from rabbit neutrophils. I. Evidence for an Ni-like protein coupled to the formyl peptide, C5a, and leukotriene B4 chemotaxis receptors. J Immunol 1986; 137:1961–70.

143. Wilde MW, Carlson KE, Manning DR, Zigmond SH. Chemoattractant-stimulated GTPase activity is decreased on membranes from polymorphonuclear leukocytes incubated in chemoattractant. J Biol Chem 1989; 264:190–6.

144. Pelz C, Matsumoto T, Molski TFP, Becker EL, Sha'afi RI. Characterization of the membrane-associated GTPase activity: Effects of chemotactic factors and toxins. J Cell Biochem 1989; 39:197–206.

145. Bokoch GM, Gilman AG. Inhibition of receptor-mediated release of arachidonic acid by pertussis toxin. Cell 1984; 39:301–8.
146. Okajima F, Ui M. ADP-ribosylation of the specific membrane protein by islet-activating protein, pertussis toxin, associated with inhibition of a chemotactic peptide-induced arachidonate release in neutrophils. Possible role of the toxin substrate in Ca^{2+}-mobilizing biosignaling. J Biol Chem 1984; 259:13863–71.
147. Becker EL, Kermode JC, Naccache PH, Yassin R, Munoz JJ, March ML, Huang CK, Sha'afi RI. Pertussis toxin as a probe of neutrophil activation. Fed Proc 1986; 45:2151–5.
148. Gireschik P, Sidiropoulos D, Spiegel A, Jakobs KH. Purification and immunochemical characterization of the major pertussis-toxin-sensitive guanine-nucleotide-binding protein of bovine-neutrophil membranes. Eur J Biochem 1987; 165:185–94.
149. Goldsmith P, Gierschik P, Milligan G, Unson CG, Vinitsky R, Malech, HL, Spiegel AM. Antibodies directed against synthetic peptides distinguish between GTP-binding proteins in neutrophil and brain. J Biol Chem 1987; 262:14683–8.
150. Uhing RJ, Polakis PG, Snyderman R. Isolation of GTP-binding proteins from myeloid HL-60 cells. Identification of two pertussis toxin substrates. J Biol Chem 1987; 262:15575–9.
151. Bokoch GM, Bickford K, Bohl BP. Subcellular localization and quantitation of the major neutrophil pertussis toxin substrate, J Cell Biol 1988; 106:1927–36.
152. Rotrosen D, Gallin JI, Spiegel AM, Malech HL. Subcellular localization of G_i-alpha in human neutrophils. J Biol Chem 1988; 263:10958–64.
153. Gierschik P, Falloon J, Milligan G, Pines M, Gallin JI, Spiegel A. Immunochemical evidence for a novel pertussis toxin substrate in human neutrophils. J Biol Chem 1986; 261:8058–62.
154. Oinuma M, Katada T, Ui M. A new GTP-binding protein in differentiated human leukemic (HL-60) cells serving as the specific substrate of islet-activating protein, pertussis toxin. J Biol Chem 1987; 262:8347–53.
155. Bokoch GM, Parkos CA. Identification of novel GTP-binding proteins in the human neutrophil. FEBS Lett 1988; 227:66–70.
156. Murphy PM, Eide B, Goldsmith P, Brann M, Gierschik P, Spiegel A, Malech HL. Detection of multiple forms of G_i-alpha in HL60 cells. FEBS Lett 1987; 221:81–6.
157. Kanaho Y, Stadel JM, Huang CK, Becker EL. Biochemical discrimination of the predominant pertussis toxin substrate of rabbit neutrophils from brain G_i and G_o: isoelectric focusing improves resolution of pertussis toxin substrates. Biochem Int 1988; 16:879–86.
158. Rudolph U, Koesling D, Hinsch K-D, Seifert R, Bigalke M, Schultz G, Rosenthal W. G-protein alpha-subunits in cytosolic and membranous fractions of human neutrophils. Mol Cell Endocrinol 1989; 63:143–53.
159. Smolen JE, Stoehr SJ. Guanine nucleotides reduce the free calcium requirement for secretion of granule constituents from permeabilized human neutrophils. Biochim Biophys Acta 1986; 889:171–8.
160. Barrowman MM, Cockcroft S, Gomperts BD. Two roles for guanine nucleotides in the stimulus-secretion sequence of neutrophils. Nature 1986; 319:504–7.
161. Mackin WM, Stevens TM. Biochemical and pharmacologic characterization of a phosphatidylinositol specific phospholipase C in rat neutrophils. J Leukocyte Biol 1988; 44:8–16.
162. Cockcroft S, Baldwin JM, Allan D. The Ca^{2+}-activated polyphosphoinositide phosphodiesterase of human and rabbit neutrophil membranes. Biochem J 1984; 221:477–82.
163. Dougherty RW, Godfrey PP, Hoyle PC, Putney JW Jr, Freer RJ. Secretagogue-induced phosphoinositide metabolism in human leucocytes. Biochem J 1984; 222:307–14.
164. Bradford PG, Rubin RP. Characterization of formylmethionyl-leucyl-phenylalanine stimulation of inositol trisphosphate accumulation in rabbit neutrophils. Mol Pharmacol 1985; 27:74–8.

165. Takenawa T, Ishitoya J, Homma Y, Kato M, Nagai Y. Role of enhanced inositol phospholipid metabolism in neutrophil activation. Biochem Pharmacol 1985; 34:1931–5.
166. Cockcroft S. Ca^{2+}-dependent conversion of phosphatidylinositol to phosphatidate in neutrophils stimulated with fMet-Leu-Phe or ionophore A23187. Biochim Biophys Acta 1984; 795:37–46.
167. Spat A, Bradford PG, McKinney JS, Rubin RP, Putney JW Jr. A saturable receptor for ^{32}P-inositol-1,4,5-trisphosphate in hepatocytes and neutrophils. Nature 1986; 319:514–6.
168. Prentki M, Wollheim CB, Lew PD. Ca^{2+} homeostasis in permeabilized human neutrophils. Characterization of Ca^{2+}-sequestering pools and the action of inositol 1,4,5-trisphosphate. J Biol Chem 1984; 259:13777–82.
169. Bradford PG, Rubin RP. Quantitative changes in inositol 1,4,5-trisphosphate in chemoattractant-stimulated neutrophils. J Biol Chem 1986; 261:15644–7.
170. Gierschik P, Jakobs KH. Receptor-mediated ADP-ribosylation of a phospholipase C-stimulating G protein. FEBS Lett 1987; 224:219–23.
171. Naccache PH, Molski MM, Volpi M, Becker EL, Sha'afi RI. Unique inhibitory profile of platelet activating factor induced calcium mobilization, polyphosphoinositide turnover and granule enzyme secretion in rabbit neutrophils towards pertussis toxin and phorbol ester. Biochem Biophys Res Commun 1985; 130:677–84.
172. Verghese MW, Charles L, Jakoi L, Dillon SB, Snyderman R. Role of a guanine nucleotide regulatory protein in the activation of phospholipase C by different chemoattractants. J Immunol 1987; 138:4374–80.
173. Smith CD, Uhing RJ, Snyderman R. Nucleotide regulatory protein-mediated activation of phospholipase C in human polymorphonuclear leukocytes is disrupted by phorbol esters. J Biol Chem 1987; 262:6121–7.
174. Strand CF, Parente JE, Wong K. Use of fluoride ion as a probe for the guanine nucleotide-binding protein involved in the phosphoinositide-dependent neutrophil transduction pathway. FEBS Lett 1986; 206:20–4.
175. Bradford PG, Rubin RP. Guanine nucleotide regulation of phospholipase C in permeabilized rabbit neutrophils. Inhibition by pertussis toxin and sensitization to submicromolar calcium concentrations. Biochem J 1986; 239:97–102.
176. Anthes JC, Billah MM, Cali A, Egan RW, Siegel MI. Chemotactic peptide, calcium and guanine nucleotide regulation of phospholipase C activity in membranes from DMSO-differentiated HL60 cells. Biochem Biophys Res Commun 1987; 145:825–33.
177. Mackin WM. Effects of GTPgammaS and fMet-Leu-Phe on rat PMN phospholipase C (PLC) activity. Agents Actions 1989; 27:407–9.
178. Pai JK, Siegel MI, Egan RW, Billah MM. Activation of phospholipase D by chemotactic peptide in HL-60 granulocytes. Biochem Biophys Res Commun 1988; 150:355–64.
179. Agwu DE, McPhail LC, Chabot MC, Daniel LW, Wykle RL, McCall CE. Choline-linked phosphoglycerides. A source of phosphatidic acid and diglycerides in stimulated neutrophils. J Biol Chem 1989; 264:1405–13.
180. Pai J-K, Siegel MI, Egan RW, Billah MM. Phospholipase D catalyzes phospholipid metabolism in chemotactic peptide-stimulated HL-60 granulocytes. J Biol Chem 1988; 263:12472–7.
181. Jackowski S, Rock CO. Stimulation of phosphatidylinositol 4,5-bisphosphate phospholipase C activity by phosphatidic acid. Arch Biochem Biophys 1989; 268:516–24.
182. Billah MM, Pai J-K, Mullmann TJ, Egan RW, Siegel MI. Regulation of phospholipase D in HL-60 granulocytes. Activation by phorbol esters, diglyceride, and calcium ionophore via protein kinase C-independent mechanisms. J Biol Chem 1989; 864:9069–76.
183. Gelas P, Ribbes G, Record M, Terce F, Chap H. Differential activation by fMet-Leu-Phe and phorbol ester of a plasma membrane phosphatidylcholine-specific phospholipase D in human neutrophil. FEBS Lett 1989; 251:213–8.
184. Anthes JC, Eckel S, Siegel MI, Egan RW, Billah MM. Phospholipase D in homogenates

from HL-60 granulocytes: implications of calcium and G protein control. Biochem Biophys Res Commun 1989; 163:657–64.

185. Billah MM, Eckel S, Mullmann TJ, Egan RW, Siegel MI. Phosphatidylcholine hydrolysis by phospholipase D determines phosphatidate and diglyceride levels in chemotactic peptide-stimulated human neutrophils. Involvement of phosphatidate phosphohydrolase in signal transduction. J Biol Chem 1989; 264:17069–77.

186. Bonser RW, Thompson NT, Randall RW, Garland LG. Phospholipase D activation is functionally linked to superoxide generation in the human neutrophil. Biochem J 1989; 264: 617–20.

187. Balsinde J, Diez E, Fernandez B, Mollinedo F. Biochemical characterization of phospholipase D activity from human neutrophils. Eur J Biochem 1989; 186:717–24.

188. Reinhold SL, Prescott SM, Zimmerman GA, McIntyre TM. Activation of human neutrophil phospholipase D by three separable mechanisms. FASEB J 1990; 4:208–14.

189. Ochs DL, Reed PW. ATP-dependent calcium transport in plasma membrane vesicles from neutrophil leukocytes. J Biol Chem 1983; 258:10116–22.

190. Ochs DL, Reed PW. Ca^{2+}-stimulated, Mg^{2+}-dependent ATPase activity in neutrophil plasma membrane vesicles. Coupling to Ca^{2+} transport. J Biol Chem 1984; 259:102–6.

191. Lagast H, Pozzan T, Waldvogel FA, Lew PD. Phorbol myristate acetate stimulates ATP-dependent calcium transport by the plasma membrane of neutrophils. J Clin Invest 1984; 73:107–15.

192. Goldman DW, Gifford LA, Olson DM, Goetzl EJ. Transduction by leukotriene B4 receptors of increases in cytosolic calcium in human polymorphonuclear leukocytes. J Immunol 1985; 135:525–30.

193. Korchak HM, Vienne K, Rutherford LE, Wilkenfeld C, Finkelstein MC, Weissmann G. Stimulus response coupling in the human neutrophil. II. Temporal analysis of changes in cytosolic calcium and calcium influx. J Biol Chem 1984; 259:4076–82.

194. Pozzan T, Lew DP, Wollheim CB, Tsein RY. Is cytosolic ionized calcium regulating neutrophil activation? Science 1983; 221:1413–5.

195. White JR, Naccache PH, Molski TFP, Borgeat, P, Sha'afi RI. Direct demonstration of increased intracellular concentration of free calcium in rabbit and human neutrophils following stimulation with chemotactic factor. Biochem Biophys Res Commun 1983; 113:44–50.

196. Volpi M, Yassin R, Tao W, Molski TFP, Naccache PH, Sha'afi RI. Leukotriene B4 mobilizes calcium without the breakdown of polyphosphoinositides and the production of phosphatidic acid in rabbit neutrophils. Proc. Natl. Acad. Sci. USA 1984; 81:5966–9.

197. Lew PD, Wollheim CB, Waldvogel FA, Pozzan T. Modulation of cytosolic-free calcium transients by changes in intracellular calcium-buffering capacity: correlation with exocytosis and O_2^- production in human neutrophils. J Cell Biol 1984; 99:1212–20.

198. Lew PD, Dayer JM, Wollheim CB, Pozzan T. Effect of leukotriene B_4, prostaglandin E_2 and arachidonic acid on cytosolic-free calcium in human neutrophils. FEBS Lett 1984; 166:44–8.

199. Kruskal BA, Shak S, Maxfield FR. Spreading of human neutrophils is immediately preceded by a large increase in cytoplasmic free calcium. Proc Natl Acad Sci USA 1986; 83:2919–23.

200. Rickard JE, Sheterline P. Evidence that phorbol ester interers with stimulated Ca^{2+} redistribution by activating Ca^{2+} efflux in neutrophil leucocytes. Biochem J 1985; 231:623–8.

201. Naccache PH, Molski MM, Volpi M, Shefcyk J, Molski TF, Loew L, Becker EL, Sha'afi RI. Biochemical events associated with the stimulation of rabbit neutrophils by platelet-activating factor. J Leuk Biol 1986; 40:533–48.

202. von Tscharner V, Prod'hom B, Baggionlini M, Reuter H. Ion channels in human neutrophils activated by a rise in free cytosolic calcium concentration. Nature 1986; 324:369–72.

203. Smolen JE, Stoehr SJ. Micromolar concentrations of free calcium provoke secretion of

lysozyme from human neutrophils permeabilized with saponin. J Immunol 1985; 134:1859–65.

204. Smolen JE, Stoehr SJ, Boxer LA. Human neutrophils permeabilized with digitonin respond with lysosomal enzyme release when exposed to micromolar levels of free calcium. Biochim Biophys Acta 1986; 886:1–17.

205. Sklar LA, Bokoch GM, Swann WN, Comstock C, Smolen JE. Ligand-receptor dynamics and signal amplification in the neutrophil. Int J Tissue React 1987; 9:277–84.

206. Smolen JE, Stoehr SJ, Bartone D. Protein kinase C is not involved in secretion by permeabilized human neutrophils. Cell Signal 1989; 1:471–81.

207. Stutchfield J, Cockcroft S. Guanine nucleotides stimulate polyphosphoinositide phosphodiesterase and exocytotic secretion from HL60 cells permeabilized with streptolysin O. Biochem J 1988; 250:375–82.

208. Gomperts BD, Barrowman MM, Cockcroft S. Dual role for guanine nucleotides in stimulus-secretion coupling. Fed Proc 1986; 45:2156–61.

209. Barrowman MM, Cockcroft S, Gomperts BD. Differential control of azurophilic and specific granule exocytosis in sendai-virus-permeabilized rabbit neutrophils. J Physiol 1987; 383:115–24.

210. Grinstein S, Furuya W. Receptor-mediated activation of electropermeabilized neutrophils. Evidence for a Ca^{2+}- and protein kinase C-independent signaling pathway. J Biol Chem 1988; 263:1779–83.

211. Smolen JE, Sandborg RR. Ca^{2+}-induced secretion by electropermeabilized human neutrophils. The roles of Ca^{2+}, nucleotides and protein kinase C. Biochim Biophys Acta 1990; 1052:133–142.

212. Lew PD, Monod A, Waldvogel FA, Dewald B, Baggiolini M, Pozzan T. Quantitative analysis of the cytosolic free calcium dependency of exocytosis from three subcellular compartments in intact human neutrophils. J Cell Biol 1986; 102:2197–204.

213. Walter A, Steer CJ, Blumenthal R. Polylysine induces pH-dependent fusion of acidic phospholipid vesicles: a model for polycation-induced fusion. Biochim Biophys Acta 1986; 861:319–30.

214. Ohki S, Duax J. Effects of cations and polyamines on the aggregation and fusion of phosphatidylserine membranes. Biochim Biophys Acta 1986; 861:177–86.

215. Duzgunes N, Straubinger RM, Baldwin PA, Friend DS, Papahadjopoulos D. Proton-induced fusion of oleic acid-phosphatidylethanolamine liposomes. Biochemistry 1985; 24:3091–8.

216. Morris SJ, Gibson CC, Smith PD, Greif PC, Stirk CW, Bradley D, Haynes DH, Blumenthal R. Rapid kinetics of Ca^{2+}-induced fusion of phosphatidylserine/phosphatidylethanolamine vesicles. The effect of bilayer curvature on leakage. J Biol Chem 1985; 260:4122–7.

217. Franson R, Patriarca P, Elsbach P. Phospholipid metabolism by phagocytic cells. Phospholipases A_2 associated with rabbit polymorphonuclear leukocyte granules. J Lipid Res 1974; 15:380–8.

218. Franson R, Weiss J, Martin L, Spitznagel JK, Elsbach P. Phospholipase A activity associated with the membranes of human polymorphonuclear leukocytes. Biochem J 1977; 167:839–41.

219. Kaplan L, Weiss J, Elsbach P. Low concentration of indomethacin inhibit phopholipase A_2 of rabbit polymorphonuclear leukocytes. Proc Natl Acad Sci USA 1978; 75:2955–8.

220. Traynor JR, Authi KS. Phospholipase A_2 activity of lysosomal origin secreted by polymorphonuclear leukocytes during phagocytosis or treatment with calcium. Biochim Biophys Acta 1981; 665:571–7.

221. Victor M, Weiss J, Klempner MS, Elsbach P. Phospholipase A_2 activity in the plasma membrane of human polymorphonuclear leukocytes. FEBS Lett 1981; 136:298–300.

222. Smith DM Jr, Waite M. Phospholipid metabolism in human neutrophil subfractions. Arch Biochem Biophys 1986; 246:263–73.
223. Clancy RM, Dahinden CA, Hugli TE. Arachidonate metabolism by human polymorphonuclear leukocytes stimulated by N-formyl-Met-Leu-Phe or complement component C5a is independent of phospholipase activation. Proc Natl Acad Sci USA 1983; 80:7200–4.
224. Bormann BJ, Huang CK, Mackin WM, Becker EL. Receptor-mediated activation of a phospholipase A_2 in rabbit neutrophil plasma membrane. Proc Natl Acad Sci USA 1984; 81:767–70.
225. Franson R, Waite M. Relation between calcium requirement, substrate charge, and rabbit polymorphonuclear leukocyte phospholipase A_2 activity. Biochemistry 1978; 17:4029–33.
226. Izumi F, Yanagihara N, Wada A, Toyohira Y, Kobayashi H. Lysis of chromaffin granules by phospholipase A_2-treated plasma membranes. A cell-free model for exocytosis in adrenal medulla. FEBS Lett 1986; 196:349–52.
227. Creutz CE, Dowling LG, Sando JJ, Villar-Palasi C, Whipple JH, Zaks WJ. Characterization of the chromobindins. Soluble proteins that bind to the chromaffin granule membrane in the presence of Ca^{2+}. J Biol Chem 1983; 258:14664–74.
228. Meers P, Ernst JD, Duzgunes N, Hong KL, Fedor J, Goldstein IM, Papahadjopoulos D. Synexin-like proteins from human polymorphonuclear leukocytes. Identification and characterization of granule-aggregating and membrane-fusing activities. J Biol Chem 1987; 262:7850–8.
229. Sato EF, Okimasu E, Takahashi R, Miyahara M, Matsuno T, Utsumi K. Lipocortin-like 33 kDa protein of guinea pig neutrophil. Its distribution and stimulation-dependent translocation detected by monoclonal anti-33 kDa protein antibody. Cell Structure Function 1988; 13:89–96.
230. Sato EF, Miyahara M, Utsumi K. Purification and characterization of a lipocortin-like 33 kDa protein from guinea pig neutrophils. FEBS Lett 1988; 227:131–5.
231. Stoehr SJ, Smolen JE, Suchard SJ. Lipocortins are major substrates for protein kinase C in extracts of human neutrophils. J Immunol 1990; 144:3936–3945.
232. Sato EF, Tanaka Y, Edashige K, Kobuchi H, Morishita S, Sugino YM, Inoue M, Utsumi K. Expression of the cDNA encoding lipocortin-like 39 kDa protein of guinea pig neutrophils in yeast. Purification and biological characterization. FEBS Lett 1989; 255:231–6.
233. Comera C, Rothhut B, Cavadore J-C, Wilgrain I, Cochet C, Chambaz E, Russo-Marie F. Further characterization of four lipocortins from human peripheral blood mononuclear cells. J Cell Biochem 1989; 40:361–70.
234. Blackwood RA, Ernst JD. Characterization of Ca^{2+}-dependent phospholipid binding, vesicle aggregation and membrane fusion by annexins. Biochem J 1990; 266:195–200.
235. Francis JW, Smolen JE, Balazovich KJ, Sandborg RR, Boxer LA. Calcium-dependent fusion of the plasma membrane fraction from human neutrophils with liposomes. Biochim Biophys Acta 1990; 1025:1–9.
236. White JR, Huang CK, Hill JM Jr, Naccache PH, Becker EL, Sha'afi RI. Effect of phorbol 12-myristate 13-acetate and its analogue 4alpha-phorbol 12,13-didecanoate on protein phosphorylation and lysosomal enzyme release in rabbit neutrophils. J Biol Chem 1984; 259:8605–11.
237. Andrews PC, Babior BM. Endogenous protein phosphorylation by resting and activated human neutrophils. Blood 1983; 61:333–40.
238. Okamura N, Ohashi S, Nagahisa N, Ishibashi S. Changes in protein phosphorylation in guinea pig polymorphonuclear leukocytes by treatment with membrane-perturbing agents which stimulate superoxide anion production. Arch Biochem Biophys 1984; 228:270–7.
239. Schneider C, Zanetti M, Romeo D. Surface-reactive stimuli selectively increase protein phosphorylation in human neutrophils. FEBS Lett 1981; 127:4-8.

240. Huang CK, Hill JM Jr, Bormann BJ, Mackin WM, Becker EL. Chemotactic factors induced vimentin phosphorylation in rabbit peritoneal neutrophil. J Biol Chem 1984; 259:1386–9.
241. Helfman DM, Applebaum BD, Volger WR, Kuo JF. Phospholipid-sensitive Ca^{2+}-dependent protein kinase and its substrates in human neutrophils. Biochem Biophys Res Commun 1983; 111:847–53.
242. Huang CK, Hill JM Jr, Bormann BJ, Mackin WM, Becker EL. Endogenous substrates for cyclic AMP-dependent and calcium-dependent protein phosphorylation in rabbit peritoneal neutrophils. Biochim Biophs Acta 1983; 760:126–35.
243. Niedel JE, Kuhn LJ, Vandenbark GR. Phorbol diester receptor copurifies with protein kinase C. Proc Natl Acad Sci USA 1983; 80:36–40.
244. Vandenbark GR, Kuhn LJ, Niedel JE. Possible mechanism of phorbol diester-induced maturation of human promyelocytic leukemia cells. Activation of protein kinase C. J Clin Invest 1984; 73:448–57.
245. Nishihira J, O'Flaherty JT. Phorbol myristate acetate receptors in human polymorphonuclear neutrophils. J Immunol 1985; 135:3439–47.
246. Deli E, Kiss Z, Wilson E, Lambeth JD, Kuo JF. Immunocytochemical localization of protein kinase C in resting and activated human neutrophils. FEBS Lett 1987; 221:365–9.
247. Shoji M, Girard PR, Mazzei GJ, Vogler WR, Kuo JF. Immunochemical evidence for phorbol ester-induced protein kinase C translocation in HL60 cells. Biochem Biophys Res Commun 1986; 135:1144–9.
248. O'Flaherty JT, Schmitt JD, Wykle RL, Redman JF Jr, McCall CE. Diacyglycerols and mezerein activate neutrophils by a phorbol myristate acetate-like mechanism. J Cell Physiol 1985; 125:192–9.
249. Berkow RL, Kraft AS. Bryostatin, a non-phorbol macrocyclic lactone, activates intact human polymorphonuclear leukocytes and binds to the phorbol ester receptor. Biochem Biophys Res Commun 1985; 131:1109–16.
250. O'Flaherty JT, Schmitt JD, Wykle RL. Interactions of arachidonate metabolism and protein kinase C in mediating neutrophil function. Biochem Biophys Res Commun 1985; 127:916–23.
251. Cooke E, Hallett MB. The role of C-kinase in the physiological activation of the neutrophil oxidase. Evidence from using pharmacological manipulation of C-kinase activity in intact cells. Biochem J 1985; 232:323–7.
252. Penfield A, Dale MM. Synergy between A23187 and 1-oleoyl-2-acetylglycerol in superoxide production by human neutrophils. Biochem Biophys Res Commun 1984; 125:332–6.
253. Dewald B, Payne TG, Baggiolini M. Activation of NADPH oxidase of human neutrophils. Potentiation of chemotactic peptide by a diacylgylcerol. Biochim Biophys Acta 1984; 125:367–73.
254. Tsung PK, Sakamoto T, Weissman G. Protein kinase and phosphatases from human polymorphonuclear leukocytes. Biochem J 1975; 145:437–48.
255. Juhl H, Esmann V. Phosphorylation of rabbit skeletal muscle glycogen synthase I by the cAMP dependent protein kinase, the cAMP independent synthase kinase and the phosvitin kinase from human polymorphonuclear leukocytes. Mol Cell Biochem 1980; 30:131–41.
256. Juhl H. Phosphorylation of glycogen synthase I from human polymorphonuclear leukocytes. Mol Cell Biochem 1981; 35:77–92.
257. Juhl H, Esmann V. Phosphorylation of glycogen synthase in a homogenate of human polymorphonuclear leukocytes. Mol Cell Biochem 1981; 35:93–101.
258. Nahas N, Juhl H, Esmann V. Chromatographic characteristics and subcellular localization of synthase phosphatase, phosphorylase phosphatase and histone phosphatase in human polymorphonuclear leukocytes. Mol Cell Biochem 1984; 58:147–56.
259. Wright CD, Hoffman MD. The protein kinase C inhibitors H-7 and H-9 fail to inhibit

human neutrophil activation. Biochem Biophys Res Commun 1986; 135:749–55.
260. Gerard C, McPhail LC, Marfat A, Stimler-Gerard NP, Bass DA, McCall CE. Role of protein kinases in stimulation of human polymorphonuclear leukocyte oxidative metabolism by various agonists. Differential effects of a novel protein kinase inhibitor. J Clin Invest 1986; 77:61–5.
261. Metchnikoff E. Immunity in infective diseases. New York: Johnson Reprint Company, 1905 (reprinted 1968).
262. Weissman G. Inflammation: historical perspectives. In: Gallin JI, ed. Inflammation: basic principles and clinical correlates. New York: Raven Press, 1985:5–8.
263. Hayashi H, Honda M, Shimakawa Y, Hirashima M. Chemotactic factors associated with leukocyte emigration in immune tissue injury: their separation, characterization and functional specificity. Int Rev Cytol 1984; 89:170–250.
264. Keller HU, Till GO (eds). Leukocyte locomotion and chemotaxis. Agents and actions. Base: Birkhauser, 1983; 12(suppl).
265. Sherry B, Cerami A. Cachectin/tumor necrosis factor exerts endocrine, paracrine and autocrine control of inflammatory responses. J Cell Biol 1988; 107:1269–77.
266. Le J, Vilcek J. Tumor necrosis factor and Interleukin 1: cytokines with multiple overlapping biological activities. Lab Invest 1987; 56:234.
267. Harlan JM. Leukocyte-endothelial interactions. Blood 1985; 65:513.
268. Bevilacqua MP, Gimbrone MA. Inducable endothelial functions in inflammation and coagulation. Seminars in thrombosis and hemostasis. 1987; 13(4):425–33.
269. Smith CW, et al. Recognition of an endothelial determinant of cD18-dependent human neutrophil adherence and transendothelial migration. J Clin Invest 1988; 82:1746–56.
270. Anderson DC, Springer TA. Leukocyte adhesion deficiency. An inherited defect in Mac-1, LFA-1, p 150, 95 glycoproteins. Ann Rev Med 1987; 38:175.
271. Nathan CV. Neutrophil activation on biological surfaces. J Clin Invest 1987; 80:1550–60.
272. Cochrane CG, Aiken BS. Polymorphonuclear leuckotyes in immunologic reactions. The destruction of vascular basement membrane in vivo and in vitro. J Exp Med 1966; 124:733–52.
273. Brigham KL, Meyrick B. Endotoxin and lung injury. Am Rev Resp Dis 1986; 133:913–27.
274. Till GO, Johnson KJ, Kunkel R, Ward PA. Intravascular activation of complement and acute lung injury: Dependency on neutrophils and toxic oxygen metabolites. J Clin Invest 1982; 69:1126–35.
275. Merrit TA, Cochrane CG, Hoolcomb K, Bohl B. Elastase and α1-proteinase inhibitor activity in tracheal aspirates during respiratory distress syndrome. J Clin Invest 1983; 72:656–66.
276. McGuire W, Spragg R, Cohen A, Cochrane CG. Studies of the pathogenesis of the adult respiratory distress syndrome. J Clin Invest 1982; 69:543–68.
277. Lee C, Fein A, Lippman M, Holtzmore H, Kimbel P, Weinbaum G. Elastoyltic activity in pulmonary lavage fluid from patients with adult respiratory disease syndrome. N Engl J Med 1981; 304:192–6.
278. Johnson KJ, Rehan A, Ward PA. The role of oxygen radicals in kidney disease. In: Halliwell I, ed. Oxygen radicals and tissue injury: proceedings of an Upjohn Symposium. Bethesda: FASEB Publications, 1988: 115–21.
279. Simpson PJ, Fantone, JC, Lucchesi BR. Myocardial ischemia and reperfusion injury. Oxygen radicals and the role of the neutrophil. In: Halliwell I, ed. Oxygen radicals and tissue injury: proceedings of an Upjohn Symposium. Bethesda: FASEB Publications, 1988:63–77.
280. Johnson KJ, Fantone JC, Kaplan J, Ward PA. In vivo damage of rat lungs by oxygen metabolites. J Clin Invest 1981; 67:983–93.

281. Tate RM, Vanbenthuysen KM, Shasby DM. Oxygen-radical-mediated permeability edema and vasoconstriction in isolated perfused rabbit lungs. Ann Rev Resp Dis 1982; 126:802–6.
282. Johnson KJ, Ward PA. Role of oxygen metabolites in immune complex injury of lung. J Immunol 1981; 126:2365–9.
283. Fligiel SE, Ward PA, Johnson KJ, Till GO. Evidence for a role of hydroxy radical in immune complex-induced vasculities. Am J Pathol 1984; 115:375–82.
284. Ward PA, Till GO, Kunkel R, Beauchamp C. Evidence for role of hydroxyl radical in complement and neutrophil-dependent tissue injury. J Clin Invest 1983; 72:789–801.
285. Till GO, Johnson KJ, Kunkel R, Ward PA. Intravascular activation of complement and acute lung injury: dependency on neutrophils and toxic oxygen metabolites. J Clin Invest 1982; 69:1126–35.
286. Till GO, Hatherill JR, Tourtellotte WW, Lutz MJ, Ward PA. Lipid peroxidation and acute lung injury after thermal trauma to skin. Evidence of a role for hydroxyl radical. Am J Pathol 1985; 119:376–84.
287. Johnson KJ, Ward PA, Kunkel RG, Wilson BS. Mediation of IgA induced lung injury in the rat. Role of macrophages and reactive oxygen products. Lab Invest 1986; 54:499–506.
288. Gramse M, Havemann K, Egbring R. Alpha-2-plasmin-inhibitor inactivation by human granulocyte elastase. Adv Exp Med Biol 1984; 167:253–61.
289. Janoff A, Carp H. Proteases, antiproteases and oxidants: pathways of tissue injury during inflammation. Monogr. Pathol. 1982; 23:62–82.
290. McDonald JA, Kelley DG. Degradation of fibronectin by human leukocyte elastase. J Biol Chem 1986; 255:8848–58.
291. Ott V, Odermatt E, Engel J, Furthmayr H, Timpl R. Protease esistance and conformation of laminin. Eur J Biochem 1982; 123:63–72.
292. Clark RA, Klebanoff SJ. Myeloperoxidase-mediated platelet release reaction. J Clin Invest 1979; 63:177.
293. Hensen PM, Henson JE, Eitlschen C, Kimani G, Bratton DL, Riches DWH. Phagocytic cells. Degranulation and secretion. In: Gallin JI, Goldstein IM, Snyderman R, eds. Inflammation: basic principles and clinical correlates. New York: Raven Press, 1988:363–80.
294. Janoff A. Elastase in tissue injury. Ann Rev Med 1986; 36:207–16.
295. Smedley LA, Tonnesen MG, Haslett G, Guthrie LA, Johnston RB, et al. Neutrophil-mediated injury to endothelial cells. J Clin Invest 1988; 77:1233–43.
296. Janoff A, Carp H, Laurent P, Raju L. The role of oxidative processes in emphysema. Am Rev Resp Dis 1983; 127:S31–8.
297. Janoff A. Elastases and emphysema. Current assessment of the protease-antiprotease hypothesis. Am Rev Resp Dis 1985; 132:417–33.
298. Damiano VV, Tsang A, Kucich V. Immunolocalization of elastase in human emphysematous lungs. J Clin Invest 1980; 78:482–93.
299. Bruce MC, Poncz L, Klinger JD, Stern RC, Tomashifski JF, Dorr DG. Biochemical and pathologic evidence for proteolytic destruction of lung connective tissue in cystic fibrosis. Am Rev Resp Dis 1985; 132:529–35.
300. Lee CT, Fein AM, Lippman M, Holtzman H, Kimbel P, Weinbaum G. Elastolytic activity in pulmonary lavage fluid from patients with adult respiratory disease syndrome. N Engl J Med 1981; 304:192–6.
301. Fritz H, Jochum M, Geiger R, Dusuald KH. Folia Histochemica et Cytobiologica 1986; 24:99–115.
302. Hock CE, Lefer AM. Beneficial effects of a neutral protease inhibitor in traumatic shock. Pharmacol Res Commun 1985; 17(3):217–226.
303. Wong PS, Travis J. Isolation and properties of oxidized alpha-1 proteinase inhibitor from human rheumatoid synovial fluid. Biochem Biophys Res Commun 1980; 96:1449–54.

304. Senior RM, Tegner H, Kuhn K, Ohlsson B, Starcher B, Pierce JA. The induction of pulmonary emphysema with human leukocyte elastase. Am Rev Resp Dis 1977; 116:469–75.
305. Janoff A, Sloan B, Weinbaum G, Damiano R, Sanahais A, Elias J, Kimbel P. Experimental emphysema induced with purified human neutrophil elastase: tissue localization of the instilled protease. Am Rev Respir Dis 1977; 115:461–78.
306. Baird BR, Cheroncis JC, Sanglhaus RA, Berger EM, White CW, Repine JC. O_2^- metabolites and neutrophil elastase synergistically cause edematous injury in isolated rat lungs. J Appl Physiol 1986; 61:2224–9.
307. Hawkins G, Cochrane GG. Glomerular basement membrane damage in immunological glomerulonephritis. J Immunol 1968; 14(5):665–81.
308. Hennette JC, Tedwell RR, Geratz JD, Bing DH, Falk RJ. Amerlioration of immune complex-mediated glomerulonephritis by synthetic protease inhibitors. Am J Pathol 1987; 127:499–506.
309. Weiss SJ, Peppin GJ. Collagenolytic metalloenzymes of the human neutrophil: characteristics, regulation and potential function in vivo. Biochem Pharmacol 1986; 35:3189–97.
310. Weiss SJ. Tissue destruction by neutrophils. N Engl J Med 1989; 320(6):365–76.
311. Sacks T, Moldow CF, Craddock PR, Bowers TK, Jacob HA. Oxygen radicals mediate endothelial cell damage by complement-stimulated granulocytes: an in vitro model of immune complex vasculitis. J Clin Invest 1978; 61:1161–7.
312. Weiss SJ, Young J, LoBuglio AF, Slivka A, Nimeh NF. Role of hydrogen peroxide in neutrophil-mediated destruction of cultured endothelial cells. J Clin Invest 1981; 68:714–20.
313. Martin WJ. Neutrophils kill pulmonary endothelial cells by a hydrogen peroxide-dependent pathway: an in vitro model of neutrophil-mediated lung injury. Am Rev Resp Dis 1984; 130:209–13.
314. Clark RA, Klebanoff SJ. Neutrophil-mediated tumor cell cytotoxicity: role of the peroxidase system. J Exp Med 1975; 141:1442–7.
315. Nathan CF, Silverstein SC, Brukner LH, Cohn ZA. Extracellular cytolysis by activated macrophages and granulocytes. II. Hydrogen peroxide as mediator of cytotoxicity. J Exp Med 1979; 149:100–13.
316. Varani J, Fligiel SEG, Till GO, Kunkel RG, Ryan US, Ward PA. Pulmonary endothelial cell killing by human neutrophils: possible involvement of hydroxyl radical. Lab Invest 1985; 53:656–63.
317. Gannon DE, Varani J, Phan SH, Ward JH, Kaplan J, Till GO, Simon RH, Ryan US, Ward PA. Source of iron in neutrophil-mediated killing of endothelial cells. Lab Invest 1987; 57:37–44.
318. Phan SH, Gannon DE, Varani J, Ryan US, Ward PA. Xanthine oxidase activity in rat pulmonary artery endothelial cells and its modulation by activated neutrophils. Am J Pathol 1989; 134:1201–11.
319. Varani J, Phan SH, Gibbs DF, Ryan US, Ward PA. H_2-mediated cytotoxicity of rat pulmonary artery endothelial cells: changes in ATP and purine products and effects of protective interventions. Lab Invest 1990; 63:683–689.
320. Rodell TC, Cheronis JC, Ohnemus CL, Piermattei DJ, Repine JE. Xanthine oxidase mediates elastase induced injury to isolated lungs and endothelium. J Appl Physiol 1987; 63:2159–63.
321. Harlan JM, Killen PD, Harker LA, Striker GE, Wright DG. Neutrophil-mediated endothelial injury in vitro: mechanisms of cell detachment. J Clin Invest 1981; 68:1394–9.
322. Harlan JM, Schwartz BR, Reidy MA, Schwartz SM, Ochs HD, Harker LA. Activated neutrophils disrupt endothelial monolayer integrity by an oxygen radical-independent mechanism. Lab Invest 1985; 52:141–50.
323. Smedly LA, Tonnesen MG, Sandhaus RA, Haslett C, Guthrie LA, Johnson RB, Henson PM, Worthen GS. Neutrophil-mediated injury to endothelial cells: enhancement by endo-

toxin and essential role of neutrophil elastase. J Clin Invest 1986; 77:1233–43.
324. Pontremoli S, Melloni E, Michetti M, Sacco O, Sparatore B, Salamino F, Damiani G, Horecker BL. Cytolytic effects of neutrophils: role for a membrane-bound neutral proteinase. Proc Natl Acad Sci USA 1986; 83:1685–9.
325. Ginsburg I, Gibbs DF, Schuger L, Johnson KJ, Ryan US, Ward PA, Varani J. Vascular endothelial cell killing by combination of membrane-active agents and hydrogen peroxide. Free Radicals Biol Med 1989; 7:369–76.
326. Ginsburg I, Borinski R, Sadovnic M, Eilam Y, Rainsford K. Poly-L-histidine, a potent stimulator of superoxide generation in human blood leukocytes. Inflammation 1987; 11:253–77.
327. Ginsburg I, Ward PA, Varani J. Lysophosphatides enhance superoxide responses of stimulated human neutrophils. Inflammation 1989; 13:163–79.
328. Varani J, Ginsburg I, Schuger L, Gibbs DF, Bromberg J, Johnson KJ, Ryan US, Ward PA. Endothelial cell killing by neutrophils: synergistic interaction of oxygen products and proteases. Am J Pathol 1989; 135:435–8.
329. Shalaby MR, Aggarwal BB, Rinderknecht E, Svedersky LP, Finkle BS, Palladino MA. Activation of human polymorphonuclear neutrophil function by interferon-γ and tumor necrosis factor. J Immunol 1985; 135:2069.
330. Larrick JW, Graham D, Toy K, Lin LS, Senyk G, Fendly BM. Recombinant tumor necrosis factor causes activation of human granulocytes. Blood 1987; 69:640.
331. Bevilacqua MP, Pober JS, Wheeler ME, Cotran RS, Gimbrone MA Jr. Interleukin I acts on cultured human vascular endothelium to increase the adhesion of polymorphonuclear leukocytes, monocytes and related leukocyte cell lines. J Clin Invest 1985; 76:2003.
332. Pober JS, Bevilacqua MP, Mendrick DL, Lapierre LA, Fiers W, Gimbrone MA. Two distinct monokines, interleukin 1 and tumor necrosis factor, each independently induce biosynthesis and transient expression of the same antigen on the surface of cultured human vascular endothelial cells. J Immunol 1986; 136:1680.
333. Schuger L, Varani J, Marks R, Kunkel SL, Johnson KJ, Ward PA. Cytotoxicity of tumor necrosis factor-α for human umbilical vein endothelial cells. Lab Invest 1989; 61:62–8.
334. Varani J, Bendelow MJ, Sealey DE, Kunkel SL, Gannon DE, Ryan US, Ward PA. Tumor necrosis factor enhances susceptibility of vascular endothelial cells to neutrophil-mediated killing. Lab Invest 1989; 59:292–4.
335. Rothestein JL, Schreiber H. Tumor necrosis factor and bacterial products synergize to induce hemorrhagic necrosis and lethal shock in normal mice. FASEB J 1988; 2:A1821.

2

The Neutrophil Respiratory Burst Mechanism

LINDA C. McPHAIL, SUSAN L. STRUM, PETER A. LEONE
Wake Forest University, Bowman Gray School of Medicine, Winston-Salem, North Carolina

SILVANO SOZZANI
Istituto di Richerche Farmacologiche Mario Negri, Milan, Italy

I. THE NEUTROPHIL RESPIRATORY BURST ENZYME

A. Function of the Respiratory Burst

Human polymorphonuclear leukocytes (neutrophils, PMNs) markedly increase their utilization of oxygen upon interaction with opsonized particles or a variety of inflammatory stimuli, a phenomenon termed the respiratory burst. Oxygen is converted by the cell to several toxic metabolites, including superoxide anion (O_2^-), hydrogen peroxide (H_2O_2), and hypochlorous acid. It has been well documented that normal production of these oxygen metabolites by blood and tissue phagocytic cells is vital for the successful resistance of individuals to bacterial infections (reviewed in 1,2). In addition, enhanced production of reactive oxygen species may be detrimental to the host in certain disease states, i.e., adult respiratory distress syndrome, arthritis, etc. (reviewed in 1,2).

B. Components of the Respiratory Burst Enzyme

The enzyme responsible for converting oxygen to toxic products is an NADPH oxidase, which catalyzes the following reaction:

$$NADPH + 2O_2 \rightarrow NADP^+ + 2O_2^- + H^+ \quad (1)$$

Evidence to date suggests that the active enzyme system is membrane bound and that at least five polypeptides are either associated with the enzyme or necessary for activity (reviewed in 3). These are summarized in Table 1 and include: a heterodimeric cytochrome b, cytochrome b_{558}, consisting of two polypeptides—one of ~22 kDa (p22-*phox*) and a glycoprotein of ~91 kDa (gp91-*phox*); a low-molecular-weight (~22 kDa) guanine nucleotide regulatory protein (G-protein), *rap*-1; and two cytosolic proteins of ~47 kDa (p47-*phox*) and ~67 kDa (p67-*phox*). Except for cytochrome b_{558},

Table 1 Components of NADPH Oxidase

Component	MW	Characteristics[a]
Membrane-associated		
gp91-*phox*	91 kDa	Glycosylated subunit of cytochrome b_{558}; defective in X-linked CGD; expression of gene is unique to phagocytic cells and B-lymphocytes
p22-*phox*	22 kDa	Nonglycosylated subunit of cytochrome b_{558}; defective in ~11% of autosomal recessive CGD cases; expression of gene, but not protein, found in many cell types
rap-1	22 kDa	*ras*-related G-protein; not defective in CGD; found in many cell types; substrate for PKA; cycles between membrane and cytosol?
Cytosolic factors		
p67-*phox*	67 kDa	Defective in ~11% of autosomal recessive CGD cases; protein is unique to phagocytic cells and B-lymphocytes; contains two SH3 regions
p47-*phox*	47 kDa	Defective in ~75% of autosomal recessive CDG cases; protein is unique to phagocytic cells and B-lymphocytes; contains two SH3 regions; substrate of PKC and PKA
"Factor 3"	?	Not characterized; present in many cell types; *rap*1?

[a] See text for references.

the function of most of these putative oxidase components is unknown. The following sections summarize the properties of each of these polypeptides, as currently understood.

1. Cytochrome b_{558}

The unique cytochrome b_{558} has an unusually low midpoint potential (−245 mV) and is thought to be the terminal electron acceptor, accepting electrons derived from NADPH and donating them directly to oxygen (reviewed in 3,4). It is hypothesized that the NADPH oxidase may be an electron-transport chain and that the initial electron acceptor interacting with NADPH is a flavoprotein, possibly of ~66 kDa or 45 kDa MW (3–5). However, none of the proteins classified thus far as oxidase components has been proven to be a flavoprotein and/or the NADPH-binding protein. Identification of the NADPH-binding protein remains an area of active research (5–14).

The genes for the two polypeptide subunits of cytochrome b_{558} have been cloned (15–18), and defects in each gene are responsible for separate forms of NADPH oxidase deficiency in patients with chronic granulomatous disease (CGD) (19). The gene for gp91-*phox* is on the X chromosome (4,15), and defects in this gene account for approximately 56% of total patient defects (19). The gene for p22-*phox* is on chromosome 16 (20), and defects in this gene account for only about 5% of patients (19). Expression of the gene for p22-*phox* is found in many cell types, while the gene for gp91-*phox* is expressed only in phagocytic cells (15,18). However, both proteins must be present in order to obtain detectable levels of either in a cell (18). Therefore, the intracellular stability of either polypeptide chain must be dependent on the presence of the other.

Evaluation of the predicted sequence for each subunit has not revealed significant sequence similarity to known proteins; nor does the sequence predict an unequivical heme-binding region on either polypeptide (4,20). It has been speculated that the heme binds partially to both polypeptides (18), although some studies suggest association of the heme with p22-*phox* (21,22). Cytochrome b_{558} may also have a noncatalytic, structural role in oxidase function. Recent studies (23–25) suggest that a site on gp91-*phox* near the carboxy terminus is required for translocation of cytosolic NADPH oxidase components. The structural feature of the holoenzyme responsible for its functions in the oxidase complex will be an important area for further study.

Studies by Jesaitis and co-workers (26), using affinity-purified antibodies and electron microscopy, have localized both cytochrome b_{558} subunits largely to lactoferrin-bearing specific granules, with about 20% of the cytochrome present in the plasma membrane, in unstimulated neutrophils. This confirms earlier subcellular fractionation studies by Borregaard et al. (27). However, the plasma membrane compartment may be partially composed of an easily mobilizable subset of cytoplasmic granules reported to contain the majority of the cytochrome not present in specific granules (28,29). The purpose of the intracellular localization of cytochrome b_{558} is unclear. Fusion of specific granule membranes with plasma membrane is not necessarily correlated with nor required for activation of NADPH oxidase (30,31). It is possible that the translocation of cytochrome b_{558} from either specific or the easily mobilizable granules functions to augment the amount of NADPH oxidase available for activation in the plasma membrane under certain conditions (29), which may play a role in the phenomenon known as priming of neutrophils.

2. *Rap*-1

A member of the *ras* proto-oncogene family, *rap*-1, has been shown by Jesaitis and co-workers (32) to co-purify with cytochrome b_{558}, and thus may be an oxidase component. In addition, preliminary evidence suggests that other polypeptides important for oxidase function (p47-*phox* and p67-*phox*) can be immunopurified with cytochrome b_{558} and *rap*-1 from stimulated neutrophils and that guanine nucleotides regulate the association between the cytochrome and the G-protein (33). These studies demonstrate that *rap*-1 is closely associated with the NADPH oxidase and could be an oxidase component with an as-yet unknown function.

It is intriguing to speculate that *rap*-1 participates in the guanine nucleotide sensitivity observed for NADPH oxidase activation in cell-free systems (34–38). In support of this is a recent report (39) that *rap*-1 has a cytosolic location in neutrophils and participates directly in the cell-free activation of NADPH oxidase. However, *rap*-1 is found in cell types other than phagocytes (40) and is therefore likely to have a generalized role in cell function. In this regard, *rap*-1 has been shown to reverse the *ras* phenotype (41). In addition, *rap*-1 can be phosphorylated by cyclic AMP-dependent protein kinase (PKA), and phosphorylation induces partial release of the G-protein from the membrane (42,43). Thus, *rap*-1 may be the site for inhibition of chemoattractant-triggered activation of NADPH oxidase by agents which increase cyclic AMP (cAMP) levels in cells (reviewed in 44, below, and in Chapter 9). Additional research is needed for understanding the precise function of *rap*-1 in regulating NADPH oxidase activation.

3. Cytosolic Factors

The development of a cell-free system for NADPH oxidase activation, by Bromberg and Pick (45) and Heyneman and Vercauteren (46) in animal phagocytes and by our laboratory (47) and that of Curnutte (48) in human neutrophils, has led to the discovery of several cytosolic proteins necessary for oxidase function. Two of these (p47-*phox* and p67-*phox*) are absent in separate forms of autosomal recessive CGD (19,49–51). The absence of p47-*phox* accounts for most of the patients with this form of the disease and is responsible for ~33% of total surveyed cases of CGD (19). Deficiency of p67-*phox* is much less prevalent, accounting for ~5% of total cases (19).

Since the deficiency of either of these proteins results in CGD, they must play an essential role in NADPH oxidase function. However, their role in either the activation or the catalytic activity of the enzyme is still obscure. The genes for both of these proteins have recently been cloned (52–55). Interestingly, analyses of the predicted amino acid sequence suggests two regions of sequence similarity in each protein to a region termed SH3 found in a variety of cytosolic proteins involved in cell signaling mechanisms (52–55). Proteins containing SH3 regions include: phospholipase $C_{-\gamma}$ (56); the *src* family of nonreceptor tyrosine kinases (56); a protein (GAP) which stimulates the GTPase activity of the G-protein *ras* (57); the cytoskeletal protein α-spectrin (58); and the yeast proteins *IRA1* (59), CDC25 (60), and STE6 (61). The SH3 region is thought to be in a noncatalytic domain of each protein, suggesting all of these proteins either share common structural features or interact with common cellular elements. Others have speculated that the SH3 region functions to promote cytoskeletal interactions (55) or interactions with low-molecular-weight G-proteins such as *rap*-1 (54). Preliminary evidence (62) suggests that elimination of the carboxyterminal SH3 region from p67-*phox* does not abrogate its ability to function in the activation of NADPH oxidase in a cell-free system. Thus, this region is either not necessary for functioning of p67-*phox* or the cell-free system bypasses the need for this regulatory site. Elucidation of the function of the SH3 regions in p47-*phox*, p67-*phox*, and other signaling proteins will be an active area of investigation.

The p47-*phox* protein has several predicted sites for phosphorylation on serine residues and one site predicted for phosphorylation on tyrosine (52–54). Phosphorylation of this protein in response to cell stimulation was initially reported to be absent in patients with the autosomal recessive form of CGD by Segal and co-workers (63). Babior and his colleagues (64,65) established that this protein was phosphorylated on multiple sites during cell stimulation, resulting in several forms with pI's ranging from ~6 to ~9 by two-dimensional electrophoresis. Our laboratory (66) reported that phosphorylation of this protein in subcellular fractions of neutrophils from patients with autosomal recessive CGD was also absent in the cell-free system for NADPH oxidase activation. These observations were understood when it was established that this phosphorylated protein is one of the cytosolic factors necessary for NADPH oxidase activation and is absent in most patients with the autosomal recessive form of the disease (19,49,50,67). Roos and co-workers have demonstrated that p47-*phox* is a substrate in vitro for both protein kinase C (PKC) (68) and PKA (69). Whether or not p47-*phox* is a substrate for a tyrosine kinase has not yet been rigorously examined. The role that phosphorylation of p47-*phox* may have in controlling NADPH oxidase activity is not yet clear and will be discussed in more detail below. However, studies of the structure and function of p47-*phox* will be facilitated by recent reports of its purification from normal PMNs (70) and expression of the functional recombinant protein in a baculovirus system (62).

At least one other cytosolic factor is necessary for activation of NADPH oxidase in the cell-free system (50,51,71). This protein or proteins has not yet been well characterized or purified, but it has been implicated in mediating the sensitivity of the cell-free system to guanine nucleotides (71). Interestingly, this factor appears to be found in a variety of nonphagocytic cell types (72), in contrast to p47-*phox* and p67-*phox*, which have been reported as present only in phagocytic cells and B lymphocytes (49,54). It is possible that this protein is *rap*-1. Available evidence suggests that the multiple cytosolic factors may form a complex or interact with one another in some way (9,49,50,72–74), and this is currently an active area of investigation.

II. ACTIVATION OF THE RESPIRATORY BURST ENZYME

A. Introduction

Although tremendous progress has been made in identification of NADPH oxidase components, the mechanism(s) by which the enzyme complex becomes activated upon cellular stimulation is still unknown. Activation presumably requires the translocation of certain components and assembly of an active complex. Activation of NADPH oxidase can be initiated at the plasma membrane of the phagocytic cell by the binding of an extracellular stimulus to its cell-surface receptor. The second messengers generated from such receptor-ligand interactions implicate a variety of signal transductional mechanisms as candidates for mediating oxidase activation. Studies in vitro using agonists which bypass receptor-ligand interactions and act at specific sites in signaling pathways have further implicated certain signaling mechanisms.

Table 2 summarizes the categories of stimuli which have been shown to activate the respiratory burst in either intact or permeabilized human neutrophils and the signaling pathways which may be involved with each. Stimuli can be classified as either *receptor-mediated* (interacting with specific cell-surface receptors) or *non-receptor-mediated* (affecting cell membranes or interacting directly with intracellular proteins). The following sections will briefly discuss the evidence supporting the participation of various signaling pathways utilized by these stimuli and also summarize the data obtained in a cell-free system for NADPH oxidase activation implicating potential activation mechanisms. Additional information can be obtained in previous reviews (1,44,75,76).

B. Receptor-Mediated Stimuli—Generation of Second Messengers

A wide variety of extracellular ligands bind to specific receptors on the surface of neutrophils, resulting in either the activation of NADPH oxidase or enhancement of activation by a second stimulus (priming). These can be categorized into four major classes: (a) *Chemoattractants* are peptides or lipids which induce chemotaxis of neutrophils, as well as triggering of the respiratory burst; (b) *phagocytic stimuli* are protein ligands that also trigger phagocytosis of particles to which they are attached; (c) *cytokines* are proteins, secreted by inflammatory cells, which are good priming agonists but which require ligation of an additional unrelated receptor for triggering of the respiratory burst; (d) *extracellular ATP* binds to P_2-purinergic cell-surface receptors (77) and primes the respiratory burst (78).

Table 2 Categories of PMN Stimuli That Activate NADPH Oxidase[a]

Category	Examples	Possible transduction pathways
Receptor-mediated		
Chemoattractants	fMLP, LTB_4, C5a	Pertussis toxin-sensitive G-protein(s), phospholipases (C, D) protein kinases (PKC, tyrosine kinases)
Phagocytic	IgG, C3b, iC3b	Pertussis toxin-insensitive and -sensitive G-protein, phospholipases (A_2, C, D), other?
Cytokine	TNF-α, GM-CSF	Dual receptors, decreased cAMP, phospholipases (A_2, D), tyrosine kinases, other?
Extracellular ATP	ATP	Same as chemoattractants?
Non-receptor-mediated		
G-protein agonists	F^-, GTP-γ-S	Various G-proteins, phospholipases (A_2, C, D?), protein kinases
PKC activators	PMA, DAG	PKC, phospholipase D
Ca^{2+} ionophores	A23187, ionomycin	Ca^{2+} influx, phospholipases (A_2, D)
"Surface active"	AA, detergents	Direct enzyme activation (PKC, phospholipases, oxidase), Other?

[a] See text for references.

1. Chemoattractants

The best-studied receptor-mediated signaling system is that triggered by the chemoattractants, with the most used ligand being the peptide formyl-methionyl-leucyl-phenylalanine (fMLP). The fMLP receptor has recently been cloned (79), as has the receptor for the chemotactic complement-derived protein C5a (80). Analysis of the predicted sequences suggests these receptors are in the superfamily of G-protein-linked receptors, typified by rhodopsin and the adrenergic receptors (81). These receptors transduce signals by coupling to and activating a G-protein, followed by G-protein-mediated activation of an effector enzyme. The G-protein(s) that are functionally linked to chemoattractant receptors have not been absolutely identified. The neutrophil contains G_{i2} as the predominant pertussis-toxin substrate (82–84), and chemoattractant-induced responses in neutrophils are pertussis-toxin sensitive (85). In addition, G_{i2} co-purifies with receptors for fMLP (86) and C5a (87). However, a portion of receptors for fMLP co-purifies with a low-molecular-weight G-protein (86), suggesting that this receptor can couple to more than one G-protein. The individual roles of these G-proteins are not yet understood.

Effector enzymes that appear to be activated by chemoattractant receptor/G-protein interaction include: a phosphatidylinositol-4,5-bisphosphate-hydrolyzing phospholipase C (82,85), phosphatidylinositol- and phosphatidylcholine-hydrolyzing phospholipases D (89–90), and phospholipases A_2 acting on choline-, ethanolamine-, and inositol-containing phospholipids (91–95). Activation of phospholipase A_2 by chemoattractants is small in the absence of a second exogenous signal, such as arachidonic acid (AA) or diacylglycerol (DAG) (92,96), or an intracellular signal generated by engagement of a second receptor, such as receptors for cytokines (97,98). The G-protein(s) responsible for activating these phospholipases have not been identified. It is possible that G_{i2} is primarily responsible, since activation of the various phospholipases is pertussis-toxin sensitive (85,90,97). Phospholipase activation produces a variety of second messengers [DAG, alkylacylglycerol, phosphatidic acid (PA), AA and its metabolites, platelet-activating factor (PAF), and inositol-1,4,5-trisphosphate (Ins 1,4,5P_3)]. In addition, chemoattractant receptors cause a transient elevation in cAMP levels (reviewed in 44,75). This elevation appears to be mediated indirectly and not by coupling of the receptor to G_s to activate adenylate cyclase (99,100). These second messengers may be generated at varying ratios, depending on the identity and concentration of the chemoattractant used as stimulus and on the time of stimulation (as an example, see Refs. 101 and 102).

The second messengers generated by phospholipases and adenylate cyclase activate various target enzymes within the cell. Cyclic AMP activates PKA (103). DAG and AA are activators of the ubiquitous enzyme PKC, while Ins 1,4,5P_3 induces release of calcium from intracellular stores (reviewed in 104 and 105). Calcium is a co-factor for activation of certain PKC isozymes (105), as well as for activation of calmodulin (106) and various phospholipases (106). PA may also be an activator of PKC (107), as well as a direct activator of NADPH oxidase (108,109). AA can also activate NADPH oxidase directly (45–48). The major metabolites of AA in neutrophils are the lipoxygenase products 5-hydroxyeicosatetraenoic acid and leukotriene B_4(LTB_4) (93). These products, as well as PAF, may interact with their specific cell-surface receptors to enhance phospholipase activation and/or to increase calcium levels (110–113). The role of second messengers and their various target enzymes in activation of the respiratory burst enzyme will be considered in more detail below.

2. *Phagocytic Ligands*

Signaling mechanisms utilized by the other classes of receptors are not as well studied. Phagocytic receptors include those for the Fc portion of IgG (FcγRII and FcγRIII) and the receptors for the complement fragment C3b (CR1) and its breakdown product iC3b (CR3). Activation of the respiratory burst by Fcγ appears to be mediated primarily by FcγRII (114,115), whose predicted sequence suggests a trasmembrane protein with an intracellular domain (116). However, recent data (117) suggest that FcγRIII also can trigger respiratory burst activation under certain conditions. These receptors mediate respiratory burst activation partially through a pertussis toxin-sensitive G-protein-dependent mechanism (116–119), and both phospholipase C acting on phosphatidylinositol bisphosphate (PIP_2) and phospholipase A_2 are activated (120,121). In addition, other, pertussis-toxin-insensitive, and as yet unidentified, mechanisms contribute to respiratory burst activation (117,119,121).

The complement receptors CR1 and CR3 mediate phagocytosis, but do not induce activation of NADPH oxidase directly (122,123). The predicted structures of both receptors are known (122,124) and are unrelated. CR3 is a member of the integrin family (124), and the signaling mechanisms triggered include activation of PIP_2-hydrolyzing phospholipase C (121), resulting in small increases in DAG and intracellular calcium levels.

Progress in understanding signaling mechanisms triggered by phagocytic receptors has been slow, primarily because most particulate stimuli used by investigators engage multiple receptors. This may be the most physiologic situation; however, contributions by individual receptors to signaling pathways are difficult to dissect under such conditions.

3. Cytokines and Bacterial Products

Neutrophils have receptors for several cytokines, including interleukin 1 [IL-1, (125)], tumor necrosis factor-α (TNF-α, 126), granulocyte/macrophage colony-stimulating factor (GM-CSF, 127), and γ-interferon (γ-IFN, 128). In addition, the bacterial product lipopolysaccharide (LPS) binds to PMNs, resulting in priming of the cell (129). None of these agonists activates the respiratory burst directly, but most can either prime the response of the cell to a second stimulus (129–132) or induce activation in conjunction with engagement of an integrin receptor (133,134). The mechanisms involved in priming are still not well understood and will not be considered in detail here. The receptors for the cytokines have been cloned (135–139), appear to be unrelated, and their predicted structures have yielded few insights into their transductional mechanisms.

Recent work has suggested that effects of cytokines on the PMN respiratory burst are independent of effects on PIP_2-hydrolyzing phospholipase C (97,140–142). However, receptor-linked G-proteins appear to be involved with effects by GM-CSF (97,143), but not effects by TNF-α (144,145). GM-CSF induces phosphorylation of proteins on tyrosine (146,147), enhances activation of phospholipases D and A_2 (148,149), and modulates cyclic nucleotide metabolism (141). TNF-α enhances activation of phospholipases D and A_2 by a second stimulus (98,150), reduces cAMP levels (151), and induces the phosphorylation of proteins (144) and the synthesis of MARCKS, a PKC substrate (152). γ-INF induces phosphorylation of proteins in macrophages (153), but this has not been examined in neutrophils. LPS enhances production of PAF and LTB_4 (154,155) and increases basal and stimulated levels of intracellular calcium (156). In addition, LPS induces the turnover of phosphatidylcholine in macrophages (157). One effect of both LPS and γ-IFN in PMNs is to enhance mRNA levels of the heavy chain of cytochrome b_{558} [gp91-*phox* (158)], suggesting that alterations in gene transcription may play a role in enhancement of NADPH oxidase activation by these agonists. Clearly, a myriad of cytokine effects can be observed in PMNs. Further studies are needed to determine the exact mechanisms involved in the priming and activation of the respiratory burst by cytokines.

4. Extracellular ATP

Initial studies of signaling via the ATP receptor suggests similarities to transductional mechanisms utilized by the chemoattractants (159–163). ATP (78), like LTB_4 (85,102), is a poor direct stimulus for the respiratory burst. This suggests that signaling mechanisms triggered by ATP and LTB_4 must differ in some respects from those triggered by chemoattractants more effective for NADPH oxidase activation (e.g., fMLP). The poor oxidative response to LTB_4 has been linked to inadequate levels of PA, but not of DAG, following cell stimulation (102). In support of this observation, LTB_4 is as effective as fMLP in triggering activation of PIP_2-hydrolyzing phospholipase C (85), but is less effective for activation of phospholipase D (110). These differences in phospholipase activation may be caused by reported differences between LTB_4 and fMLP at the level of receptor/G-protein(s) interaction (164).

C. Nonreceptor Agonists—Generation of Second Messengers

A variety of agents bypass cell-surface receptors and stimulate the respiratory burst by activating intracellular proteins or effector enzymes directly. Use of such agents has provided valuable information as to the transductional steps involved in the activation of NADPH oxidase.

1. Activators of G-Proteins

It is clear that non-receptor-mediated activation of G-proteins, by either NaF in intact cells (31,165) or nonhydrolyzable GTP analogs (e.g., GTPγS) in permeabilized cells (166), can trigger NADPH oxidase activation. Activation of G-proteins via these pharmacologic manipulators results in activation of several phospholipases, including phospholipases C, A_2, and possibly D (167–171). The second messengers (Ins 1,4,5P_3, DAG,PA,AA) generated can then activate various intermediate effector enzymes and/or induce NADPH oxidase assembly directly, as discussed in more detail below. These studies indicate that G-proteins are likely to participate in receptor-mediated signal transduction.

2. PKC Activators

Direct activation of PKC, by either phorbol diesters (172–176) or cell-permeable DAGs (177–179), stimulates the respiratory burst. Interestingly, the ability of the phorbol diester, phorbol myristate acetate (PMA), to trigger the respiratory burst was initially reported in 1974 (172), long before its mechanism of action was known. Blockage of the respiratory burst in response to phorbol diesters and DAGs by inhibitors of PKC provides further support for the participation of PKC in activation of NADPH oxidase (180–182). However, it is not clear if PKC mediates activation of NADPH oxidase by direct phosphorylation of an oxidase component (68) or indirectly via generation of PA and DAG through phospholipase D activation (90).

3. Calcium Ionophores

An increase in the intracellular concentration of calcium ($[Ca^{2+}]_i$) also results in activation of NADPH oxidase. This has been demonstrated by the ability of calcium ionophores, such as A23187 (183) and ionomycin (184), to trigger the respiratory burst. Most chemoattractant ligands induce the release of calcium from intracellular stores, via activation of PIP_2-hydrolyzing phospholipase C to form Ins 1,4,5P_3, and many agonists also trigger an influx of calcium across the plasma membrane (reviewed in 185). Nevertheless, stimulation of the respiratory burst by chemoattractants does not require a change in $[Ca^{2+}]_i$, if cells are exposed first to an activator of PKC (186–189). This suggests that the normal function of the rise in $[Ca^{2+}]_i$ may be to activate PKC. Indeed, the calcium ionophore A23187 induces the apparent translocation of PKC from cytosolic to membrane fractions in human neutrophils (190), a hallmark of PKC activation (191). However, a requirement for PKC in activation of NADPH oxidase by agonists other than direct PKC activators has not been proven (see discussion below). In addition, calcium ionophores also trigger activation of phospholipases to generate second messengers, such as PA, DAG, and AA (90,192). Therefore, the exact mechanism by which an elevation in calcium can activate NADPH oxidase is not yet clear.

4. Surface-Active Agents

The final category of nonreceptor agonists effective for activation of the respiratory burst includes agents that are termed "surface active" due to their detergent properties. Examples are fatty acids, such as AA (193,194), and anionic detergents, such as digitonin, deoxycholate, and sodium dodecyl sulfate (SDS) (195–199). Little progress has been made in determining the mechanism(s) of action of these compounds. Fatty acids (45–48) and the anionic amphiphilic detergent SDS (200) have been shown to activate NADPH oxidase in a cell-free system. However, other anionic detergents, effective in stimulating the respiratory burst in the intact cell, appear to be ineffective in the cell-free system (200), suggesting that the mechanisms operating in the two systems are not the same. This is supported by studies (201–204) showing that phospholipases appear to play a role in arachidonate-mediated stimulation of the intact cell, but not in activation of the oxidase in the cell-free system. Additional detail concerning activation mechanisms that may be operating in the cell-free system is included below.

In summary, nonreceptor agonists provide some clues as to the transductional mechanisms important for the activation of NADPH oxidase. However, it is clear that virtually all nonreceptor agonists activate phospholipases to generate the lipid second messengers PA, DAG, and AA. Therefore, it is possible that these second messengers play a more direct role in NADPH oxidase activation than has been previously appreciated. Studies in the cell-free system for NADPH oxidase activation, described later in this chapter, support this possibility.

D. Effectors of Second Messengers

Because most of the second messengers described above can activate specific protein kinases, kinases and protein phosphorylation/dephosphorylation reactions have received considerable attention as mediators of NADPH oxidase activation. The following sections discuss the roles of various protein kinases (reviewed previously in 44,75,76,205).

1. *Cyclic AMP-Dependent Protein Kinase*

PKA may be involved in down-regulating the respiratory burst, based primarily on the use of cAMP analogs and agonists to elevate cAMP levels pharmacologically (44,75,205). However, the inhibitory effects of cAMP are stimulus specific (206,207), suggesting that it influences transductional events instead of NADPH oxidase itself. This is supported by recent studies (110,208) documenting an inhibitory effect of cAMP agonists on activation of phospholipase D by chemoattractants but not by PMA. Similarly, previous studies have reported that cAMP agonists inhibit phosphoinositide metabolism triggered by chemoattractants (209,210). The specificity of cAMP agonists for inhibition of responses to calcium-mobilizing stimuli suggests a common site of action in the signaling pathways triggered. One possible site is a receptor-linked G-protein, and cAMP-mediated effects on G-proteins have been reported (42,43,211).

2. *Calmodulin*

Calmodulin and calmodulin-dependent protein kinases have been implicated in signal transduction by the ability of a variety of calmodulin antagonists to inhibit stimulation of the respiratory burst (212, reviewed in 44 and 205). Unfortunately, most calmodulin antagonists also inhibit PKC and, more recently, have been shown to inhibit calpain I (213). However, my laboratory (214) and others (215) have shown that the calmodulin antagonist *N*-(6-aminohexyl)-5-chloro-1-napthalenesulfonamide (W-7) inhibits activation of NADPH oxidase in the cell-free system without inhibition of PKC. Calcium and calmodulin were not able to substitute for SDS or AA in the activation system (215; Hendricks and McPhail, unpublished results), suggesting W-7 was not acting as a calmodulin antagonist. Modulation of NADPH oxidase activation by calpain I has not been tested in the cell-free system. It is intriguing, however, that several cell-free system activators (SDS, AA, PA) of NADPH oxidase (45–48,108,109,200) can also substitute for calcium and calmodulin in the activation of many calmodulin-dependent enzymes, and that such activation is sensitive to inhibition by calmodulin antagonists (216–218). Further study is needed to explore if the site of SDS/AA binding during the activation of NADPH oxidase has similarities to sites of amphiphile binding on calmodulin-dependent enzymes.

3. Protein Kinase C

PKC may participate in both activation and down-regulatory mechanisms (reviewed previously in 44,75,76,205). PKC is a target for most of the lipid-derived second messengers, as well as for calcium (44,104,105,190,191,219–222). Interestingly, the potential for both activation and inhibition of PKC exists, since second messengers which enhance (calcium, DAGs, PA, arachidonate, and certain lipoxygenase products) or inhibit (alkylacylglycerols, sphingosine) PKC activity are generated. It is also possible that PKC activity is down-regulated by the calcium-dependent protease calpain (223) or endogenous inhibitors other than second messengers (224). Thus, PKC activity may be very complexly regulated in PMNs.

The precise role of PKC in modulation of NADPH oxidase activation is not yet clear. Phorbol diesters and cell-permeable DAGs stimulate NADPH oxidase activity in the intact cell by an apparent PKC-dependent mechanism (175,176,178–182,225). In addition, PMA and PKC (226) or proteolytically activated PKC (227) can substitute for neutrophil cytosol in the cell-free activation of NADPH oxidase, although the level of NADPH oxidase activity obtained is much lower than with SDS or AA (228). The evidence for participation of PKC in signaling for other stimuli is less conclusive (reviewed in 75,76,205). Although most neutrophil agonists have now been shown to increase the level of membrane-associated PKC activity in correlation with stimulation of the respiratory burst (113,175,176,190,229,230), the effect of PKC inhibitors on activation of the burst by many agonists has been variable (179–182,231,232). Thus, either PKC-independent pathways exist, or there are pools of PKC inaccessible or insensitive to certain inhibitors. The existence of discrete pools of PKC in PMNs is supported by the temperature-dependent sensitivity of fMLP-stimulated superoxide release to the isoquinoline sulfonamide inhibitors H-7 and C-I (232) and the differential stimulation of the respiratory burst and degranulation by synthetic DAGs (178). In addition, conclusions based on inhibitor data are complicated by the lack of specificity of all PKC inhibitors used thus far.

It is also becoming apparent that PMNs contain more than one isozyme of PKC (190,233–235). The known PKC family consists of at least eight subspecies, designated α, β_{I}, β_{II}, γ, δ, ϵ, ζ, and η, and these appear to be differentially expressed and localized in various tissues (191,236,237). The α, β, and γ isozymes show differences in biochemical and regulatory properties (191,238–241) and appear to be regulated differently by stimulation in certain cell types (190,242–246). The δ, ϵ, ζ, and η subspecies are less well characterized, but appear to be relatively independent of calcium (236,237,247–249). PMNs contain PKC-ζ, one of the calcium-independent isozymes, as well as PKC-α and PKC-β (233–235; Sozzani, Kent, and McPhail, unpublished data). PMNs do not appear to contain PKC-γ, -δ, or -ϵ, at least in quantities detectable by immunoblotting (233–235; Sozzani, Kent, and McPhail, unpublished data). It is clear that an understanding of the role of PKC in the activation of the respiratory burst in PMNs will require characterization of the PKC isozymes present under various conditions of cellular stimulation.

4. *Tyrosine Kinases*

Recent data suggests that tyrosine kinase activity is stimulated by both receptor and nonreceptor agonists in PMNs (146,250–252) and that tyrosine kinase inhibitors block the ability of receptor agonists to stimulate the respiratory burst (146,147,253). This raises the possibility that a PKC-independent pathway for activation of NADPH oxidase may involve a tyrosine kinase. Phagocytic cells contain at least three nonreceptor tyrosine kinases, including $p55^{fgr}$, $p59^{hck}$, and $p60^{src}$ (254,255), but their individual roles in regulation of cell function have not been discerned. These cells also contain a tyrosine phosphatase, CD45, (256) which has been implicated in the regulation of PMN chemotaxis (257). Sequence analysis of the NADPH oxidase cytosolic component p47-*phox* indicates a possible tyrosine phosphorylation site (53); however, actual phosphorylation of this site has not been demonstrated. The intriguing SH3 region found in p47-*phox* and p67-*phox* implies a role for a regulatory pathway involving tyrosine kinases and phosphatases, since, as described earlier in this chapter, the SH3 region is found in both nonreceptor tyrosine kinases and in several signaling proteins regulated by tyrosine kinases. Clearly, additional work is needed to understand the contribution of tyrosine kinases to the activation of NADPH oxidase.

5. *Phosphorylation of Oxidase Components*

Presently, the best-studied phosphoprotein component of NADPH oxidase is the cytosolic protein p47-*phox*, and it can be phosphorylated on multiple sites (63–69,258). It appears that some of the sites are phosphorylated when the protein is cytosolic and some are phosphorylated once the protein has translocated to the membrane (64,65,259). It has been shown (68,69) that p47-*phox* is a substrate for both PKC and PKA, but effects of other kinases or of PKC isozymes have not been examined. The functional role of p47-*phox* phosphorylation is still unclear. Recent studies suggest that phosphorylation of p47-*phox* is neither necessary nor sufficient for oxidase activation (101,260,261). Possibly, the conformational changes induced by phosphorylation can be duplicated by other mechanisms (i.e., binding of anionic amphiphiles, such as AA or PA) and/or an additional oxidase component is regulated by a phosphorylation-dependent mechanism. Further study to explore the nature and effects of phosphorylation of p47-*phox* is needed.

Recent studies (262,264) suggest that both subunits of cytochrome b_{558} are substrates for phosphorylation and this could be an additional site in the oxidase system for regulation by either protein kinases or other mechanisms. However, more rigorous approaches must be taken to prove that the proteins observed are components of cytochrome b_{558} and are not co-migrating proteins dependent on the presence of cytochrome b_{558} in order to be phosphorylated. For example, it is now known that the phosphorylatable low-molecular-weight G-protein *rap*-1 co-migrates on SDS-PAGE with p22-*phox* and also co-purifies with cytochrome b_{558} (32). Thus, it is not clear whether the 22kDa phosphoprotein observed previously (262,263) is p22-*phox* or *rap*-1.

E. Activation of NADPH Oxidase in a Cell-Free System

Identification of proteins necessary for NADPH oxidase activity/activation was greatly advanced by the development in several laboratories of a cell-free system for NADPH oxidase activation (45–48), as discussed earlier in this chapter. Progress has been slower in using the cell-free system to understand the mechanisms controlling activation of NADPH oxidase. Effective activators (SDS, fatty acids, PA) share the property of being anionic amphiphilic compounds, but their site(s) of action have yet to be identified. It is hypothesized, since NADPH oxidase components are present in both cytosolic and membrane fractions, that one function of the activator is to induce translocation of cytosolic components for assembly with cytochrome b_{558}. Support for the existence of the active oxidase as an assembled complex comes from studies demonstrating that treatment with cross-linking agents stabilizes membrane-associated enzyme activity (264,265). Using SDS as the activator, we have shown that translocation of one of the cytosolic components, p47-*phox*, correlates with activation of NADPH oxidase (266) and depends on the presence of cytochrome b_{558} in the membrane (267). These results support a role for translocation of cytosolic components in the activation mechanism and also support the concept that cytochrome b_{558} plays a structural role in the process of NADPH oxidase assembly, as discussed earlier in the chapter.

The mechanism(s) responsible for translocation and assembly in the cell-free system is (are) still not clear. Possibilities include: (a) conformational changes induced directly by the activator in either cytosolic or membrane components or both, which allow interaction between components; (b) activation of an as-yet-unidentified intermediate effector protein, which then modifies one or more oxidase component(s) to allow assembly to occur; and (c) modification of the membrane environment to allow access and binding of cytosolic to membrane components. Studies have not yet been performed to address whether anionic amphiphiles interact directly with one or more of the identified NADPH oxidase components. Instead, most investigators have centered on the second and third possibilities, and these are summarized in the next few paragraphs.

An obvious candidate for an intermediate effector protein is PKC, based on its ability to be activated by the amphiphilic compounds effective in the cell-free NADPH oxidase system (105,219,268). SDS has been shown to induce phosphorylation of multiple proteins during cell-free NADPH oxidase activation (66), supporting a role for protein kinases. However, other studies (37,73,214,228,266–269) have clearly dissociated protein kinase, and particularly PKC, activation from activation of NADPH oxidase in the cell-free system. Therefore, if an intermediate effector protein is required for cell-free NADPH oxidase activation, it appears not to be PKC.

A more likely participant in the activation mechanism is a G-protein, potentially *rap*-1. A role for a pertussis- and cholera toxin-insensitive G-protein in the cell-free system was initially suggested by Seifert et al. in 1986 (35) and Gabig et al. in 1987 (36). Recent studies (38,71,270) support the concept that the role of the putative G-protein is to promote interaction between cytosolic and membrane NADPH oxidase components. The location of the G-protein is not yet clear, as different laboratories have reported principal effects of guanine nucleotides in either membrane fractions (71) or cytosolic fractions (38,270,271). However, Gabig et al. (39) recently provided strong evidence supporting cytosolic *rap*-1 as the G-protein participating in cell-free NADPH oxidase activation. In addition, stimulation of NADPH oxidase in intact cells before fractionation induced apparent translocation of *rap*-1 from cytosolic to membrane-containing fractions (39). Based on this observation and earlier studies (32), it would appear that *rap*-1 is localized in both cytosol and membrane or, perhaps, it can reversibly associate with the membrane. If *rap*-1 does regulate assembly of an active NADPH oxidase, the mechanism utilized may be similar to that used by other low-molecular-weight G-proteins in assembly of proteins and organelles during prokaryotic and eukaryotic transcription and secretion in yeast (272). Of primary importance now will be studies to determine if *rap*-1 is the target for anionic amphiphiles in the cell-free system.

A variety of studies have also implicated a regulatory role for the membrane environment in supporting activation of NADPH oxidase. The presence of phospholipids is necessary for NADPH oxidase activation in the cell-free system (273,274), and certain phospholipids can induce further activation in membrane fractions from prestimulated neutrophils (275). Positively charged membrane-soluble compounds inhibit NADPH oxidase activity and activation, hypothesized to be due to disruption of negative charge-dependent association between membrane and cytosolic oxidase components (276,277). PA has recently been shown to activate NADPH oxidase in the cell-free system (108,109,267), and DAG has been reported to synergize with either SDS (278) or PA (267,279). Since these lipids remain in the membrane once formed by phospholipase action, it is likely that their effects on oxidase activation are exerted there.

Based on these observations, it is intriguing to speculate that the cytosolic proteins necessary for NADPH oxidase activation belong to a newly proposed class of "membrane" proteins called amphitropic proteins (280). These proteins are thought to associate with membranes reversibly through interaction with specific lipids. The best-known example of this type of protein is PKC, which associates with membranes reversibly via interaction with phosphatidylserine and DAG. Other examples include many cytoskeletal-associated proteins, such as α-actinin, gelsolin, and spectrin, and nonreceptor tyrosine kinases, such as p60^{src}. Possibly, the SH3 region found in many of these proteins plays some role in this process, although this is sheer speculation. Studies to address the possible amphitropic nature of the oxidase cytosolic factors will be interesting to pursue.

In conclusion, many unanswered questions remain in determining the mechanism(s) of NADPH oxidase activation. It is clear that complete understanding of the assembly/activation process in the cell-free system will require both reconstitution of an active NADPH oxidase using purified components and identification of the site(s) of activator binding. In addition, the dissection of signaling mechanisms resulting in NADPH oxidase activation in intact cells is far from complete. Future research will undoubtedly focus on these issues.

ACKNOWLEDGMENTS

The authors express their sincere appreciation to Diane Qualliotine-Mann and Mary Ellenburg for excellent editorial and technical assistance. Research by the authors was supported by NIH grants AI-22564 and HL-02123. Dr. Sozzani was supported by a fellowship from L. Berti, Champion Industries, Winston-Salem, North Carolina, from 1988 to 1990.

List of Abbreviations

AA	Arachidonic acid
cAMP	Cyclic AMP
CGD	Chronic granulomatous disease
DAG	Diacylglycerol
fMLP	Formyl-methionyl-leucyl-phenylalanine

GM-CSF	Granulocyte/macrophage colony-stimulating factor
G-protein	Guanine nucleotide regulatory protein
gp91-*phox*	glycosylated 91-kDa subunit of the *ph*agocyte NADPH *ox*idase component cytochrome b_{558}
γ-IFN	γ-Interferon
$INS1,4,5P_3$	Inositol-1,4,5-trisphosphate
LPS	Lipopolysaccharide
LTB_4	Leukotriene B_4
p22-*phox*	22-kDa subunit of the *ph*agocyte NADPH *ox*idase component cytochrome b_{558}
p47-*phox*	47-kDa cytosolic component of the *ph*agocyte NADPH *ox*idase
p67-*phox*	67-kDa cytosolic component of the phagocyte NADPH oxidase
PA	Phosphatidic acid
PAF	Platelet-activating factor
PIP_2	Phosphatidylinositol bisphosphate
PKA	Cyclic AMP-dependent protein kinase
PKC	Protein kinase C
PMA	Phorbol myristate acetate
PMN	Polymorphonuclear leukocyte, neutrophil
SDS	Sodium dodecyl sulfate
TNF-α	Tumor necrosis factor-α
W-7	*N*-(6-aminohexyl)-5-chloro-1-napthalenesulfonamide

REFERENCES

1. Curnutte JT, Babior BM. Chronic granulomatous disease. In: Harris H and Hirchhorn K, eds. Advances in human genetics, vol 16. New York: Plenum Publishing, 1987: 229–97.
2. Weiss SJ. Tissue destruction by neutrophils. N Engl J Med 1989; 320:365–76.
3. Segal AW. The electron transport chain of the microbicidal oxidase of phagocytic cells and its involvement in the molecular pathology of chronic granulomatous disease. J Clin Invest 1989; 83:1785–93.
4. Clark RA. The human neutrophil respiratory burst oxidase. J Infect Dis 1990; 161:1140–7.
5. Yea CM, Cross AR, Jones OTG. Purification and some properties of the 45 kDa diphenylene iodonium-binding flavoprotein of neutrophil NADPH oxidase. Biochem J 1990; 265:95–100.
6. Umei T, Takeshige K, Minakami S. NADPH-binding component of the superoxide-generating oxidase is unstimulated neutrophils and the neutrophils from the patients with chronic granulomatous disease. Biochem J 1987; 243:467–72.
7. Kakinuma K, Fukuhara Y, Kaneda M. The respiratory burst oxidase of neutrophils: separation of an FAD enzyme and its characterization. J Biol Chem 1987; 262:12316–22.
8. Doussiere J, LaPorte F, Vignais PV. Photolabeling of a O_2^- generating protein in bovine polymorphonuclear neutrophils by an arylazido $NADP^+$ analog. Biochem Biophys Res Commun 1986; 139:85–93.
9. Sha'ag D, Pick E. Nucleotide binding properties of cytosolic components required for expression of activity of the superoxide generating NADPH oxidase. Biochim Biophys Acta 1990; 1037:405–12.
10. Smith RM, Curnutte JT, Babior BM. Affinity labeling of the cytosolic and membrane components of the respiratory burst oxidase by the 2′,3′-dialdehyde derivative of NADPH. J Biol Chem 1989; 264:1958–62.
11. Takasugi S, Ishida K, Takeshige K, Minakami S. Effect of 2′,3′-dialdehyde NADPH on activation of superoxide-producing NADPH oxidase in a cell-free system of pig neutrophils. J Biochem 1989; 105:155–7.

12. Cross AR, Jones OTG. The effect of the inhibitor diphenylene iodonium on the superoxide-generating system of neutrophils: specific labeling of a component polypeptide of the oxidase. Biochem J 1986; 237:111–6.
13. Smith RM, Curnutte JT, Mayo LA, Babior BM. Use of an affinity label to probe the function of the NADPH binding component of the respiratory burst oxidase of human neutrophils. J Biol Chem 1989; 264:12243–8.
14. Laporte F, Doussiere J, Vignais PV. Properties of the NADPH dehydrogenase component of the oxidase complex from rabbit peritoneal neutrophils: reconstitution of an oxidase activity with the dehydrogenase component and a membrane extract. Biochem Biophys Res Commun 1990; 167:790–7.
15. Royer-Pokora B, Kunkel LM, Monaco AP, Goff SC, Newburger PE, Baehner RL, Cole FS, Curnutte JT, Orkin SH. Cloning the gene for an inherited human disorder—chronic granulomatous disease—on the basis of its chromosomal location. Nature 1986; 322:32–8.
16. Dinauer MC, Orkin SH, Brown R, Jesaitis AJ, Parkos CA. The glycoprotein endcoded by the X-linked chronic granulomatous disease locus is a component of the neutrophil cytochrome *b* complex. Nature 1987; 327:717–20.
17. Teahan C, Rowe P, Parker P, Totty N, Segal AW. The X-linked chronic granulmatous disease gene codes for the beta-chain of cytochrome b_{-245}. Nature 1987; 327:720–1.
18. Parkos CA, Dinauer MC, Walker LE, Allen RA, Jesaitis AJ, Orkin SH. Primary structure and unique expression of the 22-kilodalton light chain of human neutrophil cytochrome b. Proc Natl Acad Sci USA 1988; 85:3319–23.
19. Clark RA, Malech HL, Gallin JI, Nunoi H, Volpp BD, Pearson DW, Nauseef WM, Curnutte JT. Genetic variants of chronic granulomatous disease: prevalence of deficiencies of two cytosolic components of the NADPH oxidase system. N Engl J Med 1989; 321:647–52.
20. Dinauer MC, Pierce EA, Bruns GAP, Curnutte JT, Orkin SH. Human neutrophil cytochrome *b* light chain (p22-*phox*). Gene structure, chromosomal location, and mutations in cytochrome-negative autosomal recessive chronic granulomatous disease. J Clin Invest 1990; 86:1729–37.
21. Nugent JH, Gratzer W, Segal AW. Identification of the haem-binding subunit of cytochrome b_{-245}. Biochem J 1989; 264:921–4.
22. Yamaguchi T, Hayakawa T, Kaneda M, Kakinuma D, Yoshikawa A. Purification and some properties of the small subunit of cytochrome b_{558} from human neutrophils. J Biol Chem 1989; 264:112–8.
23. Rotrosen D, Kleinburg ME, Nunoi H, Leto T, Gallin JI, Malech HL. Evidence for a functional cytoplasmic domain of phagocyte oxidase cytochrome b_{558}. J Biol Chem 1990; 265:8745–50.
24. Heyworth PG, Curnutte JT, Nauseef WM, Volpp BD, Pearson DW, Rosen H, Clark RA. Neutrophil nicotinamide adenine dinucleotide phosphate oxidase assembly. Translocation of p47-*phox* and p67-*phox* requires interaction between p47-*phox* and cytochrome b_{558}. J Clin Invest 1991; 87:352–6.
25. Kleinberg ME, Malech HL, Rotrosen D. The phagocyte 47-kilodalton cytosolic oxidase protein is an early reactant in activation of the respiratory burst. J Biol Chem 1990; 265:15577–83.
26. Jesaitis AJ, Buescher ES, Harrison D, Quinn MT, Parkos CA, Livesey S, Linner J. Ultrastructural localization of cytochrome *b* in the membranes of resting and phagocytosing human granulocytes. J Clin Invest 1990; 85:821–35.
27. Borregaard N, Heiple JM, Simons ER, Clark RA. Subcellular localization of the b-cytochrome component of the human neutrophil microbicidal oxidase. Translocation during activation. J Cell Biol 1983; 97:52–61.
28. Borregaard N, Christensen L, Bjerrum OW, Birgens HS, Clemmensen I. Identification of

a highly mobilizable subset of human neutrophil intracellular vesicles that contains tetranectin and latent alkaline phosphatase. J Clin Invest 1990; 85:408–16.

29. Bjerrum OW, Borregaard N. Dual granule localization of the dormant NADPH oxidase and cytochrome b_{559} in human neutrophils. Eur J Haematol 1989; 43:67–77.
30. Ohno Y, Seligmann BE, Gallin JI, Cytochrome *b* translocation to human neutrophil plasma membranes and superoxide release. J Biol Chem 1985; 260:2409–14.
31. Curnutte JT, Babior BM, Karnovsky ML. Fluoride-mediated activation of the respiratory burst in human neutrophils. A reversible process. J Clin Invest 1979; 63:637–47.
32. Quinn MT, Parkos CA, Walker L, Orkin SH, Dinauer MC, Jesaitis AJ. Association of a *ras*-related protein with cytochrome *b* of human neutrophils. Nature 1989; 342:198–200.
33. Jesaitis A, McPhail LC, Clark RA, Bokoch G, Quinn M. Regulatory interactions of formyl peptide receptor and cytochrome B of neutrophils. FASEB J 1990; 4:A2181.
34. Ishida K, Takeshige K, Takesugi S. Minakami S. GTP-dependent and -independent activation of superoxide producing NADPH oxidase in a neutrophil cell-free system. FEBS Lett 1989; 243:169–72.
35. Seifert R, Rosenthal W, Schultz G. Guanine nucleotides stimulate NADPH oxidase in membranes of human neutrophils. FEBS Lett 1986; 205:161–5.
36. Gabig TG, English D, Akard LP, Schell MJ. Regulation of neutrophil NADPH oxidase activation in a cell-free system by guanine nucleotides and fluoride. J Biol Chem 1987; 262:1685–90.
37. Seifert R, Schultz G. Fatty-acid-induced activation of NADPH oxidase in plasma membranes of human neutrophils depends on neutrophil cytosol and is potentiated by stable guanine nucleotides. Eur J Biochem 1987; 162:563–9.
38. Doussiere J, Pilloud M-C, Vignais PV. Activation of bovine neutrophil oxidase in a cell free system. GTP-dependent formation of a complex between a cytosolic factor and a membrane protein. Biochem Biophys Res Commun 1988; 152:993–1001.
39. Eklund EA, Marshall M, Gibbs JB, Crean CD, Gabig TG. Resolution of a low molecular weight G protein in neutrophil cytosol required for NADPH oxidase activation and reconstitution by recombinant Krev-1 protein. J Biol Chem 1991; 266:13964–70.
40. Kikuchi A, Sasaki T, Araki S, Hata Y, Takai Y. Purification and characterization from bovine brain cytosol of two GTPase-activating proteins specific for *smg* p21, a GTP-binding protein having the same effector domain as c-*ras* p21s. J Biol Chem 1989; 264:9133–6.
41. Kitayama H, Sugimoto Y, Matsuzaki T, Ikawa Y, Noda M. A *ras*-related gene with transformation suppressor activity. Cell 1989; 56:77–84.
42. Lazarowski ER, Winegar DA, Nolan RD, Oberdisse E, Lapetina EG. Effect of protein kinase A on inositide metabolism and rap 1 G-protein in human erythroleukemia cells. J Biol Chem 1990; 265:13118–23.
43. Bokoch GM, Quilliam LA. Guanine nucleotide binding properties of rap1 purified from human neutrophils. Biochem J 1990; 267:407–11.
44. McPhail LC, Snyderman R. Mechanisms of regulating the respiratory burst in leukocytes. In: R Snyderman, ed. Regulation of leukocyte function. New York: Plenum Publishing, 1984:247–81.
45. Bromberg Y, Pick E. Unsaturated fatty acids stimulate NADPH-dependent superoxide production by cell-free system derived from macrophages. Cell Immunol 1984; 88:213–21.
46. Heyneman RA, Vercauteren RE. Activation of a NADPH oxidase from horse polymorphonuclear leukocytes in a cell-free system. J Leuk Biol 1984; 36:751–9.
47. McPhail LC, Shirley PS, Clayton CC, Snyderman R. Activation of the respiratory burst enzyme from human neutrophils in a cell-free system: evidence for a soluble cofactor. J Clin Invest 1985; 75:1735–9.

48. Curnutte JT. Activation of human neutrophil nicotinamide adenine dinucleotide phosphate, reduced (triphosphopyridine nucleotide, reduced) oxidase by arachidonic acid in a cell-free system. J Clin Invest 1985; 75:1740–3.
49. Volpp BD, Nauseef WM, Clark RA. Two cytosolic neutrophil oxidase components absent in autosomal chronic granulomatous disease. Science 1988; 242:1295–7.
50. Nunoi H, Rotrosen D, Gallin JI, Malech HL. Two forms of autosomal chronic granulomatous disease lack distinct neutrophil cytosol factors. Science 1988; 242:1298–1301.
51. Curnutte JT, Scott PJ, Mayo LA. Cytosolic components of the respiratory burst oxidase: resolution of four components, two of which are missing in complementing types of chronic granulomatous disease. Proc Natl Acad Sci USA 1989; 86:825–9.
52. Lomax KJ, Leto TL, Nunoi H, Gallin JI, Malech HL. Recombinant 47-kilodalton cytosol factor restores NADPH oxidase in chronic granulomatous disease. Science 1989; 245:987–90.
53. Volpp BD, Nauseef WM, Donelson JE, Moser DR, Clark RA. Cloning of the cDNA and functional expression of the 47-kilodalton cytosolic component of human neutrophil respiratory burst oxidase. Proc Natl Acad Sci USA 1989; 86:9563–7.
54. Rodaway ARF, Teahan CG, Casimir CM, Segal AW, Bentley DL. Characterization of the 47-kilodalton autosomal chronic granulomatous disease protein: tissue-specific expression and transcriptional control by retinoic acid. Mol Cell Biol 1990; 10:5388–96.
55. Leto TL, Lomax KG, Volpp BD, Nunoi H, Sechler JMB, Nauseef WM. Clark RA, Gallin JI, Malech HL. Cloning of a 67-kD neutrophil oxidase factor with similarity to a noncatalytic region of $p60^{c\text{-}src}$. Science 1990; 248:727–30.
56. Stahl ML, Ferenz CR, Kelleher KL, Kriz RW, Knoph JL. Sequence similarity of phospholipase C with the non-catalytic region of *src*. Nature 1988; 332:269–72.
57. Vogel US, Dixon RAF, Schaber MD, Diehl RE, Marshall MS, Scolnick EM, Sigal IS, Gibbs JB. Cloning of bovine GAP and its interaction with oncogenic *ras* p21. Nature 1988; 335:90–3.
58. Wasenius V, Saraste M, Salven P, Eramaa M, Holm L, Lehto V. Primary structure of the brain α-spectrin. J Cell Biol 1989; 108:79–93.
59. Tanaka K, Matsumoto K, Toh-e A. *IRA1*, an inhibitory regulator of the *RAS*-cyclic AMP pathway in *Saccaromyces cerevisiae.* Mol Cell Biol 1989; 9:757–68.
60. Broek D, Toda T, Michaeli T, Levin L, Birchmeier C, Zollen M, Powers S, Wigler M. The *S. cerevisiae* CDC25 gene product regulates the RAS/adenylate cyclase pathway. Cell 1987; 48:789–99.
61. Hughes D, Fukui Y, Yamamoto M. Homologous activators of *ras* in fission and budding yeast. Nature (London) 1990; 344:355–7.
62. Leto TL, Garrett MC, Fujii H, Nunoi H. Characterization of the neutrophil NADPH oxidase using recombinant cytosolic factors. J Cell Biol 1990; 111:49a.
63. Segal AW, Heyworth PG, Cockcroft S, Barrowman MM. Stimulated neutrophils from patients with autosomal recessive chronic granulomatous disease fail to phosphorylate a M_r-44,000 protein. Nature 1985; 316:547–9.
64. Okamura N, Curnutte JR, Roberts RL, Babior BM. Relationship of protein phosphorylation to the activation of the respiratory burst in human neutrophils: defects in the phosphorylation of a group of closely related 48-kDa proteins in two forms of chronic granulomatous disease. J Biol Chem 1988; 263:6777–82.
65. Okamura N, Malawista SE, Roberts RL, Rosen H, Ochs HD, Babior BM, Curnutte JT. Phosphorylation of the oxidase-related 48K phosphoprotein family in the unusual autosomal cytochrome-negative and X-linked cytochrome-positive types of chronic granulomatous disease. Blood 1988; 72:811–6.
66. Caldwell SE, McCall CE, Hendricks CL, Leone PA, Bass DA, McPhail LC. Coregulation of NADPH oxidase activation and phosphorylation of 48-kD protein(s) by a cytosolic fac-

tor defective in autosomal recessive chronic granulomatous disease. J Clin Invest 1988; 81:1485–96.
67. Bolscher BGJM, van Zwieten R, Kramer IM, Weening RS, Verhoeven AJ, Roos D. A phosphoprotein of M_r 47,000, defective in autosomal chronic granulomatous disease, copurifies with one of two soluble components required for NADPH:O_2 oxidoreductase activity in human neutrophils. J Clin Invest 1989; 83:757–63.
68. Kramer IM, Verhoeven AJ, van der Bend RL, Weening RS, Roos D. Purified protein kinase C phosphorylates a 47-kDa protein in control neutrophil cytoplasts but not in neutrophil cytoplasts from patients with the autosomal form of chronic granulomatous disease. J Biol Chem 1988; 263:2352–7.
69. Kramer IM, van der Bend RL, Verhoeven AJ, Roos D. The 47-kDa protein involved in the NADPH:O_2 oxidoreductase activity of human neutrophils is phosphorylated by cyclic AMP-dependent protein kinase without induction of a respiratory burst. Biochim Biophys Acta 1988; 971:189–96.
70. Teahan CG, Totty N, Casimir CM, Segal AW. Purification of the 47 kDa phosphoprotein associated with the NADPH oxidase of human neutrophils. Biochem J 1990; 267:485–9.
71. Bolscher BGJM, Denis SW, Verhoeven AJ, Roos D. The activity of one soluble component of the cell-free NADPH:O_2 oxidoreductase of human neutrophils depends on guanosine 5′-O-(3-thio)triphosphate. J Biol Chem 1990; 265:15782–7.
72. Pick E, Kroizman T, Abo A. Activation of the superoxide-forming NADPH oxidase of macrophages requires two cytosolic components—one of them is also present in certain nonphagocytic cells. J Immunol 1989; 143:4180–7.
73. Curnutte JT, Kuver R, Scott PJ. Activation of neutrophil NADPH oxidase in cell-free system. Partial purification of components and characterization of the activation process. J Biol Chem 1987; 262:5563–9.
74. Okamura N, Babior BM, Mayo LA, Peveri P, Smith RM, Curnutte JT. The p67-*phox* cytosolic peptide of the respiratory burst oxidase from human neutrophils. Functional aspects. J Clin Invest 1990; 85:1583–87.
75. Lambeth JD. Activation of the respiratory burst oxidase in neutrophils: on the role of membrane-derived second messengers, Ca^{++}, and protein kinase C. J Bioenerg Biomembr 1988; 20:709–33.
76. Heyworth PG, Badwey JA. Protein phosphorylation associated with the stimulation of neutrophils. Modulation of superoxide production by protein kinase C and calcium. J Bioenerg Biomembr 1990; 22:1–26.
77. Dubyak GR, Cowen DS. Activation of inositol phospholipid-specific phopholipase C by P_2-purinergic receptors in human phagocytic leukocytes. Role of pertussis toxin-sensitive G protein. Annals NY Acad Sci 1990; 603:227–45.
78. Kuhns DB, Wright DG, Nath J, Kaplan SS, Basford RE. ATP induces transient elevations of $[Ca^{2+}]_i$ in human neutrophils and primes these cells for enhanced O_2^- generation. Lab Invest 1988; 58:448–53.
79. Boulay F, Tardiff M, Brouchon L, Vignais P. Synthesis and use of a novel *N*-formyl peptide derivative to isolate a human *N*-formyl peptide receptor cDNA. Biochem Biophys Res Commun 1990; 168:1103–9.
80. Gerard NP, Gerard C. The chemotactic receptor for human C5a anaphylatoxin. Nature 1991; 349:614–7.
81. O'Dowd BF, Lefkowitz RJ, Caron MG. Structure of the adrenergic and related receptors. Ann Rev Neurosci 1989; 12:67–83.
82. Snyderman R, Smith CD, Verghese MW. Model for leukocyte regulation by chemoattractant receptors: roles of a guanine nucleotide regulatory protein and polyphosphoinositide metabolism. J Leuk Biol 1986; 40:785–800.

83. Murphy PM, Eide B, Goldsmith P, Brann M, Gierschik P, Spiegel A, Malech HL. Detection of multiple forms of $G_{i\alpha}$ in HL60 cells. FEBS Lett 1987; 221:81–6.
84. Goldsmith P, Gierschik P, Milligan G, Unson CG, Vinitsky R, Malech HL, Spiegel AM. Antibodies directed against synthetic peptides distinguish between GTP-binding proteins in neutrophils and brain. J Biol Chem 1987; 262:14683–8.
85. Verghese MW, Charles L, Jakoi L, Dillon SB, Snyderman R. Role of a guanine nucleotide regulatory protein in the activation of phospholipase C by different chemoattractants. J Immunol 1987; 138:4374–80.
86. Polakis PG, Evans T, Snyderman R. Multiple chromatographic forms of the formylpeptide chemoattractant receptor and their relationship to GTP-binding proteins. Biochem Biophys Res Commun 1989; 161:276–83.
87. Rollins TE, Siciliano S, Kobayashi S, Cianciarulo DN, Bonilla-Argudo V, Collier K, Springer MS. Purification of the active C5a receptor from the human polymorphonuclear leukocytes as a receptor-G_i complex. Proc Natl Acad Sci USA 1991; 88:971–5.
88. Cockroft S, Allan D. The fatty acid composition of phosphatidylinositol, phosphatidate and 1,2-diacylglycerol in stimulated human neutrophils. Biochem J 1984; 222:557–9.
89. Pai J-K, Siegal MI, Egan RW, Billah MM. Phospholipase D catalyses phospholipid metabolism in chemotactic peptide-stimulated HL-60 granulocytes. J Biol Chem 1988; 263:12472–77.
90. Agwu DE, McPhail LC, Chabot MC, Daniel LW, Wykle RL, McCall CE. Choline-linked phosphoglycerides. A source of phosphatidic acid and diglycerides in stimulated neutrophils. J Biol Chem 1989; 264:1405–13.
91. Palmer RMJ, Salmon JA. Release of leukotriene B_4 from human neutrophils and its relationship to degranulation induced by *N*-formyl-methionyl-leucyl-phenylalanine, serum-treated zymosan and the ionophore A23187. Immunology 1983; 50:65–73.
92. Clancy RM, Dahinden CA, Hugli TE. Arachidonate metabolism by human polymorphonuclear leukocytes stimulated by *N*-formyl-met-leu-phe or complement component C5a is independent of phospholipase activation. Proc Natl Acad Sci USA 1983; 80:7200–4.
93. Salari H, Braquet P, Naccache P, Borgeat P. Characterization of effect of *N*-formyl-methionyl-leucyl-phenylalanine on leukotriene synthesis in human polymorphonuclear leukocytes. Inflammation 1985; 9:127–38.
94. Haines KA, Giedd KN, Rich AM, Korchak HM, Weissmann G. The leukotriene B_4 paradox: neutrophils can, but will not, respond to ligand-receptor interactions by forming leukotriene B_4 or its ω-metabolites. Biochem J 1987; 241:55–62.
95. Nakashima S, Suganuma A, Sato M, Tohmatsu T, Nozawa Y. Mechanism of arachidonic acid liberation in platelet-activating factor-stimulated human polymorphonuclear neutrophils. J Immunol 1989; 143:1295–1302.
96. Bauldry SA, Wykle RL, Bass DA. Phospholipase A_2 activation in human neutrophils. Differential actions of diacylglycerols and alkylacylglycerols in priming cells for stimulation by *N*-formyl-Met-Leu-Phe. J Biol Chem 1988; 263:16787–95.
97. Corey SJ, Rosoff PM. Granulocyte-macrophage colony-stimulating factor primes neutrophils by activating a pertussis toxin-sensitive G protein not associated with phosphatidylinositol turnover. J Biol Chem 1989; 264:14165–71.
98. Bauldry SA, McCall CE, Cousart SL, Bass DA. Tumor necrosis factor-α priming of phospholipase A_2 activation in human neutrophils: an alternative mechanism of priming. J Immunol 1991; 146:1277–85.
99. Verghese MW, Fox K, McPhail LC, Snyderman R. Chemoattractant-elicited alterations of cAMP levels in human polymorphonuclear leukocytes require a Ca^{2+}-dependent mechanism which is independent of transmembrane activation of adenylate cyclase. J Biol Chem 1985; 260:6769–75.
100. Iannone MA, Wolberg G, Zimmerman TP. Chemotactic peptide induces cAMP elevation

in human neutrophils by amplification of the adenylate cyclase response to endogenously produced adenosine. J Biol Chem 1989; 264:20177–80.
101. Reibman JR, Korchak HM, Vosshall LB, Haines KA, Rich AM, Weissmann G. Changes in diacylglycerol labeling, cell shape, and protein phosphorylation distinguish "triggering" from "activation" of human neutrophils. J Biol Chem 1988; 263:6322–8.
102. Korchak HM, Vosshall LB, Haines KA, Wilkenfeld C, Lundquist KF, Weissmann G. Activation of the human neutrophil by calcium-mobilizing ligands: II. Correlation of calcium, diacylglycerol, and phosphatidic acid generation with superoxide anion generation. J Biol Chem 1988; 263:11098–106.
103. Taylor SS, Buechler JA, Yonemoto W. cAMP-dependent protein kinase: framework for a diverse family of regulatory enzymes. Ann Rev Biochem 1990; 59:971–1005.
104. Berridge MJ. Inositol trisphosphate and diacylglycerol: two interacting second messengers. Ann Rev Biochem 1987; 56:159–93.
105. Huang K-P. The mechanism of protein kinase C activation. TINS 1989; 12:425–32.
106. Exton JH. Mechanisms of action of calcium-mobilizing agonists: some variations on a young theme. FASEB J 1988; 2:2670–6.
107. Takai Y, Kishimoto A, Iwasa Y, Kawahara Y, Mori T, Nishizuka Y. Calcium-dependent activation of a multifunctional protein kinase by membrane phospholipids. J Biol Chem 1979; 254:3692–5.
108. Bellavite P, Corso F, Dusi S, Grzeskowiak M, Della-Bianca V, Rossi F. Activation of NADPH-dependent superoxide production in plasma membrane extracts of pig neutrophils by phosphatidic acid. J Biol Chem 1988; 263:8210–4.
109. Agwu DE, McPhail LC, Sozzani S, Bass DA, McCall CE. Phosphatidic acid as a second messenger in human polymorphonuclear leukocytes. Effects on activation of NADPH oxidase. J Clin Invest 1991; 88:531–9.
110. Agwu DE, McCall CE, McPhail LC. Regulation of phospholipase D-induced hydrolysis of choline-containing phosphoglycerides by cyclic AMP in human neutrophils. J Immunol 1991; 146:3895–903.
111. O'Flaherty JT, Jacobson D, Redman J. Mechanism involved in the mobilization of neutrophil calcium by 5-hydroxyeicosatetraenoate. J Immunol 1988; 140:4323–8.
112. Naccache PH, Molski MM, Volpi M, Shefcyk J, Molski TFP, Loew L, Becker EL, Sha'afi RI. Biochemical events associated with the stimulation of rabbit neutrophils by platelet activating factor. J Leuk Biol 1986; 40:533–48.
113. O'Flaherty JT, Nishihira J. Arachidonate metabolites, platelet-activating factor, and the mobilization of protein kinase C in human polymorphonuclear neutrophils. J Immunol 1987; 138:1889–95.
114. Tosi MF, Berger M. Functional differences between the 40 kDa and 50 to 70 kDa IgG Fc receptors on human neutrophils revealed by elastase treatment and antireceptor antibodies. J Immunol 1988; 141:2097–103.
115. Huizinga TWJ, van Kemanade F, Koenderman L, Dolman KM, von dem Borne AEGK, Tetteroo PAT, Roos D. The 40-kDa Fcγ receptor (FcRII) on human neutrophils is essential for the IgG-receptor respiratory burst and IgG-induced phagocytosis. J Immunol 1989; 142:2365–9.
116. Stuart SG, Trounstine ML, Vaux DJT, Koch T, Martens CL, Mellman I, Moore KW. Isolation and expression of cDNA clones encoding a human receptor for IgG (FcγRII). J Exp Med 1987; 166:1668–84.
117. Crockett-Torabi E, Fantone JC. Soluble and insoluble immune complexes activate human neutrophil NADPH oxidase by distinct Fcγ receptor-specific mechanisms. J Immunol 1990; 145:3026–32.
118. Feister AJ, Browder B, Willis HE, Mohanakumar T, Ruddy S. Pertussis toxin inhibits human neutrophil responses mediated by the 42-kilodalton IgG Fc receptor. J Immunol 1988; 141:228–33.

119. Shirato M, Takahashi K, Nagasawa S, Koyama J. Different sensitivities of the responses of human neutrophils stimulated with immune complex and C5a anaphylatoxin to pertussis toxin. FEBS Lett 1988; 234:231–4.
120. Fällman M, Lew DP, Stendahl O, Andersson T. Receptor-mediated phagocytosis in human neutrophils is associated with increased formation of inositol phosphates and diacylglycerol. Elevation in cytosolic free calcium and formation of inositol phosphates can be dissociated from accumulation of diacylglycerol. J Clin Invest 1989; 84:886–91.
121. Bianca VD, Grzeskowiak M, Rossi F. Studies on molecular regulation of phagocytosis and activation of the NAPDH oxidase in neutrophils. IgG-and C3b mediated ingestion and associated respiratory burst independent of phospholipid turnover and Ca^{2+} transients. J Immunol 1990; 144:1411–7.
122. Ahearn JM, Fearon DT. Structure and function of the complement receptors, CR1 (CD35) and CR2 (CD21). Adv Immunol 1989; 46:183–219.
123. Newman SL, Johnston RB Jr. Role of binding through C3b and IgG in polymorphonuclear neutrophil function: studies with trypsin-generated C3b. J Immunol 1979; 123:1839–46.
124. Kishimoto TK, Larson RS, Corbi AL, Dustin ML, Staunton DE, Springer TA. The leukocyte integrins. Adv Immunol 1989; 46:149–82.
125. Rhyne JA, Mizel SB, Taylor RG, Chedid M, McCall CE. Characterization of the human interleukin 1 receptor on human polymorphonuclear leukocytes. Clin Immunol Immunopathol 1988; 48:354–61.
126. Shalaby MR, Palladino MA Jr, Hirabayashi SE, Eessalu TE, Lewis GD, Shepard HM, Aggarwal BB. Receptor binding and activation of polymorphonuclear neutrophils by tumor necrosis factor-alpha. J Leuk Biol 1987; 41:196–204.
127. Uzumaki H, Okabe T, Sasaki N, Hagiwara K, Takaku R, Itoh, S. Characterization of receptor for granulocyte colony-stimulating factor on human circulating neutrophils. Biochem Biophys Res Commun 1988; 156:1026–32.
128. Hansen BD, Finbloom DS. Characterization of the interaction between recombinant human interferon-γ and its receptor on human polymorphonuclear leukocytes. J Leuk Biol 1990; 47:64–9.
129. Guthrie LA, McPhail LC, Henson PM, Johnson RB Jr. Priming of neutrophils for enhanced release of oxygen metabolites by bacterial lipopolysaccharide. Evidence for increased activity of the superoxide-producing enzyme. J Exp Med 1984; 160:1656–71.
130. Berkow RL, Wang D, Larrick JW, Dodson RW, Howard TH. Enhancement of neutrophil superoxide production by preincubation with recombinant human tumor necrosis factor. J Immunol 1987; 139:3783–91.
131. Weisbart RH, Kwan L, Golde DW, Gasson JC. Human GM-CSF primes neutrophils for enhanced oxidative metabolism in response to the major physiological chemoattractants. Blood 1987; 69:18–21.
132. Berton G, Zeni L, Cassatella MA, Rossi F. Gamma interferon is able to enhance the oxidative metabolism of human neutrophils. Biochem Biophys Res Commun 1986; 138:1276–82.
133. Nathan C, Srimal S, Farber C, Sanchez E, Kabbash L, Asch A, Gailit J, Wright SD. Cytokine-induced respiratory burst of human neutrophils: dependence on extracellular matrix proteins and CD11/CD18 integrins. J Cell Biol 1989; 109:1341–9.
134. Nathan C. Respiratory burst in adherent human neutrophils: triggering by colony-stimulating factors CSF-GM and CSF-G. Blood 1989; 73:301–6.
135. Sims JE, March CJ, Cosman D, Widmer MB, MacDonald HR, McMahan CJ, Grubin CE, Wignall JM, Jackson JL, Call SM, Friend D, Alpert AR, Gillis S, Urdal DL, Dower SK. cDNA expression cloning of the IL-1 receptor, a member of the immunoglobulin superfamily. Science 1988; 241:585–9.
136. Smith CA, Davis T, Anderson D, Solam L, Beckmann MP, Jerzy R, Dower SK, Cosman D, Goodwin RG. A receptor for tumor necrosis factor defines an unusual family of cellu-

lar and viral proteins. Science 1990; 248:1019–23.
137. Gearing DP, King JA, Gough NM, Nicola NA. Expression cloning of a receptor for human granulocyte-macrophage colony-stimulating factor. EMBO J 1989; 8:3667–76.
138. Hayashida K, Kitamura T, Gorman DM, Arai, K-I, Yokota T, Miyajima A. Molecular cloning of a second subunit of the receptor for human granulocyte-macrophage colony-stimulating (GM-CSF): reconstitution of a high-affinity GM-CSF receptor. Proc Natl Acad Sci USA 1990; 87:9655–9.
139. Aguet M, Dembić Z, Merlin G. Molecular cloning and expression of the human interferon-γ receptor. Cell 1988; 55:273–80.
140. Laudanna C, Miron S, Berton G, Rossi F. Tumor necrosis factor-α/cachetin activates the O_2^- generating system of human neutrophils independently of the hydrolysis of phosphoinositides and the release of arachidonic acid. Biochem Biophys Res Commun 1990; 166:308–15.
141. Coffey RG, Davis JS, Djeu JY. Stimulation of guanylate cyclase activity and reduction of adenylate cyclase activity by granulocyte-macrophage colony-stimulating factor in human blood neutrophils. J Immunol 1988; 140:2695–2701.
142. Sullivan R, Griffin JD, Simons ER, Schafer AI, Mashulam T, Fredette JP, Maas AK, Gadenne A-S, Leavitt JL, Melnick DA. Effects of recombinant human granulocyte-macrophage colony-stimulating factor on signal transduction pathways in human granulocytes. J Immunol 1988; 139:3422–30.
143. McColl SR, Beauseigle D, Gilbert C, Naccache PH. Priming of the human neutrophil respiratory burst by granulocyte-macrophage colony-stimulating factor and tumor necrosis factor-α involves regulation at a post-cell surface receptor level. J Immunol 1990; 145:3047–53.
144. Berkow RL, Dodson MR. Biochemical mechanisms involved in the priming of neutrophils by tumor necrosis factor. J Leuk Biol 1988; 44:345–52.
145. Meurer R, MacIntyre DE. Lack of effect of pertussis toxin on TNF-α-induced formation of reactive oxygen intermediates by human neutrophils. Biochem Biophys Res Commun 1989; 159:763–9.
146. Gomez-Cambronero J, Yamazaki M, Metwally F, Molski TFP, Bonak VA, Huang C-K, Becker EL, Sha'afi RI. Granulocyte-macrophage colony-stimulating factor and human neutrophils: role of guanine nucleotide regulatory proteins. Proc Natl Acad Sci USA 1989; 86:3569–73.
147. Gomez-Cambronero J, Huang C-K, Bonak VA, Wang E, Casnellie JE, Shiaishi T, Sha'afi RI. Tyrosine phosphorylation in human neutrophil. Biochem Biophys Res Commun 1989; 162:1478–85.
148. Bourgoin S, Plante E, Gaudry M, Naccache PH, Borgeat P, Poubelle PE. Involvement of a phospholipase D in the mechanism of action of granulocyte-macrophage colony-stimulating factor (GM-CSF): priming of human neutrophils in vitro with GM-CSF is associated with accumulation of phosphatidic acid and diradylglycerol. J Exp Med 1990; 172:767–77.
149. DiPersio JF, Billing P, Williams R, Gasson JC. Human granulocyte-macrophage colony-stimulating factor and other cytokines prime human neutrophils for enhanced arachidonic acid release and leukotriene B_4 synthesis. J Immunol 1988; 140:4315–22.
150. Bauldry SA, Bass DA, Cousart SL, McCall CE. Tumor necrosis factor α priming of phospholipase D in human neutrophils: correlation between phosphatidic acid production and superoxide generation. J Biol Chem 1991; 266:4173–9.
151. Nathan C, Sanchez E. Tumor necrosis factor and CD11/CD18 ($\beta 2$) integrins act synergistically to lower cAMP in human neutrophils. J Cell Biol 1990; 111:2171–81.
152. Thelen M, Rosen A, Nairn AC, Aderem A. Tumor necrosis factor α modifies agonist–dependent responses in human neutrophils by inducing the synthesis and myristoylation of a specific protein kinase C substrate. Proc Natl Acad Sci USA 1990; 87:5603–7.

153. Weiel JE, Hamilton TA, Adams DO. LPS induces altered phosphate labeling of proteins in murine peritoneal macrophages. J Immunol 1986; 136:3012–8.
154. Worthen GS, Seccombe JF, Clay KL, Guthrie LA, Johnson RB Jr. The priming of neutrophils by lipopolysaccharide for production of intracellular platelet-activating factor: potential role in mediation of enhanced superoxide secretion. J Immunol 1988; 140:3553–9.
155. Doerfler ME, Danner RL, Shelhamer JH, Parrillo JE. Bacterial lipopolysaccharides prime human neutrophils for enhanced production of leukotriene B_4. J Clin Invest 1989; 83:970–7.
156. Forehand JR, Pabst MJ, Phillips WA, Johnston RB Jr. Lipopolysaccharide priming of human neutrophils for an enhanced respiratory burst. Role of intracellular free calcium. J Clin Invest 1989; 83:74–83.
157. Grove RI, Allegretto NJ, Kiener PA, Warr GA. Lipopolysaccharide (LPS) alters phosphatidylcholine metabolism in elicited peritoneal macrophages. J Leuk Biol 1990; 48:38–42.
158. Cassatella MA, Bazzoni F, Flynn RM, Dusi S, Trinchieri G, Rossi F. Molecular basis of interferon-γ and lipopolysaccharide enhancement of phagocyte respiratory burst capability: studies on the gene expression of several NADPH oxidase components. J Biol Chem 1990; 265:20241–6.
159. Cockroft S, Stutchfield J. The receptors for ATP and fMetLeuPhe are independently coupled to phospholipases C and A_2 via G-protein(s): relationship between phospholipase C and A_2 activation and exocytosis in HL60 cells and human neutrophils. Biochem J 1989; 263:715–23.
160. Cockroft S, Stutchfield J. ATP stimulates secretion in human neutrophils and HL60 cells via a pertussis toxin-sensitive guanine nucleotide-binding protein coupled to phospholipase C. FEBS Lett 1989; 245:25–9.
161. Seifert R, Burde R, Schultz G. Activation of NADPH oxidase by purine and pyrimidine nucleotides involves G proteins and is potentiated by chemotactic peptides. Biochem J 1989; 259:813–9.
162. Seifert R, Wenzel K, Eckstein F, Schultz G. Purine and pyrimidine nucleotides potentiate activation of NADPH oxidase and degranulation by chemotactic peptides and induce aggregation of human neutrophils via G proteins. Eur J Biochem 1989; 181:277–85.
163. Balazovich KJ, Boxer LA. Extracellular adenosine nucleotides stimulate protein kinase C activity and human neutrophil activation. J Immunol 1990; 144:631–7.
164. McLeish KR, Gierschik P, Schepers T, Sidiropoulos D, Jakobs KH. Evidence that activation of a common G-protein by receptors for leukotriene B_4 and *N*-formylmethionyl-leucyl-phenylalanine in HL-60 cells occurs by different mechanisms. Biochem J 1989; 260:427–34.
165. English D, Rizzo MT, Tricot G, Hoffman R. Involvement of guanine nucleotides in superoxide release by fluoride-treated neutrophils. Implications for a role of a guanine nucleotide regulatory protein. J Immunol 1989; 143:1685–91.
166. Lu DJ, Grinstein S. ATP and guanine nucleotide dependence of neutrophil activation. Evidence for the involvement of two distinct GTP-binding proteins. J Biol Chem 1990; 265:13721–9.
167. English D, Debono DJ, Gabid TG. Relationship of phosphatidylinositol bisphosphate hydrolysis to calcium mobilization and functional activation of fluoride-treated neutrophils. J Clin Invest 1987; 80:145–53.
168. Bokoch GM, Gilman AG. Inhibition of receptor-mediated release of arachidonic acid by pertussis toxin. Cell 1984; 39:301–8.
169. English D, Taylor GS. Divergent effects of propranolol on neutrophil superoxide release: involvement of phosphatidic acid and diacylglycerol as second messengers. Biochem Biophys Res Commun 1991; 175:423–9.
170. Cockcroft S, Gomperts BD. Role of guanine nucleotide binding proteins in the activation of polyphosphoinositide phosphodiesterase. Nature (London) 1985; 314:534–6.

171. Cockcroft S. Relationship between arachidonate release and exocytosis in permeabilized human neutrophils stimulated with formylmethionyl-leucyl-phenylalanine (fMetLeuPhe), guanosine 5′-[γ-thio]triphosphate (GTP[S]) and Ca^{2+}. Biochem J 1991; 275:127–31.
172. Repine JE, White JG, Clawson CC, Holmes BM. The influence of phorbol myristate acetate on oxygen consumption by polymorphonuclear leukocytes. J Lab Clin Med 1974; 83:911–20.
173. DeChatelet LR, Shirley PS, Johnston RB Jr. Effect of phorbol myristate acetate on the oxidative metabolism of human polymorphonuclear leukocytes. Blood 1976; 47:545–54.
174. Lehrer RI, Cohen L. Receptor-mediated regulation of superoxide production in human neutrophils stimulated by phorbol myristate acetate. J Clin Invest 1981; 68:1314–20.
175. Wolfson M, McPhail LC, Nasrallah VN, Snyderman R. Phorbol myristate acetate mediates redistribution of protein kinase C in human neutrophils: potential role in the activation of the respiratory burst enzyme. J Immunol 1985; 135:2057–62.
176. Myers MA, McPhail LC, Snyderman R. Redistribution of protein kinase C activity in human monocytes: correlation with activation of the respiratory burst. J Immunol 1985; 135:3411–6.
177. Fujita I, Irita K, Takeshige K, Minakami S. Diacylglycerol, 1-oleoyl-2-acetyl-glycerol, stimulates superoxide-generation from human neutrophils. Biochem Biophys Res Commun 1984; 120:318–24.
178. Cox CC, Dougherty RW, Ganong BR, Bell RM, Niedel JE, Snyderman R. Differential stimulation of the respiratory burst and lysosomal enzyme secretion in human polymorphonuclear leukocytes by synthetic diacylglycerols. J Immunol 1986; 136:4611–6.
179. Bass DA, Gerard C, Olbrantz P, Wilson J, McCall CE, McPhail LC. Priming of the respiratory burst of neutrophils by diacylglycerol. Independence from activation or translocation of protein kinase C. J Biol Chem 1987; 262:6643–9.
180. Naccache PH, Molski MM, Sha'afi RI. Polymyxin B inhibits phorbol 12-myristate 13-acetate, but not chemotactic factor, induced effects in rabbit neutrophils. FEBS Lett 1985; 193:227–30.
181. Gerard C, McPhail LC, Marfat A, Stimler-Gerard NP, Bass DA, McCall CE. Role of protein kinases in stimulation of human polymorphonuclear leukocyte oxidative metabolism by various agonists. Differential effects of a novel protein kinase inhibitor. J Clin Invest 1986; 77:61–5.
182. Kramer IM, van der Bend RL, Tool ATJ, van Blitterswijk WJ, Roos D, Verhoeven AJ. 1-O-hexadecyl-2-O-methylglycerol, a novel inhibitor of protein kinase C, inhibits the respiratory burst in human neutrophils. J Biol Chem 1989; 264:5876–84.
183. Schell-Frederick E. Stimulation of the oxidative metabolism of polymorphonuclear leukocytes by the calcium ionophore A23187. FEBS Lett 1974; 48:37–40.
184. Dahlgren C. Difference in extracellular radical release after chemotactic factor and calcium ionophore activation of the oxygen radical generating system in human neutrophils. Biochem Biophys Acta 1987; 930:33–8.
185. Lew DP. Receptor signaling and intracellular calcium in neutrophil activation. Eur J Clin Invest 1989; 19:338–46.
186. Della-Bianca V, Grzeskowiak M, Cassatella MA, Zeni L, Rossi F. Phorbol 12, myristate 13, acetate potentiates the respiratory burst while inhibits phosphoinositide hydrolysis and calcium mobilization by formyl-methionyl-leucyl-phenylalanine in neutrophils. Biochem Biophys Res Commun 1986; 135:556–65.
187. Grzeskowiak M, Della-Bianca V, Cassatela MA, Rossi F. Complete dissociation between activation of phosphoinositide turnover and of NADPH oxidase by formyl-methionyl-leucyl-phenylalanine in human neutrophils depleted of Ca^{2+} and primed by subthreshold doses of phorbol 12, myristate 13, acetate. Biochem Biophys Res Commun 1986; 135:785–94.

188. Rossi F, Grzeskowiak M, Della-Bianca V. Double stimulation with FMLP and Con A restores the activation of the respiratory burst but not of the phosphoinositide turnover in Ca_{2+}-depleted human neutrophils. A further example of dissociation between stimulation of the NADPH oxidase and phosphoinositide turnover. Biochem Biophys Res Commun 1986; 140:1–11.
189. Tyagi RJ, Tamura M, Burnham DN, Lambeth JD. Phorbol myristate acetate (PMA) augments chemoattractant-induced diglyceride generation in human neutrophils but inhibits phophoinositide hydrolysis. J Biol Chem 1988; 263:13191–8.
190. McPhail LC, Sozzani S, Wilson JL, Qualliotine-Mann D, Cousart S, McCall CE. Regulation of protein kinase C in human neutrophils by arachidonic acid and other lipid mediators. In: Lewis AJ, Doherty NS, Ackerman NR, eds. Therapeutic approaches to inflammatory diseases. New York: Elsevier, 1989:101–112.
191. Nishizuka Y. Studies and perspectives of the protein kinase C family for cellular regulation. Cancer 1989; 63:1891–903.
192. Walsh CE, Waite BM, Thomas MJ, DeChatelet LR. Release and metabolism of arachidonic acid in human neutrophils. J Biol Chem 1981; 256:7228–34.
193. Kakinuma K. Effects of fatty acids on the oxidative metabolism of leukocytes. Biochim Biophys Acta 1974; 348:76–85.
194. Badwey JA, Curnutte JT, Karnovsky ML. cis-Polyunsaturated fatty acid induce high levels of superoxide production by human neutrophils. J Biol Chem 1981; 256:12640–3.
195. Graham RC Jr, Karnovsky MJ, Shafer AW, Glass EA, Karnovsky ML. Metabolic and morphological observations on the effect of surface-active agents on leukocytes. J Cell Biol 1967; 32:629–47.
196. Zatti M, Rossi F. Relationship between glycolysis and respiration in surfactant-treated leukocytes. Biochim Biophys Acta 1967; 148:553–5.
197. Cohen HJ, Chovaniec ME. Superoxide generation by digitonin-stimulated guinea pig granulocytes. A basis for a continuous assay for monitoring superoxide reduction and for the study of the activation of the generating system. J Clin Invest 1977; 78:1081–7.
198. Kakinuma K, Hatae T, Minakami S. Effect of ionic sites of surfactants on leukocyte metabolism. J Biochem (Tokyo) 1976; 79:795–802.
199. Washida N, Sagawa A, Tamoto K, Koyama J. Comparative studies on superoxide anion production by polymorphonuclear leukocytes stimulated with various agents. Biochim Biophys Acta 1980; 631:371–9.
200. Bromberg Y, Pick E. Activation of NADPH-dependent superoxide production in a cell-free system by sodium dodecyl sulfate. J Biol Chem 1985; 260:13539–45.
201. Traynor AE, Scott PJ, Harris AL, Badway JA, Sklar LA, Babior BM, Curnutte JT. Respiratory burst oxidase activation can be dissociated from phosphatidylinositol bisphosphate degradation in a cell-free system from human neutrophils. Blood 1989; 73:296–300.
202. Maridonneau-Parini I, Tauber AI. Activation of NADPH-oxidase by arachidonic acid involves phospholipase A_2 in intact human neutrophils but not in the cell-free system. Biochem Biophys Res Commun 1986; 138:1099–105.
203. Naccache PH, McColl SR, Caon AC, Borgeat P. Arachidonic acid-induced mobilization of calcium in human neutrophils: evidence for a multicomponent mechanism of action. Br J Pharmacol 1989; 97:461–8.
204. McColl SR, Krump E, Naccache PH, Caon AC, Borgeat P. Activation of the human neutrophil 5-lipoxygenase by exogenous arachidonic acid: involvement of pertussis toxin-sensitive guanine nucleotide-binding proteins. Br J Pharmacol 1989; 97:1265–73.
205. Huang C-K. Protein kinase in neutrophils: a review. Membrane Biochem 1989; 8:61–79.
206. Nielson CP. β-Adrenergic modulation of the polymorphonuclear leukocyte respiratory burst is dependent upon the mechanism of cell activation. J Immunol 1987; 139:2392–7.
207. Sedgwick JB, Berube ML, Zurier RB. Stimulus-dependent inhibition of superoxide generation by prostaglandins. Clin Immunol Immunopathol 1985; 34:205–15.
208. Tyagi SR, Olson SC, Burnham DN, Lambeth JD. Cyclic AMP-elevating agents block

chemoattractant activation of diradylglycerol generation by inhibiting phospholipase D activation. J Biol Chem 1991; 266:3498–504.

209. Kato H, Ishitoya J, Takenawa T. Inhibition of inositol phospholipids metabolism and calcium mobilization by cyclic AMP-increasing agents and phorbol ester in neutrophils. Biochem Biophys Res Commun 1986; 139:1272–8.
210. Bianca VD, De Togni P, Grzeskowiak M, Vicentini LM, Di Virgilio F. Cyclic AMP inhibition of phosphoinositide turnover in human neutrophils. Biochim Biophys Acta 1986; 886:441–7.
211. Mueller H, Sklar LA. Coupling of antagonistic signalling pathways in modulation of neutrophil function. J Cell Biochem 1989; 40:287–94.
212. Wright CD, Hoffman MD. Comparison of the roles of calmodulin and protein kinase C in activation of the human neutrophil respiratory burst. Biochem Biophys Res Commun 1987; 142:53–62.
213. Brumley LM, Wallace RW. Calmodulin and protein kinase C antagonists also inhibit the Ca^{2+}-dependent protein protease, calpain I. Biochem Biophys Res Commun 1989; 159:1297–303.
214. McPhail LC, Hendricks CL, Seeds MC, Bass DA, McCall CE. A possible role for calmodulin in activation of the respiratory burst enzyme of human neutrophils. Abstr, Clin Res 1986; 34:45A.
215. Sakata A, Ida E, Tominaga M, Onoue K. Calmodulin inhibitors, W-7 and TFP, block the calmodulin-independent activation of NADPH-oxidase by arachidonate in a cell-free system. Biochem Biophys Res Commun 1987; 148:112–9.
216. Wolff DJ, Brostrom CO. Calcium-dependent cyclic nucleotide phosphodiesterase from brain: identification of phospholipids as calcium-independent activators. Arch Biochem Biophys 1976; 173:720–31.
217. Tanaka T, Hidaka H. Hydrophobic regions function in calmodulin-enzyme(s) interactions. J Biol Chem 1980; 255:11078–80.
218. Niggli V, Adunyah ES, Carafoli E. Acidic phospholipids unsaturated fatty acids, and limited proteolysis mimic the effect of calmodulin on the purified erythrocyte Ca^{2+}-ATPase. J Biol Chem 1981; 256:8588–92.
219. McPhail LC, Clayton CC, Snyderman R. A potential second messenger role for unsaturated fatty acids: activation of Ca^{2+}-dependent protein kinase. Science 1984; 224:622–5.
220. Daniel LW, Small GW, Schmitt JD. Alkyl-linked diglycerides inhibit protein kinase C activation by diacylglycerols. Biochem Biophys Res Commun 1988; 151:291–7.
221. Bass DA, McPhail LC, Schmitt JD, Morris-Natschke S, McCall CE, Wykle RL. Selective priming of rate and duration of the respiratory burst of neutrophils by 1,2-diacyl and 1-*O*-alkyl-2-acyl diglycerides: possible relation to effects on protein kinase C. J Biol Chem 1988; 263:19610–7.
222. Hunnun YA, Loomis CR, Merrill AH Jr, Bell RM. Sphingosine inhibition of protein kinase C activity and of phorbol dibutyrate binding *in vitro* and in human platelets. J Biol Chem 1986; 261:12604–9.
223. Pontremoli S, Melloni E, Salamino F, Patrone M, Michetti M, Horecker BL. Activation of neutrophil calpain following its translocation to the plasma membrane induced by phorbol ester or fMet-Leu-Phe. Biochem Biophys Res Commun 1989; 160:737–43.
224. Balazovich KJ, Smolen JE, Boxer LA. Endogenous inhibitor of protein kinase C: association with human peripheral blood neutrophils but not with specific granule-deficient neutrophils or cytoplasts. J Immunol 1986; 137:1665–73.
225. Gennaro R, Florio C, Romeo D. Co-activation of protein kinase C and NADPH oxidase in the plasma membrane of neutrophil cytoplasts. Biochem Biophys Res Commun 1986; 134:305–12.
226. Cox JA, Jeng AY, Sharkey NA, Blumberg PM, Tauber AI. Activation of the human neutrophil nicotinamide adenine dinucleotide phosphate (NADPH)-oxidase by protein kinase C. J Clin Invest 1985; 76:1932–8.

227. Tauber AI, Cox JA, Curnutte JT, Carrol PM, Nakakuma H, Warren B, Gilbert H, Blumberg PM. Activation of human neutrophil NADPH-oxidase in vitro by the catalytic fragment of protein kinase-C. Biochem Biophys Res Commun 1989; 158:884–90.
228. Cox JA, Jeng AY, Blumberg PM, Tauber AI. Comparison of subcellular activation of the human neutrophil NADPH-oxidase by arachidonic acid, sodium dodecyl sulfate (SDS), and phorbol myristate acetate (PMA). J Immunol 1987; 138:1884–8.
229. Pike MC, Jakoi L, McPhail LC, Snyderman R. Chemoattractant-mediated stimulation of the respiratory burst in human polymorphonuclear leukocytes may require appearance of protein kinase activity in the cells' particulate fraction. Blood 1986; 67:909–13.
230. Christiansen NO, Peterslund NA, Larsen CS, Esmann V. Evidence that bacteria induce translocation of protein kinase C activity in human polymorphonuclear leukocytes. Biochem 1987; 147:787–93.
231. Seifert R, Schachtele C. Studies with protein kinase C inhibitors presently available cannot elucidate the role of protein kinase C in the activation of NADPH oxidase. Biochem Biophys Res Commun 1988; 152:585–92.
232. Nath J, Powledge A, Wright DG. Studies of signal transduction in the respiratory burst-associated stimulation of fMet-Leu-Phe-induced tubulin tyrosinolation and phorbol 12-myristate 13-acetate-induced posttranslational incorporation of tyrosine into multiple proteins in activated neutrophils and HL-60 cells. J Biol Chem 1989; 264:848–55.
233. Pontremoli S, Melloni E, Sparatore B, Michetti M, Salamino F, Horecker BL. Isozymes of protein kinase C in human neutrophils and their modification by two endogenous proteinases. J Biol Chem 1990; 265:706–12.
234. Stasia MJ, Strulovici B, Daniel-Issakani S, Pelosin JM, Dianoux AC, Chambaz E, Vignais PV. Immunocharacterization of β- and ζ-subspecies of protein kinase C in bovine neutrophils. FEBS Lett 1990; 274:61–4.
235. Majumdar S, Rossi MW, Fujiki T, Phillips WA, Disa S, Queen CF, Johnston RB Jr, Rosen OM, Corkey BE, Korchak HM. Protein kinase C isotypes and signaling in neutrophils. Differential substrate specificities of a translocatable, calcium- and phospholipid-dependent β-protein kinase C and a novel calcium-independent, phospholipid-dependent protein kinase which is inhibited by long chain fatty acyl coenzyme A. J Biol Chem 1991; 266:9285–94.
236. Osada S, Mizuno K, Saido TC, Akita Y, Suzuki K, Kuroki T, Ohno S. A phorbol ester receptor/protein kinase, nPKCη, a new member of the protein kinase C family predomaninantly expressed in lung and skin. J Biol Chem 1990; 265:22434–40.
237. Bacher N, Zisman Y, Berent E, Livneh E. Isolation and characterization of PKC-L, a new member of the protein kinase C-related gene family specifically expressed in lung, skin, and heart. Mol and Cell Biol 1991; 11:126–33.
238. Shearman MS, Berry N, Oda T, Ase K, Kikkawa U, Nishizuka Y. Isolation of protein kinase C subspecies from a preparation of human T lymphocytes. FEBS Lett 1988; 234:387–91.
239. Marias RM, Parker PJ. Purification and characterization of bovine brain protein kinase C isotypes α, β, and γ. Eur J Biochem 1989; 182:129–37.
240. Jaken S, Kiley SC. Purification and characterization of three types of protein kinase C from rabbit brain cytosol. Proc Natl Acad Sci USA 1987; 84:4418–22.
241. Huang K, Nakabayashi H, Huang FL. Isozymic forms of rat brain Ca^{2+}-activated and phospholipid-dependent protein kinase. Proc Natl Acad Sci USA 1986; 83:8535–9.
242. Huang FL, Yoshida Y, Cunha-Melo JR, Beaven MA, Huang K. Differential down-regulation of protein kinase C isozymes. J Biol Chem 1989; 264:4238–43.
243. Strulovici B, Daniel-Issakani S, Oto E, Nestor J Jr, Chan H, Tsou A. Activation of distinct protein kinase C isozymes by phorbol esters: correlation with induction of interleukin 1β gene expression. Biochemistry 1989; 28:3569–76.
244. Houweling M, Vaartjes WJ, van Golde LMG. Isozymic forms of protein kinase C in regenerating rat liver. FEBS Lett 1989; 247:487–91.

245. Cooper DR, Watson JE, Acevedo-Duncan M, Pollet RJ, Standaert ML, Farese RV. Retention of specific protein kinase C isozymes following chronic phorbol ester treatment in BC3H-1 myocytes. Biochem Biophys Res Commun 1989; 161:327–34.
246. Fournier A, Hardy SJ, Clark KJ, Murray AW. Phorbol ester induces differential membrane-association of protein kinase C subspecies in human platelets. Biochem Biophys Res Commun 1989; 161:556–61.
247. Ono Y, Fujii T, Ogita K, Kikkawa U, Igarashi K, Nishizuka Y. The structure, expression, and properties of additional members of the protein kinase C family. J Biol Chem 1988; 263:6927–32.
248. Schaap D, Parker PJ, Bristol A, Kriz R, Knopf J. Unique substrate specificity and regulatory properties of PKC-ϵ: a rationale for diversity. FEBS Lett 1989; 243:351–7.
249. Ono Y, Fujii R, Ogita K, Kikkawa U, Igarashi K, Nishizuka Y. Protein kinase C ζ subspecies from rat brain: its structure, expression and properties. Proc Natl Acad Sci USA 1989; 86:3099–103.
250. Huang C, Laramee GR, Casnellie JE. Chemotactic factor induced tyrosine phosphorylation of membrane associated proteins in rabbit peritoneal neutrophils. Biochem Biophys Res Commun 1988; 151:794–801.
251. Berkow RL, Dodson RW. Tyrosine-specific protein phosphorylation during activation of human neutrophils. Blood 1990; 75:2445–52.
252. Nasmith PE, Mills GB, Grinstein S. Guanine nucleotides induce tyrosine phosphorylation and activation of the respiratory burst in neutrophils. Biochem J. 1989; 257:893–7.
253. Berkow RL, Dodson RW, Kraft AS. Human neutrophils contain distinct cytosolic and particulate tyrosine kinase activities: possible role in neutrophil activation. Biochim Biophys Acta 1989; 997:292–300.
254. Gutkind JS, Robbins KC. Translocation of the FGR protein-tyrosine kinase as a consequence of neutrophil activation. Proc Natl Acad Sci USA 1989; 86:8783–7.
255. Perlmutter RM, Marth JD, Ziegler SF, Garvin AM, Pawar S, Cooke MP, Abraham KM. Specialized protein tyrosine kinase proto-oncogenes in hematopoietic cells. Biochim Biophys Acta 1988; 948:245–62.
256. Tonks NK, Charbonneau H, Diltz CD, Fischer EH, Walsh KA. Demonstration that the leukocyte common antigen CD45 is a protein tyrosine phosphatase. Biochemistry 1988; 27:8695–701.
257. Harvath L, Balke JA, Christiansen NP, Russell AA, Skubitz KM. Selected antibodies to leukocyte common antigen (CD45) inhibit human neutrophil chemotaxis. J Immunol 1991; 146:949–57.
258. Nauseef WM, Volpp BD, Clark RA. Immunochemical and electrophoretic analyses of phosphorylated native and recombinant neutrophil oxidase component p47-*phox*. Blood 1990; 76:2622–9.
259. Rotrosen D, Leto TL. Phosphorylation of neutrophil 47-kDa cytosolic oxidase factor. Translocation to membrane is associated with distinct phosphorylation events. J Biol Chem 1990; 265:19910–5.
260. Sha'afi RI, Molski TFP, Gomez-Caronero J, Huang C-K. Dissociation of the 47-kilodalton protein phosphorylation from degranulation and superoxide production in neutrophils. J Leuk Biol 1988; 43:18–27.
261. Badwey JA, Robinson JM, Heyworth PG, Curnutte JT. 1,2-dioctanoyl-*sn*-glycerol can stimulate neutrophils by different mechanisms. Evidence for a pathway that does not involve phosphorylation of the 47-kDa protein. J Biol Chem 1989; 264:20676–82.
262. Garcia RC, Segal AW. Phosphorylation of the subunits of cytochrome b_{-245} upon triggering of the respiratory burst of human neutrophils and macrophages. Biochem J 1988; 252:901–4.
263. Heyworth PG, Shrimpton CF, Segal AW. Localization of the 47 kDa phosphoprotein involved in the respiratory-burst NADPH oxidase of phagocytic cells. Biochem J 1989; 260:243–8.

264. Tamura M, Tamura T, Burnham DN, Uhlinger DJ, Lambeth JD. Stabilization of the superoxide-generating respiratory burst oxidase of human neutrophil plasma membrane by crosslinking with 1-ethyl-3-(3-dimethylaminopropyl) carbodiimide. Arch Biochem Biophys 1989; 275:23–32.
265. Katayama T, Ohtsuka T, Wakamura K, Yoshida K, Okamura N, Ishibashi S. Effect of glutaraldehyde on NADPH oxidase system of guinea pig polymorphonuclear leukocytes. Arch Biochem Biophys 1990; 278:431–6.
266. Strum SL, Hendricks CL, McPhail LC. Cell-free activation of NADPH oxidase: mechanisms regulating translocation of the 47 kDa oxidase component. FASEB J. 1990; 4:A2181.
267. McPhail LC, Strum SL, Ellenburg M, Qualliotine-Mann D, Agwu DE, McCall, Leone PA. Molecular mechanism of activation of leukocyte superoxide production. J Cell Biochem 1991; Suppl 15C:203.
268. Seifert R, Rosenthal W, Schächtele C, Schultz G. Arachidonic acid-induced activation of NADPH oxidase in membranes of human neutrophils and HL-60 leukemic cells is regulated by guanine nucleotide-binding proteins and is independent of Ca^{2+} and protein kinase C. In: Nigam S, McBrein DC, Slater TF, eds. Eicosanoids, lipid peroxidation and cancer. Berlin, Heidelberg: Springer-Verlag, 1988; 169–79.
269. Seifert R, Rosenthal W, Schultz G, Wieland T, Gierschick P, Jakobs KH. The role of nucleoside-diphosphate kinase reactions in G protein activation of NADPH oxidase by guanine and adenine nucleotides. Eur J Biochem 1988; 175:51–5.
270. Ligeti E, Tardif M, Vignais PV. Activation of O_2^- generating oxidase of bovine neutrophils in a cell-free system. Interaction of a cytosolic factor with the plasma membrane and control by G nucleotides. Biochemistry 1989; 28:7116–23.
271. Gabig TG, Eklund EA, Potter GB, Dykes JR II. A neutrophil GTP-binding protein that regulates cellfree NADPH oxidase activation is located in the cytosolic fraction. J Immunol 1990; 145:945–51.
272. Bourne HR, Sanders DA, McCormick. The GTPase superfamily: a conserved switch for diverse cell functions. Nature 1990; 348:125–32.
273. Shpungin S, Dotan I, Abo A, Pick E. Activation of the superoxide forming NADPH oxidase in a cell-free system by sodium dodecyl sulfate. Absolute lipid dependence of the solubilized enzyme. J Biol Chem 1989; 264:9195–203.
274. Nozaki M, Takeshige K, Sumimoto H, Minakami S. Reconstitution of the partially purified membrane component of the superoxide-generating NADPH oxidase of pig neutrophils with phospholipid. Eur J Biochem 1990; 187:335–40.
275. Tamura M, Tamura T, Tyagi SR, Lambeth, JD. The superoxide-generating respiratory burst oxidase of human neutrophil plasma membrane. Phosphatidylserine as an effector of the activated enzyme. J Biol Chem 1988; 263:17621–6.
276. Miyahara M, Watanabe S, Okimasu E, Utsumi K. Charge-dependent regulation of NADPH oxidase activity in guinea-pig polymorphonuclear leukocytes. Biochim Biophys Acta 1987; 929:253–62.
277. Ohtsuka T, Hiura M, Ozawa M, Okamura N, Nakamura M, Ishibashi S. Involvement of membrane charges in constituting the active form of NADPH oxidase in guinea pig polymorphonuclear leukocytes. Arch Biochem Biophys 1990; 280:74–9.
278. Burnham DN, Uhlinger DJ, Lambeth JD. Diradylglycerol synergizes with an anionic amphiphile to activate superoxide generation and phosphorylation of $p47_{phox}$ in a cell-free system from human neutrophils. J Biol Chem 1990; 265:17550–9.
279. McPhail LC, McCall CE, Agwu DE, Qualliotine-Mann D. Synergism with phosphatidic acid and diacylglyercol for cell-free activation of neutrophil NADPH oxidase. J Cell Biol 1991; 115:362a.
280. Burn P. Amphitropic proteins: a new class of membrane proteins. TIBS 1988; 13:79–83.

3

Regulation of Lipoxygenase Enzymes in Leukocytes

JACK Y. VANDERHOEK
The George Washington University School of Medicine and Health Sciences, Washington, D.C.

I. INTRODUCTION

Lipoxygenases are one of the enzyme systems that are activated when leukocytes are stimulated by endogenous agonists or exogenous stimuli. When these enzymes act on polyunsaturated fatty acid substrates such as arachidonic acid, a variety of oxygenated products are generated, including hydroperoxyeicosanoids, leukotrienes, and lipoxins (1,2). These metabolites exhibit a broad range of biological activities such as chemotaxis and smooth muscle contraction and appear to play a significant role in the pathophysiology of immediate hypersensitivity reactions and inflammation.

Many cellular lipoxygenases exist in a cryptic state, and they have to be activated in order to metabolize substrate (3). The stimulation of these enzymes appears to be controlled by a variety of factors. Some of these factors are common to all lipoxygenases, because the general enzymology of lipoxygenase-catalyzed reactions appears to be the same whereas other factors appear to influence one lipoxygenase in a cell but not another. This chapter will first outline and review the role of enzymatic factors that are common to controlling all lipoxygenases. In the second part of the chapter, the regulatory effects of other factors on the leukocytic 5- and 15-lipoxygenases will be emphasized.

II. LIPOXYGENASE-CATALYZED REACTIONS

A. Steric Structures of Lipoxygenase Products

Lipoxygenases catalyze the dioxygenation of polyunsaturated fatty acids which contain a *cis,cis*-1,4-pentadiene system and involves the insertion of one oxygen molecule onto the carbon chain backbone.* Many studies indicate that lipoxygenases exhibit positional specificity in that they remove a specific hydrogen atom from arachidonic acid (all *cis*-5,8,11,14-eicosatetraenoic acid) and stereospecifically insert oxygen at a specific carbon atom (4). Although many polyunsaturated fatty acids have been shown to be substrates for lipoxygenases, we will restrict this discussion to studies utilizing arachidonic acid as substrate and the introduction of one oxygen molecule. The dioxygenation of polyunsaturated fatty acids by lipoxygenases involves two stages (Figure 1). These are as follows.

1. The sterospecific removal of one hydrogen atom from a double allylic methylene carbon atom and the electrophilic addition of Fe(III) to carbon to give an organoiron intermediate which is coordinated to the enzyme. This reaction sequence includes an electron rearrangement which produces a double bond with a trans configuration. As a result of the positional specificity and electron rearrangement, the 5-lipoxygenase removes the pro-S hydrogen from the C_7 atom and produces a Δ^6 trans double bond which is conjugated with the Δ^8 *cis* double bond. Similarly, the 15-lipoxygenase removes the pro-S hydrogen from the C_{13} atom, which leads to the formation of the Δ^{11}-*cis*, Δ^{13}-trans conjugated system. Hydrogen abstraction is the rate-determining step in the dioxygenation reaction (5).
2. The addition of dioxygen by σ bond insertion followed by protolytic cleavage of the Fe-oxygen bond to produce the hydroperoxide product and concomitant regeneration of the enzyme. Insertion of oxygen occurs stereospecifically with the production of a chiral center. Introduction of oxygen onto the C_5 atom produces the 5(S)-peroxy group, and the addition of oxygen at the C_{15} atom yields the 15(S)-peroxy functionality.

This scheme is attractive because it accounts for the well-known stereospecificities and regioselectivities of lipoxygenases. Evidence in support of this mechanism is based on the analysis of (a) the stereochemistry of products formed from arachidonic acid and several substrate analogs and either soybean 15-lipoxygenase or potato 5-lipoxygenase, and (b) the influence of oxygen pressure on both product formation and frequency of self-inactivation of soybean lipoxygenase (6,7). However, there is no direct evidence yet for the proposed organoiron intermediate. An alternative mechanism for lipoxygenase catalysis has also been proposed and involves free radicals and a cycling of the iron between two different oxidation states. This second mechanism suggests that, after binding to the enzyme, substrate fatty acid is oxidized to a pentadienyl radical intermediate with concomitant reduction of lipoxygenase iron from Fe(III) to Fe(II). The free radical then interacts with oxygen to produce a peroxyl radical, which reoxidizes Fe(II) to Fe(III) with the formation of the peroxy anion. Experimental support for this mechanism was recently obtained by analyzing reaction mixtures of soybean lipoxygenase and linoleic acid by EPR and Mossbauer spectroscopy (8,9).

It should be noted that lipoxygenase-catalyzed dioxygenation is antarafacial in that hydrogen removal and dioxygen insertion take place from opposite sides of the *cis,cis*-

*The number of the carbon atom in arachidonic acid which is oxygenated is used to identify lipoxygenases. Thus, the 5- and 15- lipoxygenases (the two major lipoxygenases present in human leukocytes) are enzymes that produce metabolites in which the 5 and 15 carbon atoms (respectively) of arachidonic acid are oxygenated.

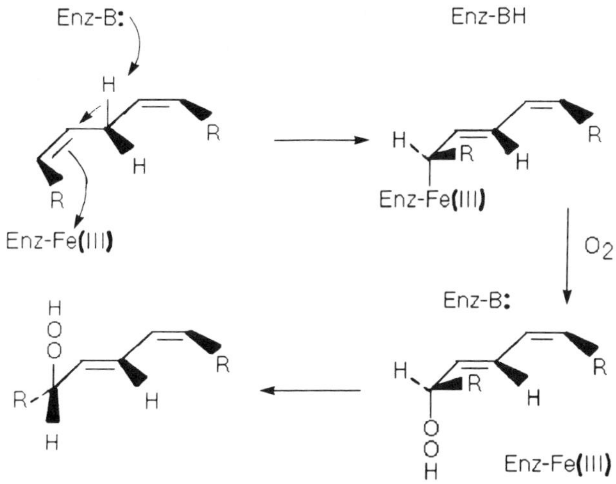

Figure 1 Proposed scheme for the enzymatic lipoxygenation of a *cis,cis*-1,4-pentadiene system.

1,4-pentadiene system that is oxygenated. In addition, observations that these dioxygenation reactions do not always produce metabolites with complete positional specificity or stereospecificity can be explained by a reversible dissociation of intermediates from the lipoxygenase enzyme (10).

B. Kinetics of Lipoxygenase Catalysis

Most of the kinetic studies with lipoxygenases to date have utilized the soybean 15-lipoxygenase and the rabbit reticulocyte 15-lipoxygenase because of the relative ease of obtaining the purified enzymes, and the discussion in this section will be based on the findings with these enzymes.

The kinetic behavior of lipoxygenases exhibits several unusual features (11–13). The early phase of the lipoxygenase-catalyzed dioxygenation reaction is characterized by a lag phase and nonlinear kinetics. This lag phase can be eliminated by addition of lipid hydroperoxide or extended by the addition of glutathione peroxidase. Furthermore, this hydroperoxide must be continuously present during oxygenation of substrate, because peroxide removal by glutathione peroxidase stops the oxygenation process. In other words, this lag phase is overcome by an autoactivation process.

15-Lipoxygenases are nonheme iron-containing enzymes, and iron is essential for enzyme activity (14,15). Treatment of native soybean lipoxygenase Fe(II) with product hydroperoxide produces the catalytically active Fe(III)-containing species (16,17). This shift in iron valence state can explain the requirement for hydroperoxide activator.

Smith and Lands reported that the soybean lipoxygenase became irreversibly inactivated during the oxygenation of substrate in a time-dependent manner (11). The kinetics of self-inactivation was first order with respect to enzyme concentration, and this self-limiting feature was not due to a lack of substrate or to product inhibition but was a result of the "suicide substrate" nature of the fatty acid substrate. It appears that a distinct methionine residue is monooxygenated during inactivation of the reticulocyte 15-

lipoxygenase, which would explain the fatty acid hydroperoxide requirement for the inactivation process (18). However, other inactivation mechanisms are probably also operating. Polyunsaturated fatty acids differ in their ability to catalyze this self-inactivation, and this observation could represent an unusual type of metabolic control of lipoxygenases (11). Since many studies indicate that a variety of these fatty acids are released as a result of the action of acylhydrolases on cellular lipids (19), it is quite possible that the fatty acid content of cellular lipids can ultimately affect the amount of product formed by lipoxygenases.

Other features common to all lipoxygenases include observations that enzyme activities depend on the concentration of oxygen, the second substrate, that high concentrations of substrate inhibit the reaction, and that the presence of product induces a progressive loss of enzyme activity (11–13).

A kinetic model for the lipoxygenase-catalyzed aerobic dioxygenation of polyunsaturated fatty acids that fits all these experimental observations is shown in Figure 2 (12,13,20). The lag phase indicates that the enzyme has to be autoactivated by fatty acid hydroperoxide P. Furthermore, it is assumed that lipoxygenases exist in differing

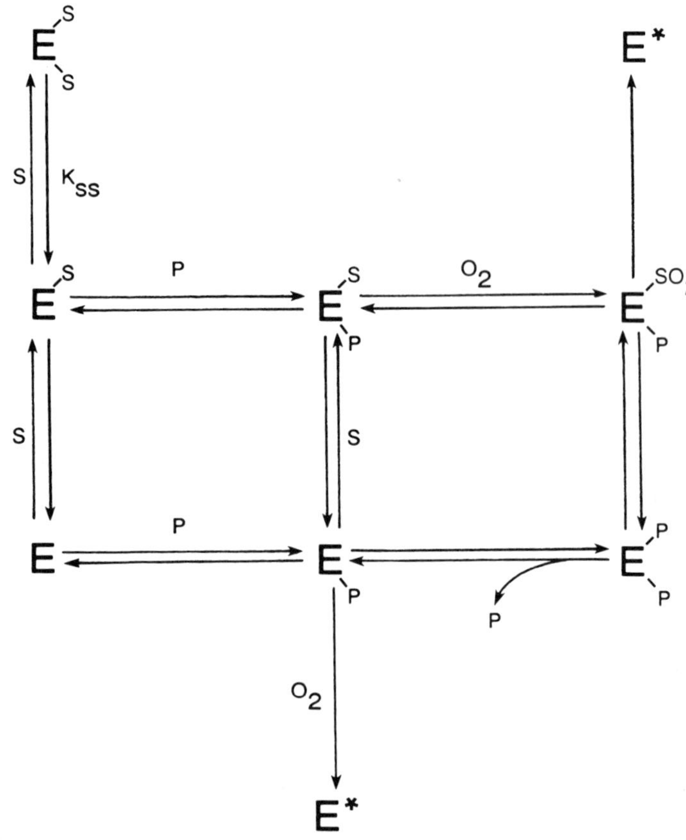

Figure 2 A kinetic model for the lipoxygenase-catalyzed dioxygenation of the *cis,cis*-1,4-pentadiene system in polyunsaturated fatty acids. E, lipoxygenase; S, substrate; P, product; E*, inactive enzyme.

redox states, a native state (E) and an activated form (EP) which is produced by the putative action of product P. Both fatty acid substrate S and product P are competitive inhibitors of the enzyme and appear to have different binding sites. In addition, it is proposed that the inhibitory effect of high concentrations of substrate is the result of the formation of an ESS complex which competes with EPS production. Once EPS is formed, hydrogen abstraction, electron rearrangement, and oxygen addition yields $EPSO_2$ which is then transformed to EPP. Lowering the concentration of oxygen increases the extent of substrate inhibition (increased $EPSO_2$ dissociation), which is accompanied by decreased regio- and stereospecificities of the dioxygenation reaction.

III. THE LEUKOCYTE 5-LIPOXYGENASE

The 5-lipoxygenase, which converts arachidonic acid to 5(S)-hydroperoxy-eicosatetraenoic acid (5-HPETE), is the seminal enzyme in the conversion of arachidonic acid to the biologically active leukotrienes (1). The human leukocyte enzyme is a cytosolic protein with a molecular weight of 80,000 Da, whereas the 5-lipoxygenases isolated from other cells appear to be somewhat smaller (73,000-76,000 Da) (21–23). The enzyme has a pH optimum of 7.5–8.0; its K_m for arachidonic acid is 12.2 $\pm$4.5 μM with a V_{max} = 2.8 $\pm$0.9 nmol/min/mg protein (24). Observations that the mechanism of purified 5-lipoxygenase action was in agreement with the general lipoxygenase mechanism included a lag phase, product inhibition, self-inactivation during the course of the dioxygenation reaction (25), and the requirement for fatty acid hydroperoxides. The latter was noted when the 5-lipoxygenase purification procedures were carried out in the presence of sulfhydryl reagents (26). Presumably these sulfhydryl reagents either could stimulate peroxidases to remove endogenous hydroperoxides necessary for 5-lipoxygenase activity or could reduce the nonheme iron of the 5-lipoxygenase to the inactive form and thus exogenous fatty acid hydroperoxides had to be added to overcome either or both of these effects.

Various studies have shown that the pure enzyme is strongly dependent on calcium, which appears to be tightly bound to the enzyme since 5-lipoxygenase activity was not affected by the presence of EDTA (27,28). The half-maximal response was observed at calcium concentrations of 30–50 μM (24,28), and a kinetic analysis with purified guinea pig 5-lipoxygenase indicated that calcium activated the enzyme by (a) decreasing the lag phase from 1–3 min (without calcium) to 10–20 s, (b) increasing the V_{max} from 4.2 $\pm$0.4 (without calcium) to 24 $\pm$2 nmol 5-HETE formed/min/mg protein, (c) decreasing the K_m from 25 $\pm$4 (without calcium) to 7.7 $\pm$1.7 μM, (d) increasing the extent of product formation, and (e) changing the mechanism to one involving substrate inhibition (K_{SS} = 13 $\pm$1μM), where the substrate increasingly binds to a regulatory site rather than the catalytic site (28).

It had previously been observed that the 5-lipoxygenase was stimulated by several nucleotides, most strongly by ATP (29). In the presence of saturating concentrations of calcium, ATP (half-maximal response was observed at 31 $\pm$7 μM) reduced the lag phase to less than 5 s, increased both the V_{max} (to 30 $\pm$4 nmol 5-HETE formed/min/mg protein) as well as the extent of product formation, but did not affect either the K_m or the K_{SS}, indicating that ATP did not influence the enzyme's affinity for arachidonic acid (28). Since neither arachidonic acid methyl ester nor arachidonol was a substrate for the 5-lipoxygenase, Aharony and Stein suggested that calcium interacts with the free carboxyl group of arachidonic acid to produce a form of substrate that is easily bound to and used by the 5-lipoxygenase, although the induction of a more catalytically active conformation of the protein could not be ruled out. No amino acid sequence in the 5-lipoxygenase has yet been identified that corresponds to known binding regions for either calcium or ATP (30).

In trying to purify the human leukocyte 5-lipoxygenase, Rouzer and co-workers reported that three other cellular factors were important to the cellular activity of the enzyme (31). In the presence of calcium and ATP, these factors were able to maximally stimulate the cytosolic 5-lipoxygenase present in the 100,000 × g supernatant. The three factors consisted of a microsomal membrane factor found in the 100,000 × g pellet and two high-molecular-weight cytosolic factors: (a) a pass-through fraction obtained after mono-Q chromatography (MQ-PTF) and (b) an activity isolated from the resuspension of the precipitate obtained when the 30–60% ammonium sulfate supernatant was saturated to 90% ammonium sulfate. The interaction of these factors with the 5-lipoxygenase was strongly influenced by calcium. Both the MQ-PTF factor and the cytosolic 5-lipoxygenase become associated with the microsomal membrane fraction in a calcium-dependent manner (32,33). Once formed, the 5-lipoxygenase-membrane complex appears to be used preferentially for leukotriene synthesis prior to suicide inactivation. Recently, an 18,000-MW membrane protein (FLAP) was isolated and characterized which was essential for complete leukotriene synthesis (34). It is possible that the MQ-PTF factor is involved in the translocation of the 5-lipoxygenase to the membrane, and that FLAP is the membrane target to which the 5-lipoxygenase binds once it arrives from the cytosol (34).

Phosphatidylcholine vesicles (but not other phospholipids) or isolated human neutrophil plasma membranes were as effective as the 100,000 × g pellet fraction in stimulating the human leukocyte 5-lipoxygenase (35). These stimulatory effects were calcium dependent, and possible explanations for these observations are that phosphatidylcholine has a direct stimulatory effect on the enzyme, or calcium enhances the binding of the 5-lipoxygenase to phosphatidylcholine-rich regions in membranes, which results in the stimulation of the enzyme; or phosphatidylcholine vesicles enhance the solubility of the enzyme, thereby making it more accessible to a calcium-substrate complex (35,36).

So far this chapter has reviewed the effects of various factors that stimulate the 5-lipoxygenase when the enzyme is either in a purified state or when it is present in a cytosolic milieu. It appears that in intact leukocytes additional mechanisms may be involved in the activation of the 5-lipoxygenase. A recent study indicates that pertussis toxin interferes with the arachidonic acid-induced activation of the 5-lipoxygenase in intact human leukocytes, which suggests that guanine nucleotide-binding proteins are also involved in the activation of this enzyme (37). When intact leukocytes were treated with agents that decrease cellular glutathione levels, increased cellular 5-lipoxygenase activity was observed (38). The most likely explanation for this observation was that these agents inhibited glutathione peroxidases, thereby making more peroxides available for lipoxygenase activation. Enhancement of peroxide tone could also explain the stimulatory effect of 12-HPETE on the 5-lipoxygenase present in human leukocytes (39).

Although the emphasis of this chapter is primarily on reviewing the stimulatory effects of various cellular factors on the leukocyte 5-lipoxygenase, it should also be noted that certain cellular metabolites or conditions can regulate the 5-lipoxygenase by turning it off. For example, both 15-HPETE and its reduced hydroxy analog 15-HETE, products of the 15-lipoxygenase pathway, inhibited the leukocyte 5-lipoxygenase (40). This report was the first indication of a regulatory interrelationship between a product of the 15-lipoxygenase pathway and the 5-lipoxygenase. In addition, treatment of cell homogenates with agents that decrease glutathione levels inhibited 5-lipoxygenase activity, presumably by interacting with essential SH groups on the enzyme (38). Other examples have recently been reviewed (41).

IV. THE LEUKOCYTE 15-LIPOXYGENASE

The leukocyte 15-lipoxygenase dioxygenates arachidonic acid to 15(S)-HPETE, which is either reduced to 15-HETE or is further metabolized to the lipoxins (2). The pure human leukocyte 15-lipoxygenase appears to be a cytosolic, cationic (at pH 7) protein which was less hydrophobic than the 5-lipoxygenase. The protein had an apparent MW of 70,000 and a pH optimum in the range of 7–8.5 (42). It presumably is a nonheme iron protein, and a histidine-rich region has been identified that may be involved in the binding of iron (43). The enzyme exhibited a K_m for arachidonic acid of 63–68 μM and a V_{max} of 5.3–8.6 nmol/min/mg protein (24,42).

The effect of calcium on the 15-lipoxygenase appears to be somewhat paradoxical. The activity of the pure enzyme was unchanged in the absence or presence of calcium (44,45). However, when the 15-lipoxygenase was in a cytosolic milieu, the enzyme activity increased progressively when the calcium concentration was increased from 0.1 nM to 50 μM but decreased at higher calcium concentrations (46). Others also have observed a calcium dependence in crude enzyme preparations (24,45). It is possible that nM-μM concentrations of calcium stabilize the protein or enhance the interaction with a calcium-dependent cofactor (46).

The effects of several cellular factors or conditions on the leukocyte 15-lipoxygenase contrasted directly with their effects on the 5-lipoxygenase. Thus, ATP inhibited the 15-lipoxygenase, whereas agents that interact with sulfhydryl groups were reported to stimulate the 15-lipoxygenase activity in leukocyte homogenates (38,42). We recently observed that phosphatidylserine and phosphatidylcholine inhibited the cytosolic 15-lipoxygenase (46). These observations contrasted with a report that phosphatidylcholine stimulated the partially purified eosinophilic 15-lipoxygenase (42), and it is possible that differences in calcium levels and/or cytosolic factors can account for these discrepancies. These results suggest that certain cellular conditions can differentially regulate these enzymes.

The effects of various agents on the 15-lipoxygenase activity in intact leukocytes have also been investigated. Another indication of reciprocal regulatory interrelationships between the 5- and 15-lipoxygenases was our observation that 5-hydroxyeicosanoids can selectively stimulate the 15-lipoxygenase (relative to the 5-lipoxygenase) in unstimulated leukocytes (47). 12-HETE and 15-HETE were much less effective activators of the 15-lipoxygenase. Interestingly, the differences in stimulatory potencies of the monoHETE isomers disappeared when activated leukocytes were used (48). Treatment of intact leukocytes with agents that reduce glutathione levels resulted in a doubling of the 15-lipoxygenase activity. These cellular conditions probably lead to increased peroxide tone, which can stimulate the enzyme (38).

V. CONCLUSION

Many studies indicate that the 5- and 15-lipoxygenases in unstimulated leukocytes exist in an inactive or cryptic state. Before these enzymes can metabolize substrate fatty acids, they have to be activated. During inflammation and other pathophysiological conditions, resting leukocytes are stimulated. Since cell activation is accompanied by a variety of changes, it is now clear that some of these changes are essential to the formation of active lipoxygenases. This chapter has reviewed some of the cellular factors and conditions that are believed to be involved in the conversion of these cryptic lipoxygenases to active species.

REFERENCES

1. Samuelsson B. Leukotrienes: mediators of immediate hypersensitivity reactions. Science 1983; 220: 568–75.
2. Serhan CN, Samuelsson B. Lipoxins: a new series of eicosanoids. Adv Exp Med Biol 1988; 229:1–14.
3. Vanderhoek JY, Bailey JM. Postphospholipase activation of lipoxygenase/leukotriene systems. In: Bailey JM, ed. Prostaglandins, leukotrienes, and lipoxins. New York: Plenum Press 1985; 133–46.
4. Kuhn H, Schewe T, Rapoport SM. The stereochemistry of the reactions of lipoxygenases and their metabolites. Proposed nomenclature of lipoxygenases and related enzymes. Adv Enzymol 1986; 58:273–311.
5. Egmond MR, Veldink GA, Vliegenthart JFG, Boldingh J. C-11 H-Abstraction from linoleic acid, the rate-limiting step in lipoxygenase catalysis. Biochem Biophys Res Commun 1973; 54:1178–84.
6. Corey EJ, Nagata R. Evidence in favor of an organoiron-mediated pathway for lipoxygenation of fatty acids by soybean lipoxygenase. J Am Chem Soc 1987; 109:8107–8.
7. Corey EJ, Wright SW, Matsuda SPT. Stereochemistry and mechanism of the biosynthesis of leukotriene A_4 from 5(S)hydroperoxy-6(E), 8,11,14(Z)-eicosatetraenoic acid. Evidence for an organoiron intermediate. J Am Chem Soc 1989; 111:1452–5.
8. Funk MO, Carroll RT, Thompson JF, Sands RH, Dunham WR. Role of iron in lipoxygenase catalysis. J Am Chem Soc 1990; 112:5375–6.
9. Nelson MJ, Seitz SP, Cowling RA. Enzyme-bound pentadienyl and peroxyl radicals in purple lipoxygenase. Biochemistry 1990; 29:6897–903.
10. Funk MO, Andre JC, Otsuki T. Oxygenation of trans polyunsaturated fatty acids by lipoxygenase reveals steric features of the catalytic mechanism. Biochemistry 1987; 26:6880–4.
11. Smith WL, Lands WEM. Oxygenation of unsaturated fatty acids by soybean lipoxygenase. J Biol Chem 1972; 247:1038–47.
12. Cook HW, Lands WEM. Further studies of the kinetics of oxygenation of arachidonic acid by soybean lipoxygenase. Can J Biochem 1975; 53:1220–31.
13. Ludwig P, Holzhutter HG, Colosimo A, Silvestrini MC, Schewe T, Rapoport SM. A kinetic model for lipoxygenases based on experimental data with the lipoxygenase of reticulocytes. Eur J Biochem 1987; 168:325–37.
14. Pistorius EK, Axelrod B. Iron, an essential component of lipoxygenase. J Biol Chem 1974; 249:3183–6.
15. Veldink GA, Vliegenthart JFG. Lipoxygenases, non heme iron-containing enzymes. Adv Inorg Chem 1984; 6:139–61.
16. Slappendel S, Malmstrom BG, Petersson L, Ehrenberg A, Veldink GA, Vliegenthart JFG. On the spin and valence state of iron in native soybean lipoxygenase-1. Biochem Biophys Res Commun 1982; 108:673–7.

17. Cheesbrough TM, Axelrod B. Determination of the spin state of iron in native and activated soybean lipoxygenase-1 by paramagnetic susceptibility. Biochemistry 1983; 22:3837–40.
18. Rapoport S, Hartel B, Hausdorf G. Methionine sulfoxide formation: the cause of self-inactivation of reticulocyte lipoxygenase. Eur J Biochem 1984; 139:573–6.
19. Van den Bosch H. Intracellular phospholipases A. Biochim Biophys Acta 1980; 604:191–246.
20. Lands WEM. Biological consequences of fatty acid oxygenase reaction mechanisms. Prostaglandins, Leukotrienes and Medicine 1984; 13:35-46.
21. Rouzer CA, Samuelsson B. On the nature of the 5-lipoxygenase reaction in human leukocytes: enzyme purification and requirement for multiple stimulatory factors. Proc Natl Acad Sci USA 1985; 82:6040–4.
22. Goetze AM, Fayer L, Bouska J, Bornemeier D, Carter GW. Purification of a mammalian 5-lipoxygenase from rat basophilic leukemia cells. Prostaglandins 1985; 29:689–701.
23. Hogaboom GK, Cook M, Newton JF, Varrichio A, Shorr GL, Sarau HM, Crooke ST. Purification, characterization, and structural properties of a single protein from rat basophilic leukemia (RBL-1) cells possessing 5-lipoxygenase and leukotriene A_4 synthetase activities. Mol Pharm 1986; 30:510–9.
24. Soberman RJ, Harper TW, Betteridge D, Lewis RA, Austen KF. Characterization and separation of the arachidonic acid 5-lipoxygenase and linoleic acid ω-6 lipoxygenase (arachidonic acid 15-lipoxygenase) of human polymorphonuclear leukocytes. J Biol Chem 1985; 260:4508–15.
25. Ueda N, Kaneko S, Yoshimoto T, Yamamoto S. Purification of arachidonate 5-lipoxygenase from porcine leukocytes and its reactivity with hydroperoxyeicosatetraenoic Acids. J Biol Chem 1986; 261:7982–8.
26. Rouzer CA, Samuelsson B. The importance of hydroperoxide activation for the detection and assay of mammalian 5-lipoxygenase. FEBS Lett 1986; 204:293–6.
27. Jakschik BA, Sun FF, Lee L-H, Steinhoff MM. Calcium stimulation of a novel lipoxygenase. Biochem Biophys Res Commun 1980; 95:103–10.
28. Aharony D, Stein RL. Kinetic mechanism of guinea pig neutrophil 5-lipoxygenase. J Biol Chem 1986; 261:11512–9.
29. Ochi K, Yoshimoto T, Yamamoto S, Taniguchi K, Miyamoto T. Arachidonate 5-lipoxygenase of guinea pig peritoneal polymorphonuclear leukocytes. J Biol Chem 1983; 258:5754–8.
30. Dixon RAF, Jones RE, Diehl RE, Bennett CD, Kargman S, Rouzer CA. Cloning of the cDNA for human 5-lipoxygenase. Proc Natl Acad Sci USA 1988; 85:416–20.
31. Rouzer CA, Shimizu T, Samuelsson B. On the nature of the 5-lipoxygenase reaction in human leukocytes: characterization of a membrane-associated stimulatory factor. Proc Natl Acad Sci USA 1985; 82:7505–9.
32. Rouzer CA, Samuelsson B. Reversible, calcium-dependent membrane association of human leukocyte 5-lipoxygenase. Proc Natl Acad Sci USA 1987; 84:7393–7.
33. Rouzer CA, Kargman S. Translocation of 5-lipoxygenase to the membrane in human leukocytes challenged with ionophore A23187. J Biol Chem 1988; 263:10980–8.
34. Miller DK, Gillard JW, Vickers PJ, Sadowski S, Leveille C, Mancini JA, Charleson P, Dixon RAF, Ford-Hutchinson, AW, Fortin R, Gauthier JY, Rodkey J, Rosen R, Rouzer C, Sigal IS, Strader CD, Evans JF. Identification and isolation of a membrane protein necessary for leukotriene production. Nature 1990; 343:278–81.
35. Puustinen T, Scheffer MM, Samuelsson B. Regulation of the human leukocyte 5-lipoxygenase: stimulation by micromolar Ca^{2+} levels and phosphatidylcholine vesicles. Biochem Biophys Acta 1987; 960:261–7.
36. Wong A, Hwang SM, Cook MN, Hogaboom K, Crooke ST. Interactions of 5-lipoxygenase with membranes: studies on the association of soluble enzyme with membranes and alterations in enzyme activity. Biochemistry 1988; 27:6763–9.

37. McColl SR, Krump E, Naccache PH, Caon AC, Borgeat P. Activation of the human neutrophil 5-lipoxygenase by exogenous arachidonic acid: involvement of pertussis toxin-sensitive guanine nucleotide-binding proteins. Br J Pharmacol 1989; 97:1265–73.
38. Hatzelmann A, Ullrich V. Regulation of 5-lipoxygenase activity by the glutathione status in human polymorphonuclear leukocytes. Eur J Biochem 1987; 169:175–84.
39. Maclouf J, Fructeau deLaclos B, Borgeat P. Stimulation of leukotriene biosynthesis in human blood leukocytes by platelet-derived 12-hydroperoxy-icosatetraenoic acid. Proc Natl Acad Sci USA 1982; 79:6042–6.
40. Vanderhoek JY, Bryant RW, Bailey JM. Inhibition of leukotriene biosynthesis by the leukocyte product 15-hydroxy-5,8,11,13-eicosatetraenoic acid. J Biol Chem 1980; 255:10064–6.
41. Lagarde M, Gualde N, Rigaud M. Metabolic interactions between eicosanoids in blood and vascular cells. Biochem J 1989; 257:313–20.
42. Sigal E, Grunberger D, Cashman JR, Craik CS, Caughey GH, Nadel JA. Arachidonate 15-lipoxygenase from human eosinophil-enriched leukocytes: partial purification and properties. Biochem Biophys Res Commun 1988; 150:376–83.
43. Sigal E, Craik CS, Highland E, Grunberger D, Costello LL, Dixon RAF, Nadel JA. Molecular cloning and primary structure of human 15-lipoxygenase. Biochem Biophys Res Commun 1988; 157:457–64.
44. Narumiya S, Salmon JA, Cottee FH, Weatherley BC, Flower RJ. Arachidonic acid 15-lipoxygenase from rabbit peritoneal polymorphonuclear leukocytes. J Biol Chem 1981; 256:9583–92.
45. Sigal E, Grunberger D, Craik CS, Caughey GH, Nadel JA. Arachidonate 15-lipoxygenase (w-6 lipoxygenase) from human leukocytes. J Biol Chem 1988; 263:5328–32.
46. Nichols RC, Vanderhoek JY. Calcium Regulation of the Human PMN Cytosolic 15-Lipoxygenase. Biochim. Biophys. Acta 1991; 1085:77–81.
47. Nichols RC, Vanderhoek JY. 5-Hydroxyeicosanoids selectively stimulate the human neutrophil 15-lipoxygenase to use endogenous substrate. J Exp Med 1990; 171:367–75.
48. Vanderhoek JY, Wilhelmi LL, Ekborg SL, Karmin MT. Stimulation of the 15-lipoxygenase in activated polymorphonuclear neutrophils. Eicosanoids 1990; 3:181–5.

4

Activation of Leukotriene Production in Granulocytes: Effects on Cell Activation

ANTHONY W. FORD-HUTCHINSON
Merck Frosst Centre for Therapeutic Research, Pointe Claire-Dorval, Quebec, Canada

I. INTRODUCTION

Arachidonic acid, a C_{20} polyunsaturated fatty acid, is extensively incorporated in cell membranes at the *sn*-2 position of membrane phospholipids. In the resting state the concentration of free arachidonic acid in the cell is low, well below the K_m for metabolic enzymes such as 5-lipoxygenase. A variety of pathological and physiological stimuli are known to cause cell activation, a rise in intracellular calcium and the release of free arachidonic acid through the action of either a Ca^{2+}-dependent phospholipase A_2 or a phosphatidylinositol-specific phospholipase C and diacyl/monoacylglycerol lipases. In cells containing 5-lipoxygenase, such as the polymorphonuclear leukocyte, the basophil and the eosinophil, the elevation in intracellular calcium also results in the activation of 5-lipoxygenase and the generation of 5-lipoxygenase products—namely, the leukotrienes (see Figure 1 for pathway). Polymorphonuclear leukocytes can convert the key intermediate, leukotriene A_4, to leukotriene B_4, a potent stimulator of leukocyte function. On the other hand, eosinophils convert leukotriene A_4 to the peptidolipid conjugate, leukotriene C_4, which in turn can be rapidly metabolized to leukotrienes D_4 and E_4. The peptidolipid leukotrienes are potent smooth muscle contracting agents which are thought to be important mediators of human bronchial asthma. Thus, following activation, granulocytes produce 5-lipoxygenase metabolites, and one of the products, leukotriene B_4, in turn induces granulocyte activation.

II. PRODUCTION OF LEUKOTRIENES

A. 5-Lipoxygenase

The first step in the formation of leukotrienes involves the conversion of arachidonic acid to 5S,6S-oxido-7,9,11,14-(E,E,Z,Z)-eicosatetraenoic acid (leukotriene A_4) via 5S-hydroperoxy-6,8,11,14-(E,E,Z,Z)-eicosatetraenoic acid (5-HPETE). The addition of

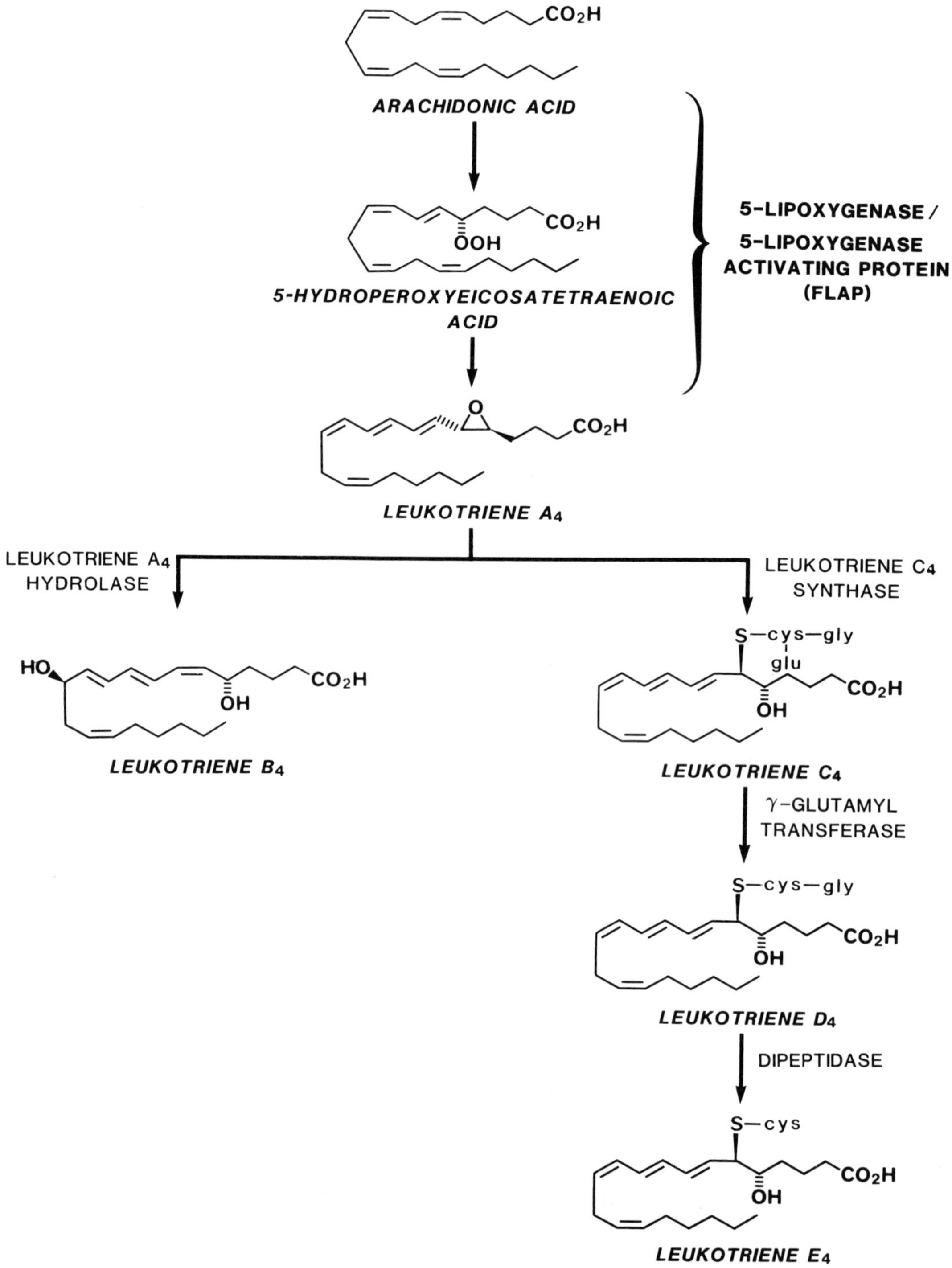

Figure 1 Pathways of arachidonic acid metabolism to leukotrienes.

molecular oxygen leads to the formation of a 1–4-*cis,cis*-pentadiene moiety which is converted to a 1-hydroperoxy-2,4-*trans,cis* pentadiene unit through the removal of the pro-S-hydrogen from C_7 of arachidonic acid. The same enzyme then catalyzes a dehydration step involving stereospecific removal of a pro-R-hydrogen from position C_{10} (1,2).

5-Lipoxygenase has been characterized in a number of granulocyte populations, including human (3), porcine (4), rat (5), and guinea-pig polymorphonuclear leukocytes (6), and rat basophil leukemia (RBL-1) cells (7). All these preparations show certain characteristic properties. These include a requirement for Ca^{2+}; involvement of ATP and other nucleotides in activation of the enzyme; activation by hydroperoxides; characteristic lag phase and self-catalyzed inactivation (8–10). The human enzyme has been purified to homogeneity (8–10) and is a highly unstable 78-kDa protein which catalyzes the conversion of arachidonic acid to both 5-HPETE and leukotriene A_4. The human enzyme, in addition to requiring Ca^{2+} and ATP, also requires other undefined protein and membrane factors for optimal activity in a cell-free system (8–10). The gene for the human enzyme has recently been cloned (11) and expressed in an osteosarcoma cell line (12), the expressed enzyme having all the characteristics of the original purified enzyme from human leukocytes.

B. 5-Lipoxygenase Activating Protein (FLAP)

As outlined above, the activity of 5-lipoxygenase is highly dependent on a number of factors, including calcium, phosphatidylcholine vesicles, and undefined protein and membrane fractions (8–10). The fact that leukotriene synthesis occurs only in intact cells following exposure to defined stimuli which cause a considerable elevation in intracellular Ca^{2+} is consistent with the suggestion that there is a regulatory process for activation of 5-lipoxygenase. A number of observations have indicated a potential role for membranes in such an activation process. First, the enzyme is stimulated by either membrane fractions or phosphatidylcholine vesicles. Second, the substrate arachidonic acid is derived from membrane phospholipids through the action of a specific phospholipase A_2. Third, there are sequence homologies on 5-lipoxygenase with the interfacial binding domains of lipases which are suggestive of membrane interactions (11).

Direct evidence that, following activation of human polymorphonuclear leukocytes with ionophore A23187, 5-lipoxygenase undergoes an activation step has been obtained in experiments reported by Rouzer and Kargman (13). They showed a correlation between the loss of 5-lipoxygenase activity from the supernatant, loss of 5-lipoxygenase protein from the cytosol, and appearance of an active 5-lipoxygenase protein in the $100{,}000 \times g$ membrane, consistent with the hypothesis that enzyme activation involves translocation to the membrane where the enzyme becomes activated, synthesizes leukotrienes, and undergoes suicide inactivation. Other evidence supporting this hypothesis was the fact that cytosolic 5-lipoxygenase retained its activity, suggesting that this enzyme pool was not used for leukotriene synthesis, and the fact that varying the ionophore concentration resulted in varying amounts of leukotriene synthesis which could be correlated with varying amounts of enzyme translocation. Finally, terminating leukotriene synthesis during ongoing cell activation by addition of excess EDTA resulted in termination of enzyme translocation.

Further elucidation of the mechanism of 5-lipoxygenase activation has come from studies on the leukotriene biosynthesis inhibitor MK-886 (L-663,536; 3-[1-(4-chlorobenzyl)-3-*t*-butyl-thiol-5-isopropylindole-2-yl]-2,2-dimethyl propanoic acid) (14). This compound is a potent inhibitor of leukotriene biosynthesis in a variety of intact leukocyte preparations and is highly selective for the 5-lipoxygenase pathway, having no effect on either cyclooxygenase or 15- or 12-lipoxygenase (14). These potent in-vitro effects on leukotriene biosynthesis are also observed in vivo, both biochemically—through inhibition of leukotriene levels in inflammatory exudates and rat bile—and functionally—through inhibition of antigen-induced bronchoconstriction in the rat and the squirrel monkey (14). However, when this compound was studied in either broken cell preparations or purified enzyme preparations, no inhibition of 5-lipoxygenase was observed. In addition, compounds such as MK-886 inhibit leukotriene synthesis in neutrophils but do not inhibit arachidonic acid release, implying that they have no effect on phospholipases (Ham and Soderman, unpublished results).

A clue to the mechanism of action of MK-886 came from studies in intact human polymorphonuclear leukocytes in which the compound caused a concentration-dependent inhibition of the translocation of 5-lipoxygenase to the membrane which could be correlated with inhibition of leukotriene biosynthesis (15). Using a range of structural analogs of MK-886, it was possible to inhibit the membrane translocation of 5-lipoxygenase in a rank order of potency that correlated with the potencies of the compounds as inhibitors of leukotriene biosynthesis. It could be argued that translocation is not connected with cell activation but simply reflects deposition of inactive enzyme after leukotriene biosynthesis. However, evidence against this was obtained in experiments in which addition of MK-886, after cellular activation with ionophore A23187, and thus after enzyme translocation has occurred, resulted in the release back into the cytosol of inactivated, translocated enzyme. Experiments attempting to demonstrate the effects of MK-886 on the association of 5-lipoxygenase with membrane and cell-free preparations failed due to a nonspecific Ca^{2+}-dependent sedimentation of the enzyme.

The fact that 5-lipoxygenase underwent a translocation to the membrane following cellular activation suggested that the membrane may contain a "docking" protein or 5-lipoxygenase-activating protein (FLAP) which would be the target binding site for drugs such as MK-886. In order to investigate this further, a number of experimental approaches were carried out.

The first of these involved the preparation of an analog of MK-886 labeled with ^{125}I and containing a photoactivatable azido group (^{125}I-L-669,083) (16). Incubation of this photoaffinity probe with neutrophils, followed by irradiation with ultraviolet light, resulted in the labeling of a number of proteins. However, the labeling was specifically inhibited by MK-886 only in the case of a single membrane protein of molecular weight 18 kDa. This protein was present only in the membrane (100,000 $\times$ g pellet) of leukocytes and was not present in a variety of other cell lines known not to have 5-lipoxygenase.

The second step was to isolate this protein by passing solubilized extracts of neutrophil membranes over affinity columns prepared from analogs of MK-886 (16). Using this technique, an 18-kDa protein was found in both rat and human neutrophils which could be selectively eluted from the column by MK-886, this protein co-migrating with the photoaffinity-labeled protein. The rat protein was then purified to homogeneity by chromatography on Superose 12 and TSK-3000 columns, and sequence information from the native protein, cyanogen bromide cleavage, and tryptic cleavage products was obtained. Immunoprecipitation experiments using a polyclonal rabbit antibody to the N-terminal sequence of the rat 18-kDa protein demonstrated that the protein identified by the photoaffinity probe was the same as that purified by the affinity column.

Using the partial amino acid sequence of purified rat FLAP, cDNA clones were isolated from both rat RBL-1 and human HL60 cell-line cDNA libraries (17). Both cDNA clones encoded proteins of 161 amino acids which were 92% identical and contained all the peptide sequence derived from the purified rat protein (16). Hydropathy plots have indicated that the proteins are very hydrophobic, consistent with their membrane localization and three hydrophobic transmembrane spanning regions were predicted by hydrophobic moment analysis. Thus, the proposed structure of the protein consists of three transmembrane domains connected by two hydrophilic loops with the N and C termini on opposite sides of the membrane (see Figure 2).

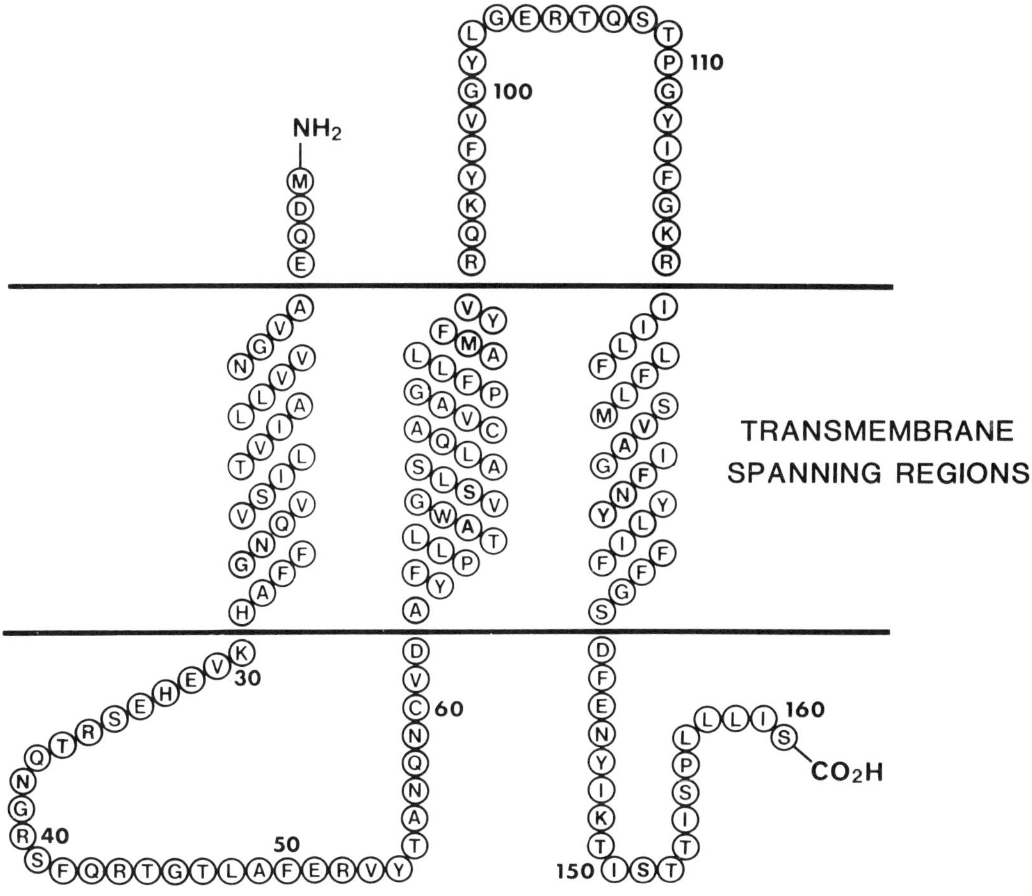

Figure 2 Proposed structure of human 5-lipoxygenase activating protein (FLAP).

Comparison of the sequences of other proteins with those of FLAP revealed that this protein is not identical to any other known protein but does show some similarities to several integral membrane proteins. These similarities are with hydrophobic residues in the putative transmembrane regions rather than significant primary sequence identity.

In order to determine whether FLAP is required for cellular leukotriene synthesis, human osteosarcoma cells were transfected with either 5-LO or FLAP alone or co-transfected with 5-lipoxygenase and FLAP (17). When cells containing either 5-LO or FLAP alone were treated with ionophore A23187, no arachidonic acid metabolites were detected. In contrast, treatment of lines co-expressing both 5-lipoxygenase and FLAP with ionophore A23187 resulted in the release of significant quantities of 5-lipoxygenase products, the production of which could be inhibited by MK-886.

The above experiments clearly demonstrate that the expression of FLAP together with 5-lipoxygenase is essential for cellular leukotriene biosynthesis (17). The binding of MK-886 to FLAP thus explains the mechanisms of inhibition of leukotriene biosynthesis by this compound. The current hypothesis is shown in Figure 3. Activation of 5-lipoxygenase, by elevation of intracellular calcium following receptor activation, causes the enzyme to translocate to the membrane and attach to the "docking" protein, FLAP. In this model, a stable complex would be required to form at the membrane between activated 5-lipoxygenase and FLAP as well as possibly other components of the leukotriene synthetic pathway, such as phospholipase A_2. The formation of this complex

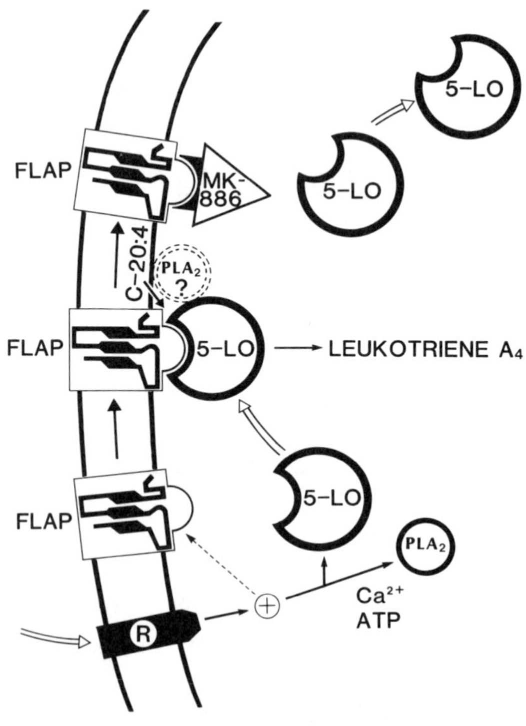

Figure 3 Hypothetical scheme for the involvement of 5-lipoxygenase (5LO), 5-lipoxygenase activating protein (FLAP), and phospholipase $A_2(PLA_2)$ in cellular leukotriene biosynthesis and its inhibition by MK-886.

could regulate the interaction of 5-lipoxygenase with its substrate, arachidonic acid, and the attachment of MK-886 to FLAP could prevent this association. This proposed mechanism is of interest because other enzymes such as protein kinase C (18) and phospholipase C (19) undergo membrane translocation from the cytosol to the membrane following cellular activation. Thus, protein interactions of this type could represent a general mechanism for regulating enzymes that act on membrane-associated substrates, and such membrane proteins could serve as novel therapeutic targets, as is the case with MK-886.

C. Leukotriene A_4 Hydrolase

Cells such as polymorphonuclear leukocytes contain the enzyme leukotriene A_4 hydrolase, which catalyzes the enzymatic hydrolysis of leukotriene A_4 to the biologically active dihydroxy fatty acid, leukotriene B_4 (5S,12R-dihydroxy-6,8,10,14(Z,E,E,Z) eicosatetraenoic acid). Leukotriene A_4 hydrolase has been purified from a number of sources, including human (20) and rat polymorphonuclear leukocytes (21). The enzyme is quite distinct from human liver epoxide hydrolase. Thus, substrate specificity is entirely different, as is the quaternary structure and molecular size, the molecular weights of leukotriene A_4 hydrolase from human and rat leukocytes being 70 and 68 kDa, respectively.

The enzyme appears to be the key enzyme for regulation of leukotriene B_4 production in granulocytes as it undergoes suicide inactivation by the substrate with covalent coupling of the epoxide to the inactivated enzyme (22). There are variabilities in the efficiency of suicide inhibition by alternative leukotriene epoxides, such as leukotriene A_3 and A_5 (22,23). These variations have been correlated with inhibition of leukotriene B_4 production following dietary supplementation with eicosapentanoic acid (24). It should be noted, however, that polymorphonuclear leukocytes, in addition to metabolizing leukotriene A_4 to leukotriene B_4, may also release leukotriene A_4. This unstable intermediate is stabilized through binding to serum albumin (25) and may undergo efficient transcellular metabolism by other cellular sources of either leukotriene A_4 hydrolase or leukotriene C_4 synthase (26,27).

D. Leukotriene C_4 Synthase

In cells such as eosinophils, leukotriene A_4 undergoes enzymatic conjugation with glutathione to produce 5-S-hydroxy-6R,S-glutathionyl-7,9,11,14-(E,E,Z,Z)-eicosatetraenoic acid (leukotriene C_4). The enzyme responsible, leukotriene C_4 synthase, catalyzes the stereospecific opening of the epoxide, leukotriene A_4, through *sn*-2 attack of glutathione at position C_6. Leukotriene C_4 synthase has been solubilized and partially purified from RBL-1 cells (28,29). The fact that the enzyme is membrane-bound, rather than a soluble enzyme, distinguishes it from the abundant cytosolic glutathione-S-transferases found, for example, in liver (30). The enzyme is also quite distinct from membrane-bound glutathione-S-transferases. Enzymatic metabolism of leukotriene C_4, probably outside the eosinophil, involves the cleavage of glutamic acid by a specific membrane-bound γ-glutamyl transferase to produce leukotriene D_4 (31–33), the most important of the biologically active peptidolipid leukotrienos. Further metabolism of leukotriene D_4 to leukotriene E_4 occurs through a specific membrane-bound dipeptidase with loss of L-glycine, this process occurring in a variety of systems (34–39).

E. Modulation of Leukotriene Production by Cytokines

A number of studies have examined whether various cytokines can either directly stimulate arachidonic acid release and the subsequent activation of 5-lipoxygenase and synthesis of leukotrienes or can "prime" granulocyte populations so that enhanced leukotriene synthesis can be demonstrated following exposure to stimuli such as ionophore A23187, zymosan, and the synthetic chemotactic peptide, fMet-Leu-Phe. The only cytokine for which there is convincing evidence for a direct effect on leukotriene biosynthesis is interleukin-8 (IL-8 or monocyte-derived neutrophil-activating peptide). IL-8 is similar to other chemotactic factors, such as C_{5a}, fMet-Leu-Phe, and platelet-activating factor, in that it induces a direct activation of the 5-lipoxygenase in human polymorphonuclear leukocytes (40). In the same study (h)rIL-1α had no effect on leukotriene biosynthesis consistent with the failure of (h)rIL-1α or (h)rIL-1β to activate neutrophil function (41). A reported positive effect of biologically derived IL-2 (a mixture containing 90% IL-1β and 10% IL-1α) on arachidonic acid lipoxygenation in human neutrophils (42) can probably be accounted for by the presence of IL-8 in such preparations (40). Similarly, a T-lymphocyte-derived factor that enhances IgG-dependent release of leukotriene B_4 from human neutrophils may be related to IL-8 (43). In the same study γ-interferon and IL-2 were shown to have no effect on leukotriene biosynthesis.

A number of studies have suggested that human recombinant granulocyte-macrophage colony-stimulating factor (GM-CSF) can "prime" neutrophils and enhance arachidonic acid release and leukotriene B_4 synthesis. Thus, GM-CSF has been shown to enhance the synthesis of leukotriene B_4 following exposure of neutrophils to ionophore A23187, fMet-Leu-Phe, platelet-activating factor, and zymosan (44–46) and enhance the synthesis of leukotriene C_4 in human eosinophils following exposure to ionophore A23187 (47). In contast, conflicting results have been obtained with tumor necrosis factor (TNF). Luedke and Humes (48) showed no effect of $rTNF_\alpha$ or $rTBF_\beta$ on leukotriene B_4 production by human neutrophils, and TNF was shown to have no effect on ionophore A23187-induced synthesis of leukotriene C_4 by eosinophils (47). Roubin et al. (49), however, reported that human $rTNF_\alpha$ had no direct effect on leukotriene release by either neutrophils or eosinophils, but that it did enhance leukotriene production in response to challenge with ionophore A23187. In contrast, Camussi et al. (50) have reported that human rTNF had a direct effect on the synthesis of leukotriene B_4 by neutrophils.

It is clear that certain cytokines may modulate the synthesis of 5-lipoxygenase products and that such a modulation may have either pathological or physiological effects. However, the mechanisms of these effects are not understood, and it will be of interest to determine whether they involve either increased release of arachidonic acid, increased activation of 5-lipoxygenase, or effects on FLAP. Furthermore, all the above effects are observed in short-term incubations, and it will be important to determine if cytokines can modulate either the transcriptional or translational control of the synthesis of either 5-lipoxygenase or FLAP.

III. LEUKOTRIENE B_4 RECEPTORS ON GRANULOCYTES

As will be described in Section IV, leukotriene B_4 is a potent activator of leukocyte function. The activities of leukotriene B_4 are expressed at nanomolar concentrations in a stereospecific fashion, suggesting the presence of high-affinity, structurally specific receptor sites (51). Leukotriene B_4 receptors have been characterized on granulocytes through radioligand binding studies using the tritiated leukotriene. Such studies have demonstrated that binding to either intact cell or membrane preparations of either human or rat neutrophils is both saturable and reversible (52–55). As shown in Table 1, human neutrophils contain two classes of receptors, which have been associated with separate biological activities. Rat neutrophils, in contast, possess only a high-affinity receptor population (54). Consistent with this is the fact that a tight correlation has been observed between receptor binding of analogs of leukotriene B_4 and their ability to stimulate either the chemokinesis of human polymorphonuclear leukocytes or the aggregation of rat neutrophils (55,56).

Granulocyte populations contain receptors for a number of chemotactic ligands, including C_{5a}, fMet-Leu-Phe, PAF, and presumably IL-8. These receptors share many common properties, all being G-protein-linked receptors which generate inositol(1,4,5)-P_3 as a second messenger for intracellular Ca^{2+} mobilization (57). Some early work had suggested that leukotriene B_4 might act as a naturally occurring ionophore capable of transporting Ca^{2+} across lipid bilayers with no increases in pI breakdown occurring following stimulation with the autocoid (58,59). It now seems that this is not correct and that leukotriene B_4 is coupled to a pertussis toxin-sensitive G-protein, stimulation of which leads to the formation of inositol (1,4,5)-P_3 (60–64). This results in an elevation of intracellular calcium and activation of the cellular contractile mechanisms (65–68).

The leukotriene B_4 receptor has been solubilized with detergents, indicating that purification is possible (69). The appearance of the receptor has been demonstrated during differentiation of the promyelocytic cell line, HL-60 (70–71). It is not clear whether the high- and low-affinity receptors for leukotriene B_4 on neutrophils are different forms of the same receptor. However, one study has suggested that a portion of high-affinity leukotriene B_4 receptors could be converted to the low-affinity state by GTP and nonhydrolysable GTP analogs in a concentration-dependent, nucleotide-specific, and reversible manner without altering the intrinsic binding affinities of either class (72).

Other points that need to be clarified include the exact nature of the G-protein linked to the leukotriene B_4 receptor; whether the receptor is always linked to the same G-protein; and whether the G-protein used is common to other chemotactic receptors. In this context, it has been suggested that in HL-60 cells the receptors for both leukotriene

Table 1 Leukotriene B_4 Receptors on Polymorphonuclear Leukocytes

Human cells	Affinity	K_D	Functional response
Whole cells	High	3.9×10^{-10} M	Chemotaxis, chemokinesis
	Low	1.0×10^{-7} M	Lysosomal enzyme release, superoxide anion production
Membranes	High	1.9×10^{-9} M	
	Low	7.9×10^{-8} M	
Rat cells			
Whole cells	High	4.5×10^{-9} M	Aggregation
Membranes	High	2.4×10^{-9} M	

B_4 and fMet-Leu-Phe share a common G-protein (73). This was based on the fact that leukotriene B_4 stimulated a dose-dependent increase in GTP hydrolysis and guanosine 5′-(γ-thio)triphosphate (GTP[S]) binding, and that both pertussis toxin and cholera toxin inhibited stimulation of GTPase activity and GTP[S] binding by either leukotriene B_4 or fMet-Leu-Phe. fMet-Leu-Phe was shown to enhance cholera toxin-induced inhibition of GTPase activity stimulated by either fMet-Leu-Phe or leukotriene B_4, indicating that the two receptors share a common G-protein. However, leukotriene B_4 did not enhance cholera toxin-induced inhibition of GTPase activity, indicating that the receptors interact differently with the G-protein. This difference was confirmed by showing that fMet-Leu-Phe, but not leukotriene B_4, stimulated receptor-specific [^{32}P]ADP-ribosylation of the 40-kDa α-subunit. The authors have therefore concluded, first, that although both receptors may be coupled to common G proteins, the receptor-G protein interaction is different for the two receptors and, second that G-proteins not coupled to both receptors may account for the additive response (73). It is clear from this type of study that there is considerable room for further study to elucidate the precise secondary transduction mechanisms involved with both the leukotriene B_4 and other chemotactic receptors as well as to determine whether there are receptor subtypes or different forms of the same receptor.

IV. LEUKOTRIENE ACTIVATION OF GRANULOCYTES

A. In-Vitro Actions of Leukotriene B_4

Leukotriene B_4 is a potent chemotactic and chemokinetic agent for leukocytes (74–76), these effects being mediated through high-affinity receptor sites as described in Section III. Leukotriene B_4 shares many properties with other potent chemotactic factors such as C_{5a} and fMet-Leu-Phe. Thus it stimulates a variety of leukocyte functions. These include aggregation (74); enhancement of lysosomal enzyme release (76–78); stimulation of ion fluxes (65–68,79); enhanced superoxide anion production (80); enhancement of C_{3b} receptor site expression (81); stimulation of adherence (82,83); enhancement of the expression of integrins (84,85); and enhancement of complement-dependent cytotoxicity reactions (86). These actions of leukotriene B_4 on neutrophils and eosinophils are summarized in Table 2.

In addition to promoting the movement of leukocytes, it has been hypothesized that a major role for leukotriene B_4 is to promote leukocyte adherence to the endothelium (87). Thus pretreatment of endothelial cells, but not neutrophils, with leukotriene B_4 resulted in an increase in neutrophil/endothelial adhesion at relevant concentrations of the autocoid. This is consistent with in-vivo observations which have shown that exogenous leukotriene B_4 can enhance the sticking of circulating leukocytes to the walls of postcapillary venules (88,89). Recently, integrins involved in the transient adhesion of polymorphonuclear leukocytes to the endothelium have been identified. On the leukocyte cell surface these include the CD18 family of leukocyte receptors, namely, the CD11a/CD18(LFA-1), CD11b/CD18(CR3,Mac-1), and CD11c/CD18(p150,95) (84, 85,90). Thus leukotriene B_4, along with other chemotactic factors such as C_{5a}, greatly increased the expression of CD11/18 components, in particular, Mac-1 (84,85). At the same time, neutrophils shed another surface receptor, gp100^{MEL-14}, from the cell surface within 4 min after activation with leukotriene B_4 and other chemotactic factors, releasing a 96-kDa fragment of the antigen into the supernatant (84,85).

Table 2 Effects of Leukotriene B_4 on Leukocyte Function in Vivo

Target cell	Biological activity	Reference
Polymorphonuclear leukocyte, eosinophil	Chemotaxis	74–76
Polymorphonuclear leukocyte, eosinophil, macrophage, monocyte	Chemokinesis	74
Polymorphonuclear leukocyte	Aggregation	74
Polymorphonuclear leukocyte	Enhancement of lysosomal enyzme release	76–78
Polymorphonuclear leukocyte	Superoxide anion production	80
Polymorphonuclear leukocyte, eosinophil	Enhancement of C3b receptor expression	81
Polymorphonuclear leukocyte, eosinophil	Enhancement of complement-dependent cytotoxicity	86
Polymorphonuclear leukocyte	Enhancement of expression of integrins (Mac-1, MEL-14)	84,85

It has been suggested that both the MEL-14 antigen and Mac-1/LFA-1 are important factors in promoting neutrophil localization to inflamed sites in vivo, but that their roles in endothelial cell interactions are distinct. In particular, the rapid shedding of MEL-14 may prevent extravasation into and damage of normal tissues by activated neutrophils.

B. In-Vivo Actions of Leukotriene B_4

The in-vitro actions of leukotriene B_4 on leukocyte activation can be observed in vivo through induction of leukocyte migration. Thus, leukocyte accumulation has been observed following injection of leukotriene B_4 into rabbit skin (89), rabbit eye (91), and the guinea-pig peritoneal cavity (75), and leukocyte movement through and adherence to the endothelium has been visualized directly in a hamster cheek pouch preparation (88,89). In humans, the effects of leukotriene B_4 on leukocyte accumulation have been studied in three experimental systems. These were chambers containing either buffer alone or buffer and leukotriene B_4 applied over abrasions on the human forearm (89), intradermal injection of leukotriene B_4 directly into the skin, and topical application of leukotriene B_4 (92–94). Significant neutrophil accumulation in the skin was observed with all three systems. In addition, following topical application, intradermal micro-abscesses containing a mixed perivascular neutrophil and mononuclear cell infiltrate could be observed following histological analysis (92). It is important to realize that there may be species differences in the chemotactic activity of leukotriene B_4. Thus, leukotriene B_4 can induce leukocyte infiltration to the skin of the mouse, the rabbit, the guinea pig, the hamster, and humans, but it is not an important mediator of leukocyte accumulation in the rat (95–98) despite the presence of high-affinity receptors for leukotriene B_4 on rat neutrophils (54). This is of particular importance because many models of inflammation have been developed in the rat, and thus caution needs to be taken in evaluating the role of leukotriene B_4 as a mediator of inflammatory events in this species.

In addition to inducing leukocyte accumulation, leukotriene B_4 also causes changes in vascular permeability in the skin of the rabbit (99,100), the rat (99,101), the guinea pig (99), and humans (94), as well as when applied topically to the hamster cheek pouch (88,102). This increase in vascular permeability can be enhanced by administration of either prostaglandin E_2 or other vasodilators (99,100), and the changes in vascular permeability appear to be dependent on the presence of neutrophils (88,100,101). From these observations it has been proposed that the actual permeability changes are mediated through a neutrophil-derived mediator released following induction of neutrophil adhesion to the endothelium and cellular activation in response to chemotactic factors such as leukotriene B_4. There is some evidence that under certain circumstances leukotriene B_4 may also induce vasodilatation directly—for example, in porcine skin (103)—although this is not the case in the rabbit skin (99).

There is some evidence to suggest that leukotriene B_4 may also modulate inflammatory pain reactions, as has been demonstrated for prostaglandins. The first study to demonstrate such an effect was in the rat, in which either leukotriene B_4 or prostaglandins E_1, when co-injected with brewer's yeast into the rat paw, prevented the initial hypoalgesia and significantly reduced the latency and development of the subsequent hyperalgesia (104). No synergy was observed between the two autocoids, suggesting that both leukotriene B_4 and prostaglandin E_1 work through a common mechanism. Subsequently, leukotriene B_4 has been shown to have a direct hyperalgesic action in the rat paw similar in magnitude to that produced by either prostaglandin E_2 or bradykinin (105). The hyperalgesic effect of leukotriene B_4 was independent of the production of cyclooxygenase products, as evidenced by the failure of indomethacin to inhibit the response, but was dependent on the presence of polymorphonuclear leukocytes (106). As similar effects have been observed with other chemotactic factors, it has been suggested that this mechanism may involve the release of a neutrophil-derived mediator. In contrast to the results observed in the rat, leukotriene B_4 failed to potentiate bradykinin-induced nociception in the dog (107), and in humans the intradermal injection of leukotriene B_4 alone does not result in the induction of pain responses (93,94). Clearly, other studies will have to be carried out, in species other than the rat, to further assess the potential role of leukotriene B_4 as a modulator of pain responses.

C. Other Lipoxygenase Products

While it is clear that the principal route of arachidonic acid metabolism in the granulocyte is through 5-lipoxygenase, other pathways of arachidonic acid metabolism exist, including 12-lipoxygenase, 15-lipoxygenase, double lipoxygenase pathways, and cytochrome P-450-dependent pathways. Such pathways may also generate products that may have effects on leukocyte activation. Thus 5- and 12-hydroxyeicosatetraenoic (HETE) acids stimulate PMN degranulation, and both 5- and 15-HETE enhance platelet-activating factor-induced degranulation (108–110). Whether such effects occur at concentrations that can be achieved physiologically is questionable. Other products of the 15-lipoxygenase pathway, in particular, 8(S),15(S)-dihydroxy-5,11-*cis*-9,13-*trans*-eicosatetraenoic acid, prepared by treating arachidonic acid with soybean lipoxygenase or generated by mixed human leukocytes after stimulation with ionophore A23187 and arachidonic acid, have been proposed as potent chemotactic agents, comparable to leukotriene B_4 (111). However, studies with various synthetic isomers of 8,15-dihydroxyeicosatetraenoic acid failed to detect significant chemokinetic or aggregatory activity (112).

The principal product of the 12-lipoxygenase pathway is 12(S)-HETE, which has little effect on leukocyte function. However, the enantiomer, 12(R)-HETE, has significant activity in inducing leukocyte activation and has been found to bind to the leukotriene B_4 receptor, indicating that the 12(R) group is an important determinant for receptor recognition (113). 12R-HETE has also been detected in psoriatic lesions (114), and a mechanism for its synthesis from arachidonic acid via cytochrome P-450-dependent pathways has been proposed (115). Other eicosanoids may also have effects on leukocyte function through interaction with the leukotriene B_4 receptor. An example of this may be the lipoxins, tetraene products produced in polymorphonuclear leukocytes through double lipoxygenation reactions (116,117). Thus, both lipoxin A and lipoxin B have been shown to induce granulocyte chemotaxis and aggregation, probably through a weak interaction with the leukotriene B_4 receptor (118).

V. CONCLUSIONS

Activation of granulocytes results in a Ca^{2+}-dependent activation of 5-lipoxygenase in combination with 5-lipoxygenase activating protein (FLAP). This results in the synthesis of leukotrienes, in particular, leukotriene B_4. Leukotriene B_4 shows similarities to other chemotactic factors such as C_{5a}, fMet-Leu-Phe, PAF, and IL-8 and induces leukocyte activation, adherence, and stimulated movement at low concentrations. Leukotriene B_4 differs from these other chemotactic factors in that it is produced by the neutrophils themselves, can be rapidly metabolized by these cells, and is of low molecular weight and thus could be an endogenous modulator of leukocyte function upregulating the activity of other leukocyte activators. It is of interest that biologically significant amounts of leukotriene B_4 can be detected in psoriatic lesions and inflammatory bowel disease mucosa, pathological conditions in which extensive neutrophil infiltration occurs. Thus it has been proposed that leukotriene B_4 may be an important pathological mediator of these diseases (119). However, whether leukotriene B_4 has an important role in normal physiological processes and in host defense mechanisms remains to be determined.

REFERENCES

1. Mass RL, Ingram CD, Taber DF, Oates JA, Brash AR. Stereospecific removal of the D_R hydrogen atom at the 10-carbon of arachidonic acid in the biosynthesis of leukotriene A_4 by human leukocytes. J Biol Chem 1982; 257:13515–9.
2. Panossian AA, Hamberg M, Samuelsson B. On the mechanism of biosynthesis of leukotrienes and related compounds. FEBS Lett 1982; 150:511–3.
3. Rouzer CA, Matsumoto T, Samuelsson B. Single protein from human leukocytes possesses 5-lipoxygenase and leukotriene A_4 synthase activities. Proc Natl Acad Sci USA 1986; 83:857–61.

4. Ueda N, Kaneko S, Yoshimoto T, Yamamoto S. Purification of arachidonate 5-lipoxygenase from porcine leukocytes and its reactivity with hydroperoxyeicosatetraenoic acids. J Biol Chem 1986; 261:7982–8.
5. Skoog MT, Nichols JS, Wiseman JS. 5-lipoxygenase from rat PMN lysate. Prostaglandins 1986; 31:561–76.
6. Aharony D, Stein RL. Kinetic mechanism of guinea pig neutrophil 5-lipoxygenase. J Biol Chem 1986; 261:11512–9.
7. Cook M, Hogaboom GK, Sarau HM, Foley JJ, Crooke ST. Characterization of arachidonate 5-lipoxygenase and leukotriene A_4 synthase from RBL-1 cells. Fed Proc 1986; 45:1935.
8. Rouzer CA, Samuelsson B. On the nature of the 5-lipoxygenase reaction in human leukocytes: enzyme purification and requirement for multiple stimulatory factors. Proc Natl Acad Sci USA 1985; 82:6040–4.
9. Rouzer CA, Samuelsson B. The importance of hydroperoxide activation for the detection and assay of mammalian 5-lipoxygenase. FEBS Lett 1986; 204:293–6.
10. Rouzer CA, Shimizu T, Samuelsson B. On the nature of the 5-lipoxygenase reaction in human leukocytes: characterization of a membrane-associated stimulatory factor. Proc Natl Acad Sci USA 1985; 82:7505–9.
11. Dixon RAF, Jones RE, Diehl RE, Bennett CD, Kargman S, Rouzer CA. Cloning of the cDNA for human 5-lipoxygenase. Proc Natl Acad Sci USA 1988; 85:416–20.
12. Rouzer CA, Rands E, Kargman S, Jones RE, Register RB, Dixon RAF. Characterization of cloned human leukocyte 5-lipoxygenase expressed in mammalian cells. Cloned human leukocyte 5-lipoxygenase. J Biol Chem 1988; 263:10135–40.
13. Rouzer CA, Kargman S. Translocation of 5-lipoxygenase to the membrane in human leukocytes challenged with ionophore A23187. J Biol Chem 1988; 263:10980–8.
14. Gillard J, Ford-Hutchinson AW, Chan C, Charleson S, Denis D, Foster A, Fortin R, Leger S, McFarlane CS, Morton H, Piechuta H, Riendeau D, Rouzer CA, Rokach J, Young R, MacIntyre DE, Peterson L, Bach T, Eiermann G, Hopple S, Humes J, Hupe L, Luell S, Metzger J, Meurer R, Miller DK, Opas E, Pacholok S. L-663,536 (MK-886) (3-[1-(4-chlorobenzyl)-3-*t*-butyl-thio-5-isopropylindol-2-yl]-2,2-dimethylpropanoic acid), a novel, orally active leukotriene biosynthesis inhibitor. Can J Physiol Pharmacol 1989; 67:456–64.
15. Rouzer CA, Ford-Hutchinson AW, Morton HE, Gillard JW. MK-886 a potent and specific leukotriene biosynthesis inhibitor blocks and reverses the membrane association of 5-lipoxygenase in ionophore-challenged leukocytes. J Biol Chem 1990; 265:1436–42.
16. Miller DK, Gillard JW, Vickers PJ, Sadowski S, Lévellé C, Mancini JA, Charleson P, Dixon RAF, Ford-Hutchinson AW, Fortin R, Gauthier J-Y, Rodkey J, Rozen R, Rouzer C, Sigal IS, Strader CD, Evans JF. Identification and isolation of a membrane protein necessary for leukotriene production. Nature 1990; 343:278–81.
17. Dixon RAF, Diehl RE, Opas E, Rands E, Vickers PJ, Evans JF, Gillard JW, Miller DK. Requirement of a 5-lipoxygenase-activating protein for leukotriene synthesis. Nature 1990; 343:282–4.
18. Melloni E, Pontremoli S, Michetti M, Sacco O, Sparatore B, Salamino F, Horecker BL. Binding of protein kinase C to neutrophil membranes in the presence of Ca^{2+} and its activation by a Ca^{2+}-requiring proteinase. Proc Natl Acad Sci USA 1985; 82:6435–9.
19. Creutz CE, Dowling LG, Kyger EM, Franson RC. Phosphatidylinositol-specific phospholipase C activity of chromaffin granule-binding proteins. J Biol Chem 1985; 260:7171–3.
20. Radmark O, Shimizu T, Jornvall H, Samuelsson B. Leukotriene A_4 hydrolase in human leukocytes. Purification and properties. J Biol Chem 1984; 259:12339–45.
21. Evans JF, Dupuis P, Ford-Hutchinson AW. Purification and characterization of leukotriene A_4 hydrolase from rat neutrophils. Biochim Biophys Acta 1985; 840:43–50.

22. Evans JF, Nathaniel DJ, Zamboni RJ, Ford-Hutchinson AW. Leukotrienes A_3. A poor substrate but a potent inhibitor of rat and human neutrophil leukotriene A_4 hydrolase. J Biol Chem 1985; 260:10966–70.
23. Nathaniel DJ, Evans JF, Leblanc Y, Lévellé C, Fitzsimmons BJ, Ford-Hutchinson AW. Leukotriene A_5 is a substrate and an inhibitor of rat and human neutrophil LTA_4 hydrolase. Biochem Biophys Res Commun 1985; 131:827–35.
24. Ford-Hutchinson AW. Alternative fatty acids and the production and action of leukotriene B. Transplantation Proc 1986; 18:33–6.
25. Maycock AL, Anderson MS, DeSousa DM, Kuehl FA Jr. Leukotriene A_4: preparation and enzymatic conversion in a cell-free system to leukotriene B_4. J Biol Chem 1982; 257:13911–4.
26. Dahinden CA, Clancy RM, Gross M, Chiller JM, Hugli TE. Leukotriene C_4 production by murine mast cells: evidence of a role for extracellular leukotriene A_4. Proc Natl Acad Sci USA 1985; 82:6632–6.
27. Marcus AJ. Transcellular metabolism of eicosanoids. Prog Hemost Thromb 1986; 8:127–42.
28. Bach MK, Brashler JR, Peck RE, Morton DR Jr. Leukotriene C synthetase, a special glutathione S-transferase: properties of the enzyme and inhibitor studies with special reference to the mode of action of U-60,257, a selective inhibitor of leukotriene synthesis. J Allergy Clin Immunol 1984; 74:353–7.
29. Bach MK, Brashler JR, Morton DR Jr. Solubilization and characterization of the leukotriene C_4 synthetase of rat basophil leukemia cells: a novel, particulate glutathione S-transferase. Arch Biochem Biophys 1984; 230:455–65.
30. Jakschik BA, Harper T, Murphy RC. Leukotriene C_4 and D_4 formation by particulate enzymes. J Biol Chem 1982; 257:5346–9.
31. Orning L, Hammarstrom S. Inhibition of leukotriene C and leukotriene D biosynthesis. J Biol Chem 1980; 255:8023–6.
32. Tate S. Enzymes of mercapturic acid formation. In: Jakoby W, ed. Enzymatic basis of detoxication, vol. 2. New York: Academic Press, 1980:95–120.
33. Meister A, Tate S, Ross L. Membrane-bound γ-glutamyl transpeptidase. In: Martonosi A, ed. The enzymes of biological membranes, vol. 3 New York: Plenum Press, 1976:315–47.
34. Bernstrom K, Hammarstrom S. Metabolism of leukotriene D by porcine kidney. J Biol Chem 1981; 256:9579–82.
35. Kuo CG, Lewis MT, Jakschik BA. Leukotriene D_4 and E_4 formation by plasma membrane bound enzymes. Prostaglandins 1984; 28:929–38.
36. Anderson ME, Allison RD, Meister A. Interconversion of leukotrienes catalyzed by purified γ-glutamyl transpeptidase: concomitant formation of leukotriene D_4 and γ-glutamyl amino acids. Proc Natl Acad Sci USA 1982; 79:1088–91.
37. Yokota K, Shono F, Yamamoto S, Kominami E, Katunuma N. Transformation of leukotriene D_4 catalyzed by lysosomal cathepsin H of rat liver. J Biochem (Tokyo) 1983; 94:1173–8.
38. Lee CW, Lewis RA, Corey EJ, Austen KF. Conversion of leukotriene D_4 to leukotriene E_4 by a dipeptidase released from the specific granule of human polymorphonuclear leukocytes. Immunology 1983; 48:27–35.
39. Parker C, Falkenhein S, Huber M. Sequential conversion of the glutathionyl side chain of slow reacting substance (SRS) to cysteinyl-glycine and cysteine in rat basophilic leukemia cells stimulated with A23187. Prostaglandins 1980; 20:863–86.
40. Schroder J-M. The monocyte-derived neutrophil activating peptide (NAP/interleukin 8) stimulates human neutrophil arachidonate-5-lipoxygenase, but not the release of cellular arachidonate. J Exp Med 1989; 170:847–63.

41. Georgilis K, Schaefer C, Dinarello CA, Klempner MS. Human recombinant interleukin 1β has no effect on intracellular calcium or on functional response of human neutrophils. J Immunol 1987; 138:3403–7.
42. Smith, RJ, Epps DE, Justen JM, Sam LM, Wynalda MA, Fitzpatrick FA, Yein FS. Human neutrophil activation with Interleukin-1. A role for intracellular calcium and arachidonic acid lipoxygenation. Biochem Pharmacol 1987; 36:3851–8.
43. Tsai J-J, Maestrelli P, Cromwell O, Moqbel R, Fitzharris P, Kay AB. A T-lymphocyte-derived factor that enhances IgG-dependent release of leukotriene $B_4(LTB_4)$ from human neutrophils. Immunology 1988; 65:449–56.
44. DiPersio JF, Billing P, Williams R, Gasson JC. Human granulocyte-macrophage colony-stimulating factor and other cytokines prime human neutrophils for enhanced arachidonic acid release and leukotriene B_4 synthesis. J Immunol 1988; 140:4315–22.
45. DiPersio JF, NAccache PH, Borgeat P, Gasson JC, Nguyen M-H, McColl SR. Characterization of the priming effects of human granulocyte-macrophage colony-stimulating factor on human neutrophil leukotriene synthesis. Prostaglandins 1988; 36:673–91.
46. Poubelle PE, Bourgoin S, Naccache PH, Borgeat P. Granulocyte-macrophage colony-stimulating factor (GM-CSF) and opsonization synergistically enhance leukotriene B_4 (LTB_4) synthesis induced by phagocytosis in human neutrophils. Agents Actions 1989; 27:388–90.
47. Silberstein DS, Owen WF, Gasson JC, DiPersio JF, Golde DW, Bina JC, Soberman R, Austen KF, David JR. Enhancement of human eosinophil cytotoxicity and leukotriene synthesis by biosynthetic (recombinant) granulocyte-macrophage colony-stimulating factor. J Immunol 1986; 137:3290–4.
48. Luedke ES, Humes JL. Effect of tumor necrosis factor on granule release and LTB_4 production in adherent human polymorphonuclear leukocytes. Agents Actions 1989; 27:451–4.
49. Roubin R, Elsas PP, Fiers W. Dessein AJ. Recombinant human tumour necrosis factor $(rTNF)^2$ enhances leukotriene biosynthesis in neutrophils and eosinophils stimulated with Ca^{2+} ionophore A23187. Clin Exp Immunol 1987; 70:484–90.
50. Camussi G, Tetta C, Bussolino F, Baglioni C. Tumor necrosis factor stimulates human neutrophils to release leukotriene B_4 and platelet activating factor. Induction of phospholipase A_2 and acetyl-CoA:1-alkyl-*sn*-glycero-3-phosphocholine O_2-acetyltransferase activity and inhibition by antiproteinase. Eur J Biochem 1989; 182:661–6.
51. Ford-Hutchinson AW. The role of leukotriene B_4 as a mediator of leukocyte function. Agents Actions [Suppl] 1983; 12:154–66.
52. Goldman DW, Goetzl EJ. Specific binding of leukotriene B_4 to receptors on human polymorphonuclear leukocytes. J Immunol 1982; 129:1600–4.
53. Goldman DW, Goetzl EJ. Heterogeneity of human polymorphonuclear leukocyte receptors for leukotriene B_4: identification of a subset of high affinity receptors that transduce the chemotactic response. J Exp Med 1984; 159:1027–41.
54. Charleson S, Evans JF, Zamboni RJ, Leblanc Y, Fitzsimmons BJ, Leveillé C, Dupuis P, Ford-Hutchinson AW. Leukotriene B_3, Leukotriene B_4 and Leukotriene B_5: binding to Leukotriene B_4 receptors on rat and human leukocyte membranes. Prostaglandins 1986; 32:503–16.
55. Ford-Hutchinson AW, Charleson S, Evans JF. Leukotriene B_4 receptors in rat and human neutrophil membranes. Methods Enzymol 1988; 163:340–3.
56. Ford-Hutchinson AW, Evans JF. Neutrophil aggregation and chemokinesis assays. Methods Enzymol 1988; 162:72–8.
57. Berridge MJ and Irvine RF. Inositol trisphosphate, a novel second messenger in cellular signal transduction. Nature (Lond), 1984; 312–5.

58. Serhan CN, Fridovich J, Goetzl EJ, Dunham PB, Weissman G. Leukotriene B_4 and phosphatidic acid are calcium ionophores: studies employing arsenazo III in liposomes. J Biol Chem 1982; 257:4746–52.
59. Volpi M, Yassin R, Tao W, Molski TFP, Naccache PH, Sha'afi RI. Leukotriene B_4 mobilizes calcium without the breakdown of polyphosphoinositides and the production of phosphatidic acid in rabbit neutrophils. Proc Natl Acad Sci USA 1984; 81:5966–9.
60. Andersson T, Schlegel W, Monod A, Krause K-H, Stendahl O, Lew DP. Leukotriene B_4 stimulation of phagocytes results in the formation of inositol 1,4,5-triphosphate; a second messenger for Ca^{2+} mobilization. Biochem J 1986; 240:333–40.
61. Goldman DW, Chang F-H, Gifford LA, Goetzl EJ, Bourne HR. Pertussis toxin inhibition of chemotactic factor-induced calcium mobilization and function in human polymorphonuclear leukocytes. J Exp Med 1985; 162:145–56.
62. Feltner DE, Smith RH, Marasco WA. Characterization of the plasma membrane bound GTPase from rabbit neutrophils; I. Evidence for an N_i-like protein coupled to the formyl peptide, C_{5a}, and leukotriene B_4 chemotaxis receptors. J Immunol 1986; 137:1961–70.
63. Shefcyk J, Yassin R, Volpi M, Molski TFP, Naccache PH, Munoz JJ, Becker EL, Feinstein MB, Sha'afi RI. Pertussis but not cholera toxin inhibits the stimulated increase in actin association with the cytoskeleton in rabbit neutrophils: role of the "G proteins" in stimulus-response coupling. Biochem Biophys Res Commun 1985; 126:1174–81.
64. Mong S, Chi-Rosso G, Miller J, Hoffman K, Razgaitis KA, Bender P, Crooke ST. Leukotriene B_4 induces formation of inositol phosphates in rat peritoneal polymorphonuclear leukocytes. Mol Pharmacol 1986; 30:235–42.
65. Naccache PH, Faucher N, Therrien S, Borgeat P. Calcium mobilization, actin polymerization and right-angle light scatter responses to leukotriene B_4, 12(R)- and 12(S)-hydroxyeicosatetraenoic acid in human neutrophils. Life Sci 1988; 42:727–33.
66. Naccache PH, Molski TFP, Becker EL, Borgeat P, Picard S, Vallerand P, Sha'afi RI. Specificity of the effect of lipoxygenase metabolites of arachidonic acid on calcium homeostasis in neutrophils; correlation with functional activity. J Biol Chem 1982; 257:8608–11.
67. Lew PD, Dayer J-M, Wollheim CB, Pozzan T. Effect of leukotriene B_4, protaglandin E_2 and arachidonic acid on cytosolic-free calcium in human neutrophils. FEBS Lett 1984; 166:44–8.
68. Goldman DW, Gifford LA, Olson DM, Goetzl EJ. Transduction by leukotriene B_4 receptors of increases in cytosolic calcium in human polymorphonuclear leukocytes. J Immunol 1985; 135:525–30.
69. Lin AH, Ruppel PL, Gorman RR. Detergent solubilization of human neutrophil leukotriene B_4 receptors. Biochem Biophys Res Commun 1985; 128:878–83.
70. Benjamin CW, Rupple PL, Gorman RR. Appearance of specific leukotriene B_4 binding sites in myeloid differentiated HL-60 cells. J Biol Chem 1985; 260:14208–13.
71. Goldman DW, Olson DM, Payan DG, Gifford LA, Goetzl EJ. Development of receptors for leukotriene B_4 on HL-60 cells induced to differentiate by 1α,25-dihydroxyvitamin D_3. J Immunol 1986; 136:4631–6.
72. Sheman JW, Goetzl EJ, Koo CH. Selective modulation by guanine nucleotides of the high affinity subset of plasma membrane receptors for leukotriene B_4 in human polymorphonuclear leukocytes. J Immunol 1988; 140:3900–4.
73. Mcleish KR, Gierschik P, Schepers T, Sidiropoulos P, Jakobs KH. Evidence that activation of a common G-protein by receptors for leukotriene B_4 and N-formylmethionyl-leucyl-phenylalanine in HL-60 cells occurs by different mechanisms. Biochem J 1989; 260:427–34.

74. Ford-Hutchinson AW, Bray MA, Doig MV, Shipley ME, Smith MJH. Leukotriene B: a potent chemokinetic and aggregating substance released from polymorphonuclear leukocytes. Nature 1980; 286:264–5.
75. Smith MJH, Ford-Hutchinson AW, Bray MA. Leukotriene B: a potential mediator of inflammation. J Pharm Pharmacol 1980; 32:517–8.
76. Goetzl EJ, Pickett WC. The human PMN leukocyte chemotactic activity of complex hydroxy-eicosatetraenoic acids (HETEs). J Immunol 1980; 125:1789–91.
77. Rollins TE, Zanolari B, Springer MS, Guindon Y, Zamboni R, Lau C-K, Rokach J. Synthetic leukotriene B_4 is a potent chemotaxin but a weak secretagogue for human PMN. Prostaglandins 1983; 25:281–9.
78. Rae SA, Smith MJH. The stimulation of lysosomal enzyme secretion from human polymorphonuclear leucocytes by leukotriene B_4. J Pharm Pharmacol 1981; 33:616–7.
79. Molski TFP, Naccache PH, Borgeat P, Sha'afi RI. Similarities in the mechanisms by which formyl-methionyl-leucyl-phenylalanine, arachidonic acid and leukotriene B_4 increase calcium and sodium influxes in rabbit neutrophils. Biochem Biophys Res Commun 1981; 103:227–32.
80. Serhan CN, Radin A, Smolen JE, Korchak H, Samuelsson B, Weissmann G. Leukotriene B_4 is a complete secretagogue in human neutrophils: a kinetic analysis. Biochem Biophys Res Commun 1982; 107:1006–12.
81. Nagy L, Lee TH, Goetzl EJ, Pickett WC, Kay AB. Complement receptor enhancement and chemotaxis of human neutrophils and eosinophils by leukotrienes and other lipoxygenase products. Clin Exp Immunol 1982; 47:541–7.
82. McMillan RM, Foster SJ. Leukotriene B_4 and inflammatory disease. Agents Actions 1988; 24:114–9.
83. Gimbrone MA Jr, Brock AF, Schafer AI. Leukotriene B_4 stimulates polymorphonuclear leukocyte adhesion to cultured vascular endothelial cells. J Clin Invest 1984; 74:1552–5.
84. Jutila MA, Rott L, Berg EL, Butcher EC. Function and regulation of the neutrophil MEL-14 antigen in vivo: comparison with LFA-1 and Mac-1. J Immunol 1989; 143:3318–24.
85. Kishimoto TK, Jutila MA, Berg EL, Butcher EC. Neutrophil Mac-1 and MEL-14 adhesion proteins inversely regulated by chemotactic factors. Science 1989; 245:1238–41.
86. Moqbel R, Sass-Kuhn SP, Goetzl EJ, Kay AB. Enhancement of neutrophil and eosinophil-mediated complement-dependent killing of schistosomula of *Schistosoma mansoni* in vitro by leukotriene B_4. Clin Exp Immunol 1983; 52:519–27.
87. Hoover RL, Karnovsky MJ, Austen KF, Corey EJ, Lewis RA. Leukotriene B_4 action on endothelium mediates augmented neutrophil/endothelial adhesion. Proc Nat Acad Sci USA 1984; 81:2191–3.
88. Dahlen S-E, Bjork J, Hedqvist P, Arfors K-E, Hammarstrom S, Lindgren J-A, Samuelsson B. Leukotrienes promote plasma leakage and leukocyte adhesion in postcapillary venules: in vivo effects with relevance to the acute inflammatory response. Proc Natl Acad Sci USA 1981; 78:3887–91.
89. Bray MA, Ford-Hutchinson AW, Smith MJH. Leukotriene B_4: an inflammatory mediator in vivo. Prostaglandins 1981; 22:213–22.
90. Lo SK, Van Seventer GA, Levin SH, Wright SD. Two leukocyte receptors (CD11a/CD18 and CD11b/CD18) mediate transient adhesion to endothelium by binding to different ligands. J Immunol 1989; 143:3325–9.
91. Bhattacherjee P, Hammond B, Salmon JA, Stepney R, Eakins KE. Chemotactic response to some arachidonic acid lipoxygenase products in the rabbit eye. Eur J Pharmacol 1981; 73:21–8.
92. Camp R, Jones RR, Brain S, Woollard P, Greaves M. Production of intraepidermal microabscesses by topical application of leukotriene B_4. J Invest Dermatol 1984; 82:202–4.

93. Camp RDR, Coutts AA, Greaves MW, Kay AB, Walport MJ. Responses of human skin to intradermal injection of leukotrienes C_4, D_4 and B_4. Br J Pharmacol 1983; 80:497–502.
94. Soter NA, Lewis RA, Corey EJ, Austen KF. Local effects of synthetic leukotrienes (LTC_4, LTD_4, LTE_4 and LTB_4) in human skin. J Invest Dermatol 1983; 80:115–9.
95. Thieroff R, Frohlich W, Ekerdt R. Chemotactic activity of LTB_4 in the skin of different laboratory animals in vivo. J Invest Dermatol 1988; 90:254.
96. Ford-Hutchinson AW, Brunet G, Savard P, Charleson S. Leukotriene B_4, polymorphonuclear leukocytes and inflammatory exudates in the rat. Prostaglandins 1984; 28:13–27.
97. Foster SJ, McCormick ME, Howarth A, Aked D. Leukocyte recruitment in the subcutaneous sponge implant model of acute inflammation in the rat is not mediated by leukotriene B_4. Biochem Pharmacol 1986; 35:1709–17.
98. Kopp DE, Esser B, Tashoff T, Goldman DW, Goetzl EJ, Lemanske RF Jr. In vivo and in vitro assessment of the role of leukotriene B_4 as a mediator of rat cutaneous late-phase reactions. J Allergy Clin Immunol 1986; 77:302–8.
99. Bray MA, Cunningham FM, Ford-Hutchinson AW, Smith MJH. Leukotriene B_4: a mediator of vascular permeability. Br J Pharmacol 1981; 72:483–6.
100. Wedmore CV, Williams TJ. Control of vascular permeability by polymorphonuclear leukocytes in inflammation. Nature 1981; 289:646–50.
101. Stenson WF, Chang K, Williamson JR. Tissue differences in vascular permeability induced by leukotrienes B_4 and prostaglandin E_2 in the rat. Prostaglandins 1986; 32:5–17.
102. Bjork J, Hedqvist P, Arfors KE. Increase in vascular permeability induced by leukotrienes B_4 and the role of polymorphonuclear leukocytes. Inflammation 1982; 6:189–200.
103. Chan C-C, Ford-Hutchinson A. Effects of synthetic leukotrienes on local blood flow and vascular permeability in porcine skin. J Invest Dermatol 1985; 84:154–7.
104. Rackham A, Ford-Hutchinson AW. Inflammation and pain sensitivity: effects of leukotrienes D_4, B_4 and prostaglandin E_1 in the rat paw. Prostaglandins 1983; 25:193–203.
105. Levine JD, Lau W, Kwiat G, Goetzl EJ. Leukotriene B_4 produced hyperalgesia that is dependent on polymorphonuclear leukocytes. Science 1984; 225:743–6.
106. Levine JD, Gooding J, Donatoni P, Borden L, Goetzl EJ. The role of the polymorphonuclear leukocyte in hyperalgesia. J Neurosci 1985; 5:3025–9.
107. Hori Y, Katori M, Harada Y, Uchida Y, Tanaka K. Potentiation of bradykinin-induced nociceptive response by arachidonate metabolites in dogs. Eur J Pharmacol 1986; 132:47–52.
108. O'Flaherty JT, Thomas MJ. Effect of 15-lipoxygenase-derived arachidonate metabolites on human neutrophil degranulation. Prostaglandins Leukotrienes and Medicine 1985; 17:199–212.
109. O'Flaherty JT, Thomas MJ, McCall CE, Wykle RL. Potentiating actions of hydroxyeicosatetraenoates on human neutrophil degranulation responses to leukotriene B_4 and phorbol myristate acetate. Res Commun Chem Pathol Pharmacol 1983; 40:475–87.
110. O'Flaherty JT, Thomas MJ, Hammett MJ, Caroll C, McCall CE, Wykle RL. 5-L-hydroxy-6,8,11,14-eicosatetraenoate potentiates the human neutrophil degranulating action of platelet-activating factor. Biochem Biophys Res Commun 1983; 111:1–7.
111. Shak S, Perez HO, Goldstein IM. A novel dioxygenation product of arachidonic acid possesses potent chemotactic activity for human polymorphonuclear leukocytes. J Biol Chem 1983; 258:14948–53.
112. Evans JF, Ford-Hutchinson AW, Fitzsimmons B, Rokach J. Biological activities of isomers of 8,15-dihydroxyeicosatetraenoic acid. Prostaglandins 1984; 28:435–8.
113. Evans JF, Leblanc Y, Fitzsimmons BJ, Charleson S, Nathaniel D, Léveillé C. Activation of leukocyte movement and displacement of [^{3}H]leukotriene B_4 from leukocyte membrane preparations by (12R)- and (12S)-hydroxyeicosatetraenoic acid. Biochim Biophys Acta 1987; 917:406–10.

114. Wollard PM. Stereochemical difference between 12-hydroxy-5,8,10,14-eicosatetraenoic acid in platelets and psoriatic lesions. Biochem Biophys Res Commun 1986; 136:169–76.
115. Murphy RC, Folck JF, Lumin S, Yadagin P, Zirrolli JA, Balazy M, Masferrer JL, Abraham NG, Schwartzman ML. 12(R)-hydroxyeicosatetraenoic acid: a vasodilator cytochrome P-450-dependent arachidonate metabolite from bovine corneal epithelium. J Biol Chem 1988; 263:17197–202.
116. Serhan CN, Hamberg M, Samuelsson B. Trihydroxytetraenes: a novel series of compounds formed from arachidonic acid in human leukocytes. Biochem Biophys Res Commun 1984; 118:943–9.
117. Serhan CN, Hamberg M, Samuelsson B. Lipoxins: novel series of biologically active compounds formed from arachidonic acid in human leukocytes. Proc Natl Acad Sci USA 1984; 81:5335–9.
118. Palmblad J, Gyllenhammar H, Ringertz B, Serhan CN, Samuelsson B, Nicolaou KC. The effects of lipoxin A and lipoxin B on functional responses of human granulocytes. Biochem Biophys Res Commun 1987; 145:168–75.
119. Ford-Hutchinson AW. Evidence for the involvement of leukotrienes and other lipoxygenase products in disease states. In: Rokach J, ed. Leukotrienes and lipoxygenases. Chemical, biological and clinical aspects. (Bioactive molecules II). Amsterdam: Elsevier, 1989:405–25.

5

G-Proteins and the Role of Second Messengers in the Regulation of the Human Neutrophil

PRAMOD M. LAD, JOHN S. KAPTEIN, CHING-KOW E. LIN,
COSMAS I. KALUNTA, STEPHEN J. SCOTT, and DAVID GUOQING GU
Kaiser Foundation Hospitals, Los Angeles, California

I. INTRODUCTION

A. Role of the Neutrophil in Health and Disease

The human neutrophil plays an important role in host defense. It moves to sites of infection along gradients of chemical mediators (chemotaxis) and destroys the infecting organism by ingestion (phagocytosis) and release of free radicals and proteases (superoxide generation and enzyme release). The neutrophil also plays a significant adverse role in disease processes, being a centrally important cell in inflammation. Here, inappropriately triggered responses of cell recruitment and degranulation can cause damage to tissues, a reaction found to contribute to multiple disease states including rheumatoid arthritis and asthma (1,2).

B. Chemoattractant Receptors and Neutrophil Function

Neutrophil functions are initiated by cell surface receptors. The most prominant among these, which will be the focus here, is the receptor for the chemoattractant, formyl-Met-Leu-Phe (FMLP) (3) one of the major peptides secreted from *E. coli* (4). Other chemoattractants include the peptide C5a (5), which is generated during complement activation in both the alternate and classical pathways, platelet-activating factor (PAF) (6), a lipid derived from a 1-alkyl-2-acyl-phosphatidyl choline, and leukotriene B_4 (LTB_4) (7), an eicosanoid generated from arachidonate (8). A number of other molecules have been mentioned as chemoattractants and may serve in this capacity. However, the molecular events associated with receptors for these agents have not been defined.

Although FMLP, PAF, C5a, LTB_4, and other agents are referred to as "chemoattractants," they cause multiple reactions in neutrophils. The earliest among these are the reactions of shape change, subsequent orientation in a chemical gradient, and aggregation (9,10). These constitute early cellular responses to chemoattractants; however, quantitative measures of these reactions have been difficult. For example, the measurement of aggregation depends not only on the nature of the chemoattractant, but also on the physical conditions of mixing, vessel configuration, and mode of ligand addition, rendering a reproducible measurement difficult.

To measure the neutrophil's response to chemotactic agents, studies have concentrated on measurements such as polymerization of actin, for which indirect assays based on inhibition of DNase activity (11), or light scattering and flow cytometry (12–15), have been proposed. Novel biophysical approaches such as the "cell-stiffening" assay developed by Elson (16) may point the way to more objective biophysical measures of these early reactions.

1. Indirect Measurement of Neutrophil Responses in Neutrophil Function

Under artificial conditions, which include the addition of cytochalasin B, reactions which are usually intracellular can be rendered extracellular (17,18). For example, release of lysosomal enzymes and the generation of superoxide and other free radicals generally occurs only upon the fusion of the lysosomal membrane with the phagosome. Here the addition of FMLP together with cytochalasin B causes extracellular release of enzymes from both primary and secondary granules. The reaction is readily observed by assaying both beta glucuronidase, a constituent of primary granules, and lysozyme, located predominantly in secondary granules. Release of other constituents (lactoferrin, elastase, and other enzymes) can also be utilized to assess degranulation. Similarly, superoxide generation can be observed extracellularly by electron transfer to cytochrome C and its reduction. Without cytochalasin B, externalization of intracellular reactions cannot be produced (17,18). These assays are thus particularly useful, since they are less time consuming than chemotaxis or bactericidal assays, the true counterparts of the in-vivo reaction, which are less readily evaluated. To summarize, shape change, aggregation changes, degranulation and superoxide generation, and various methods to measure motility in chemical gradients form the bulk of the functional measurements of the neutrophil's responses to chemoattractant stimulation.

C. Receptors That Mediate Phagocytosis

A different set of receptors mediates phagocytosis. These include the C3bi receptor (CR3) (19) and $Fc_{\gamma}R$ (I-III) (20,21). The coating of foreign particles by antibodies and complement (a process referred to as opsonization) is followed by the binding of these opsonized particles to the Fc and C3bi (CR3) receptors and their phagocytosis into the cells via structures known as phagosomes. As will be evident later, the molecular pathways associated with chemotaxis and phagocytosis are different (see Section II.B.9).

D. Receptors That Inhibit Chemoattractant Receptor Responses

Another group of receptors which has been studied includes the receptors for various regulatory molecules which serve predominantly to inhibit the reactions which are initiated by chemoattractants (22–30). These receptors, generally linked to adenylate cyclase and the generation of cyclic AMP, are the β-adrenergic, prostaglandin, and adenosine receptors (31–33).

E. Receptors That Augment Chemoattractant Receptor Responses

A separate group of receptors exists on neutrophils which seem not to initiate either chemotaxis or phagocytosis but serve instead to potentiate these responses. Notable among these are receptors for GM-CSF, substance P, and the muscarinic cholinergic receptors as well as receptors for newly discovered lymphokines such as tumor necrosis factor, transforming growth factor β, γ-interferon, and interleukins 1, 2, 4, and 8. The transduction mechanisms involved in these priming reactions, which render neutrophils more responsive to chemoattractants, is the subject of intense study in several laboratories (34). Various aspects of cytokine action on neutrophils are reviewed in other chapters in this volume.

II. ASSOCIATION OF CELL SURFACE RECEPTORS WITH G-PROTEINS

A. Introduction

An important question which is common to all the receptor studies mentioned above concerns the intracellular signal which is generated upon receptor occupancy. Studies in systems other than the neutrophil had already pointed to the existence of a family of "GTP-binding transducer proteins" which mediate the transduction of signal from the hormone-stimulated receptor to the specific target enzyme activated in response to the stimulation (34–36). These proteins, once referred to as N-proteins (for nucleotide binding), are now referred to as G-proteins (for GTP-binding). Table 1 summarizes the different types of G-proteins that have been detected thus far, the methods for their detection, and the target enzymes with which they are associated. The biochemical reactions which occur at G-proteins have been summarized elsewhere (34–36). The salient features are noted here.

Table 1 Family of G-Proteins and Target Enzymes in the Neutrophil System

G-protein	Toxin for which G-protein is a substrate	Target enzyme	Receptor association
G_s	Cholera toxin	Adenylate cyclase	B-adrenergic prostaglandin
G_i	Pertussis toxin	Adenylate cyclase	(?)
"G_i" or G_c	Pertussis toxin and cholera toxin (?)	PIP_2 lipase C	FMLP, PAF, LTB_4
"G_i/G_c" (insens)	Not ADP-ribosylated by toxins	(?)	(?)
G_{PLA_2}	Relationship to G_i or "G_i/G_c" unclear		
G_o	Not reported for neutrophils		

1. The G-proteins belong to a family of proteins which bear differing degrees of homology to one another. Small changes in the primary structure can differentiate between G-proteins which activate different types of enzymes (e.g., adenylate cyclase versus phospholipases). How such small changes determine drastically different enzymatic associations is unclear.

2. The nomenclature for G-proteins is still in a state of evolution. Systems for nomenclature are based in part on the action of the G-protein on a particular enzyme (for example, G_s is stimulatory for adenylate cyclase and G_i is inhibitory to adenylate cyclase) and partly on the type of toxin which can modify the G-protein. The rapidly growing number of these proteins, and their diverse regulatory roles, suggest that a carefully revised classification and nomenclature system needs to be developed.

3. The G-proteins consist of three subunits, termed α, β, and γ. Activation of the G-protein upon binding GTP (or GTP analogs) involves dissociation of the β-γ complex from the α-subunit. The β-γ subunits remain tightly associated with each other. The receptor G-protein α-subunit complex then associates with the target enzyme, causing activation.

4. The G-proteins bind guanine nucleotides. GTP is stimulatory, while GDP is inhibitory to hormone activation. Activation and inhibition of adenylate cyclase require the simultaneous presence of both hormone/receptor complex and GTP.

5. GTP is hydrolyzed by a GTPase activity associated with the G-protein. The product of the reaction, GDP, is rapidly exchanged for GTP upon hormone stimulation. This reaction is referred to as hormone-induced nucleotide exchange.

6. Guanine nucleotide analogs such as Gpp(NH)p bind tightly to G-proteins and induce persistent changes in the activity of the target enzymes such as adenylate cyclase.

7. The α-subunits of the G-proteins are substrates for various toxins. These include cholera toxin- and pertussis toxin-sensitive substrates, a group of proteins modified by both toxins (37), and a new class of proteins modified by botulinum toxins (see section II.B.8). This property has been helpful in identifying broad subtypes of G-proteins.

8. A novel group of G-proteins of small molecular weight (20–25 kDa) clearly different from the α- and β-subunits of adenylate cyclase-activating enzyme have been identified (38,39). Their role in cellular regulation is not altogether clear, although certain trends are beginning to emerge and are discussed later.

B. Identification of G-Proteins in the Human Neutrophil

1. The G_s Protein and cAMP Signaling

For the human neutrophil the first G-protein to be identified was G_s, which was shown to be associated with stimulation of adenylate cyclase following ligand binding to the β-adrenergic or prostaglandin receptors (Figure 1). G_s was shown to be a substrate for modification by cholera toxin (31,32), which catalyzed ADP ribosylation of the α-subunit. In the whole cell, stimulation by prostaglandins and β-receptor agonists resulted in an increase in intracellular cyclic AMP. The order of potency of various GTP analogs on cyclic AMP elevation in whole cells paralleled the activation of adenylate cyclase in isolated plasma membrane. More recently, the purinergic receptor for adenosine has been shown to be another member of the G_s-linked family of receptors.

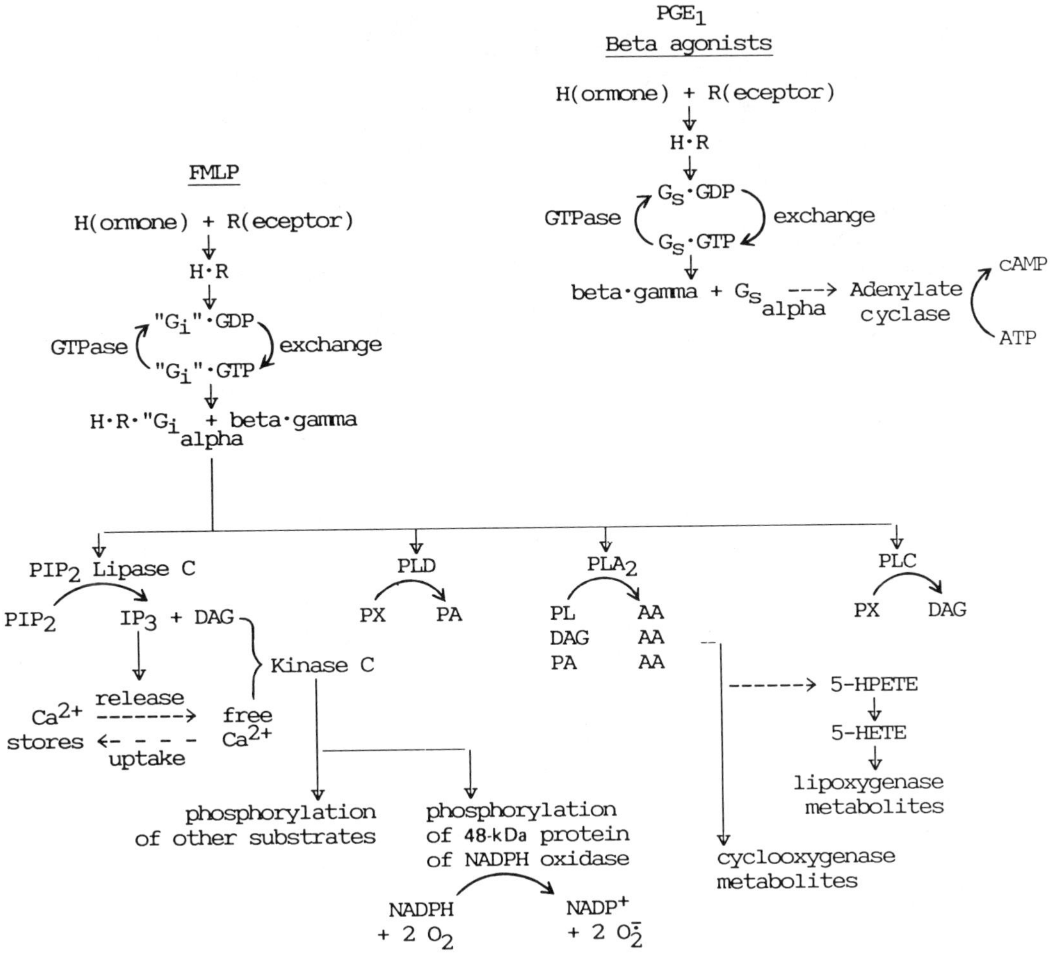

Figure 1 Activation of multiple enzymes through G-proteins. Activation of adenyl cyclase following stimulation of the PGE_1 receptor is illustrated on the upper right. This pathway is mediated via the G_s protein and leads to increases in the second messenger cAMP. The remainder of the figure illustrates proposed pathways by which various enzymes of lipid metabolism may be activated following stimulating of the cell by FMLP. These pathways are activated by a G_i protein. Activation of these pathways may lead to multiple second messengers being generated, including PIP_2, IP_3, DAG, Ca^{2+}, phosphatidic acid, arachidonic acid, HETE, and metabolites of the cyclooxygenase and lipoxygenase pathways.

The G_s-protein is identified by cholera toxin-mediated ADP-ribosylation of the α-subunit. We note, parenthetically, the mode of action of toxin. The toxin itself consists of two subunits, a B-subunit, which binds ganglioside GM3, and an A-subunit, which contains the ADP-ribosyl transferase activity. Using labeled NAD as substrate, a 42- to 45-kDa α-subunit of G_s is ADP-ribosylated. The ADP ribosylation inhibits GTPase activity, accelerates the rate of nucleotide exchange, and renders GTP a potent hormone-independent stimulator of the adenylate cyclase system (34–36).

Speculation arose that the FMLP receptor too may be coupled to G_s and thus to adenylate cyclase (40,41). This was based on the observation that, in whole neutrophils, exposure of the cells to FMLP caused a transient rise in cyclic AMP. The reason for this rise in cyclic AMP is not apparent. It is clear, however, that stimulation of adenylate cyclase is not observed in intact membranes. Indeed, very high concentrations of FMLP (10,000 times the levels required for cell function enhancement) cause paradoxically a slight inhibition of the enzyme (42). It is possible that the rise in cyclic AMP stems from an effect on phosphodiesterase. The transience of this effect is probably related to the transient rise in calcium which accompanies FMLP stimulation of neutrophils. This would bind to the calcium-binding protein calmodulin, which is known to regulate phosphodiesterase activity. This hypothesis remains to be completely validated.

1. The G_i Protein

The nature of the G-protein associated with the FMLP receptor thus remained unknown. An important tool became available in the form of pertussis toxin, which was shown by Ui to be a modifier of the G-protein associated with inhibition of adenylate cyclase (G_i) (43–50). Work in 1984–1985 from several laboratories showed that in neutrophils, pertussis toxin treatment caused a complete abolition of the multiple responses associated with the FMLP receptor (43–55). These included chemotaxis, aggregation, superoxide generation, enzyme release, shape change, actin polymerization, and capping. Furthermore, this effect was shown to be general, in that other receptors for PAF (56,57) and LTB_4 (36) were also shown to be inhibited by pertussis toxin modification.

That the effects are due to a protein which is structurally associated with the FMLP receptor has been demonstrated by the finding that guanine nucleotide exchange as well as GTPase (58) activities mediated by FMLP stimulation of the FMLP receptor were abolished following pertussis toxin treatment (54,55). Abolition was associated with the ADP-ribosylation of a 41 kDa protein. This substrate was shown to be distinct from the cholera toxin substrate (46–50). More recently, this G-protein has been purified, its distribution in the cell has been determined, and the protein has been reconstituted in phospholipid vesicles with the "purified" FMLP receptor (59,60).

a. Calcium Signaling via G_i. Previous studies had shown that one of the major consequences of FMLP occupancy of its receptor was a rise in calcium concentration inside neutrophils (61). With the development of calcium-binding dyes, it was shown that FMLP induced a rapid rise in intracellular Ca^{2+} concentration followed by a sharp decline back to baseline, the entire response being over within a time period of about 20–50 s. This was followed by a slower rise in steady-state levels of intracellular calcium. Pertussis toxin treatment of neutrophils abolishes the rise in intracellular calcium, suggesting that the FMLP receptor-G_i complex is involved in calcium-related transduction. Calcium levels inside neutrophils and other cells are regulated by diverse systems (calcium influx, efflux). Other ionic events, most prominently the sodium proton antiport system, are also regulated by the FMLP receptor (see Section III.I). For the purpose of continuity, the emphasis here is on the mobilization of calcium from intracellular stores; other systems are considered later.

2. The G_i-Protein and Regulation of the PI Cycle

Studies in systems other than the neutrophil, by Berridge and co-workers (62–65), showed that other events intervened between hormone-receptor stimulation of G-proteins and the subsequent Ca^{2+} mobilization. The rise in intracellular calcium was due to the formation and release into the cytoplasm of inositol trisphosphate (IP_3), which functioned as an intracellular ionophore to release calcium from intracellular stores. The IP_3 was derived from a complex series of related enzymatic reactions which are shown in Figure 2. Phosphorylation of PI results in the formation of PIP and PIP_2. Hydrolysis of PIP_2 results in the formation of IP_3, which acts upon intracellular calcium stores to release calcium. Diacylglycerol is also released during these reactions, and the combined action of diacylglycerol with calcium results in the activation of protein kinase C. The relevance of this overall pathway in neutrophils has been explored by various investigators (66–68). As a result of these studies, it became clear that FMLP activates a PIP_2 lipase C to produce IP_3. Pertussis toxin treatement leads to a loss of PIP_2 lipase C activation. Put together with previous studies, the overall pathways for activation by the FMLP receptor now reads as follows: FMLP receptor $\rightarrow$ G_i $\rightarrow$ PIP_2 lipase C $\rightarrow$ IP_3 $\rightarrow$ Ca^{2+}.

4. Lipases Without G-Proteins

The initial clarity of these observations has, however, grown murkier in the last three years. An important observation made by Crockroft and others is that FMLP receptor occupancy caused hydrolysis of other lipids, and this occurred in much larger measures than did the hydrolysis of PI (66,67,69–90). Activation of phospholipase A_2, C, and D have now been shown to occur. In addition, release of arachidonate from neutrophils loaded with labeled arachidonate has also been noted. This led to the hypothesis that, in addition to PIP_2 lipase C, phospholipases C, D, and A_2 were also involved in the actions of the FMLP receptor (Figure 1). However, the direct link of these enzymes to the FMLP receptor and evidence that their activation involves an FMLP receptor-G protein complex is far from clear. Phospholipases have been noted in the cytosol as

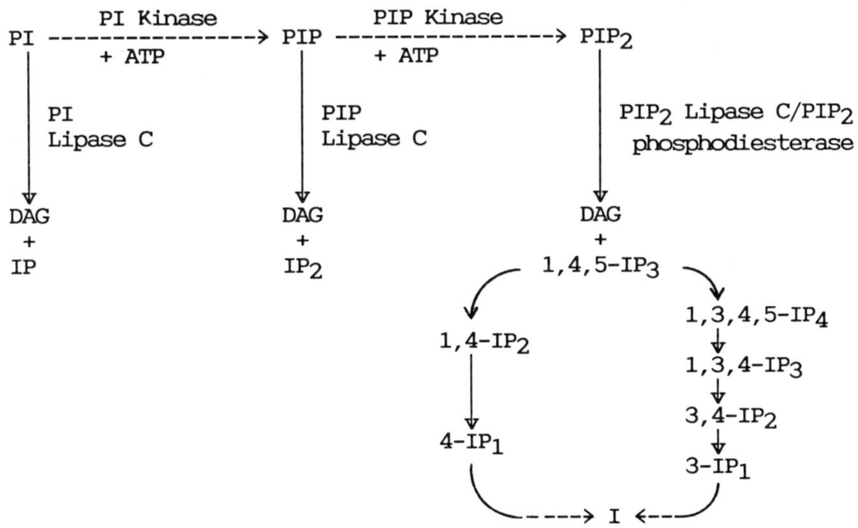

Figure 2 PI and IP_3 metabolism: the pathways by which the inositol phospholipids can be interconverted.

well as in the plasma membrane, thus complicating the interpretation of these results. Several of these enzymes are also regulated by calcium, raising the possibility that calcium release from intracellular stores activates these enzymes, in a fashion rather analogous to that noted for cyclic AMP phosphodiesterase mentioned earlier. Also, the problem of whether the PI kinases are under the control of G-proteins remains unresolved. This seems particularly important, since the formation of PIP and PIP_2 are among the earliest measurable biochemical reactions in neutrophils. In short, an abundance of phospholipases with no clear link to G-proteins seems to contribute to phospholipid metabolism in the neutrophil system.

5. *Recent Views of G-Proteins in Human Neutrophils*

After the initial identification of the major pertussis toxin substrate in human neutrophils, it was shown that this protein is also a substrate for cholera toxin. On the basis of this experiment a "novel" pertussis toxin/cholera toxin-sensitive G_i type of protein has been proposed distinct from the G_i-protein which is a substrate for pertussis toxin alone. The results remain ambiguous, since labeling with cholera toxin is weak (91). The presence of contaminating cytosolic factors which may enhance ADP ribosylation and which are termed ARF can augment the labeling of several proteins in plasma membranes; the significance of these substrates for ADP-ribosyl transferases remains unknown. The amount of toxin needed, and the particular conditions of ADP ribosylation, may determine whether modification by cholera toxin is observed. Certainly the functional effects of pertussis toxin in abolishing neutrophil functions are far more rapidly observable than those with cholera toxin, casting doubt on the significance of the labeling patterns noted.

Analysis of HL-60 cells points to two closely coupled proteins, only one of which purifies with the FMLP receptor. Immunochemical differentiation of this protein from the "G_i alpha"-protein is also implied (92,93). On balance, however, the following questions remain: (a) Are there two pertussis toxin substrates present in the neutrophil membrane? (b) Is only one of these proteins a substrate for both cholera and pertussis toxins? Is the pattern of labeling by both toxins reflective of complex and possibly nonspecific labeling condition, or truly indicative of structural differences which permit unique labeling? (c) The relationship of cholera toxin modification of membrane protein to alterations of FMLP-related activities such as guanine nucleotide exchange or GTPase has not been demonstrated thus far. (d) What are the enzymatic targets for these two substates? Are they exclusive for PIP_2 lipase C or PLC or PLA_2 or PLD, all of which have been shown to be linked to the FMLP receptor? (e) Since cloning of the G-proteins from HL-60 cells points to only small differences in sequence from the G_i-proteins identified in other cells, the question arises as to how these small differences might determine complete changes in enzymatic targets. These questions still remain to be resolved.

The suggestion that the G-protein may itself be part of a heterogeneous family of proteins suggests that a definitive delineation of structure and function is likely to be forthcoming. A summary of the G-protein family related to receptor regulation and signal transduction is provided in Table 1.

6. *Low-Molecular-Weight G-Proteins*

An exciting finding relates to small-molecular-weight G-proteins (in the range of 20–26 kDa) which have been found in the human neutrophil. Using an overlay of labeled GTP on blots of "denatured" proteins, Bokoch and others have been able to detect three proteins whose subunits are 26 kDa, 24 kDa, and 22 kDa (94–98). Crossreactivity with a monoclonal antibody to the gene product of *ras* was also observed, implying that these proteins may be in part homologous to the *ras* family of GTP-binding proteins.

The functional role for these proteins is being explored. Burgoyne, who has examined similar proteins in chromaffin granule-containing cells, suggests that they may be involved in exocytosis (39). Studies by Jesaitis point to the possibility that a 22-kDa protein may be the GTP-binding protein which is involved in conferring GTP sensitivity to the NADPH oxidase complex (99). By analogy with *ras*, a role for these proteins in the regulation of transcriptionally significant events has also been proposed (39); this possibility is not unlikely in neutrophils, since it has recently been shown that the neutrophil does indeed have inducible mRNAs for a number of proteins and, though "fully" differentiated, still retains some potential for transductional regulation of nuclear events.

7. *G-Proteins Related to NADPH Oxidase*

A problem with the family of small-molecular-weight G-proteins which have been identified thus far has been that these G-proteins have not been associated with any particular function. An exception, however, is offered by the newly discovered small-molecular-weight G-protein which co-purifies with the cytochrome that is essential in the functioning of the NADPH oxidase system (100,101). This system is central to the production of superoxide ion and consists of multiple components including a cytochrome, NADPH-binding proteins, flavo proteins, and other constituents. Recently, progress has been made in the definition of a membrane preparation in which this enzyme system can be studied (101–103). Work with this form of the system showed a requirement for GTP in the activation of the oxidase. The GTP activation of the oxidase was insensitive to cholera and pertussis toxins. Uncoupling of the GTP-sensitive oxidase from the FMLP receptor-G_i proteins could also be demonstrated, suggesting that a novel form of G-protein might be present. This has been borne out by the studies of the purified cytochrome which co-purifies with a GTP-binding protein of low molecular weight. Preliminary indications (99) are that this protein is partially analogous to the *ras* G-protein and may be identical to a G-protein termed *rap-1* (also *Krev-1*), a *ras*-related protein which has recently been shown to be associated with the *Drosophila Dras 3* gene, which has also been isolated from a human fibroblast cDNA library.

8. *Botulinum Toxin Substrates*

An emerging area of research is the role of botulinum C2 toxin-mediated potentiation of the neutrophil oxidase system. A role for actin polymerization is thought to be involved and ADP ribosylation of actin has been observed (97). The toxin produces "mixed" effects (96) on neutrophil function, enhancing superoxide generation and enzyme release, but inhibiting chemotaxis. *Rho,* a GTP-binding protein, has also been shown to be a substrate for the toxin (95). The mechanisms which relate ADP ribosylation to regulation of cell function are being examined further.

9. *Distinct Pathways for Chemotaxis and Phagocytosis*

While G-proteins are involved in the actions of chemoattractants, they do not play a direct role in the action of receptors involved in phagocytosis. Thus pertussis toxin does not affect phagocytosis, while it clearly inhibits chemotaxis and receptor capping (104). A selective role for G-proteins in cellular regulation is indicated by these findings.

Recent observations (105,106) suggest that cytokine-mediated stimulation of phagocytosis may be mediated by pertussis toxin-sensitive G-protein. Stimulation of phagocytosis by cytokines should be distinguished from the primary phagocytic process, however.

These observations also relate to the Fc receptor-mediated action in neutrophils. FcγR III is present in neutrophils (100-200 × 10^3 sites/cell). FcγR I and II are present in smaller amounts. Although a role for PI cycle-related effects has been proposed by analogy with the IgE receptor, this has not been convincingly demonstrated (20,21).

In short, signaling pathways in phagocytosis remain controversial. "Local" rises of calcium have been proposed, but their relevance for cellular activation is unclear (107).

III. SECOND MESSENGERS

A. Introduction

Tremendous advances in the understanding of transduction pathways have led to a rapid increase in the number of known second messengers which can be generated inside the cell (see Figure 1). The simplest set of criteria originally proposed by Sutherland (108,109) for the definition of a second messenger—that it can mimic completely the hormone system which produces it—has suffered in the process, however. For example, calcium is produced by the action of IP_3 on intracellular stores. IP_3 itself is produced by the hydrolysis of PIP_2, which also produces diacylglycerol; however, diacylglycerol can also be produced by the hydrolysis of other lipids through the action of diverse phospholipase C activities. The diacylglycerol which is required for the sustained metabolic effects in neutrophils is almost certainly derived not from PIP_2 but from other sources. Furthermore, diacylglycerol is itself converted to other metabolites, which could themselves act as second messengers. The action of diacylglycerol lipase produces arachidonate; phosphorylation generates phosphatidic acid. Both of these can exert effects independent of diacylglycerol. These examples illustrate some conceptual features about second messengers which are summarized below:

1. Combined action of multiple messengers may be required to generate the effect of the hormone.
2. Degeneracy in production makes it difficult to ascribe a second messenger to a particular reaction or hormone system. Diacylglycerol is produced by a number of different enzymatic steps. Which is proximal to hormone action and which is secondary is unclear.
3. Second messengers can generate other messengers or other hormones. Diacylglycerol can be converted to arachidonate, and arachidonate can be metabolized by the cyclooxygenase and lipoxygenase pathways to produce many different hormones.
4. Reconstitution of a complete transduction system in the membrane itself to verify a tightly linked transduction system, as for the case of adenylate cyclase, may not be possible in many instances. IP_3 stores do not exist in the plasma membranes, and calcium generation cannot be reproduced in plasma membrane preparations alone.
5. Second messengers without function are being identified at a rapid rate. Intracellular pH, regulated by hormone through the action on the sodium/proton antiport system, is one such system. Its precise function remains unknown in

neutrophils, although the mechanisms for its generation have been studied intensively. Cyclic GMP production has been examined in some detail in neutrophils, but its role in the function of most cells including granulocytes remains poorly understood.

6. Precursors to second messengers can turn out to be "second messengers." PIP_2, the precursor to IP_3, is now suspected of having a role in the control of actin polymerization at least as important as that for IP_3.
7. G-proteins may themselves be messengers. A soluble α-subunit of a G-protein is found in the cytosol, as is a subunit analogous to the β-subunit. This group of proteins may turn out to be middle messengers, i.e., proteins involved in signal transduction and in hormone action in the cytosol and in the nucleus.

The above considerations point to several complexities in the interpretation of the nature of second messengers, a situation far more complex than when the term was introduced 30 years ago. Figure 1 summarizes the different G-protein-related pathways for enzyme activation.

B. Cyclic AMP as a Second Messenger

Agents which are linked with the activation of adenylate cyclases in isolated neutrophil membranes and cause elevation of intracellular cyclic AMP in whole neutrophils inhibit neutrophil functions (22–30,110,111). PGE_1, β-adrenergic agonists, and most recently adenosine have all been shown to inhibit various neutrophil functions. That the effect is in fact due to cyclic AMP was verified by the fact that cyclic AMP analogs such as Br-cAMP and dibutyryl-cAMP are inhibitory to multiple neutrophil functions (22). The question of the specificity of this inhibition was considered next. Our own work has shown that receptor-specific threshold effects of cyclic AMP are involved in the inhibition of neutrophil functions (23). Accordingly, the type of receptor occupied and the level of cyclic AMP that is produced are both important in determining which particular function is inhibited and to what extent. A potency series for the activation of adenylate cyclase is $PGE_1 >> \beta$-adrenergic agonists $>$ adenosine. Comparisons of the effects of PGE_1 and beta agonists shows that (a) either agent will inhibit superoxide generation without the presence of a phosphodiesterase inhibitor; (b) inhibition of phosphodiesterase is obligatory to the inhibition of enzyme release by cylic AMP; and (c) under conditions of PDE inhibition, only PGE_1, the most potent stimulator of adenylate cyclase, is effective in the attenuation of enzyme release. These results suggest that the potency series observed in the activation of adenylate cyclase and elevation of cyclic AMP are both relevant to the specificity of the neutrophil function that is inhibited. The sensitivity of superoxide generation to inhibition by low levels of cyclic AMP is in agreement with the observations made recently that a phosphoprotein subunit of 47 kDa (probably a substrate for kinase A), is involved in the action of the NADPH oxidase which is involved in superoxide generation (102). In contrast to the inhibition of enzyme release and superoxide generation, relatively little information is available for the inhibition of aggregation and chemotaxis. The latter is particularly difficult to study, since the assay itself spans several hours—a time frame in which steady-state cyclic AMP levels cannot be maintained. Specificity of inhibition is observed relative to the type of stimulant that is used for neutrophil activation (23). Observations here again point to considerable specificity in that stimuli such as FMLP are more readily inhibited than is the activation by opsonized zymosan or immune complexes.

C. Cyclic GMP as a Second Messenger (26–29,112)

Cyclic GMP is altered by various agents acting on the neutrophil. Early observations indicated that stimulation of the muscarinic cholinergic receptor caused an elevation of cyclic GMP levels in neutrophils, and direct stimulation of guanylate cyclase was demonstrated to occur predominantly via indirect mechanisms involving the cyclooxygenase and lipoxygenase pathways. More recently, Coffey has demonstrated a modulation of guanylate cyclase activity by GM-CSF (113,114). The matter is reviewed by Coffey in greater detail in a later chapter in this volume.

The functional significance of cGMP in neutrophil action is not known. A potentiation of various neutrophil functions is indicated, an effect opposite to that of cAMP.

D. PIP_2 as a Second Messenger

Since the discoveries of the PI cycle and the realization that IP_3 is a second messenger (Figure 2), the prevailing assumption has been that calcium generated from intracellular stores by the action of IP_3 serves to initiate most cellular processes. However, this view has been increasingly called into question by a number of studies. At least two investigators have noted that actin polymerization does not require calcium mobilization (115,116). In our own work (see Section 4) we have shown that desensitization of cell function can be achieved without perturbations of calcium mobilization. These observations suggest the following possibilities: (a) Calcium is not required for initiation of cell function; (b) calcium is required for the initiation of some but not all cellular processes; (c) calcium-dependent action of kinase C and other enzymes serves predominantly to inhibit rather than initiate cell function; (d) degeneracy is noted with respect to calcium mobilization in that only a very small portion of strategically distributed calcium finds a role in cell function. Evidence thus far suggests that calcium is required for the initiation of some but not all cellular responses (115,116). For example, the phenomenon of degranulation depends on the level of calcium generated inside the cell, higher levels being required for release from secondary granules than from primary granules (117–119). It is equally clear, however, that little or no calcium is required for initiating the process of aggregation and the associated processes of cell shape change and actin polymerization.

The question posed by these observations is simple enough. If calcium is not the second messenger, then what is the likely messenger for cellular control of early reactions which involve actin polymerization? The answer, which seems to be emerging from a number of studies, is that PIP_2 itself may serve as a regulator of actin polymerization, and that this action may not require bulk calcium mobilization, or, in the extreme, may be independent of the subsequent mobilization of calcium from intracellular stores. Such a role for PIP_2 is becoming evident from the studies of Yin and colleagues, and others (120–123), who have shown that the actin-binding proteins contain specific regions which bind PIP_2. Such PIP_2-binding regions may function to alter the polymerization properties of actin without the requirement for calcium. Conversely, the conversion of PIP_2 to IP_3 may alter the properties of actin-binding proteins, not by virtue of the calcium-mobilizing properties of IP_3, but by virtue of the diminution in the levels of PIP_2 and the alteration in the state of actin-binding proteins stabilized by PIP_2. Since PIP_2 is generated in low amounts in the cell, progress in understanding its role in actin polymerization is likely to come primarily from the study of isolated cytoskeleton and from the study of the interactions of purified actin-binding proteins with actin.

E. Inositol Phosphates as Second Messengers

The evidence is clear that IP_3 is a second messenger in human neutrophils. In permeabilized cells, IP_3 can function as a second messenger, causing elevations in intracellular calcium and potentiating various cellular functions (37). It is clear that extracellular calcium is not required for the production of IP_3. Thus, the sequence that PIP_2 lipase C results in IP_3 production, which causes release of intracellular calcium, seems reasonably certain. An intracellular receptor for IP_3 has been reported, and a calcium-sequestering domain which is thought to account for the bulk of the calcium mobilized by chemoattractant has been located (117–119).

A number of enzyme systems have been identified which catalyze the rapid conversion of IP_3 to other metabolites (85,86,124). The interconversions which are shown in Figure 2 indicate that 1,4,5-IP_3 undergoes two reactions, conversion by a kinase to 1,3,4,5-IP_4 and a dephosphorylation reaction to 1,4-IP_2. The 1,4-IP_2 is further dephosphorylated to 4-IP_1 and subsequently to inositol. A similar pathway of dephosphorylation is observed for the tetraphosphate derivative of inositol. 1,3,4,5-IP_4 is rapidly converted to 1,3,4-IP_3 and then to 3,4-IP_2 and subsequently to 3-IP_1.

With such a complex array of metabolites being rapidly induced (125), the question which remains is the significance of the metabolites other than 1,4,5-IP_3 and possible regulation of the enzymes which cause these interconversions. The latter is important because the enzymes involved in the interconversions are specific. Work in platelets indicates that a specific phosphatase is responsible for dephosphorylation of 1,4,5-IP_3 and 1,3,4,5-IP_4 (126,127). Lithium-sensitive enzymes specific for 1,3,4-IP_3 and 1,4-IP_2, and for 3,4-IP_2 and 4-IP_1 dephosphorylation, have been noted (62,63).

The role of inositol phosphates other than the 1,4,5-IP_3 is as yet unclear in the neutrophil system. The tetraphosphate is thought to promote calcium influx, a process which is itself augmented by rises in intracellular calcium (62,63,128). The lithium sensitivity of the inositol phosphatases has been noted previously. In addition, studies of the conversion of 1,4,5-IP_3 to IP_2 show that PMA activates the phosphatase that converts 1,4,5-IP_3 to the IP_2. Others have reported that the IP_3 kinase is also paradoxically activated by PMA pretreatment (129). Involvement of a calmodulin-dependent kinase in the regulation of IP_3 kinase has also been proposed (130). The relevance of these systems for the neutrophil is as yet unclear.

Further progress in this area will probably address such unanswered questions as the nature of the IP_3 receptor, the exact specificities of the enzymes involved in inositol phosphate interconversions, the significance for cellular regulation of the individual inositol phosphates, and the influence of the activation of individiual kinases (kinase A and kinase C) on the activities of these enzymes.

F. Calcium as a Second Messenger

Stimulation of neutrophils with FMLP causes a number of changes in calcium movements. The major changes include mobilization of intracellular calcium, initiation of calcium influx, and a late phase of calcium efflux. Increases in the levels of intracellular calcium have been the most intensely studied, and, as described above, the sequence of events leading up to the mobilization of intracellular calcium (PIP_2 conversion to IP_3) has been relatively well established. Some interest surrounds the temporal sequence of these three movements of calcium. As discussed below, it is now thought that the mobilization of intracellular calcium is the earliest of the three events, and that elevated levels of intracellular calcium may prime the cells for calcium influx and efflux (37,131,132).

In addition to the movement of calcium, changes in membrane potential have been observed in neutrophils after FMLP receptor occupancy, and increases in alkalinization of the cytoplasm due to the activation of the sodium proton antiport system have also been noted (132,133). The relationship of these events to calcium movements is as yet unclear.

A detailed model which explains the ionic movements and ties them into the biochemical events has not been forthcoming. Proceeding by analogy to other systems, the following picture seems to be emerging. FMLP occupancy of its receptor causes a rise in intracellular calcium levels via the hydrolysis of PIP_2 and the generation of IP_3. The mobilized calcium causes an increase in the influx of calcium, a process that may itself be potentiated by both IP_4 as well as calcium itself. Finally, calcium efflux is activated, probably as a result of the activation of kinase C by calcium and diacylglycerol. It is unclear whether the calcium magnesium ATPase, which may regulate calcium efflux, is under the control of FMLP or a G-protein. A direct role of an FMLP receptor-G protein complex in the regulation of calcium influx and efflux is implied by the literature but is not proven (8,118,119,131).

The possible connection of the membrane depolarization to calcium movements has been examined (134). The results thus far indicate that while a mediation of a G-protein sensitive to pertussis toxin seems likely, membrane depolarization can for the most part be separated from calcium mobilization and calcium influx. It has been suggested that voltage-gated calcium channels are not involved in the depolarization events. The most compelling argument comes from kinetic studies in which depolarization events occur after the mobilization of intracellular calcium. The data point to the hypothesis that intracellular calcium mobilization precedes the influx of calcium from external sources; whether a discrete coupling of released calcium to distinct kinase C isoenzymes or to different phases of neutrophil activation mediated by the same isoenzyme occurs as suggested is still unclear.

G. Arachidonate as a Second Messenger

Arachidonate is a centrally important agent in the generation of inflammatory mediators. It is the precursor to prostaglandin, thromboxane, and leukotriene generation. All of these agents are known to affect neutrophil functions. In addition, arachidonate exercises independent influences on neutrophil function. It is a regulator of enzyme release and superoxide generation (135,136). For these reasons the generation of arachidonate, its regulation, and significance for neutrophil function have been the subject of considerable study.

Arachidonate is generated by the action of phospholipase A_2 on phospholipids (Figure 1). The position of hydrolysis has been established as the 2-position, and the enzyme involved has been identified as a phospholipase A_2. Of obvious interest is which of the phospholipids can serve as a generator of arachidonate. The studies of Takenawa are pertinent (79). Studies of ^{32}P incorporation suggest that the phosphate is incorporated predominantly into PI and PA upon FMLP stimulation. The levels of incorporation into other phospholipids are substantially lower. When the calcium ionophore A23187 is examined as a stimulus, ^{32}P is incorporated into PI and PA (due to de-novo synthesis of phospholipid), but incorporation into PC, PE, and PS is paradoxically inhibited. Incorporation of ^{3}H-arachidonate suggests also that the phospholipid which is notably remodeled as a result of FMLP stimulation is PI. The arachidonate that is released from neutrophils prelabeled with ^{3}H-arachidonate is derived from PI (137,138). In ionophore-stimulated neutrophils, by contrast, hydrolysis of PC, PE, and PI is also observed and is verified by the independent measurement of the corresponding lysophospholipids. The temporal sequence suggests that the hydrolysis of PI precedes the hydrolysis of other phospholipids. Other investigators (100,102) have noted that arachidonate can be generated indirectly as follows: The first step is the hydrolysis of PI by a specific phospholipase C; the second is conversion of DAG to PA by a DAG kinase; the third consists of arachidonate being released by the action of a PA-specific phospholipase A_2. The indirect activation of a DAG-specific phospholipase has also been described. The stimulation of PLA_2 by kinase C has also been proposed based on the finding that PMA stimulates arachidonate release, a reaction blocked by H-7. The various reactions are summarized in Figure 1.

An important question is whether arachidonate release, which is stimulated by FMLP, is under the regulation of a G-protein. Certainly the evidence is clear that pertussis toxin treatment abolishes the release of arachidonate. Thus an FMLP-dependent and a pertussis toxin-sensitive substrate (probably a G_i type of protein) are involved. The next question concerns the target enzyme which this complex might activate. The answer to this is far from clear. If the data for the participation of PIP_2 lipase C are somewhat unclear, the situation with PLA_2 seems frankly contradictory. A direct relationship of FMLP to a PLA_2 has been noted by Bormann (77) but has been questioned by other investigators (139). The alternative view is that the FMLP receptor-G_i complex is linked to a phospholipase C and arachidonate generation is a distal step which is activated indirectly through the action of DAG lipase or PA-directed lipase A_2. Since neutrophils are important cells in the generation of inflammation and arachidonate is central to pathways of inflammation, this rather confusing picture needs to be corrected. The isolation and definitive characterization of phospholipases and their relationship to G-proteins needs to be explored directly.

Metabolism of arachidonate by neutrophils has also been studied intensively. The major conclusions are that both cyclooxygenase and lipoxygenase pathways are stimulated in neutrophils by FMLP. Conversion of arachidonate to prostaglandins E_2, $F_{2\alpha}$, thromboxane B_2, and monohydroxyeicosatetraenoic acid has been shown. Most important, however, the conversion of arachidonate to leukotriene B_4 has been documented (80,81). Since LTB_4 is a chemoattractant for neutrophils, this observation may have significance for a positive-feedback cycle in the inflammatory process. However, an argument against a prominent role for LTB_4 is that its effects on neutrophils, though observed at low concentrations, are weak in their magnitude. In addition, claims about the isolation of the LTB_4 receptors are somewhat difficult to evaluate, probably because of their low receptor density.

Generation of arachidonate does not always lead to its metabolism (80,81). An interesting finding is that calcium mobilized from intracellular stores does not correlate with the amount of arachidonate that is released and does not ensure its subsequent conversion into 5-HETE or leukotrienes. For example, immune complexes and opsonized zymosan produce local enhancement of calcium levels and are still potent stimulators of arachidonate release. Thus, indirect mechanisms which require modulation of intracellular calcium as a precursor to PLA_2 activation are not supported by this data. The exception here is that ionophore causes a stimulation of both arachidonate release and its subsequent metabolism.

The data on the metabolism of arachidonate in neutrophils remains a little controversial. Clancy (80) suggests that the production of arachidonate metabolites requires the activation of a lipoxygenase which can be dissociated from the activation of phospholipase A_2; by contrast, the studies of Bokoch and Reed (81) imply that direct activation without the supply of exogenous arachidonate are sufficient to produce arachidonate metabolism (140). The matter is as yet unresolved.

H. HETE as a Second Messenger (102,141)

Activation of phospholipase A_2 causes release of arachidonate from the 2-position of phospholipids; the lipoxygenase then converts the arachidonate to an intermediate 5-HPETE which is subsequently converted to 5-HETE by glutathione peroxidase. Collectively these reactions are part of what is referred to as the lipoxygenase pathway, which terminates with the production of various leukotrienes (Figure 1). Multiple enzymes of the pathway are either dependent on or are activated by calcium. Thus any role for 5-HETE as a messenger constitutes a potential feedback cycle in which its production is amplified by the pathway on which the metabolite itself might act.

Unlike other "second messengers," the action of 5-HETE is essentially completely dependent on the co-activation of kinase C, either with PMA or with DAG. Since the action of both PMA and DAG depends on the co-presence of calcium, it is possible that the effect of 5-HETE may rest in part on its functioning as a facilitator of calcium entry. Whether this action requires a specific interaction with a channel or more generally by membrane perturbation remains to be elucidated. The concept has precedence, since it has been proposed that prostaglandins may in part activate the neutrophil at low concentrations by functioning as an ionophore rather than by specific action through cell surface receptors linked to G-proteins and the activation of adenylate cyclase. Complete nonspecificity of the membrane perturbing action of the 5-HETE seems unlikely in view of the fact that 5-HETE is ineffective in promoting kinase C potentiation of either superoxide generation or calcium influx.

The difficulties encountered above are typical of the problems encountered in determining the role of metabolites which are both made by and act on neutrophils. Arachidonate, prostaglandins, phosphatidic acid, and diacylglycerol are all examples of such compounds. Although these agents are frequently thought to be second messengers, or at least mimic the role, they do not fit the usual conditions for such a definition. They do not mimic independently the action of a defined hormone acting at the cell surface, they require cofactors, and their interconversion to hormones renders a definitive assessment of their cell-activating capacity difficult.

I. Intracellular pH as a Second Messenger (133,142–144)

Work by several investigators has shown that the sodium-proton antiport system is activated by the FMLP receptor. Techniques for measurement of the system include sodium transport and the use of fluorescent dyes sensitive to pH changes. Using both techniques, it has been shown that alkalinization of the cytoplasm occurs within 5 min of FMLP receptor occupancy. Involvement of a pertussis toxin substrate ("G_i") is suspected, since the toxin abolishes stimulation. The reaction has particular relevance for cytokine research, since GM-CSF has been shown to be an activator of this system. Furthermore, GM-CSF activation of the antiport system "interferes" with the FMLP-mediated activation of the antiporter.

In the overall sequence of transduction-related and cellular events, the antiport activation occurs slowly relative to multiple changes observed within the first minute of FMLP receptor occupancy. A role for the antiport system in such events as aggregation, shape change, superoxide generation, and enzyme release seems unlikely. Similarly, phospholipase activation and IP_3 generation and calcium mobilization are not dependent on antiport activation. However, the converse proposition, namely, a role of the calcium- and diacylglycerol-mediated activation of kinase C, or cyclic AMP-mediated kinase A stimulation in the activation of the antiport seems probable.

An important area of research is the role of antiport activation in neutrophil regulation. The prevailing and somewhat general view is that membrane traffic-related phenomena are likely affected. Receptor recycling and sequestration and phenomena related to expression of cryptic receptors may be controlled by the antiport system.

IV. DESENSITIZATION OF RECEPTOR AND G-PROTEINS

We have considered above the processes which are involved in the initiation of cellular responses in human neutrophils. The results presented here are directed at understanding the converse process, whereby cell surface transduction is switched off—namely, desensitization. Early studies indicate that desensitization (145) and sensitization (146) of the FMLP receptor occurs in granulocytes. The work of O'Flaherty and colleagues has shown that prior exposure of granulocytes to FMLP causes a loss of aggregation responses to a subsequent challenge with FMLP and diminished enzyme release (145). Studies by Sha'afi and colleagues pointed out that the desensitization phenomenon is in part dependent on the experimental conditions which are utilized to study the process (147,148). As noted previously, degranulation and superoxide generation are observed only in the presence of cytochalasin B. Differences are noted in the desensitization pattern observed in the presence and absence of this agent, although the significance of this observation at the molecular level is not clear. An important observation is that of O'Flaherty, that desensitization of the responses for one agent can occur without the desensitization of other receptors (145). Thus homologous rather than heterologous desensitization seems to be the predominant pattern in neutrophils. This is evidenced by the fact that PAF pretreatment causes a diminution in the subsequent calcium activation by PAF but does not affect the calcium mobilization observed in the presence of FMLP. Work on the FMLP receptor suggests that pretreatment with FMLP causes a diminution in the number of FMLP receptors. The diminution in receptor number has been related to two phenomena: The first is the formation of a high-affinity, slow-dissociation state of the receptor, in which the receptor probably becomes associated with the cytoskeleton (149,150). The second relates to the internalization of the receptor and the appearance of "recycled" receptors on specific granule membranes (151–153). Both phenomena contribute to a net "down-regulation" of the receptor (10,110).

Several aspects of desensitization remained to be clarified, however. For example, it is unclear from the above studies whether the multiple reactions initiated by a single cell surface receptor are desensitized simultaneously and whether the predominant transduction response (calcium mobilization) is desensitized in these cells. Our recent studies have approached this question, and the answer seems to be that desensitization is definitely not a one-step, global reaction in which all cellular responses are terminated simultaneously (154). For example, complete desensitization of aggregation is observed at very low levels of FMLP; higher levels of ligand and repetitive exposure are required to desensitize partially to degranulation, while superoxide generation (observed in the presence of cytochalasin B) is not desensitized. A study of calcium mobilization in these cells suggests that it is largely unaffected in cells which are desensitized to aggregation, implying that either a very low level of total IP_3 is released or that calcium is not required or that calcium mobilization is associated, not with the origination of aggregation, but with its termination. Other investigators have noted recently that calcium mobilization is not required for actin polymerization, implying that another pathway may be involved (115). The possibility is emerging that this other pathway may represent the direct action of PIP_2 or other metabolites of the PI pathway on actin-binding proteins (122,123). Recent studies have shown that actin-binding proteins have specific binding domains for PIP_2 (120,121). Thus a role for PIP_2 as a second messenger may be in the stimulation of early reactions such as actin polymerization; IP_3-mediated calcium mobilization may serve predominantly to modulate their duration via kinase C activation.

V. NEW RECEPTORS ASSOCIATED WITH UNKNOWN G-PROTEINS OR SECOND MESSENGERS

A. Substance P and Neutrophil Activation (155–160)

Considerable interest has centered around the actions of substance P on human neutrophils. This is in part due to the emerging picture that the nervous system can influence the actions of the immune system. A discussion of this aspect of the nervous-immune systems interactions can be found in an excellent article by Coquelin and Gorski (161). Probably the first observation concerning substance P was that it could potentiate phagocytosis, an activity thought to reside in the N-terminal tetrapeptide sequence. A paradoxical finding which followed was that substance P could bind competitively to receptors for FMLP, a finding which is perplexing in that independent receptors for substance P have since been documented in leukocytes. Recent studies of the action of substance P have suggested that it can cause phosphoinositide hydrolysis and calcium mobilization. The relationship of this pathway to the potentiation of FMLP responses is obscure. The involvement of kinase C is ritually proposed. A very different mechanism (possibly unrelated to polyphosphoinositide hydrolysis) is that substance P potentiation of FMLP-associated functions may be due to an increase in the number of receptors for FMLP, a process which is thought to be similar to that proposed for the action of GM-CSF (113,114,155–160). This mechanism needs to be verified by direct binding studies. An intriguing aspect of future studies is to see whether the increased antibody-dependent cytotoxicity observed in neutrophils in response to several mediators including substance P is due to the up-regulation of $Fc\gamma$ receptors.

B. Cytokines and Neutrophil Activation

An area of increasing interest concerns the influence of cytokines discovered in the last several years on granulocyte function. Unfortunately, the effects of different cytokines seem to be very divergent and far more heterogeneous than the effects of chemoattractants. Table 2 (adapted from Ref. 162) summarizes the salient features of the effects of cytokines on neutrophil functions. Some of the more striking observations are emphasized here, and ambiguities and future directions are indicated. GM-CSF and

Table 2 Effects of Cytokines on Cellular Responses

	Cytokine					
	GM-CSF	G-CSF	IL-1-α/β	TNF-α/β	IFN-γ	IFN-α
Cellular Function						
Adherence	None		↓	↑		
Aggregation						
Superoxide generation						
Primary	None	None	None	↑(weak)	↑(?)	None
Secondary	↑	↑	↑	↑(weak)	↑(?)	None
Phagocytosis	↑		↑(weak)	↑	↑(?)	↑
Enzyme release (degranulation)						
Primary	↑		↑(weak)	↑(weak)		
Secondary	None	None	↑(weak)	↑(weak)		
Bactericidal activity (or H_2O_2/MPO-H_2O_2 halide reactivity)	↑		↑(weak)	↑		↑
Chemotaxis						
Primary	None(?)		None		↓	
Secondary		None	None	↓	↓	
Cytotoxicity (ADCC)	↑			↑	↑	↑(?)
Second messenger generation/action						
Arachidonate release	↑(weak)	↑(?)				
IP_3 generation	None					
Intracellular cAMP	↓					
Intracellular cGMP	↑					
Calcium mobilization	None	None	None	None		
Na^+/H^+ antiport activation	↑	None				
Membrane depolarization		↑				
G-protein involvement	Yes					
Cell surface antigen expression						
CRI/CR2/CR3			None	↑	None	None
GFA-1, GFA-2, Mol	↑					
Fc_{γ}R I< II, III/TFR				None	↑	None

TNF-α are among the most intensively studied of the cytokines. The effects of GM-CSF are predominantly to enhance the effects of chemoattractants on neutrophil function and in part to stimulate neutrophils by themselves. The direct effects, though reported, seem difficult to reconcile with the observation that calcium mobilization is not observed, or seems to be variable with this agent.

The effects of interleukin-1 (IL-1) seem to indicate that priming of chemotactic receptors is the primary response that is observed with this agent. A recent review of the transduction mechanism associated with IL-1 points out that while many transduction mechanisms have been proposed, none has been definitively proven. The marginal cellular effects observed and the controversies surrounding the second messengers which might be generated suggest a very tenuous regulatory role or the possibility that other agents as yet undefined may be required for IL-1 to exert its effects.

A somewhat less controversial profile is observed with γ-interferon. The most prominent role for this agent would seem to be in the potentiation of cytotoxicity reactions, particularly the subset which would be antibody dependent. An observation in agreement with the above is that the Fc receptors are up-regulated after treatment with γ-interferon and that corresponding increases in cytotoxicity are observed (163). These observations have to be balanced by other observations which suggest that the ADCC reaction in neutrophils is highly dependent on the stoichiometry of cells and antibody and the nature of the cellular target (20,21). The extensive use of the chicken erythrocyte as a target, the generally low levels of lysis observed, and the lack of efficacy of lysis with tumor cell lines and other targets complicate the interpretation of these results. At the level of second messenger generation, virtually no information is available in the context of the human neutrophil, although numerous second messengers have been proposed as candidates for mediating the action of γ-interferon (162,163). The observations made with α-interferon are similarly diverse. It is interesting to note that both interferons seem to exert similar effects on neutrophils. This seems puzzling in view of the sharp segregation of priming responses that is observed between interferons in their action on monocytes and lymphocytes, i.e., γ-interferon being selective for monocytes and α-interferon for lymphocytes.

VI. SUMMARY

The ideas discussed above clearly point to increasingly complex and interactive transduction mechanisms for the regulation of the neutrophil. The central challenges to be met include the following:

1. Better assays are needed for the study of physiological parameters such as adherence, aggregation, shape change, and cytoskeletal rearrangements, assays which are not prohibitively complex and expensive while still allowing for more detailed physiological observations.
2. The neutrophil receptors need to be characterized in greater detail at the molecular level. Protein purification, sequencing, and cloning approaches are needed. Given the inherent shortcomings of working with the neutrophil system due to the presence of proteases and the problems of obtaining sufficient amounts of plasma membranes as source material for receptor purification, this is a difficult task. Advances in micropurification and sequencing may alleviate some of the difficulties here.

3. The size and complexity of the G-protein family continue to expand. However, as pointed out earlier, stimulus-responsive enzymes without G-protein-associated regulation, and G-proteins without clearly identified targets, remain. A better definition and description of the G-protein family will be required if cellular regulation is to be understood at the molecular level.

In terms of second messengers and their role in cellular regulation, the main questions which remain to be answered concern identification of the precise pathways which are important to cellular regulation. In order to understand the complex cascades of arachidonate metabolism, phospholipid turnover, and calcium homeostasis, it is all the more important that the manner in which second messengers may regulate particular cell functions be better understood. An omission in this review is the role of kinases in cellular regulation. Activation of kinase C (through calcium and diacylglycerol) and kinase A (through cAMP) has been demonstrated. The substrates for these kinases have been described by various investigators. However, relating phosphorylation changes in a particular protein to the activity of the protein, and assignment of activity to particular physiological roles, has not been satisfactorily accomplished and remains a challenge for the future.

ACKNOWLEDGMENTS

Some of the work from our group, which is described here, was supported by a Biomedical Research Support Grant RR-05521-19 and grants from the National Institutes of Health, AM30878 and AM34550.

REFERENCES

1. Snyderman R, Pike MC. Chemoattractant receptors on phagocytic cells. Ann Rev Immunol 1984; 2:257–81.
2. Klebanoff SJ, Clark RA. In: The neutrophil: functions and clinical disorders. Amsterdam: North Holland, 1978:239–40.
3. Becker E, Ward P. Chemotaxis. In: Parker C, ed. Clinical immunology. New York: Academic Press, 1980:272–9.
4. Aswanikumar S, Corcoran B, Schiffmann E, Day AR, Freer RJ, Showell HJ, Becker EL, Pert CB. Demonstration of a receptor on rabbit neutrophils for chemotactic peptides. Biochem Biophys Res Commun 1977; 74:810–7.
5. Chenoweth DE, Hugli TE. Demonstration of a specific C5a receptor on intact human polymorphonuclear leukocytes. Proc Natl Acad Sci USA 1978; 75:3943–7.
6. Henson PM. Platelet-activation factor as a mediator of neutrophil-platelet interactions in inflammation. Agents and Actions 1981; 11:545–6.
7. Goldman DW, Goetzl, EJ. Specific binding of leukotriene B_4 to receptors on human polymorphonuclear leukocytes. J Immunol 1982; 129:1600–4.
8. Sha'afi R, Molski TFP. Activation of the neutrophil. Prog Allergy 1988; 42:1–64.
9. Sklar LA. Ligand receptor dynamics and signal amplification in the neutrophil. Adv Immunol 1986; 39:95–143.
10. Sklar LA, Jesaitis AJ, Painter RG, Cochrane CG. Ligand/receptor internalization: a spectroscopic analysis and a comparison of ligand binding, cellular response and internalization by human neutrophils. J Cell Biochem 1982; 20:193–202.
11. Rao KMK, Varani J. Actin polymerization induced by chemotactic peptide and concanavalin A in rat neutrophils. J Immunol 1982; 129:1605–7.

12. Sklar LA, Oades ZG, Jesaitis AJ, Painter RG, Cochrane CG. Fluoresceinated chemotactic peptide and high-affinity antifluorescein antibody as a probe of the temporal characteristics of neutrophil stimulation. Proc Natl Acad Sci USA 1981; 78:7540–4.
13. Sklar LA, McNeil VM, Jesaitis AJ, Painter RG, Cochrane CG. A continuous, spectroscopic analysis of the kinetics of elastase secretion by neutrophils. The dependence of secretion upon receptor occupancy. J Biol Chem 1982; 257:5471–5.
14. Sklar LA, Finney DA, Oades ZG, Jesaitis AJ, Painter RG, Cochrane CG. The dynamics of ligand-receptor interactions. Real-time analyses of association, dissociation, and internalization of an N-formyl peptide and its receptors on the human neutrophil. J Biol Chem 1984; 259:5661–9.
15. Sklar LA, Hyslop PA, Oades ZG, Omann GM, Jesaitis AJ, Painter RG, Cochrane CG. Signal transduction and ligand-receptor dynamics in the human neutrophil. Transient responses and occupancy-response relations at the formyl peptide receptor. J Biol Chem 1985; 260:11461–7.
16. Liu ZY, Young JI, Elson EL. Rat basophilic leukemia cells stiffen when they secrete. J Cell Biol 1987; 105:2933–43.
17. Zurier RB, Weissman G, Hoffstein S, Kammerman S, Tai HH. Mechanisms of lysosomal enzyme release from human leukocytes. II. Effects of cAMP and cGMP, autonomic agonists, and agents which affect microtubule function. J Clin Invest 1974; 53:297–309.
18. Simchowitz L, Spilberg I. Chemotactic factor-induced generation of superoxide radicals by human neutrophils: evidence for the role of sodium. J Immunol 1979; 123:2428–35.
19. Fearon DT. The human C_{3b} receptor. In: Muller HJ, Miescher PA, eds. Complement. New York: Springer-Verlag, 1984: 101–14.
20. Fanger MW, Shen L, Graziano RF, Guyre PM. Cytotoxicity mediated by human Fc receptors for IgG. Immunology Today 1989; 10:92–9.
21. Fanger MW, Graziano RF, Shen L, Guyre PM. $Fc_{\gamma}R$ in cytotoxicity exerted by mononuclear cells. Chem Immunol 1989; 47:214–53.
22. Hill HR. Cyclic nucleotides as modulators of leukocyte chemotaxis. In: Gallin JI, Quie PG, eds. Leukocyte chemotaxis. New York: Raven Press, 1978:193–9.
23. Lad PM, Goldberg BJ, Smiley PA, Olson CV. Receptor-specific threshold effects of cyclic AMP are involved in the regulation of enzyme release and superoxide production from human neutrophils. Biochim Biophys Acta 1985; 846:286–95.
24. Bourne HR, Lehrer RI, Cline MJ, Melmon KL. Cyclic 3′5′-adenosine monophosphate in the human leukocyte: synthesis, degradation, and effects on neutrophil candidacidal activity. J Clin Invest 1971; 50:920–9.
25. Weissmann G, Kukor P, Zurier RB. Effects of cyclic AMP on release of lysosomal enzyme from phagocytes. Nature New Biol 1971; 231:131–3.
26. Ignarro LJ, Cech SY. Bidirectional regulation of lysosomal enzyme secretion and phagocytosis in human neutrophils by guanosine 3′,5′-monophosphate and adenosine 3′,5′-monophosphate. Proc Soc Exp Biol Med 1976; 151:448–52.
27. Ignarro LJ, George WJ. Hormonal control of lysosomal enzyme release from human neutrophils: elevation of cyclic nucleoside levels by neurohormones. Proc Natl Acad Sci USA 1974; 71:2027–31.
28. Ignarro LJ, George WJ. Mediation of immunologic discharges of lysosomal enzymes from human neutrophils by guanosine 3′,5′-monophosphate. Requirement of calcium, and inhibition by adenosine 3′,5′-monophosphate. J Exp Med 1974; 140:225–38.
29. Smith RJ, Ignarro LJ. Bioregulation of lysosomal enzyme secretion from human neutrophils: roles of guanosine 3′,5′-monophosphate and calcium stimulus-secretion coupling. Proc Natl Acad Sci USA 1975; 72:108–12.
30. Hill HR, Estensen RD, Quie PG, Hogan NA, Goldberg ND. Modulation of human neutrophil chemotactic responses by cyclic 3′,5′-guanosine monophosphate and cyclic 3′,5′-adenosine monophosphate. Metabolism 1975; 24:447–56.

31. Lad PM, Glovsky MM, Smiley PA, Klempner M, Reisinger DM, Richards JH. The beta adrenergic receptor in the human neutrophil plasma membrane: receptor-cyclase uncoupling is associated with amplified GTP activation. J Immunol 1984; 132:1466–71.
32. Lad PM, Glovsky MM, Richards JH, Smiley PA, Reisinger DM, Learn DB. Identification of receptor regulatory proteins, membrane glycoproteins, and functional characteristics of adenylate cyclase in vesicles derived from the human neutrophil. Mol Immunol 1984; 21:627–39.
33. Cronstein BN, Rosenstein ED, Kramer SB, Weissmann G, Hirschhorn R. Adenosine; a physiologic modulator of superoxide anion generation by human neutrophils. Adenosine acts via an A2 receptor on human neutrophils. J Immunol 1985; 135:1366–71.
34. Gilman AG. G proteins: transducers of receptor-generated signals. Ann Rev Biochem 1987; 56:615–49.
35. Stryer L, Bourne HR. G proteins: a family of signal transducers. Ann Rev Cell Biol 1986; 2:391–419.
36. Becker EL, Kanaho Y, Kermode JC. Nature and functioning of the pertussis toxin-sensitive G protein of human neutrophils. Biomed Pharmacother 1987; 41:289–97.
37. Dillon SB, Verghese MW, Snyderman R. Signal transduction in cells following binding of chemoattractants to membrane receptors. Virchows Archiv B Cell Pathol 1988; 55:65–80.
38. Burgoyne RD, Morgan A. Low molecular mass GTP-binding proteins of adrenal chromaffin cells are present on the secretory granule. FEBS Lett 1989; 245:122–6.
39. Burgoyne RD. Small GTP-binding proteins. Trends Biol Sci 1989; 14:394–5.
40. Simchowitz L, Fischbein LC, Spilberg I, Atkinson JP. Induction of a transient elevation in intracellular levels of adenosine-3′,5′-cyclic monophosphate by chemotactic factors: An early event in human neutrophil activation. J Immunol 1980; 124:1482–91.
41. Simchowitz L, Atkinson JP, Spilberg I. Stimulus-specific deactivation of chemotactic factor-induced cyclic AMP response and superoxide generation by human neutrophils. J Clin Invest 1980; 66:736–47.
42. Lad PM, Olson CV, Smiley PA. Association of the f-met-leu-phe receptor in human neutrophils with a GTP-binding protein sensitive to pertussis toxin. Proc Natl Acad Sci USA 1985; 82:869–73.
43. Nakamura T, Ui M. Simultaneous inhibitions of inositol phospholipid breakdown, arachidonic acid release, and histamine secretion in mast cells by islet-activating protein, pertussis toxin. A possible involvement of the toxin-specific substrate in the Ca^{2+} mobilizing receptor-mediated biosignaling system. J Biol Chem 1985; 260:3584–93.
44. Okajima F, Ui M. ADP-ribosylation of the specific membrane protein by islet-activating protein, pertussis toxin, associated with inhibition of a chemotactic peptide-induced arachidonate release in neutrophils. A possible role of the toxin substrate in Ca^{2+}-mobilizing biosignaling. J Biol Chem 1984; 259:13863–71.
45. Okajima F, Katada T, Ui M. Coupling of the guanine nucleotide regulatory protein to chemotactic peptide receptors in neutrophil membranes, and its uncoupling by islet-activating protein, pertussis toxin. A possible role of the toxin substrate in Ca^{2+}-mobilizing receptor-mediated signal transduction. J Biol Chem 1985; 260:6761–8.
46. Lad PM, Reisinger DM, Smiley PA. Ligand requirements for the relaxation of adenylate cyclase from activated and inhibited states. Biochemistry 1983; 22:3278–84.
47. Lad PM, Olson CV, Grewal IS, Scott SJ. A pertussis-toxin sensitive GTP-binding protein in the human neutrophil regulates multiple receptors, calcium mobilization and lectin-induced capping. Proc Natl Acad Sci USA 1985; 82:8643–7.
48. Lad PM, Olson CV, Grewal IS, Frolich MF, Scott SJ. Role of GTP binding proteins in the regulation of the human neutrophil. In: Oppenheim JJ, ed. Leukocytes and host defense. New York: Alan R. Liss, 1986:373–8.
49. Scott SJ, Olson CV, Lad PM. Peptide mapping studies of the pertussis toxin substrate in human neutrophils, platelets and erythrocytes. Mol Immunol 1988; 25:305–11.

50. Lad PM, Grewal I, Olson C, Lee D, Niedzin H. Regulation of cap formation in neutrophils: role of ion channels. J Leukocyte Biol 1987; 42:339.
51. Bokoch GM, Gilman AG. Inhibition of receptor mediated release of arachidonic acid by pertussis toxin. Cell 1984; 39:301–8.
52. Brandt SJ, Dougherty RW, Lapetina EG, Niedel JE. Pertussis toxin inhibits chemotactic peptide stimulated generation of inositol phosphates and lysosomal enzyme secretion in human leukemic (HL60) cells. Proc Natl Acad Sci USA 1985; 82:3277–80.
53. Koo C, Lefkowitz RJ, Snyderman R. Guanine nucleotides modulate the binding affinity of the oligopeptide chemoattractant receptor on human polymorphonuclear leukocytes. J Clin Invest 1983; 72:748–53.
54. Volpi M, Naccache PH, Molski TFP, Shefcyk J, Huang C-K, Marsh ML, Munoz J, Becker EL, Sha'afi RI. Pertussis toxin inhibits fMet-Leu-Phe- but not phorbol ester-stimulated changes in rabbit neutrophils: role of G proteins in excitation response coupling. Proc Natl Acad Sci USA 1985; 82:2708–12.
55. Becker EL, Kermode JC, Naccache PH, Yassin R, Marsh ML, Munoz JJ, Sha'afi RI. The inhibition of neutrophil granule enzyme secretion and chemotaxis by pertussis toxin. J Cell Biol 1985; 100:1641–6.
56. Lad PM, Olson CV, Grewal IS. Platelet activating factor mediated effects on human neutrophil function are inhibited by pertussis toxin. Biochem Biophy Res Commun. 1985; 129:632–8.
57. Lad PM, Olson CV, Grewal IS, Scott SJ, Frolich M. Molecular mechanisms in the action of platelet activation factor and other mediators of inflammation. In: Winslow CM, Lee ML, eds. New Horizons in PAF Research. New York: Wiley, 1987:103–22.
58. Hyslop PA, Oades ZG, Jesaitis AJ, Painter RG, Cochrane CG, Sklar LA. Evidence for N-formyl chemotactic peptide-stimulated GTPase activity in human neutrophil homogenates. FEBS Lett 1984; 166:165–9.
59. Bokoch GM, Bickford K, Bohl BP. Subcellular localization and quantitation of the major neutrophil pertussis toxin substrate, G_i. J Cell Biol 1988; 106:1927–36.
60. Kikuchi A, Kozawa O, Kaibuchi K, Katada T, Ui M, Takai Y. Direct evidence for involvement of a guanine nucleotide-binding protein in chemotactic peptide-stimulated formation of inositol biphosphate and trisphosphate in differentiated human leukemic (HL-60) cells. Reconstitution with Gi or Go of the plasma membranes ADP-ribosylated by pertussis toxin. J Biol Chem 1986; 261:11558–62.
61. Korchak NM, Rutherford LE, Weissmann G. Stimulus response coupling in the human neutrophil: temporal analysis of changes in cytosolic calcium and calcium efflux. J Biol Chem 1984; 259:4070–4.
62. Berridge MJ. Inositol trisphosphate and diacylglycerol: two interacting second messengers. Ann Rev Biochem 1987; 56:159–93.
63. Berridge MJ. The molecular basis of communication within the cell. Sci Am 1985; 253:142–52.
64. Berridge MJ, Irvine RF. Inositol trisphosphate and calcium mobilization. In: Bleasdale JE, Eichberg J, Hauser G, eds. Inositol and phosphoinositides: metabolism and regulation. Clifton, NJ: Humana Press, 1985:351–66.
65. Berridge MJ, Taylor CW. Inositol trisphosphate and calcium signaling. Cold Spring Harbor Symp Quant Biol 1988; 53:927–33.
66. Cockcroft S. The dependence on Ca^{2+} of the guanine-nucleotide-activated polyphosphoinositide phosphodiesterase in neutrophil plasma membranes. Biochem J 1986; 240:503–7.
67. Cockcroft S, Gomperts BD. Role of guanine nucleotide binding protein in the activation of polyphosphoinositide phosphodiesterase. Nature (Lond) 1985; 314:534–6.
68. Smolen JE, Stoehr SJ. Guanine nucleotides reduce the free calcium requirement for secre-

tion of granule constituents from permeabilized human neutrophils. Biochim Biophy Acta 1986; 889:171–8.

69. Smith CD, Lane BC, Kusaka I, Verghese MW, Snyderman R. Chemoattractant receptor-induced hydrolysis of phosphatidylinositol 4,5-bisphosphate in human polymorphonuclear leukocyte membranes. Requirement for a guanine nucleotide regulatory protein. J Biol Chem 1985; 260:5875–8.
70. Bradford PG, Rubin RP. Characterization of formylmethionyl-leucyl-phenylalanine stimulation of inositol trisphosphate accumulation in rabbit neutrophils. Mol Pharmacol 1985; 27:74–8.
71. Burgess GM, McKinney JS, Irvine RF, Berridge MJ, Hoyle PC, Putney JW. Inositol 1,4,5-trisphosphate may be a signal for f-Met-Leu-Phe induced intracellular Ca mobilisation in human leukocytes (HL-60 cells). FEBS Lett 1984; 176:193–6.
72. Cockcroft S. Ca^{2+}-dependent conversion of phosphatidylinositol to phosphatidate in neutrophils stimulated with fMet-Leu-Phe or ionophore A23187. Biochim Biophys Acta 1984; 795:37–46.
73. Yano K, Hattori H, Imai A, Nozawa Y. Modification of positional distribution of fatty acids in phosphatidylinositol of rabbit neutrophils stimulated with formyl-methionyl-leucyl-phenylalanine. Biochim Biophys Acta 1983; 752:137–44.
74. Cockcroft S, Barrowman MM, Gomperts BD. Breakdown and synthesis of polyphosphoinositides in fMet-Leu-Phe stimulated neutrophils. FEBS Lett 1985; 181:259–63.
75. Bradford PG, Rubin RP. Pertussis toxin inhibits chemotactic factor-induced phospholipase C stimulation and lysosomal enzyme secretion in rabbit neutrophils. FEBS Lett 1985; 183:317–20.
76. Matsumoto T, Tao W, Sha'afi RI. Demonstration of calcium-dependent phospholipase A_2 activity in a membrane preparation of rabbit neutrophils: absence of activation by f-met-leu-phe, phorbol 12-myristate 13-acetate and A-kinase. Biochem J 1988; 250:343–8.
77. Bormann BJ, Huang C-K, Mackin WM, Becker EL. Receptor-mediated activation of a PLA_2 in rabbit neutrophil plasma membrane. Proc Natl Acad Sci USA 1984; 81:767–70.
78. McPhail LC, Shirley PS, Clayton CC, Snyderman R. Activation of the respiratory burst enzyme from human neutrophils in a cell-free system. Evidence for a soluble factor. J Clin Invest 1985; 75:1735–9.
79. Takenawa T, Homma Y, Nagai Y. Role of calcium in phosphatidylinositol response and arachidonate release in formylated tripeptide- or calcium ionophore A23187-stimulated guinea pig neutrophils. J Immunol 1983; 130:2849–55.
80. Clancy RM, Dahinden CA, Hugli TE. Arachidonate metabolism by human polymorphonuclear leukocytes stimulated by N-formyl-met-leu-phe or complement component C5a is independent of phospholipase activation. Proc Natl Acad Sci USA 1983; 80:7200–4.
81. Bokoch GM, Reed PW. Stimulation of arachidonic acid metabolism in the polymorphonuclear leukocyte by an N-formylated peptide. Comparison with ionophore A23187. J Biol Chem 1980; 255:10223–6.
82. Jelsema CL. Light activation of phospholipase A_2 in rod outer segments of bovine retina and its modulation by GTP-binding proteins. J Biol Chem 1987; 262:163–8.
83. Jelsema CL, Axelrod J. Stimulation of phospholipase A_2 activity in bovine rod outer segments by the beta-gamma subunits of transducin and its inhibition by the alpha subunit. Proc Natl Acad Sci USA 1987; 84:3623–7.
84. Borgeat P, Samuelson B. Arachidonic acid metabolism in polymorphonuclear leukocytes: effects of ionophore A23187. Proc Natl Acad Sci USA 1979; 76:2148–52.
85. Dillon SB, Murray JJ, Verghese MW, Snyderman R. Regulation of inositol phosphate metabolism in chemoattractant-stimulated human polymorphonuclear leukocytes. J Biol Chem 1987; 262:11546–52.

86. Dillon SB, Murray JJ, Uhing R, Snyderman R. Regulation of inositol phospholipid and inositol phosphate metabolism in chemoattractant-activated human polymorphonuclear leukocytes. J Cell Biochem 1987; 35:345–9.
87. Billah MM, Eckel S, Mullmann TJ, Egan RW, Siegel MI. Phosphatidylcholine hydrolysis by phospholipase D determines phosphatidate and diglyceride levels in chemotactic peptide-stimulated human neutrophils. Involvement of phosphatidate phosphohydrolase in signal transduction. J Biol Chem 1989; 264:17069–77.
88. Anthes JC, Eckel S, Siegel MI, Egan RW, Billah MM. Phospholipase D in homogenates from HL-60 granulocytes: implications of calcium and G protein control. Biochem Biophys Res Commun 1989; 163:657–64.
89. Billah MM, Pai JK, Mullmann TJ, Egan RW, Siegel MI. Regulation of phospholipase D in HL-60 granulocytes. Activation by phorbol esters, diglyceride, and calcium ionophore via protein kinase-independent mechanisms. J Biol Chem 1989; 264:9069–76.
90. Pai JK, Siegel MI, Egan RW, Billah MM. Activation of phospholipase D by chemotactic peptide in HL-60 granulocytes. Biochem Biophys Res Commun 1988; 150:355–64.
91. Verghese M, Uhing RJ, Snyderman R. A pertussis/cholera-toxin-sensitive N protein may mediate chemoattractant receptor signal transduction. Biochem Biophys Res Commun 1986; 138:887–94.
92. Gierschik P, Falloon J, Milligan G, Pines M, Gallin JI, Speigel A. Immunochemical evidence for a novel pertussis toxin substrate in human neutrophils. J Biol Chem 1986; 261:8058–62.
93. Gierschik P, Sidiropoulos D, Spiegel A, Jakobs KH. Purification and immunochemical characterization of the major pertussis-toxin-sensitive guanine-nucleotide-binding protein of bovine-neutrophil membranes. Eur J Biochem 1987; 165:185–94.
94. Bokoch GM, Parkos CA. Identification of novel GTP-binding proteins in the human neutrophil. FEBS Lett 1988; 227:66–70.
95. Quilliam LA, Lacal JC, Bokoch GM. Identification of *rho* as a substrate for botulinum toxin C-3-catalyzed ADP-ribosylation. FEBS Lett 1989; 247:221–6.
96. Norgauer J, Kounatzki E, Seifert R, Aktories K. Botulinum-C2 ADP ribosylates actin and enhances O_2^- production and secretion but inhibits migration of activated human neutrophils. J Clin Invest 1988; 82:1376–82.
97. Al-Mohanna FA, Ohishi I, Hallett MB. Botulinum C2 toxin potentiates activation of the neutrophil oxidase. Further evidence of a role for actin polymerization. FEBS Lett 1987; 219:40–4.
98. Gomez-Cambronero J, Yamazaki M, Metwally F, Molski TFP, Bonak VA, Huang CK, Becker EL, Sha'afi RI. Granulocyte-macrophage colony stimulating factor and human neutrophils: role of guanine nucleotide regulatory proteins. Proc Natl Acad Sci USA 1989; 86:3569–73.
99. Quinn MT, Parkos CA, Walker L, Orkin SH, Dinnaer MC, Jesaitis AJ. Association of a Ras-related protein with cytochrome b of human neutrophils. Nature (Lond) 1989; 342:198–200.
100. Lambeth JD. Activation of the respiratory burst oxidase in neutrophils: on the role of membrane-derived second messengers, Ca^{++} and protein kinase C. J Bioenerg Biomembr 1988; 20:709–33.
101. Allen RA, Traynor AE, Omann GM, Jesaitis AJ. The chemotactic peptide receptor: a model for future understanding of chemotactic disorders. Hematol Oncol Clin N Am 1988; 2:33–60.
102. Sadler KL, Badwey JA. Second messengers involved in superoxide production by neutrophils: function and metabolism. Hematol Oncol Clin N Am 1988; 2:185–200.
103. Rossi F. The O_2^--forming NADPH oxidase of the phagocytes: nature, mechanisms of activation and function. Biochim Biophys Acta 1986; 853:65–89.
104. Lad PM, Olson CV, Grewal IS. A step sensitive to pertussis toxin and phorbol ester in

human neutrophils regulates chemotaxis and capping but not phagocytosis. FEBS Lett 1986; 200:91–6.

105. Gresham HD, Clement LT, Volanakis JE, Brown EJ. Cholera toxin and pertussis toxin regulate the Fc receptor-mediated phagocytic response of human neutrophils in a manner analogous to regulation by monoclonal antibody 1C2. J Immunol 1987; 139:4159–66.
106. Brown EJ, Newell AM, Gresham HD. Molecular regulation of phagocyte function. Evidence for involvement of a guanosine triphosphate-binding protein in opsonin-mediated phagocytosis by monocytes. J Immunol 1987; 139:3777–82.
107. DiVirgilio F, Meyer BC, Greenberg S, Silverstein SC. Fc receptor-mediated phagocytosis occurs in macrophages at exceedingly low cytosolic Ca^{2+} levels. J Cell Biol 1988; 106:657–66.
108. Sutherland EW. An introduction. In: Robison GA, Butcher RW, Sutherland EW, eds. Cyclic AMP. New York: Academic Press, 1971:1–16.
109. Sutherland EW, Robison GA, Butcher RW. Cyclic AMP and hormone action. In: Robison GA, Butcher RW, Sutherland EW, eds. Cyclic AMP. New York: Academic Press, 1971:17–47.
110. Zigmond SH. Consequences of chemotactic peptide receptor modulation for leukocyte orientation. J Cell Biol 1981; 88:644–7.
111. Busse WW, Sosman JM. Isoproterenol inhibition of isolated human neutrophil function. J Allergy Clin Immunol 1984; 73:404–10.
112. Lad PM, Glovsky MM, Richards JH, Backstrom B, Smiley PA. Regulation of human neutrophil guanylate cyclase by metal ions, free radicals and the muscarinic cholinergic receptor. Mol Immunol 1985; 22:731–9.
113. Coffey RG. Mechanism of GM-CSF stimulation of neutrophils. Immunol Res 1989; 8:236–48.
114. Coffey RG, Davis JS, Djeu JY. Stimulation of guanylate cyclase activity and reduction of adenylate cyclase activity by granulocyte-macrophage colony-stimulating factor in human blood neutrophils. J Immunol 1988; 140:2695–701.
115. Sha'afi RI, Shefcyk J, Yassin R, Molski TFP, Volpi M, Naccache PH, White JR, Feinstein MB, Becker EL. Is a rise in intracellular concentration of free calcium necessary or sufficient for stimulated cytoskeletal-associated actin? J Cell Biol 1986; 102:1459–63.
116. Al-Mohanna FA, Hallett MB. Actin polymerization in neutrophils is triggered without a requirement for a rise in cytoplasmic Ca^{2+}. Biochem J 1990; 266:669–74.
117. Lew PD, Monod A, Walkvogel FA, Dewald B, Baggiolini M, Pozzan T. Quantitative analysis of the cytosolic free calcium dependency of exocytosis from three subcellular compartments in intact human neutrophils. J Cell Biol 1986; 102:2197–204.
118. Lew DP. Receptor signalling and intracellular calcium in neutrophil activation. Eur J Clin Invest 1989; 19:338–46.
119. Krause KH, Pittet D, Volpe P, Pozzan T, Meldolesi J, Lew DP. Calciosome, a sarcoplasmic reticulum-like organelle involved in intracellular Ca^{2+}-handling by non-muscle cells: studies in human neutrophils and HL-60 cells. Cell Calcium 1989; 10:351–61.
120. Yin HL, Iida K, Janmey PA. Identification of a polyphosphoinositide-modulated domain in gelsolin which binds to the sides of actin filaments. J Cell Biol 1988; 106:805–12.
121. Hartwig JH, Yin HL. The organization and regulation of the macrophage actin skeleton. Cell Motility and the Cytoskeleton 1988; 10:117–25.
122. Anderson RA, Marchesi VT. Regulation of the association of membrane skeletal protein 4.1 with glycophorin by a polyphosphoinositide. Nature (Lond) 1985; 318:295–8.
123. Lassing I, Lindberg U. Specific interaction between phosphatidylinositol 4,5-bisphosphate and profilactin. Nature (Lond) 1985; 314:472–4.
124. Dillon SB, Murray JJ, Snyderman R. Identification of a novel inositol bisphosphate isomer formed in chemoattractant stimulated human polymorphonuclear leukocytes. Biochem Biophys Res Commun 1987; 144:264–70.

125. Frolich M, Olson CV, Lad PM. Distinct sites in the PI cycle are involved in the inhibition of calcium mobilization by phorbol ester and prostaglandins. Fed Proc 1987; 46:606.
126. Connolly TM, Lawing WJ Jr, Majerus PW. Protein kinase C phosphorylates human platelet inositol trisphosphate 5′-phosphomonoesterase, increasing the phosphatase activity. Cell 1986; 46:951–8.
127. Connolly TM, Bansal VS, Bross TE, Irvine RF, Majerus PW. The metabolism of tris- and tetraphosphates of inositol by 5′-phosphomonoesterase and 3′-kinase enzymes. J Biol Chem 1987; 262:2146–9.
128. Irvine RF, Moor RM. Inositol (1,3,4,5) tetrakisphosphate-induced activation of sea urchin eggs requires the presence of inositol trisphosphate. Biochem Biophys Res Commun 1987; 146:284–90.
129. Imboden JB, Pattison G. Regulation of inositol 1,4,5-trisphosphate kinase activity after stimulation of human T cell antigen receptor. J Clin Invest 1987; 79:1538–41.
130. Biden TJ, Comte M, Cox JA, Wollheim CB. Calcium-calmodulin stimulates inositol 1,4,5-trisphosphate kinase activity from insulin-secreting RINm5F cells. J Biol Chem 1987; 262:9437–40.
131. Rasmussen H. The calcium messenger system (parts I and II). New Engl J Med 1986; 314:1094–101 and 314:1164–70.
132. Naccache PH, Sha'afi RI. Biochemical events associated with the mobilization of calcium. Surveys in Immunol Res 1984; 3:288–95.
133. Grinstein S, Furuya W. Characterization of the amiloride-sensitive Na^+/H^+ anti-port of human neutrophils. Am J Physiol 1986; 250:C283–91.
134. Berger M, Birx DL. Relationship between membrane depolarization and extracellular calcium influx during neutrophil activation. J Lab Clin Med 1988; 111:384–92.
135. Curnutte JT. Activation of human neutrophil nicotinamide adenine dinucleotide phosphate, reduced (triphosphopyridine nucleotide, reduced) oxidase by arachidonic acid in a cell free system. J Clin Invest 1985; 75:1740–3.
136. Curnutte JT, Badwey JA, Robinson JM, Karnovsky MJ, Karnovsky ML. Studies on the mechanism of superoxide release from human neutrophils stimulated with arachidonate. J Biol Chem 1984; 259:11851–7.
137. Volpi M, Molski TFP, Naccache PH, Feinstein MB, Sha'afi RI. Phorbol 12-myristate, 13-acetate potentiates the action of the calcium ionophore in stimulating arachidonic acid release and production of phosphatidic acid in rabbit neutrophils. Biochem Biophys Res Commun 1985; 128:594–600.
138. Godfrey RW, Manzi RM, Clark MA, Hoffstein ST. Stimulus-specific induction of phospholipid and arachidonic acid metabolism in human neutrophils. J Cell Biol 1987; 104:925–32.
139. Tao W, Molski TFP, Sha'afi RI. Arachidonic acid release in rabbit neutrophils. Biochem J 1989; 257:633–7.
140. Lee TH, Mencia-Huerta J-M, Shih C, Corey EJ, Lewis RA, Austen KF. Effects of exogenous arachidonic eicosapentanoic and docosahexanoic acids on the generation of 5-lipoxygenase pathway products by ionophore-activated human neutrophils. J Clin Invest 1984; 74:1922–33.
141. Naccache PH, Sha'afi RI, Borgeat P, Goetzl EJ. Mono- and dihydroxyeicosatetraenoic acids alter calcium homeostasis in rabbit neutrophils. J Clin Invest 1981; 67:1584–7.
142. Simchowitz L, Roos A. Regulation of intracellular pH in human neutrophils. J Gen Physiol 1985; 85:443–70.
143. Grinstein S, Cohen S, Goetz JD, Rothstein A. Osmotic and phorbol ester-induced activation of Na^+/H^+ exchange: possible role of protein phosphorylation in lymphocyte volume regulation. J Cell Biol 1985; 101:269–76.

144. Molski TFP, Ford C, Weisman SJ, Sha'afi RI. Cell alkalinization is not necessary and increased sodium influx is not sufficient for stimulated superoxide production. FEBS Lett 1986; 203:267–72.
145. O'Flaherty JT, Lees CJ, Miller CH, McCall CE, Lewis JC, Love SH, Wykle RL. Selective desensitization of neutrophils: further studies with 1-O-alkyl-*sn*-glycero-3-phosphocholine analogues. J Immunol 1981; 127:731–7.
146. Fletcher MP, Gallin JI. Degranulating stimuli increase the availability of receptors on human neutrophils for the chemoattractant f-met-leu-phe. J Immunol 1980; 124:1585–8.
147. Showell HJ, Williams D, Becker EL, Naccache PH, Sha'afi R. Desensitization and deactivation of the secretory responsiveness of rabbit neutrophils induced by the chemotactic peptide, formyl-methionyl-leucyl-phenylalanine. J Reticuloendothelial Soc 1979; 25:139–50.
148. O'Flaherty JT, Kreutzer DL, Showell HJ, Vitkauskas G, Becker EL, Ward PA. Selective neutrophil desensitization to chemotactic factors. J Cell Biol 1979; 80:564–72.
149. Jesaitis AJ, Naemura JR, Painter RG, Schmitt M, Sklar LA, Cochrane CG. The fate of the N-formyl-chemotactic peptide receptor in stimulated human granulocytes: subcellular fractionation studies. J Cell Biochem 1982; 20:177–91.
150. Jesaitis AJ, Naemura JR, Cochrane CG, Painter RG. Rapid modulation of N-formyl chemotactic peptide receptors on the surface of human granulocytes: formation of high-affinity ligand-receptor complexes in transient association with cytoskeleton. J Cell Biol 1984; 98:1378–87.
151. Jesaitis AJ, Naemura JR, Painter RG, Sklar LA, Cochrane CG. Intracellular localization of N-formyl chemotactic receptor and magnesium dependent ATPase in human granulocytes. Biochim Biophys Acta 1982; 719:556–68.
152. Jesaitis AJ, Tolley JO, Allen RA. Receptor-cytoskeleton interactions and membrane traffic may regulate chemoattractant-induced superoxide production in human neutrophils. J Biol Chem 1986; 261:13662–9.
153. Jesaitis AJ, Naemura JR, Painter RG, Sklar LA, Cochrane CG. The fate of an N-formylated chemotactic peptide in stimulated human granulocytes: subcellular fractionation studies. J Biol Chem 1983; 258:1969–77.
154. Lee G-HD, Kaptein JS, Scott SJ, Niedzin H, Kalunta CI, Lad PM. Desensitization of calcium mobilization and cell function in human neutrophils. Biochem J 1989; 262:165–72.
155. Wozniak A, McLennan G, Betts WH, Murphy GA, Scicchitano R. Activation of human neutrophils by substance P: effect on FMLP-stimulated oxidative and arachidonic acid metabolism and on antibody-dependent cell-mediated cytotoxicity. Immunology 1989; 68:359–64.
156. Hafstrom I, Gyllenhammar H, Palmblad J, Ringertz B. Substance P activates and modulates neutrophil oxidative metabolism and aggregation. J Rheumatol 1989; 16:1033–7.
157. Wiedermann CH, Wiedermann FJ, Apperl A, Kieselbach G, Konwalinka G, Braunsteiner H. In vitro human polymorphonuclear leukocyte chemokinesis and human monocyte chemotaxis are different activities of aminoterminal and carboxyterminal substance P. Naunyn Schmiedebergs Arch Pharmacol 1989; 340:185–90.
158. Goldman R, Bar-Shavit Z. On the mechanism of the augmentation of the phagocytic capability of phagocytic cells by Tuftsin, substance P, neurotensin, and kentsin and the interrelationship between their receptors. Ann NY Acad Sci 1983; 419:143–55.
159. Marasco WA, Showell HJ, Becker EL. Substance P binds to the formylpeptide chemotaxis receptor on the rabbit neutrophil. Biochem Biophys Res Commun 1981; 99:1065–72.
160. Bar-Shavit Z, Goldman R, Stabinsky Y, Gottlieb P, Fridken M, Teichberg VI, Blumberg S. Enhancement of phagocytosis—a newly found activity of substance P residing in its N-terminal tetrapeptide sequence. Biochem Biophys Res Commun 1980; 94:1445–51.

161. Coquelin AW, Gorski RA. Neuroendocrine control, stress, and immunity. In: Cooper EL, ed. Stress, immunity, and aging. Immunology series, vol 24. New York: Marcel Dekker, 1984: 27–40.
162. Steinbeck MJ, Roth JA. Neutrophil activation by recombinant cytokines. Rev Inf Dis 1989; 11:549–68.
163. Becker EL. The cytotoxic action of neutrophils on mammalian cells in vitro. Prog Allergy 1988; 40:183–208.

6

Eosinophil Activation and Function in Health and Disease

RANDA I. ABU-GHAZALEH, HIROHITO KITA and GERALD J. GLEICH
Mayo Clinic and Mayo Foundation, Rochester, Minnesota

I. INTRODUCTION

A. The Eosinophil

T.W. Jones (1) probably described the eosinophil for the first time in 1846 as a "coarse granular cell." Ehrlich in 1879 (2) noted the affinity of this cell for acid aniline dyes, such as eosin, and coined the term eosinophil. Knowledge of eosinophils and their functions has expanded rapidly, especially over the last decade (3–10). Eosinophilia is associated with allergic diseases (11–14), parasitic infections (15–18), syndromes associated with cutaneous edema (19–21), neoplastic conditions (22–25), and various diseases (26–29). Eosinophil granulocytes are formed in the bone marrow (30), and their life cycle then continues through blood and finally tissues (31). Circulating eosinophils represent from 0 to 5% of the peripheral white blood count in normal, healthy individuals (32). The normal range of the eosinophil count in adults is between 0 and 600 cells/mm^3 (33). In this chapter, eosinophil differentiation, activation, degranulation, and involvement in different diseases will be reviewed.

B. Eosinophil Granules and Their Protein Contents

Eosinophils contain three different types of granules: (a) the specific (or secondary) granule with its characteristic core, (b) the small granule, and (c) the primary granule (7–9).

1. Specific Granule Proteins

The specific human eosinophil granule contains four major proteins (7,8), the major basic protein (MBP) (34), eosinophil cationic protein (ECP) (35), eosinophil peroxidase (EPO) (36), and the eosinophil-derived neurotoxin (EDN) (37,38). The molecular weight of human MBP is 14,000, and in the guinea pig MBP constitutes more than

50% of the granule's protein content (7,34). ECP has a molecular weight ranging from 18,600 to 21,000 (7,37); EDN has a molecular weight of 18,600 (7,37,38); and both proteins possess RNase activity. EPO has a molecular weight of 71–77,000 and is made up of two polypeptides, a heavy chain (molecular weight 57,000) and a light chain (molecular weight 11,000) (39,40). A detailed description of the structure and function of these proteins is presented elsewhere (7,8).

a. MBP. MBP was localized to the eosinophil granule core as shown by biochemical analysis (41) and immunoelectron microscopy (42,43). MBP is present in the sputum (12) and is deposited in the bronchial tissues of patients with asthma (11,13). In-vitro experiments established that MBP is cytotoxic to bronchial epithelial cells in guinea pig tracheal rings (44,45), as well as rat and human pneumocytes (46). Moreover, the addition of MBP to mammalian ciliated cells decreases their ciliary activity, presumably as a consequence of inhibition of their axonemal ATPase (47). MBP also alters ion transport in dog tracheal epithelium (48). In addition, MBP is capable of inducing guinea pig (49) and canine (50) bronchial smooth muscle hyperreactivity. MBP is also capable of inducing superoxide anion generation in and the degranulation of neutrophils (51), inducing histamine release from basophils and mast cells (52–54), inducing EDN release from eosinophils (55), activating platelets (56), and regulating complement (57). The effect of MBP on neutrophils, basophils, mast cells, eosinophils, and platelets is inhibited by EDTA (51–56). MBP is toxic to helminths (58) and is localized on the surface of damaged parasites in vivo (59). MBP has also been localized to human and primate term placentae (60), where its function is yet to be determined. Of interest, serum levels of MBP are elevated during pregnancy and seem to predict the onset of labor (61).

MBP has recently been cloned from the cDNA library of promyelocytic cell line, HL-60 (62), and a cDNA library of human polymorphonuclear cells (63). It has a very high pI as judged by its amino acid sequence [pI 10.6 (62–64)]. The cationic nature of MBP could explain its wide range of toxicity for both helminths and mammalian cells. The cDNA sequence predicts the presence of a precursor molecule with an acidic N-terminal peptide [pI 3.9 (62)]. The proprotein could neutralize the charge of MBP intracellularly [predicted pI of 6.2 for the whole molecule "proMBP" (62)] and could possibly moderate its toxicity to eosinophils within the eosinophil granule itself. This "proMBP" protein, however, has not been isolated.

b. EDN. EDN is a powerful neurotoxin with the ability to selectively destroy Purkinje cells in the cerebellum and to cause paralysis in experimental animals if injected intrathecally (the Gordon phenomenon) (38). EDN is localized to the eosinophil granule matrix. Based on biochemical and functional similarities, EDN and another eosinophil granule protein, eosinophil protein X, are likely the same molecule (65). In addition, EDN is a potent ribonuclease (66). The cDNA for EDN has been cloned and sequenced (67,68).

c. ECP. ECP represents a group of eosinophil granule proteins localized to the eosinophil granule matrix (42,43). ECP is one of the most potent eosinophil granule protein helminthotoxins (69–71) and is found deposited on dead parasites in vivo (72). Furthermore, ECP, like EDN, possesses ribonuclease activity (66,73) and induces the Gordon phenomenon (7); it also possesses antibacterial properties (74). Two forms of ECP can be distinguished by the use of monoclonal antibodies, a secreted and a stored form (75). The secreted form of ECP was found deposited in tissues of patients with different allergic conditions in association with activated eosinophils (76). ECP probably mediates its cytotoxic effect by causing membrane damage in its target (77). The cDNA for ECP has also been cloned (78,79). The homology between the EDN, ECP, secretory human and rat pancreatic ribonucleases, bovine seminal ribonuclease, and angiogenin suggests that they belong to a ribonuclease "super family" of proteins having evolved from a common ancestral gene (67,68,78,79).

d. EPO. EPO is also localized to the granule matrix (43). It is composed of a light and a heavy chain (36,39,40,80) and a prosthetic heme group (81). The heavy chain of the molecule is glycosylated (80) and tends to form aggregates. EPO has the ability to oxidize halides and produce hypohalous acids (82–85), with bromides used preferentially (85). EPO is a helminthotoxin (86,87). It also augments both neutrophil- (88) and mast cell- (89) mediated toxicity to schistosomula of *Schistosoma mansoni.* In addition, a mixture of EPO and MBP is cytotoxic to different mammalian cell lines (90). EPO cDNA been has also cloned (39,40) and EPO is strikingly homologous to myeloperoxidase and thyroid peroxidase. A few patients with EPO deficiency have been reported (91,92).

2. *Small Granule Proteins*

The small eosinophil granules have been reported to contain acid phosphatase and aryl sulfatase (93). It has also been suggested that small granules in human eosinophils are the remains of crystalloid granules which have secreted most of their contents (9).

3. *Primary Granule Proteins*

By immunoelectron microscopy, primary granules are round, uniformly electron dense, and characteristically seen in eosinophilic promyelocytes (94). Another of the eosinophil proteins, the Charcot-Leyden crystal (CLC) protein, has also been localized to a minor population ($\sim 5\%$) of the eosinophil granules that are large and membrane bound (95). These granules appear to be the primary eosinophil granules (95). CLC was first described in 1853 and later in 1872 (95,96) and appears as hexagonal bipyramidal crystals (8). Biochemical analysis of CLC showed that it is a single protein of 17,400 MW (95,97) which possesses lysophospholipase activity (98,99). Human basophils are also able to form CLC (100).

C. Eosinophil Membrane Proteins

Eosinophils possess a number of membrane proteins, some of which serve as receptors. The functions of others are unknown. The membrane proteins acting as receptors are described below.

1. *Complement Receptors*

Eosinophils adhere to and degranulate on large serum-coated surfaces via complement or Fc receptors or a combination of the two. Evidence for complement (C3b) receptors on eosinophils comes from rosetting techniques with C3b and with the use of anti-C3b receptor monoclonal antibodies (101–105). Evidence for C5a receptors comes from Scatchard analysis of radiolabeled C5a binding to eosinophils (106).

2. *Immunoglobulin Receptors*

Fc gamma receptors on the eosinophil have also been extensively studied by rosetting techniques and by their ability to mediate eosinophil function (101,107–110). Eosinophils have also been reported to possess low-affinity IgE Fc receptors (111,112), which were found to play a role in the hypodense eosinophil effector function (113–120). Evidence from fluorocytometric analysis (121) and degranulation studies (122) suggests that eosinophils also have IgA receptors. IgA receptors were detected both in patients with hypereosinophilic syndrome (121) and in normal individuals (122). After comparing IgE, IgG, IgA, and sIgA, sIgA was the most potent immunoglobulin stimulant for in-vitro eosinophil degranulation (122). This, along with the localization of eosinophils at epithelial surfaces (123,124), where they carry out their effector function, suggests an important role for sIgA in mediating the eosinophil effector function.

3. Cytokine Receptors

Eosinophils are known to possess receptors for and respond to interleukin (IL)-5 (125). Human eosinophils were also found to express a single class of high-affinity receptors for IL-3 and GM-CSF (126). The role that cytokines play in eosinophil biology will be described in a separate section.

4. Receptor for Platelet-Activating Factor (PAF)

The study of the surface expression of the PAF receptor on eosinophils utilizing ^{3}H-PAF has been complicated by nonspecific binding, metabolism, and uptake of the radioligand (127). Therefore, a PAF antagonist, WEB 2086, was utilized to study the expression of this receptor. The receptor was found to possess a dissociation constant of 16.1 nM (127).

5. Surface Antigens

More recently, eosinophils cultured with human granulocyte macrophage colony-stimulating factor (hGM-CSF) and murine 3T3 fibroblasts were found to express CD4 (128); eosinophils cultured in a similar manner express HLA-DR (129) as well. At this writing, the role that these receptors might play in eosinophil function is obscure.

D. Eosinophil Variability

Ehrlich was the first to describe eosinophil variability in his presentation to the Physiologic Society in 1879 (130). Later, eosinophils with fewer granules and with vacuoles were described (131–133) in the blood of patients with eosinophilia associated with an allergic condition or a parasitic infection (8,9). This population of vacuolated eosinophils seemed to represent a more mature form as judged by nuclear segmentation. In those reports, vacuolated eosinophils disappeared after eosinophil counts became normal. In discontinuous Percoll density gradients, a vacuolated population of eosinophils with a lighter buoyant density than normal eosinophils, as well as a higher level of oxygen consumption and higher number of Fc gamma receptors, was described (134). This eosinophil population has been called hypodense, in contrast to eosinophils from normal individuals, which separate at a higher buoyant density and are referred to as normodense (134–136). These two eosinophil populations were also found using metrizamide discontinuous density gradients for eosinophil purification (135,136). In addition, hypodense eosinophils were observed in bronchial lavage fluids from patients with pulmonary eosinophilia and from pleural fluids of patients with eosinophilic pleural effusion (135). Furthermore, eosinophils from nasal washings of two patients with allergic rhinitis were of the hypodense population as well (137).

Two reports suggest that hypodense eosinophils represent a more active cell than normodense cells with regard to parasite killing (116) and leukotriene release (138). A relationship may exist between these two types of eosinophils in vivo. However, most of the work to study this relationship has been done in vitro. For example, incubation of normal eosinophils with serum treated with cobra venom, or with concanavalin A, induced the formation of vacuolated eosinophils; this effect was inhibited by cytochalasin B (132). More recent work in vitro suggests another relationship between the hypodense and normodense eosinophils. For example, incubation of normodense eosinophils, either with IL-5 (139), IL-5 and 3T3 fibroblasts (140), GM-CSF in the presence of fibroblasts (141), or with IL-3 alone or in the presence of fibroblasts (142), prolongs the survival of eosinophils and induces them to become hypodense. Of even greater interest is the finding that infection of normal volunteers with the hookworm larvae *Necator americanus* elevates their peripheral eosinophil count (143), and their peripheral blood eosinophils become hypodense (from 34 $\pm 13\%$ to 80 $\pm 7\%$). Furthermore, hyodense eosinophils from patients with eosinophilia were found to contain two proteins (identified by two-dimensional gel electrophoresis) not found in their normodense counterparts, suggesting additional protein synthesis in those cells (144). The hypodense eosinophil in vivo could represent: (a) a more mature, activated form of eosinophils induced by lymphokines; (b) a more immature form of eosinphils; (c) a separate lineage of eosinophils induced by the need for the cell in an immune response; or (d) some combination of the above possibilities. A more detailed analysis of the differences between those two populations is reviewed in Ref. 145.

II. CONDITIONS ASSOCIATED WITH EOSINOPHILIA

A. Parasitic Infections

The association of helminth infections with eosinophilia has been known since the turn of this century (2,7,8,15,31,146). In-vitro studies have shown the ability of eosinophils to kill different parasites (15). This ability of eosinophils to kill in vivo likely requires either the presence of a specific antiparasite antibody, complement, or both (147). Furthermore, purified eosinophil cationic proteins, when added to parasites in vivo, are by themselves toxic to those targets (87).

Analyses of the interactions between eosinophils and various parasites including schistosomula of *Schistosoma mansoni* (148–152), *Trichinella spiralis* larvae (153–156), and others (157,158), have been studied in vitro. In vivo these parasites induce eosinophilia (140,159,160) in their host which appears to be protective, because the use of anti-eosinophilic serum inhibits this protective effect (161–163). Furthermore, deposition of the eosinophil granule proteins on the surface of dead parasites has been documented (16–18,59,164,165).

B. Allergic Diseases

1. Bronchial Asthma

Bronchial asthma is associated with eosinophilia (4,7–11). This association was found to be useful in the management of bronchial asthma because peripheral blood eosinophil counts were found to be inversely related to airway conductance (166) and nonspecific bronchial responsiveness (167). Bronchial asthma is also associated with significant bronchoalveolar eosinophilia (168–170), elevated levels of MBP in serum and lavage fluid, as well as elevated levels of arylsulfatase in lavage fluids (170). The elevations of MBP and arylsulfatase are correlated with the extent of eosinophilia. Elevated levels of MBP in sputum from patients with asthma have also been reported (12). Furthermore, in tissue specimens of lungs from patients with bronchial asthma, MBP deposition occurs on damaged bronchial epithelium (13). Finally, patients with asthma have an increased number of hypodense eosinophils (136). The in-vitro destructive effects of MBP on tracheal epithelium, as well as the action of MBP on tracheal smooth muscle (49,50), strongly suggest that eosinophils play a major role in the pathophysiology of asthma (11).

2. *Dermatologic Conditions*

Eosinophil infiltration and degranulation, as evidenced by MBP deposition, is observed in a number of dermatologic conditions including atopic dermatitis (18), eosinophilic pustular folliculitis (171), cutaneous edema (172), facial edema (173), and solar urticaria (174).

3. *Drug Reactions*

Eosinophilia can be associated both with immediate hypersensitivity and with chronic or delayed hypersensitivity responses. Many different types of drugs can induce eosinophilia (175). The target organs affected include the skin, lung, heart, kidney, and liver; however, the roles of eosinophils in these responses are not known. The most recent and dramatic to be described is the outbreak of the eosinophilia-myalgia syndrome (EMS), which is associated with the ingestion of L-tryptophan (176). Although EMS was initially characterized by eosinophilia and myalgia, it has become clear that many organs are involved, especially the skin, which becomes diffusely fibrotic (177).

C. Neoplastic Diseases

1. *Hodgkin's Disease*

Eosinophil infiltration in the lymph nodes of patients with Hodgkin's disease has been reported since the turn of the century (25). More recent evidence shows that not only do eosinophils infiltrate the lymph nodes of those patients (25,178,179), they also degranulate as shown by the extracellular deposition of MBP (25) and EPO (178,179) in the tissues. Furthermore, in 21% of Hodgkin's patients, bone marrow eosinophilia is observed (180); in 15% of patients, peripheral blood eosinophilia is observed (181). However, neither bone marrow eosinophilia nor peripheral blood eosinophilia, as a component of general leukocytosis, had prognostic significance in the disease. In contrast, selective peripheral blood eosinophilia was associated with a survival advantage (181).

2. *Leukemias*

Eosinophilia has been reported in a number of patients with acute leukemia (182–191). In a number of those patients, chromosomal abnormalities involving chromosome 16 (183,185,186,188,189) or other chromosomes have been reported.

3. *Other Tumor-Associated Eosinophils*

Eosinophilia has been reported in a number of other neoplastic states and termed tumor-associated eosinophilia (192,193). Those carcinomas have involved the lung (192,194), cervix (192), nasopharynx (193), stomach (195), rectum (196), and others (192).

D. Other Conditions

1. Idiopathic Hypereosinophilic Syndrome

Idiopathic hypereosinophilic syndrome refers to a number of conditions associated with eosinophilia of unknown etiology. Patients suffering from this syndrome have multisystem involvement including neurologic, dermatologic, cardiovascular, spleen, pulmonary, hepatic, and other organs (197,198). Eosinophils from these patients were found to be of the hypodense variety (199).

2. Episodic Angioedema Associated with Eosinophilia

Another syndrome with idiopathic eosinophilia is the episodic angioedema associated with eosinophilia (19,28,200). This syndrome is characterized by cyclical eosinophilia associated with angioedema.

3. Cardiovascular Involvement

Cardiovascular involvement is one of the manifestations of the idiopathic hypereosinophilic syndrome. Eosinophil degranulation (15,201) is seen in cardiac tissue specimens from patients with eosinophilic endomyocardial disease and eosinophilic myocarditis. This involvement with infiltration and degranulation suggests a role for the eosinophil in the pathophysiology of cardiac damage in those conditions.

4. Renal Conditions

Eosinophilia is associated with a number of renal conditions (202–205), and appears to be useful in the diagnosis of acute interstitial nephritis, although it is not specific for this diagnosis (205). It may also be characteristic of athero-embolic renal disease (206). The most useful association between eosinophilia and renal disease, however, is in renal allograft rejection (207–211), where an increase in the level of MBP in urine is detected (211).

5. Liver Transplant Rejection

Peripheral blood eosinophilia has been reported to be associated with the rejection of human liver transplants (212). However, the association of graft eosinophilia with acute rejection appears to be much more sensitive and specific (27). Eosinophilia, therefore, appears to be a good predictor of hepatic allograft rejection.

6. Eosinophilic Gastroenteritis

Eosinophilic gastroenteritis is a condition in which eosinophils infiltrate the gastrointestinal tract (213). Patients have variable presentations of the disease depending on which layer of the gut is infiltrated with eosinophils (214). Ultrastructural evidence suggests the release of MBP into the tissues infiltrated with eosinophils (215), which could explain the tissue damage observed.

7. Acquired Immune Deficiency Syndrome (AIDS)

Patients with AIDS suffering from *Pneumocystis carinii* pneumonitis were found to have bronchoalveolar eosinophilia (216), not seen otherwise in patients with AIDS nor in those with *Pneumocystis carinii.* Furthermore, eosinophilic pustular folliculitis has been reported to be associated with AIDS as well (217), and is proposed as an early sign of infection with the human immunodeficiency virus (HIV) (218).

8. Complications of Pregnancy

A protein immunochemically similar to MBP is elevated in serum during pregnancy (61); MBP is localized to the placenta (60), to the placental X-cells, and the placental-site giant cells. Elevations in the serum levels of MBP were found to predict the onset of labor (219).

For an excellent and a more extensive review of different diseases associated with eosinophilia consult Ref. 9.

III. EOSINOPHIL DIFFERENTIATION

A. Eosinophil-Thymic Lymphocyte Interaction in Vivo

The role of T-lymphocytes in the regulation of the eosinophil response emerged in the early 1970s. One of the earliest reports on this subject (220) suggested that, in mice, a thymic-derived mononuclear cell population is necessary for optimal development of eosinophilia in response to parasite antigens. Others (221,222) reported a decrease in the eosinophilic response to parasitic infections in nude mice. Of interest, nude rats were reported to respond to a parasitic infection with eosinophilia (223). A number of factors produced by mononuclear cells acting on eosinophils have been described (224–231) in mice, humans, rats, and guinea pigs, both in vivo and in vitro.

In addition, a number of factors produced by mononuclear cells and T-cells in the mouse, guinea pig, and human enhance eosinophil cytotoxicity (232–239). It was also reported that serum from a patient with chronic pruritus (240) induced both eosinophil and neutrophil degranulation in vivo and in vitro. Furthermore, a study on an eosinophil granuloma (241) reported the presence of OKT6- (subsequently called CD1a) (242) positive cells within the granuloma. A significantly high number of CD3- and CD4-positive T-cells that express IL-2 receptors were found in the skins of patients after intradermal allergen challenge (243). These cells were adjacent to eosinophils expressing the eosinophil activation marker EG2. From all the above, it is concluded that T-cells (in addition to other mononuclear cells) play an important role in the regulation of eosinophilopoiesis, eosinophil activation, and probably degranulation as well.

B. In-Vitro Models

1. Bone Marrow

A factor now known as IL-5 produced by a mouse T-cell hybrid (235,244,245) was found to stimulate eosinophil differentiation in vitro. This factor was cloned (246,247), studied (139,248–250), and found to induce eosinophilopoiesis (251). Injection of a monoclonal antibody to IL-5 in mice inhibited *Nippostrongylus brasilienis*-induced eosinophilia (252). Other soluble products, including IL-3 and GM-CSF, also influence eosinophil function. Both IL-3 and GM-CSF play roles in eosinophil differentiation, eosinophilopoiesis (253,254), increase the ability of eosinophils to kill parasites, and prolong eosinophil survival in vitro (141,142,245). Tumor necrosis factor (TNF) has also been reported to enhance the ability of eosinophils to kill parasites (255).

2. Cord Blood

The ability to generate eosinophils in vitro from cord-blood mononuclear cells (256) using IL-5 provides further support for the primary role of IL-5 in inducing eosinophil differentiation. Eosinophils derived by IL-5 stimulation in this procedure are morphologically similar to peripheral blood eosinophils (257).

IV. EOSINOPHIL FUNCTION

A. Regulation of the Inflammatory Response: A Historical Perspective

The exact role the eosinophil plays in vivo is unknown. At the turn of the century (2), Ehrlich reported an increase in eosinophil number in the healing phase of inflammatory reactions. Since then, it was commonly held that the eosinophil plays a regulatory role in the inflammatory response (3–5,258). However, more recent evidence suggests otherwise.

B. In-Vitro Models for Studying Eosinophil Function

1. Helminthotoxicity

It was not until the last decade that a helminthotoxic role for the eosinophil was described (15,147). Eosinophils are capable of both inducing ^{51}Cr release (148) from and inflicting gross damage to schistosomula of *S. mansoni* in vitro as judged by microscopy (149–151). This process is antibody dependent and involves adherence of the eosinophil to the schistosomule (148,152). Such a mechanism has also been described in the killing of *Trichinella spiralis* larvae by both eosinophils and neutrophils in the presence of stage-specific antibodies (153).

The eosinophil-parasite interaction is bidirectional, as evidenced from the ability of schistosomules of *S. mansoni* (259), *T. spiralis* (260), and *Toxocara canis* larvae (261,262) to produce soluble antigens that chemoattract and/or activate eosinophils. This chemoattraction/activation property is likely one of the steps enhancing parasite killing by eosinophils. This mechanism ends in eosinophil degranulation on the parasite's surface, as Ehrlich hypothesized in his review of 1900 (130), and as observed in more recent experiments (16,17). The degranulation events are mediated through eosinophil receptors as discussed earlier.

2. The Importance of a Large Surface

The models used to study eosinophil function in vitro in the absence of a parasite have usually used a large, nonphagocytosable surface. These models are based, in part, on the observation (6) that homogenized *T. spiralis* (no large surface) did not induce eosinophilia as did its intact counterpart. This result suggested a need for a large parasite surface to induce eosinophilia in vivo, and several studies have been based on this concept. One study included incubation of human eosinophils with agar surfaces coated with antigen-antibody complexes (263–265). Here, eosinophils spread out on the agar surface and subsequently degranulated. In another study, eosinophils were incubated with serum-coated Sepharose beads (266), and the eosinophils adhered to the beads. This interaction induced superoxide production in eosinophils, and the effect was enhanced by coating the beads with phorbol myristate acetate. In a third study, eosinophils and neutrophils were incubated with opsonized zymosan particles, and the two cell types generated comparable amounts of H_2O_2 (267). In a fourth study, eosinophils stimulated by IgG-coated Sepharose beads generated leukotriene C_4 (138). In a fifth study, eosinophils were incubated with serum-coated Sephadex particles and ECP was released (268). This inducible effect was lost after heat inactivation of serum, suggesting a requirement for complement. In a sixth study, various immunoglobulin isotypes coupled to Sepharose 4B beads were employed as targets for eosinophil degranulation as judged by the release of EDN (122). Here, sIgA was found to be the most potent immunoglobulin inducing eosinophil degranulation (122). Finally, anti-IgA-induced eosinophil degranulation has also been reported (121) to induce EPO release.

In addition, a study with rat eosinophils (269) showed that only IgE and IgG_{2a} were able to induce EPO release, not the other IgG subclasses or IgM. These authors suggested (269,270) that eosinophils release EPO only in response to IgE and the other cationic eosinophil proteins in response to the other immunoglobulins.

From all the above reports, one concludes that large immunoglobulin- or complement-coated surfaces provided by parasites or even tissues in allergic reactions induce eosinophil adherence and perhaps even degranulation. Not all degranulation models, however, utilized a large surface to activate eosinophils. In one study, aggregated immunoglobulins seemed to be sufficient to induce degranulation (112).

The inconsistencies in degranulation responses to immunoglobulin stimulation may arise from species differences or from the density of the eosinophils used. For example, in one study, neither eosinophil binding nor degranulation on exposure to IgE-coated beads was found (122); however, normodense human eosinophils, which may not express the IgE receptor (119,120), were tested. Furthermore, in five experiments using hypodense human eosinophils and IgE-coated beads, eosinophil degranulation was observed only once (unpublished results). The finding that IgA causes eosinophil degranulation is at variance with a report that murine IgA proteins do not promote eosinophil binding to or lysis of coated erythrocytes and that human eosinophils do not form rosettes with sheep erythrocytes coated with IgA1 and IgA2 myeloma proteins (271). However, sIgA was not tested in these latter experiments.

Eosinophils and sIgA could play an important role in immunity at mucosal surfaces, both in the case of intestinal helminths and in the pathogenesis of bronchial asthma, especially idiopathic cases or those precipitated by viral infections. Studies of patients with asthma have shown the presence of IgA antibodies to various antigens (272–274). Indeed, in a patient with asthma, IgA2 deposition was observed on alveolar membranes in association with eosinophils and viral particles (275).

IL-5, initially described as possessing eosinophil differentiating activity (248,249), has now been shown to exert its effects on both eosinophils and on lymphocytes involved in IgA synthesis. It induces eosinophil activation (250) and is chemotactic for eosinophils (139). IL-5 also induces the production of murine IgA (139,276,277), although its effects on IgA production in humans are still controversial (278–280). Thus, IL-5 may orchestrate the interaction of eosinophils and IgA, which together may play an important role in mucosal immunity and possibly in human disease.

3. *Calcium Ionophores*

Other degranulation models included the use of calcium ionophores to study eosinophil degranulation (281–283). In these studies the degranulation of horse (281) and human (282,283) eosinophils was studied in the presence of A23187, a potent calcium ionophore. The results from these reports demonstrate that A23187 is a potent inducer of eosinophil degranulation.

C. Chemotaxis

A number of eosinophil chemotactic factors are known. Some are parasite products, or bacterial peptides, others are soluble mediators produced in vivo.

1. Parasite Products

Parasite-derived factors can act as chemoattractants for eosinophils, and a number of such factors have been described (284–289). These factors could also activate the eosinophil (290–293).

2. Soluble Mediators

A number of mediators have been described as eosinophilotactic factors. Among the earliest described are the low-molecular-weight tetrapeptides referred to as the eosinophil chemotactic factors of anaphylaxis (294). Other eosinophil chemotactic factors include C5a (295–297), N-formyl-methionyl-leucyl-phenylalanine (FMLP) (296,297), histamine (295), monohydroxy-eicosatetraenoic acids (HETEs) (295,298), and leukotriene B_4 (LTB_4), both in vitro (299) and in vivo (300,301).

One of the most recently described eosinophil chemotactic factors is PAF (302–307). Its chemotactic activity is seen both in vitro (302–305) and in vivo (306,307). In fact, in one study where the potencies of different eosinophil chemotactic factors were compared, PAF was equivalent to C5a and they were both more potent than LTB_4 and FMLP (304). The role PAF plays as a chemoattractant in vivo, however, might be mediated by a secondary mediator as suggested by a study in rats (308). In this study (308), the ability of PAF to act as an eosinophil chemoattractant in pleural fluids was transferable by the pleural fluid 6 h after intrapleural injection of PAF, at which time the injected PAF would be inactivated. Furthermore, the administration of the protein synthesis inhibitor cycloheximide abolished the generation of this transferable chemotactic activity in rats receiving PAF and not in those receiving the chemotactic activity induced by PAF. In a different report (309), an antagonist of PAF did not inhibit airway eosinophilia.

A serum factor inducing eosinophil differentiation has also been described in *Mesocestoides corti*-infected mice (310); this factor is now known as IL-5. More recent evidence suggested that IL-5, the eosinophil differentiation and activation factor (248–250), is an eosinophil chemotactic factor as well (139). Not only that, it is also a selective eosinophil chemoattractant (311).

V. THE ROLE OF SOLUBLE MEDIATORS IN MODULATING EOSINOPHIL FUNCTION

The eosinophil effector function can be modulated by different interleukins, colony stimulating factors, and lipid mediators (312). This section will review some of those factors and their effects in eosinophil function.

A. Interleukins

1. IL-1

IL-1 represents a group of interleukins that has a multitude of effects on many targets in vivo (313,314). The ability of IL-1 to modulate the eosinophil's release of arylsulfatase and β-glucuronidase has been studied (315,316). Purified monocyte IL-1 and recombinant IL-1β (rIL-1β) are capable of inducing the release of both arylsulfatase and β-glucuronidase (315). IL-1β did not, however, stimulate superoxide anion production by eosinophils (315). Furthermore, the addition of IL-1 to phorbol myristic acetate (TPA) enhanced the TPA-induced superoxide anion generation (315). The ability of IL-1 to modulate eosinophil enzyme release appears to be due mainly to IL-1β, not IL-1α (316). In contrast, rIL-1β was not capable of modulating Ig-induced EDN release (317). Murine IL-1 was found to play a role in eosinophil differentiation (253); in humans, however, rIL-1α does not play a role in eosinophil differentiation (251).

2. IL-2

IL-2, originally called the T-cell growth factor, plays an important role in cellular interactions in the immune system (318). In vitro, IL-2 does not seem to directly modulate eosinophil degranulation (317), nor does it play a direct role in eosinophil differentiation (251). However, patients who received IL-2 treatment for metastatic cancer (319,320) developed eosinophilia. Likewise, rats on IL-2 treatment developed eosinophilia, among other changes (321). The induced human eosinophils (320) became hypodense, developed hypersegmented nuclei, and changed their ECP from the storage to the secretory form. They also become more cytotoxic to *S. mansoni* larvae (320). This, however, does not seem to be due to the direct effect of IL-2 on eosinophils (320) and is probably mediated indirectly by induction of IL-5 production from T-cells or other eosinophil differentiation/growth-promoting factors, as has been described earlier (322,323). In contrast, the human eosinophilic leukemia cell lines, EoL-1 and EoL-3 (324–327), express the IL-2 receptor (Tac/p55) on their surfaces (328). IL-2 receptor expression in those cell lines is upregulated by interferon-γ (IFN-γ) (328).

6. IL-3

a. Hematopoietic Activity. IL-3 has multiple hematopoietic activities (329–332). It supports the growth and differentiation of progenitor cells committed to megakaryocytic, erythroid, monocytic, and different granulocytic cell lineages (329–331). IL-3 is able to support an early stage of eosinophil differentiation in both bone marrow (253,254) and cord blood cultures (256,257).

b. Effect on Basophils, Eosinophils, and Mast Cells. IL-3 enhances human basophil mediator release induced by IgE (333,334) and C5a (335). This effect is probably mediated via high-affinity IL-3 receptors on basophils (336). IL-3 also enhances immunoglobulin-induced eosinophil degranulation (317). This effect is also probably mediated via the IL-3 receptors on human eosinophils (126). IL-3 is also capable of the prolongation of eosinophil survival in vitro (142). The ability of IL-3 to cause mast cells to release other interleukins that could in turn affect the allergic response is also of interest (337). Those varied effects of IL-3 suggest that it plays a central role in the allergic response.

4. IL-5

IL-5 was initially described as the eosinophil differentiation factor (248,249). It was also found to be a selective activator of eosinophil function (250) and enhanced immunoglobulin-induced eosinophil degranulation (317). Eosinophils express IL-5 receptors (125). In addition, IL-5 is chemotactic for eosinophils (311). IL-5 also prolongs eosinophil survival in vitro (139) and induces normodense eosinophils to become hypodense and more active in their cytotoxic abilities (140). In a number of reports (278–280), IL-5 was found to enhance IgA production from B-cells. This, with the finding that sIgA is the most potent signal for eosinophil degranulation (122), suggests an important role for IL-5 in orchestrating the eosinophil function at mucosal surfaces, where eosinophils carry out their effector function.

B. Granulocyte-Macrophage Colony-Stimulating Factor (GM-CSF)

GM-CSF has the ability to induce the differentiation of a number of cell lineages in culture (338), and is believed to act on early progenitor cells in the bone marrow (339). It is capable of inducing eosinophil differentiation (254), prolonging eosinophil survival in vitro (141), and enhancing immunoglobulin induced eosinophil degranulation (317). Eosinophils possess GM-CSF receptors (126).

C. Interferon-γ

The role of INF-γ in modulating eosinophil function has not been studied extensively. In one report (317), INF-γ was found to inhibit sIgA-induced eosinophil degranulation without affecting IgG-induced degranulation.

D. Lipid Mediators

1. PAF

PAF (340) is one of the most potent eosinophil chemotactic factors, as discussed above (304–310,341). It also induces leukotriene C_4 generation from eosinophils (342) and stimulates eosinophil degranulation (343). PAF also causes the elevation of intracellular calcium concentrations in eosinophils (344). Furthermore, when normodense eosinophils are incubated with PAF, they become hypodense (345).

VI. SUMMARY AND CONCLUSIONS

The emerging picture regarding the role of eosinophils in the immune response appears to be the following: IL-3 [in humans, (251)], and/or IL-1 [in the mouse system, (253)], then IL-5 and GM-CSF [which are secreted from activated T-cells at the inflammation sites or even from activated mast cells (346–348)] induce differentiation and proliferation of eosinophils in bone marrow. Other factors, such as PAF (303–309), C5a, soluble parasite products (259–261), or even IL-5 (139), serve as chemoattractants for eosinophils to the sites of allergic inflammation, usually around mucosal surfaces. Eosinophil survival and state of activation is enhanced by IL-5 (139). Eosinophils degranulate, thus releasing their toxic granule proteins by cross-linking Ig receptors, the most potent of which is sIgA, and the degranulation is enhanced by IL-5, IL-3, GM-CSF, and other factors or parasite products. Eosinophil degranulation can also be induced by complement, as well as PAF.

The interplay of all these different mediators, and their effects on eosinophil function, is an integral part of the eosinophil's involvement in different disease conditions. Eosinophils appear to be involved in the pathophysiology of different diseases, in part, by releasing their toxic granule contents in tissues and causing tissue damage.

ACKNOWLEDGMENTS

We would like to thank Cheryl Adolphson for editorial review and Linda H. Arneson for excellent secretarial assistance.

REFERENCES

1. Jones TW. The blood corpuscle considered in its different phases of development in the animal series. Memoir, I.—Vertebrata. Phil Trans R Soc Lond 1846; 136:63–87.
2. Cline MJ. The white cell. Cambridge, MA: Harvard University Press, 1975:104–22.
3. Weller PF, Goetzl EJ. The regulatory and effector roles of eosinophils. Adv Immunol 1979: 27:339–71.
4. Kay AB. The role of the eosinophil. J Allergy Clin Immunol 1979; 64:90–104.
5. Sullivan TJ. The role of eosinophils in inflammatory reactions. Prog Hematol 1979; 11:65–82.
6. Beeson PB, Bass DA. The eosinophil. In: Smith LH, Jr, ed. Major problems in internal medicine, vol. XIV. Philadelphia: WB Saunders, 1977:161–89.
7. Gleich GJ, Loegering DA. Immunobiology of eosinophils. Ann Rev Immunol 1984; 2:429–59.
8. Gleich GJ, Adolphson CR. The eosinophilic leukocyte: structure and function. Adv Immunol 1986; 39:177–253.
9. Spry CJF. Eosinophils. A comprehensive review and guide to the scientific and medical literature. New York: Oxford University Press, 1988.
10. Slifman NR, Adolphson CR, Gleich GJ. Eosinophils: biochemical and cellular aspects. In: Middleton E Jr, Reed CE, Ellis EF, Adkinson NF Jr, Yunginger JW, eds. Allergy Principles and Practice, vol. 1, 3d ed., St. Louis: CV Mosby, 1988:179–205.
11. Frigas E, Gleich GJ. The eosinophil and the pathophysiology of asthma. J Allergy Clin Immunol 1986; 77:527–37.
12. Frigas E, Loegering DA, Solley GO, Farrow GM, Gleich GJ. Elevated levels of the eosinophil granule major basic protein in the sputum of patients with bronchial asthma. Mayo Clin Proc 1981; 56:345–53.
13. Filley WV, Holley KE, Kephart GM, Gleich GJ. Identification by immunofluorescence of eosinophil granule major basic protein in lung tissues of patients with bronchial asthma. Lancet 1982; 2:11–6.
14. Yoshida H, Sadao A, Hori M, Akiyama T, Ushijima N, Tanaka M. Ultrastructural studies of eosinophils in passive cutaneous anaphylaxis. Arch Dermatol Res 1982; 272:197–200.
15. Butterworth AE. Cell mediated damage to helminths. Adv Parasitol 1984; 23:143–235.
16. Kephart GM, Gleich GJ, Connor DH, Gibson DW, Ackerman SJ. Deposition of eosinophil granule major basic protein onto microfilariae of *Onchocerca volvulus* in the skin of patients treated with diethylcarbamazine. Lab Invest 1984; 50:51–61.
17. Li Hsu SY, Hsu HF, Mitros FA, Helms CM, Solomon RI. Eosinophils as effector cells in the destruction of *Schistosoma mansoni* eggs in granulomas. Ann Trop Med Parasitol 1980; 74:179–83.
18. Leiferman KM, Ackerman SJ, Sampson HA, Haugen HS, Venencie PY, Gleich GJ. Dermal deposition of eosinophil-granule major basic protein in atopic dermatitis: comparison with onchocerciasis. N Engl J Med 1985; 313:282–5.
19. Gleich GJ, Schroeter AL, Marcoux JP, Sachs MI, O'Connell EJ, Kohler PF. Episodic angioedema associated with eosinophilia. N Engl J Med 1984; 310:1621–6.
20. Kim CH, Vlietstra RE, Edwards WD, Reeder GS, Gleich GJ. Steroid-responsive eosinophilic myocarditis: diagnosis by endocardial biopsy. Am J Cardiol 1984; 53:1472–3.
21. Stern JB, Sobel HJ, Rotchford JP. Well's syndrome: is there collagen damage in the flame figures? J Cutan Pathol 1984; 11:501–5.

22. Lowe D, Jorizzo J, Hutt MSR. Tumor associated eosinophilia: a review. J Clin Pathol 1981; 34:1343–8.
23. Slungaard A, Ascensao J, Zanjani E, Jacob HS. Pulmonary carcinoma with eosinophilia: demonstration of a tumor-derived eosinophilopoietic factor. N Engl J Med 1983; 309:778–81.
24. Mulligan MJ, Vasu R, Grossi CE, Prasthofer EF, Griffin FM, Kapila A, Trupp JM, Barton JC. Case report: Neoplastic meningitis with eosinophilic pleocytosis in Hodgkin's disease: a case with cerebellar dysfunction and a review of the literature. Am J Med Sci 1988; 296:322–6.
25. Butterfield JH, Kephart GM, Banks PM, Gleich GJ. Extracellular deposition of eosinophil granule major basic protein in lymph nodes of patients with Hodgkin's disease. Blood 1986; 68:1250–6.
26. Harlin SL, Ansel DG, Lane SR, Myers J, Kephart GM, Gleich GJ. A clinical and pathologic study of chronic sinusitis: the role of the eosinophil. J Allergy Clin Immunol 1988; 81:867–75.
27. Foster PF, Sankary HN, Hart M, Ashmann M, Williams JW. Blood and graft eosinophilia as predictors of rejection in human liver transplantation. Transplantation 1989; 47:72–4.
28. Wolf C, Pehamberger H, Breyer S, Leiferman KM, Wolff K. Episodic angioedema with eosinophilia. J Am Acad Dermatol 1989; 20:21–7.
29. Badesch DB, King TE, Schwarz MI. Acute eosinophilic pneumonia: a hypersensitivity phenomenon? Am Rev Resp Dis 1989; 139:249–52.
30. Goldman JM. Normal leukocytes. In: Hoffbrand AV, Lewis SM, eds. Postgraduate hematology, 2d ed. London: William Heinemann, 1981:381–430.
31. Nuttman TB, Ottesen RA, Cohen SG. Eosinophilia and eosinophil-related disorders. In: Middleton E Jr, Reed CE, Ellis EF, Adkinson NF Jr, Yunginger JW, eds. Allergy: principles and practice, 3d ed., vol. 2. St. Louis: CV Mosby, 1988:861–90.
32. Ravel R. Clinical laboratory medicine, clinical application of laboratory data, 3d ed. Chicago: Year Book Medical Publishers, 1978:39–44.
33. Smith JM. Epidemiology and natural history of asthma, allergic rhinitis and atopic dermatitis (eczema). In: Middleton E Jr, Reed CE, Ellis EF, Adkinson NF Jr, Yunginger JW, eds. Allergy: principles and practice, 3d ed., vol. 2. St. Louis: CV Mosby, 1988:891–929.
34. Gleich GJ, Loegering DA, Frigas E, Wassom DL, Solley GO, Mann KG. The major basic protein of the eosinophil granule: physicochemical properties, localization, and function. In: Mahmoud AAF, Austen KF, eds. The eosinophil in health and disease. New York: Grune & Stratton, 1980;79–92.
35. Olsson I, Venge P, Spitznagel JK, Lehrer RI. Arginine-rich cationic proteins of human eosinophil granules. Lab Invest 1977; 36:493–500.
36. Carlson MGCh, Peterson CGB, Venge P. Human eosinophil peroxidase: purification and characterization. J Immunol 1985; 134:1875–9.
37. Ackerman SJ, Loegering DA, Venge P, Olsson I, Harley JB, Fauci AS, Gleich GJ. Distinctive cationic proteins of the human eosinophil granule: major basic protein, eosinophil cationic protein, and eosinophil-derived neurotoxin. J Immunol 1983; 131:2977–82.
38. Durack DT, Ackerman SJ, Loegering DA, Gleich GJ. Purification of human eosinophil-derived neurotoxin. Proc Natl Acad Sci USA 1981; 78:5165–9.
39. Ten RM, Pease LR, McKean DJ, Bell MP, Gleich GJ. Molecular cloning of the human eosinophil peroxidase. Evidence for the existence of a peroxidase multigene family. J Exp Med 1989; 169:1757–9.
40. Sakamaki K, Tomonaga M, Tsukui K, Nagata S. Molecular cloning and characterization of a chromosomal gene for human eosinophil peroxidase. J Biol Chem 1989; 264:16828–36.
41. Lewis DM, Lewis JC, Loegering DA, Gleich GJ. Localization of the guinea pig eosinophil major basic protein to the core of the granule. J Cell Biol 1978; 77:702–13.

42. Peters MS, Rodriguez M, Gleich GJ. Localization of human eosinophil granule major basic protein, eosinophil cationic protein, and eosinophil-derived neurotoxin by immunoelectron microscopy. Lab Invest 1986; 54:650–62.
43. Egesten A, Alumets J, Von Mecklenburg C, Palmegren M, Olsson I. Localization of eosinophil cationic protein, major basic protein, and eosinophil peroxidase in human eosinophils by immunoelectron microscopic technique. J Histochem Cytochem 1986; 34:1399–1403.
44. Frigas E, Loegering DA, Gleich GJ. Cytotoxic effects of the guinea pig eosinophil major basic protein on tracheal epithelium. Lab Invest 1980; 42:35–43.
45. Motojima S, Frigas E, Loegering DA, Gleich GJ. Toxicity of eosinophil cationic proteins for guinea pig tracheal epithelium in vitro. Am Rev Resp Dis 1989; 139:801–5.
46. Ayars GH, Altman LC, Gleich GJ, Loegering DA, Baker BS. Eosinophil- and eosinophil granule-mediated pneumocyte injury. J Allergy Clin Immunol 1985; 76:595–604.
47. Hastie AT, Loegering DA, Gleich GJ, Kueppers F. The effect of purified human eosinophil major basic protein on mammalian ciliary activity. Am Rev Resp Dis 1987; 135:848–53.
48. Jacoby DB, Ueki IF, Widdicombe JH, Loegering DA, Gleich GJ, Nadel JA. Effect of human major basic protein on ion transport in dog tracheal epithelium. Am Rev Resp Dis 1988; 137:13–6.
49. Flavahan NA, Slifman NR, Gleich GJ, Vanhoutte PM. Human eosinophil major basic protein causes hyperreactivity of respiratory smooth muscle. Role of the epithelium. Am Rev Resp Dis 1988; 138:685–8.
50. Brofman JD, White SR, Blake JS, Munoz NM, Gleich GJ, Leff A. Epithelial augmentation of trachealis contraction caused by major basic protein of eosinophils. J Appl Physiol 1989; 66:1867–73.
51. Moy JN, Gleich GJ, Thomas LL. Noncytotoxic activation of neutrophils by eosinophil granule major basic protein: effect on superoxide anion generation and lysosomal enzyme release. J Allergy Clin Immunol 1989; 83:194 (abstr).
52. O'Donnell MC, Ackerman SJ, Gleich GJ, Thomas LL. Activation of basophil and mast cell histamine release by eosinophil granule major basic protein. J Exp Med 1983; 157:1981–91.
53. Thomas LL, Zheultin LM, Gleich GJ. Pharmacological control of human basophil histamine release stimulated by eosinophil granule major basic protein. Immunology 1989; 66:611–5.
54. Espiritu BR, Haskell MD, Gleich GJ, Thomas LL. Stimulation of basophil and neutrophil leukotriene (LT) production by major basic protein (MBP). J Allergy Clin Immunol 1990; 85:216 (abstr).
55. Abu Ghazaleh RI, Gleich GJ. The effect of major basic protein on eosinophils. Fed Proc 1987; 46:988 (abstr).
56. Rohrbach MS, Wheatley CL, Slifman NR, Gleich GJ. Activation of platelets by eosinophil granule proteins. J Exp Med 1990; 172:1271–4.
57. Weiler JM, Gleich GJ. Eosinophil granule major basic protein regulates the generation of classical and alternative-amplification pathway C3 convertases in vitro. J Immunol 1988; 140:1605–10.
58. Butterworth AE, Wassom DL, Gleich GJ, Loegering DA, David JR. Damage to schistosomula of *Schistosoma mansoni* induced directly by eosinophil major basic protein. J Immunol 1979; 122:221–9.
59. Ackerman SJ, Kephart GM, Francis H, Awadzi K, Gleich GJ, Ottesen EA. Eosinophil degranulation. An immunologic determinant in the pathogenesis of the Mazzotti reaction in human onchocerciasis. J Immunol 1990; 144:3961–6.

60. Maddox DE, Kephart GM, Coulam CB, Butterfield JH, Benirschke K, Gleich GJ. Localization of a molecule immunochemically similar to eosinophil major basic protein in human placenta. J Exp Med 1984; 160:29–41.
61. Maddox DE, Butterfield JH, Ackerman SJ, Coulam CB, Gleich GJ. Elevated serum levels in human pregnancy of a molecule immunochemically similar to eosinophil major basic protein. J Exp Med 1983; 158:1211–26.
62. Barker RL, Gleich GJ, Pease LR. Acidic precursor revealed in human eosinophil granule major basic protein cDNA. J Exp Med 1988; 168:1493–8.
63. McGrogan M, Simonsen C, Scott R, Griffith J, Ellis N, Kennedy J, Campanelli D, Nathen C, Gabay J. Isolation of a complementary DNA clone encoding a precursor to human eosinophil major basic protein. J Exp Med 1988; 168:2295–308.
64. Wasmoen TL, Bell MP, Loegering DA, Gleich GJ, Prendergast FG. Biochemical and amino acid sequence analysis of human eosinophil granule major basic protein. J Biol Chem 1988; 263:12559–63.
65. Slifman NR, Venge P, Peterson CGB, McKean DJ, Gleich GJ. Human eosinophil-derived neurotoxin and eosinophil protein X are likely the same protein. J Immunol 1989; 143:2317–22.
66. Slifman NR, Loegering DA, McKean DJ, Gleich GJ. Ribonuclease activity associated with human eosinophil-derived neurotoxin and eosinophil cationic protein. J Immunol 1986; 137:2913–7.
67. Rosenberg HF, Tenen DG, Ackerman SJ. Molecular cloning of the human eosinophil-derived neurotoxin: a member of the ribonuclease gene family. Proc Natl Acad Sci USA 1989; 86:4460–4.
68. Hamann KJ, Barker RL, Loegering DA, Pease LR, Gleich GJ. Sequence of human eosinophil-derived neurotoxin cDNA: identity of deduced amino acid sequence with human nonsecretory ribonucleases. Gene 1989; 83:161–7.
69. Ackerman SJ, Gleich GJ, Loegering DA, Richardson BA, Butterworth AE. Comparative toxicity of purified human eosinophil granule cationic proteins for schistosomula of *Schistosoma mansoni.* Am J Trop Med Hyg 1985; 34:735–45.
70. Yazdanbakhsh M, Tai P-C, Spry CJF, Gleich GJ, Roos D. Synergism between eosinophil cationic protein and oxygen metabolites in killing of schistosomula of *Schistosoma mansoni.* J Immunol 1987; 138:3443–7.
71. Hamann KJ, Barker RL, Loegering DA, Gleich GJ. Comparative cytotoxicity of purified human eosinophil granule proteins for newborn larvae of *Trichinella spiralis.* J Parasitol 1987; 73:523–9.
72. Kierszenbaum F, Villata F, Tai P-C. Role of inflammatory cells in Chagas' disease. J Immunol 1986; 136:662–6.
73. Gullberg U, Widegren B, Arnason U, Egesten A, Olsson I. The cytotoxic eosinophil cationic protein (ECP) has ribonuclease activity. Biochem Biophys Res Commun 1986; 139:1239–42.
74. Lehrer RI, Szklarek D, Barton A, Ganz T, Hamann KJ, Gleich GJ. Antibacterial properties of eosinophil major basic protein and eosinophil cationic protein. J Immunol 1989; 142:4428–34.
75. Tai P-C, Spry CJF, Peterson C, Venge P, Olsson I. Monoclonal antibodies distinguish between storage and secreted forms of eosinophil cationic protein. Nature 1984; 309:182–4.
76. Spry CJF, Tai P-C, Barkans J. Tissue localization of human eosinophil cationic protein in allergic diseases. Int Arch Allergy Appl Immunol 1985; 77:252–4.
77. Young JD-E, Peterson CGB, Venge P, Cohn ZA. Mechanism of membrane damage mediated by human eosinophil cationic protein. Nature 1986; 321:613–6.

78. Rosenberg HF, Ackerman SJ, Tenen DG. Human eosinophil cationic protein, molecular cloning of a cytotoxin and a helminthotoxin with ribonuclease activity. J Exp Med 1989; 170:163–76.
79. Barker RL, Loegering DA, Ten RM, Hamann KJ, Pease LR, Gleich GJ. Eosinophil cationic protein cDNA: comparison with other toxic granule proteins. J Immunol 1989; 143:952–5.
80. Olsen RL, Syse K, Little C, Christensen TB. Further characterization of human eosinophil peroxidase. Biochem J 1985; 229:779–84.
81. Klebanoff SJ, Henderson WR Jr, Jong EC, Jorg A, Locksley RM. Role of peroxidase in eosinophil function. In: Yoshida T, Torisu M, eds. Immunobiology of the eosinophil. New York: Elsevier, 1983:261–82.
82. Bos AJ, Wever R, Hamers MN, Roos D. Some enzymatic characteristics of eosinophil peroxidase from patients with eosinophilia and from healthy donors. Infect Immun 1981; 32:427–31.
83. Weiss SJ, Test ST, Eckmann CM, Roos D, Regiani S. Brominating oxidants generated by human eosinophils. Science 1986; 234:200–3.
84. Kanofsky JR, Hoogland H, Wever R, Weiss SJ. Singlet oxygen production by human eosinophils. J Biol Chem 1988; 263:9692–6.
85. Mayeno AN, Curran AJ, Roberts RL, Foote CS. Eosinophils preferentially use bromide to generate halogenating agents. J Biol Chem 1989; 264:5660–8.
86. Jong EC, Mahmoud AAF, Klebanoff SJ. Peroxidase-mediated toxicity to schistosomula of *Schistosoma mansoni.* J Immunol 1981; 126:468–71.
87. Hamann KJ, Gleich GJ. Eosinophil structure and function: roles in host defense, pathogenesis and disease. In: Natural resistance to infection, Sorg C (ed). Stuttgart: Gustav Fischer Verlag, 1990, Local Immunity 1990; 6:60–88.
88. Jong EC, Chi EY, Klebanoff SJ. Human neutrophil-mediated killing of schistosomula of *Schistosoma mansoni:* augmentation by schistosomal binding of eosinophil peroxidase. Am J Trop Med Hyg 1984; 33:104–15.
89. Henderson WR, Chi EY, Jong EC, Klebanoff SJ. Mast cell-mediated toxicity to schistosomula of *Schistosoma mansoni:* potentiation by exogenous peroxidase. J Immunol 1986; 137:2695–9.
90. Samoszuk MK, Petersen A, Gidanian F, Rietveld C. Cytophilic and cytotoxic properties of human eosinophil peroxidase plus major basic protein. Am J Pathol 1988; 132:455–60.
91. Presentey B. Partial and severe peroxidase and phospholipid deficiency in eosinophils. Cytochemical and genetic considerations. Acta Haematol 1970; 44:345–54.
92. Hoffman JJML, Tielens AGWM. Partial deficiency of eosinophil peroxidase. Blut 1987; 54:165–69.
93. Parmley RT, Spicer SS. Cytochemical and ultrastructural identification of a small type granule in human late eosinophils. Lab Invest 1974; 30:557–67.
94. Zucker-Franklin D. Eosinophil structure and maturation. In: Mahmoud AAF, Austen KF, eds. The eosinophil in health and disease. New York: Grune & Stratton, 1980;43–59.
95. Dvorak AM, Letourneau L, Login GR, Weller PF, Ackerman SJ. Ultrastructural localization of the Charcot-Leyden crystal protein (lysophospholipase) to a distinct crystalloid-free granule population in mature human eosinophils. Blood 1988; 72:150–8.
96. Samter M. Eosinophils: the first 90 years. In: Mahmoud AAF, Austen KF, eds. The eosinophil in health and disease. New York: Grune & Stratton, 1980:25–42.
97. Gleich GJ, Loegering DA, Mann KG, Maldonado JE. Comparative properties of the Charcot-Leyden crystal protein and the major basic protein from human eosinophils. J Clin Invest 1976; 57:633–40.
98. Weller PF, Bach DS, Austen KF. Biochemical characterization of human eosinophil Charcot-Leyden crystal protein (lysophospholipase). J Biol Chem 1984; 259:15100–5.

99. Ackerman SJ, Weil GJ, Gleich GJ. The Charcot-Leyden crystal protein (lysophospholipase): biochemical characteristics, measurement by radioimmunoassay and detection in human basophils. In: Yoshida T, Torismu M, eds. Immunobiology of the eosinophil. New York: Elsevier, 1983:121–44.
100. Ackerman SJ, Weil GJ, Gleich GJ. Formation of Charcot-Leyden crystals by human basophils. J Exp Med 1982; 155:1597–609.
101. Rabellino EM, Metcalf D. Receptors for C3 and IgG on macrophage, neutrophil and eosinophil colony cells grown in vitro. J Immunol 1975; 115:688–92.
102. Anwar ARE, Kay AB. Enhancement of human eosinophil complement receptors by pharmacologic mediators. J Immunol 1978; 121:1245–50.
103. Lopez AF, Strath M, Sanderson CJ. IgG and complement receptors on purified mouse eosinophils and neutrophils. Immunology 1981; 43:779–86.
104. Nagy L, Lee TH, Goetzl EJ, Pickett WC, Kay AB. Complement receptor enhancement and chemotaxis of human neutrophils and eosinophils by leukotrienes and other lipoxygenase products. Clin Exp Immunol 1982; 47:541–7.
105. Capron M, Kazatchkine MD, Fischer E, Joseph M, Butterworth AE, Kusnierz J-P, Prin L, Papin J-P, Capron A. Functional role of the alpha-chain of complement receptor type 3 in human eosinophil-dependent antibody-mediated cytotoxicity against schistosomes. J Immunol 1987; 139:2059–65.
106. Gerard NP, Hodges MK, Drazen JM, Weller PF, Gerard C. Characterization of a receptor for C5a anaphylatoxin on human eosinophils. J Biol Chem 1989; 264:1760–6.
107. DiPrisco-de-Feunmayor MC. Fc receptors for human, rabbit and pig antibodies on human eosinophils from normal persons and patients with atopic dermatitis. Int Arch Allergy Appl Immun 1979; 59:249–55.
108. Thorne, KJI, Franks D. Surface proteins of the human eosinophil. I. Isolation of eosinophil IgG binding proteins. Clin Exp Immunol 1984; 56:464–72.
109. Kulczycki A. Human neutrophils and eosinophils have structurally distinct Fc-gamma receptors. J Immunol 1984; 133:849–54.
110. Lopez AF, Battye FL, Vadas MA. Fc receptors on mouse neutrophils and eosinophils: antigenic characteristics, isotype specificity and relative cell membrane density measured by flow cytometry. Immunology 1985; 55:125–33.
111. Spiegelberg HL. Structure and function of Fc receptors for IgE on lymphocytes, monocytes and macrophages. Adv Immunol 1984; 35:61–88.
112. Capron M, Capron A, Dessain J-P, Torpier G, Johansson SGO, Prin L. Fc receptors for IgE on human and rat eosinophils. J Immunol 1981; 126:2087–92.
113. Capron M, Bazin H, Joseph M, Capron A. Evidence for IgE-dependent cytotoxicity by rat eosinophils. J Immunol 1981; 126:1764–8.
114. Lopez AF, Strath M, Sanderson CJ. Mouse immunoglobulin isotypes mediating cytotoxicity of target cells by eosinophils and neutrophils. Immunology 1983; 48:503–9.
115. Capron M, Nogueira-Queiroz JA, Papin JP, Capron A. Interactions between eosinophils and antibodies: in vivo protective role against rat schistosomiasis. Cell Immunol 1984; 83:60–72.
116. Capron M, Spiegelberg HL, Prin L, Bennich H, Butterworth AE, Pierce RJ, Ali Quaissi M, Capron A. Role of IgE receptors in effector function of human eosinophils. J Immunol 1984; 132:462–8.
117. Moqbel R, MacDonald AJ, Kay AB. Enhancement of human eosinophil- and neutrophil-mediated killing of schistosomula of *Schistosoma mansoni* by reversed type (IgE-mediated) anaphylaxis in vitro. Clin Exp Immunol 1985; 59:577–84.
118. Khalife J, Dunne DW, Richardson BA, Mazza G, Thorne KJI, Capron A, Butterworth AE. Functional role of human IgG subclasses in eosinophil-mediated killing of schistosomula of *Schistosoma mansoni.* J Immunol 1989; 142:4422–7.

119. Capron M, Kusnierz JP, Prin L, Spiegelberg HL, Ovlaque G, Gosset P, Tonnel AB, Capron A. Cytophilic IgE on human blood and tissue eosinophils: detection by flow microfluorometry. J Immunol 1985; 134:3013–8.
120. Capron M, Jouault T, Prin L, Joseph M, Ameisen J-C, Butterworth AE, Papin J-P, Kusnierz J-P, Capron A. Functional study of a monoclonal antibody to IgE Fc receptor (Fc_eR2) of eosinophils, platelets, and macrophages. J Exp Med 1986; 164:72–89.
121. Capron MC, Tomassin M, Voist EVD, Kuznierz J-P, Papin J-P, Capron A. Existence and functions of a receptor for immunoglobulin A on human eosinophils. CR Acad Sci Paris 1988; 307:397–402.
122. Abu-Ghazaleh RI, Fujisawa T, Mestecky J, Kyle RA, Gleich GJ. IgA-induced eosinophil degranulation. J Immunol 1989; 142:2393–400.
123. Rytomaa T. Organ distribution and histochemical properties of eosinophil granulocytes in rats. Acta Pathol Microbiol Scand 1960; 50(Suppl 140):1–118.
124. Osgood EE. Number and distribution of human hemic cells. Blood 1954; 9:1141–54.
125. Mita S, Harada N, Naomi S, Hitoshi Y, Sakamoto K, Akagi M, Tominaga A, Takatsu K. Receptors for T cell-replacing factor/interleukin 5. Specificity, quantitation, and its implication. J Exp Med 1988; 168:863–78.
126. Lopez AF, Eglinton JM, Gillis D, Park LS, Clark S, Vada MA. Reciprocal inhibition of binding between interleukin 3 and granulocyte-macrophage colony-stimulating factor to human eosinophils. Proc Natl Acad Sci USA 1989; 86:7022–6.
127. Ukena D, Krogel C, Dent G, Yukawa T, Sybrecht G, Barnes PJ. PAF-receptors on eosinophils: identification with a novel ligand, [^{3}H]WEB 2086. Biochem Pharmacol 1989; 38:1702–5.
128. Lucey DR, Dorsky DI, Nicholson-Weller A, Weller PF. Human eosinophils express CD4 protein and bind human immunodeficiency virus 1 gp120. J Exp Med 1989; 169:327–32.
129. Lucey DR, Nicholson-Weller A, Weller P. Mature human eosinophils have the capacity to express HLA-DR. Proc Natl Acad Sci USA 1989; 86:1348–51.
130. Hirsch JG, Hirsch BI. Paul Ehrlich and the discovery of the eosinophil. In: Mahmoud AAF, Austen KF, Simon AS, eds. The eosinophil in health and disease. New York: Grune & Stratton, 1980:3–23.
131. Tai P-C, Spry CJF. Studies on blood eosinophils. I. Patients with a transient eosinophilia. Clin Exp Immunol 1976; 24:415–22.
132. Tai P-C, Spry CJF. The mechanisms which produce vacuolated and degranulated eosinophils. Br J Haematol 1981; 49:219–26.
133. Acharya U, Saxena S. Estimation of total and vacuolated eosinophil counts in childhood asthma. Indian J Pediatr 1983; 50:635–7.
134. Winqvist I, Olofsson T, Olsson I, Persson A-M, Hallberg T. Altered density, metabolism and surface receptors of eosinophils in eosinophilia. Immunology 1982; 47:531–9.
135. Prin L, Charon J, Capron M, Gosset P, Taelman H, Tonnel AB, Capron A. Heterogeneity of human eosinophils. II. Variability of respiratory burst activity related to cell density. Clin Exp Immunol 1984; 57:735–42.
136. Fukuda T, Dunnette SL, Reed CE, Ackerman SJ, Peters MS, Gleich CJ. Increased numbers of hypodense eosinophils in the blood of patients with bronchial asthma. Am Rev Resp Dis 1985; 132:981–5.
137. Masuyama K, Samejima Y, Ishikawa T. Eosinophils in nasal secretion. Acta Otolaryngol (Stockh) Suppl 1988; 458:181–9.
138. Shaw RJ, Walsh GM, Cromwell O, Moqbel R, Spry CJF, Kay AB. Activated human eosinophils generate SRS-A leukotrienes following physiological (IgG-dependent) stimulation. Nature 1985; 316:150–2.
139. Yamaguchi Y, Hayashi Y, Sugama Y, Miura Y, Kasahara T, Kitamura S, Torisu M, Mita S, Tominaga A, Takatsu K, Suda T. Highly purified murine interleukin 5 (IL-5) stimulates eosinophil function and prolongs in vitro survival. IL-5 as an eosinophil chemotactic factor. J Exp Med 1988; 167:1737–42.

140. Rothenberg ME, Peterson J, Stevens RL, Silberstein DS, McKenzie DT, Austen KF, Owen WF Jr. IL-5 dependent conversion of normodense human eosinophils to the hypodense phenotype uses 3T3 fibroblasts for enhanced viability, accelerated hypodensity and sustained antibody-dependent cytotoxicity. J Immunol 1989; 143:2311–6.
141. Owen WF, Rothenberg ME, Silberstein DS, Gasson JC, Stevens RL, Austen KF, Soberman RJ. Regulation of human eosinophil viability, density, and function by granulocyte/macrophage colony-stimulating factor in the presence of 3T3 fibrobasts. J Exp Med 1987; 166:129–41.
142. Rothenberg MC, Owen WF, Silberstein DS, Woods J, Soberman RJ, Austen KF, Stevens RL. Human eosinophils have prolonged survival, enhanced functional properties, and become hypodense when exposed to human interleukin 3. J Clin Invest 1988; 81:1986–92.
143. Jo White C, Maxwell CJ, Gallin JI. Changes in the structural and functional properties of human eosinophils during experimental hookworm infection. J Infect Dis 1986; 154:778–83.
144. Gruart V, Balloul J-M, Prin L, Tamassini M, Loiseau S, Capron A, Capron M. Variations in protein expression related to human eosinophil heterogeneity. J Immunol 1989; 142:4416–21.
145. Fukuda T, Gleich GJ. Heterogeneity of human eosinophils. J Allergy Clin Immunol 1989; 83:369–73.
146. Dessein AJ, David JR. The eosinophil in parasitic diseases. In: Gallin JI, Fauci AS, eds. Advances in host defense mechanisms, phagocytic cells, vol. 1. New York: Raven Press, 1982; 243–68.
147. Butterworth AE, Vadas MA, David JR. Mechanisms of eosinophil mediated helminthotoxicity. In: Mahmoud AAF, Austen KF, Simon AS, eds. The eosinophil in health and disease. New York: Grune & Stratton, 1980: 253–73.
148. Butterworth AE, Remold HG, Houba V, David JR, Franks D, David PH, Sturrock RF. Antibody-dependent eosinophil-mediated damage to ^{51}Cr-labelled schistosomula of *Schistosoma mansoni:* mediation by IgG and inhibition by antigen antibody complexes. J Immunol 1977; 118:2230–6.
149. Vadas MA, Butterworth AE, Sherry B, Dessein A, Hogan M, Bout D, David JR. Interactions between human eosinophils and schistosomula of *Schistosoma mansoni.* I. Stable and irreversible antibody-dependent adherence. J Immunol 1980; 124:1441–8.
150. Butterworth AE, Sturrock RF, Houba V, Mahmoud AAF, Sher A, Rees PH. Eosinphils as mediators of antibody-dependent damage to schistosomula. Nature 1975; 256:727–9.
151. Vadas MA, David JR, Butterworth AE, Pisani NT, Siongok TA. A new method for the purification of human eosinophils and neutrophils, and a comparison of the ability of these cells to damage schistosomula of *Schistosoma mansoni.* J Immunol 1979; 122:1228–36.
152. Butterworth AE, Vadas MA, Wassom DL, Dessein A, Hogan M, Sherry B, Gleich GJ, David JR. Interactions between human eosinophils and schistosomula of *Schistosoma mansoni.* II. The mechanism of irreversible adherence. J Exp Med 1979; 150:1456–71.
153. Kazura JW. Host defense mechanisms against nematode parasites: destruction of newborn *Trichinella spiralis* larvae by human antibodies and granulocytes. J Infect Dis 1981; 143:712–8.
154. Bass DA, Szejda P. Mechanisms of killing of newborn larvae of *Trichinella spiralis* by neutrophils and eosinophils. Killing by generators of hydrogen peroxide in vitro. J Clin Invest 1979; 64:1558–64.
155. Pincus SH, Cammarata P. Eosinophil adherence to infective larvae of *Trichinella spiralis:* quantification and modulation. Immunology 1985; 56:219–25.
156. Ortega-Pierres G, Mackenzie CD, Parkhouse RME. Protection against *Trichinella spiralis* induced by a monoclonal antibody that promotes killing of newborn larvae by granulocytes. Parasite Immunol 1984; 6:275–84.
157. Waters LS, Taverne J, Tai P-C, Spry CJF, Targett GAT, Playteur JHL. Killing of *Plasodium falciparim* by eosinophil secretory products. Infect Immun 1987; 55:877–81.

158. Villalta F, Pankratz HS, Kierszenbaum F. Extracellular killing of *Trypanosoma cruzi* amastigotes by human eosinophils. J Protozool 1987; 34:285–90.
159. Gill GV, Bailey JW. Eosinophilia as a marker for chronic strongyloidiasis—use of a serum ELISA test to detect asymptomatic cases. Ann Trop Med Parasitol 1989; 83:249–52.
160. Sugane K, Oshima T. Induction of peripheral blood eosinophilia in mice by excretory and secretory antigen of *Toxocara canis* larvae. J Helminthol 1984; 58:143–7.
161. Mahmoud AAF, Warren KS, Boros DL. Production of a rabbit antimouse eosinophil serum with no cross-reactivity to neutrophils. J Exp Med 1973; 137:1526–31.
162. Mahmoud AAF, Warren KS, Peters PA. A role for the eosinophil in acquired resistance to *Schistosoma mansoni* infection as determined by anti-eosinophil serum. J Exp Med 1975; 142:805–13.
163. Goven AJ. Effect of anti-eosinophil serum in phospholipase B activity in mice infected with *Trichinella spiralis*. J Parasitol 1988; 69:88–90.
164. Kephart GM, Andrade ZA, Gleich GJ. Localization of eosinophil major basic protein onto eggs of *Schistosoma mansoni* in human pathologic tissue. Am J Pathol 1989; 133:389–96.
165. Hamann KJ, Kephart GM, Kazacos KR, Gleich GJ. Immunofluorescent localization of eosinophil granule major basic protein in fatal human cases of *Baylisascaris procyonis* infection. Am J Trop Med Hyg 1989; 40:291–7.
166. Horn BR, Robin ED, Theodore J, van Kessel A. Total eosinophil counts in the management of bronchial asthma. N Engl J Med 1975; 292:1152–5.
167. Taylor KJ, Luksza AR. Peripheral blood eosinophil counts and bronchial responsiveness. Thorax 1987; 42:452–6.
168. de Monchy JGR, Kauffman HF, Venge P, Koeter GH, Jansen H, Sluiter HJ, De Vries K. Bronchoalveolar eosinophilia during allergen-induced late asthmatic reactions. Am Rev Resp Dis 1985; 131:373–6.
169. Wardlaw AJ, Dunnette S, Gleich GJ, Collins JV, Kay AB. Eosinc .ils and mast cells in bronchoalveolar lavage subjects with mild asthma: relationship to bronchial hyperreactivity. Am Rev Resp Dis 1988; 137:62–9.
170. Tanizaki Y, Sudo M, Kitani H, Araki H, Oki K, Tsuji M, Takahashi K, Kimura I. Eosinophilic leukocytes and arylsulfatase activity in bronchoalveolar lavage fluid of patients with bronchial asthma. Acta Med Okayama 1988; 42:227–30.
171. Takematsu H, Tagami H. Eosinophilic pustular folliculitis. Studies on possible chemotactic factors involved in the formation of pustules. Br J Dermatol 1986; 114:209–15.
172. Leiferman KM, Peters MS, Gleich GJ. The eosinophil and cutaneous edema. J Am Acad Dermatol 1986; 15:513–7.
173. Songsiridej V, Peters MS, Dor PJ, Ackerman SJ, Gleich GJ, Busse WW. Facial edema and eosinophilia. Evidence for eosinophil degranulation. Ann Intern Med 1985; 103:503–6.
174. Leiferman KM, Norris PG, Murphy GM, Hawk JLM, Winkelmann RK. Evidence for eosinophil degranulation with deposition of granule major basic protein in solar urticaria. J Am Acad Dermatol 1989; 21:75–80.
175. Spry CJ. Eosinophilia and allergic reaction to drugs. Clin Haematol 1981; 9:521–34.
176. Hertzman PA, Blevins WL, Mayer J, Greenfield B, Ting M, Gleich GJ. Association of the eosinophilia-myalgia syndrome with the ingestion of tryptophan. N Engl J Med 1990; 322:869–73.
177. Silver RM, Heyes MP, Maize JC, Quearry B, Viomet-Fausset M, Sternberg EM. Scleroderma, faciitis, and eosinophilia associated with the ingestion of tryptophan. N Engl J Med 1990; 322:874–81.
178. Samoszuk MK, Nathwani BN, Lukes RJ. Extensive deposition of eosinophil peroxidase in Hodgkin's and non-Hodgkin's lymphomas. Am J Pathol 1986; 125:426–9.
179. Samoszuk MK, Sholly S, Epstein AL. Eosinophil peroxidase is detectable with a monoclonal antibody in collagen bands of nodular sclerosis Hodgkin's disease. Lab Invest 1987; 56:394–400.

180. MacIntyre EA, Vaughan Hudson B, Vaughan Hudson G, Jellife AM, Linch DC. Incidence and clinical importance of bone marrow eosinophilia in Hodgkin's disease (BNLI report no. 29). J Clin Pathol 1987; 40:245–6.
181. Vaughan Hudson B, Linch DC, MacIntyre EA, Bennett MH, MacLennan KA, Vaughan Hudson G, Jelliffe AM. Selective peripheral blood eosinophilia associated with survival advantage in Hodgkin's disease (BNLI report no. 31). J Clin Pathol 1987; 40:247–50.
182. DeKorte D, Haverkort WA, Behrendt H, Roos D, Van Gennip AH. Abnormal nucleotide pattern in the eosinophils of a patient with acute lymphoblastic leukemia associated with eosinophilia. Leukemia Res 1986; 10:1419–24.
183. Mecucci C, Bosly A, Michaux J-L, Broeckaert-Van Orshoven A, Van Den Berghe H. Acute nonlymphoblastic leukemia with bone marrow eosinophilia and structural anomaly of chromosome 16. Cancer Genet Cytogenet 1985; 17:359–63.
184. Ishibashi T, Kimura H, Abe R, Matsuda S, Uschida T, Kariyone S. Involvement of eosinophils in leukemia: cytogenetic study of eosinophilic colonies from acute myelogenous leukemia associated with translocation (8;21). Cancer Genet Cytogenet 1986; 22:189–94.
185. Larson RA, Williams SF, LeBeau MM, Bitter MA, Vardiman JW, Rowley JD. Acute myelomonocytic leukemia with abnormal eosinophils and inv(16) or t(16;16) has a favorable prognosis. Blood 1986; 68:1242–9.
186. Extra JM, Marty M, Calvo F, Daniel MT, Berger R, Boiron M. Abnormal eosinophils in acute myelomonocytic leukemia. Nouv Rev Fr Hematol 1987; 29:73–6.
187. Keene P, Mendelono B, Pinto MR, Bezwoda W, McDougall L, Falkson G, Ruff P, Bernstein R. Abnormalities of chromosome 12;13 and malignant proliferation of eosinophils: a nonrandom association. Br J Haematol 1987; 67:25–31.
188. Bhambhani K, Inoue S, Tyrkus M, Gohle N. Acute myelomonocytic leukemia type M4 with bone marrow eosinophilia and t(5;16)(q33;q22). Cancer Genet Cytogenet 1986; 20:187–8.
189. Hollings PE, Rosman I, Beard MEJ, Fitzgerald PH. Abnormal chromosome 16 in clonogenic eosinophils from a case of acute myeloid leukemia (FAB,M2). Cancer Genet Cytogenet 1988; 31:217–26.
190. Ghosh K, Varma N, Dash S. Dysplastic eosinophils in three patients with acute promyelocytic leukaemia. Leukemia Res 1988; 12:963–7.
191. Vukelja SJ, Weiss RB, Perry DJ, Longo DL. Eosinophilia associated with adult T-cell leukemia/lymphoma. Cancer 1988; 62:1527–30.
192. Lowe D, Jorizzo J, Huh M. Tumor associated eosinophilia: a review. J Clin Pathol 1981; 34:1343–8.
193. Looi L-M. Tumor-associated tissue eosinophilia in nasopharyngeal carcinoma. A pathologic study of 422 primary and 138 metastatic tumors. Cancer 1987; 59:466–70.
194. Slungaard A, Ascensao J, Zanjani E, Jacob HS. Pulmonary carcinoma with eosinophilia. Demonstration of a tumor-derived eosinophilopoietic factor. N Engl J Med 1983; 309:778–81.
195. Fredens K, Tottrup A, Kristensen IB, Dahl R, Jacobsen NO, Funch-Jensen P, Thommesen P. Severe destruction of esophageal nerves in a patient with achalasia secondary to gastric cancer. A possible role of eosinophil neurotoxic proteins. Dig Dis Sci 1989; 34:297–303.
196. Fisher ER, Palk SM, Rockette H, Jones J, Caplan R, Fisher B, Other NSABP Collaborators. Prognostic significance of eosinophils and mast cells in rectal cancer: findings from the national surgical adjuvant breast and bowel project (Protocol R-01). Human Pathol 1989; 20:159–63.
197. Fauci AS, Harley JB, Roberts WC, Ferrans VJ, Gralnick HR, Bjornson BH. The idiopathic hypereosinophilic syndrome. Clinical, pathophysiologic, and therapeutic considerations. Ann Intern Med 1982; 97:78–92.
198. Leiferman KM, O'Duffy JD, Perry HO, Greipp PR, Giuliani ER, Gleich GJ. Recurrent incapacitating mucosal ulcerations: a prodrome of the hypereosinophilic syndrome. JAMA 1982; 247:1018–20.

199. Peters MS, Gleich GJ, Dunnette SL, Fukuda T. Ultrastructural study of eosinophils from patients with hypereosinophilic syndrome: a morphological basis of hypodense eosinophils. Blood 1988; 71:780–5.
200. Davies JR, Gaery CG, Testa NG, Pumphrey RSH. Cyclical eosinophilia: a manifestation of haemopoiesis? Br J Haematol 1985; 61:65–70.
201. Tai P-C, Ackerman SJ, Spry CJF, Dunnette S, Olsen EGJ, Gleich GJ. Deposits of eosinophil granule proteins in cardiac tissues of patients with eosinophilic endomyocardial disease. Lancet 1987; 1:643–7.
202. Sutton JM. Urinary eosinophils. Arch Intern Med 1986; 146:2243–4.
203. Nolan CR, Anger MS, Kelleher SP. Eosinophiluria—a new method of detection and definition of the clinical spectrum. N Engl J Med 1986; 315:1516–9.
204. Corwin HL, Bray RA, Haker MH. The detection and interpretation of urinary eosinophils. Arch Pathol Lab Med 1989; 113:1256–8.
205. Ten RM, Torres VE, Milliner DS, Schwab TR, Holley KE, Gleich GJ. Acute interstitial nephritis: immunologic and clinical aspects. Mayo Clin Proc 1988; 63:921–30.
206. Kasinath BS, Lewis EJ. Eosinophilia as a clue to the diagnosis of atherembolic renal disease. Arch Intern Med 1987; 147:1384–5.
207. Lautenschlager I, von Willebrand E, Hayry P. Blood eosinophilia, steroids, and rejection. Transplantation 1985; 40:354–7.
208. Weir MR, Hall-Craggs M, Shen SY, Posner JN, Algoni SV, Dagher FJ, Sadler JH. The prognostic value of the eosinophil in acute renal allograft rejection. Transplantation 1986; 41:709–12.
209. Perorella I, Ciardi A, Pretagostin R, Caricato M, Forti A, Berloco P, Alfani D, DiTondo U, Cortesini R. Blood eosinophilia and major histocompatibility complex II expression in renal allograft rejection. Transplant Proc 1988; 20:606–7.
210. Kormendi F, Gupta R, Bagor G, Miller SM, Belilsky P. Eosinophil cells in dog kidney transplants during rejection. Transplantation 1989; 47:919–20.
211. Ten RM, Gleich GJ, Holley KE, Perkins JD, Torres VE. Eosinophil granule major basic protein in acute renal allograft rejection. Transplantation 1989; 47:959–63.
212. Foster PF, Sankary H, Williams JW. Study of eosinophilia and hepatic dysfunction as a predictor of rejection in human liver transplantation. Transplant Proc 1988; 20:676–7.
213. Trounce JQ, Tanner MS. Eosinophilic gastroenteritis. Arch Dis Child 1985; 60:1186–8.
214. Moots RJ, Prouse P, Gumpel JM. Near fatal eosinophilic gastroenteritis responding to oral sodium chromoglycate. Gut 1988; 29:1282–5.
215. Torpier G, Colombel JF, Mathieu-Chandelier C, Capron M, Dessaint JP, Cortot A, Paris JC, Capron A. Eosinophilic gastroenteritis: ultrastructural evidence for a selective release of eosinophil major basic protein. Clin Exp Immun 1988; 74:404–8.
216. Fleury-Feith J, Van Nhieu JT, Picard C, Escudier E, Bernaudin J-F. Bronchoalveolar lavage eosinophilia associated with *Pneumocystis carinii* pneumonitis in AIDS patients. Comparative study with non-AIDS patients. Chest 1989; 95:1198–201.
217. Buchness MR, Lim HW, Hatcher VA, Sanchez M, Soter NA. Eosinophilic pustular folliculitis in the acquired immunodeficiency syndrome. Treatment with ultraviolet B phototherapy. N Engl J Med 1988; 318:1183–6.
218. Frentz G, Niordson A-M, Thomsen K. Eosinophilic pustular dermatosis: an early skin marker of infection with human immunodeficiency virus? Br J Dermatol 1989; 121:271–4.
219. Wasmoen TL, Coulam CB, Leiferman KM, Gleich GJ. Increases of plasma eosinophil major basic protein levels late in pregnancy predict onset of labor. Proc Natl Acad Sci USA 1987; 84:3029–32.
220. McGarry MP, Speirs RS, Jenkins VK, Trentin JJ. Lymphoid cell dependence of eosinophil response to antigen. J Exp Med 1971; 134:801–14.
221. Nielsen K, Fogh L, Andersen S. Eosinophil response to migrating *Ascaris suum* larvae in normal and congenitally thymusless mice. Acta Path Microbiol Scand 1974; 82(Sect. B):919–20.

222. Hsu C-K, Hsu SH, Whitney RA, Hansen CT. Immunopathology of schistosomiasis in athymic mice. Nature 1976; 262:397–9.
223. Doy TG, Hughes DL. The role of the thymus in the eosinophil response of rats infected with *Fasciola hepatica*. Clin Exp Immunol 1982; 47:74–6.
224. Ruscetti FW, Cypess RH, Chervenick PA. Specific release of neutrophilic- and eosinophilic-stimulating factors from sensitized lymphocytes. Blood 1976; 47:757–65.
225. Basten A, Beeson PB. Mechanisms of eosinophilia. II. Role of the lymphocyte. J Exp Med 1970; 131:1288–305.
226. Bartelmez SH, Dodge WH, Mahmoud AAF, Bass DA. Stimulation of eosinophil production in vitro by eosinophilopoietin and spleen-cell-derived eosinophil growing-stimulating factor. Blood 1980; 56:706–11.
227. Metcalf D, Cutler RL, Nicola NA. Selective stimulation by mouse spleen cell conditioned medium of human eosinophil colony formation. Blood 1983; 61:999–1005.
228. Czarnetzki BM, Pawelzik B. The effect of eosinophil chemotactic factors on in vitro eosinopoiesis in the guinea pig. Blut 1983; 47:287–96.
229. Bjornson BH, Andre-Schwartz J, Desforges JF. In vitro culture of circulating CFU_{eos} from normal donors. Exp Hematol 1982; 10:271–6.
230. Heilmann E, Burkart M, Czarnetzki B. In vitro studies to prove the effect of sera on eosinophilia in colony formation. Folia Haematol Leipzig 1983; 110:503–9.
231. Enokihara H, Hamaguchi H, Sakamaki H, Hazama S, Saito K, Furusawa S, Shishido H. Specific production of eosinophil colony stimulating factor from sensitized T cells from a patient with allergic eosinophilia. Br J Haematol 1985; 59:85–91.
232. Dessein AJ, Lenzi HL, David JR. Modulation of the cytotoxicity of human blood eosinophils by factors secreted by monocytes and T lymphocytes. Monogr Allergy 1983; 18:45–51.
233. Veith M, Taylor DW, Thorne K, Richardson BA, Butterworth AE. Studies on the enhancement of human eosinophil function by mononuclear cell products in vitro. Clin Exp Immunol 1984; 58:603–10.
234. Veith MC, Butterworth AE. Enhancement of human eosinophil-mediated killing of *Schistosoma mansoni* larvae by mononuclear cell products in vivo. J Exp Med 1983; 157:1828–43.
235. Sanderson CJ, Warren DJ, Strath M. Identification of a lymphokine that stimulates eosinophil differentiation in vitro. Its relationship to interleukin 3, and functional properties of eosinophils produced in cultures. J Exp Med 1985; 162:60–74.
236. Rand TH, Colley DG. Influence of a lymphokine fraction containing eosinophil stimulation promoter (ESP) on oxidative and degranulation responses of murine eosinophils. Cell Immunol 1982; 71:334–45.
237. Dessein AJ, Vadas MA, Nicola NA, Metcalf D, David JR. Enhancement of human blood eosinophil cytotoxicity by semi-purified eosinophil colony-stimulating factor(s). J Exp Med 1982; 156:90–103.
238. Tai P-C, Bakes DM, Barkans JR, Spry CJF. Plasma membrane antigens on light density and activated human blood eosinophils. Clin Exp Immunol 1985; 60:427–36.
239. Tashiro K, Sakata K, Hirashima M, Hayashi H. The regulation of tissue eosinophilia. III. In vitro production of eosinophil-directed chemotactic inhibitory factor by T lymphocytes of complete Freund's adjuvant-treated guinea pigs. Immunology 1985; 55:115–24.
240. Venge P, Boberg M, Hakansson L, Peterson C. Identification of a serum-derived promoter of granulocyte granule secretion: study on a patient with chronic pruritus. Immunology 1982; 45:521–9.
241. Hashimoto K, Takahashi S, Fligiel A, Savoy B. Eosinophilic granuloma. Presence of OKT6-positive cells and good response to intralesional steroid. Arch Dermatol 1985; 121:770–4.
242. Knapp W, Rieber P, Dorken B, Schmidt RE, Stein H, Borne AEGKrvd. Towards a better definition of human leukocyte surface molecules. Immunology Today 1989; 10:253–8.

243. Frew AJ, Kay AB. The relationship between infiltrating $CD4^+$ lymphocytes, activated eosinophils, and the magnitude of the allergen-induced late phase cutaneous reaction in man. J Immunol 1988; 141:4158–64.
244. Warren DJ, Sanderson CJ. Projection of a T-cell hybrid producing a lymphokine stimulating eosinophil differentiation. Immunology 1985; 54:615–23.
245. Lopez AF, Begley CG, Williamson DJ, Warren DJ, Vadas MA, Sanderson CJ. Murine eosinophil differentiation factor. An eosinophil-specific colony-stimulating factor with activity for human cells. J Exp Med 1986; 163:1085–99.
246. Azuma C, Tanabe T, Konishi M, Noma T, Matsuda F, Yaoita Y, Takatsu K, Hammarstrom L, Edvard Smith CI, Seveinson E, Honjo T. Cloning of cDNA for human T-cell replacing factor (interleukin-5) and comparison with the murine homologue. Nucleic Acids Res 1986; 14:9149–58.
247. Campbell HD, Tucker WQJ, Hort Y, Martinson ME, Mayo G, Clutterbuck EJ, Sanderson CJ, Young IG. Molecular cloning, nucleotide sequence, and expression of the gene encoding human eosinophil differentiation factor (interleukin 5). Proc Natl Acad Sci USA 1987; 84:6629–33.
248. Sanderson CJ, Campbell HD, Young IG. Molecular and cellular biology of the eosinophil differentiation factor (interleukin-5) and its effects on human and mouse B cells. Immunol Rev 1988; 102:29–50.
249. Yamaguchi Y, Suda T, Suda J, Eguchi M, Miura Y, Harada N, Tominaga A, Takatsu K. Purified interleukin 5 supports the terminal differentiation and proliferation of murine eosinophilic precursors. J Exp Med 1988; 167:43–56.
250. Lopez AF, Sanderson CJ, Gamble JR, Campbell HD, Young IG, Vadas MA. Recombinant human interleukin 5 is a selective activator of human eosinophil function. J Exp Med 1988; 167:219–24.
251. Clutterbuck EJ, Sanderson CJ. Human eosinophil hematopoiesis studied in vitro by means of murine eosinophil differentiation factor (IL-5): production of functionally active eosinophils from normal human bone marrow. Blood 1988; 71:646–51.
252. Coffman RL, Seymour BWP, Hudak S, Jackson J, Rennick D. Antibody to interleukin-5 inhibits helminth-induced eosinophilia in mice. Science 1989; 245:308–10.
253. Warren DJ, Moore MAS. Synergism among interleukin 1, interleukin 3, and interleukin 5 in the production of eosinophils from primitive hemopoietic stem cells. J Immunol 1988; 140:94–9.
254. Sonoda Y, Arai N, Ogawa M. Humoral regulation of eosinophilopoiesis in vitro: analysis of the targets of interleukin-3, granulocyte/macrophage colony-stimulating factor (GM-CSF), and interleukin-5. Leukemia 1989; 3:14–8.
255. Silberstein DS, David JR. Tumor necrosis factor enhances eosinophil toxicity to *Schistosoma mansoni* larvae. Proc Natl Acad Sci USA 1986; 83:1055–9.
256. Saito H, Hatake K, Dvorak AM, Leiferman KM, Donnenberg AD, Arai N, Ishizaka K, Ishizaka T. Selective differentiation/proliferation of hematopoietic cells by recombinant human interleukins. Proc Natl Acad Sci USA 1988; 85:2288–92.
257. Dvorak AM, Saito H, Estrella P, Kissell S, Arai N, Ishizaka T. Ultrastructure of eosinophils and basophils stimulated to develop in human cord blood mononuclear cell cultures containing recombinant interleukin-5 or interleukin-3. Lab Invest 1989; 61:116–32.
258. Hubscher T. Role of the eosinophil in the allergic reactions. I. EDI- an eosinophil-derived inhibitor of histamine release. J Immunol 1975; 114:1379–88.
259. Auriault C, Capron M, Capron A. Activation of rat and human eosinophils by soluble factor(s) released by *Schistosoma mansoni* schistosomula. Cell Immunol 1982; 66:59–69.
260. Warren KS, Karp R, Pelley RP, Mahmoud AAF. The eosinophil stimulation promoter test in murine and human *Trichinella spiralis* infection. J Infect Dis 1976: 134:277–80.
261. Badley JE, Greive RB, Rockey JH, Glickman LT. Immune-mediated adherence of eosinophils to *Toxocara canis* infective larvae: the role of excretory-secretory antigens. Parasite Immunol 1987; 9:133–43.

262. Sugane K, Oshima T. Induction of peripheral blood eosinophilia in mice by excretory and secretory antigen of *Toxocara canis* larvae. J Helminthol 1984; 58:143–7.
263. Thorne KJ, Oliver RC, Glauert AM. Eosinophil interaction with antibody coated, non-phagocytosable surfaces: changes in cell surface proteins. J Cell Sci 1980; 42:367–78.
264. Oliver RC, Glauert AM, Thorne KJI. Mechanism of Fc-mediated interaction of eosinophils with immobilized immune complexes. I. Effects of inhibitors and activators of eosinophil function. J Cell Sci 1982; 56:337–56.
265. Thorne KJI, Free J, Franks D, Oliver R. The mechanism of Fc-mediated interaction of eosinophils with immobilized immune complexes. II. Identification of two membrane proteins, modified by the interaction. J Cell Sci 1982; 56:357–69.
266. Pincus SH. Eosinophil-particle interactions: a model system for study of cellular adherence and activation. Cell Immunol 1984; 86:460–71.
267. Yazdanbakhsh M, Eckmann CM, Roos D. Characterization of the interaction of human eosinophils and neutrophils with opsonized particles. J Immunol 1985; 135:1378–84.
268. Winqvist I, Olofsson T, Olsson I. Mechanism for eosinophil degranulation: release of the eosinophil cationic protein. Immunology 1984; 51:1–8.
269. Khalife J, Capron M, Crzych J-M, Bazin H, Capron A. Extracellular release of rat eosinophil peroxidase (EPO). I. Role of anaphylactic immunoglobulins. J Immunol 1985; 134:1968–74.
270. Capron A, Dessaint JP, Capron M, Joseph M, Ameisen JC, Tonnel AB. From parasites to allergy: a second receptor for IgE. Immunology Today 1986; 7:15–8.
271. Walsh GM, Kay AB. Binding of immunoglobulin classes and subclasses to human neutrophils and eosinophils. Clin Exp Immunol 1986; 63:466-72.
272. Kitani S, Ito K, Miyamoto T. IgG, IgA, and IgM antibodies to mite in sera and sputa from asthmatic patients. Ann Allergy 1985; 55:612–20.
273. Gutt L, Greenberger PA, Liotta JL. Serum IgA antibodies to *Aspergillus fumigatus* in various stages of allergic bronchopulmonary aspergillosis. J Allergy Clin Immunol 1986; 78:98–101.
274. Vanto T, Viander M, Koivikko A. Humoral and cell mediated immune responses to dog dander and hair in asthmatic children. Allergy 1983; 38:103–12.
275. Popper H, Pongratz M, Lanzer G. IgA_2-alveolitis and eosinophilic pneumonia—a possibly virus-triggered allergy. Allergol Immunopathol 1982; 10:177–84.
276. Coffman RL, Shrader B, Carty J, Mosmann TR, Bond MW. A mouse T cell product that preferentially enhances IgA production. I. Biologic characterization. J Immunol 1987; 139:3685–90.
277. Bond MW, Shrader B, Mosmann TR, Coffman RL. A mouse T cell product that preferentially enhances IgA production. II. Physicochemical characterization. J Immunol 1987; 139:3691–6.
278. Yokota T, Coffman RL, Hagiwara H, Rennick DM, Takebe Y, Yokota K, Gemmell L, Shrader B, Yang G, Meyerson P, Luh J, Hoy P, Pene J, Briere F, Spits H, Banchereau J, de Vries J, Lee FD, Arai N, Arai K. Isolation and characterization of lymphokine cDNA clones encoding mouse and human IgA-enhancing factor and eosinophil colony-stimulating factor activities: relationship to interleukin 5. Proc Natl Acad Sci USA 1987; 84:7388–92.
279. Clutterbuck E, Shields JG, Gordon J, Smith SH, Boyd A, Callard RE, Campbell HD, Young IG, Sanderson CJ. Recombinant human interleukin 5 is an eosinophil differentiation factor but has no activity in standard human B cell growth factor assays. Eur J Immunol 1987; 17:1743–50.
280. Beagley KW, Eldridge JH, Lee F, Kiyono H, Everson MR, Koopman WJ, Hirano T, Kishimoto T, McGhee JR. Interleukins and IgA synthesis. Human and murine IL-6 induce high rate IgA secretion in IgA-committed B cells. J Exp Med 1989; 169:2133–48.
281. Henderson WR, Chi EY, Jorg A, Klebanoff SJ. Horse eosinophil degranulation induced by the ionophore A23187. Am J Path 1983; 111:341–9.

282. Henderson WR, Chi E. Ultrastructural characterization and morphometric analysis of human eosinophil degranulation. J Cell Sci 1985; 73:33–48.
283. Fukuda T, Ackerman SJ, Reed CE, Peters MS, Dunnette SL, Gleich GJ. Calcium ionophore A23187 calcium-dependent cytolytic degranulation in human eosinophils. J Immunol 1985; 135:1349–56.
284. Horii Y, Owhashi M, Fujita K, Nakanishi H, Ishii A. A comparative study on eosinophil and neutrophil chemotactic activities of various helminth parasites. Parasitol Res 1988; 75:76–8.
285. Owhashi M, Horii Y, Ishii A, Nawa Y. Low molecular weight eosinophil chemotactic factor (ECF) in the serum of murine *Schistosomiasis japonica.* Int Arch Allergy Appl Immun 1986; 79:178–81.
286. Horii Y, Fujita K, Owhashi M. Partial purification and characterization of eosinophil chemotactic factors from soluble extract of *Fasciola* species. Am J Vet Res 1986; 47:123–6.
287. Owhashi M, Nawa Y. Eosinophil chemotactic lymphokine produced by spleen cells of *Schistosoma japonicum*-infected mice. III. Isolation and characterization of two distinctive eosinophil chemotactic lymphokines directed against different maturation stages of eosinophils. Int Arch Allergy Appl Immun 1987; 84:185–9.
288. Tanaka J, Baba T, Torisu M. Ascaris and eosinophils. II. Isolation and characterization of eosinophil chemotactic factor and neutrophil chemotactic factor of parasite in *Ascaris* antigen. J Immunol 1979; 122:302–8.
289. Potter KA, Wes Leid R. Isolation and partial characterization of an eosinophil chemotactic factor from metacestodes of *Taenia taeniaeformis* (EF-Tt). J Immunol 1986; 136:1712–7.
290. Musgrove NRJ, Cook RM. Effect of chemotactic agents on rat and guinea pig eosinophil cytotoxicity in vitro. Int Arch Allergy Appl Immun 1988; 86:319–24.
291. Kowalski JC, Thorson RE. Immunization of laboratory mice against tetrathyridia of *Mesocestoides corti* (cestoda) using a secretory and excretory antigen and a soluble somatic antigen. J Parasitol 1972; 58:732–4.
292. Sogandares-Bernal F, Race MC, Dennis MV, Voge M. Circulating antigens in infections of mice by tetrathyridia of *Mesocestoides corti* Hoeppli, 1925. Z Parasitenkd 1981; 64:157–67.
293. Washington EA, Barton AM, Nicholas WL. *Mesocestoides corti* in the rat: the cellular response in the peritoneal cavity of rats infected with *Mesocestoides corti.* Int J Parasitol 1984; 14:395–9.
294. Goetzl EJ, Austen KF. Natural eosinophilotactic peptides: evidence of heterogeneity and studies of structure and function. In: Mahmoud AAF, Austen KF, Simon AS, eds. The eosinophil in health and disease. New York: Grune & Stratton, 1980:149–65.
295. Goetzl EJ. The unique roles of monohydroxy-eicosatetraenoic acids (HETEs) in the regulation of eosinophil function. In: Mahmoud AAF, Austen KF, Simon AS, eds. The eosinophil in health and disease. New York: Grune & Stratton, 1979:167.
296. Ogawa H, Kunkel SL, Fantone JC, Ward PA. Comparative study of eosinophil and neutrophil chemotaxis and enzyme release. Am J Pathol 1981; 105:149–55.
297. Czarnetzki BM, Pawelzi KB. The effect of eosinophil chemotactic factors on in vitro eosinopoiesis in the guinea pig. Blut 1983, 47:287–96.
298. Goetzl EJ, Weller PF, Sun FF. The regulation of human eosinophil function by endogenous mono-hydroxy-eicosatetraenoic acids (HETEs). J Immunol 1980; 124:926–33.
299. Palmblad J, Uden A-M, Friberg I, Ringertz B, Radmark O, Lindgren J-A, Hansson G, Malmsten CL. Effects of novel lipoxygenase products on neutrophil and eosinophil functions in vitro. In: Samuelsson B, Paoletti R, Ramwell P, eds. Advances in prostaglandin, thromboxane, and leukotriene research, vol. 21. New York: Raven Press, 1983:25.
300. Spada CS, Woodward DF, Hawley SB, Nieves AL. Leukotrienes cause eosinophil emigration into conjunctival tissue. Prostaglandins 1986; 31:795–809.

301. Spada CS, Woodward DF, Hawley SB, Nieves AL, Williams LS, Feldmann BJ. Synergistic effects of LTB_4 and LTD_4 on leukocyte emigration into the guinea pig conjunctiva. Am J Pathol 1988; 130:354–68.
302. Wardlaw AJ, Moqbel R, Cromwell O, Kay AB. Platelet-activating factor. A potent chemotactic and chemokinetic factor for human eosinophils. J Clin Invest 1986; 78:1701–6.
303. Tamura N, Agarwal DK, Suliaman FA, Townley RG. Effects of platelet activating factor on the chemotaxis of normodense eosinophils from normal subjects. Biochem Biophys Res Commun 1987; 142:638–44.
304. Sigal CE, Valone FH, Holtzman MJ, Goetzl EJ. Preferential human eosinophil chemotactic activity of the platelet-activating factor (PAF) 1-o-hexadecyl-2-acetyl-sn-glyceryl-3-phosphocholine (AGEPC). J Clin Immunol 1987; 7:179–84.
305. Hakansson L, Westerlund D, Venge P. New method for the measurement of eosinophil migration. J Leukocyte Biol 1987; 42:689–96.
306. Arnoux B, Denjean A, Page CP, Nolibe D, Morley J, Benveniste J. Accumulation of platelets and eosinophils in baboon lung after Paf-acether challenge. Am Rev Resp Dis 1988; 137:855–60.
307. Lellouch-Tubiana A, Lefort J, Simon M-T, Pfister A, Vargaftig B. Eosinophil recruitment into guinea pig lungs after PAF-acether and allergen administration. Am Rev Resp Dis 1988; 137:948–54.
308. Silva PMR, Martins MA, Cordeiro RSB, Vargaftig BB. Late mobilization induced by PAF-acether in the pleural cavity of rats. Brazil J Med Biol Res 1989; 22:1281–5.
309. Ishida K, Thomson RJ, Beattie LL, Wiggs B, Schellenberg RR. Inhibition of antigen-induced airway hyperresponsiveness, but not acute hypoxia nor airway eosinophilia, by an antagonist of platelet-activating factor. J Immunol 1990; 144:3907–11.
310. Strath M, Sanderson CJ. Detection of eosinophil differentiation factor and its relationship to eosinophilia in *Mesocestoides corti*-infected mice. Exp Hematol 1986; 14:16–20.
311. Wang JM, Rambaldi A, Biondi A, Chen ZG, Sanderson CJ, Mantovani A. Recombinant human interleukin 5 is a selective eosinophil chemoattractant. Eur J Immunol 1989; 19:701–5.
312. Silberstein DS, David JR. The regulation of eosinophil function by cytokines. Immunology Today 1987; 8:380–5.
313. Dinarello CA. Interleukin-1. Rev Infect Dis 1984; 6:51–95.
314. Oppenheim JJ, Kovacs EJ, Matsushima K, Durum SK. There is more than one interleukin 1. Immunology Today 1986; 7:45–56.
315. Pincus SH, Whitcomb EA, Dinarello CA. Interaction of IL1 and TPA in modulation of eosinophil function. J Immunol 1986; 137:3509–14.
316. Whitcomb EA, Dinarello CA, Pincus SH. Differential effects of interleukin-1 alpha and interleukin-1 beta on human peripheral blood eosinophils. Blood 1989; 73:1904–8.
317. Fujisawa T, Abu-Ghazaleh R, Kita H, Sanderson CJ, Gleich GJ. Regulatory effect of cytokines on eosinophil degranulation. J Immunol 1990; 144:642–6.
318. Robb RJ. Interleukin 2: the molecule and its function. Immunology Today 1984; 5:203–9.
319. Rosenberg SA, Lotze MT, Muul LM, Leitman S, Chang AE, Ellinghausen SE, Matory YL, Skibber JM, Shiloni E, Veto JT, Seipp CA, Simpson C, Reichert CM. Observations on the systemic administration of autologous lymphokine-activated killer cells and recombinant interleukin-2 to patients with metastatic cancer. N Engl J Med 1985; 313:1485–92.
320. Silberstein DS, Schoof DD, Rodrick ML, Tai P-C, Spry CJF, David JR, Eberlein TJ. Activation of eosinophils in cancer patients treated with IL-2 and IL-2-generated lymphokine-activated killer cells. J Immunol 1989; 142:2162–7.
321. Anderson TD, Hayes TJ. Toxicity of human recombinant interleukin-2 in rats. Lab Invest 1989; 60:331–46.
322. Enokihara H, Furusawa S, Kajitani H, Hamaguchi H, Saito K, Fukuda T. Interleukin 2

stimulates the T-cells from patients with eosinophilia to produce CFU-Eo growth stimulating factor. Br J Haematol 1988; 69:431–6.

323. Enokihara H, Furusawa S, Nakakubo H, Kajitani H, Nagashima S, Saito K, Shishid H, Hitoshi Y, Takatsu K, Noma T, Shimizu A, Honjo T. T cells from eosinophilia patients produce interleukin-5 with interleukin-2 stimulation. Blood 1989; 73:1809–13.
324. Saito H, Bourinbaiar A, Ginsburg M, Minato K, Ceresi E, Yamada K, Machover D, Breard J, Matine G. Establishment and characterization of a new human eosinophilic leukemia cell line. Blood 1985; 66:1233–40.
325. Yokota A, Kikutani H, Tanaka T, Sato R, Barsumia EL, Suemura M, Kishimoto T. Two species of human Fcϵ receptor II (FcϵRII/CD23): tissue-specific and IL-4-specific regulation of gene expression. Cell 1988; 55:611–8.
326. Yoshie O, Majima T, Saito H. Membrane oxidative metabolism of human eosinophilic cell line EoL-1 in response to phorphol diester and formyl peptide: synergistic augmentation by interferon-gamma and tumor necrosis factor. J Leukocyte Biol 1989; 45:10–20.
327. Tanaka M, Lee K, Yodoi J, Saito H, Iwai Y, Kim K-M, Morita M, Mayumi M, Mikawa H. Regulation of Fc_ϵ receptor 2 (CD23) expression on a human eosinophilic cell line EoL3 and a human monocytic cell line CL937 by transforming growth factor β. Cell Immunol 1989; 122:96–107.
328. Hosoda M, Makino S, Kawabe T, Maeda Y, Satoh S, Takami M, Mayumi M, Arai K-I, Saitoh H, Yodoi J. Differential regulation of the low affinity Fc receptor for IgE (FCER2/CD23) and the IL-2 receptor (Tac/p55) on eosinophilic leukemia cell line (EoL-1 and EoL-3). J Immunol 1989; 143:147–52.
329. Schrader JW. The panspecific hemopoietin of activated T lymphocytes (interleukin-3). Ann Rev Immunol 1986; 4:205–30.
330. Lopez AF, To LB, Yang Y-C, Gamble JR, Shannon MF, Burns GF, Dyson PG, Juttner CA, Clark S, Vadas MA. Stimulation of proliferation, differentiation, and function of human cells by primate interleukin 3. Proc Natl Acad Sci USA 1987; 84:2761–5.
331. Prystowsky MB, Otten G, Naujokas MF, Vardiman J, Ihle JN, Goldwasser E, Fitch FW. Multiple hemopoietic lineages are found after stimulation of mouse bone marrow precursor cells with interleukin 3. Am J Pathol 1984; 117:171–9.
332. Ihle JN, Keller J, Oroszlan S, Henderson LE, Copeland TD, Fitch F, Prystowsky MB, Goldwasser E, Schrader JW, Palaszynski E, Dy M, Lebel B. Biologic properties of homogeneous interleukin 3. I. Demonstration of WEHI-3 growth factor activity, mast cell growth factor activity, P cell-stimulating factor activity, colony-stimulating factor activity, and histamine-producing cell-stimulating factor activity. J Immunol 1983; 131:282–7.
333. MacDonald SM, Schleimer RP, Kagey-Sobotka A, Gillis S, Lichtenstein LM. Recombinant IL-3 induces histamine release from human basophils. J Immunol 1989; 142:3527–32.
334. Schleimer RP, Derse CP, Friedman B, Gillis S, Plaut M, Lichtenstein LM, MacGlashan DW Jr. Regulation of human basophil mediator release by cytokines. I. Interaction with antiinflammatory steroids. J Immunol 1989; 143:1310–7.
335. Kurimoto Y, de Weck AL, Dahinden CA. Interleukin 3-dependent mediator release in basophils triggered by C5a. J Exp Med 1989; 170:467–79.
336. Valent P, Besemer J, Muhm M, Majdic O, Lechner K, Bettelheim P. Interleukin 3 activates human blood basophils via high-affinity binding sites. Proc Natl Acad Sci USA 1989; 86:5542–6.
337. Burd PR, Rogers HW, Gordon JR, Martin CA, Jayaraman S, Wilson SD, Dvorak AM, Galli SJ, Dorf ME. Interleukin 3-dependent and -independent mast cells stimulated with IgE and antigen express multiple cytokines. J Exp Med 1989; 170:245–57.

338. Metcalf D, Begley CG, Johnson GR, Nicola NA, Vadas MA, Lopez AF, Williamson DJ, Wong GG, Clark SC, Wang EA. Biologic properties in vitro of a recombinant human granulocyte-macrophage colony-stimulating factor. Blood 1986; 67:37–45.
339. Clark SC, Kamen R. The human hematopoietic colony-stimulating factors. Science 1987; 236:1229–37.
340. Henson PM. PAF-A perspective. Am J Resp Cell Mol Biol 1989; 1:263–5.
341. Wardlaw AJ, Moqbel R, Cromwell O, Kay AB. Platelet-activating factor. A potent chemotactic and chemokinetic factor for human eosinophils. J Clin Invest 1986; 78:1701–6.
342. Bruynzeel PLB, Koenderman L, Kok PTM, Hameling ML, Verhagen J. Platelet-activating factor (PAF-acether) induced leukotriene C_4 formation and luminal dependent chemiluminescence by human eosinophils. Pharmacol Res Commun 1986; 18(Suppl):61–9.
343. Kroegel C, Yukawa T, Dent G. Venge P, Fan Chung K, Barnes PJ. Stimulation of degranulation from human eosinophils by platelet-activating factor. J Immunol 1989; 142:3518–26.
344. Kroegel C, Pleass R, Yukawa T, Fan Chung K, Westwick J, Barnes PJ. Characterization of platelet-activating factor-induced elevation of cytosolic free calcium concentration in eosinophils. Fed Eur Biochem Soc 1989; 243:41–6.
345. Yukawa T, Kroegel C, Evans P, Fukuda T, Chung KF, Barnes PJ. Density heterogeneity of eosinophil leukocytes: induction of hypodense eosinophils by platelet-activating factor. Immunology 1989; 68:140–3.
346. Plaut M, Pierce JH, Watson CJ, Hanley-Hyde J, Nordan RP, Paul WE. Mast cell lines produce lymphokines in response to cross-linkage of FcϵRI or to calcium ionophores. Nature 1989; 339:64–7.
347. Wodnar-Filipowicz A, Heusser CH, Moroni C. Production of the haemopoietic growth factors GM-CSF and interleukin-3 by mast cells in response to IgE receptor-mediated activation. Nature 1989; 339:150–2.
348. Burd PR, Rogers HW, Gordon JR, Martin CA, Jayaraman S, Wilson SD, Dvorak AM, Galli SJ, Dorf ME. Interleukin 3-dependent and -independent mast cells stimulated with IgE and antigen express multiple cytokines. J Exp Med 1989; 170:245–57.

7

Basophils and Mast Cells: Piecemeal Degranulation in Situ and ex Vivo: A Possible Mechanism for Cytokine-Induced Function in Disease

ANN M. DVORAK
Beth Israel Hospital and Harvard Medical School, Boston, Massachusetts

I. INTRODUCTION

Basophils and mast cells, initially described by Ehrlich using light microscopic morphologic techniques (1,2), are cells with functional and anatomical similarities and differences. Ultrastructural morphology provides the means for definitive identification of, and distinction between, basophils and mast cells in in-situ and ex-vivo circumstances and models in multiple species. We provide the general and specific morphological rules for doing so in six species with which we are familiar: human (Figure 1), guinea pig (Figure 2), mouse (Figure 3), rat, monkey (Figure 4), and rabbit (Figure 5). Both basophils and mast cells are distinguished by high-affinity IgE receptors on their surfaces which, when bound to IgE, cause biochemical and anatomical changes that place stored and newly generated cellular products into the extracellular milieu. Key, stored biochemical mediators of inflammation (such as histamine) and newly generated products of arachidonic acid metabolism (such as prostaglandins and leukotrienes) are released in this manner. The anatomic process by which these release events occur is termed anaphylactic degranulation (AND). Careful study of basophils and mast cells of multiple species has shown overall similarities as well as discrete differences in this anatomic process. Mast cells of three species (human, mouse, and rat) and basophils of one species (guinea pig) have been shown to recover from the massive release reaction termed AND. The anatomic events associated with the recovery of mast cells and basophils from AND provide insight into the complex capabilities of these similar cells.

Basophils and mast cells may also have a role in cell-mediated disease. This role is suggested by the widespread presence of basophils and mast cells in diseases of multiple etiologies, in diseases of unknown etiology, and in host defense and healing processes. Little is known about whether the role(s) is beneficial, detrimental, or both. Virtually nothing is known regarding the biochemistry of release of cell constituents

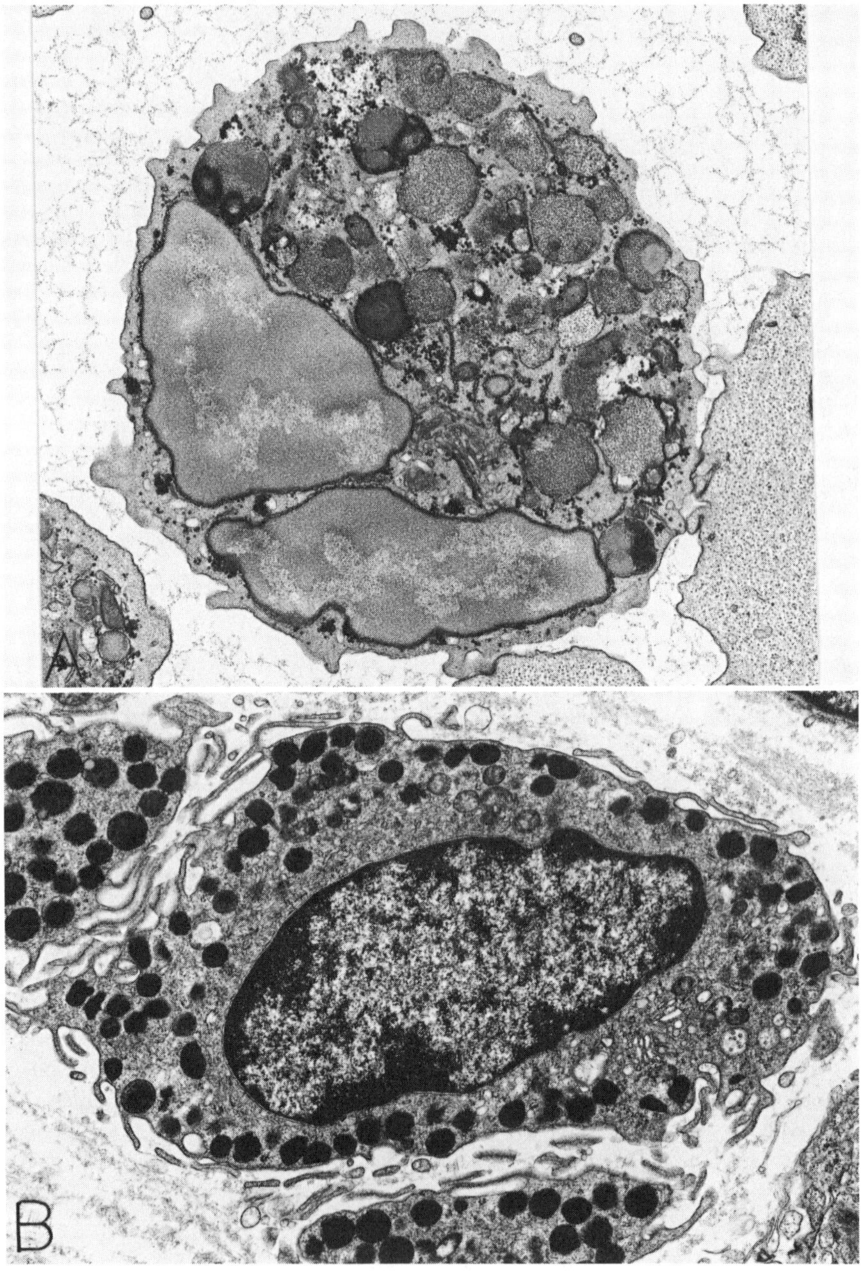

Figure 1 Human peripheral blood basophil (A) and ileal mast cell (B) show essential features of two cell types. The basophil (A) has a polylobed nucleus, irregular, short, broad cell surface processes, cytoplasmic glycogen, and large granules filled with particles. The mast cell (B) has a single nucleus, slender, elongated surface folds, and numerous, small dense granules. A ×18,800; B, ×9,000.

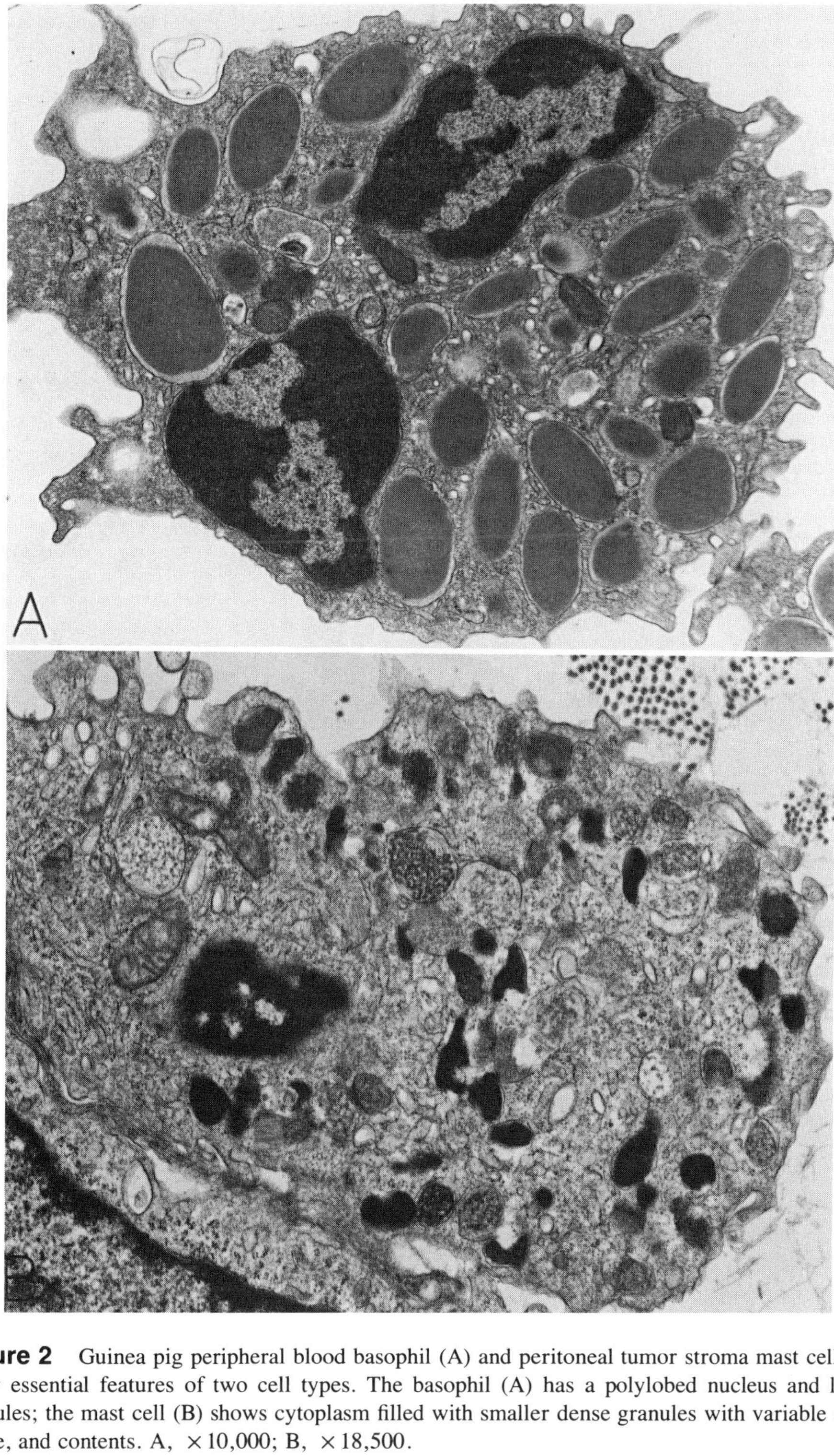

Figure 2 Guinea pig peripheral blood basophil (A) and peritoneal tumor stroma mast cell (B) show essential features of two cell types. The basophil (A) has a polylobed nucleus and large granules; the mast cell (B) shows cytoplasm filled with smaller dense granules with variable size, shape, and contents. A, ×10,000; B, ×18,500.

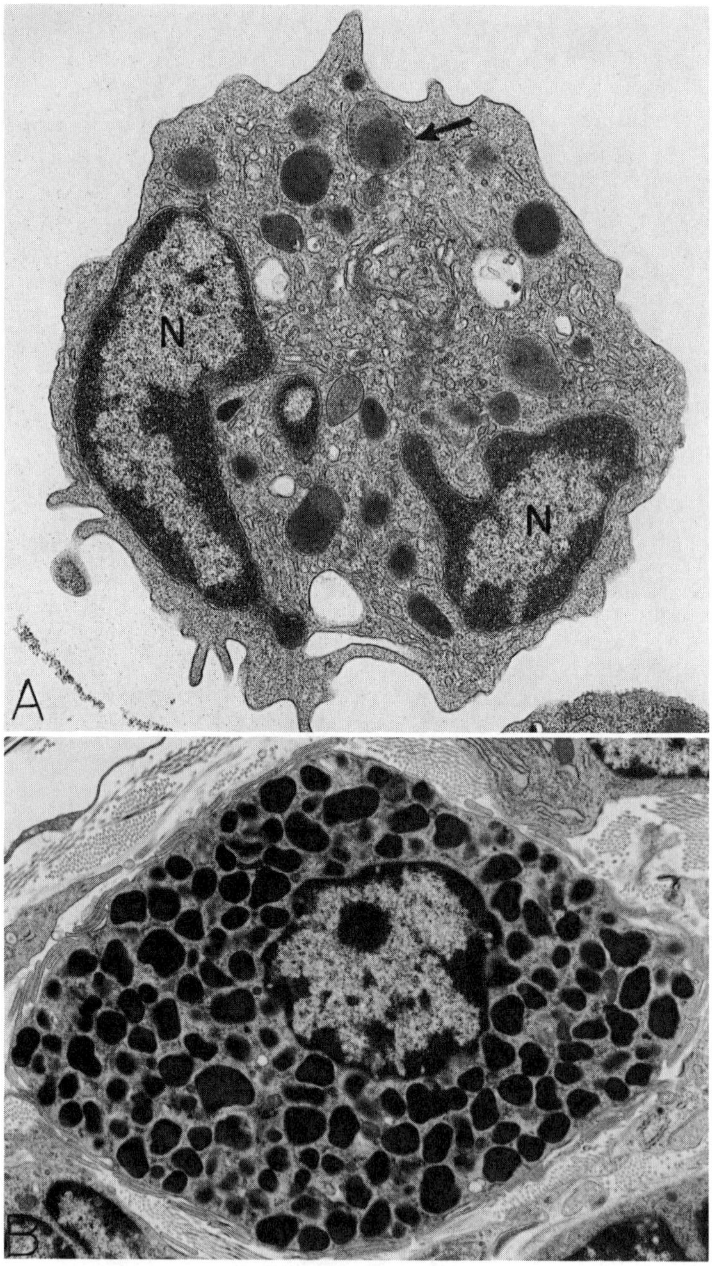

Figure 3 Mouse basophil cultured from bone marrow (A) and skin mast cell from a chronically inflamed ear of a mast cell-deficient mouse (W/W^v) (B) show essential features of two cell types. The basophil has a polylobed nucleus (N), irregular, short, broad cell surface processes, and small numbers of large dense granules. One immature granule contains numerous vesicles (arrow). The mast cell (B) has a single nucleus, narrow surface folds and is filled with dense granules. A, ×17,000; B, ×31,500. (A, from Ref. 41, with permission.)

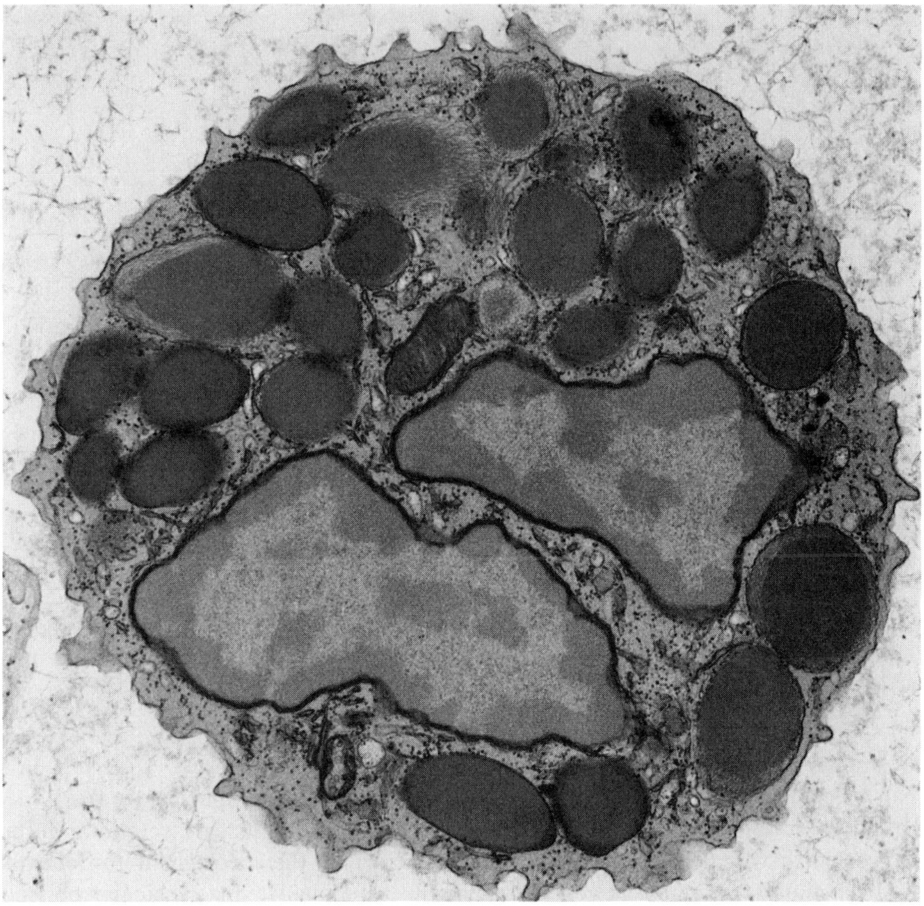

Figure 4 Monkey peripheral blood basophil has polylobed nucleus, blunt, short surface processes, monoparticulate glycogen, and large dense granules. ×26,500. (From Ref. 88, with permission.)

from basophils and mast cells in these tissue sites in situ. Ultrastructural morphology has, however, consistently identified a nonanaphylactic release response, termed piecemeal degranulation (PMD), in basophils and mast cells in tissues in a wide variety of circumstances in several species. Similar to the recovery potential which basophils and mast cells display in response to AND, recovery from losses sustained by the nonanaphylactic process, PMD, may also be possible. Despite these advances in our knowledge of the role of basophils and mast cells in disease, we still do not know the function(s) of these cells in health.

Secretion is an essential physiologic cellular process that is up-regulated in basophils and mast cells in disease. For example, AND is an example of regulated secretion, a property of all granulated secretory cells, for many of which physiological functions are known. In addition to IgE-mediated mechanisms for stimulating AND, numerous other triggers can be shown to induce anaphylacticlike degranulation. We refer to all

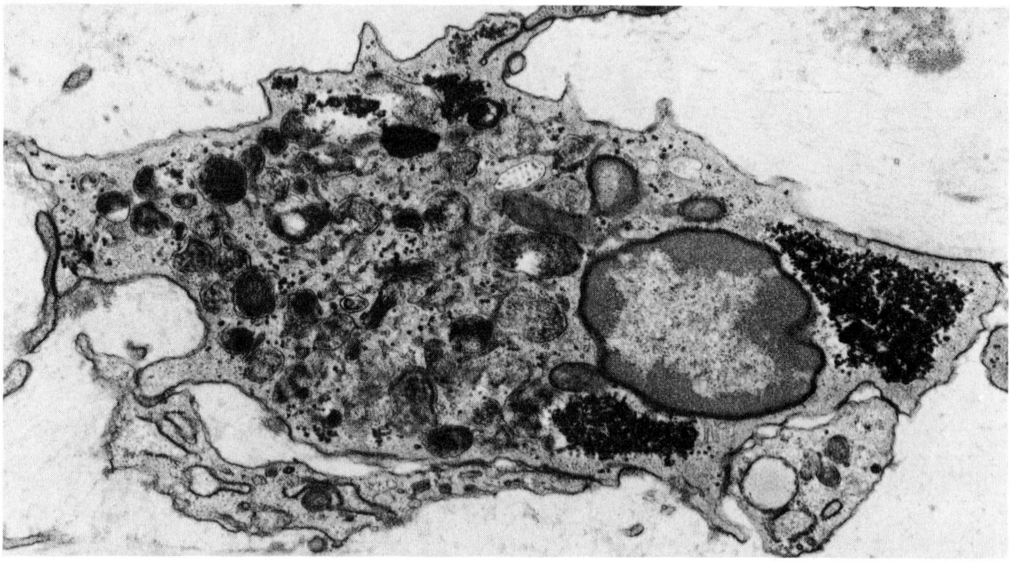

Figure 5 Rabbit tumor-containing corneal pocket stromal basophil shows only one lobe of a heavily chromatin-condensed nucleus, large cytoplasmic aggregates of glycogen, irregular, blunt surface processes, and numerous dense granules with heterogeneous contents. ×17,000.

such similar morphologies, by analogy, as AND. PMD, a process widely seen in human basophils and mast cells in situ, may represent an up-regulated expression of constitutive secretion, or a down-regulated expression of regulated secretion. Certain evidence exists which implicates vesicular transport as the mechanism for effecting PMD. Constitutive secretion is generally thought to be mediated by vesicular transport that bypasses storage organelles, such as secretory granules. If PMD represents up-regulated constitutive secretion, albeit from storage depots in granules, triggers which regulate this process must exist. Morphological analysis, using electron microscopic techniques, has recently provided certain clues to possible triggers. Whether release of all granule biochemical mediators, or differential release of selected ones, is a product of PMD is entirely unknown. Nor do we know the ultimate result on tissue pathologies and reaction responses to etiologic agents or injuries of basophil and mast cell products released by either constitutive secretion or PMD into tissues. Losses sustained by basophils and mast cells from PMD may be repaired in certain circumstances, as visualized by electron microscopy in in-situ graft rejection and wound healing. Ultrastructural analysis of the release and recovery responses, of which basophils and mast cells are capable, led us, in 1975, to propose a general model for degranulation (3). Additions to this scheme have resulted in a general scheme for the various forms of AND and PMD and their recovery responses which can be observed using ultrastructural methods.

Cytokines, interleukins, and tumor and bacterial products are all possible candidates for regulation of basophil and mast cell function(s) in vivo. For years, some [i.e., f-Met peptide(s), a bacterial product] have been demonstrated to do so in in-vitro systems. Others, such as interleukin 3, have only recently been implicated in release reactions from basophils. The potential complexities of these interactions are considerable. For example, interleukin 3 and other as-yet-unidentified growth factors are now known to stimulate the differentiation and maturation of basophils and mast cells of human, guinea pig, mouse, and monkey origin, and recombinant human interleukin 3 is associated with the ultrastructural morphology of PMD in human basophils in vitro and monkey basophils in vivo. Recovery from secretory processes visually resembles certain aspects of the initial differentiation and maturation of basophils and mast cells. Therefore, it seems certain that these recovery reactions may also be regulated by cytokines, interleukins, etc. It is now certain that mast cells themselves produce cytokines, a process which is up-regulated in the wake of IgE-stimulated secretion. The potential role(s) of these mast cell-derived products in autoregulatory loops, as well as in regulation of the various functions of other inflammatory cells (lymphocytes, macrophages, eosinophils, neutrophils), in regulation of barrier functions of epithelial and endothelial cells, and in regulation of integrated units of messages and motion (nerves and muscles) and in repair processes in wound healing (fibroblasts), is considerable.

In this review, we cannot address all of the numerous areas of potential interactions among basophils, mast cells, cytokines, and their intercellular associations. Our point of view, based on ultrastructural studies, provides important signposts for consideration of these events. This presentation will provide guidelines for the correct identification of basophils and mast cells and their release and recovery reactions. The possible role of basophils and mast cells in various pathologies will be presented. Recent experience in the identification of factor-driven, cultured basophils and mast cells will be reviewed. These studies provide a morphologic window into the possibilities for interactions between basophils and mast cells and their environment that may be mediated by cytokines and interleukins, as well as by tumor and bacterial products.

II. DISTRIBUTION OF BASOPHILS AND MAST CELLS IN HEALTH AND DISEASE

Basophils are the least numerous of human granulocytes, accounting for 0.5–1% of circulating leukocytes and 0.33% of nucleated cells in the bone marrow (4). Modest variations in basophil frequency have been reported with age (5), and young adult women have slightly higher basophil counts than men or older women (6). The frequency of basophils in most mammalian species approximates that of humans, although rabbits have 5 to 10 times this number. In lower vertebrates, basophils are considerably more abundant and, in some instances (e.g., reptiles) may account for more than half of the leukocytes (7). Surveying the animal kingdom as a whole, there is a striking, although not invariant, inverse relationship between the frequency of basophils and of fixed tissue mast cells within different species. Thus, rats, mice, and many types of fishes, in which basophils are vanishingly rare, have extremely numerous tissue mast cells. This relationship supports the widely held view that basophils and mast cells supplement each other and have similar or even identical functions.

Blood basophil frequency may be altered by adrenal, thyroid, and sex hormones (8). Injections of cortisone (or of ACTH in individuals with functioning adrenal glands) depress the level of circulating basophils. Thyrotropic hormone and L-thyroxine depress basophils, whereas the metabolically inert D-thyroxine increases basophil levels, possibly by inhibiting TSH secretion. Basophils are elevated in myxedema and lowered in thyrotoxicosis. Basophil elevation by estrogens and depression by progesterones have been reported, as have decreased basophils in pregnancy and alterations in basophil frequency with the menstrual cycle. The blood basophil count falls significantly on the day of ovulation in women and rabbits.

Variations in circulating basophil levels have been reported in a variety of disease states. Basophilia is not uncommon in myeloproliferative disorders, particularly chronic granulocytic leukemia, where basophils may number more than $90{,}000/mm^3$ (9) and can account for 90% or more of circulating leukocytes. Basophilia may be among the earliest signs of developing myelogenous leukemia (10). Total blood histamine rises, roughly in proportion to basophil number, to the highest levels reported in human disease. Youman et al. (9) report a patient with a blood histamine content of 5 mg%. Elevated basophil levels have also been reported in polycythemia vera, ulcerative colitis, and in various allergic states including atopy (11–13). By contrast, the peripheral basophil count is low in urticaria (14) and immediately following anaphylaxis (15).

Mature mast cells are widespread in the connective tissues of virtually all organs of the body (16,17). They are concentrated in organs (skin, lung, and gut) that are potential portals of entry for foreign agents. Mast cells also tend to be localized to perivascular structures in these organs. They can, however, be found throughout the tissues, including within epithelia.

Mast cells are found in increased numbers in the tissues of patients with a wide variety of diseases, including primary mast cell disorders (16). These include chronic inflammatory disorders, cell-mediated immunologic disorders (contact allergy), neoplastic events, and urticaria pigmentosa and systemic mastocytosis.

Basophils may also be found in tissue sites following migration from the vascular space. This may occur in the absence of peripheral blood basophilia. Infiltrations of basophils may occur in the skin in the absence of a peripheral basophilia. Basophils are characteristically present in reactions of delayed-type hypersensitivity, including allergic contact dermatitis, hypersensitivity to protein antigens, and skin allograft rejection (18–21). They also appear in several other skin diseases whose pathogenesis may include a component of cell-mediated hypersensitivity. These include various types of eczema, psoriasis, drug reactions, erythema multiforme, dermatitis herpetiformis, epidermolysis bullosa, discoid lupus erythematosus, insect bites, pemphigus, Behçet's syndrome, alopecia areata, and photo-contact dermatitis (22–25).

Basophil infiltration is not confined to the skin. Basophils have been found in tissues obtained from a wide variety of circumstances (Table 1) in humans and animals. In some of these circumstances, both tissue basophils and mast cells are readily found. For example, biopsies of bullous pemphigoid-involved skin or Crohn's disease-involved ileum (both inflammatory disorders of uncertain etiology) contain basophils and mast cells (26–28). Basophils are also regular components of the inflammatory infiltrate in renal allografts undergoing active cellular rejection during the first 6 weeks after transplant (29). Interestingly, rejection episodes at later intervals after transplantation are characterized by mast cell hyperplasia and fewer basophils. These data support the hypothesis that basophils—preformed, quickly mobilized, and relatively short-lived cells—participate in sensitized hosts in the initial cell-mediated response to antigenic challenge, whereas in more chronic processes, basophils give way and are replaced by mast cells (30).

III. ULTRASTRUCTURAL MORPHOLOGY. THE MEANS FOR DEFINITIVE IDENTIFICATION OF, AND DISTINCTION BETWEEN, BASOPHILS AND MAST CELLS IN SITU AND EX VIVO

Basophilic leukocytes are granulocytes. They are produced in the bone marrow from committed granulocyte precursors and undergo several rounds of mitoses, followed by postmitotic maturation prior to release into the circulation as mature granulocytes (31,32). Mast cells are not granulocytes. Mast cell precursors originate in the bone marrow and circulate as nongranulated mononuclear cells that do not display a differentiated phenotype sufficient for morphologic identification (16,33–36). These precursors regularly leave the circulation and mature within tissues into recognizable mast cells filled with typical secretory granules. Basophilic leukocytes (like all granulocytes) generally remain within the vascular compartment until special circumstances induce their migration into tissue spaces (30,33,37–40).

The differentiation and maturation of basophils in the bone marrow have been described in several species (31,32,41–44). Like all granulocytes, immature basophils are large, granulated, mononuclear cells highly endowed with the synthetic machinery for protein production. Thus, basophilic myelocytes (Figure 6) have large, single nuclei with dispersed chromatin, active, large Golgi structures, numerous filled cisterns of rough endoplasmic reticulum, and variable mixtures of immature and mature secretory granules (31,32,41–44). These secretory storage organelles are sufficiently distinctive in myelocytes to identify those of basophilic, neutrophilic, and eosinophilic origin in most species. The surface architecture of myelocytes is also distinctive. Broad, irregular cytoplasmic processes characterize myelocytes of all three types and differ from the narrow surface folds generally found on mast cells.

Postmitotic myelocytes mature by identical processes—i.e., by nuclear size reduction, condensation, and segmentation, by cytoplasmic size reduction, and by reduction in the synthetic machinery of the cytoplasm (31,32,41–44). Basophilic myelocytes undergo maturational changes of their immature granules to produce typical mature granules. These changes include condensation of contents, reduction in granule size, and the appearance of definitive substructural patterns.

Maturation of mast cells (Figure 7) also involves cell, nuclear, cytoplasmic, and granule size changes as well as condensation and organization of secretory granule contents (16,33). While these maturational changes have been described in rodents in vivo (45–47), descriptions of human mast cell maturation in vivo are less complete. Recently we have identified mast cells developing in cultures of human cord blood cells (48), a model system which, in future studies, will provide ideal circumstances for defining the maturational events of human mast cells.

Mature basophils and mast cells are identifiable by general ultrastructural criteria, considered together with the distinctiveness of their secretory granules (Table 2). The electron-dense, membrane-bound granules of human basophils contain particles (Figure 8a), focal, multiple, concentric membrane arrays (Figure 8b), and Charcot-Leyden crystals (Figure 8b) (32,33,49–60). Rarely, large or small, homogeneously dense granules are also present. Secretory granules of human mast cells contain scrolls (Figure 9a), crystals (Figure 9b), particles (Figure 9c), and mixtures of these patterns. Some granules are homogeneously dense (Figure 9d) (16,33,50,61–67). Guinea pig basophils have granules displaying regular crystalline arrays (Figure 10a) or finely

Table 1 Circumstances in Which Basophilic Leukocytes Have Been Identified in Extravascular Tissues and Fluids

Species	Circumstance	References
Human	Crohn's disease	26, 27, 32, 33, 39, 50, 128, 193, 195–198, 404, 405
	Bullous pemphigoid	25, 28, 33, 39, 50, 404
	Drug-related allergic interstitial nephritis	406
	Renal allograft rejection	29
	Allergic contact dermatitis	8, 18–21, 25, 30–33, 37–39, 49, 50, 177, 188, 407–409
	Skin reactivity in atopic disease	25, 410–413
	Photo contact dermatitis	22–24
	Ulcerative colitis, colon or skin window fluid	19, 414; Dvorak AM, unpublished data
	Skin allograft rejection	33, 39, 50, 178, 192, 415
	Insect bite	22, 23, 25
	Alopecia areata	22, 23, 25
	Behçet's syndrome	22, 23, 25
	Pemphigus	22, 23, 25
	Discoid lupus erythematosus	22, 23, 25
	Dermatitis herpetiformis	22, 23, 25
	Erythema multiforme	22, 23, 25
	Drug-induced skin reactions	22, 23, 25
	Eczema	22, 23, 25, 413
	Psoriasis	22, 23, 25
	Hodgkin's disease	416, 417; Dvorak AM, unpublished data
	Hypersensitivity to microbial antigens	18
	Delayed hypersensitivity	3, 18–20, 37–39, 40, 418–423
	Hypersensitivity to protein antigens	19
	Tuberculin test reactions	424–427
	Breast cancer, skin window fluid	428
	Lung, Legionnaire's disease	429, 430
	Late-phase reaction	431–434
	Cutaneous and nasal ragweed allergy	435
	Allergic rhinitis	436–438
	Allergic conjunctivitis	439, 440
	Interstitial fibrosis of lung	441; Dvorak AM, unpublished data
	Peritoneal dialysis fluid	51
	Familial polyposis of colon	Dvorak AM, unpublished data
	Lung adenocarcinoma	32; Dvorak AM, unpublished data
	Gastric lymphoma	32
	Metastatic esthesioneuroblastoma	Dvorak AM, unpublished data
	Skin reactions of experimentally produced lymphocyte transfer test	25, 419
	Lymphoma	Dvorak AM, unpublished data
	Cutaneous necrotizing angiitis	444, 445
	Skin hypersensitivity reactions to insulin	446

Table 1 Continued

Species	Circumstance	References
	Skin hypersensitivity reactions to fire ants	434
	Porphyria	25
	Darier's disease	25
	Sarcoidosis	25
	Tinea circinata	25
	Dermatomyositis	25
	Scabies	25
	Herpes zoster	25
	Herpes simplex	25
	Vaccinia	25
	Lichen planus bullosus	25
	Interstitial cystitis	414
	Insulinoma	Dvorak AM, unpublished data
Guinea pig	The late reaction	447
	Vaccinia virus infection	448
	Solid and ascites tumor rejection	33, 178, 186, 187, 449–451
	Cutaneous basophil hypersensitivity	3, 31, 33, 37–40, 144–146, 177, 179–182, 211, 212, 215–217, 220, 404, 405, 420, 422, 423, 447, 452–468
	Contact allergy	216, 455
	Reaction to antigen-antibody complexes	216
	Delayed hypersensitivity	180, 182, 216, 454, 456, 469
	Allograft rejection	178, 470
	Immunity to ticks	39, 147, 471–475
	Protein injection site	39, 476
	Antigen injection site	477
	Delayed hypersensitivity, eye	478
	Contact allergen, colon	479
	Nematode (*Trichostrongylus colubriformis*) infection	480–483
	Schistosomiasis	467
	Mitogens	484
Chicken	Mitogens	485
	Rouse sarcoma virus infection	486
Rabbit	Ovary, fallopian tubes at ovulation	487–489
	3T3 fibroblast tumors in corneal pockets	Dvorak AM, unpublished data
	Bronchial epithelium, healthy rabbits	490
	Antigen injection sites	477
	CBH	491
Rat	Experimental allergic encephalomyelitis	81
	Ovary	492
	Irradiation-induced lung fibrosis	493

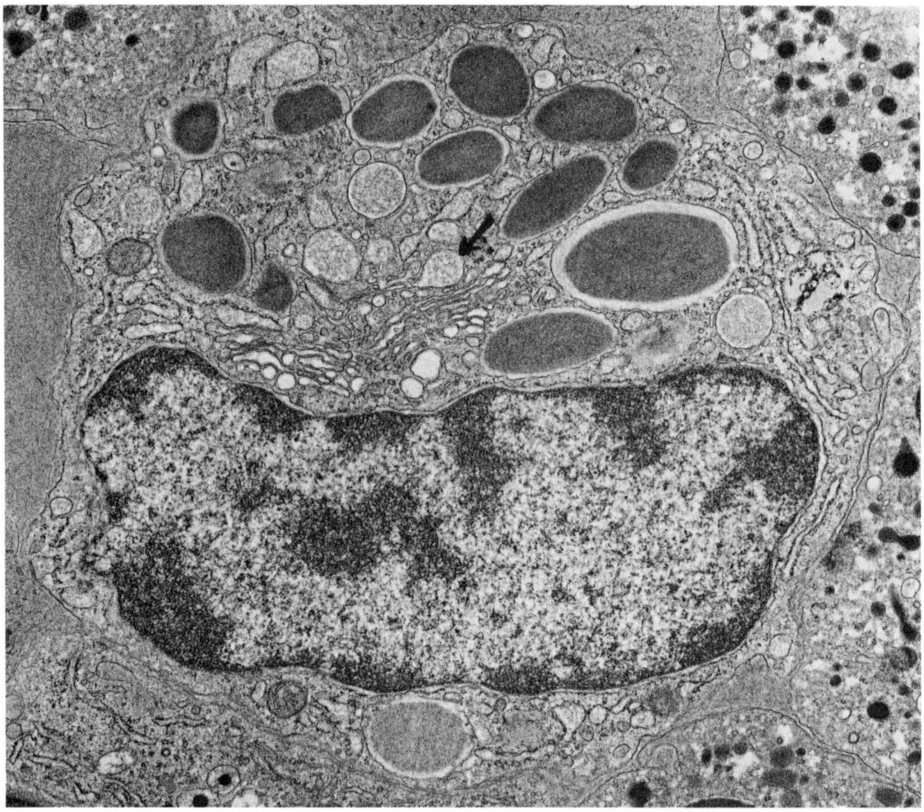

Figure 6 Guinea pig bone marrow basophilic myelocyte shows large single nucleus with partially dispersed chromatin, numerous dilated cisterns of membrane-bound ribosomes, mature and immature granules; one of the latter is budding from an enlarged Golgi area (arrow). ×13,500. (From Ref. 43, with permission.)

granular dense contents (31,57,63,68–76). Guinea pig mast cells contain granules that have particles, crystals, irregular thickened threads, regular arrays of 12-nm tubules, homogeneously dense material, and mixtures of these patterns (Figure 10b) (33,42,71,77–80). Mature granules of mouse (41,57) and rat basophils (57,81–84) and mast cells (Figure 11a) (41,45,46,85–87) are characteristically homogeneously dense, as are the granules of monkey basophils (Figure 11b) (57,88). Monkey mast cells, however, display heterogeneous patterns which include particles, threads, and crystals (89–91). Rabbit basophil granules contain particles, concentric and tangled thick threads, and finely granular dense contents (92–96; Dvorak AM, unpublished data); rabbit mast cell granules are generally homogeneously dense (97; Dvorak AM, unpublished data).

While the exact patterns that exist in the granules of basophils and mast cells in these various species assist us in cell identification, we do not yet know whether these special patterns reflect the biochemical contents of the stored secretory products of basophils and mast cells. Despite the individual differences noted in the ultrastructural

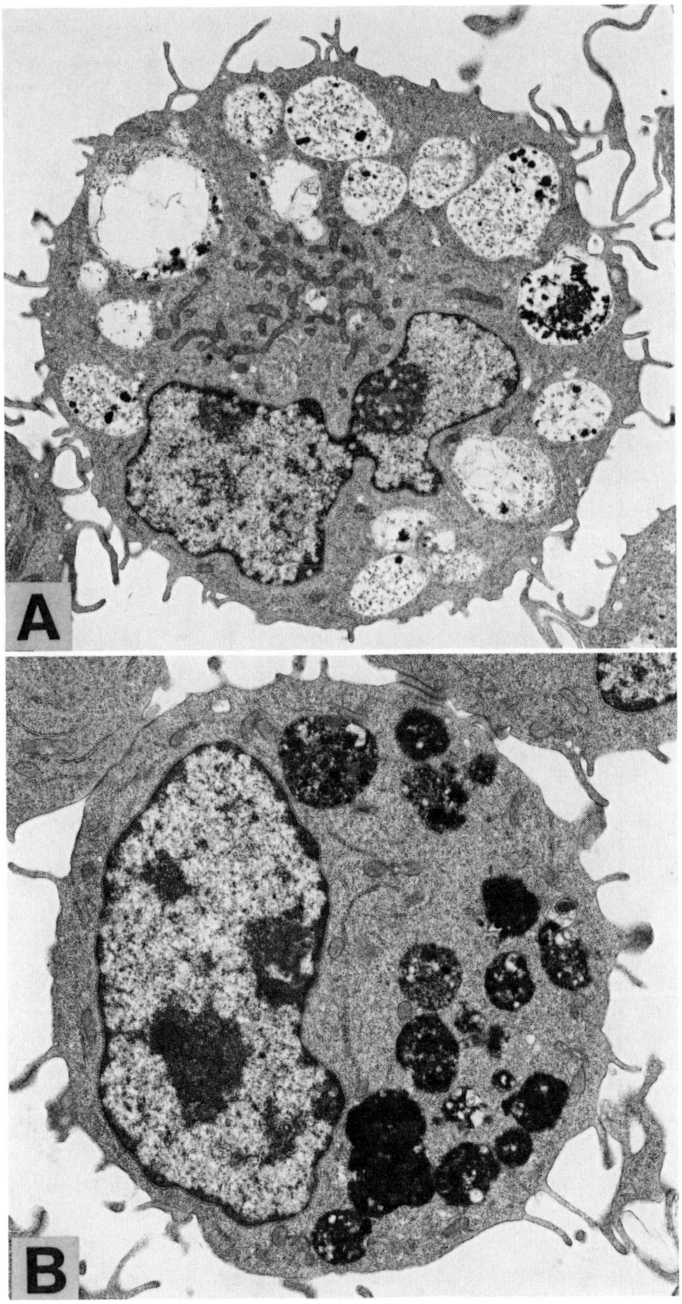

Figure 7 Immature, factor-dependent, cultured mouse mast cell (A) shows single lobular nucleus, narrow surface folds, numerous immature granules with many vesicles and few dense contents, and many mitochondria. In (B), a similar cell cultured in 1-mM sodium butyrate for 4 days shows cytoplasmic granules nearly filled with dense contents. A, ×6,000; B, ×8,500. (From Ref. 155, with permission.)

Table 2 Substructural Architecture of Human, Guinea Pig, Mouse, Rat, Monkey, and Rabbit Basophil and Mast Cell Granules

Species	Mature basophil granule patterns	Mature mast cell granule patterns
Human (16, 32, 33, 49–59, 61–67)	1. Particles 2. Multiple concentric membrane arrays 3. Charcot-Leyden crystals 4. Homogeneously dense	1. Scrolls 2. Crystals 3. Particles 4. Concentric and tangled thick threads 5. Homogeneously dense
Guinea pig (31, 33, 42, 57, 63, 68–80)	1. Crystals 2. Finely granular 3. Homogeneously dense	1. Crystals 2. Particles 3. Homogeneously dense 4. Irregular thick threads 5. Regular arrays of 12-nm tubules
Mouse (33, 41, 57, 86, 87)	1. Homogeneously dense	1. Homogeneously dense
Rat (45, 46, 57, 81–85)	1. Homogeneously dense	1. Homogeneously dense
Monkey (57, 88–90)	1. Homogeneously dense	1. Particles 2. Concentric and irregular threads 3. Homogeneously dense
Rabbit (92–96; Dvorak AM, unpublished data)	1. Particles 2. Concentric and tangled thick threads 3. Finely granular 4. Homogeneously dense	1. Homogeneously dense

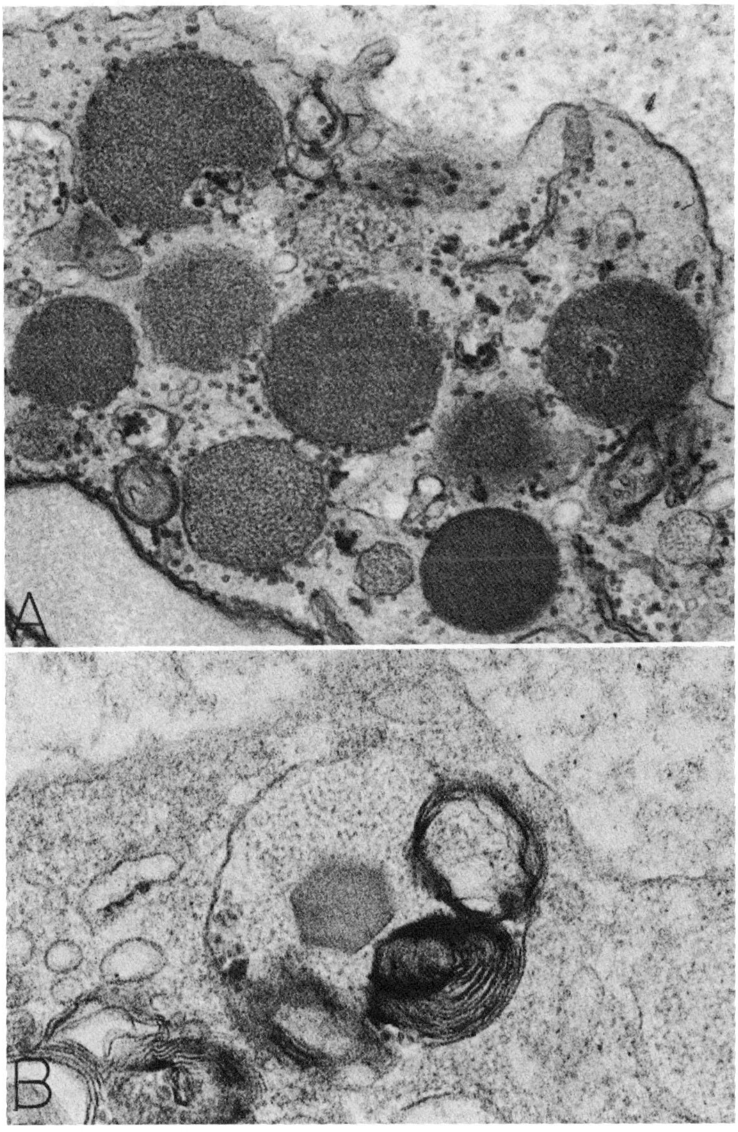

Figure 8 Human peripheral blood basophils show typical particle-filled granules (A) and a particle-depleted granule containing a hexagonal Charcot-Leyden crystal and multiple dense membrane arrays (B). A, ×37,500; B, ×48,000. (B, from Ref. 58 with permission.)

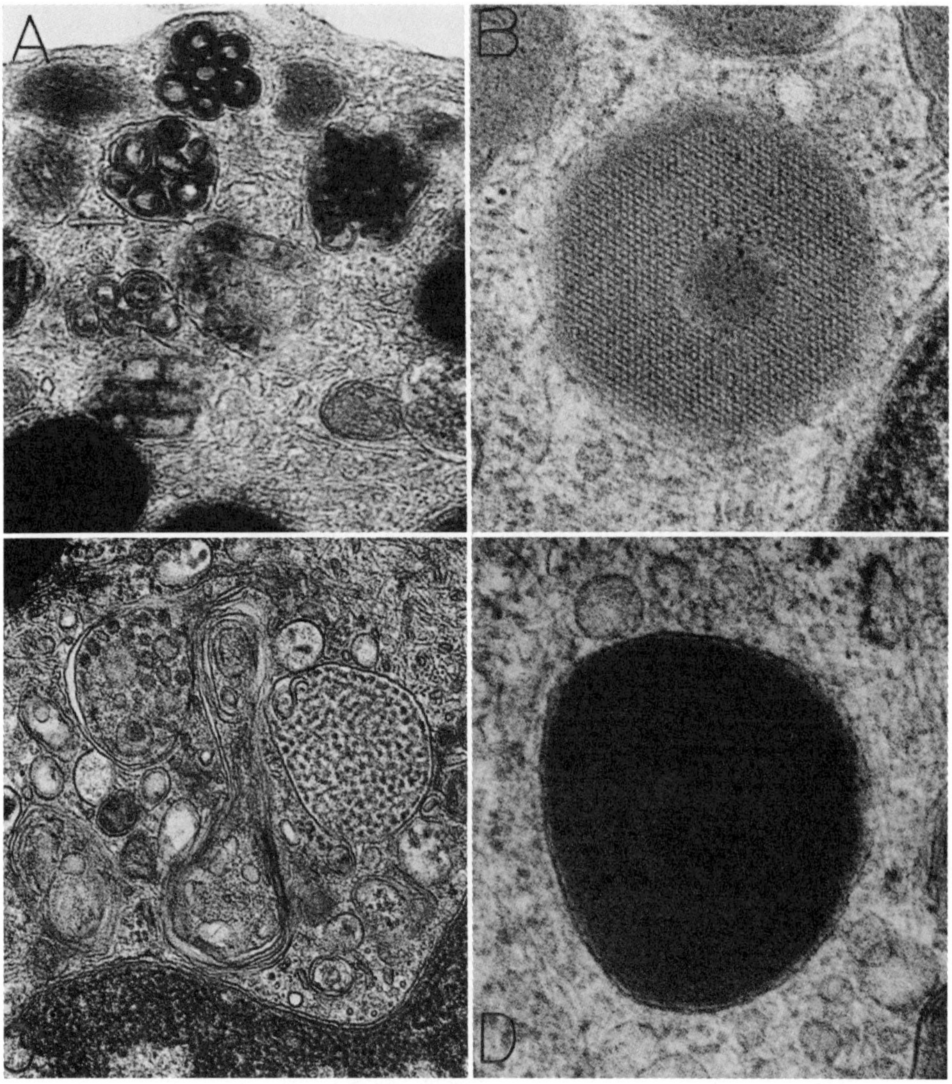

Figure 9 Human mast cell granules from lung cultured for 36 h show scrolls (A), from ileal biopsy show crystalline structure in cross section (B), from lung cultured for 6 h after degranulation show particles (C), from ileal biopsy show homogeneously dense contents (D). A, ×40,000; B, ×88,500; C, ×35,500; D, ×73,000. (B & C from Ref. 33 with permission.)

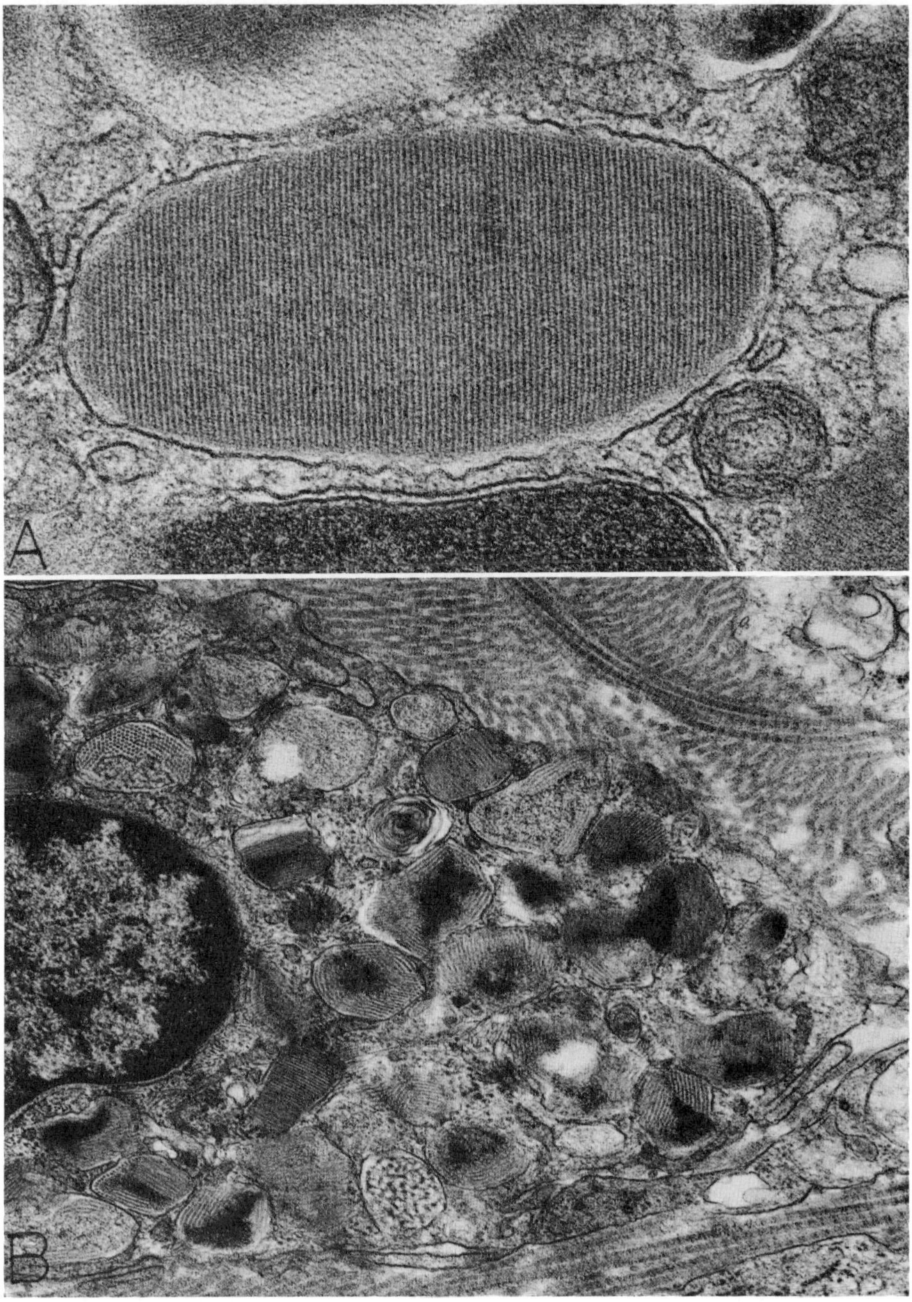

Figure 10 Guinea pig peripheral blood basophil granule shows regular parallel array (A), and lung mast cell granules show a heterogeneous collection of particles, crystals, regular 12-nm tubular arrays, and homogeneously dense material (B). A, ×68,000; B, ×26,000. (B from Ref. 33 with permission.)

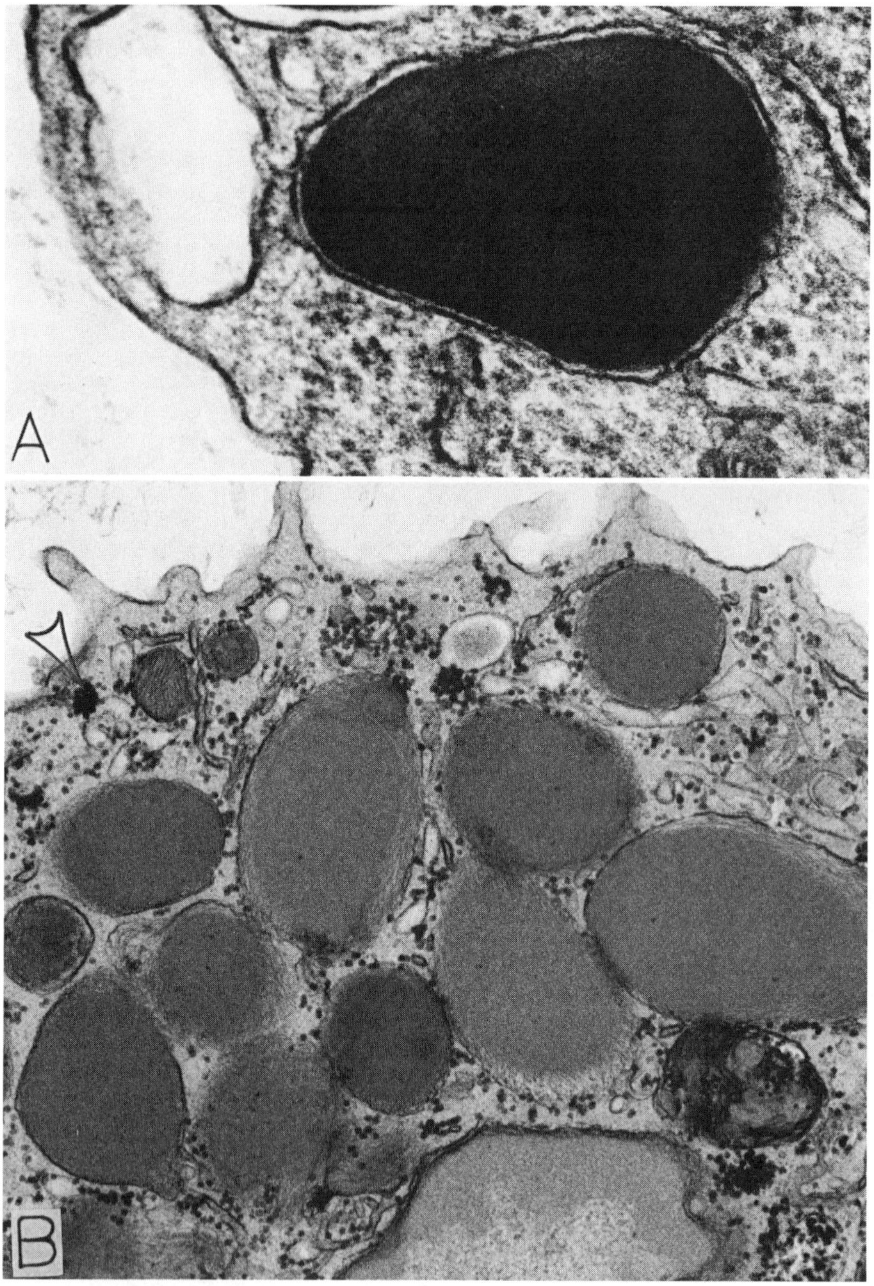

Figure 11 Mouse peritoneal mast cell granule has homogeneously dense contents (A). Monkey basophil granules are also homogeneously dense (B). Processing method for (B) allows demonstration of glycogen (arrowhead) in monkey basophil cytoplasm. A, ×93,000; B, ×34,500. (A from Ref. 33 with permission; B, from Ref. 88, with permission.)

patterns of basophils and mast cells of various species, the similarities of these patterns in the granules of basophils and mast cells exceed those of similarities with granules of other secretory cells, including those of neutrophils and eosinophils.

IV. ROLE OF BASOPHILS AND MAST CELLS IN IMMUNOGLOBULIN E-MEDIATED DISEASE

A. Anaphylactic Degranulation

Basophils and mast cells undergo a biochemical cascade when stimulated by an IgE-mediated triggering event that results in the rapid release of potent biochemical mediators of inflammation into the extracellular milieu. A new class of immunoglobulin E (IgE) was determined to have reagenic antibody activity in 1967 (98,99). IgE was visually determined to be present on the surface of basophils by immunoelectron microscopy (100–102), a process mediated by binding to a high-affinity receptor for IgE ($Fc_\epsilon R$) (99,103). Cross-linking of adjacent IgE receptors on the surfaces of basophils and mast cells is a critical event in triggering histamine release (104–107). In addition to IgE-mediated mechanisms for stimulating these rapid release reactions, a large number of stimulating agents also effect similar release (33,108–110). The mediators released include well-known, preformed mediators (such as histamine) as well as those generated from lipid compartments of the cell that are cyclooxygenase and lipoxygenase metabolites of arachidonic acid (such as prostaglandins and leukotrienes) (33,111–116).

The anatomical counterpart of these biochemical events in basophils and mast cells is termed anaphylactic degranulation (AND) (16,31–33,39,50,117). AND, viewed by electron microscopic examination of releasing basophils and mast cells in multiple species, shares considerable similarities as well as differences (Table 3). While the kinetics of these release reactions differ, these differences all occur within ~30 min of initial stimulation, depending on the individual trigger used and cell studied. Thus, they all qualify as rapid release reactions in contrast to release events developing over days in basophils within contact allergy skin reactions in humans (18,49).

1. *Human Basophil*

Anaphylactic degranulation of human basophils stimulated by either antigen, anti-IgE, mannitol, C5A peptide(s), histamine-releasing activity or f-Met peptide is characterized primarily by extrusion of individual membrane-free granules through multiple plasma membrane pores (Figures 12 and 13) (52,118–124). Rarely, intracytoplasmic degranulation chambers are formed by fusion of granule membranes. These chambers contain membrane-free granules which are ultimately released from the cell through a plasma membrane pore. These intracytoplasmic events were rarely seen in basophils stimulated by a hyperosmolar agent, mannitol, and more frequently as a later event in the continuum of release events stimulated by f-Met peptidc (119,122). Recently, we have also noted extrusion of intragranular Charcot-Leyden crystals and dense concentric membranes through degranulation pores stimulated to form in human basophils by f-Met peptide (122). In the latter case, it was noted that release of intragranular, dense concentric membranes overlapped with the kinetics of leukotriene (LTC_4) release stimulated by f-Met peptide, whereas a continuum of PMD → AND characterized the morphology of the interval of maximum histamine release, a more rapid event than the generation and release of LTC_4 (108) by this trigger.

Table 3 Ultrastructure of Anaphylactic Degranuation in Basophils and Mast Cells

Species	Cell	Triggers	Structural events
Human	Basophil	Antigen, C5a peptide(s), histamine-releasing activity, mannitol, anti-IgE, f-Met peptide	1. Extrusion of individual granules through multiple plasma membrane pores (32, 50, 52, 117–124)
		Mannitol, f-Met peptide	2. Multiple or single intracytoplasmic degranulation chambers (119, 122)
Human	Mast cell	Anti-IgE	1. Multiple intracytoplasmic degranulation chambers (16, 33, 61, 117, 125, 126, 129)
		Anti-IgE	2. Extrusion of individual granules through multiple plasma membrane pores (126, 138–143, 494)
Guinea pig	Basophil	Antigen, lectin, ionophore	1. Single intracytoplasmic degranulation chambers (31, 68, 117, 145, 149–154)
			2. Extrusion of multiple granules through a single plasma membrane pore (31, 68, 117, 148–152)
Mouse	Mast cell	Anti-DNP IgE	1. Multiple intracytoplasmic degranulation chambers (157)
			2. Extrusion of individual granules through multiple plasma membrane pores (33, 42, 155–157)
Rat	Mast cell	Antigen, 48/80, polymyxin B	1. Multiple intracytoplasmic degranulation chambers (33)
			2. Extrusion of individual granules through multiple plasma membrane pores (33, 158–160)

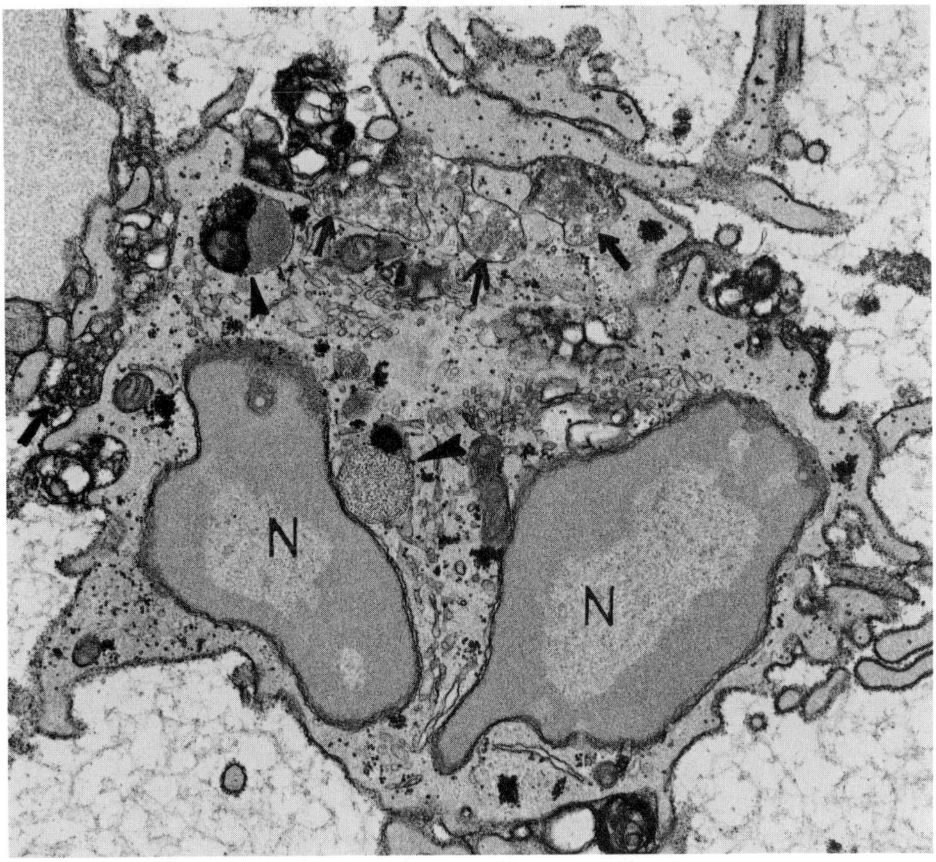

Figure 12 Human peripheral blood basophil exposed to C5 peptide(s) for 5 min shows AND characterized by extrusion of individual granules and granule membranes at multiple points around the perimeter of the cell (arrows). Particulate, membrane-free granule masses remain attached to the cell surface. These are labeled on their surfaces with cationized ferritin to which the cells were exposed after fixation. Only two unaltered granules (arrowheads) remain in the cytoplasm. N = nucleus. ×20,000. (From Ref. 120, with permission.)

2. *Human Mast Cell*

We have examined the ultrastructure of AND induced in human mast cells isolated from lung and skin (16,33,61,117,125,126). We also have noted AND in human mast cells in situ in heart and ileal biopsies (127,128). Anti-IgE was used to induce AND in isolated cells. When mast cells of lung origin were examined by electron microscopy, the primary morphologic event was the formation of multiple intracytoplasmic degranulation chambers within which membrane-free granules solubilized (Figure 14) (16,33,61,117,125,129). These chambers eventually either opened to the cell surface (Figure 15) or resolved within the cytoplasm. We rarely noted extrusion of individual membrane-free granules through multiple membrane pores in mast cells of lung origin

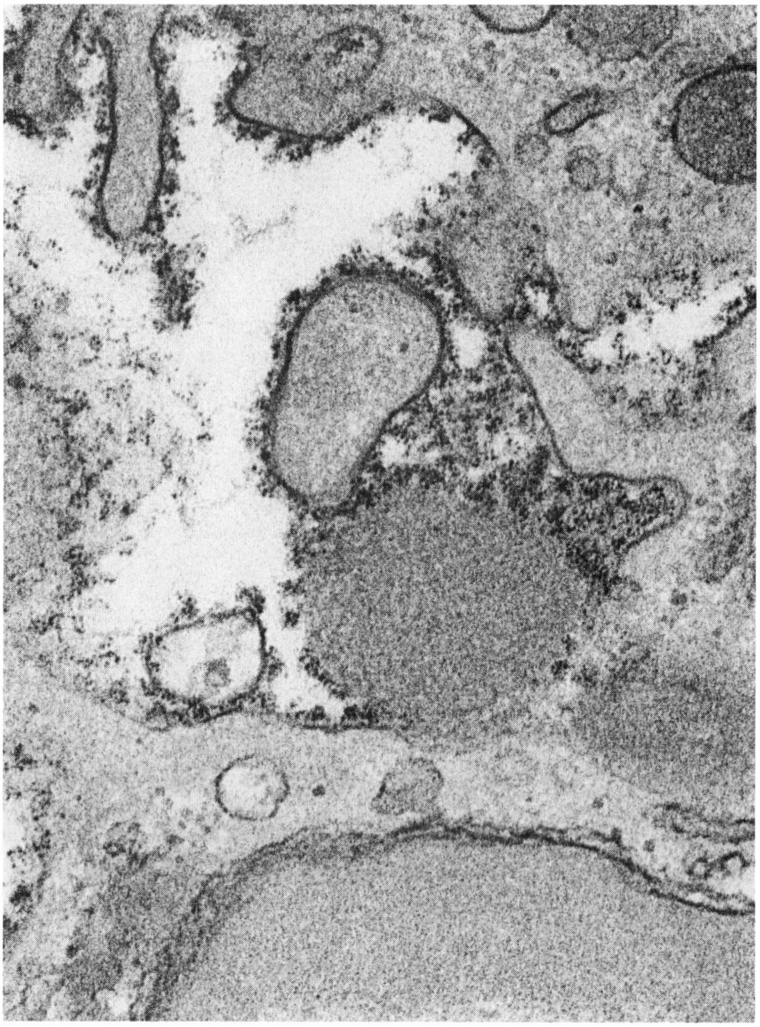

Figure 13 Human peripheral blood basophil exposed to C5 peptide(s) for 2 min shows extruded membrane-free granule, typical for AND. The granule surface and plasma membrane stain with cationized ferritin. ×74,000. (From Ref. 120, with permission.)

(Figure 16) (125). By contrast, skin mast cells of human origin primarily utilized granule extrusion and, less frequently, formed intracytoplasmic granule membrane fusions to produce degranulation chambers (126). The differences we noted between the primary anatomic mechanism(s) of AND in mast cells of lung or skin origin are only some of many differences between the mast cells of these two organs. For example, differences in the triggers that will produce mediator release, in the optimal temperature for release, in the kinetics of release, and in the protease contents have been described between mast cells of lung or skin origin in humans (130–137).

We have also found AND images in mast cells examined by electron microscopy of heart and ileal biopsies (127,128). In both cases, extrusion of granules to the cells' exte-

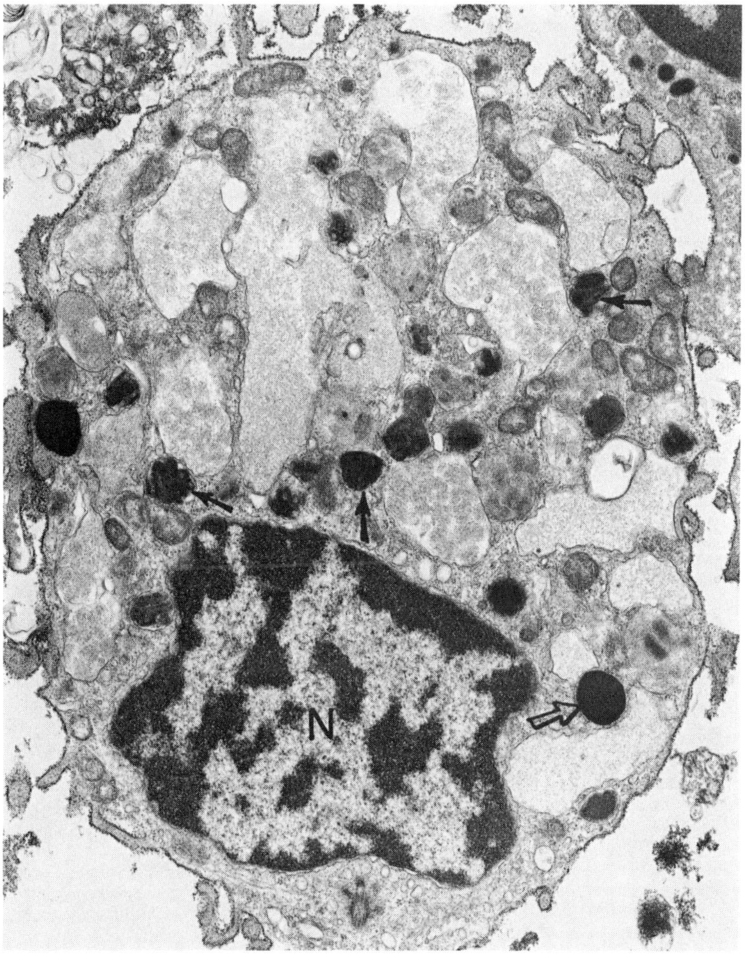

Figure 14 Isolated human lung mast cell 5 min after exposure to anti-IgE in vitro shows AND. Note numerous cytoplasmic degranuation channels filled with altered granule matrix material. Unaltered scroll granules remain (closed arrows), as do a few lipid bodies (open arrow). Cationized ferritin stains the cell surface but has not entered the degranulation channels, indiçating that these were not open to the exterior at the time of fixation. N = nucleus. ×14,000. (From Ref. 39, with permission.)

rior was noted (Figure 17), but intracytoplasmic degranulation chamber formation was also found in ileal mucosal mast cells (128). Others have studied the stimulated release of mast cells in situ using various triggers injected into normal skin or urticaria pigmentosa skin, prior to biopsy (138–143). In all such circumstances, and like our observations of isolated skin mast cells, AND was characterized by extrusion of granules through multiple membrane pores in skin mast cells stimulated in situ.

3. Guinea Pig Basophil

AND of guinea pig basophils is initially characterized by fusion of granule membranes, to form large cytoplasmic degranulation chambers, or sacs, within which insoluble

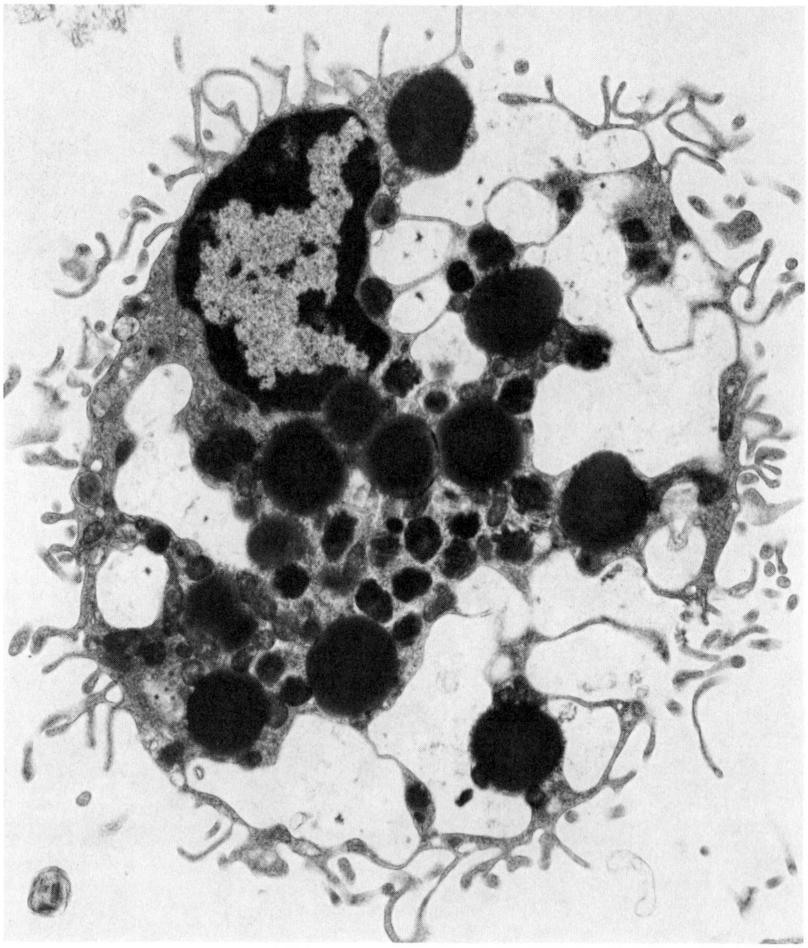

Figure 15 Isolated human lung mast cell 10 min after exposure to anti-IgE in vitro shows AND. Empty degranulation channels permeate the cytoplasm and open to the exterior. Small, unaltered scroll granules and large lipid bodies remain in the cytoplasm. ×7,500. (From Ref. 32, with permission.)

membrane-free granules reside. These granules are eventually released through a single membrane degranulation pore by extrusion (Figures 18 and 19). This process has been studied in vitro as well as in various in-situ circumstances, and all such studies are in agreement regarding the morphology of AND in basophils of this species (31, 39,68,117,144–154).

4. *Mouse Mast Cell*

Cloned and highly pure immature mast cells from normal or Beige mice undergo AND when sensitized and stimulated to do so by antigen (33,42,155,156). In these circumstances, AND is characterized by release of the heterogeneous contents of immature granules through multiple membrane pores (Figure 20); formation of intracytoplasmic degranulation chambers is not a characteristic feature of AND in immature

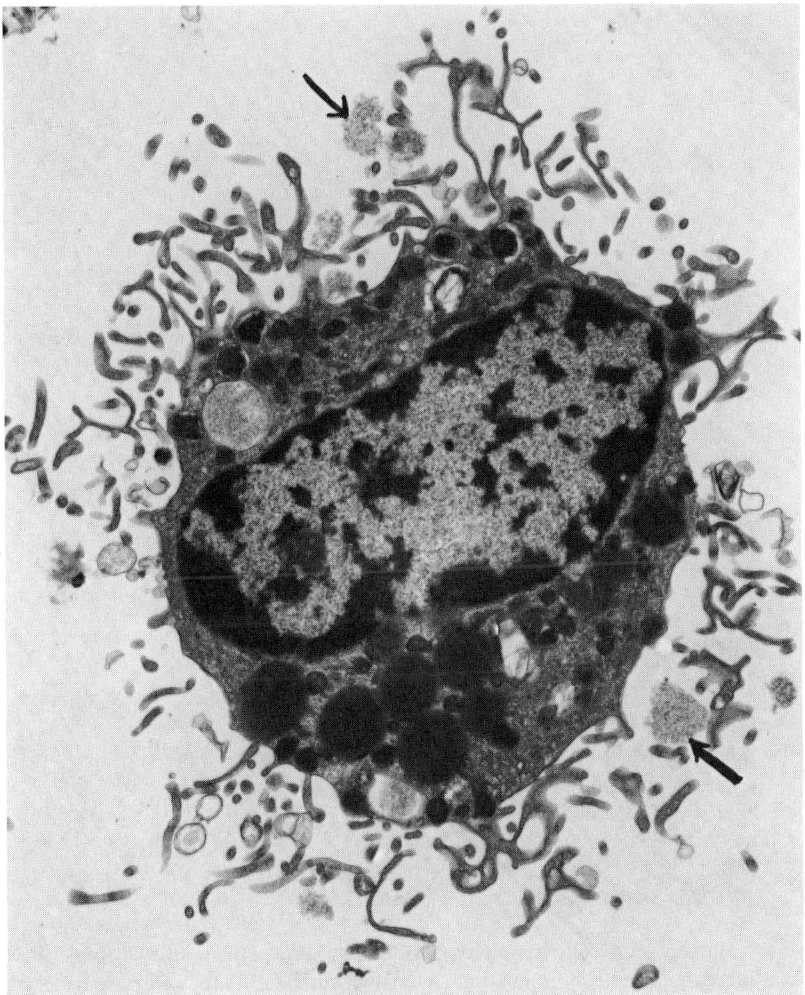

Figure 16 Isolated human lung mast cell 20 min after exposure to anti-IgE shows AND characterized by extrusion of membrane-free swollen granules (arrows) among markedly elongated and shed surface folds. ×10,000. (From Ref. 50, with permission.)

mouse mast cells in vitro. Similar studies have not yet been accomplished using mature cells in vitro. Mature mast cells challenged in vivo by IgE-mediated mechanisms show intracytoplasmic degranulation channels and alteration of granules within these chambers, as well as extrusion of granules to the extracellular domain through multiple pores in the plasma membrane (157).

5. Rat Mast Cells

The rat mast cell has been the prototype cell used for ultrastructural studies of AND (158–160, and reviewed in 33). All such studies are essentially in agreement—i.e., that extrusion of individual membrane-free granules through multiple membrane pores and the formation of multiple intracytoplasmic degranulation chambers both characterize AND in mature rat peritoneal mast cells. While these studies can be done within the

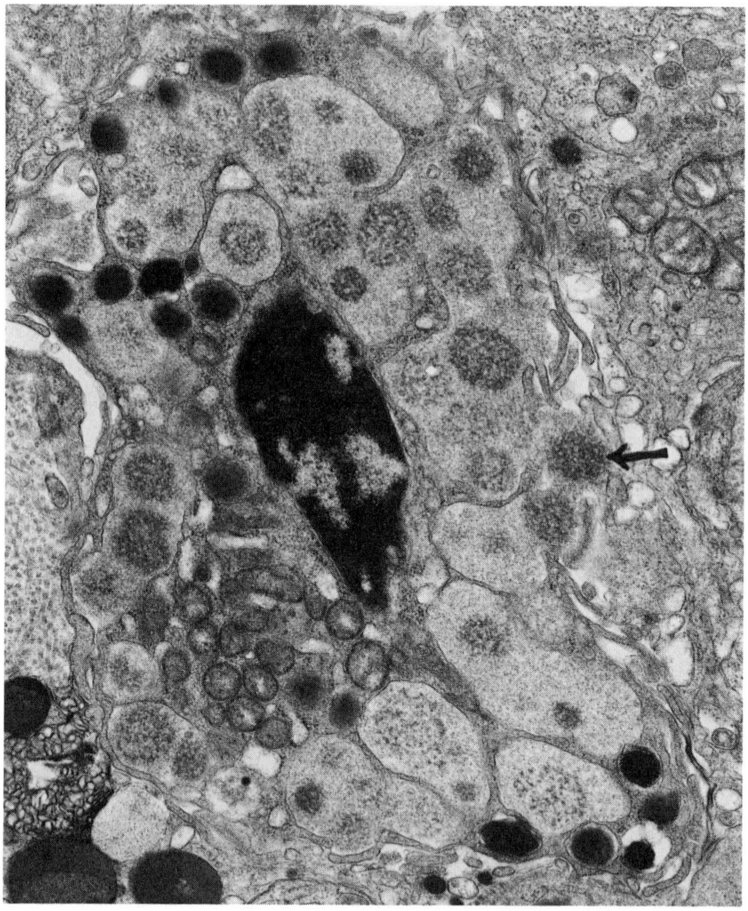

Figure 17 Human mast cell in an ileostomy biopsy of a patient with Crohn's disease shows AND. Note intracytoplasmic degranulation channels formed by fusion of granule membranes that contain altered, swollen granule matrix material. Some altered, membrane-free granules have been extruded to the exterior through openings in the plasma membrane (arrow). Some unaltered, dense cytoplasmic granules remain. ×27,000. (From Ref. 128 with permission.)

peritoneal cavity, most have been generally done in vitro. (Similar studies of rat mast cells in situ or ex vivo, using cells from other sites, are not available.)

In summary, AND in basophils and mast cells in these circumstances is characterized by either extrusion of granules, formation of intracytoplasmic degranulation chambers, or a combination of both. What determines the regulation of these various morphologies in individual cells from various organs in individual species ex vivo or in situ is entirely unknown.

B. Recovery from Anaphylactic Degranulation

The recovery of basophils and mast cells from AND has been studied in basophils of guinea pigs and mast cells in three species: human, mouse, and rat (Table 4; reviewed in Ref. 33). These recovery reactions have been studied in vitro in guinea pig basophils

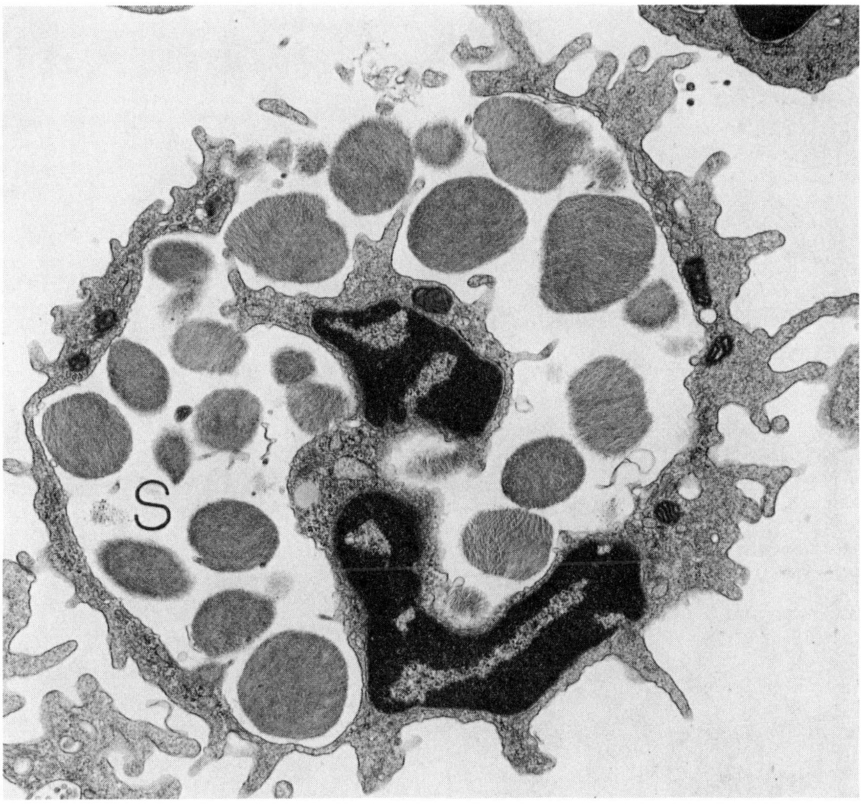

Figure 18 Guinea pig basophil 20 min after antigen shows AND characterized by a large cytoplasmic degranulation sac (S) containing membrane-free granules. The degranulation sac is open widely to the exterior through one degranulation pore. ×10,000. (From Ref. 68, with permission.)

(149,151,152), human and mouse mast cells (16,33,161–164; Dvorak AM and Galli SJ, unpublished data), and in mast cells either in rat peritoneal cavities or in vitro (158,165–176). In all of these circumstances, synthesis of new granules associated with the expansion of synthetic organelles—i.e., Golgi apparatus and membrane-free or membrane-bound ribosomes—was noted (Figures 21–23). This response was more prevalent following AND characterized by granule extrusion events, regardless of the trigger or cell. When AND is characterized by the formation of degranulation chambers within the cytoplasm, two resolution possibilities are apparent. For example, these chambers can open to the exterior and resolve by flow of membrane from chamber to external plasma membrane, or they can seal and partition to form new containers within which granule structures recondense and crystallize (Figures 24–27).

We have studied the recovery process extensively in isolated human lung mast cells stimulated to undergo AND by anti-IgE (16,33,161–164). In total, these studies have provided considerable details of the morphologic recovery events of which these cells are capable. For example, we noted variable perturbation of lung mast cells during isolation procedures, as compared to lung mast cells in situ not exposed to isolation pro-

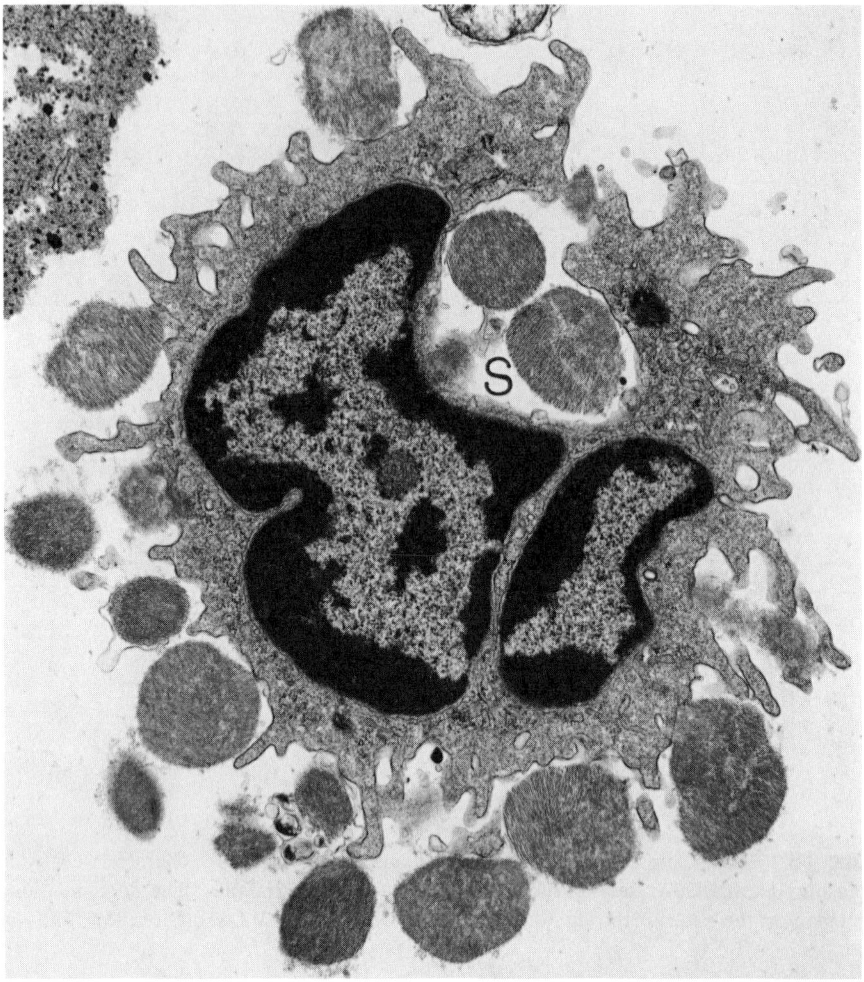

Figure 19 Guinea pig basophil 20 min after lectin (concanavalin A) shows AND characterized by nearly complete resolution of the small degranulation sac (S) and numerous extruded, membrane-free granules associated with the cell surface. ×10,000.

cedures (17,125,164). These changes did not affect all cells, nor were all granules perturbed. The changes included granule swelling and granule matrix alterations in the absence of granule-plasma membrane fusions and in the absence of morphological criteria for cell injury. When such perturbed cells are placed in culture media overnight, all granule swelling and matrix alterations are replaced by normal condensed granule patterns indicating complete reversibility (125,164). Similarly, some recovering mast cells with intracytoplasmic degranulation chambers re-formed cytoplasmic granules by reversal of chamber formation (Figures 24–27) (161). That is, membrane partitions compartmentalized the condensing, crystallizing granule domains. Recovery from AND, characterized by extrusion of degranulation chamber contents and the chamber itself, was characterized by expansion of plasma membrane folds followed by shedding

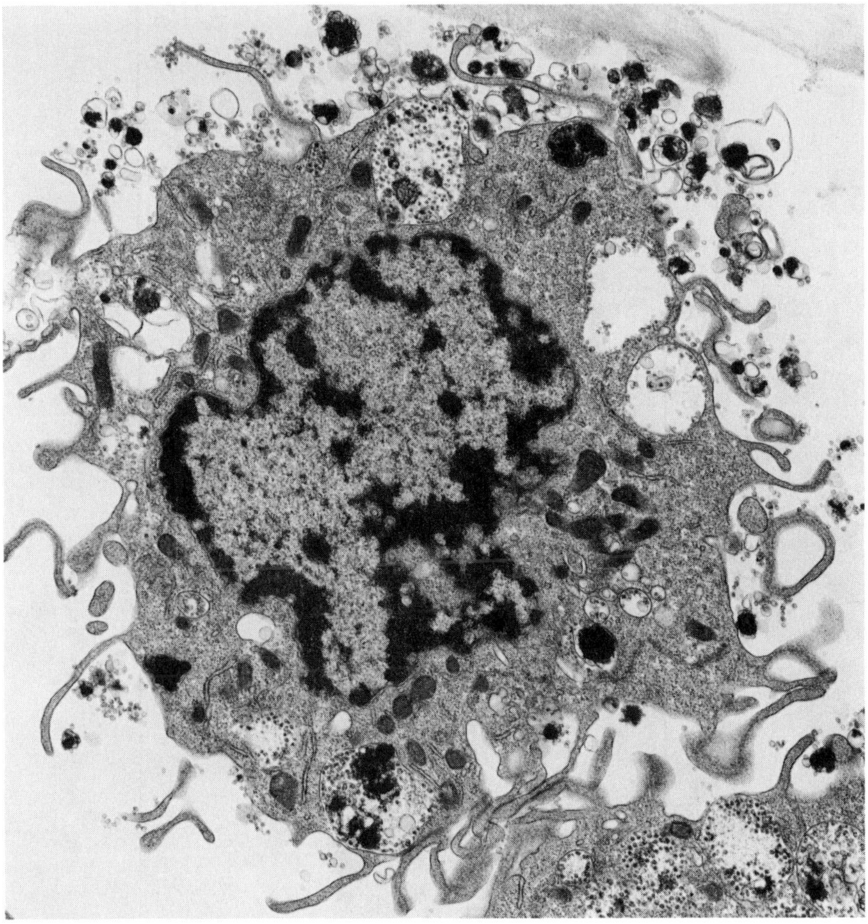

Figure 20 Cultured, immature, mouse bone marrow mast cell stimulated with antigen after sensitization shows AND characterized by extrusion of dense and vesicular contents of immature granules at numerous points in the cell membrane. ×12,000. (From Ref. 42, with permission.)

or internalization of plasma membrane and surface processes and synthesis of new granules (Figure 28) (162,163). Thus, in human mast cells recovering from AND, a mixture of conservation and synthesis mechanisms prevails (33,164).

V. ROLE OF BASOPHILS AND MAST CELLS IN CELL-MEDIATED DISEASE

Cell-mediated immunity, or delayed hypersensitivity, classically is a category of disease which can be transferred by cells (lymphocytes) but not serum, whereas immediate hypersensitivity is transferred by serum (177–180). Cell-mediated immunity has been implicated (or suggested) as a mechanism for disease in a large number of disorders. In 1970, we described a distinct category of cell-mediated hypersensitivity, characterized by large numbers of basophilic leukocytes in appropriately sensitized and challenged

Table 4 Ultrastructure of Basophils and Mast Cells Recovering from Anaphylactic Degranulation

Species	Cell	Trigger	Structural events
Guinea pig	Basophil (33,149,151,152)	Antigen, lectin	1. Closure of degranulation sacs 2. Expansion of secretory organelles, Golgi and rough endoplasmic reticulum 3. Synthesis of new granules
Human	Mast cell (16,33,161–164)	Anti-IgE	1. Condensation, crystallization, and partitioning of cytoplasmic degranulation chambers 2. Expansion of Golgi and free polysomes 3. Synthesis of new granules
Rat	Mast cell (33,158,165–176)	Multiple	1. Closure of degranulation chambers 2. Expansion of synthetic structures 3. Synthesis of new granules
Mouse	Mouse cell (Dvorak AM and Galli SJ, unpublished data)	Multiple	1. Expansion of Golgi, membrane-bound, and free ribosomes 2. Synthesis of new granules

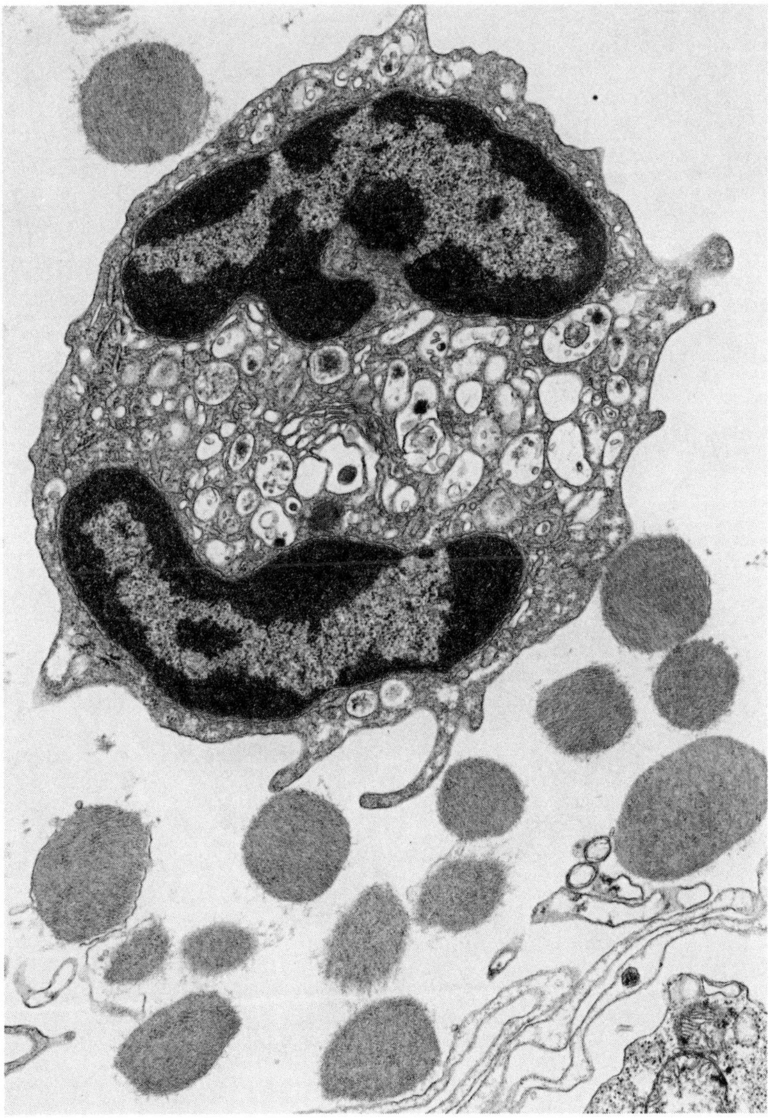

Figure 21 Guinea pig basophil recovered 5 h after stimulation with antigen shows markedly expanded Golgi area where immature granules with a mixture of vesicles and dense materials are being produced. Note large number of extruded, membrane-free granules nearby. ×18,000. (From Ref. 33 with permission.)

skin test sites in guinea pigs. We called this category of cell-mediated hypersensitivity "cutaneous basophil hypersensitivity" (CBH) to delineate the presence of blood basophils in the reactions (181). Subsequently, basophil-rich, cell-mediated reactions were found in multiple species and circumstances (Table 1).

The presence of basophils which migrated from the blood vascular space into tissues in CBH alerted us to the possibility that basophils might be functionally active in these sites by secreting stored mediators of inflammation. Histamine values are increased in

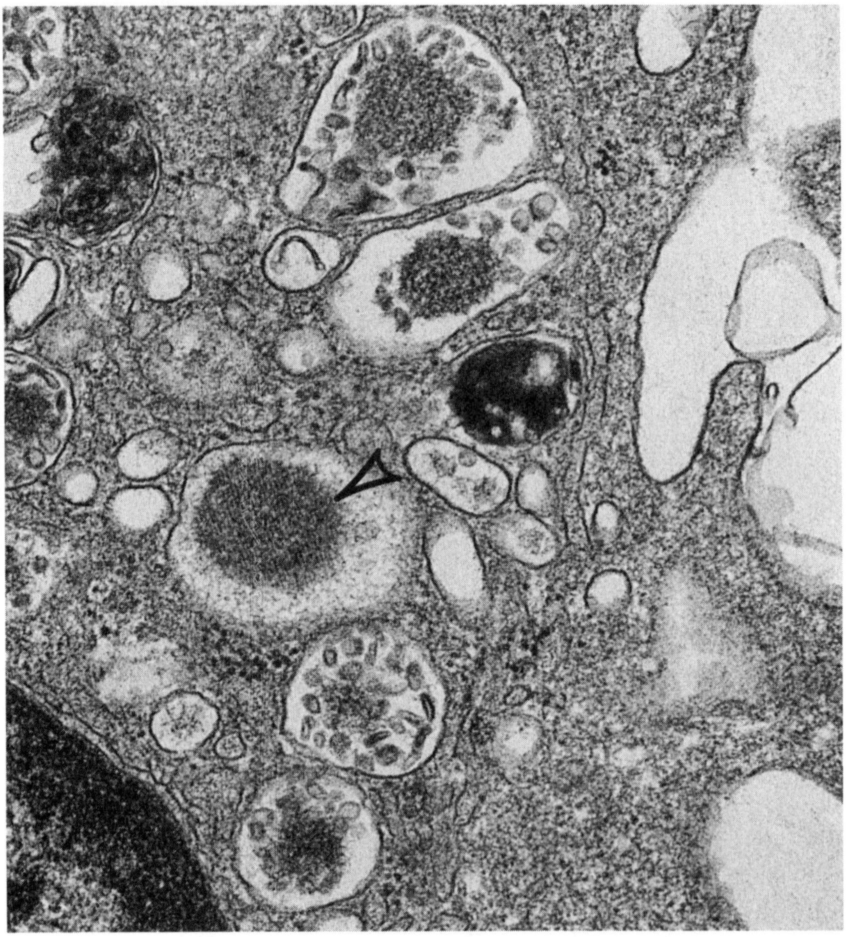

Figure 22 Guinea pig basophil recovered 24 h after antigen shows a cluster of five immature granules containing a mixture of vesicles and dense material. One of these shows a characteristic parallel array centrally (arrowhead). ×42,000. (From Ref. 149, with permission.)

skin biopsies of CBH reactions. This reflects increased numbers of histamine-containing cells over controls (182). It has not been possible to determine by biochemical means whether release of histamine by tissue basophils (or mast cells) has occurred in situ. Anatomic studies, by contrast, have been useful to determine the possibility that in-situ release from tissue basophils and mast cells has occurred (reviewed in Ref. 33). For example, we initially noted a uniquely rich complement of small (100- to 150-nm) smooth vesicles in the cytoplasm of guinea pig bone marrow and peripheral blood basophils in situ (Figure 2a) (31,183). These structures suggested the possibility that basophils were engaged in endocytosis and perhaps secretion, using these vesicles as transport vehicles. Initially, we demonstrated the uptake function of these structures using an intravenous tracer, horseradish peroxidase, which is rendered electron-dense by a cytochemical procedure (183). These studies clearly showed uptake and transport of

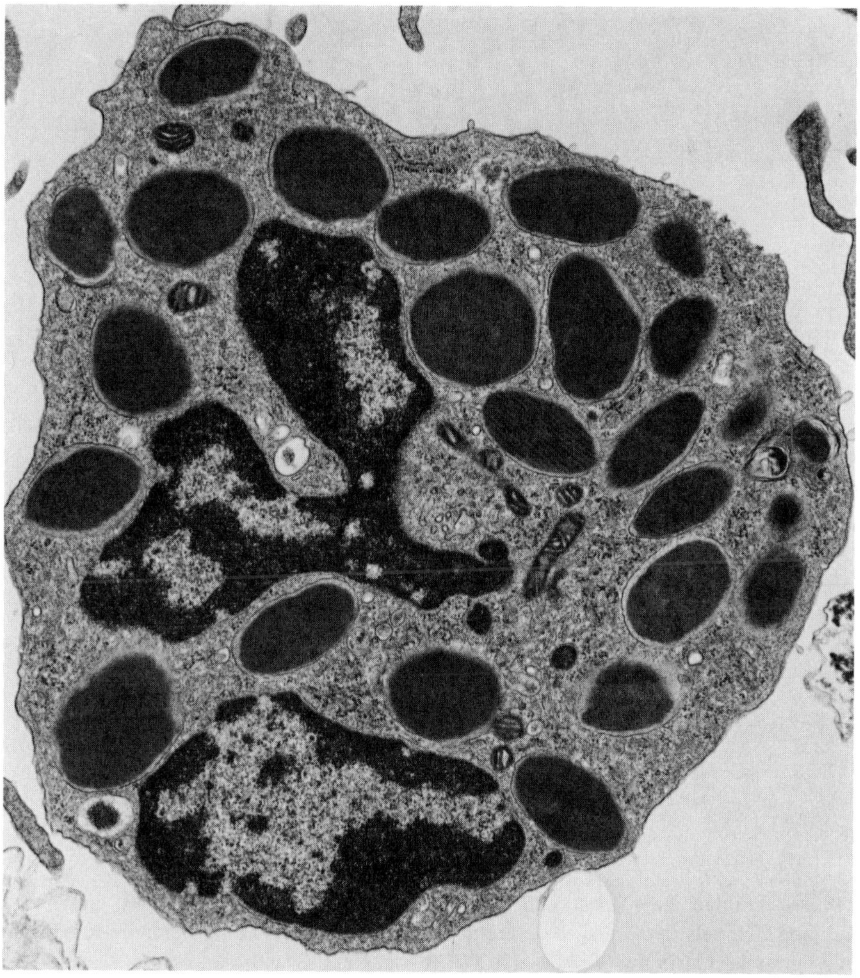

Figure 23 Guinea pig basophil recovered 11 h after antigen shows reconstitution of a full complement of mature granules. ×16,500. (From Ref. 33 with permission.)

this protein to granules in vivo (Figures 29 and 30). Subsequently, using purified guinea pig basophils in vitro and washing experiments, we were able to show transport of horseradish peroxidase in vesicles in the reverse direction, such as cellular secretion might utilize in certain circumstances (Figure 31) (184). These studies of vesicular transport were extended to include uptake and transport to granules of exogenous eosinophil peroxidase by guinea pig basophils (Figures 32 and 33) and mouse mast cells in vitro (Figure 34), thereby documenting a role for vesicular transport of a biologically important protein released in eosinophil-rich inflammatory reactions and extending this uptake mechanism to mast cells (33,185).

We next examined tissue reactions to a number of stimuli by electron microscopy in several species. Initially, we noted a process, which we termed piecemeal degranulation (PMD), in guinea pig basophils infiltrating subcutaneous growths of experimentally

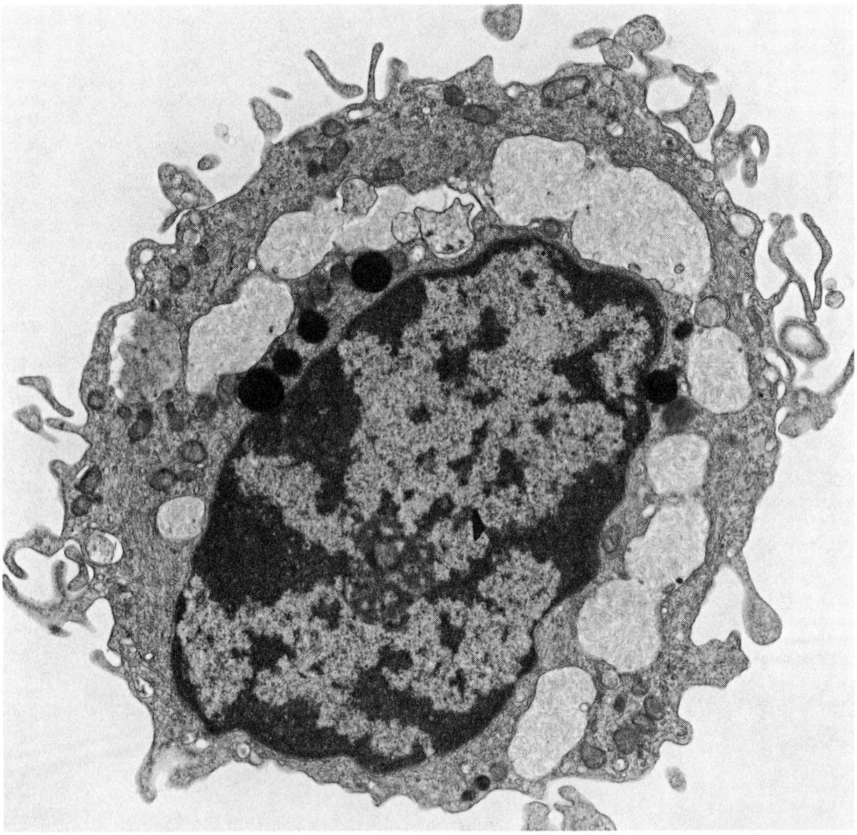

Figure 24 Human lung mast cell recovered 6 h after anti-IgE shows conservation of degranulation channels. Note that these are now partially partitioned into granule-sized containers containing granule matrix materials. ×12,000. (From Ref. 33 with permission.)

implanted tumors of bile duct origin and in basophils migrating into the peritoneal ascites fluid containing similar tumors (186,187). A similar event was present in basophils infiltrating virus-induced fibrosarcomas in guinea pig skin (Dvorak AM and Galli SJ, unpublished data). Light microscopy and electron microscopy of plastic sections revealed decreased granule contents in the absence of granule fusions. This was illustrated by focal losses and by emptying of entire individual granules. Smooth vesicles were found attached to granules. These were either filled with dense material or were apparently empty.

Identical findings were observed in basophils entering skin lesions of contact allergy in humans (18,30,49,188,189). In this instance, quantitation of sequential biopsies by light microscopy after specific stimuli clearly showed the time dependence of PMD. That is, the number of basophils showing granule losses increased to peak levels at 3 days poststimulus (Figure 35). Over this time course, electron microscopic studies showed progressive losses of granule particles, budding of particle-filled vesicles from granules, and progressive increases in empty granule containers (Figure 36). PMD

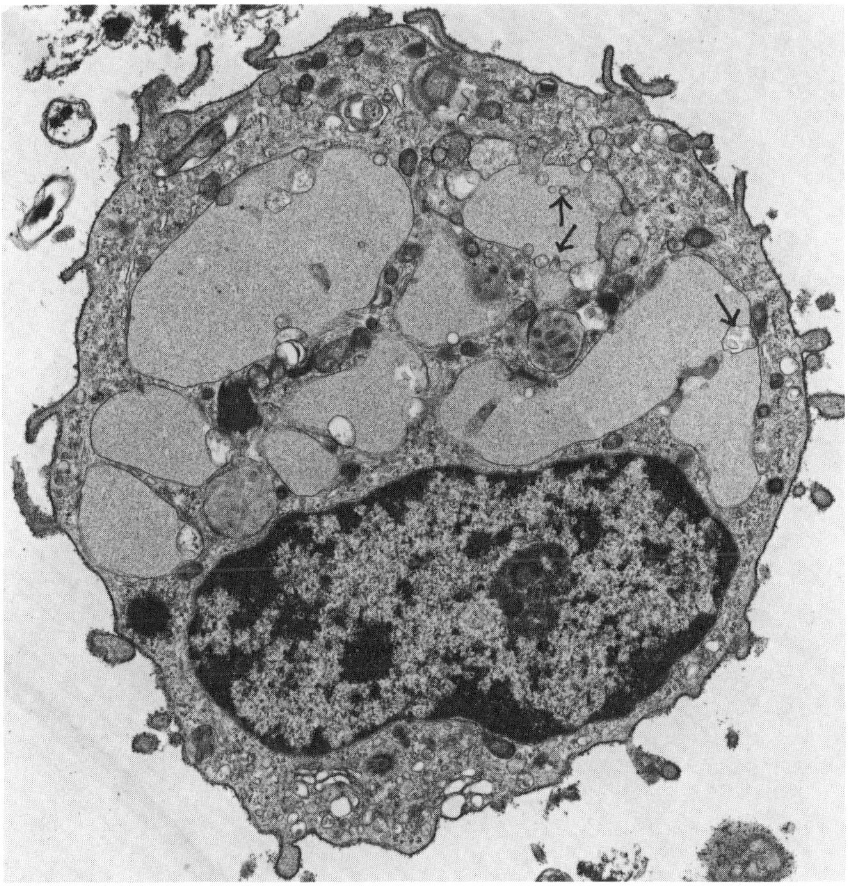

Figure 25 Human lung mast cell recovered 24 h after anti-IgE shows partitioning channels with more concentrated contents than in Figure 24. These channels contain numerous vesicles (arrows) and crystallization foci. Golgi area expansion is present, and the immature nucleus contains a large nucleolus. ×11,000. (From Ref. 50, with permission.)

characteristically occurs over a long time (~days relative to losses stimulated by IgE ~minutes), and empty granule chambers do not fuse and are not externalized. Subsequently, we have identified PMD of basophils and mast cells in vivo in a wide variety of human diseases and in experimental models of several species (Table 5). In humans, the diseases include chronic glomerulonephritis and pyelonephritis (190), delayed hypersensitivity to microbial antigens (18,49,189), allergic contact dermatitis (Figure 36) (18,49,189), basophil leukemia (191), allograft rejection (192), Crohn's disease (Figure 37a) (16,26,27,58,128,193–198), ulcerative colitis (Dvorak AM, unpublished data), melanoma (199), peritoneal dialysis fluid (51), bullous pemphigoid (Figure 37b) (28,62), renal cell adenoma (200), gastric lymphoma (16,32,33,50), lung adenocarcinoma (Figure 38) (16,32,33,50), metastatic adenocarcinoma (16,32,33,50), interstitial fibrosis of the lung (Dvorak AM, unpublished data), Whipple's disease (194), and Sézary's syndrome (Dvorak AM, unpublished data). This response pattern, viz., PMD,

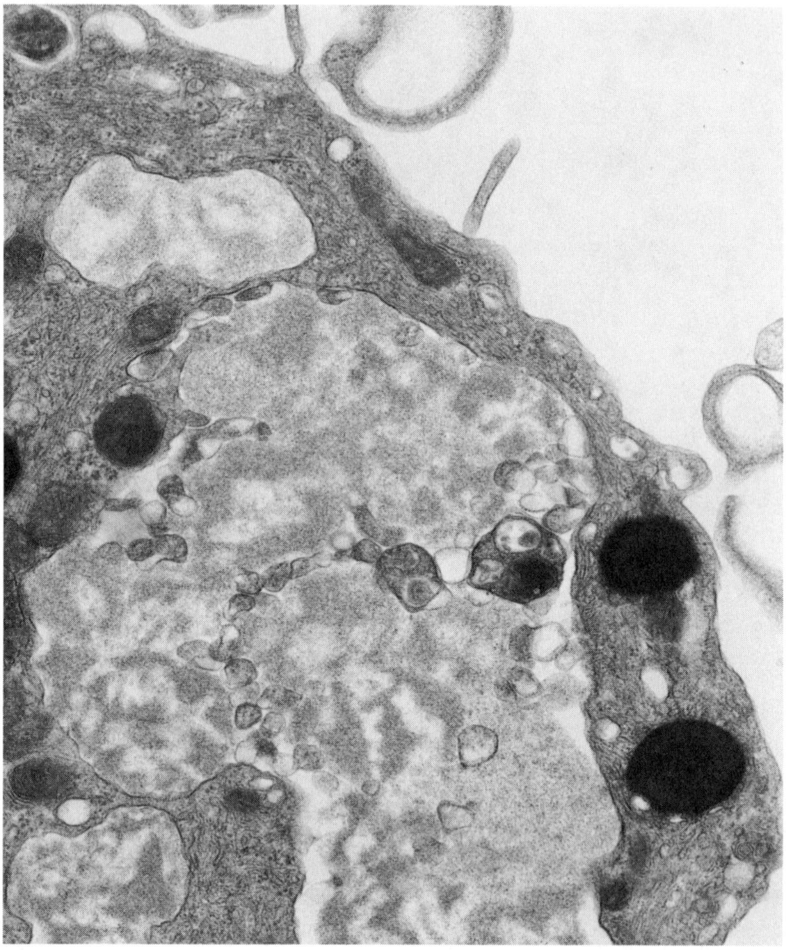

Figure 26 Human lung mast cell recovered 6 h after anti-IgE shows recovering channels at higher magnification. Note strings of vesicles bridging the interior of channels in approximate sizes of granule domains and focally condensed contents. Two lipid bodies enmeshed in intermediate filaments are nearby. ×33,000. (From Ref. 33 with permission.)

clearly represents the most frequently encountered functional event discernible by morphologic analysis of basophils and mast cells in pathologic lesions (reviewed in Ref. 33).

Several experimental models have also recently been useful in establishing the potential relevance of PMD as a mechanism for release of granule contents from basophils and mast cells. Human unbilical cord blood mononuclear cells cultured in growth factor-containing media (44,118) or in rhIL-3 (59) develop into basophilic leukocytes in large numbers. We have identified PMD in mature basophils produced in this fashion (Figure 39) (59). We have also identified the uptake of eosinophil peroxidase in basophil vesicles with subsequent transport to granules for storage (Figures 40 and 41) (44). The morphologic evidence for PMD is present in basophils stimulated to develop in

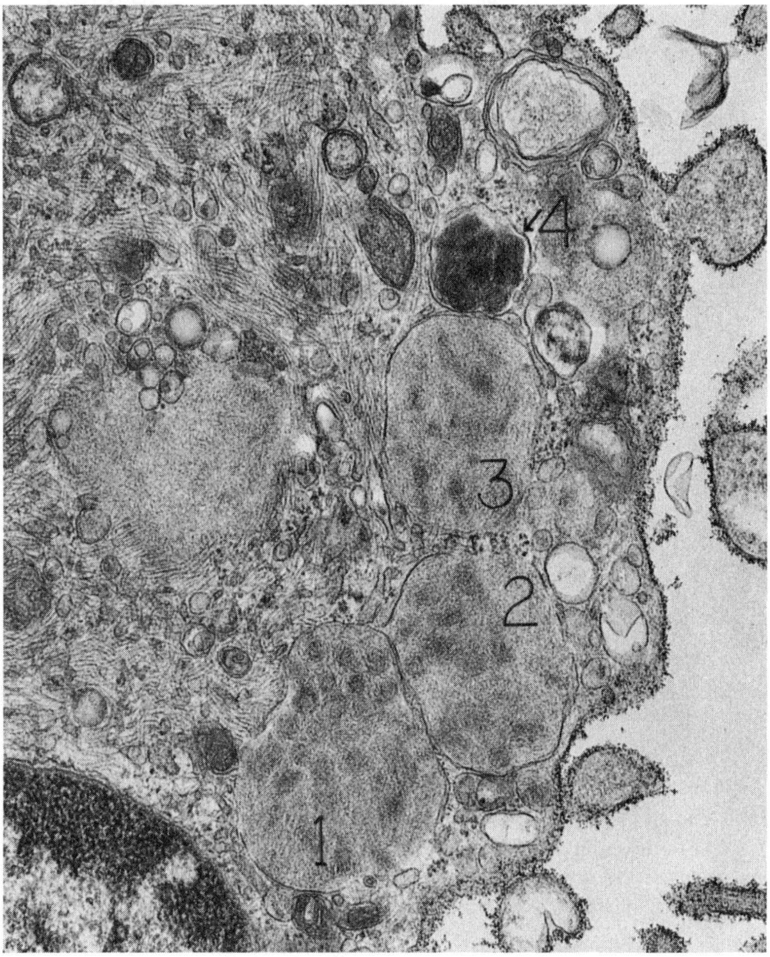

Figure 27 Human lung mast cell recovered 12 h after anti-IgE shows recovering degranulation channel-granules at higher magnification. Note that granule domains are now separated by membranes and contain scroll foci that become more dense as granules diminish in size. Compare granule 1 with granule 4. ×28,000. (From Ref. 33 with permission.)

vivo in large numbers during intravenous infusion of rhIL-3 in monkeys (Figure 42) (88); and both mast cells (Figure 43) and basophils (Figure 44) show extensive granule content losses typical for PMD in rabbit corneal pockets containing experimentally placed fibroblast tumors (Dvorak AM, unpublished data). Thus, PMD is a prevalent event in many biologically important circumstances, some of which may be directly or indirectly related to cytokines such as interleukin-3.

We are certain that the empty granules which characterize PMD do not result from artifactual solubilization of basophil and mast cell granule contents in processing fluids, as was claimed in certain older ultrastructural literature (reviewed in 32,33), for several important reasons. These are that (a) individual cells in the same section often show adjacent, partially empty, empty, and full granules (Figures 36a and 37), and (b) cells

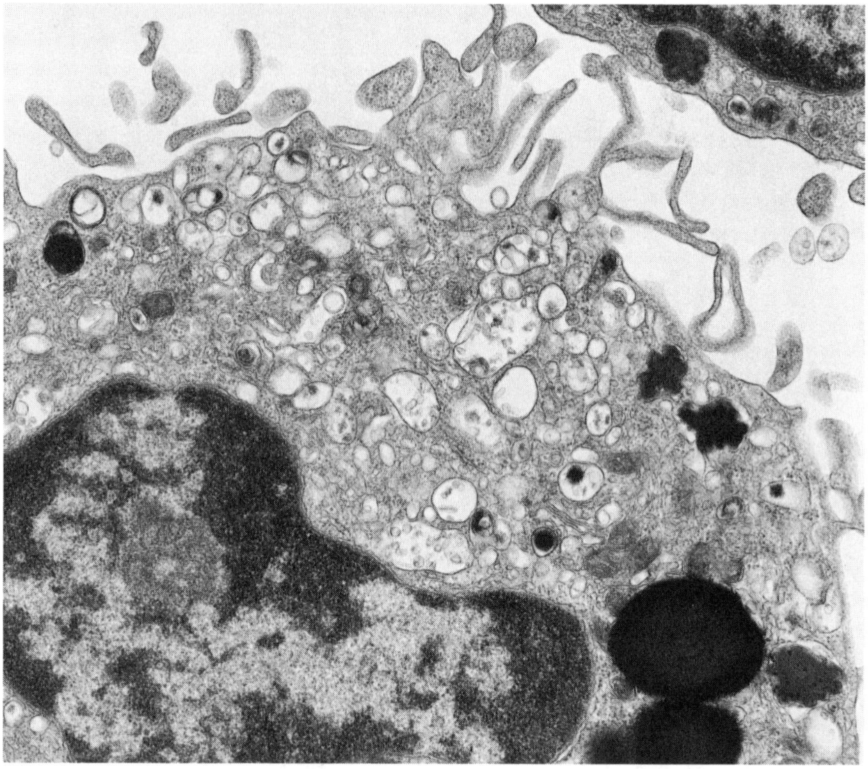

Figure 28 Human lung mast cell recovered 24 h after anti-IgE shows large numbers of Golgi area vesicles and vacuoles involved in synthesis of new granules. Some contain dense material; most contain vesicles; a few with scrolls are present in the more peripheral areas. The nucleus has a large nucleolus. Several large lipid bodies are also seen. ×18,500. (From Ref. 33 with permission.)

that extrude membrane-free granules when stimulated to undergo AND in vitro often have these granules attached to their surface. While such granule contents may be altered in appearance, they are identifiable and do not immediately solubilize in processing fluids, regardless of their more exposed position (Figures 12, 13, 16, 17, and 19–21).

Since mast cells and basophils undergo recovery following AND, it seems reasonable that they might also recover from granule losses sustained during PMD, where empty granule containers are not extruded from cells. We have recently found images that are consistent with refilling of empty containers in human mast cells during wound healing in vivo (62). In this circumstance, re-excision of a previously operated site for removal of melanoma provided material to examine wound healing in the aftermath of a skin tumor in which PMD of mast cells has been shown to occur (199). This tissue reaction contained large numbers of synthetic fibroblasts, angiogenesis, and mast cells, but no residual tumor. Nearly all mast cells showed increased focal densities of unusual as well as typical granule content configurations within granule containers (62). We also noted similar granule content increases in some human skin allograft basophils in a

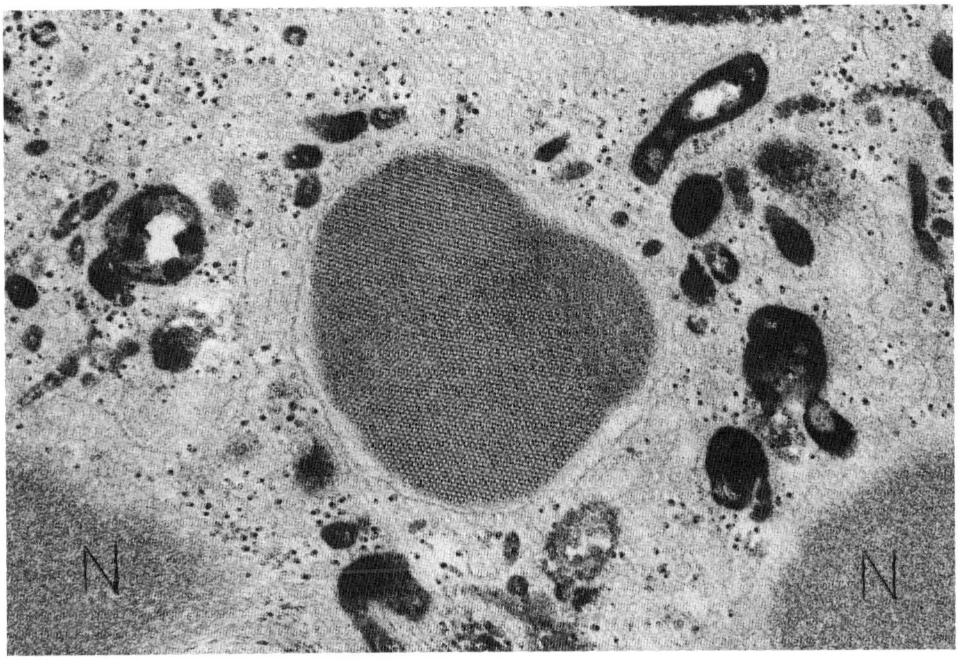

Figure 29 Guinea pig basophil, incubated in vitro in 10 mg of horseradish peroxidase (HRP) and prepared with a cytochemical procedure to demonstrate this enzyme, shows numerous endocytotic tubules and vesicles filled with HRP adjacent to a negative granule. Note that this granule displays a hexagonal array. N = nucleus. ×48,000. (From Ref. 33 with permission.)

study done some years ago (Figure 45) (Dvorak AM, unpublished data). In both circumstances, we believe the best interpretation of such visual evidence is that previously emptied containers are recovering their dense contents in wound healing. The actual mechanism of such recovery is not known. Two possibilities exist—i.e., Golgi-derived synthetic vesicles filled with dense materials could refill empty granules, or uptake and transport of extracellular dense materials by vesicles could refill empty granules.

VI. SECRETION: AN ESSENTIAL PHYSIOLOGICAL PROCESS THAT MAY BE UP-REGULATED IN BASOPHILS AND MAST CELLS IN DISEASE

It is clear that basophils and mast cells have a role in mediating immediate hypersensitivity reactions or allergic diseases. It also seems clear that PMD of basophils and mast cells may provide materials important to the onset, sustenance, or healing of a wide variety of disorders collectively involved with cell-mediated immunity. It is not clear, however, what role(s) these cells have in normal physiology, i.e., in health.

Secretion biologists categorize release mechanics from the various secreting cells in the body (the normal functions for most of which are known) as regulated or constitutive (201–205). Regulated secretion, put simply, means an episodic, triggered release of stored cellular synthetic products; constitutive secretion means a continuous flow of synthetic cellular products. Regulated secretion utilizes classic exocytosis of membrane-free granules; constitutive secretion occurs by vesicular transport. Anaphylactic

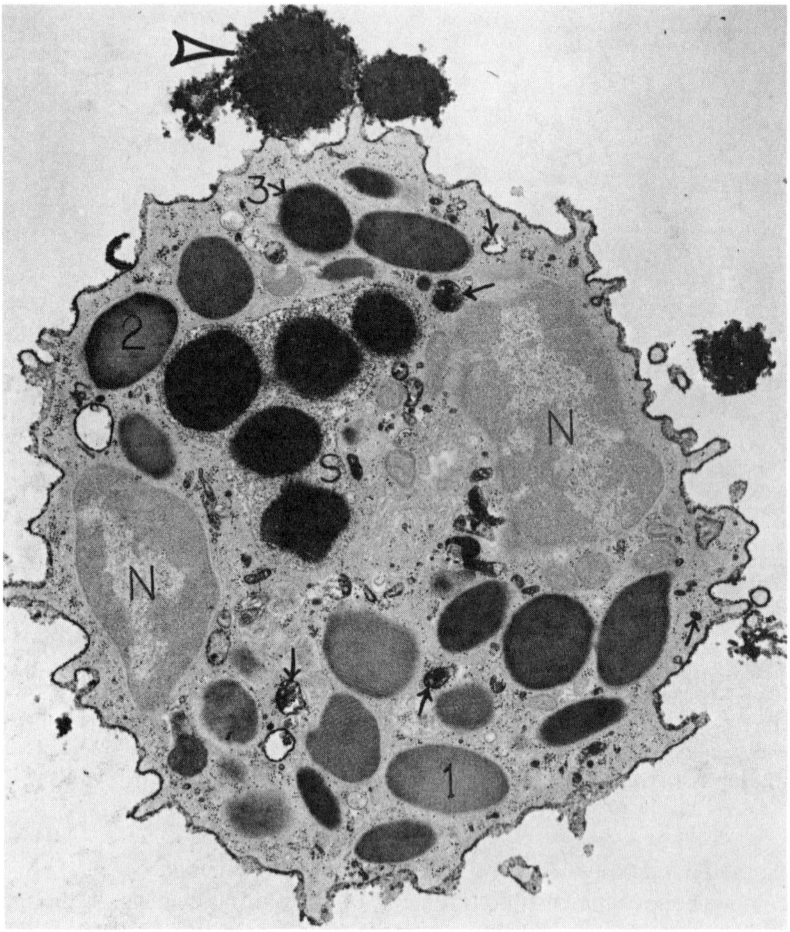

Figure 30 Guinea pig basophil incubated in vitro in 10 mg of HRP for 30 min. Reaction product fills a degranulation sac (S) and binds to the membrane-free granules within, indicating that these granules, like those extruded to the exterior (arrowhead), are in open continuity with the extracellular space. Numerous peroxidase-positive endocytotic vesicles fill the cytoplasm (arrows). Cytoplasmic granules are either completely negative (1), partially positive (2), or completely positive (3). N = nucleus. ×11,500. (From Ref. 33 with permission.)

degranulation of basophils and mast cells, then, is an example of regulated secretion; piecemeal degranulation of basophils and mast cells is similar to, and perhaps an example of, up-regulated constitutive secretion.

In 1975, we proposed a general model of basophil degranulation (Figure 46), based on our studies of guinea pig and human basophils, to account for the varied rates of granule substance release occurring under a variety of physiological and pathological circumstances (3,33). The model (3) holds that PMD occurs by means of exocytotic vesicles which bud from the granule membrane, carrying with them small quanta of intact or dissolved granule material, and which flow to the cell surface where they fuse with the plasma membrane and discharge their contents into the extracellular space.

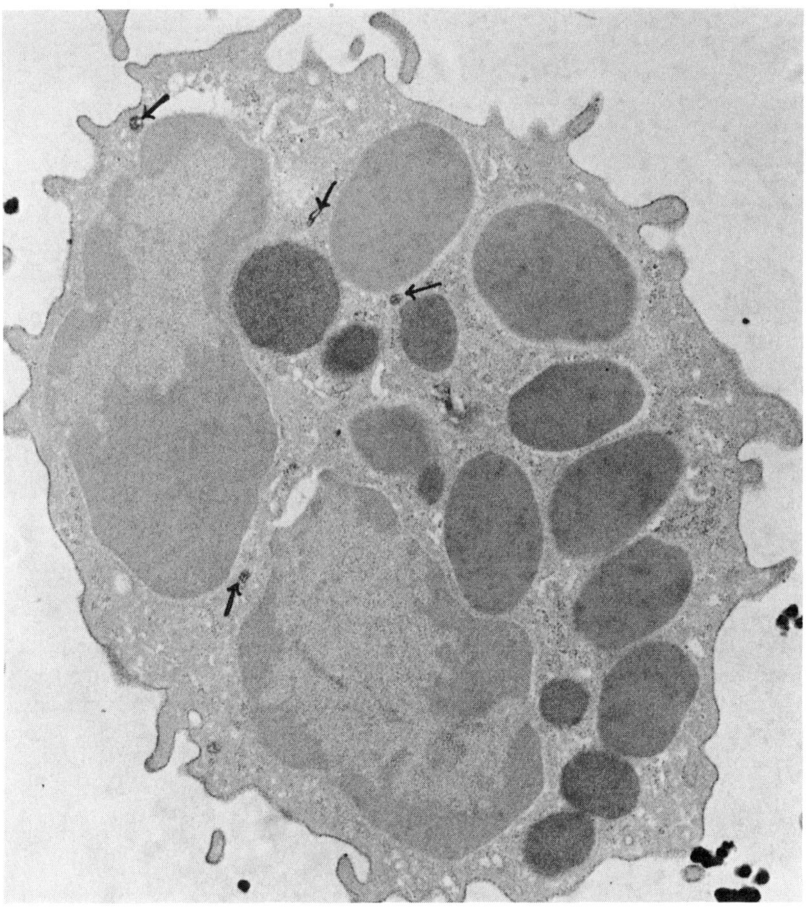

Figure 31 Guinea pig basophil, incubated for 30 min in 10 mg of HRP followed by a 10-min washout period in the presence of a nondegranulating dose of the lectin, concanavalin A (0.1 μg), shows essentially peroxidase-negative granules in the cytoplasm. A few positive exocytotic vesicles in the cytoplasm are still visible (arrows). ×18,000.

The glycogen aggregates closely associated with granules at sites of vesicle attachment may afford an energy supply for vesicle budding. Once separation of vesicles from the granule membrane is complete, transport of vesicles may proceed at random. A net flux of granule contents out of the cell will result from random vesicle movement if, for reasons of chemical structure, vesicles are able to fuse only with each other and with the membranes of other granules and the plasma membrane but not with the membranes limiting other cellular organelles.

It is useful to postulate a closely coupled transport of endocytotic (pinocytotic) vesicles migrating from the cell surface to the cytoplasmic granules associated with vesicular exocytosis. Coupled endocytosis is necessary to account for the undiminished (actually, slightly increased) size of granules which are releasing their contents and hence are continuously losing portions of their enveloping membranes. An imbalance in the

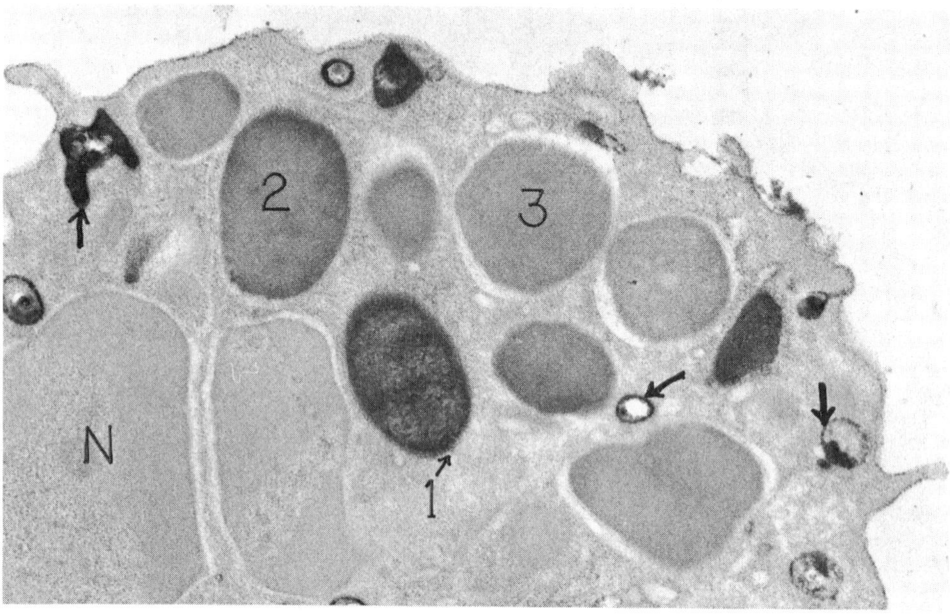

Figure 32 Guinea pig basophil incubated for 30 min in eosinophil peroxidase shows enzyme-positive cytoplasmic endocytotic vesicles and tubules (arrows), one completely positive granule (1), several partially positive granules (2), and completely negative granules (3). N = nucleus. ×19,000.

amount of vesicular traffic would result in changes in granule size. For example, excess efflux would produce smaller granules, and excess influx would produce larger granules. We have recently identified such a circumstance in f-Met peptide-stimulated human basophils in vitro (see later) (122). The extracellular fluid transported to the granules by endocytotic vesicles may provide solvent for the partial dissolution of granules regularly observed, for example, in the basophils infiltrating the reactions of allergic contact dermatitis (49). Conceivably, the extra membranes accumulating within these basophil granules may be derived from those of the endocytotic vesicles, also indicating an imbalance between vesicular influx and efflux. In our vesicular transport model, the release of granule contents ordinarily proceeds at a rate governed by the frequency of discharge of microvesicles from the granule membrane. The frequency of exocytosis possibly is determined by the rate of endocytosis which, in turn, may be controlled and modified by agents (antibodies, and probably other materials, such as cytokines, lymphokines, interleukins, bacterial peptides, etc.) acting at the cell surface.

Based on the occasional granule alterations observed in "normal" circulating basophils, it is likely that a slow release of granule substance occurs under physiological conditions. In delayed-type reactions, degranulation apparently proceeds at a substantially greater pace. At still faster rates of degranulation, a threshold would eventually be reached, above which there would be insufficient time between successive discharges to permit complete separation of individual vesicles from the plasma or granule membranes or from each other. Under these conditions, endocytotic and/or exocytotic vesicles budding from the plasma or granule membranes would not form discrete, spherical

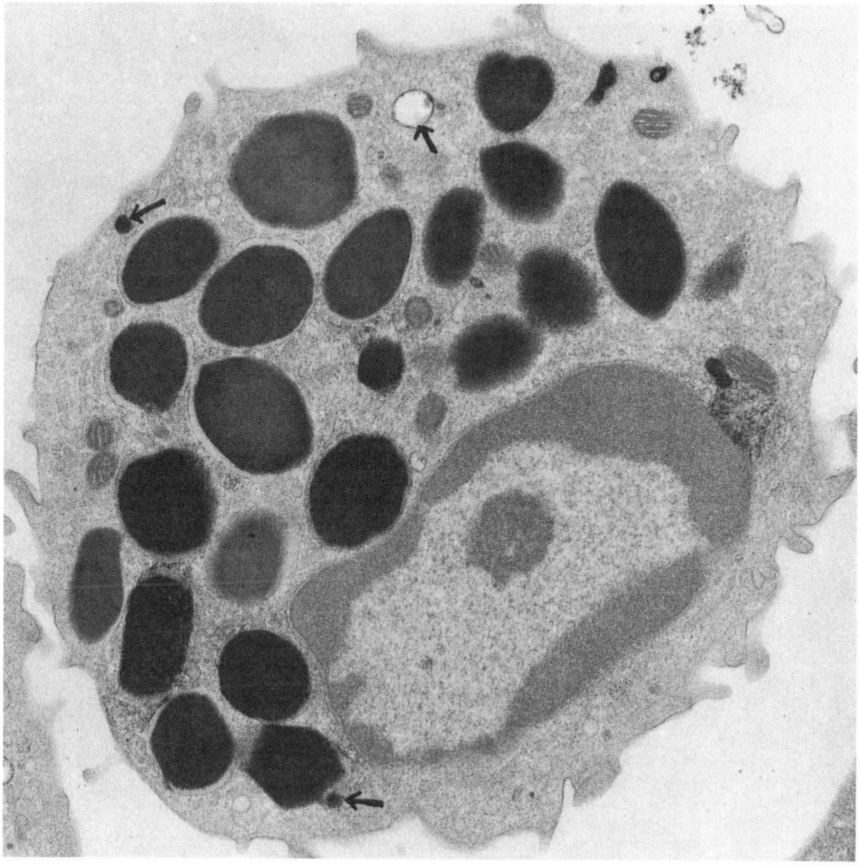

Figure 33 Guinea pig basophil incubated for 60 min in eosinophil peroxidase shows all cytoplasmic granules to be positive. A few cytoplasmic vesicles are also filled with eosinophil peroxidase (arrows). ×15,000.

structures; rather, they would coalesce to form continuous channels. In fact, segments of tubulovesicular structures are observed in basophils participating in allergic contact dermatitis or endocytosing horseradish peroxidase (HRP) (31). Better-developed channels might link the cell surface with granules and/or interconnect neighboring granules, depending on random collisions with either the plasma or granule membranes. Continuous channels of this sort would lead to fusion of granule membranes with each other and with the plasma membrane, characteristic features of AND.

In an ultrastructural kinetic analysis of human basophils stimulated to release histamine and leukotriene C_4 by the bacterial peptide, f-Met peptide, in vitro, we identified a morphologic continuum, predicted by this general degranulation model, where PMD → AND (122). Samples of basophils from normal donors were prepared for electron microscopy at 0, 10, 20, 30 s and 1, 2, 5, and 10 min poststimulation with f-Met peptide. We found that this bacterial peptide induced a unique sequence of morphologic events, which included morphologies that we have previously identified and termed

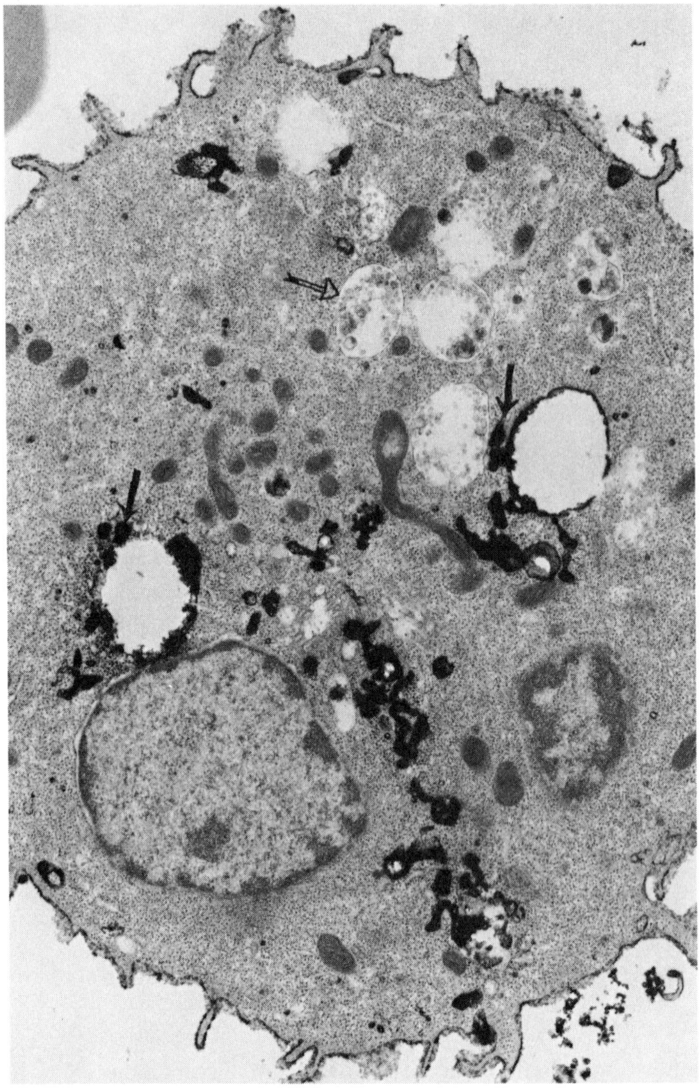

Figure 34 Immature mouse mast cell exposed to eosinophil peroxidase for 5 min shows extensive binding of enzyme to the plasma membrane and internalization in numerous tubules and vesicles. A number of positive vesicles have fused to peroxidase-containing immature granules (arrows). Other immature granules (open arrow) do not contain eosinophil peroxidase. ×16,000. (From Ref. 185, with permission.)

piecemeal degranulation in human basophils in situ, as well as those induced by IgE mechanisms ex vivo and termed anaphylactic degranulation. In addition to this degranulation continuum, we found that releasing granule chambers underwent extraordinary increases in size as their contents solubilized and prior to their resolution by extrusion. The enlarging granule chambers accumulated numerous concentric dense membranes, vesicles, and Charcot-Leyden crystals, and decreased granule particle contents. These

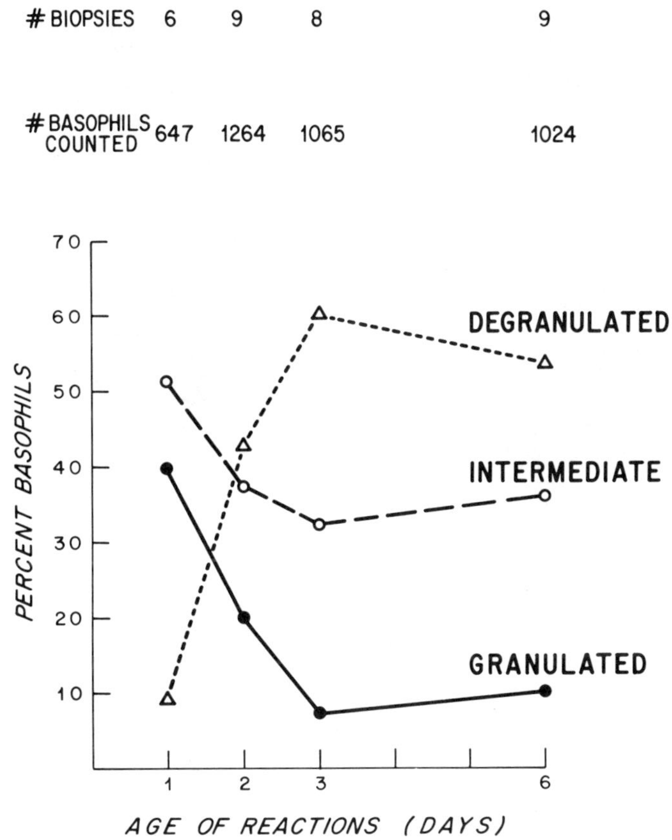

Figure 35 Piecemeal degranulation of basophils in allergic contact dermatitis reactions with time after skin test to dinitrochlorobenzene (DNCB) in nine volunteers or Urushiol (one volunteer). Granulated basophils had a complete complement of metachromatic granules; intermediate basophils had a mixture of metachromatic granules and empty granules; degranulated basophils contained nearly all empty granules. The changes between days 1 and 2 and between days 2 and 3 were highly significant ($p<0.001$, chi square). Changes between days 3 and 6 after skin test were also significant (at $p = 0.05$ but not at $p = 0.02$). (From Ref. 49, with permission.)

early changes generally preceded half-maximum histamine release, whereas the later extrusion of full granules, emptied granules, and their membranous contents coincided with half-maximum histamine release. Extraordinary membrane shifts were generated and persisted over the 10-min period examined and coincided with the later time frame within which LTC_4 was generated and released from f-Met peptide-stimulated basophils (108,122).

While these findings substantially support our original degranulation model (Figure 46) and for the first time provide a documentation of this degranulation continuum ex vivo, as well as a trigger for its induction, it is also true that limited data currently exist that definitively implicate triggers for PMD in vivo, and no data are available which implicate actual release of granule or cellular mediators in situ via this route.

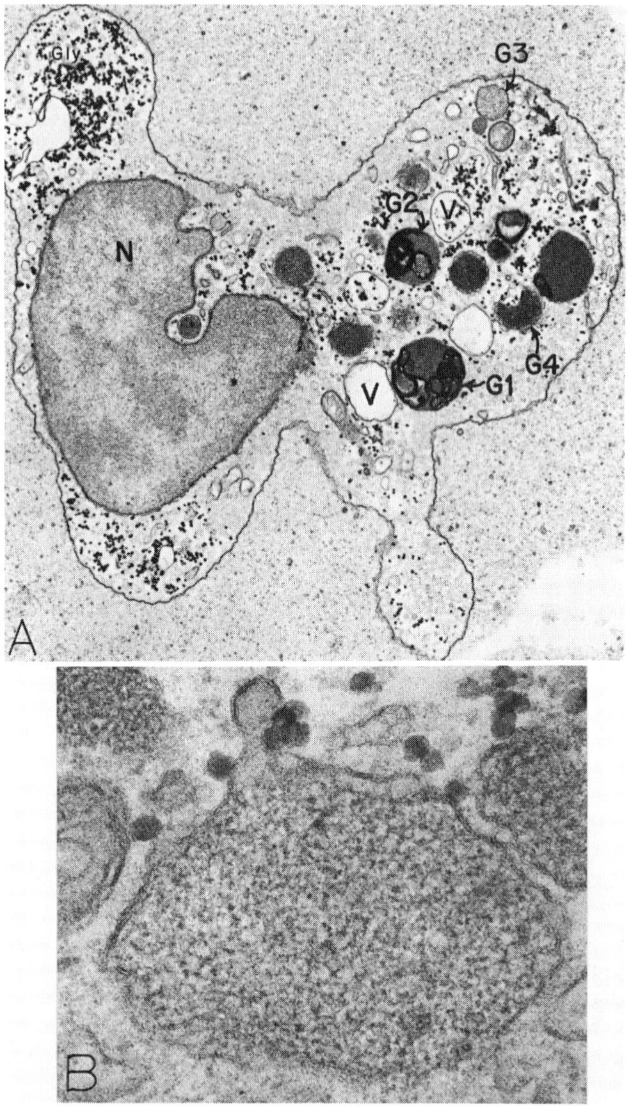

Figure 36 A. Human basophil within an epidermal vesicle in a 3-day lesion of allergic contact dermatitis. Granules contain variable numbers of particles. Granule G3 has greatly reduced particle content. Several granules contain multiple myelin concentric membranes (G1). Granule G4 exhibits focal complete loss of granule particles. Numerous small vesicles in the cytoplasm contain granule particles; others appear empty. Several large, empty, granule-sized vacuoles (V), representing granules which have lost their contents, are present. B. High-magnification electron micrograph of human basophil granule in the skin lesion of allergic contact dermatitis shows reduced particle content. A vesicle containing finely granular material is attached to the granule. Dense, rounded glycogen particles are closely associated with this attached vesicle. A, ×19,000; B, ×103,500. (A, from Ref. 18, with permission; B, from Ref. 3, with permission.)

Table 5 Ultrastructural Identification of Piecemeal Degranulation in Basophils and Mast Cells

Disease/circumstance	Species	Basophil	Mast cell	Anatomic location
Vesicular transport of exogenous HRP (31,183,184)	Guinea pig	+		Bone marrow in vivo Blood basophils in vitro
Immunologic tumor rejection (186,187)	Guinea pig	+		Subcutaneous tissue, peritoneal cavity
Virus-induced fibrosarcoma (Dvorak AM and Galli SJ, unpublished data)	Guinea pig	+		Skin
Vesicular transport of eosinophil peroxidase (185)	Guinea pig	+		Blood basophils in vitro
Chronic glomerulonephritis and pyelonephritis (190)	Human		+	Renal tubular epithelium
Allergic contact dermatitis (18,49)	Human	+		Skin
Delayed hypersensitivity to microbial antigens (18, 49, 189)	Human	+	+	Skin
Basophil leukemia (191)	Human	+		Blood
Allograft rejection (192, 415)	Human	+		Skin
Crohn's disease (16, 26, 27, 58, 128, 193–198)	Human	+	+	Ileum, peripheral blood
Ulcerative colitis (Dvork AM, unpublished data)	Human		+	Colon
Melanoma (199)	Human		+	Skin
Bullous pemphigoid (28, 62)	Human	+	+	Skin
Peritoneal dialysis fluid (51)	Human	+		Peritoneal fluid
Vesicular transport of eosinophil peroxidase (44)	Human	+		Umbilical cord blood cultures
Renal cell adenoma (200)	Human		+	Kidney
Gastric lymphoma (16, 32, 33, 50)	Human	+		Stomach
Adenocarcinoma (16, 32, 33, 50)	Human	+		Lung
Adenocarcinoma (16, 32, 33, 50)	Human		+	Lymph node metastasis
rhIL-3-containing cultures (59)	Human	+		Umbilical cord blood cultures
f-Met peptide stimulation in vitro (122)	Human	+		Peripheral blood
Interstitial fibrosis (Dvorak AM, unpublished data)	Human		+	Lung
Whipple's disease (194)	Human		+	Small Intestine
Sézary's syndrome (Dvorak AM, unpublished data)	Human	+		Peripheral blood
rhIL-3 infusion in vivo (88)	Monkey	+		Peripheral blood
3T3 fibroblast tumors Dvorak AM, unpublished data)	Rabbit	+	+	Corneal pocket
Vesicular transport of eosinophil peroxidase (185)	Mouse		+	Cultured immature mast cells from fetal liver
Picryl chloride-induced contact sensitivity (157)	Mouse		+	Skin

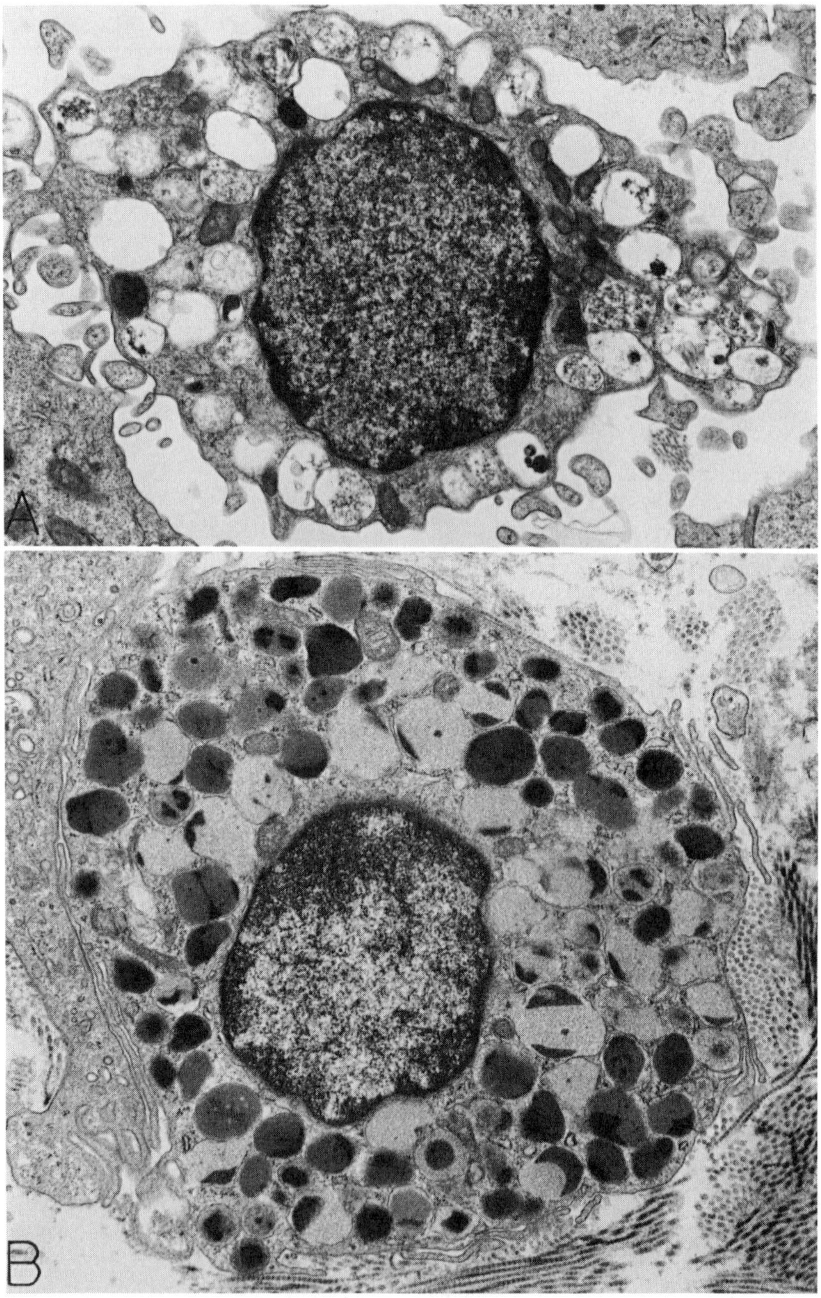

Figure 37 Human mast cells in biopsies of Crohn's disease ileum (A) and bullous pemphigoid skin (B) show granule losses characteristic for piecemeal degranulation. Many granules in A are completely empty; many granules in B show partial granule losses. In both cells, several completely unaltered granules remain. A, ×27,000; B, ×13,500. (B, from Ref. 33 with permission.)

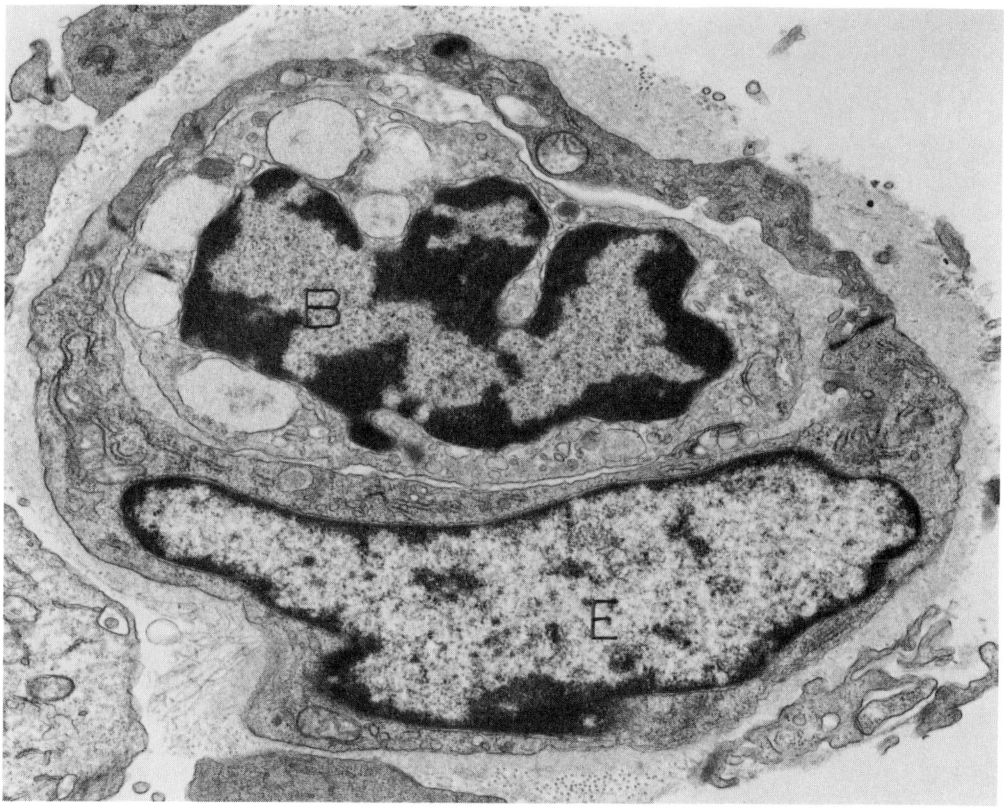

Figure 38 Human basophil (B) in biopsy of lung adenocarcinoma shows piecemeal degranulation characterized by empty, nonfused granules. The basophil is within a capillary. E = endothelial cell. ×13,500. (From Ref. 32, with permission.)

VII. CYTOKINES, INTERLEUKINS, TUMOR AND BACTERIAL PRODUCTS AS CANDIDATES FOR REGULATION OF BASOPHIL AND MAST CELL FUNCTION(S)

There is now ultrastructural evidence that documents the anatomy of AND and PMD and their individual recovery reactions in basophils and mast cells of several species, in several circumstances. These events are represented schematically in Figure 47. There is also evidence that, in a variety of circumstances, cytokines, interleukins, tumor and bacterial products are involved in the regulation of basophils and mast cells and their functions. These events may be due to direct or indirect effects of basophils and mast cells; they may result in up-regulation or down-regulation of basophil and mast cell functions; some factors may act synergistically with others, or alone; effects on differentiation, maturation, and function of basophils and mast cells are possible; regulation of intercellular interactions among basophils, mast cells, and other inflammatory, barrier, or mesenchymal cells could be important; simulation of secretion by PMD and recovery from PMD in basophils and mast cells by these products are likely; such products may originate from other cells or from basophils, and mast cells themselves to participate in autoregulatory loops.

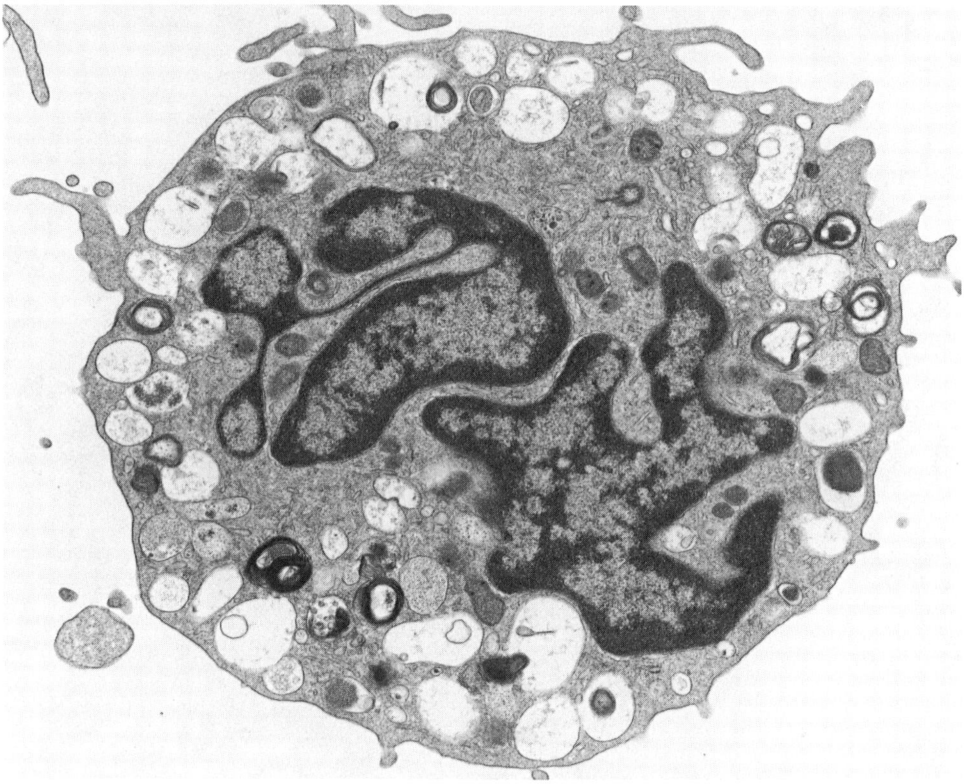

Figure 39 Mature human basophil which developed from human cord blood mononuclear cells cultured in basophil growth factor-containing media shows a full complement of empty, nonfused granule chambers characteristic for piecemeal degranulation. ×13,000. (From Ref. 32, with permission.)

A form of cellular immunity that was delayed in onset, characterized by an extensive infiltration of basophilic leukocytes, and mediated by lymphocytes was designated cutaneous basophil hypersensitivity (CBH), to distinguish it from classic delayed hypersensitivity (179,181). Basophil function in immediate hypersensitivity reactions is regulated by cell surface-bound homocytotropic antibodies whose interactions lead to the release by AND of basophil granules and their pharmacological contents (206–210). Basophils participating in CBH-type reactions do not have specificity for sensitizing antigen (37,38,40,181,211,212). Typical CBH reactions may be elicited at 4 days after sensitization, before antibodies can be detected. In fact, intravenous or local injections of sensitizing antigens into guinea pigs bearing mature (24-h), basophil-rich CBH reactions to human serum albumin or to ovalbumin failed to induce vascular permeability alterations characteristic of histamine release, nor did they lead to overt basophil degranulation. Using a sensitive rosetting technique, the overwhelming majority (93–99%) of basophils circulating in the blood or accumulating in skin reactions of CBH failed to form rosettes, indicating a lack of surface specificity for antigens (212). Finally, animals sensitized with keyhole limpet hemocyanin (KLH) in saline developed

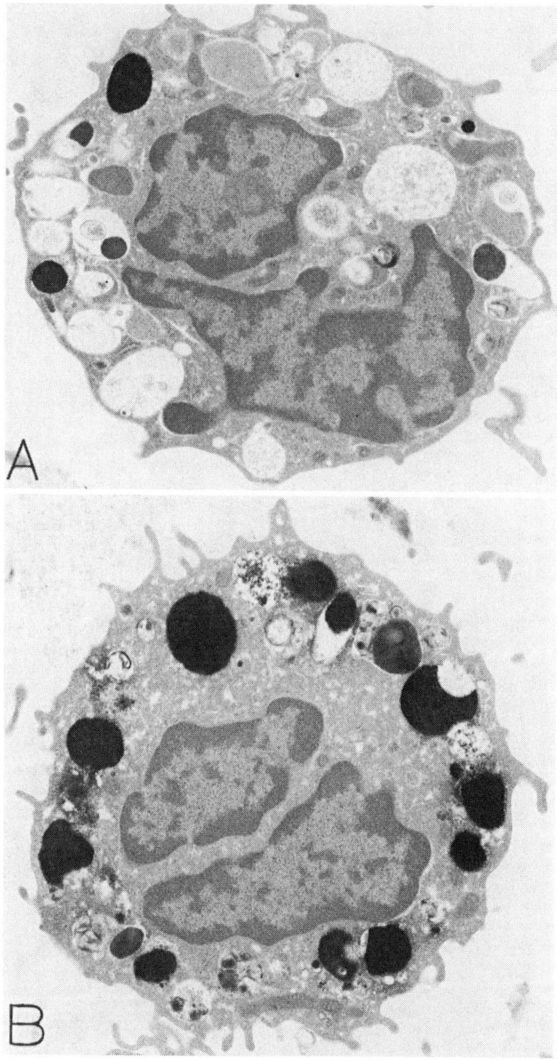

Figure 40 Mature human basophils, which developed from human cord blood mononuclear cells cultured in basophil growth factor-containing media and prepared to demonstrate peroxidase by electron microscopy, show several positive granules and many negative granules in (A) and nearly all positive granules and positive endocytotic vesicles in (B). The source of peroxidase in these experiments was released eosinophil peroxidase from damaged and dying eosinophils also present in these cultures. A, B, $\times 12{,}000$. (From Ref. 44, with permission.)

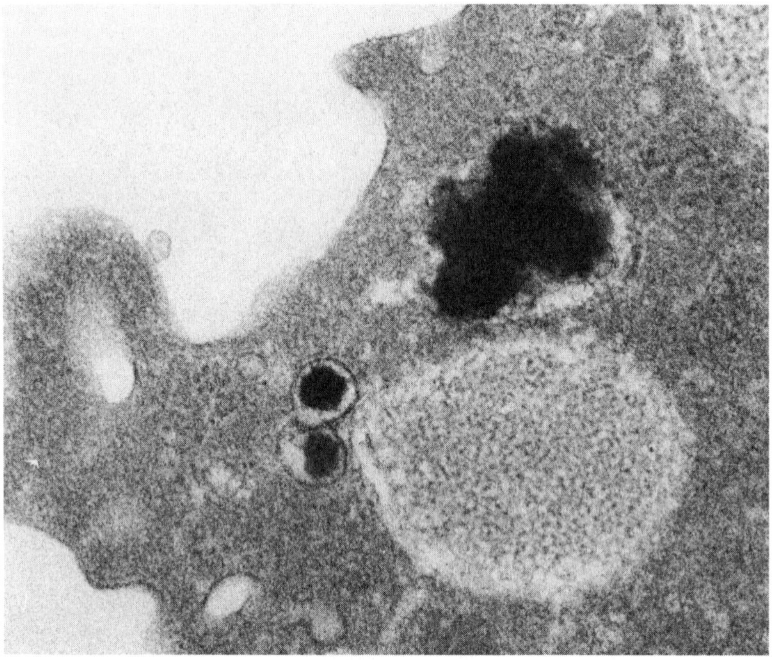

Figure 41 Higher-magnification view of mature human basophil, developed in culture under circumstances similar to those of Figures 39 and 40 and prepared to demonstrate peroxidase, shows two eosinophil peroxidase-positive vesicles adjacent to a particle-filled, peroxidase-negative basophil granule. A positive granule is also present. ×60,000.

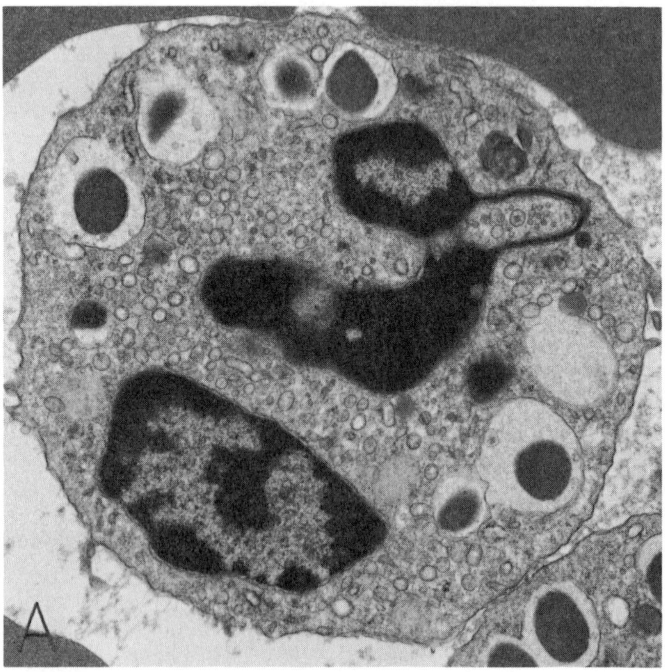

Figure 42 Monkey peripheral blood basophil, which appeared in response to rhIL-3 administration in vivo, shows piecemeal degranulation characterized by focal losses from normally completely dense granules and markedly increased numbers of small, smooth, membrane-bound cytoplasmic vesicles. ×12,000. (From Ref. 88, with permission.)

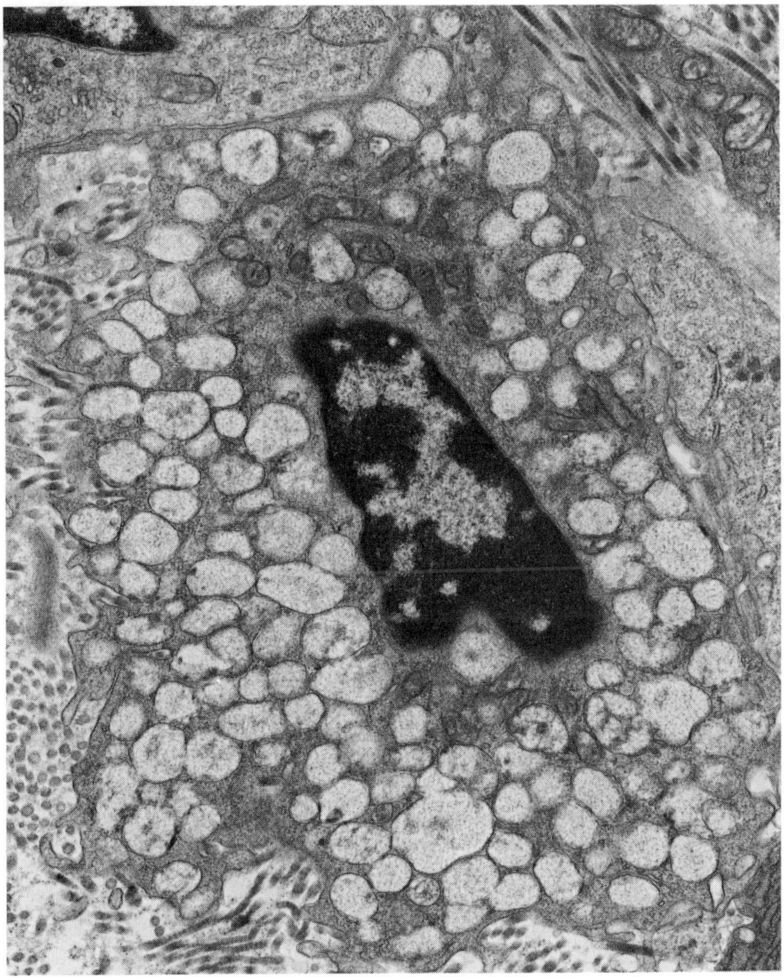

Figure 43 Rabbit mast cell, in a corneal pocket containing an experimentally placed fibroblast tumor, shows piecemeal degranulation characterized by numerous nearly empty, nonfused cytoplasmic granules. ×14,500.

excellent CBH reactions at 8 days, but basophils from these animals did not release histamine in response to antigen (213). On the other hand, occasional basophils participating in CBH reactions to purified protein antigens do exhibit anaphylactic-type degranulation. Moreover, Askenase (214) has demonstrated that injection of a potent immunogen, KLH, into mature (24-h) CBH reactions to that antigen provokes both basophil degranulation and histamine release. Finally, it is probable that the anaphylactic changes described in cutaneous and intestinal basophils (214) in parasite-infected guinea pigs also reflect a two-stage mechanism in which cellular immunity and immediate hypersensitivity cooperate in a synergistic fashion. According to this view, lymphocytes or their products bring sensitized basophils to a site of antigenic accumulation where their surface homocytotropic antibody reacts with such antigen (212), triggering AND and mediator release.

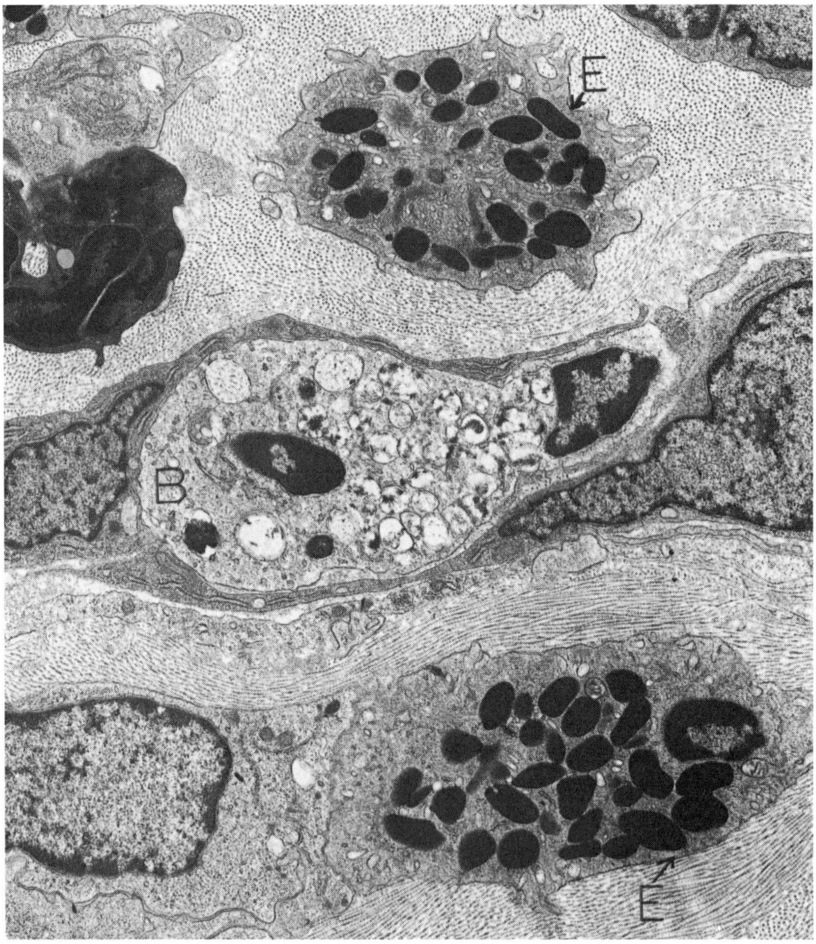

Figure 44 Rabbit basophil (B) and eosinophils (E), in a corneal pocket containing an experimentally placed fibroblast tumor, show piecemeal degranulation of the basophil characterized by empty and partially empty, nonfused granule chambers. The eosinophils are unaltered. ×9,000.

While basophils are a prominent component of CBH reactions, lymphocytes are essential to the induction and expression of this form of hypersensitivity, just as they are in classic delayed hypersensitivity. Animals primed for CBH exhibit an expansion of the thymus-dependent paracortical zones of draining lymph nodes (215); reactivity may be inhibited by antilymphocyte serum, and reactions may be passively transferred to normal recipients by viable lymphoid cells (211,216).

We have proposed (30), and it has been shown in certain circumstances, that sensitized lymphocytes produced in CBH-sensitized animals, upon exposure to specific antigen, are capable of secreting mediators that affect basophil function(s) (217). By analogy, similar lymphocyte products (lymphokines, interleukins) might be expected to interact with mast cells and basophils in other circumstances. In this section, we review some of these possible interactions under several categories of function.

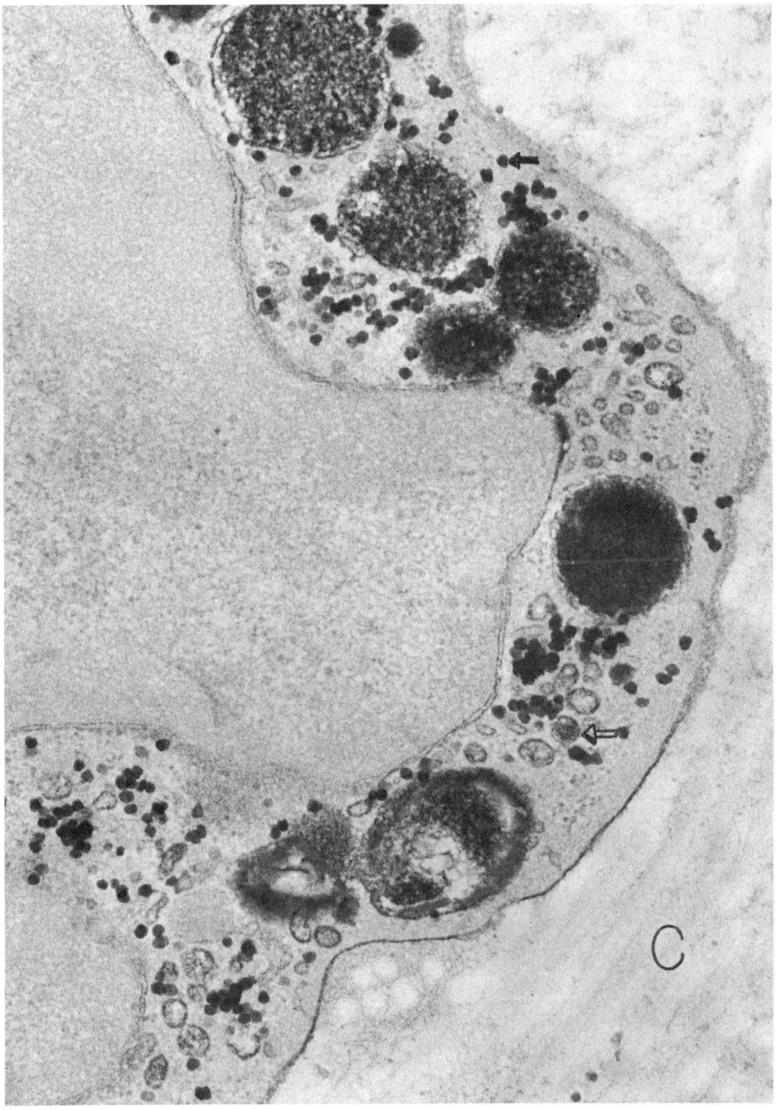

Figure 45 High-magnification view of human basophil in a skin allograft that shows increased and very dense granule particle contents. The cytoplasm has numerous dense glycogen particles (closed arrow) and a mixture of particle-filled (open arrow) and empty vesicles. C = collagen. ×50,000.

A. Cellular Motility

Chemotactic factors for guinea pig basophils include a lymphokine present in culture fluids from antigen-stimulated lymphocytes, a material generated in zymosan-activated guinea pig serum, a C5 cleavage factor, and a bacterial factor (217). Other reports have described chemotactic factors for human basophils (218,219). We noted, by ultrastruc-

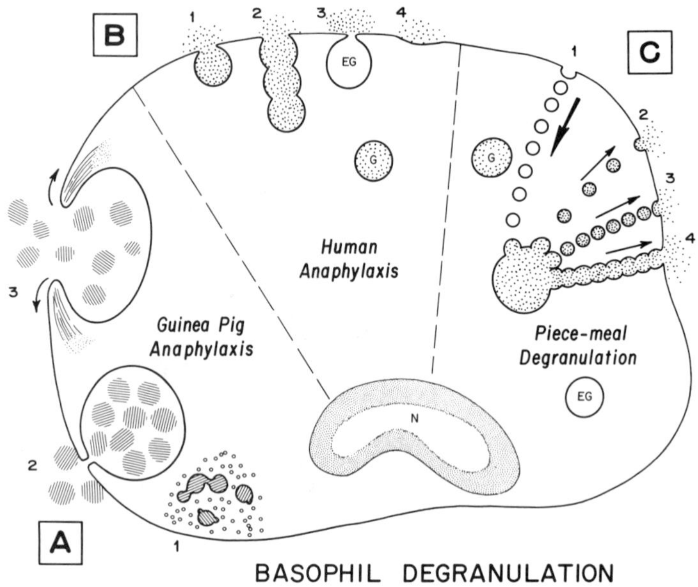

Figure 46 Schematic diagram of AND and PMD in basophils. A. Anaphylactic degranulation of guinea pig basophils. (1) Increased cytoplasmic vesicles 1 min after triggering with concanavalin A. Vesicles have fused with some granules; one has formed a bridge joining adjacent granules. (2) At 5–20 min, membranes of granules and cytoplasmic vesicles have fused with each other and with the plasma membrane, forming a "degranulation sac" containing membrane-free granules that open to the cell exterior by a narrow pore. Only occasional granules have escaped outside the cell, and many of these remain adherent to the cell surface. (3) Filaments have become prominent in the cytoplasmic processes embracing the degranulation sac. Over a period of hours, these processes retracted, as indicated by arrows, presumably powered by the filaments, opening the degranulation sac to the exterior and permitting granule escape. B. Anaphylactic degranulation of human basophils. (1, 2) Fusion of membranes of individual or joined granules directly with plasma membrane, with resulting discharge of granule contents. (3) Empty granule (EG) membranes eventually become part of plasma membrane as in (4). Note that portions of granule matrix remain adherent to plasma membrane. C. Piecemeal degranulation of human (or guinea pig) basophils as in certain cell-mediated immune reactions. (1) Endocytotic vesicles travel from plasma membrane through the cytoplasm to basophilic granules, with which they fuse. (2) Exocytotic vesicles, containing bits of granule matrix, bud from granule membrane, pass through the cytoplasm, and fuse with the plasma membrane, discharging their contents to the extracellular space. (3) Same as (2), but budding proceeds at a faster rate. (4) Still more rapid exocytosis, in which vesicles bud from granule at so fast a rate that they do not separate from each other and form a channel joining the granule with the extracellular space. This is equivalent to anaphylaxis. N = nucleus. (From Orenstein NS, Galli SJ, Dvorak AM, Dvorak HF. Glycosaminoglycans and proteases of guinea pig basophilic leukocytes. In: Becker EL, Simon AS, Austen KF, eds. Biochemistry of the acute allergic reactions: Fourth International Symposium. New York: Alan R. Liss, 1981:123–43, with permission.)

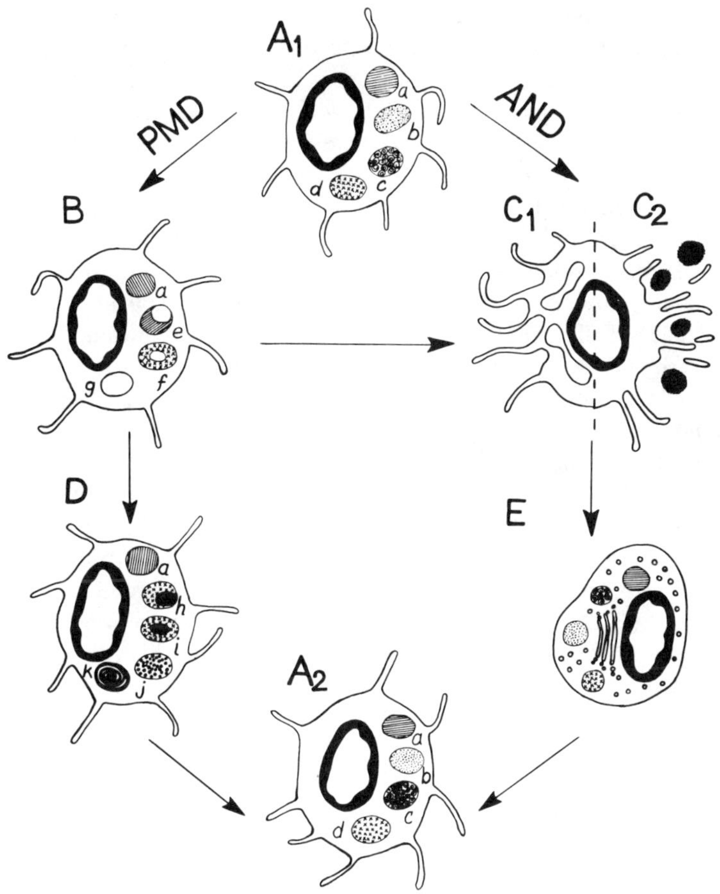

Figure 47 Schematic diagram summarizes release and recovery reactions of which human mast cells are capable. Mature mast cells (A1) with full complement of granules displaying crystal (a), particle (b), scroll (c), and mixed (d) patterns. Given appropriate stimuli to produce AND, mast cells develop intracytoplasmic channels which permeate the cytoplasm. Granule patterns are altered and solubilized within the intracytoplasmic channels (C1). Degranulation pores open these channels to the exterior; individual membrane-free granules with swollen, altered matrices, free membranes, and cell processes are shed from actively degranulating cells (C2). Recovery from fully expressed AND requires synthesis of new containers and granule contents (E). These actively synthesizing cells are filled with expanded Golgi structures, cytoplasmic vesicles, progranules, and newly forming granules (E) to produce a fully recovered mature mast cell with a full complement of granules (A2). PMD of mast cells (B), identified in situ in numerous human diseases, for which specific stimuli are not yet known, is characterized by cells with unaltered granules (a), granules with focal losses of contents (e, f), and empty granule containers (g). Increasing the rate of vesicular transport of granule materials in PMD (B) could result in AND (C1). Recovery from PMD, seen in mast cells in wound healing (D), shows increasing, complex focal (h, i), particulate (j), homogeneous, or scroll and threadlike (k) densities in empty or partially empty granule containers to produce a fully recovered mature mast cell with a full complement of filled granules (A2) displaying crystal (a), particle (b), scroll (c), and mixed (d) patterns. (From Ref. 62 with permission.)

tural studies, that lymphokine-containing lymphocyte culture supernatants caused guinea pig basophils to develop typical motile configurations, termed "uropods" (220), an effect that was also evident in lesser numbers by addition of normal serum protein or by allowing continuous contact of basophils with plastic surfaces in culture tubes (Figure 48) (221). The lymphokine-enhanced development of these motile structures could provide the mechanism for migration of normally rounded, circulating basophils into appropriate tissue reactions. Motile basophils are elongate, bipolar cells characterized upon scanning and transmission electron microscopy by (a) veil-like surface ruffles or folds devoid of villi at one cell pole, and (b) a relatively thin, tail-like structure at the opposite cell pole, covered with short villi and similar in appearance to lymphocyte uropods (221,222). Tails generally excluded cytoplasmic granules and other organelles but were packed with microfilaments as well as with glycogen particles, empty vesicles, and some strands of rough endoplasmic reticulum (148,220,221). Observations of living cells demonstrated that many uropod-bearing basophils were engaged in locomotion, with the uropod generally posterior (221).

We also noted, in ultrastructural studies, the formation of uropods by human basophils (Figure 49) (52,120,121). Initially, we found small numbers of cells with motile structures in samples stimulated by antigen E or C5A peptide(s) (52,120). These motile basophils were fully granulated and did not participate in granule release. Histamine-releasing activity (HRA) is a ~10,000- to 15,000-Da protease-sensitive factor which induces histamine release from human basophils (223,224). This lymphokine was found by electron microscopy to induce ~83% of the responding basophils to assume motile configurations, or uropods, by 10 min (121). Again, all such uropod-containing human basophils showed no evidence of either AND or PMD and were fully granulated. AND was also stimulated, in conjunction with histamine release, by this lymphokine (see later), but only at early time intervals after stimulation in that portion of basophils that did not develop uropods. Subsequently, enhancement of human basophil chemotaxis has been shown to occur in vitro when cells are exposed to virus-stimulated leukocyte culture supernatants containing a lymphokine identical to interferon (225,226). Sensitized rat basophilic leukemia cells have been shown to migrate toward specific antigen (227), and augmentation of basophil chemotaxis by a factor from stimulated lymphocyte cultures has been established (218,228).

Mast cells also may move within tissues through the development of motile structures. Rarely, we have noted mast cells with polarized, uropodlike structures in electron microscopic samples of skin (28). More frequently, generally rounded mast cells assume elongate spindle shapes in tissues (62) similar to bipolar, spindle-shaped, actively migrating fibroblasts in in-vitro model systems (Dvorak AM and Dvorak HF, unpublished data). Recently, stimulation of rat peritoneal mast cell migration by tumor-derived peptides (229), or normal migration of mastocytoma cells in vitro (230), has been shown. In the latter case, exposure to sensitized lymphocyte supernatants containing macrophage migration-inhibiting factor (MIF), a lymphokine known to inhibit macrophage migration (231), was also shown to inhibit mastocytoma migration in a similar in-vitro assay (230). Peritoneal mast cells from mice have been shown to move toward a gradient of interleukin-3 of either purified natural spleen cell or recombinant murine origin (232), clearly establishing a role for this lymphocyte product in mast cell motion. Cultured mouse mast cells and the mouse mast cell line PT18 have been shown

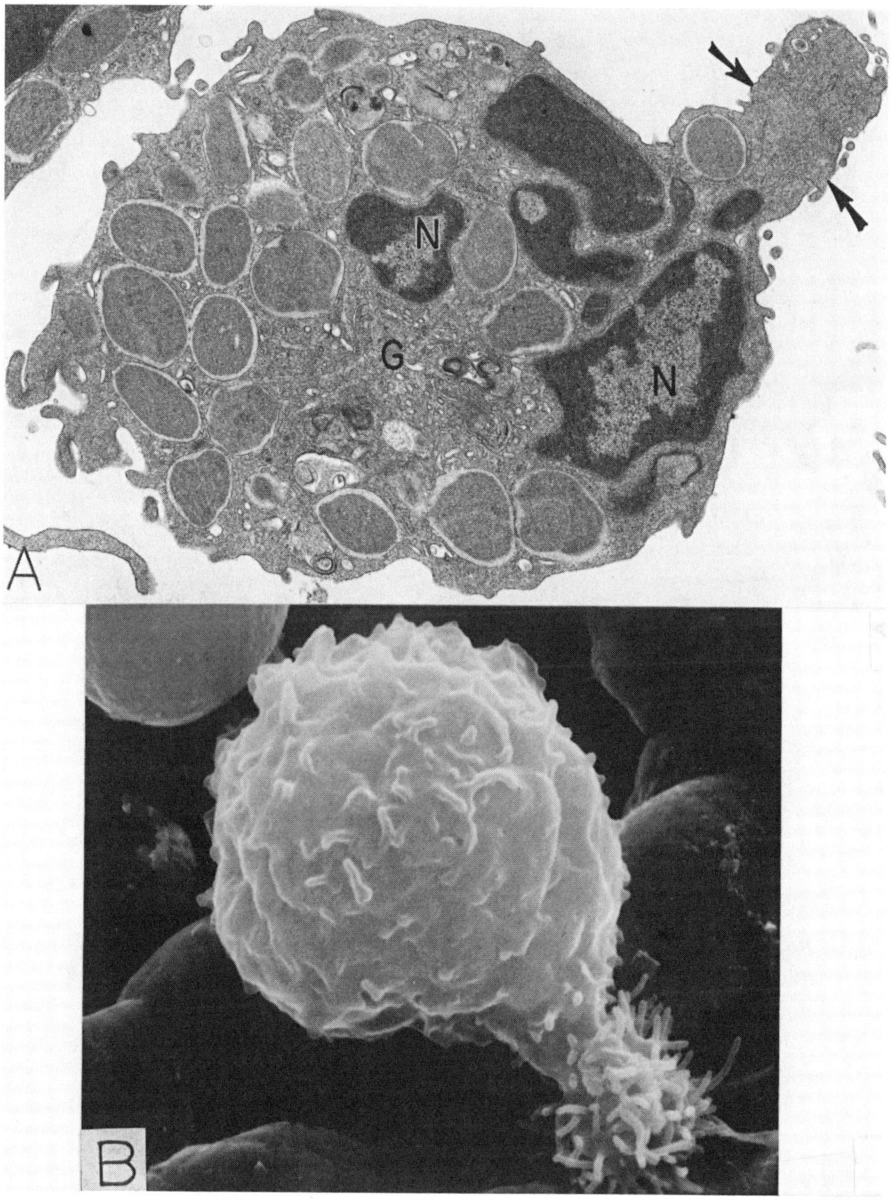

Figure 48 A. Transmission electron micrograph of guinea pig basophil cultured 20 h in Eagle's minimal essential media with Earle's salts, 10% guinea pig serum, and lymphocyte culture supernatant containing macrophage inhibition factor. Note typical filament-containing uropod (arrows). B. Scanning electron micrograph of guinea pig basophil cultured 1 h in Eagle's media with 10% guinea pig serum shows the anterior cell surface covered with short folds, ridges, and microvilli and the posterior narrow uropod covered with numerous microvilli. G = Golgi region; N = nucleus. A, ×14,500; B, ×12,000. (From Ref. 221, with permission.)

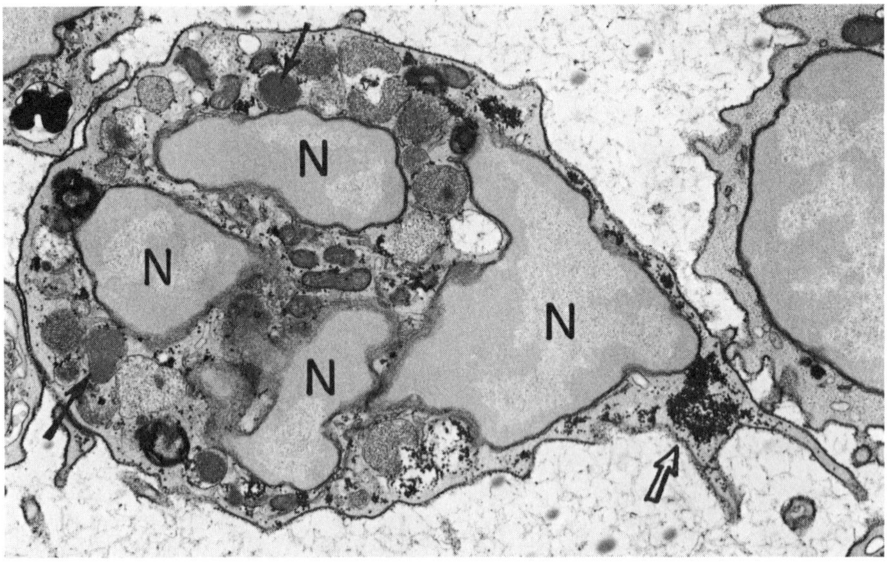

Figure 49 Uropod formation (open arrow) in human peripheral blood basophil exposed to C5 peptide(s) for 5 min. The cell surface is uniformly stained by cationized ferritin. Closed arrows = full granules; N = nucleus. ×7,000. (From Ref. 120, with permission.)

to migrate toward laminin in chemotaxis assays. This migration is enhanced after IgE-mediated activation, an enhancement which is independent of concomitant histamine release (233).

B. Cellular Differentiation and Maturation

Evidence for factor stimulation of cellular differentiation and maturation of basophils and mast cells exists for several species (Table 6). Some of the earliest indications supporting this mechanism were obtained in the peripheral blood of rabbits (234) and guinea pigs (235) stimulated with foreign proteins. Basophilia was produced by injection of foreign proteins in these two species. This principle was utilized initially by Winqvist (236) and subsequently by others (43,70,73,153) to produce large numbers of basophils in guinea pigs for functional and structural studies (Figures 2a, 6, 10a, 18, 19, 21–23, 29–33, and 48) (31,68–70,72,73,148–153,183,184,237,238). The factor dependence of basophil production in guinea pigs was established in vitro by culturing bone marrow cells from normal animals with conditioned media from cultures of either antigen- or mitogen-stimulated guinea pig spleen cells (239). Basophilic leukocytes regularly developed in these cultures, establishing the existence of a basophil growth factor(s) in the conditioned media from guinea pig lymphocytes (239).

There is evidence for the factor dependence of rat basophils as well (240). For example, early studies of a chemically induced basophil leukemia in rats revealed a factor present in normal rat serum and in rat serum of animals with basophil leukemia that stimulated increased numbers of circulating basophils (240). This factor did not increase bone marrow mast cells, however, suggesting that factors stimulatory for these two readily identified cells differ in rats (240). Additional evidence for factor-driven basophilia in rats is found in parasite models (241–243). At least two groups have shown elevation of peripheral blood basophils in rats infected with either *Nippostrongylus brasiliensis* or *Trichinella spiralis* (241–243). By analogy to the in-vitro studies in guinea pigs (239), it is possible that parasite stimulation of rat lymphocytes results in the production of a basophilopoietin responsible for increasing circulating basophils from bone marrow progenitors. Rats ordinarily have extremely small numbers of circulating basophils; but in parasite models, circulating basophils increase dramatically to ~4.5% of the leukocytes, an 80-fold increase compared to control rats (241).

In recent years, a number of investigations have implicated factor stimulation as a basis for increasing basophil numbers in humans (reviewed in Ref. 32). Initially, elevated blood basophils in myelogenous leukemia patients suggested the possibility that a basophilopoietin might exist in humans (10). We demonstrated that mature basophils developed in cultures of human cord blood mononuclear cells grown in supernatants from mitogen-stimulated T-cells (Figures 39–41) (118). Basophil growth factor-containing conditioned media obtained from a variety of sources have similarly been shown to encourage the development of basophils in various in-vitro systems (244). For example, the source of progenitors, in addition to cord blood cells (118,244), can be from fetal liver, leukemia cell line HL-60, peripheral blood or bone marrow, from normal or allergic donors, and sources of factor-containing conditioned media include mitogen-stimulated lymphocytes, antigen-stimulated lymphocytes, the MOT leukemia cell line, human placenta, and murine T-cell factor(s) (44,118,244–255). In an ultrastructural study of human basophils developing in vitro in either human basophil growth factor-containing conditioned media or murine mast cell growth factor-containing conditioned media, we noted that fetal cord blood cells grown in the mature conditioned media did not develop beyond the immature, large mononuclear cells characteristic for basophilic myelocytes, in contrast to the development of small, mature, polynuclear basophils in the human conditioned media (Figures 39 and 40) (44). Subsequently, we sequenced the conditioned media so that large basophilic myelocytes forming in the murine conditioned media developed into mature basophils when murine conditioned media were replaced by human conditioned media. These data clearly indicated the necessity for a factor(s) present in the human T-cell conditioned media for the complete differentiation and maturation of the basophil lineage from human cord blood progenitors in vitro (44).

We next investigated human basophilogenesis in vitro using recombinant human interleukin-3 (rhIL-3) (256) or recombinant human interleukin-5 (rhIL-5) (59,257,258). Human cord blood mononuclear cells cultured with either of these interleukins for 3 weeks developed into mixtures of basophils and eosinophils. Immature myelocytes predominated in 3-week cultures (258). Nearly all of these were of the eosinophil lineage in rhIL-5-supplemented cultures (258); larger numbers of basophilic myelocytes developed in rhIL-3 (258). Longer culture intervals in either of these interleukins (up to 5 weeks) resulted in the development of mature basophils and eosinophils (59). Others have also demonstrated the effectiveness of interleukin 3 (IL-3) as an important factor in the development of human basophils (259–261).

Continuous infusion of rhIL-3 (262) elicits basophilia in primates (88,263,264). Monkey basophils have been proven difficult to demonstrate by morphologic methods, despite evidence for IgE-mediated histamine release from monkey peripheral blood cells (265). Infusion of rhIL-3 into monkeys produced a significant increase in circulating peripheral blood basophils, providing sufficient material for us to define clearly the

Table 6 Evidence for Factor Stimulation of Basophil and Mast Cell Differentiation and Maturation

Cell	Circumstance	System/location	Species/cell	References
Basophil	Antigen	Peripheral blood	Guinea pig basophil	43, 70, 73, 183, 235, 236, 239, 465
Basophil	Antigen	Peripheral blood	Rabbit basophil	234
Basophil	Parasite infection	Peripheral blood	Rat basophil	241–243
Basophil	β-Chlorethylamine-induced leukemia	Peripheral blood, skin	Rat basophil	240
Basophil	PHA-stimulated T-cell supernatant	Cord blood mononuclear cell suspension culture	Human basophil	44, 118, 244, 245, 495
Basophil	rhIL-3	Cord blood mononuclear cell suspension culture	Human basophil	59, 258, 496
Basophil	Conditioned media—allergen-stimulated cells or MO T cell leukemia line	Peripheral blood	Human basophil	253
Basophil	MO-conditioned media	HL-60 cell line	Human basophil	246
Basophil	Conditioned media	Peripheral blood	Human basophil	254
Basophil	Complete media, 10% fetal calf serum	Fetal liver cells	Human basophil	247
Basophil	Conditioned medium from MO cell line or from lectin-stimulated peripheral blood mononuclear murine T-cells	Bone marrow	Human basophil	248, 249, 252, 255
Basophil	Conditioned media from human T-cell leukemia cell line, from PHA-stimulated normal blood lymphocytes, from human placenta	Peripheral blood	Human basophil	250, 251
Basophil	rhIL-3	Peripheral blood	Monkey basophil	88, 263, 264

Mast cell	Cloned Ly 1^+2^- inducer T-cell supernatants; mast cell growth factor; mitogen-activated T-cell supernatant; WEHI-3B tumor cell supernatants; rmIL-3	Suspension cultures of fetal liver, bone marrow, lymph node, or spleen cells	Mouse mast cell	39, 155, 269, 270, 272–277, 279, 305, 497, 498
Mast cell	Fibroblast monolayers	Lymph nodes, thoracic duct, thymus	Mouse mast cell	266, 268
Mast cell	Chronic dermatitis in genetically mast cell-deficient W/W^v mice	Skin	Mouse mast cell	87
Mast cells	Agar cultures supplemented with Con-A-stimulated mouse spleen cell conditioned media	Bone marrow from genetically mast cell-deficient W/W^v and congenic normal mice	Mouse mast cell	281
Mast cell	PMA induction in genetically mast cell-deficient W/W^v mice in vivo	Skin	Mouse mast cell	303
Mast cell	Methylcellulose cultures supplemented with erythropoietin and PWM spleen cell-conditioned media	Bone marrow	Mouse mast cell	302
Mast cell	Cultured, bone marrow-derived, factor-dependent mast cells injected into W/W^v mast cell-deficient mice	Peritoneal cavity in vivo	Mouse mast cell	288
Mast cell	Co-cultured with 3T3 fibroblasts	Spleen cell-derived, factor-dependent mast cells	Mouse mast cell	289
Mast cell	Methylcellulose cultures, pokeweed mitogen, spleen cell-conditioned media	Peritoneal cells	Mouse mast cell	290, 291

Table 6 Continued

Cell	Circumstance	System/location	Species/cell	References
Mast cell	Co-cultured with KiSV retrovirus-producing fibroblasts	Spleen cells	Mouse mast cell	292
Mast cell	Human synovial fluid from chronic inflammatory synovitis cases	Bone marrow cells	Mouse mast cell	314
Mast cell	Cultures	Thymus	Rat mast cell	306, 499
Mast cell	Conditioned media from antigen-, parasite-, or mitogen-stimulated lymphoid cell cultures	Spleen, bone marrow, thymus, lymph node, bone marrow cells	Rat mast cell	307–311
Mast cell	3T3 fibroblast monolayer	Cord blood mononuclear cell suspension culture	Human mast cell	48

ultrastructural features of this lineage in monkeys (Figures 4, 11b, and 42) (88). Thus, factor dependence of basophil production in another species was demonstrated in an in-vivo model (88).

Mouse mast cells have been the subject of a number of in-vivo and in-vitro studies, initially suggestive of, and ultimately providing proof for, the factor dependence of their development (reviewed in Ref. 39). In 1963, mast cells were seen to develop in cultures of thymus cells on embryonic fibroblast monolayers (266,267). Later, Ginsburg and Lagunoff reported that mast cells developed from sensitized lymph node or thoracic duct cells cultured on embryonic monolayers (268). The ultrastructure of the development of these mouse mast cells was described in detail by Combs (47). The basis for the stimulation of mast cell differentiation was not defined in these studies. However, subsequent studies (269) suggested that a factor(s) produced by lymphocytes and/or fibroblasts in these systems induced mast cell progenitors from the lymphoid organs to differentiate fully into mature mast cells (266–268).

A decade later (in 1980), Hasthorpe identified a cell line with mast cell features (including IgE receptors and granules) which were suggestive of the mast cell lineage (270). This continuously growing cell line evolved from spleen cells cultured in pokeweed mitogen-stimulated, spleen cell-conditioned media, where both cells and pokeweed mitogen-conditioned media were obtained from a mouse injected previously with the Friend erythroleukemia virus. This mast cell-like line was cloned by limiting dilution and was factor dependent for its growth (270). Also in 1980, the in-vitro characterization of the P-cell by Schrader and Nossal implicated the necessity for a growth factor in concanavalin-A-stimulated, spleen cell-conditioned media (271). These cells of spleen or bone marrow origin were termed P-cells for their growth characteristic of long-termed persistence in these factor-containing cultures.

In 1981, simultaneous reports from five laboratories (269,272–276) described factor-dependent cultures of mouse mast cells. While differing terminology was given to the cells so produced, it is now clear that all reports were of cells of the mast cell lineage in mice (269). We recognized that these cells were immature mast cells using ultrastructural criteria (269), based on previous descriptions of maturing mast cells in this species (Figures 7, 20, and 34) (47). The cells that we described were cloned by single cell micromanipulation from mouse fetal liver cells and were dependent on mast cell growth factor produced by cloned murine inducer T-lymphocytes (269). Subsequently, we defined the histamine content (269), high-affinity IgE receptor status (277), proteoglycan composition (277), serotonin content and synthetic capability (278), ultrastructure of AND (155), butyrate-induced maturation (Figure 7) (277,279), production of cytokines (280), and growth and maturation of mast cells from genetically mast cell-deficient W/W^v mice and congenic normal mice in soft agar cultures (281), of mast cells which developed from fetal liver, bone marrow, or lymph node cells cultured in mast cell growth factor-containing conditioned media from concanavalin-A-stimulated spleen cells or from WEHI tumor cells. Other groups that described the development of factor-dependent mast cells in 1981 variously termed them basophil/mast cells (272), P-cells with mast cell-like granules (273), and mast cells (274,275). Subsequently, we defined the ultrastructure of mouse basophils (Figure 3a), and compared them with mature mast cells, providing an unequivocal basis for the identification of cells of these two lineages in mice (41).

Factor-dependent mouse mast cells have been responsible for a renewal of studies of mast cell biology in this species using a combination of in-vitro and in-vivo methods, individually or in combination (39). Highlights of some of these investigations are included here. Recent extensive reviews can be used to obtain in-depth information regarding the current status of investigations made possible by the development of factor-dependent mouse mast cells (282–284). We and others noted the absence of heparin in immature, factor-dependent mast cells (277,285). Rather, the glycosaminoglycan side chains of the proteoglycans synthesized by these factor-dependent mouse mast cells were chondroitin sulfates (277,285). By analogy with rat mucosal mast cells, which also lack heparin (286,287), it was suggested that the immature, factor-dependent mouse mast cells might also be like mast cells derived from mucosal sites (277,285). Subsequently, using several approaches, it was determined that the morphologically immature mouse mast cells could undergo maturational changes of varying degrees that also resulted in progressive production of heparin by these immature mast cells (288,289). Such a transition in proteoglycan content was demonstrated using intraperitoneal transfer of cultured bone marrow-derived mast cells into the peritoneal cavities of genetically mast cell-deficient W/W^v mice (288), as well as co-cultures of factor-dependent, bone marrow-derived mast cells with 3T3 fibroblasts (289). Mast cells residing in the connective tissues of many organs in most species contain heparin (39). Mouse mast cells with the connective tissue phenotype, or those that contain heparin using berberine sulfate binding for this identification, have been shown to proliferate in methylcellulose cultures (290,291). These cells, derived from the peritoneal cavity, are also factor dependent. However, a factor(s) other than, or in addition to, interleukin-3 is necessary for their proliferation and function in vitro (290). More recently, co-culture of mouse splenocytes with Kirsten sarcoma virus-producing fibroblasts resulted in the development and persistence of a continuum of mouse mast cell phenotypes characterized by variable amounts of heparin and chondroitin sulfate proteoglycans (292). Such variability in proteoglycan content corresponded to ultrastructural changes characteristic of immature mast cells with immature granules containing heterogeneous contents and mature mast cells with homogeneously dense mature granules characteristic of the phenotype of mast cells present in mouse connective tissues (292).

The identification of factor-dependent mouse mast cells was instrumental to the ultimate purification, cloning, and automated chemical synthesis of the murine growth factor for mast cells, variously termed mast cell growth factor, WEHI-3 growth factor activity, P-cell-stimulating factor activity, colony-stimulating factor activity, histamine-producing cell-stimulating activity, multi-CSF, and, by consensus, interleukin-3 (269,276,293–300). Consequently, injections of bacterially synthesized mouse IL-3 were shown to induce increased numbers of mast cells in mesenteric lymph nodes, skin, and gut of normal mice, thus confirming the in-vivo relevance of this factor in the development of tissue mast cells (301). Similarly, genetically mast cell-deficient mice, using either in-vitro (281,302) or in-vivo (87,303) systems, have provided opportunities to show the factor-dependent development of mast cells in W/W^v mice. For example, methylcellulose cultures of W/W^v mouse bone marrow cells, containing pokeweed mitogen (PWM) spleen cell-conditioned media (302), or agar cultures of bone marrow cells, containing concanavalin-A, spleen cell-conditioned media (281), allowed growth of morphologically mature mouse mast cells; and either chronic inflammation (Figure

3b) (87) or PMA injection (303) facilitated the growth of morphologically mature mouse mast cells in the skin of W/W^v mice. In both circumstances, a lymphocyte-derived factor(s) produced in the microenvironment by either chronic inflammation or mitogens was probably responsible for the local maturation of mast cell precursors in mast cell-deficient mice.

Neoplastic transformation of mast cells by the transforming retrovirus, Abelson murine leukemia virus (Ab-MuLV), has been shown to abrogate the factor dependence (IL-3) of mouse mast cell growth (304). Moreover, these virus-transformed, mutant mast cells did not express or secrete detectable levels of IL-3, thereby obviating an autocrine mechanism for the loss of the requirement of exogenously added growth factor, or IL-3. Not all viral-infected murine mast cells, however, lose their factor dependence, illustrating that this finding cannot necessarily be generalized to other viruses (277,279,292,304,305).

The differentiation and maturation of rat mast cells have also been shown to be factor dependent (306–311). Initially, mast cells were developed by culturing thymus cells on rat embryonic fibroblasts (306). Subsequently, conditioned media from antigen, mitogen, and parasite-stimulated lymphoid cells were shown to provide the stimulation for growth of mast cells in cultures of bone marrow, spleen, and thymus lymph node cells from normal or nude rats. Both suspension and soft agar cultures were utilized in these studies (307–311).

Human lung-derived mast cells, partially purified from surgical specimens of lung, were shown to survive for up to 13 days when co-cultured with 3T3 fibroblasts (312). Previously, we had shown that similarly isolated human lung mast cells survived in cultures without fibroblasts or growth factors for several days (Figures 9a, 9c, 14–16, and 24–28) (16,33,61,313). Subsequently, survival and ultrastructural integrity of human lung mast cells co-cultured with 3T3 fibroblasts were confirmed (500). Very recently, we have observed the development of human mast cells in vitro from cultured human cord blood mononuclear cells (48). These mast cells were similar to human skin mast cells by ultrastructural criteria and developed in long-term, co-cultured 3T3 mouse fibroblasts and human cord blood cells (48). Presently, the factor dependence of these newly described human mast cells is under investigation. However, experiments using recombinant IL-1, IL-2, IL-3, IL-4, IL-5, IL-6, and GM-CSF (individually and in combinations) did not facilitate the development of human mast cells in cultures of cord blood or bone marrow cells (Ishizaka T, unpublished results). Recently, a novel mast cell growth factor has been described in rheumatoid synovitis (314). This newly described factor differs from IL-3 and was shown to be active using mouse bone marrow-derived mast cells. Since mast cells are increased in chronically inflamed synovial tissues in humans (315), this growth factor might be important to the development of human mast cells in vitro.

C. Cellular Secretion

Piecemeal degranulation is the uniform ultrastructural expression of human basophils which have infiltrated tissues in pathological lesions of varied origin (Figures 35, 36, and 38) (32). These include those associated with inflammatory reactions to bacteria, viruses, and tumors, as well as with diseases of unknown etiology. Specific triggering events for PMD are just being identified. Likely candidates include various cytokines or bacterial and viral products associated with inflammation. Similarly, human mast cells, present in tissues and involved with a wide variety of pathologies, express the morphology of PMD (Figure 37) (16). Recently, we have identified a morphologically unique continuum, spanning PMD to AND, in human peripheral blood basophils stimulated with the bacterial peptide, f-Met peptide (122). Also, in a number of biopsies of patients with inflammatory bowel disease, the continuum spanning PMD to AND is present in human mast cells (Dvorak AM, unpublished data). In the latter case, specific triggers for the morphologically determined events are not known. We have observed the morphology of PMD in two circumstances where IL-3 might be responsible, either directly or indirectly. For example, we have observed PMD (characterized by nonenlarged, empty granule containers) in the cytoplasm of basophils, which developed in rhIL-3-containing cultures of human cord blood mononuclear cells (59), and in circulating mature basophils, which developed in monkeys infused with rhIL-3 (Figure 42) (88). There is also evidence which implicates IL-3 in the activation of basophils, as determined biochemically (316–319). While the triggers for PMD are not yet known, we think non-IgE-mediated or IgE-assisted triggers, which include various cytokines, viral products, bacterial products, and tumor products, will ultimately be found to produce the ultrastructural morphology of PMD (316–336).

Cytokines with HRA for human basophils have been identified from a variety of sources. Initially, Thueson et al. found such activity in the supernatant fluids from mitogen- and antigen-stimulated, cultured human mononuclear cells and termed this material histamine-releasing activity (223,224), a finding confirmed by others later (337). Ultrastructural studies of several donor basophil preparations revealed AND as the mechanism for the histamine release reaction induced by HRA (121). Subsequently, more detailed ultrastructural analyses of multiple doses and times will be necessary to evaluate completely the ultrastructural release reaction induced by HRA. For example, in this study, evidence for PMD was absent in two donors at the single dose tested at two times poststimulus. Others have confirmed the mononuclear cell origin of HRA (326,337,338). Peripheral blood T-lymphocytes stimulated with phytohemagglutinin (PHA) or streptokinase-streptodornase (SK-SD) produced a factor that released histamine from human basophils (339). This factor was termed basophil-activating factor (BAF) (339). It was later shown that various subpopulations of peripheral blood mononuclear cells, including $CD4^-$ T-cells, $CD8^-$ T-cells, B-cells, and monocytes, all produced variable quantities of histamine-releasing factor (HRF) (340).

The IgE dependency of histamine release from human peripheral blood basophils was shown to be important in several circumstances (341–343). For example, human lung macrophage-derived HRA and HRF, generated in cutaneous IgE-mediated late-phase reactions, are both examples of such IgE-dependent factors (341,342). Similarly, nasal wash fluids contain an HRF that is IgE-dependent but is active only in some donors (343). Schulman et al. cultured human peripheral blood monocytes and demonstrated a potent HRA for human basophils in the supernatant within 24 h of culture (344). A role for food hypersensitivity in the generation of HRF from mononuclear cells was demonstrated by Sampson et al. (345). These authors also showed that this activity provoked release from basophils of food-sensitive individuals but not from normal controls, and that this activity was IgE dependent (345).

Other cells also generate cytokines with histamine-releasing properties, as assayed with human basophils. For example, platelets stimulated to undergo release reactions by a variety of triggers produce an HRF that stimulates human basophil release either by IgE-associated mechanisms or alone (333,346). Neutrophils also release a histamine-releasing activity (HRA-N) into supernatant fluids (336,346). This material has been assayed on human peripheral blood basophils (336,346) and on rat basophil leukemia cells (336). Generation of neutrophil supernatants containing the HRA occurred in the absence of granule secretion induced by several secretogogues and was detectable between 15 and 60 min of incubation of neutrophils in buffer and protein at 37°C (336,346). Recently, recombinant human neutrophil-activating peptide from *Escherichia coli* has been shown to induce histamine and leukotriene release by interleukin-3-primed basophils (347).

Early studies implicated interferon in the enhancement of IgE-mediated release from human basophils (324,325,348). Initially, this augmentation of histamine release was shown when certain viruses were incubated with human leukocytes and was also shown to require new RNA synthesis (324). Examination of supernatant fluids from antigen-containing, sensitized leukocyte cultures showed a correlation between histamine release-enhancing activity and interferon (348). Further studies showed that the soluble factor responsible for stimulating human basophils to release histamine was indeed interferon (325). Recently, the effect of interferon on basophil releasability was evaluated using short-term basophil cultures of mature basophils purified from the peripheral blood (349). In this case, enhancement of IgE-mediated histamine release (~200% of control) was established (349). These studies, in aggregate, demonstrate the involvement of this cytokine, interferon, in increased release of mediators from human basophils, an event of possible importance in viral disorders.

The advent of the application of molecular biology techniques to the field of cytokine research has been instrumental in providing pure recombinant materials in quantity for experimentation. A number of these have now been evaluated for secretogogue action in human basophils purified from blood (316–319,349,350), monkey basophils in vivo (88,264), and human basophils developing from cultured cord blood cells (59). There is now evidence regarding the capability of inducing histamine release by a number of interleukins and cytokines. The biochemical studies of mediator release show that rhIL-3 stimulates histamine release from human basophils (316–319,349,350). Recombinant human IL-3 enhanced IgE-mediated release (349,350) but, in some studies (317), also stimulated histamine release in the absence of cooperating triggers given simultaneously. Recombinant human IL-3 enhanced human basophil histamine release induced with other secretogogues as well. For example, f-Met peptide-mediated (349,350) and ionophore A23187-mediated (350) histamine release were enhanced. Basophils from patients with atopic disease responded to a greater extent to rhIL-3 than did basophils from nonatopic basophil donors (319). A novel function in the secretory processes of human basophils was demonstrated by the release of newly generated LTC_4 in large quantities when rhIL-3 and C5a were used to trigger cells (318). This established that the mediators released can be modified by this cytokine, since neither IL-3 nor C5a alone stimulates the release of LTC_4 from human basophils (318). In these studies, it was also found that IL-3 enhanced the release of histamine by other stimuli, but that IL-3 alone did not cause significant release over that of control spontaneous release (318). Interestingly, however, it was also noted in this study that IL-3 caused a low, continuous release of histamine over several hours in basophils from some atopic donors (318). To us, this profile for histamine release suggests a biochemical correlate of PMD (see later). Human recombinant GM-CSF was shown to be an effective releaser of histamine from human basophils by several groups (316,317,350);

but another group did not confirm this (349). The circumstances of study differed, however, in that basophils were used either immediately (316,317,350) or after 24 h in culture (349).

Recombinant human IL-5 was also tested for secretogogue activity and was found to release histamine from basophils in 2 of 14 donors tested (317), whereas tests of rhIL-3 and GM-CSF given together released histamine in 8 of 10 and 12 of 14 donors, respectively (317).

Interleukin-1 has also been found to have histamine-releasing capabilities (335,351,352). Different sources of IL-1 were tested on isolated human peripheral blood basophils or mast cells from adenoids (335). These included purified IL-1 from stimulated human monocytes and rhIL-1. Both were found to induce histamine release from basophils and mast cells (335). Studies from Lichtenstein's laboratory (351) showed that either rhIL-1a or rhIL-1b potentiated IgE-mediated histamine release from human peripheral blood basophils. Potentiation of histamine release by IL-1 or other secretogogues, such as f-Met peptide and the calcium ionophore, also occurred, but direct stimulation of histamine release alone was not demonstrated in this study (351). Others have shown that basophils released histamine when stimulated by IL-1 in the presence of D_2O, a histamine release-enhancing factor (316).

We recently found ultrastructural evidence for PMD in association with rhIL-3 in two circumstances (59,88). Recombinant human IL-5 was also found to be associated with images of PMD in human basophils (59). The studies of human basophils were done on cells that developed from human cord blood mononuclear cell cultures containing rhIL-3 or rhIL-5. In both cases, the ultrastructural correlate of PMD degranulation was present in viable, mature basophils (59). We next examined peripheral blood basophils which were induced to increase by continuous infusion of rhIL-3 in a monkey (88). Images consistent with PMD were also present in these circulating mature basophils in vivo (Figure 42) (88). Recently, Mayer et al. showed that monkeys infused with either rhIL-3 or rhGM-CSF (individually or combined) had elevated plasma histamine levels (264). Values for the combined infusion of rhIL-3 or rhGM-CSF exceeded those recorded for either cytokine alone (264).

Cytokines which inhibit the release of histamine from human basophils may also be produced in inflammatory reactions. For cxample, Alam et al. have identified such a factor which is produced when peripheral blood mononuclear cells are stimulated with histamine or mitogens, such as concanavalin-A (353,354). These investigators found that this histamine release inhibitory factor (HRIF) was produced by both B- and T-cells as well as monocytes (354). Both $CD4^-$ and $CD8^-$ T-cell subsets produced the factor (354). A similar HRIF has also been identified in supernatants of cultured, sensitized spleen cells (354). These studies all together (Table 7) clearly show that cytokines can stimulate, enhance, or inhibit the secretion of histamine from human basophils.

D. Cellular Recovery from Secretion

We have seen (Section IV.B) that mast cells and basophils can recover from their non-cytotoxic secretory processes. We have studied these events in detail in vitro using guinea pig basophils (Figures 21–23) and human lung mast cells (Figures 24–28) previously stimulated to undergo AND (149,151,152,161–164). In certain circumstances, we have shown that recovery of human mast cells is simply a reversal of the anatomy of some of the secretory processes (164). Recently, we have also identified recovery

Table 7 Evidence for Factor Involvement in Basophil Secretion

Cellular source of factor	Secreting cell	Factor	Species	References
Mitogen- or antigen-stimulated human mononuclear cells	Peripheral blood (PB) basophil	HRA	Human	223, 224, 337
Streptokinase-streptodornase-activated human mononuclear cells	PB basophil	HRF	Human	326, 337, 338, 346
Peripheral blood T-cells, $CD4^-$ and $CD8^-$ T-cells, B-cells, monocytes	PB basophil	HRF	Human	340
Peripheral blood T-cells stimulated with PHA or streptokinase-streptodornase	PB basophil	BAF	Human	339
Lung macrophages, skin, late-phase blister fluid	PB basophil	HRF IgE-dependent histamine-releasing activity	Human	341, 342
Cultured human peripheral blood monocytes	PB basophil	HRA	Human	344
Mononuclear cells, food allergy	PB basophil	HRF	Human	345
Stimulated platelets	PB basophil	HRA	Human	333, 346
Nasal fluid	PB basophil	HRF	Human	343
Nasal wash fluid	PB basophil	HRA-NW	Rat	346
Neutrophil	PB basophil	HRA-N	Human/rat	336, 346
rhIL-3	PB basophil	IL-3	Monkey	88, 264
rhGM-CSF	PB basophil	IL-3, GM-CSF	Monkey	264
rhIL-3	PB basophil	IL-3	Human	316, 317, 319, 349, 350
rhGM-CSF	PB basophil	GM-CSF	Human	316, 317, 350
rhIL-3	Cord blood cultured basophils	IL-3	Human	59
rhIL-3 + C5a	PB basophil	IL-3 + C5a	Human	318
rhIL-5	Cultured cord blood basophils	IL-5	Human	59
rhIL-5	PB basophil	IL-5	Human	317
rhIL-1	PB basophil	IL-1	Human	335, 352
rhIL-1 + IgE	PB basophil	IL-1	Human	351
IL-1 + D_2O	PB basophil	IL-1	Human	316
Interferon + IgE	PB basophil	Interferon	Human	324, 325, 348
γ-IFN	PB basophil, cultured overnight	γ-IFN	Human	349

human skin mast cells in vivo during wound healing (62). The best interpretation of the images obtained in this study is that human mast cells can also recover from PMD—that is, individual empty containers (granules) accumulate dense materials of diverse morphologies in a wound healing site that was excised for residual melanoma (62). Previous studies have documented PMD of mast cells in superficial spreading melanomas (199). [Also, PMD is a regular finding in tumor stroma mast cells (Dvorak AM, unpublished data).] In Section V, the extensiveness of PMD of tissue mast cells and basophils which infiltrate tissues during pathologic events is documented.

It is clear that the differentiation and maturation of mast cells and basophils are factor dependent in many circumstances (Section VII.B). Moreover, the same factors can independently stimulate, or prime for, or collaborate with IgE, f-Met peptide, C5a, or ionophore to induce release reactions in basophils (Section VII.C). The newly described monokine, monocyte histamine-inhibiting factor (353,354), may be present in circumstances where they effectively abrogate or shut down release of mediators from basophils and mast cells. Because of the unfolding facts implicating cytokines in many stages of basophil and mast cell growth and function, we think that recovery from PMD in vivo may also be under the control of similar (or the same) cytokines. That is, granule rebuilding de novo and granule container refilling, following AND and PMD release reactions, may require cytokines for these processes to occur.

Experiments to evaluate the possibility of factor-dependent recovery from degranulation (either AND or PMD) of basophils and mast cells have not yet been done. Using morphological criteria, we have noted increases in progranule formation of Golgi structures, cytoplasmic immature granule contents, and numbers of mature granules between 30 min and 3 h after degranulating stimuli in factor-dependent mouse mast cells in vitro (Figures 50–52) (Dvorak AM, Galli SJ, unpublished data). These cells have also been shown to express multiple cytokines within the same time frame following stimulation with IgE and antigen (280; see later). It is possible that these recovery changes are facilitated by the cytokines produced by the degranulated cells—i.e., an autoregulatory circuit for repairing granule losses may be factor dependent. Confirmation of these events should soon be possible. Further support for these ideas comes from the work of two groups, which have recently shown that the proliferative potential of degranulated mouse peritoneal mast cells is not reduced by degranulation (355), and that crosslinking of cell-bound IgE on mouse mature peritoneal mast cells stimulates their proliferation (356).

In summary, recovery of basophils and mast cells from degranulation is a combination of the reversal of anatomic secretory events and de-novo synthesis; recovery is analogous, in part, to maturation; some mast cell and basophil differentiation, maturation, and secretion events are under factor (cytokine) control; recovery from degranulation (AND or PMD) may also be under cytokine control; such cytokines may originate from other cells or from mast cells and basophils themselves in autoregulatory circuits stimulated by the release reactions of which these cells are capable and from which they must recover.

E. Cellular Cytokine Production

Support for the possible role of cytokines in recovery events of basophils and mast cells poststimulation was recently obtained by several groups (280,357–363). Ample evidence now exists for the production of a variety of cytokines by mast cells and, in one circumstance, by basophils (Table 8). Some of the cytokines produced by mast cells

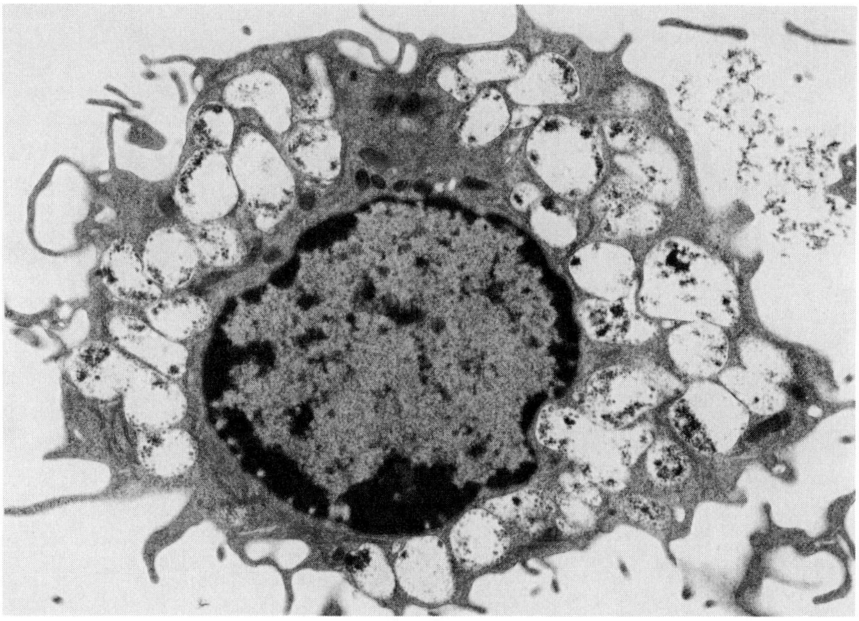

Figure 50 Unstimulated, bone marrow-derived, cultured mouse mast cell shows numerous nearly electron-lucent immature granules containing some vesicles and dense material. ×10,000.

could be directly involved with recovery events by analogy to their known effects on mast cell and basophil differentiation and maturation. For example, IL-3 (294–301) has been shown by five groups to be produced by mouse mast cells (280,357–359,363). In several circumstances, the mast cells producing IL-3 were Ab-MuLV-transformed, mast cell lines (357,359); others showed IL-3 production by nontransformed, IL-3-dependent and -independent mast cells (280,358,363). Production of IL-3 by mast cells was facilitated by an activation signal known to stimulate AND—viz., IgE and antigen. In contrast to the kinetics of histamine secretion and AND occurring within minutes of stimulation by cross-linkage of the $Fc_{\epsilon}R$ (155), IL-3 was detected between 30 min and 1 h poststimulus (358,363). In one study, IL-3 levels decreased thereafter (363), and in another study, it reached maximal levels at 2–6 h poststimulus (358). The time frame of IL-3 production by mouse mast cells poststimulus corresponds to the time frame within which early morphologic recovery events postsecretion occur in human and mouse mast cells (Figure 52) (Dvorak AM and Galli SJ, unpublished data; 164).

Other cytokines are also produced by stimulated mast cells. Several secretory stimuli responsible (in addition to IgE and antigen) include the calcium ionophore A23187, phorbol 12-myristate 13-acetate (PMA), concanavalin-A, and PMA-concanavalin-A combined (280,358,363). Cytokines produced under these circumstances include IL-1 (280), IL-4 (358,359), IL-5 (280,358), IL-6 (280,357,358), granulocyte/macrophage colony-stimulating factor (GM-CSF) (280,357,359,360,363), γ-interferon (γ-IFN) (280), tumor necrosis factor-α (TNF-α) (361,362), TCA3 (280), JE (280), and macrophage inflammatory protein (MIP)-1α and MIP-1β (280). Rat basophil leukemia cells have also been shown to produce TNF-α (362).

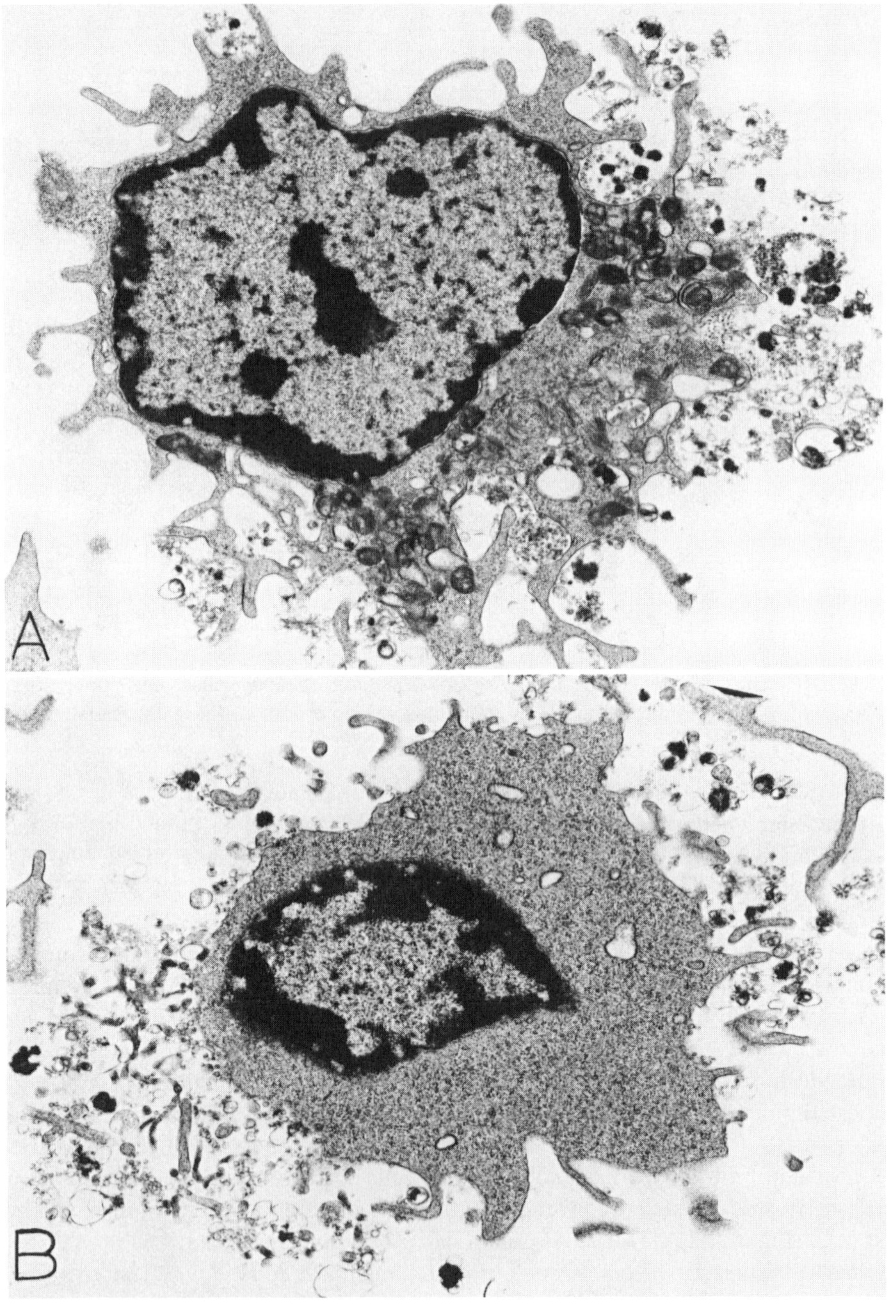

Figure 51 Bone marrow-derived, cultured mouse mast cells, sensitized with IgE and stimulated with antigen, show AND characterized by extruded immature granule vesicular and dense contents (A, B) associated with massive shedding of surface processes (B). A, ×11,000; B, ×13,000.

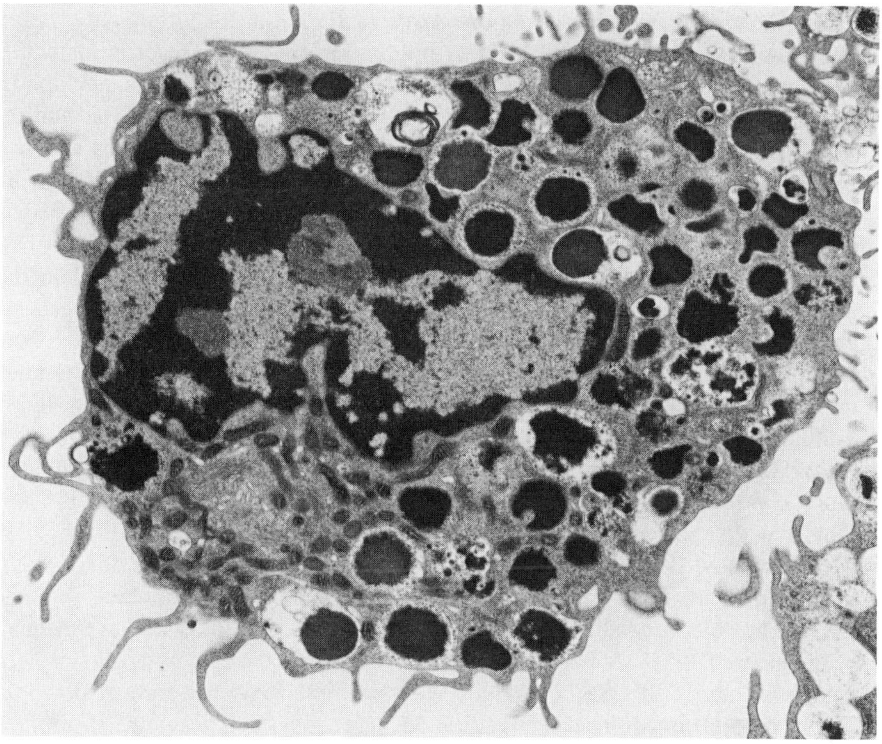

Figure 52 Thirty minutes following stimulation with antigen of IgE-sensitized cells, this bone marrow-derived, cultured mouse mast cell shows recovery of homogeneously dense granule contents in nearly all granules. Some immature granules with vesicles and dense progranules remain. The immature nucleus is increased in size and has a prominent nuclear matrix and large nucleoli. ×10,000.

Table 8 Expression of Cytokines by Mast Cells and Basophils

Cell	Species	Cytokine	References
Mast cell	Mouse	IL-1	280
Mast cell	Mouse	IL-3	280, 357–359, 363
Mast cell	Mouse	IL-4	358, 359
Mast cell	Mouse	IL-5	280, 358
Mast cell	Mouse	IL-6	280, 357, 358
Mast cell	Mouse	GM-CSF	280, 357, 359, 360, 363
Mast cell	Mouse	γ-IFN	280
Mast cell	Mouse	TNF-α	361, 362
Mast cell	Mouse	MIP-1α, MIP-1β	280
Mast cell	Mouse	JE	280
Mast cell	Mouse	TCA3	280
Basophil	Rat	TNF-α	362

Activated macrophages are the major source of IL-1, but numerous other cell types are also known to produce this ubiquitous interleukin (364). These cells include fibroblasts, endothelial cells, Langerhans' cells, mesangial cells, B- and T-lymphocytes, natural killer (NK) cells, astrocytes and microglial cells, corneal, gingival, and thymic epithelial cells, keratinocytes, and smooth muscle cells (364). Mast cells can now be added to this list (280). This widespread cellular array results in the appearance of IL-1 in a wide variety of pathological processes, including those induced by exogenous infectious agents, injury, and immunologic mechanisms.

Interleukin-4 is produced by a subset of T-helper cells and is involved in the up-regulation of IgE production by B-cells (365–372). IL-4 also enhances mast cell growth and induces T-cell activation and proliferation (365,373–376). Mast cells, by their activation-regulated production of IL-4 (358,359), may also participate in autoregulatory or intercellular processes through the known functions of IL-4 (365–376). Interleukin-5 induces eosinophil differentiation, maturation, and activation (59, 258,377,378,501). Production of IL-5 by mast cells (280,358) can now be implicated in regulatory control of these eosinophil events by mast cells. Interleukin-6 is also produced by a wide spectrum of cell types [including tumor cells (379–381)], to which mast cells can now be added (280,357,358). IL-6 is a growth factor for B cells and plasmacytomas, and it has a wide target spectrum of activity in multiple pathologies (379–381). The role of production of this interleukin by mast cells in these events must now be considered.

γ-Interferon and GM-CSF, cytokines with multiple activities, are also within the production repertoire of mast cells (280,357,359,360,363). Review of the myriad activities of these cytokines is not possible here. However, γ-IFN can act to antagonize IgE production (382) and, in these circumstances, could act to down-regulate an IgE-mediated secretory event in mast cells and basophils. GM-CSF is a growth factor for granulocytes and macrophages, as assayed by colonies stimulated to grow in soft agar or methylcellulose cultures (383–387).

A new family of cytokines includes those designated as TCA3, JE, MIP-1α, MIP-1β (280,388–393). These novel cytokines have now been shown to be produced by mast cells (280) as well as by fibroblasts, lymphocytes, and macrophages (388–393). The multiple activities of these cytokines are under investigation (393). Macrophage inflammatory proteins 1 and 2 are pro-inflammatory proteins which attract neutrophils to local sites and activate them (392,393). They also have an enhancing effect on colony formation in vitro by human and murine bone marrow granulocyte/macrophage progenitor cells (394).

TNF-α has been shown to be produced by mouse mast cells (361,362) and rat basophil leukemia cells (362). Factor-dependent, cultured mouse mast cells were initially shown by Galli et al. to be devoid of NK-like activity in tumor cytotoxicity assays (277). More recently, natural cytotoxic (NC) activity of similarly derived mouse mast cells and rat basophil leukemia cells has been demonstrated (395,396). This activity was shown to resemble that of TNF, and could be triggered to be released by IgE-dependent mechanisms (362,396). Previously, in in-vivo models of tumor rejection in guinea pigs, we demonstrated the participation of basophilic leukocytes in this process (186,187). TNF production by activated mast cells and basophils may be, in part, responsible for these interactions.

F. Intercellular Interactions

From the previous sections, the potential for intercellular interactions of basophils and mast cells can be seen to be extensive. These interactions include those with other inflammatory cells, such as lymphocytes, macrophages, eosinophils, platelets, neutrophils, as well as with cells comprising external and internal barriers (epithelium, endothelium) to the environment and cells of mesenchymal origin involved either in integrated units of motion and messages, as seen in muscle and nerves, or in repair processes involving fibroblasts in wound healing. It is not possible to review these interactions in detail. Nor is it possible to identify all possible roles for cytokines in the mechanisms involved with these interactions. Cytokines produced by, and/or acting on, basophils and mast cells almost certainly are involved in many of the possible intercellular interactions of which basophils and mast cells are capable.

We call attention to the wide range of possible mast cell-basophil intercellular events by reviewing a sample of these events here. Effects of mast cells on lymphocyte functions are exemplified by a role which mast cell granules play in lymphocyte biology. For example, Frieri and Metcalfe (397) showed first that mast cell granules, and subsequently the native heparin within them, modulate lymphocyte blastogenesis by inhibiting mitogen induction of activation of lymphocytes. Mast cell-macrophage interactions include those related to arachidonic acid metabolism. For example, although both cells are known to produce key metabolites of arachidonic acid important to inflammatory processes, Salari and Chan-Yeung showed increased mediator production as well as a change in the profile of arachidonic acid metabolism when purified cells of both types were co-incubated in the presence of activation signals (398). Mast cell products (e.g., heparin) have also been shown to increase a mononuclear cell factor similar to IL-1 when peripheral blood mononuclear cells were cultured with mast cell products or heparin (399).

Possibilities for mast cell-eosinophil interactions are many. One recent example illustrates an interesting potential interaction (400). Eosinophils were shown to transform exogenous PGD_2 to PGF_2 but produced very small quantities of PGD_2 themselves, when appropriately activated. These studies, showing the ability to use exogenous PGD_2 to produce another prostaglandin group, PGF_2, with different functional activities, by eosinophils, might be important in inflammation. Mast cells, when stimulated, generate and release PGD_2 which could be utilized by subjacent eosinophils for this purpose.

Important mast cell effects on noninflammatory cells are shown in two recent studies. For example, human mast cell granule tryptase was shown to activate a latent collagenase in rheumatoid synoviöcytes (401), and co-culture of mouse mast cells and fibroblasts resulted in stimulation of synthesis of the Forssman glycolipid by fibroblasts (402). These examples of important intercellular interactions among mast cells and basophils (or their products) and other cells have generally been assayed in in-vitro circumstances. What information exists from in-vivo experiments to implicate important interactions of mast cells and basophils with other cells in disease? Galli has recently reviewed uses of the genetically mast cell-deficient mouse strains and their reconstitution with cloned mast cells in attempts to answer these questions in in-vivo models (282–284). One example of such a model is in the study of acute inflammation (403). In this case, the data clearly show the necessity for mast cells for the full expression of the acute inflammatory response induced in mouse skin by PMA in vivo, thus implicating mast cells in pro-inflammatory events of nonimmunological origin.

VIII. CONCLUDING REMARKS

The similarities and differences between basophils and mast cells are evident using ultrastructural tools. These likenesses and differences extend to multiple species, to anatomic release and recovery reactions, to possible regulation of differentiation, maturation and functional properties, as well as to the generation of cytokines.

A continuum of anatomic release reactions exists which spans the extensive morphologies associated with AND to the more subtle morphologies associated with PMD. AND is regularly expressed in appropriate ex-vivo experimental systems; PMD has been regularly identified in tissue mast cells and basophils in multiple circumstances.

Anatomic mechanisms by which recovery from AND takes place in human mast cells involve two distinct processes—i.e., recovery (reversing the steps of degranulation) and regranulation (de-novo synthesis of new granules). In recovery, individual granules that have not gone beyond the swelling phase (i.e., to fusion with other granules) may revert to a normal appearance; thus, the first phase of degranulation is reversible. Subsequent steps involving granule fusion and partial granule content discharge may also be reversible—i.e., degranulation channels may repartition into granule-sized compartments with recovery of granule contents that have not yet been discharged. This recovery mechanism leads to repackaging of granules by recovering their unspent contents and recycling their membrane containers.

The regranulation steps taken by fully degranulated cells are much more complex and require nuclear and cytoplasmic changes that result in forms which resemble immature cells. Following completion of the acute phase of AND, after granule contents have been discharged from the cells, granule membranes become incorporated as part of the cell's plasma membrane. Subsequently, large portions of the cell's plasma membrane are apparently shed, resulting in smaller but still viable cells. Such degranulated cells subsequently synthesize new granule membranes and fill these with tightly packaged, newly synthesized granule contents. These events point to mechanisms by which mature cells (particularly cells such as mature basophilic leukocytes which have been thought to be terminally differentiated "end" cells in vivo) may dedifferentiate and be renewed within a matter of days under defined conditions in vitro.

We think it is entirely possible that the morphologies associated with factor-dependent differentiation and maturation of basophils and mast cells in vitro, as well as similar developmental processes in vivo, are recapitulated in the recovery of basophils and mast cells from the explosive morphologies associated with AND and the refilling of emptied, discrete containers associated with PMD. These recovery possibilities may well be regulated by cytokines, as are various differentiation and maturation events. Such regulatory cytokines may originate from basophils and mast cells, or a wide variety of other environmental circumstances and cells, in the milieu of basophils and mast cells.

ACKNOWLEDGMENTS

We thank Peter K. Gardner for editorial assistance, and Ellen Morgan, Rita Monahan-Earley, Patricia Estrella, Linda Letourneau, and Susan Kissell for expert technical assistance.

This work was supported by USPHS grant CA-28834.

REFERENCES

1. Ehrlich P. Beiträge zur Kenntnis der Anilinfärbungen und ihrer Verwendung in der mikroskopischen Technik. Arch Mikrosk Anat 1877; 13:263–77.
2. Ehrlich P. Beiträge zur Kenntnis der granulierten Bindegewebszellen und der eosinophilen Leukocyten. Arch Anat Physiol 1879; 3:166–9.
3. Dvorak HF, Dvorak AM. Basophilic leukocytes: structure, function, and role in disease. In: Lichtman MA, ed. Clinics in hematology. Granulocyte and monocyte abnormalities, vol. 4. London: WB Saunders, 1975:651–83.
4. Juhlin L. Basophil leukocyte differential in blood and bone marrow. Acta Haematol 1963; 29:89–95.
5. Mitchell RG. Basophilic leukocytes in children in health and disease. Arch Dis Child 1958; 33:193–201.
6. Thonnard-Neumann E. Studies of basophils. Variations with age and sex. Acta Haematol 1963; 30:221–8.
7. Michels NA. The mast cells. In: Downey H, ed. Handbook of haematology, vol. 1. New York: Paul B. Hoeber, 1938:232–372 [reprinted in Ann NY Acad Sci 1963; 103(App):1–372].
8. Boseila A-WA. Hormonal influence on blood and tissue basophilic granulocytes. Ann NY Acad Sci 1963; 103:394–408.
9. Youman JD, Taddeini L, Cooper T. Histamine excess symptoms in basophilic chronic granulocytic leukemia. Arch Intern Med 1973; 131:560–2.
10. Maloney WC, Lange RD. Cytologic and biochemical studies on granulocytes in early leukemia among atomic bomb survivors. Tex Rep Biol Med 1954; 12:887–97.
11. Juhlin L. Basophil and eosinophil leukocytes in various internal disorders. Acta Med Scand 1963; 174:249–55.
12. Shelley WB, Parnes HM. The absolute basophil count. JAMA 1965; 192:108–10.
13. Djalali A, Hunziker N, Jadassohn W. Untersuchungen über die Zahl der basophilen Leukocyten im Blut des Menschen und des Meerschweinchens. Hautarzt 1968; 18:150–2.
14. Rorsman H. Studies on basophil leukocytes with special reference to urticaria and anaphylaxis. Acta Derm Verereol 1962; 42[Suppl 48]:1–20.
15. Shelley WB, Juhlin L. New test for detecting anaphylactic sensitivity: basophil reaction. Nature 1961; 191:1056–8.
16. Dvorak AM. Human mast cells. In: Beck F, Hild W, Kriz W, Ortmann R, Pauly JE, Schiebler TH, eds. Advances in anatomy embryology and cell biology, vol. 114. Berlin: Springer-Verlag, 1989:1–107.
17. Peters SP, Dvorak AM, Schulman ES. Mast cells. In: Massaro D, ed. Lung cell biology, vol. 41. Series: Lung biology in health and disease (Lenfant C, series ed). New York: Marcel Dekker, 1989:345–99.
18. Dvorak HF, Mihm MC Jr, Dvorak AM, Johnson RA, Manseau EJ, Morgan E, Colvin RB. Morphology of delayed type hypersensitivity reactions in man. I. Quantitative description of the inflammatory response. Lab Invest 1974; 31:111–30.

19. Wolf-Jürgensen P. Basophilic leukocytes in delayed hypersensitivity. Experimental studies in man using the skin window technique. Copenhagen: Munksgaard, 1966.
20. Dvorak HF, Mihm MC Jr. Basophilic leukocytes in allergic contact dermatitis. J Exp Med 1972; 135:235–54.
21. Klausner E, Kreibich C. Über den Mastzellengehalf vesikulöser Hauteffloreszenzen. Folia Haematol 1913; 15:347–50.
22. Juhlin L. Basophil leukocytes in blood and inflammatory exudate. Acta Derm Venereol 1963; 43:528–43.
23. Aspegren N, Fregert S, Rorsman H. Basophil leukocytes in lesions of various dermatoses. Acta Derm Venereol 1963; 43:544–7.
24. Fregert S, Rorsman H. Basophil leukocytes in photo contact dermatitis. J Invest Dermatol 1964; 42:405–6.
25. Juhlin L, Ohman S. Basophil and eosinophil leukocytes in cantharidin blisters of patients with various dermatoses. Acta Derm Venereol 1964; 44:403–14.
26. Dvorak AM, Monahan RA, Osage JE, Dickersin GR. Crohn's disease: transmission electron microscopic studies. II. Immunologic inflammatory response. Alterations of mast cells, basophils, eosinophils, and the microvasculature. Hum Pathol 1980; 11:606–19.
27. Dvorak AM, Dickersin GR. Crohn's disease, electron microscopic studies. In: Sommers SC, Rosen PP, eds. Pathology annual—Part 2, vol. 14. New York: Appleton-Century-Crofts, 1979:259–306.
28. Dvorak AM, Mihm MC Jr, Osage JE, Kwan TH, Austen KF, Wintroub BU. Bullous pemphigoid, an ultrastructural study of the inflammatory response: eosinophil, basophil and mast cell granule changes in multiple biopsies from one patient. J Invest Dermatol 1982; 78:91–101.
29. Colvin RB, Dvorak HF. Basophils and mast cells in renal allograft rejection. Lancet 1974; i:212–4.
30. Dvorak HF, Dvorak AM. Basophils, mast cells and cellular immunity in animals and man. Hum Pathol 1972; 3:454–6.
31. Dvorak AM. Biology and morphology of basophilic leukocytes. In: Bach MK, ed. Immediate hypersensitivity—modern concepts and developments. Immunology series, vol. 7. New York: Marcel Dekker, 1978:369–405.
32. Dvorak AM. Morphologic and immunologic characterization of human basophils, 1879 to 1985. Riv Immunol Immunofarmacol 1988; 8:50–82.
33. Dvorak AM. Blood cell biochemistry, vol. 4: Basophil and mast cell degranulation and recovery. London: Plenum Publishing, 1991: 1–415. Series ed. Harris JJ, vol. Ed. Dvorak AM.
34. Hatanaka K, Kitamura Y, Nishimune Y. Local development of mast cells from bone marrow-derived precursors in the skin of mice. Blood 1979; 53:142–7.
35. Kitamura Y, Shimada M, Hatanaka K, Miyano Y. Development of mast cells from grafted bone marrow cells in irradiated mice. Nature 1977; 268:442–3.
36. Kitamura Y, Hatanaka K, Murakami M, Shibata H. Presence of mast cell precursors in peripheral blood of mice demonstrated by parabiosis. Blood 1979; 53:1085–8.
37. Dvorak HF, Dvorak AM. Cutaneous basophil hypersensitivity. In: Brent L, Holborow EJ, eds. Progress in immunology II, vol. 3. Amsterdam: North-Holland, 1974:171–81.
38. Dvorak HF, Orenstein NS, Galli SJ, Dvorak AM. Cutaneous basophil hypersensitivity. In: Pepys J, Edwards AM, eds. The mast cell. Its role in health and disease. Kent: Pitman Medical Publishing, 1979:76–82.
39. Galli SJ, Dvorak AM, Dvorak HF. Basophils and mast cells: morphologic insights into their biology, secretory patterns, and function. In: Ishizaka K, ed. Progress in allergy. Mast cell activation and mediator release, vol. 34. Basel, Switzerland: S Karger, 1984:1–141.
40. Dvorak HF, Dvorak AM. Basophilic leukocytes in delayed-type hypersensitivity reactions in experimental animals and man. In: Jankovic BD, Isakovic K, eds. Microenvironmental aspects of immunity. New York: Plenum Publishing, Adv Exp Med Biol 1973; 29:573–9.

41. Dvorak AM, Nabel G, Pyne K, Cantor H, Dvorak HF, Galli SJ. Ultrastructural identification of the mouse basophil. Blood 1982; 59:1279–85.
42. Dvorak AM. Morphologic expressions of maturation and function can affect the ability to identify mast cells and basophils in man, guinea pig and mouse. In: Befus AD, Bienenstock J, Denburg JA, eds. Mast cell differentiation and heterogeneity. New York: Raven Press, 1986:95–114.
43. Dvorak AM, Monahan RA. Guinea pig bone marrow basophilopoiesis. J Exp Pathol 1985; 2:13–24.
44. Dvorak AM, Ishizaka T, Galli SJ. Ultrastructure of human basophils developing in vitro. Evidence for the acquisition of peroxidase by basophils and for different effects of human and murine growth factors on human basophil and eosinophil maturation. Lab Invest 1985; 53:57–71.
45. Combs JW. Maturation of rat mast cells. An electron microscope study. J Cell Biol 1966; 31:563–75.
46. Combs JW, Lagunoff D, Benditt EP. Differentiation and proliferation of embryonic mast cells of the rat. J Cell Biol 1965; 25:577–92.
47. Combs JW. An electron microscope study of mouse mast cells arising in vivo and in vitro. J Cell Biol 1971; 48:676–84.
48. Furitsu T, Saito H, Dvorak AM, Schwartz LB, Irani A-MA, Burdick JF, Ishizaka K, Ishizaka T. Development of human mast cells in vitro. Proc Natl Acad Sci USA 1989; 86:10039–43.
49. Dvorak AM, Mihm MC Jr, Dvorak HF. Degranulation of basophilic leukocytes in allergic contact dermatitis reactions in man. J Immunol 1976; 116:687–95.
50. Dvorak AM. The fine structure of human basophils and mast cells. In: Holgate ST, ed. Mast cells, mediators and disease. Lancaster: Kluwer Academic Publishers, 1988:29–97.
51. Fox CC, Dvorak AM, MacGlashan DW Jr, Lichtenstein LM. Histamine-containing cells in human peritoneal fluid. J Immunol 1984; 132:2177–9.
52. Dvorak AM, Newball HH, Dvorak HF, Lichtenstein LM. Antigen-induced IgE-mediated degranulation of human basophils. Lab Invest 1980; 43:126–39.
53. Dvorak AM, Ackerman SJ. Ultrastructural localization of the Charcot-Leyden crystal protein (lysophospholipase) to granules and intragranular crystals in mature human basophils. Lab Invest 1989; 60:557–67.
54. Zucker-Franklin D. Electron microscopic study of human basophils. Blood 1967; 29:878–90.
55. Hastie R. A study of the ultrastructure of human basophil leukocytes. Lab Invest 1974; 31:223–31.
56. Parmley RT, Ogawa M, Spicer SS, Wright NJ. Ultrastructure and cytochemistry of bone marrow granulocytes in culture. Exp Hematol 1976; 4:75–89.
57. Wetzel B. The comparative structure of normal and diseased mammalian granulocytes. In: Gordan AS, ed. Regulation of hematopoiesis, vol. 12. New York: Appleton-Century-Crofts, 1970;819–72.
58. Dvorak AM, Monahan RA. Crohn's disease. Ultrastructural studies showing basophil leukocyte granule changes and lymphocyte parallel tubular arrays in the peripheral blood. Arch Pathol Lab Med 1982; 106:145–9.
59. Dvorak AM, Saito H, Estrella P, Kissell S, Arai N, Ishizaka T. Ultrastructure of eosinophils and basophils stimulated to develop in human cord blood mononuclear cell cultures containing recombinant human interleukin-5 or interleukin-3. Lab Invest 1989; 61:116–32.
60. Ackerman SJ, Weil GJ, Gleich GJ. Formation of Charcot-Leyden crystals by human basophils. J Exp Med 1982; 155:1597–609.
61. Dvorak AM, Hammel I, Schulman ES, Peters SP, MacGlashan DW Jr, Schleimer RP, Newball HH, Pyne K, Dvorak HF, Lichtenstein LM, Galli SJ. Differences in the behavior of cytoplasmic granules and lipid bodies during human lung mast cell degranulation. J Cell Biol 1984; 99:1678–87.

62. Dvorak AM, Kissell S. Granule changes of human skin mast cells characteristic of piecemeal degranulation and associated with recovery during wound healing in situ. J Leukocyte Biol 1991; 49:197–210.
63. Fedorko ME, Hirsch JG. Crystalloid structure in granules of guinea pig basophils and human mast cells. J Cell Biol 1965; 26:973–6.
64. Kobayasi T, Midtgård K, Asboe-Hansen G. Ultrastructure of human mast-cell granules. J Ultrastruct Res 1968; 23:153–65.
65. Ts´'ao C-h, Patterson R, McKenna JM, Suszko JM. Ultrastructural identification of mast cells obtained from human bronchial lumens. J Allergy Clin Immunol 1977; 59:320–6.
66. Fox B, Bull TB, Guz A. Mast cells in the human alveolar wall: an electron microscopic study. J Clin Pathol 1981; 34:1333–42.
67. Orr TSC. Fine structure of the mast cell with special reference to human cells. Scand J. Resp Dis 1977; 98[suppl]:1–12.
68. Dvorak AM, Galli SJ, Morgan E, Galli AS, Hammond ME, Dvorak HF. Anaphylactic degranulation of guinea pig basophilic leukocytes. I. Fusion of granule membranes and cytoplasmic vesicles: formation and resolution of degranulation sacs. Lab Invest 1981; 44:174–91.
69. Winqvist G. Electron microscopy of the basophilic granulocyte. Ann NY Acad Sci 1963; 103:352–75.
70. Terry RW, Bainton DF, Farquhar MG. Formation and structure of specific granules in basophilic leukocytes of the guinea pig. Lab Invest 1969; 21:65–76.
71. Murata F, Spicer SS. Ultrastructural comparison of basophilic leukocytes and mast cells in the guinea pig. Am J Anat 1974; 139:335–52.
72. Winqvist G. The ultrastructure of the granules of the basophil granulocyte. Zeitschrift für Zellforschung mikroskopische Anatomie 1960; 52:475–81.
73. Chan BST, Yoffey JM. The basophil cells of guinea pig bone marrow and their response to horse serum. Immunology 1960; 3:237–43.
74. Terry RW, Bainton DF, Farquhar MG. Formation and structure of "crystalline" granules in basophilic leukocytes of the guinea pig. Anat Rec 1968; 160:440 [abstr].
75. Watanabe Y. An electron microscopic study of the leukocytes in bone marrow of guinea pig. J Electron Microsc [Tokyo] 1954; 2:34–9.
76. Hebert H, Lindberg M. Granules in basophil leukocytes from guinea pig dermis and granules isolated from basophil leukocytes in guinea pig blood and bone marrow: a structural study by electron microscopy and optical diffraction. J Ultrastruct Res 1982; 78:215–25.
77. Pearce FL, Behrendt H, Blum U, Poblete-Freundt G, Pult P, Stang-Voss CH, Schmutzler W. Isolation and study of functional mast cells from lung and mesentery of guinea pig. Agents Actions 1977; 7:45–56.
78. Taichman NS. Ultrastructure of guinea pig mast cells. J Ultrastruct Res 1970; 32:284–92.
79. Taichman NS. Ultrastructural alterations in guinea pig mast cells during anaphylaxis. Int Arch Allergy Appl Immunol 1971; 40:934–42.
80. Stock EL, Hill, RA, Boyle-Vaura S, Roth SI. Eosinophil and mast cell homogeneity of the guinea pig eyelid, skin, conjunctiva and ileum. Am J Anat 1989; 186:359–68.
81. Hoenig EM, Levine S. Three localized forms of experimental allergic encephalomyelitis: an ultrastructural comparison. J Neuropathol Exp Neurol 1974; 33:251–9.
82. Palade GE. Studies on the endoplasmic reticulum. II. Simple dispositions in cells in situ. J Biophys Biochem Cytol 1955; 1:567–601.
83. Bentfeld-Barker ME, Bainton DF. Cytochemical localization of arylsulfatase B in rat basophils and mast cells. J Histochem Cytochem 1980; 28:1055–61.
84. Bentfeld ME, Nichols BA, Bainton DF. Ultrastructural localization of peroxidase in leukocytes of rat bone marrow and blood. Anat Rec 1977; 187:219–40.
85. Login GR, Galli SJ, Morgan E, Arizono N, Schwartz LB, Dvorak AM. Rapid microwave fixation of rat mast cells. I. Localization of granule chymase with an ultrastructural pos-

tembedding immunogold technique. Lab Invest 1987; 57:592–9.
86. Hammel I, Dvorak AM, Galli SJ. Defective cytoplasmic granule formation. I. Abnormalities affecting tissue mast cells and pancreatic acinar cells of beige mice. Lab Invest 1987; 56:321–8.
87. Galli SJ, Arizono N, Murakami T, Dvorak AM, Fox JG. Development of large numbers of mast cells at sites of idiopathic chronic dermatitis in genetically mast cell-deficient $WBB6F_1$-W/W^v mice. Blood 1987; 69:1661–6.
88. Dvorak AM, Monahan-Earley RA, Estrella P, Kissell S, Donahue RE. Ultrastructure of monkey peripheral blood basophils stimulated to develop in vivo by recombinant human interleukin 3. Lab Invest 1989; 61:677–90.
89. Ts´'ao C-h, Metzger J, Patterson R, Suszko JM. Histamine-containing cells in bronchial lavage fluid. I. Ultrastructural characterization and comparison with mast cells in three types of tissues of Rhesus monkeys. Int Arch Allergy Appl Immunol 1976; 52:315–24.
90. Patterson R, Ts´'ao C-h, Suszko IM. Heterogeneity of bronchial lumen mast cells which are homogeneous by electron microscopy. J Allergy Clin Immunol 1980; 65:278–84.
91. Barrett KE, Metcalfe DD. The histologic and functional characterization of enzymatically dispersed intestinal mast cells of non-human primates: effects of secretogogues and anti-allergic drugs on histamine secretion. J Immunol 1985; 135:2020–6.
92. Wetzel BK, Horn RG, Spicer SS. Fine structural studies on the development of heterophil, eosinophil and basophil granulocytes in rabbits. Lab Invest 1967; 16:349–82.
93. Benveniste J, Henson PM, Cochrane CG. Leukocyte-dependent histamine release from rabbit platelets. J Exp Med 1972; 136:1356–77.
94. Hardin JH, Spicer SS. Ultrastructural localization of dialyzed iron-reactive mucosubstance in rabbit heterophils, basophils, and eosinophils. J Cell Biol 1971; 48:368–86.
95. Komiyama A, Spicer SS. Ultrastructural localization of a characteristic acid phosphatase in granules of rabbit basophils. J Histochem Cytochem 1974; 22:1092–104.
96. Horn RG, Spicer SS. Sulfated mucopolysaccharide and basic protein in certain granules of rabbit leukocytes. Lab Invest 1964; 13:1–15.
97. Bauer H, Zvaifler NJ, Robinson JO. IgE immunoglobulin in the rabbit. The histopathology of the homologous passive cutaneous anaphylaxis reaction. Lab Invest 1972; 26:448–58.
98. Ishizaka K, Ishizaka T. Identification of gamma-E-antibodies as a carrier of reaginic activity. J Immunol 1967; 99:1187–98.
99. Ishizaka T, Ishizaka K. Activation of mast cells for mediator release through IgE receptors. Prog Allergy 1984; 34:188–235.
100. Becker KE, Ishizaka T, Metzger H, Ishizaka K, Grimley PM. Surface IgE on human basophils during histamine release. J Exp Med 1973; 138:394–409.
101. Sullivan AL, Grimley PM, Metzger H. Electron microscopic localization of immunoglobulin E on the surface membrane of human basophils. J Exp Med 1971; 134:1403–16.
102. van Elven EH, Stallman PJ, Bruhl PC. Electron microscopic studies on human basophils from atopic and non-atopic subjects, using horse radish peroxidase labelled anti-IgE. Int Arch Allergy Appl Immunol 1977; 54:560–7.
103. Ishizaka T, Ishizaka K. Biology of immunoglobulin E. Molecular basis of reaginic hypersensitivity. Prog Allergy 1975; 19:60–121.
104. Dembo M, Goldstein B, Sobotka AK, Lichtenstein LM. Histamine release due to bivalent penicilloyl haptens: control by the number of cross-linked IgE antibodies on the basophil plasma membrane. J Immunol 1978; 121:354–8.
105. Isersky C, Taurog JD, Poy G, Metzger H. Triggering of cultured neoplastic mast cells by antibodies to the receptor for IgE. J Immunol 1978; 121:549–58.
106. Ishizaka T, Ishizaka K, Conrad DH, Froese A. A new concept of triggering mechanisms of IgE-mediated histamine release. J Allergy Clin Immunol 1978; 61:320–30.
107. Siraganian RP, Hook WA, Levine BB. Specific in vitro histamine release from basophils by bivalent haptens: evidence for activation by simple bridging of membrane-bound antibody. Immunochemistry 1975; 12:149–57.

108. Warner JA, Peters SP, Lichtenstein LM, Hubbard W, Yancey KB, Stevenson HC, Miller PJ, MacGlashan DW Jr. Differential release of mediators from human basophils: differences in arachidonic acid metabolism following activation by unrelated stimuli. J Leukocyte Biol 1989; 45:558–71.
109. Smith PL, Kagey-Sobotka A, Bleecker ER, Traystman R, Kaplan AP, Gralnick H, Valentine MD, Permutt S, Lichtenstein LM. Physiologic manifestations of anaphylaxis. J Clin Invest 1980; 66:1072–80.
110. Siraganian RP, Hook WA. Complement-induced histamine release from human basophils. II. Mechanism of the histamine release reaction. J Immunol 1976; 116:639–46.
111. Needleman P, Turk J, Jakschik BA, Morrison AR, Lefkowith JB. Arachidonic acid metabolism. Ann Rev Biochem 1986; 55:69–102.
112. Orange RP, Austen KF. Slow reacting substance of anaphylaxis. Adv Immunol 1969; 10:105–44.
113. Samuelsson B. Leukotrienes: mediators of immediate hypersensitivity reactions and inflammation. Science 1983; 220:568–75.
114. Samuelsson B, Granstrom E, Green K, Hamberg M, Hammarstrom S. Prostaglandins. Ann Rev Biochem 1975; 44:669–95.
115. MacGlashan DW Jr, Schleimer RP, Peters SP, Schulman ES, Lichtenstein LM. Generation of leukotrienes by purified human lung mast cells. J Clin Invest 1982; 70:747–51.
116. Peters SP, MacGlashan DW Jr, Schulman ES, Schleimer RP, Hayes EC, Rokach J, Adkinson NF Jr, Lichenstein LM. Arachidonic acid metabolism in purified lung mast cells. J Immunol 1984; 132:1972–9.
117. Dvorak AM, Galli SJ, Schulman ES, Lichtenstein LM, Dvorak HF. Basophil and mast cell degranulation: ultrastructural analysis of mechanisms of mediator release. Fed Proc 1983; 42:2510–5.
118. Ishizaka T, Dvorak AM, Conrad DH, Niebyl JR, Marquette JP, Ishizaka K. Morphologic and immunologic characterization of human basophils developed in cultures of cord blood mononuclear cells. J Immunol 1985; 134:532–40.
119. Findlay SR, Dvorak AM, Kagey-Sobotka A, Lichtenstein LM. Hyperosmolar triggering of histamine release from human basophils. J Clin Invest 1981; 67:1604–13.
120. Dvorak AM, Lett-Brown M, Thueson D, Grant JA. Complement-induced degranulation of human basophils. J Immunol 1981; 126:523–8.
121. Dvorak AM, Lett-Brown MA, Thueson DO, Pyne K, Raghuprasad PK, Galli SJ, Grant JA. Histamine-releasing activity (HRA). III. HRA induces human basophil histamine release by provoking noncytotoxic granule exocytosis. Clin Immunol Immunopathol 1984; 32:142–50.
122. Dvorak AM, Warner JA, Kissell S, Lichtenstein LM, MacGlashan DW Jr. f-Met peptide-induced degranulation of human basophils. Lab Invest 1991; 64;234–53.
123. Hastie R, Levy DA, Weiss L. The antigen-induced degranulation of basophil leukocytes from atopic subjects studied by electron microscopy. Lab Invest 1977; 36:173–82.
124. Pruzansky JJ, Ts´'ao C-h, Krajewski DV, Zeiss CR, Patterson R. Quantification of ultrastructural variations in enriched blood basophils: correlation of morphological changes and antiqen-induced histamine release. Immunology 1982; 47:41–7.
125. Dvorak AM, Schulman ES, Peters SP, MacGlashan DW Jr, Newball HH, Schleimer RP, Lichtenstein LM. Immunoglobulin E-mediated degranulation of isolated human lung mast cells. Lab Invest 1985; 53:45–56.
126. Dvorak AM, Massey W, Warner J, Kissell S, Kagey-Sobotka A, Lichtenstein LM. IgE-mediated anaphylactic degranulation of human skin mast cells. Blood 1991; 77:569–78.
127. Dvorak AM. Mast cell degranulation in human hearts. N Engl J Med 1986; 315:969–70.
128. Dvorak AM. Ultrastructure of human gastrointestinal system. Interactions among mast cells, eosinophils, nerves and muscle in human disease. In: Snape WJ Jr, Collins SM, eds. Effects of immune cells and inflammation on smooth muscle and enteric nerves. Boca Raton, FL: CRC Press Inc., 1991; 139–68.

129. Caulfield JP, Lewis RA, Hein A, Austen KF. Secretion in dissociated pulmonary mast cells. J Cell Biol 1980; 85:299–312.
130. Benyon RC, Lowman MA, Church MK. Human skin mast cells: their dispersion, purification, and secretory characterization. J Immunol 1987; 138:861–7.
131. Lawrence ID, Warner JA, Cohan VL, Hubbard WC, Kagey-Sobotka A, Lichtenstein LM. Purification and characterization of human skin mast cells. Evidence for human mast cell heterogeneity. J Immunol 1987; 139:3062–9.
132. Lawrence ID, Warner JA, Cohan VL, Lichtenstein LM, Kagey-Sobotka A, Vavrek RJ, Stewart JM, Proud D. Induction of histamine release from human skin mast cells by bradykinin analogs. Biochem Pharmacol 1989; 38:227–33.
133. Irani AA, Schechter NM, Craig S, DeBlois G, Schwartz LB. Two human mast cell subsets with different neutral protease compositions (abstr). J Allergy Clin Immunol 1986; 77(#1, part 2) (suppl):247.
134. Irani AA, Schechter NM, Craig SS, DeBlois G, Schwartz LB. Two types of human mast cells that have distinct neutral protease compositions. Proc Natl Acad Sci USA 1986; 83:4464–8.
135. Craig SS, Schechter NM, Schwartz LB. Ultrastructural analysis of human T and TC mast cells identified by immunoelectron microscopy. Lab Invest 1988; 58:682–91.
136. Craig SS, Schechter NM, Schwartz LB. Ultrastructural analysis of maturing human T and TC mast cells in situ. Lab Invest 1989; 60:147–57.
137. Tharp MD, Kagey-Sobotka A, Fox CC, Marone G, Lichtenstein LM, Sullivan TJ. Functional heterogeneity of human mast cells from different anatomic sites: in vitro responses to morphine sulfate. J Allergy Clin Immunol 1987; 79:646–53.
138. Kobayasi T, Asboe-Hansen G. Degranulation and regranulation of human mast cells. An electron microscopic study of the whealing reaction in urticaria pigmentosa. Acta Derm Venereol 1969; 49:369–81.
139. Swerlick RA, Yancey KB, Lawley TJ. A direct in vivo comparison of the inflammatory properties of human $C5_a$ and $C5_a$ desArg in human skin. J Immunol 1988; 140:2376–81.
140. Yancey KB, Hammer CH, Harvath L, Renfer L, Frank MM, Lawley TJ. Studies of human $C5_a$ as a mediator of inflammation in normal skin. J Clin Invest 1985; 75:486–95.
141. Hashimoto K, Gross BG, Lever WF. An electron microscopic study of the degranulation of mast cell granules in urticaria pigmentosa. J Invest Dermatol 1966; 46:139–49.
142. Moriyasu S, Yamura T. Electron microscopic studies of mast cell degranulation. Acta Derm Venereol Suppl 1973; 53(suppl 73):149–56.
143. Friedman MM, Kaliner M. Ultrastructural changes in human skin mast cells during antigen-induced degranulation in vivo. J Allergy Clin Immunol 1988; 82:998–1005.
144. Askenase PW, Haynes JD, Hayden BJ. Antibody-mediated basophil accumulations in cutaneous hypersensitivity reactions in guinea pigs. J Immunol 1976; 117:216–24.
145. Mitchell EB, Brown SJ, Askenase PW. IgG_1 antibody-dependent mediator release after passive systemic sensitization of basophils arriving at cutaneous basophil hypersensitivity reactions. J Immunol 1982; 129:1663–9.
146. Askenase PW, Debernardo R, Tauben D, Kashgarian M. Cutaneous basophil anaphylaxis. Immediate vasopermeability increases and anaphylactic degranulation of basophils at delayed hypersensitivity reactions challenged with additional antigen. Immunology 1978; 35:741–55.
147. Brown SJ, Galli SJ, Gleich GJ, Askenase PW. Ablation of immunity to *Amblyomma americanum* by anti-basophil serum: cooperation between basophil and eosinophils in expression of immunity to ectoparasites (ticks) in guinea pigs. J Immunol 1982; 129:790–6.
148. Dvorak AM, Osage JE, Dvorak HF, Galli SJ. Surface membrane alterations in guinea pig basophils undergoing anaphylactic degranulation: a scanning electron microscopic study. Lab Invest 1981; 45:58–66.
149. Dvorak AM, Galli SJ, Morgan E, Galli AS, Hammond ME, Dvorak HF. Anaphylactic

degranulation of guinea pig basophilic leukocytes. II. Evidence for regranulation during recovery from degranulation in vitro. Lab Invest 1982; 46:461–75.
150. Dvorak AM, Dvorak HF, Galli SJ. Surface membrane traffic in guinea pig basophils exposed to cationic ferritin. Int Arch Allergy Appl Immunol 1985; 77:267–73.
151. Dvorak AM, Colvin RB, Monahan RA. Immunoferritin electron microscopic studies with antibasophil serum of guinea pig basophil degranulation and regranulation in vitro. Clin Immunol Immunopathol 1985; 37:63–76.
152. Dvorak AM, Monahan-Earley RA, Dvorak HF, Galli SJ. Ultrastructural cytochemical and autoradiographic demonstration of nonspecific esterase(s) in guinea pig basophils. J Histochem Cytochem 1987; 35:351–60.
153. Chan BST. Ultrastructural changes in guinea-pig bone marrow basophils during anaphylaxis. Immunology 1972; 23:215–24.
154. McLaren DJ, Worms MJ, Askenase PW. Cutaneous basophil associated resistance to ectoparasite ticks. Electron microscopy of *Rhipicephalus appendiculatus* larval feeding sites in actively sensitized guinea pigs and recipients of immune serum. J Pathol 1983; 139:291–308.
155. Dvorak AM, Galli SJ. Antigen-induced, IgE-mediated degranulation of cloned immature mast cells derived from normal mice. Am J Pathol 1987; 126:535–45.
156. Dvorak AM, Hammel I, Galli SJ. Beige mouse mast cells generated in vitro: ultrastructural analysis of maturation induced by sodium butyrate and of IgE-mediated, antigen-dependent degranulation. Int Arch Allergy Appl Immunol 1987; 82:261–8.
157. Kops SK, Loveren HV, Rosenstein RW, Ptak W, Askenase PW. Mast cell activation and vascular alterations in immediate hypersensitivity-like reactions induced by a T cell-derived antigen-binding factor. Lab Invest 1984; 50:421–34.
158. Fawcett DW. An experimental study of mast cell degranulation and regeneration. Anat Rec 1955; 121:29–52.
159. Lagunoff D, Benditt EP. Mast cell degranulation and histamine release observed in a new in vitro system. J Exp Med 1960; 112:571–80.
160. Röhlich P, Anderson P, Uvnäs B. Electron microscopic observations on compound 48/80-induced degranulation in rat mast cells: evidence for sequential exocytosis of storage granules. J Cell Biol 1971; 51:465–83.
161. Dvorak AM, Schleimer RP, Schulman ES, Lichtenstein LM. Human mast cells use conservation and condensation mechanisms during recovery from degranulation. In vitro studies with mast cells purified from human lungs. Lab Invest 1986; 54:663–78.
162. Dvorak AM, Schleimer RP, Lichtenstein LM. Human mast cells synthesize new granules during recovery from degranulation. In vitro studies with mast cells purified from human lungs. Blood 1988; 71:76–85.
163. Dvorak AM, Schleimer RP, Lichtenstein LM. Morphologic mast cell cycles. Cell Immunol 1987; 105:199–204.
164. Dvorak AM. Recovery of human lung mast cells from anaphylactic degranulation utilizes a mixture of conservation and synthetic mechanisms. In: Galli SJ, Austen KF, eds. Mast cell and basophil differentiation and function in health and disease. New York: Raven Press, 1989:119–48.
165. Berlin G, Enerbäck L. Mast cell secretion. Rapid sealing of exocytotic cavities demonstrated by cytofluorometry. Int Arch Allergy Appl Immunol 1984; 73:256–62.
166. Burwen SJ. Recycling of mast cells following degranulation in vitro: an ultrastructural study. Tissue Cell 1982; 14:125–34.
167. Bytzer P, Nielsen EH, Clausen J. Surface morphology of rat peritoneal mast cells during in vitro regeneration after histamine secretion. Cell Tissue Res 1981; 216:647–54.
168. Krüger PG, Lagunoff D. Mast cell restoration. A study of rat peritoneal mast cells after depletion with polymyxin B. Int Arch Allergy Appl Immunol 1981; 65:278–90.
169. Lagunoff D. Vital staining of mast cells with ruthenium red. J Histochem Cytochem 1972; 20:938–44.
170. Meyer SL, Saunders AM. Cytofluorometric study of mast cell polyanions. II. Adult rat

peritoneal mast cells regenerating after polymyxin treatment. J Histochem Cytochem 1969; 17:56–61.
171. Nemeth A, Röhlich P. Early membrane retrieval following exocytosis in rat mast cells. Eur J Cell Biol 1982; 28:39–46.
172. Nielsen EH, Clausen J. Electron microscopic study of the regeneration in vivo of rat peritoneal mast cells after secretion. Cell Tissue Res 1982; 224:465–8.
173. Nielsen EH, Bytzer P, Clausen J, Chakravarty N. Electron microscopic study of the regeneration in vitro of rat peritoneal mast cells after histamine secretion. Cell Tissue Res 1981; 216:635–45.
174. Nielsen EH, Clausen J, Bytzer P. Membrane retrieval in non-exocytic and exocytic rat peritoneal mast cells. Exp Cell Res 1981; 135:291–8.
175. Thilo L. Selective internalization of granule membrane after secretion in mast cells. Proc Natl Acad Sci USA 1985; 82:1711–5.
176. Weil BJ, Renoux ML. Study of granule reappearance and histamine synthesis in rat mast cells maintained in short-term cultures. Cell Immunol 1982; 68:220–33.
177. Dvorak HF, Galli SJ, Dvorak AM. Cellular and vascular manifestations of cell-mediated immunity. Hum Pathol 1986; 17:122–37.
178. Dvorak HF. Introduction—heterogeneity of the cellular immune response. In: Müller-Rucholtz W, Müller-Hermelink HK, eds. Function and structure of the immune system. New York: Plenum Publishing, 1979:369–74.
179. Dvorak HF. Delayed hypersensitivity. In: Zweifach B, Grant L, McCluskey RT, eds. The inflammatory process, 2d ed., vol. 3. New York: Academic Press, 1974:291–345.
180. Dvorak HF, Galli SJ, Dvorak AM. Expressions of delayed hypersensitivity. In: Henocq E, ed. Lymphocytes et immune-allergologie. Journées d'études. Laboratoires SA Fissons, 1980:91–9.
181. Dvorak HF, Dvorak AM, Simpson BA, Richerson HB, Leskowitz S, Karnovsky MJ. Cutaneous basophil hypersensitivity. II. A light and electron microscopic description. J Exp Med 1970; 132:558–82.
182. Goldman MA, Simpson BA, Dvorak HF. Histamine and basophils in delayed-type hypersensitivity reactions. J Immunol 1973; 110:1511–7.
183. Dvorak AM, Dvorak HF, Karnovsky MJ. Uptake of horseradish peroxidase by guinea pig basophilic leukocytes. Lab Invest 1972; 26:27–39.
184. Dvorak AM, Hammond ME, Morgan E, Orenstein NS, Galli SJ, Dvorak HF. Evidence for a vesicular transport mechanism in guinea pig basophilic leukocytes. Lab Invest 1980; 42:263–76.
185. Dvorak AM, Klebanoff SJ, Henderson WR, Monahan RA, Pyne K, Galli SJ. Vesicular uptake of eosinophil peroxidase by guinea pig basophils and by cloned mouse mast cells and granule-containing lymphoid cells. Am J Pathol 1985; 118:425–38.
186. Dvorak HF, Dvorak AM, Churchill WH. Immunologic rejection of diethylnitrosamine-induced hepatomas in strain 2 guinea pigs. Participation of basophilic leukocytes and macrophage aggregates. J Exp Med 1973; 137:751–75.
187. Dvorak AM, Galli SJ, Galli AS, Hammond ME, Churchill WH, Dvorak HF. Tumor-basophil interactions in vitro—a scanning and transmission electron microscopic study. J Immunol 1979; 122:2447–57.
188. Dvorak HF, Mihm MC Jr, Dvorak AM. Morphology of delayed-type hypersensitivity reactions in man. J Invest Dermatol 1976; 67:391–401.
189. Dvorak AM, Mihm MC Jr, Dvorak HF. Morphology of delayed-type hypersensitivity reactions in man. II. Ultrastructural alterations affecting the microvasculature and the tissue mast cells. Lab Invest 1976; 34:179–91.
190. Colvin RB, Dvorak AM, Dvorak HF. Mast cells in the cortical tubular epithelium and interstitium in human renal disease. Hum Pathol 1974; 5:315–26.
191. Dvorak AM, Dickersin GR, Connell AB, Carey RW, Dvorak HF. Degranulation mechanisms in human leukemic basophils. Clin Immunol Immunopathol 1976; 5:235–46.
192. Dvorak HF, Mihm MC Jr, Dvorak AM, Barnes BA, Manseau EJ, Galli SJ. Rejection of

first set skin allografts in man. The microvasculature is the critical target for the immune response. J Exp Med 1979; 150:322–37.
193. Dvorak AM, Monahan RA. Chronic abdominal pain, malaise, constipation and diarrhea in a forty year old woman: Crohn's disease. Norelco Reporter 1984; 31:18–44.
194. Dvorak AM, Monahan-Earley RA. Diagnostic ultrastructural pathology. EM Pathology Monograph, no. 1, vol. 1. Mahwah, NJ: Electron Optics Publishing Group, 1986:1–98.
195. Dvorak AM. Ultrastructural pathology of Crohn's disease. In: Goebell H, Peskar BM, Malchow M, eds. Inflammatory bowel disease—basic research and clinical applications. Lancaster: MTP Press, 1988:3–41.
196. Dvorak AM, Monahan RA, Osage JE, Dickersin GR. Mast cell degranulation in Crohn's disease. Lancet 1978; i:498 (letter).
197. Dvorak AM. Mast cell hyperplasia and degranulation in Crohn's disease. In: Pepys J, Edwards AM, eds. The mast cell. Its role in health and disease. Kent: Pitman Medical Publishing, 1979:657–62.
198. Dvorak AM, Silen W. Differentiation between Crohn's disease and other inflammatory conditions by electron microscopy. Ann Surg 1985; 201:53–63.
199. Dvorak AM, Mihm MC Jr, Osage JE, Dvorak HF. Melanoma. An ultrastructural study of the host inflammatory and vascular responses. J Invest Dermatol 1980; 75:388–93.
200. Dvorak AM, Monahan RA. Abdominal pain, hepatomegaly and weight loss in a fifty four year old man: renal cell carcinoma and adenoma. Norelco Reporter 1985; 32:61–6.
201. Lacy PE. Endocrine secretory mechanisms. A review. Am J Pathol 1975; 79:170–87.
202. Orci L, Malaisse-Lagae F, Ravazzola M, Amherdt M, Renold AE. Exocytosis-endocytosis coupling in the pancreatic beta cell. Science 1973; 181:561–2.
203. Palade G. Intracellular aspects of the process of protein synthesis. Science 1975; 189:347–58.
204. Jamieson JD, Palade GE. Synthesis, intracellular transport and discharge of secretory proteins in stimulated pancreatic exocrine cells. J Cell Biol 1971; 50:135–58.
205. Kelly RB. Pathways of protein secretion in eukaryotes. Science 1985; 230:25–32.
206. Bloch KJ, Angevine C. Mast cells and mast cell-sensitizing (homocytotropic) antibodies. Rheumatology 1970; 3:169–93.
207. Lichtenstein LM. The immediate allergic response: in vitro separation of antigen activation, decay and histamine release. J Immunol 1971; 107:1122–30.
208. Lichtenstein LM. Mechanisms of allergic histamine release from human leukocytes. In: Austen KF, Becker EL, eds. Biochemistry of the acute allergic reactions. Philadelphia: FA Davis, 1968:153–71.
209. Lichtenstein LM. The mechanism of basophil histamine release induced by antigen and by the calcium ionophore A23187. J Immunol 1975; 114:1692–9.
210. MacGlashan DW Jr, Schleimer RP, Peters SP, Schulman ES, Adams GK, Sobotka AK, Newball HH, Lichtenstein LM. Comparative studies of human basophils and mast cells. Fed Proc 1983; 42:2504–9.
211. Richerson HB, Dvorak HF, Leskowitz S. Cutaneous basophil hypersensitivity. I. A new look at the Jones-Mote reaction, general characteristics. J Exp Med 1970; 132:546–57.
212. Dvorak HF, Colvin RB, Churchill WH. Specificity of basophils and lymphocytes in cutaneous basophil hypersensitivity. J Immunol 1975; 114:507–11.
213. Lett-Brown MA, Thueson DO, Grant AJ. Dissociation between basophil sensitization and cutaneous basophil hypersensitivity. Fed Proc 1979; 38:1221.
214. Askenase PW. Role of basophils, mast cells, and vasoamines in hypersensitivity reactions with a delayed time course. Prog Allergy 1977; 23:199–320.
215. Dvorak AM, Bast RC Jr, Dvorak HF. Morphologic changes in draining lymph nodes and in lymphocyte cultures after sensitization with complete or incomplete Freund's adjuvant. Correlation with immunologic events in vivo and in culture. J Immunol 1971; 107:422–35.

216. Dvorak HF, Simpson BA, Bast RC, Leskowitz S. Cutaneous basophil hypersensitivity. III. Participation of the basophil in hypersensitivity to antigen-antibody complexes, delayed hypersensitivity, and contact allergy. Passive transfer. J Immunol 1971; 107:138–48.
217. Ward PA, Dvorak HF, Cohen S, Yoshida T, Data R, Selvaggio SS. Chemotaxis of basophils by lymphocyte-dependent and lymphocyte-independent mechanisms. J Immunol 1975; 114:1523–31.
218. Boetcher DA, Leonard EJ. Basophil chemotaxis: augmentation by a factor from stimulated lymphocyte cultures. Immunol Commun 1973; 2:421–9.
219. Kay AB, Austen KF. Chemotaxis of human basophil leucocytes. Clin Exp Immunol 1972; 11:557–63.
220. Dvorak AM, Galli SJ, Galli AS, Hammond ME, Dvorak HF. Lymphocyte mediator modulation of basophil motile structures. In: de Weck A, Kristensen F, Landy M, eds. Biochemical characterization of lymphokines. New York: Academic Press, 1980:205–7.
221. Galli SJ, Dvorak AM, Hammond ME, Morgan E, Galli AS, Dvorak HF. Guinea pig basophil morphology in vitro. I. Ultrastructure of uropod-bearing (motile) basophils and modulation of motile structures by serum and substrate effects. J Immunol 1981; 126:1066–74.
222. McFarland W, Heilman DH, Moorhead JF. Functional anatomy of the lymphocyte in immunological reactions in vitro. J Exp Med 1966; 124:851–8.
223. Thueson DO, Speck LS, Lett-Brown MA, Grant JA. Histamine-releasing activity (HRA). I. Production by mitogen- or antigen-stimulated human mononuclear cells. J Immunol 1979; 123:626–32.
224. Thueson DO, Speck LS, Lett-Brown MA, Grant JA. Histamine-releasing activity (HRA). II. Interaction with basophils and physicochemical characterization. J Immunol 1979; 123:633–9.
225. Lett-Brown MA, Aelvoet M, Hooks JJ, Georgides JA, Thueson DO, Grant JA. Enhancement of basophil chemotaxis in vitro by virus-induced interferon. J Clin Invest 1981; 67:547–52.
226. Lett-Brown MA, Hooks JJ, Georgides JA, Thueson DO, Grant JA. Modulation of human basophil migration in vitro by a soluble factor from virus-stimulated leukocytes. Clin Immunol Immunopathol 1981; 20:179–87.
227. Orida N, Feldman JD, Katz DH, Liu FT. IgE-mediated chemotaxis of rat basophilic leukemia cells towards specific antigen. J Exp Med 1983; 157:2166–71.
228. Lett-Brown MA, Boetcher DA, Leonard EJ. Chemotactic responses of normal human basophils to C5a and to lymphocyte-derived chemotactic factor. J Immunol 1976; 117:246–52.
229. Poole TJ, Zetter BR. Stimulation of rat peritoneal mast cell migration by tumor-derived peptides. Cancer Res 1983; 43:5857–61.
230. Cohen MC, Zeschke R, Bigazzi PE, Yoshida T, Cohen S. Mastocytoma cell migration in vitro: inhibition by MIF-containing supernatants. J Immunol 1975; 114:1641–3.
231. Dvorak AM, Hammond ME, Dvorak HF, Karnovsky MJ. Loss of cell surface material from peritoneal exudate cells associated with lymphocyte-mediated inhibition of macrophage migration from capillary tubes. Lab Invest 1972; 27:561–74.
232. Matsuura N, Zetter BR. Stimulation of mast cell chemotaxis by interleukin 3. J Exp Med 1989; 170:1421–6.
233. Thompson HL, Burbelo PD, Yamada Y, Kleinman HK, Metcalfe DD. Mast cells chemotax to laminin with enhacement after IgE-mediated activation. J Immunol 1989; 143:4188–92.
234. Levaditi C. Contribution à l'études des Mastzellen et de la Mastezellen Leucocytose. Thèse No. 183. In: Naud C, ed. Paris Thèses, 1901–1902. Paris: LeRoy à Limasset, 1902:1–80.
235. Schlecht H. Über die Einwirkung von Seruminjektionen auf die Eosinophilen und Mastzellen des menschlichen und tierischen Blutes. Deutsches Archiv für klinische

Medizin (Leipzig) 1910; 98:308–29.
236. Winqvist G. Experimental production of basophilic granulocytes in the guinea pig. Exp Cell Res 1960; 19:7–12.
237. Dvorak HF, Orenstein NS, Dvorak AM, Hammond ME, Roblin RO, Feder J, Schott CF, Goodwin J, Morgan E. Isolation of the cytoplasmic granules of guinea pig basophilic leukocytes: identification of esterase and protease activities. J Immunol 1977; 119:38–46.
238. Dvorak AM, Galli SJ, Dvorak HF. A role for cytoplasmic vesicles in anaphylactic degranulation of guinea pig basophils. Int Arch Allergy Appl Immunol 1981; 66(suppl 1):234–8.
239. Denburg JA, Davidson M, Bienenstock J. Basophil production. J Clin Invest 1980; 65:390–9.
240. Eccleston E, Leonard BJ, Lowe JS, Welford HJ. Basophilic leukemia in the albino rat and a demonstration of the basopoietin. Nature New Biol 1973; 244:73–6.
241. Ogilvie BM, Hesketh PM, Rose ME. *Nippostronglyus brasiliensis:* peripheral blood leucocyte response of rats, with special reference to basophils. Exp Parasitol 1978; 46:20–30.
242. Ogilvie BM, Askenase PW, Rose ME. Basophils and eosinophils in three strains of rats and in athymic (nude) rats following infection with the nematodes *Nippostrongylus brasiliensis* or *Trichinella spiralis.* Immunology 1980; 39:385–9.
243. Roth RL, Levy DA. *Nippostronglyus brasiliensis:* peripheral leukocyte responses and correlation of basophils with blood histamine concentration during infection in rats. Exp Parasitol 1980; 50:331–41.
244. Ogawa M, Nakahata T, Leary AG, Sterk AR, Ishizaka Y, Ishizaka T. Suspension culture of human mast cells/basophils from umbilical cord blood mononuclear cells. Proc Natl Acad Sci USA 1983; 80:4494–8.
245. Ishizaka T, Conrad DH, Huff TF, Metcalfe DD, Stevens RL. Unique features of human basophilic granulocytes developed in in vitro culture. Int Arch Allergy Appl Immunol 1985; 77:137–43.
246. Hutt-Taylor SR, Harnish D, Richardson M, Ishizaka T, Denburg JA. Sodium butyrate and a T lymphocyte cell line-derived differentiation factor induce basophilic differentiation of the human promyelocytic leukemia cell line HL-60. Blood 1988; 71:209–15.
247. Razin E, Rifkind AB, Cordon-Cardo C, Good RA. Selective growth of a population of human basophils in vitro. Proc Natl Acad Sci USA 1981; 78:5793–6.
248. Tadokoro K, Stadler BM, de Weck AL. Factor-dependent in vitro growth of human normal bone marrow-derived basophil-like cells. J Exp Med 1983; 158:857–71.
249. Hirai K, de Weck AL, Stadler BM. Characterization of human basophil-like cell promoting activity. J Immunol 1988; 140:221–7.
250. Denburg JA, Richardson M, Telizyn S, Bienenstock J. Basophil/mast cell precursors in human peripheral blood. Blood 1983; 61:775–9.
251. Denburg JA, Messner H, Lim B, Jamal N, Telizyn S, Bienenstock J. Clonal origin of human basophil/mast cells from circulating multipotent hemopoietic progenitors. Exp Hematol 1985; 13:185–8.
252. Seldin DC, Caulfield JP, Hein A, Osathanondh R, Nabel G, Schlossman SF, Stevens RL, Austen KF. Biochemical and phenotypic characterization of human basophilic cells derived from dispersed fetal liver with murine T cell factors. J Immunol 1986; 136:2222–30.
253. Ahlstedt S, Hammarström I, Into-Malmberg MB, Bjorksten B, Denburg J. In vitro appearance of large human histamine-containing basophilic cells. Int Arch Allergy Appl Immunol 1986; 79:33–7.
254. Ahlstedt S, Bjorksen B, Borwell J, Hammarström I, Nybacka J-O. Appearance of basophilic cells/mast cells and IgE antibodies in liquid human cell cultures. Int Arch Allergy Appl Immunol 1985; 77:238–40.
255. Stadler BM, Hirai K, Tadokoro K, de Weck AL. Distinction of the human basophil pro-

moting activity from human interleukin-3. Int Arch Allergy Appl Immunol 1985; 77:151–4.

256. Otsuka T, Miyajima A, Brown N, Otsu K, Abrams J, Saeland S, Caux C, de Waal Malefijt R, de Vries J, Meyerson P, Yokota K, Gemmel L, Rennick DM, Lee FD, Arai N, Arai K, Yokota T. Isolation and characterization of an expressible cDNA encoding human IL-3. Induction of IL-3 mRNA in human T cell clones. J Immunol 1988; 140:2288–95.
257. Yokota T, Coffman RL, Hagiwara H, Rennick DM, Takebe Y, Yokota K, Gemmell L, Schrader B, Yang G, Meyerson P, Luh J, Hoy P, Pene J, Briere F, Branchereau J, DeVries J, Lee FD, Arai N, Arai K-I. Isolation and characterization of lymphokine cNDA clones encoding mouse and human IgA-enhancing factor and eosinophil colony-stimulating factor activities: relationship to interleukin 5. Proc Natl Acad Sci USA 1987; 84:7388–92.
258. Saito H, Hatake K, Dvorak AM, Leiferman KM, Donnenberg AD, Arai N, Ishizaka K, Ishizaka T. Selective differentiation and proliferation of hematopoietic cells induced by recombinant human interleukins. Proc Natl Acad Sci USA 1988; 85:2288–92.
259. Abboud M, Moore MAS. Recombinant human IL-3 is a basophil/mast cell growth factor. Exp Hematol 1988; 16:489.
260. Kirshenbaum AS, Goff JP, Dreskin SC, Irani AM, Schwartz LB, Metcalfe DD. IL-3-dependent growth of basophil-like cells and mastlike cells from human bone marrow. J Immunol 1989; 142:2424–9.
261. Valent P, Schmidt G, Besemer J, Mayer P, Zenke G, Liehl E, Hinterberger W, Lechner K, Maurer D, Bettelheim P. Interleukin-3 is a differentiation factor for human basophils. Blood 1989; 73:1763–9.
262. Yang Y-C, Ciarletta AB, Temple PA, Chung MP, Kovacic S, Witek-Giannotti JS, Leary AC, Kriz R, Donahue RE, Wong GG, Clark SC. Human IL-3 (multi-CSF): identification by expression cloning of a novel hematopoietic growth factor related to murine IL-3. Cell 1986; 47:3–10.
263. Donahue RE, Seehra J, Metzger M, Lefebvre D, Rock B, Carbone S, Nathan DG, Garnick M, Sehgal PK, Laston D, Lavallie E, McCoy J, Schendel PF, Norton C, Turner K, Yang Y-C, Clark SC. Human IL-3 and GM-CSF act synergistically in stimulating hematopoiesis in primates. Science 1988; 241:1820–3.
264. Mayer P, Valent P, Schmidt G, Liehl E, Bettelheim P. The in vivo effects of recombinant human interleukin-3. Demonstration of basophil differentiation factor, histamine producing activity, and priming of GM-CSF responsive progenitors in non-human primates. Blood 1989; 74:613–21.
265. Patterson R, Chakrin LW, Suszko IM, Mengel J, Wardell JR Jr. IgE-mediated histamine and SRS-A release from respiratory cells and peripheral blood leukocytes of rhesus monkeys. J Lab Clin Med 1976; 87:1016–24.
266. Ginsburg H. The in vitro differentiation and culture of normal mast cells from the mouse thymus. Ann NY Acad Sci 1963; 103:20–39.
267. Ginsburg H, Sachs L. Formation of pure suspensions of mast cells in tissue culture by differentiation of lymphoid cells from the mouse thymus. J Natl Cancer Inst 1963; 31:1–39.
268. Ginsburg H, Lagunoff D. The in vitro differentiation of mast cells. Cultures of cells from immunized mouse lymph nodes and thoracic duct on fibroblast monolayers. J Cell Biol 1967; 35:685–97.
269. Nabel G, Galli SJ, Dvorak AM, Dvorak HF, Cantor H. Inducer T lymphocytes synthesize a factor that stimulates proliferation of cloned mast cells. Nature 1981; 291:332–4.
270. Hasthorpe S. A hemopoietic cell line dependent upon a factor in pokeweek mitogen-stimulated spleen cell conditioned medium. J Cell Physiol 1980; 105:379–84.
271. Schrader JW, Nossal GJV. Strategies for the analysis of accessory-cell function: the in vitro cloning and characterization of the P cell. Immunol Rev 1980; 53:61–85.

272. Nagao K, Yokoro K, Aaronson SA. Continuous lines of basophil/mast cells derived from normal mouse bone marrow. Science 1981; 212:333–5.
273. Schrader JW. The in vitro production and cloning of the P cell, a bone marrow-derived null cell that expresses H-2 and Ia-antigens, has mast cell-like granules, and is regulated by a factor released by activated T cells. J Immunol 1981; 126:452–8.
274. Tertian G, Yung Y-P, Guy-Grand D, Moore MAS. Long-term in vitro culture of murine mast cells. I. Descrption of a growth-factor dependent culture technique. J Immunol 1981; 127:788–94.
275. Razin E, Cordon-Cardo C, Good RA. Growth of a pure population of mouse mast cells in vitro with conditioned medium derived from concanavalin A-stimulated splenocytes. Proc Natl Acad Sci USA 1981; 28:2559–61.
276. Yung Y-P, Eger R, Tertian G, Moore MAS. Long-term in vitro culture of murine mast cells. II. Purification of a mast cell growth factor and its dissociation from TCGF. J Immunol 1981; 127:794–9.
277. Galli SJ, Dvorak AM, Marcum JA, Ishizaka T, Nabel G, Der Simonian H, Pyne K, Goldin JM, Rosenberg RD, Cantor H, Dvorak HF. Mast cell clones: a model for the analysis of cellular maturation. J Cell Biol 1982; 95:435–44.
278. Weitzman G, Galli SJ, Dvorak AM, Hammel I. Cloned mouse mast cells and normal mouse peritoneal mast cells. Determination of serotonin content and ability to synthesize serotonin in vitro. Int Arch Allergy Appl Immunol 1985; 77:189–91.
279. Galli SJ, Dvorak AM, Marcum JA, Nabel G, Goldin JM, Rosenberg RD, Cantor H, Dvorak HF. Mouse mast cell clones: modulation of functional maturity in vitro. In: Ricci M, Marone G, eds. Monographs in allergy, vol. 18. Basel: S Karger, 1983:166–70.
280. Burd PR, Rogers HW, Gordon JR, Martin CA, Jayaraman S, Wilson SD, Dvorak AM, Galli SJ, Dorf ME. Interleukin 3-dependent and -independent mast cells stimulated with IgE and antigen express multiple cytokines. J Exp Med 1989; 170:245–57.
281. Dvorak AM, Wiberg L, Monahan-Earley RA, Galli SJ. A simple technique to facilitate the ultrastructural analysis of cells in soft agar culture systems: Demonstration of the development in vitro of morphologically mature mast cells and phagocytic macrophages from the bone marrow cells of genetically mast cell-deficient W/W^v or congenic normal mice. Lab Invest 1990; 62:774–781.
282. Galli SJ. New approaches for the analysis of mast cell maturation, heterogeneity and function. Fed Proc 1987; 46:1906–14.
283. Galli SJ. Biology of disease—new insights into "the riddle of the mast cells": microenvironmental regulation of mast cell development and phenotypic heterogeneity. Lab Invest 1990; 62:5–33.
284. Galli SJ, Kitamura Y. Genetically mast cell-deficient W/W^v and Sl/Sl^d mice. Their value for the analysis of mast cells in biological responses in vivo. Am J Pathol 1987; 127:191–8.
285. Sredni B, Friedman MM, Bland CE, Metcalfe DD. Ultrastructural, biochemical, and functional characteristics of histamine-containing cells cloned from mouse bone marrow: tentative identification as mucosal mast cells. J Immunol 1983; 131:915–22.
286. Tas J, Berndsen RG. Does heparin occur in mucosal mast cells of the rat small intestine? J Histochem Cytochem 1977; 25:1058–62.
287. Befus AD, Pearce FL, Gauldie J, Horsewood P, Bienenstock J. Mucosal mast cells. I. Isolation and functional characteristics of rat intestinal mast cells. J Immunol 1982; 128:2475–80.
288. Otsu K, Nakano T, Kanakura Y, Asai H, Katz HR, Austen KF, Stevens RL, Galli SJ, Kitamura Y. Phenotypic changes of bone marrow-derived mast cells after intraperitoneal transfer into W/W^v mice that are genetically deficient in mast cells. J Exp Med 1987; 165:615–27.
289. Dayton ET, Pharr P, Ogawa M, Serafin WE, Austen KF, Levi-Schaffer F, Stevens RL. 3T3 fibroblasts induce cloned interleukin 3-dependent mouse mast cells to resemble con-

nective tissue mast cells in granular constituency. Proc Natl Acad Sci USA 1988; 85:569–72.

290. Nakahata T, Kobayashi T, Ishiguro A, Tsuji K, Naganuma K, Ando O, Yagi Y, Tadokoro K, Akabane T. Extensive proliferation of mature connective-tissue type mast cells in vitro. Nature 1986; 324:65–7.

291. Kobayashi T, Nakano T, Nakahata T, Asai H, Yagi Y, Tsuji K, Komiyama A, Akabane T, Kojima S, Kitamura Y. Formation of mast cell colonies in methylcellulose by mouse peritoneal cells and differentiation of these cloned cells in both the skin and the gastric mucosa of W/W^v mice: evidence that a common precursor can give rise to both "connective tissue-type" and "mucosal" mast cells. J Immunol 1986; 136:1378–84.

292. Reynolds DS, Serafin WE, Faller DV, Wall DA, Abbas AK, Dvorak AM, Austen KF, Stevens RL. Immortalization of murine connective tissue-type mast cells at multiple stages of their differentiation by coculture of splenocytes with fibroblasts that produce Kirsten Sarcoma Virus. J Biol Chem 1988; 263:12783–91.

293. Yung Y-P, Moore MAS. Long-term in vitro culture of murine mast cells. III. Discrimination of mast cell growth factor and granulocyte CSF. J Immunol 1982; 129:1256–61.

294. Yokota T, Lee F, Rennick D, Hall C, Arai N. Mosmann T, Nabel G, Cantor H, Arai K-I. Isolation and characterization of a mouse cDNA clone that expresses mast-cell growth-factor activity in monkey cells. Proc Natl Acad Sci USA 1984; 81:1070–4.

295. Rennick DM, Lee FD, Yokota T, Arai K-I, Cantor H, Nabel GJ. A cloned MCGF cDNA encodes a multilineage hematopoietic growth factor: multiple activities of interleukin 3. J Immunol 1985; 134:910–4.

296. Fung MC, Hapel AJ, Ymer S, Cohen DR, Johnson RM, Campbell HD, Young IG. Molecular cloning of cDNA for murine interleukin-3. Nature 1984; 307:233–7.

297. Ymer S, Tucker WQJ, Sanderson CJ, Hapel AJ, Campbell HD, Young IG. Constitutive synthesis of interleukin-3 by leukemia cell line WEHI-3B is due to retroviral insertion near the gene. Nature 1985; 317:255–8.

298. Clark-Lewis I, Aebersold R, Ziltener H, Schrader JW, Hood LE, Kent SBH. Automated chemical synthesis of a protein growth factor for hematopoietic cells, interleukin-3. Science 1986; 231:134–9.

299. Ihle JN, Keller J, Oroszlan S, Henderson LE, Copeland TD, Fitch F, Prystowsky MB, Goldwasser E, Schrader JW, Palazynski E, Dy M, Lebel B. Biological properties of homogeneous interleukin-3. I. Demonstration of WEHI-3 growth factor activity, mast cell growth factor activity, P cell-stimulating factor activity, colony-stimulating factor activity and histamine-producing cell-stimulating factor activity. J Immunol 1983; 131:282–7.

300. Hapel AJ, Fung RM, Johnson RM, Young IG, Johnson G, Metcalf D. Biologic properties of molecularly cloned and expressed murine interleukin-3. Blood 1985; 65:1453–9.

301. Metcalf D, Begley CG, Johnson GR, Nicola NA, Lopez AF, Williamson DJ. Effects of purified bacterially synthesized murine multi-CSF (IL-3) on hematopoiesis in normal adult mice. Blood 1986; 68:46–57.

302. Suda T, Suda J, Spicer SS, Ogawa M. Proliferation and differentiation in culture of mast cell progenitors derived from mast cell-deficient mice of genotype W/W^v. J Cell Physiol 1985; 122:187–92.

303. Gordon JR, Galli SJ. Phorbol 12-myristate 13-acetate-induced development of functionally active mast cells in W/W^v but not Sl/Sl^d genetically mast cell-deficient mice. Blood 1990; 75:1637–45.

304. Pierce JH, DiFiore PP, Aaronson SA, Potter M, Pumphrey J, Scott A, Ihle JN. Neoplastic transformation of mast cells by Abelson-MuLV: abrogation of IL-3 dependence by a nonautocrine mechanism. Cell 1985; 41:685–93.

305. Galli SJ, Dvorak AM, Dvorak HF. Mouse mast cells and other granulated leukocyte clones. In: Ricci M, Marone G, eds. Monographs in allergy, vol. 18. Basel: S Karger, 1983:129–37.

306. Ishizaka T, Okudaira H, Mauser LE, Ishizaka K. Development of rat mast cells in vivo. I.

Differentiation of mast cells from thymus cells. J Immunol 1976; 116:747–54.
307. Haig DM, McKee TA, Jarrett EEE. Generation of mucosal mast cells is stimulated in vitro by factors derived from T cells of helminth-infected rats. Nature 1982; 300:188–90.
308. Haig DM, McMenamin C, Gunneberg C, Woodbury R, Jarrett EEE. Stimulation of mucosal mast cell growth in normal and *nude* rat bone marrow cultures. Proc Natl Acad Sci USA 1983; 80:4499–503.
309. Haig DM, Jarrett EEE, Tas J. In vitro studies on mast cell proliferation in *N. brasiliensis* infection. Immunology 1984; 51:643–51.
310. Shanahan F, Lee TDG, Denburg JA, Bienenstock J, Befus AD. Functional characterization of mast cells generated in vitro from the mesenteric lymph nodes of rats infected with *Nippostrongylus brasiliensis*. Immunology 1986; 57:455–9.
311. Brodie DH, Metcalfe DD, Wasserman SI. Functional and biochemical characterization of rat bone marrow-derived mast cells. J Immunol 1988; 141:4298–305.
312. Levi-Schaffer F, Austen KF, Caulfield JP, Hein A, Gravallese PM, Stevens RL. Coculture of human lung-derived mast cells with mouse 3T3 fibroblasts: morphology and IgE-mediated release of histamine, prostaglandin D_2 and leukotrienes. J Immunol 1987; 139:494–500.
313. Dvorak AM, Dvorak HF, Peters SP, Schulman ES, MacGlashan DW Jr, Pyne K, Harvey VS, Galli SJ, Lichtenstein LM. Lipid bodies: cytoplasmic organelles important to arachidonate metabolism in macrophages and mast cells. J Immunol 1983; 131:2965–76 (republished in J Immunol 1984; 132:1586–97).
314. Firestein GS, Xu W-D, Townsend K, Broide D, Alvaro-Gracia J, Glasebrook A, Zvaifler NJ. Cytokines in chronic inflammatory arthritis. I. Failure to detect T cell lymphokines (interleukin 2 and interleukin 3) and presence of macrophage colony-stimulating factor (CSF-1) and a novel mast cell growth factor in rheumatoid synovitis. J Exp Med 1988; 168:1573–86.
315. Kopicky-Burd JA, Kagey-Sobotka A, Peters SP, Dvorak AM, Lennox DW, Lichtenstein LM, Wigley FM. Characterization of human synovial mast cells. J Rheumatol 1988; 15:1326–33.
316. Alam R, Welter JB, Forsythe PA, Lett-Brown MA, Grant JA. Comparative effect of recombinant IL-1, -2, -3, -4, and -6, IFN-γ, granulocyte-macrophage colony-stimulating factor, tumor necrosis factor-α, and histamine-releasing factors on the secretion of histamine from basophils. J Immunol 1989; 142:3431–5.
317. Haak-Frendscho M, Arai N, Arai K-I, Baeza ML, Finn A, Kaplan AP. Human recombinant granulocyte-macrophage colony-stimulating factor and interleukin 3 cause basophil histamine release. J Clin Invest 1988; 82:17–20.
318. Kurimoto Y, de Weck AL, Dahinden CA. Interleukin 3-dependent mediator release in basophils triggered by C5a. J Exp Med 1989; 170:467–79.
319. MacDonald SM, Schleimer RP, Kagey-Sobotka A, Gillis S, Lichtenstein LM. Recombinant IL-3 induces histamine release from human basophils. J Immunol 1989; 142:3527–32.
320. Brindley LL, Sweet JM, Goetzl EJ. Stimulation of histamine release from human basophils by human platelet factor 4. J Clin Invest 1983; 72:1218–23.
321. Clementsen P, Jensen CB, Jarlov JO, Hannoun C, Norn S. Virus enhances histamine release from human basophils. Agents Actions 1988; 23:165–7.
322. Espersen F, Jarlov JO, Jensen C, Skov PS, Norn S. *Staphylococcus aureus* peptidoglycan induces histamine release from basophil human leukocytes in vitro. Infect Immun 1984; 46:710–4.
323. Haak-Frendscho M, Dinarello C, Kaplan AP. Recombinant human interleukin-1 beta causes histamine release from human basophils. J Allergy Clin Immunol 1988; 82:218–23.
324. Hernandez-Asensio M, Hooks JJ, Ida S, Siraganian RP, Notkins AL. Interferon induced enhancement of IgE-mediated histamine release from human basophils requires new RNA synthesis. J Immunol 1979; 122:1601–3.

325. Ida S, Hooks JJ, Siraganian RP, Notkins AL. Enhancement of IgE-mediated histamine release from human basophils by viruses: role of interferon. J Exp Med 1977; 145:892–906.
326. Kaplan AP, Haak-Frendscho M, Fauci A, Dinarello C, Halbert E. A histamine releasing factor from activated human mononuclear cells. J Immunol 1985; 135:2027–32.
327. Lichtenstein LM. Histamine-releasing factors and IgE heterogeneity. J Allergy Clin Immunol 1988; 81:814–20.
328. MacDonald SM, Kagey-Sobotka A, Proud D, Naclerio RM, Lichtenstein LM. Histamine releasing factor: release mechanism and responding population. J Allergy Clin Immunol 1987; 79:248.
329. Marone G, Tamburini M, Giudizi MG, Biagiotti R, Almerigogna F, Romagnani S. Mechanism of activation of human basophils by *Staphylococcus aureus* Cowan I. Infect Immunol 1987; 55:803–9.
330. Martin RR, White A. The in vitro release of leukocyte histamine by staphylococcal antigens. J Immunol 1969; 102:437–41.
331. Norn S, Jensen C, Dahl BT, Stahl Skov P, Baek L, Permin H, Jarlov JO, Sorensen H. Endotoxins release histamine by complement activation and potentiate bacteria-induced histamine release. Agents Actions 1986; 18:149–52.
332. Okuda Y, Tsuyuguchi I, Yamatodani A. Histamine release from human leukocytes by platelet-activating factor. Int Arch Allergy Appl Immunol 1988; 85:341–5.
333. Orchard MA, Kagey-Sobotka A, Proud D, Lichtenstein LM. Basophil histamine release induced by a substance from stimulated human platelets. J Immunol 1986; 136:2240–4.
334. Smith TF, Aelvoet M, Morrison DC. The effect of bacterial lipopolysaccharide (LPS) on histamine release from human basophils. I. Enhancement of immunologic release by LPS. Clin Immunol Immunopathol 1985; 34:355–65.
335. Subramian N, Bray M. Interleukin-1 releases histamine from human basophils and mast cells in vitro. J Immunol 1987; 138:271–5.
336. White MV, Kaliner MA. Neutrophils and mast cells. I. Human neutrophil-derived histamine-releasing activity. J Immunol 1987; 139:1624–30.
337. Kaplan AP, Sheikh I, Frendscho MH. Assessment of histamine release and kinin formation in man: identification of kinin degradation products and characterization of a lymphocyte-dependent histamine releasing factor. Int Arch Allergy Appl Immunol 1985; 77:64–8.
338. Raeza ML, Haak-Frendscho M, Satnick S, Kaplan AP. Responsiveness to human mononuclear cell-derived histamine-releasing factor. Studies of allergic status and the role of IgE. J Immunol 1988; 141:2688–92.
339. Goetzl EJ, Foster DW, Payan DG. A basophil-activating factor from human T lymphocytes. Immunology 1984; 53:227–34.
340. Alam R, Forsythe PA, Lett-Brown MA, Grant JA. Cellular origin of histamine-releasing factor produced by peripheral blood mononuclear cells. J Immunol 1989; 142:3951–6.
341. Liu MC, Proud D, Lichtenstein LM, MacGlashan DW Jr, Schleimer RP, Adkinson NF Jr, Kagey-Sobotka A, Schulman ES, Plaut M. Human lung macrophage-derived histamine-releasing activities due to IgE-dependent factors. J Immunol 1986; 136:2588–95.
342. Warner JA, Pienkowski MM, Plaut M, Norman PS, Lichtenstein LM. Identification of histamine releasing factor(s) in the late phase of cutaneous IgE-mediated reactions. J Immunol 1986; 136:2583–7.
343. MacDonald SM, Lichtenstein LM, Proud D, Plaut M, Naclerio RM, MacGlashan DW Jr, Kagey-Sobotka A. Studies of IgE-dependent histamine releasing factors: heterogeneity of IgE. J Immunol 1987; 139:506–12.
344. Schulman ES, McGettigan MC, Post TC, Vigderman RJ, Shapiro SS. Human monocytes generate basophil histamine-releasing activities. J Immunol 1988; 140:2369–75.
345. Sampson HA, Broadbent KR, Bernhisel-Broadbent J. Spontaneous release of histamine from basophils and histamine-releasing factor in patients with atopic dermatitis and food

hypersensitivity. N Engl J Med 1989; 321:228–32.
346. White MV, Kaplan AP, Haak-Frendscho M, Kaliner M. Neutrophils and mast cells. Comparison of neutrophil-derived histamine-releasing activity with other histamine-releasing factors. J Immunol 1988; 141:3575–83.
347. Dahinden CA, Kurimoto Y, De Weck AL, Lindley I, Dewald B, Baggiolini M. The neutrophil-activating peptide NAF/NAP-1 induces histamine and leukotriene release by interleukin 3-primed basophils. J Exp Med 1989; 170:1787–92.
348. Ida S, Hooks JJ, Siraganian RP, Notkins AL. Enhancement of IgE-mediated histamine release from human basophils by immune-specific lymphokines. Clin Exp Immunol 1980; 41:380–7.
349. Schleimer RP, Derse CP, Friedman B, Gillis S, Plaut M, Lichtenstein LM, MacGlashan DW Jr. Regulation of human basophil mediator release by cytokines. I. Interaction with anti-inflammatory steroids. J Immunol 1989; 143:1310–7.
350. Hirai K, Morita Y, Misaki Y, Ohta K, Takaishi T, Suzuki S, Motoyoshi K, Miyamoto T. Modulation of human basophil histamine release by hemopoietic growth factors. J Immunol 1988; 141:3958–64.
351. Massey WA, Randall TC, Kagey-Sobotka A, Warner JA, MacDonald SM, Gillis S, Allison AC, Lichtenstein LM. Recombinant human IL-1a and -1b potentiate IgE-mediated histamine release from human basophils. J Immunol 1989; 143:1875–80.
352. Haak-Frendscho M, Dinarello C, Kaplan AP. Recombinant interleukin 1 beta causes histamine release from human basophils. J Allergy Clin Immunol 1988; 82:18.
353. Alam R, Forsythe PA, Lett-Brown MA, Grant JA. Study of the cellular origin of histamine release inhibitory factor using highly purified subsets of mononuclear cells. J Immunol 1989; 143:2280–4.
354. Alam R, Grant JA, Lett-Brown MA. Identification of a histamine release inhibitory factor produced by human mononuclear cells in vitro. J Clin Invest 1988; 82:2056–62.
355. Kuriu A, Sonoda S, Kanakura Y, Jozaki K, Yamatodani A, Kitamura Y. Proliferative potential of degranulated murine peritoneal mast cells. Blood 1989; 74:925–9.
356. Takagi M, Nakahata T, Koike K, Kobayashi T, Tsuji K, Kojima S, Hirano T, Miyajima A, Arai K-I, Akabane T. Stimulation of connective tissue-type mast cell proliferation by crosslinking of cell-bound IgE. J Exp Med 1989; 170:233–44.
357. Humphries RK, Abraham S, Krystal G, Lansdorp P, Lemoine F, Eaves CJ. Activation of multiple hemopoietic growth factor genes in Abelson virus-transformed myeloid cells. Exp Hematol 1988; 17:774–81.
358. Plaut M, Pierce JH, Watson CJ, Hanley-Hyde J, Nordan RP, Paul WE. Mast cell lines produce lymphokines in response to cross-linkage of $Fc_{\epsilon}RI$ or to calcium ionophores. Nature 1989; 339:64–7.
359. Brown MA, Pierce JH, Watson CJ, Falco J, Ihle JN, Paul WE. B cell stimulatory factor-1/interleukin-4 mRNA is expressed by normal and transformed mast cells. Cell 1987; 50:809–18.
360. Chung SW, Wong PMC, Sheng-Ong G, Ruscetti S, Ishizaka T, Eaves CJ. Production of granulocyte-macrophage colony-stimulating factor by Abelson virus-induced tumorigenic mast cell lines. Blood 1986; 68:1074–81.
361. Young JD-E, Liu C-C, Butler G, Cohn ZA, Galli SJ. Identification, purification, and characterization of a mast cell-associated cytolytic factor related to tumor necrosis factor. Proc Natl Acad Sci USA 1987; 84:9175–9.
362. Richards AL, Okuno T, Takagaki Y, Djeu JY. Natural cytotoxic cell-specific cytotoxic factor produced by IL-3-dependent basophilic/mast cells. Relationship to TNF. J Immunol 1988; 141:3061–6.
363. Wodnar-Filipowicz A, Heusser CH, Moroni C. Production of the haemopoietic growth factors GM-CSF and interleukin-3 by mast cells in response to IgE receptor-mediated activation. Nature 1989; 339:150–2.

364. Dinarello CA. Biology of interleukin 1. FASEB J 1988; 2:108–115.
365. Paul WE, Ohara J. B-cell stimulatory factor-1/interleukin 4. Ann Rev Immunol 1987; 5:429–59.
366. Paul WE. Interleukin 4/B cell stimulatory factor 1: one lymphokine, many functions. FASEB J 1987; 1:456–61.
367. DeKruyff RH, Turner T, Abrams JS, Palladino MA, Umetsu DT. Induction of human IgE synthesis by $CD4^+$ T cell clones. Requirement for interleukin 4 and low molecular weight B cell growth factor. J Exp Med 1989; 170:1477–93.
368. Snapper CM, Finkelman FD, Paul WE. Differential regulation of IgG1 and IgE synthesis by interleukin 4. J Exp Med 1988; 167:183–96.
369. Jabara HH, Ackerman SJ, Vercelli D, Yokota T, Arai K-I, Abrams J, Dvorak AM, Lavigne MC, Banchereau J, DeVries J, Leung DYM, Geha RS. Induction of interleukin 4-dependent IgE synthesis and interleukin 5-dependent eosinophil differentiation by supernatants of a human helper T cell clone. J Clin Immunol 1988; 8:437–46.
370. Del Prete G, Maggi E, Parronchi P, Chrétien I, Tiri A, Macchia D, Ricci M, Banchereau J, DeVries J, Romagnani S. IL-4 is an essential factor for the IgE synthesis induced in vitro by human T cell clones and their supernatants. J Immunol 1988; 140:4193–8.
371. Conrad DH, Keegan AD, Kalli KR, Van Dusen R, Rao M, Levine AD. Superinduction of low affinity IgE receptors on murine B lymphocytes by lipopolysaccharide and IL-4. J Immunol 1988; 141:1091–7.
372. Defrance T, Aubry JP, Rousset F, Vandervliet B, Bonnefoy JY, Arai N, Takebe Y, Yokota T, Lee F, Arai K, DeVries J, Banchereau J. Human recombinant interleukin 4 induces Fc_ϵ receptors (CD 23) on normal human lymphocytes. J Exp Med 1987; 165:1459–67.
373. Smith CA, Rennick DM. Characterization of a murine lymphokine distinct from interleukin 2 and interleukin 3 (IL-3) possessing a T-cell growth factor activity and a mast cell growth factor activity that synergizes with IL-3. Proc Natl Acad Sci USA 1986; 83:1857–61.
374. Mosmann TR, Bond MW, Coffman RL, Ohara J, Paul WE. T-cell and mast cell lines respond to B-cell stimulatory factor 1. Proc Natl Acad Sci USA 1986; 83:5654–8.
375. Lee F, Yokota T, Otsuka T, Meyerson P, Villaret D, Coffman R, Mosmann T, Rennick D, Roehm N, Smith C, Zlotnik A, Arai K-I. Isolation and characterization of a mouse interleukin cDNA clone that expresses B-cell stimulatory factor 1 activities and T-cell- and mast-cell-stimulating activities. Proc Natl Acad Sci USA 1986; 83:2061–5.
376. Hamaguchi Y, Kanakura Y, Fujita J, Takeda S-I, Nakano T, Tarui S, Honjo T, Kitamura Y. Interleukin 4 as an essential factor for in vitro clonal growth of murine connective tissue-type mast cells. J Exp Med 1987; 165:268–73.
377. Sanderson CJ, Campbell HD, Young IG. Molecular and cellular biology of eosinophil differentiation factor (interleukin 5) and its effects on human and mouse B cells. Immunol Rev 1988; 102:29–50.
378. Dvorak AM, Furitsu T, Letourneau L, Ishizaka T, Ackerman SJ. Mature eosinophils stimulated to develop in human cord blood mononuclear cell cultures supplemented with recombinant human interleukin-5. I. Piecemeal degranulation of specific granules and distribution of Charcot-Leyden crystal protein. Am J Pathol 1991; 138:69–82.
379. Mizel SB. The interleukins. FASEB J 1989; 3:2379–88.
380. Le J, Vilce K. Biology of disease—interleukin 6: a multifunctional cytokine regulating immune reactions and the acute phase protein response. Lab Invest 1989; 61:588–602.
381. Everson MP, Lilly MB. Interleukin-6 and granulocyte-macrophage colony-stimulating factor are candidate growth factors for chronic myelogenous leukemia cells. Blood 1989; 74:1472–6.
382. Coffman RL, Carty J. A T cell activity that enhances polyclonal IgE production and its inhibition by interferon-γ. J Immunol 1986; 136:949–54.
383. Willman CL, Stewart CC, Miller V, Yi T-L, Tomasi TB. Regulation of MHC class II

gene expression in macrophages by hematopoietic colony-stimulating factors (CSF). J Exp Med 1989; 170:1559–67.

384. Vadhan-Raj S, Broxmeyer HE, Spitzer G, LeMaistre A, Hultman S, Ventura G, Tigard J-D, Cork MA, Trujillo JM, Gutterman JU, Hittelman WN. Stimulation of nonclonal hematopoiesis and suppression of the neoplastic clone after treatment with recombinant human granulocyte-macrophage colony-stimulating factor in a patient with therapy-related myelodysplastic syndrome. Blood 1989; 74:1491–8.
385. Parker JW, Metcalf D. Production of colony-stimulating factor in mitogen-stimulated lymphocytes. J Immunol 1974; 112:502–10.
386. Bradley TR, Metcalf D. The growth of mouse bone marrow cells in vitro. Aust J Exp Biol Med Sci 1966; 44:287–99.
387. Ichikawa Y, Pluznik DH, Sachs L. In vitro control of the development of macrophage and granulocyte colonies. Proc Natl Acad Sci USA 1966; 56:488–95.
388. Rollins BJ, Morrison ED, Stiles CD. Cloning and expression of JE, a gene inducible by platelet-derived growth factor and whose product has cytokine-like properties. Proc Natl Acad Sci USA 1988; 85:3738–42.
389. Burd PR, Rollins BJ, Wilson SD, Billings PR, Stiles CD, Dorf ME. Comparison of fibroblast and T-cell activation genes. Cell Immunol 1988; 115:481–3.
390. Brown KD, Zurawski SM, Mosmann TR, Zurawski G. A family of small inducible proteins secreted by leukocytes are members of a new superfamily that includes leukocyte and fibroblast-derived inflammatory agents, growth factors, and indicators of various activation processes. J Immunol 1989; 142:679–87.
391. Sherry B, Tekamp-Olson P, Gallegos C, Bauer D, Davatelis G, Wolpe SD, Masiarz F, Coit D, Cerami A. Resolution of the two components of macrophage inflammatory protein 1, and cloning and characterization of one of those components, macrophage inflammatory protein 1beta. J Exp Med 1988; 168:2251–9.
392. Wolpe SD, Davatelis G, Sherry B, Beutler B, Hesse DG, Nguyen HT, Moldawer LL, Nathan CF, Lowry SF, Cerami A. Macrophages secrete a novel heparin-binding protein with inflammatory and neutrophil chemokinetic properties. J Exp Med 1988; 167:570–81.
393. Wolpe SD, Cerami A. Macrophage inflammatory proteins 1 and 2: members of a novel superfamily of cytokines. FASEB J 1989; 3:2565–73.
394. Broxmeyer HE, Sherry B, Lu L, Cooper S, Carow C, Wolpe SD, Cerami A. Myelopoietic enhancing effects of murine macrophage inflammatory proteins 1 and 2 on colony formation in vitro by murine and human bone marrow granulocyte/macrophage progenitor cells. J Exp Med 1989; 170:1583–94.
395. Ghiara P, Boraschi D, Villa L, Scapigliati G, Taddei C, Tagliabue A. In vitro generated mast cells express natural cytotoxicity against tumour cells. Immunology 1985; 55:317–24.
396. Okuno T, Takagaki Y, Pluznik DH, Djeu JY. Natural cytotoxic (NC) cell activity in basophilic cells: release of NC-specific cytotoxic factor by IgE receptor triggering. J Immunol 1986; 136:4652–8.
397. Frieri M, Metcalfe DD. Analysis of the effect of mast cell granules on lymphocyte blastogenesis in the absence and presence of mitogens: identification of heparin as a granule-associated suppressor factor. J Immunol 1983; 131:1942–8.
398. Salari H, Chan-Yeung M. Mast cell mediators stimulate synthesis of arachidonic acid metabolites in macrophages. J Immunol 1989; 142:2821–7.
399. Yoffe JR, Taylor DJ, Woolley DE. Mast-cell products and heparin stimulate the production of mononuclear-cell factor by cultured human monocyte/macrophages. Biochem J 1985; 230:83–8.
400. Parsons WG III, Roberts LI II. Transformation of prostaglandin D_2 to isomeric prostaglandin F_2 compounds by human eosinophils. A potential mast cell-eosinophil interaction. J Immunol 1988; 141:2413–9.

401. Gruber BL, Schwartz LB, Ramamurthy NS, Irani A-M, Marchese MJ. Activation of latent rheumatoid synovial collagenase by human mast cell tryptase. J Immunol 1988; 140:3936–42.
402. Katz HR, Dayton ET, Levi-Schaffer F, Benson AC, Austen KF, Stevens RL. Coculture of mouse IL-3-dependent mast cells with 3T3 fibroblasts stimulates synthesis of globopentaosylceramide (Forssman glycolipid) by fibroblasts and surface expression on both populations. J Immunol 1988; 140:3090–7.
403. Wershil BK, Murakami T, Galli SJ. Mast cell-dependent amplification of an immunologically nonspecific inflammatory response. Mast cells are required for the full expression of cutaneous acute inflammation induced by phorbol 12-myristate 13-acetate. J Immunol 1988; 140:2356–60.
404. Galli SJ, Dvorak AM, Dvorak HF. Morphology, biochemistry, and function of basophils. In: Williams WJ, Beutler E, Erslev AJ, Lichtman MA, eds. Hematology, 3d ed. New York: McGraw-Hill, 1983:820–5.
405. Galli SJ, Dvorak AM, Dvorak HF. Morphology, biochemistry, and function of basophils and mast cells. In: Williams WJ, Beutler E, Erslev AJ, Lichtman MA, eds. Hematology, 4th ed. New York: McGraw-Hill, 1990:840–5.
406. Colvin RB, Burton JR, Hyslop NE, Spitz L, Lichtenstein NS. Penicillin associated interstitial nephritis. Ann Intern Med 1974; 81:404–5.
407. Aspegren N, Fregert S, Rorsman H. Basophil leukocytes in allergic eczematous contact dermatitis. Int Arch Allergy 1963; 23:150–6.
408. Fregert S, Rorsman H. Basophil leukocytes in intracutaneous test reactions to metals. J Invest Dermatol 1963; 41:361–7.
409. Dvorak HF, Mihm MC Jr. Basophilic leukocytes in a case of poison ivy. N Engl J Med 1971; 285:54–5.
410. Felarca AB, Lowell FC. The accumulation of eosinophils and basophils at skin sites as related to intensity of skin reactivity and symptoms in atopic disease. J Allergy Clin Immunol 1971; 48:125–33.
411. Henocq E, Gaillard J. Cutaneous basophil hypersensitivity in atopic dermatitis. Clin Allergy 1981; 11:13–20.
412. Mitchell EB, Crown J, Chapman MD, Jouhal SS, Pope FM, Platts-Mills TAE. Basophils in allergen-induced patch test sites in atopic dermatitis. Lancet 1982; i:127–30.
413. Mihm MC Jr, Soter NA, Dvorak HF, Austen KF. The structure of normal skin and the morphology of atopic eczema. J Invest Dermatol 1976; 67:305–12.
414. Rebuck JW, Hodson JM, Priest RJ, Barth CL. Basophilic granulocytes in inflammatory tissues of man. Ann NY Acad Sci 1963; 103:409–26.
415. Dvorak HF, Mihm MC Jr, Dvorak AM, Barnes BA, Galli SJ. The microvasculature is the critical target of the immune response in vascularized skin allograft rejection. J Invest Dermatol 1980; 74:280–4.
416. Parmley RT, Spicer SS, Wright NJ. The ultrastructural identification of tissue basophils and mast cells in Hodgkin's disease. Lab Invest 1975; 32:469–75.
417. Harris NL, Dvorak AM, Smith J, Dvorak HF. Fibrin deposits in Hodgkin's disease. Am J Pathol 1982; 108:119–29.
418. Askenase PW, Atwood JE. Basophils in tuberculin and Jones-Mote delayed reactions of humans. J Clin Invest 1976; 58:1145–54.
419. Wolf-Jürgensen P, Schwartz M. Normal lymphocyte transfer in man. Basophil leukocytes in delayed skin reaction. Lancet 1964; 2:388–90.
420. Dvorak HF. Cutaneous basophil hypersensitivity. J Allergy Clin Immunol 1976; 58:229–40.
421. Colvin RB, Mosesson MW, Dvorak HF. Delayed-type hypersensitivity skin reactions in congenital afibrinogenemia lack fibrin deposition and induration. J Clin Invest 1979; 63:1302–6.

422. Adelman NE, Hammond ME, Cohen S, Dvorak HF. Lymphokines as inflammatory mediators. In: Pick E, Oppenheimer J, Cohen S, eds. Biology of the lymphokines. New York: Academic Press, 1979:13–58.
423. Galli SJ, Dvorak HF. Basophils and mast cells: structure, function and role in hypersensitivity. In: Gupta S, Good RA, eds. Cellular, molecular and clinical aspects of allergic disorders. New York: Plenum Publishing, 1979:1–53.
424. Aspegren N, Fregert S, Rorsman H. Basophil leukocytes at sites of intracutaneous tuberculin test reactions. Int Arch Allergy 1964; 24:35–8.
425. Aspegren N, Fregert S, Rorsman H. Basophil leukocytes in nonvesicular allergic patch test reactions. J Invest Dermatol 1963; 41:107–8.
426. Fulton JE, Derbes VJ. Basophil leukocyte infiltration in the positive tuberculin skin test in man. J Invest Dermatol 1964; 43:125–8.
427. Askenase PW, Atwood JE. Basophils in tuberculin and Jones-Mote delayed reactions of humans. J Clin Invest 1976; 58:1145–54.
428. Black MM, Leis HP Jr. Cellular responses to autologous breast cancer tissue. Sequential observations. Cancer 1973; 32:384–9.
429. Dvorak AM. Legionnaires' disease. Arch Pathol Lab Med 1980; 104:336–7.
430. Katz SM, Brodsky I, Kahn SB. Legionnaire's disease: ultrastructural appearance of the agent in a lung biopsy specimen. Arch Pathol Lab Med 1979; 103:261–4.
431. deShazo RD, Levinson AI, Dvorak HF, Davis RW. The late phase skin raction. Evidence for activation of the coagulation system in an IgE-dependent reaction in man. J Immunol 1979; 122:692–8.
432. Dolovich J, Hargreave FE, Chalmers R, Shier KJ, Gauldie J, Bienenstock J. Late cutaneous allergic responses in isolated IgE-dependent reactions. J Allergy Clin Immunol 1973; 52:38–46.
433. Solley GO, Gleich GJ, Jordan RE, Schroeter AL. The late phase of the immediate wheal and flame skin reaction. J Clin Invest 1976; 58:408–20.
434. deShazo RD, Griffing C, Kwan TH, Banks WA, Dvorak HF. Dermal hypersensitivity reactions to imported fire ants. J Allergy Clin Immunol 1984; 74:841–7.
435. Richerson HB, Rajtora DW, Penick GD, Dick FR, Yoo TJ, Kammermeyer JK, Anuras JS. Cutaneous and nasal allergic responses in ragweed hay fever: lack of clinical and histopathological correlations with late phase reactions. J Allergy Clin Immunol 1979; 64:67–77.
436. Hastie R, Heroy JH III, Levy DA. Basophil leukocytes and mast cells in human nasal secretions and scrapings studied by light microscopy. Lab Invest 1979; 40:554–61.
437. Okuda M, Kawabori S, Otsuka H. Electron microscope study of basophilic cells in allergic nasal secretions. Arch Otorhinolaryngol 1978; 221:215–20.
438. Okuda M, Otsuka H. Basophilic cells in allergic nasal secretions. Arch Otorhinolaryngol 1977; 214:283–9.
439. Allansmith MR, Baird RS, Greiner JV. Vernal conjunctivitis and contact lens-associated giant papillary conjunctivitis compared and contrasted. Am J Ophthalmol 1979; 87:544–55.
440. Collin HB, Allansmith MR. Basophils in vernal conjunctivitis in humans. An electron microscopic study. Invest Ophthalmol Vis Sci 1977; 16:858–64.
441. Kawanami O, Ferrans VJ, Fulmer JD, Crystal RG. Ultrastructure of pulmonary mast cells in patients with fibrotic lung disorders. Lab Invest 1979; 40:717–35.
442. Kaung DT. Periodic acid-Schiff reaction in human basophilic leucocytes. Acta Haematol 1969; 42:269–74.
443. Goodman JR, Reilly EB, Moore RE. Electron microscopy of formed elements of normal human blood. Blood 1957; 12:428–42.
444. Soter NA, Mihm MC Jr, Gigli I, Dvorak HF, Austen KF. Two distinct cellular patterns in cutaneous necrotizing angiitis. J Invest Dermatol 1976; 66:344–50.

445. Soter NA, Mihm MC Jr, Dvorak HF, Austen KF. Cutaneous necrotizing venulitis: a sequential analysis of the morphological alterations occurring after mast cell degranulation in a patient with a unique syndrome. Clin Exp Immunol 1978; 32:46–58.
446. deShazo RD, Boehm TM, Kumar D, Galloway JA, Dvorak HF. Dermal hypersensitivity reactions to insulin: correlations of three patterns to their histopathology. J Allergy Clin Immunol 1982; 69:229–37.
447. Colvin RB, Pinn VW, Simpson BA, Dvorak HF. Cutaneous basophil hypersensitivity. IV. The "late reaction": sequel to Jones-Mote type hypersensitivity. Comparison with rabbit arthus reaction. Effect of passive antibody on induction and expression of Jones-Mote hypersensitivity. J Immunol 1973; 110:1279–89.
448. Dvorak HF, Hirsch MS. Role of basophilic leukocytes in cellular immunity to vaccinia virus infection. J Immunol 1971; 107:1576–82.
449. Dvorak HF, Dvorak AM. Immunohistologic characterization of inflammatory cells that infiltrate tumors. In: Haskill S, ed. Tumor immunity in prognosis. The role of mononuclear cell infiltration. Immunology series, vol. 18. New York: Marcel Dekker, 1982:279–307.
450. Galli SJ, Bast RC, Jr, Bast BS, Isomura T, Zbar B, Rapp HJ, Dvorak HF. Bystander suppression of tumor growth. Evidence that specific targets and bystanders are damaged by injury to a common microvasculature. J Immunol 1982; 129:1790–9.
451. Dvorak HF, Dvorak AM, Manseau EJ, Wiberg L, Churchill WH. Fibrin-gel investment associated with line 1 and line 10 solid tumor growth. Angiogensis and fibroplasia in guinea pigs. Role of cellular immunity, myofibroblasts, microvascular damage, and infarction in line 1 tumor regression. J Natl Cancer Inst 1979; 62:1459–72.
452. Kimura M, Takaya K. Ultrastructure of basophilic leukocytes and mast cells in normal and cutaneous basophil hypersensitivity-reacted guinea pig dermis. Int Arch Allergy Appl Immunol 1979; 60:383–9.
453. Richerson HB, Dvorak HF, Leskowitz S. Cutaneous basophilic hypersensitivity: a new interpretation of the Jones-Mote reaction. J Immunol 1969; 103:1431–4.
454. Dvorak AM, Galli SJ, Dvorak HF. Basophilic leukocytes in cell-mediated hypersensitivity: possible non-anaphylactic mechanisms of mediator release. In: Oehling A, Glazer I, Mathov E, Arbesman C, eds. Advances in allergology and immunology. Oxford: Pergamon Press, 1980:215–22.
455. Askenase PW. Cutaneous basophil hypersensitivity in contract-sensitized guinea pigs. I. Transfer with immune serum. J Exp Med 1973; 138:1144–55.
456. Askenase PW. Cutaneous basophil hypersensitivity uncovered in the cell transfer of classical tuberculin hypersensitivity. J Immunol 1976; 117:741–7.
457. Bast RC, Simpson BA, Dvorak HF. Heterogeneity of the cellular immune response. II. The role of adjuvant lymphocyte stimulation in cutaneous basophil hyersensitivity. J Exp Med 1971; 133:202–15.
458. Dvorak HF, Hammond ME, Colvin RB, Manseau EJ, Goodwin J. Systemic expression of cutaneous basophil hypersensitivity. J Immunol 1977; 118:1549–57.
459. Stadecker MJ, Leskowitz S. Genetic control of cutaneous basophil hypersensitivity. J Exp Med 1976; 143:206–10.
460. Stadecker MJ, Leskowitz S. The inhibition of basophil-rich delayed skin reactions by a heterologous anti-guinea pig T cell serum. J Immunol 1976; 116:1646–51.
461. Richerson HB. Cutaneous basophil (Jones-Mote) hypersensitivity after "tolerogenic" doses of intravenous ovalbumin in the guinea pig. J Exp Med 1971; 134:630–41.
462. Colvin RB, Dvorak HF. Role of the clotting system in cell-mediated hypersensitivity. II. Kinetics of fibrinogen/fibrin accumulation and vascular permeability changes in tuberculin and cutaneous basophil hypersensitivity reactions. J Immunol 1975; 114:377–87.
463. Stadecker MJ, Leskowitz S. The cutaneous basophil response to particulate antigens. Proc Soc Exp Biol Med 1973; 142:150–4.

464. Dvorak HF, Hammond ME. Cutaneous basophil hypersensitivity. In: Bach MK, ed. Modern concepts and developments in immediate hypersensitivity, vol. 7. New York: Marcel Dekker, 1978:369–405.
465. Galli SJ, Colvin RB, Verdeber E, Galli AS, Monahan RA, Dvorak AM, Dvorak HF. Preparation of a rabbit anti-guinea pig basophil serum: in vitro and in vivo characterization. J Immunol 1978; 121:1157–66.
466. Colvin RB, Dvorak HF. Role of granulocytes in cell-mediated immunity. In: Ward P, McCluskey RT, Cohen S, eds. Mechanisms of immunopathology. New York: Wiley, 1979:69–89.
467. Askenase PW, Hayden B, Higashi G. Cutaneous basophil hypersensitivity (CBH) and macrophage migration inhibition (MMI) in guinea pigs with schistosomiasis. J Allergy Clin Immunol 1975; 55:111.
468. Stashenko PP, Bhan AK, Schlossman SF, McCluskey RT. Local transfer of delayed hypersensitivity and cutaneous basophil hypersensitivity. J Immunol 1977; 119:1987–93.
469. Katz S, Heather CJ, Parker D, Turk JL. Basophilic leukocytes in delayed hypersensitivity reactions. J Immunol 1974; 113:1073–8.
470. Dvorak HF. Role of basophilic leukocytes in allograft rejection. J Immunol 1971; 106:279–81.
471. Allen JR. Tick resistance: basophils in skin reactions of resistant guinea pigs. Int J Parasitol 1973; 3:195–200.
472. Brown SJ, Askenase PW. Cutaneous basophil responses and immune resistance of guinea pigs to ticks. Passive transfer with peritoneal exudate cells or serum. J Immunol 1981; 127:2163–7.
473. Brown SJ, Knapp FW. Response of hypersensitized guinea pigs to the feeding of *Amblyomma americanum* ticks. Parasitology 1981; 83:213–23.
474. Wikel SK, Allen JR. Acquired resistance to ticks. I. Passive transfer of resistance. Immunology 1976; 30:311–26.
475. Brown SJ, Askenase PW. Rejection of ticks from guinea pigs by anti-hapten-antibody-mediated degranulation of basophils at cutaneous basophil hypersensitivity sites: role of mediators other than histamine. J Immunol 1985; 134:1160–5.
476. Ringoen A. The mast leukocytes in the adult guinea pig under experimental conditions. Am J Anat 1923; 31:319–37.
477. Plimpton NC Jr. Basophilic leukocytes after local injection of ventriculin. Anat Rec 1940; 76:475–83.
478. Friedlaender MH, Dvorak HF. Morphology of delayed-type hypersensitivity reactions in guinea pig cornea. J Immunol 1977; 118:1558–63.
479. Askenase PW, Boone WT, Binder HJ. Colonic basophil hypersensitivity. J Immunol 1978; 120:198–201.
480. Rothwell TLW. Studies of the responses of basophil and eisonophil leukocytes and mast cells to the nematode *Trichostrongylus colubriformis.* I. Observations during the expulsion of the first and second infections by guinea pigs. J Pathol 1975; 116:51–60.
481. Rothwell TLW, Love RJ. Studies of the responses of basophil and eosinophil leukocytes and mast cells to the nematode *Trichostrongylus colubriformis.* II. Changes in cell numbers following infection of thymectomized and adoptively or passively immunized guinea pigs. J Pathol 1975; 116:183–94.
482. Huxtable CR, Rothwell TLW. Studies of the responses of basophil and eosinophil leukocytes and mast cells to the nematode *Trichostrongylus colubriformis.* Ultrastructural changes in basophils and eosinophils at the sites of infection. Aust J Exp Biol Med Sci 1975; 53:437–45.
483. Rothwell TLW, Dineen JK. Cellular reactions in guinea pigs following primary and challenge infection with *Trichostrongylus colubriformis* with special reference to roles played by eosinophils and basophils in rejection of the parasite. Immunology 1972; 22:733–45.

484. Stadecker MJ, Leskowitz S. The cutaneous basophil response to mitogens. J Immunol 1974; 113:496–500.
485. Stadecker MJ, Lukic M, Dvorak AM, Leskowitz S. The cutaneous basophil response to phytohemagglutinin in chickens. J Immunol 1977; 118:1564–8.
486. Burton AL, Higginbotham RD. Response of blood basophils to Rous sarcoma virus infection in chicks and its significance. J Reticuloendothelial Soc 1966; 3:314–26.
487. Thonnard-Neumann E. Studies of basophils. Basophilic leukocytes and gonadal activity in the rabbit. Acta Haematol 1964; 32:358–67.
488. Zachariae F, Asboe-Hansen G, Boseila A-WA. Studies on the mechanism of ovulation. Acta Endocrinol 1948; 28:547–52.
489. Mettler L, Shirwani D. Direct basophil count for timing ovulation. Fertil Steril 1974; 25:718–23.
490. Bienenstock J, Johnston N. A morphologic study of rabbit bronchial lymphoid aggregates and lympho-epithelium. Lab Invest 1976; 35:343–8.
491. Clark JB, Altman G, Fromowitz FB. Basophil hypersensitivity response in rabbits. Infect Immun 1977; 15:305–12.
492. Sotelo TR, Porter KR. An electron microscopic study of the rat ovary. J Biophys Biochem Cytol 1959; 5:327–41.
493. Watanabe S, Watanabe K, Oishi T, Aiba M, Kageyama K. Mast cells in the rat alveolar septa undergoing fibrosis after ionizing irradiation. Ultrastructural and histochemical studies. Lab Invest 1974; 31:555–67.
494. Behrendt H, Rosenkranz U, Schmutzler W. Ultrastructure of isolated human mast cells during histamine release induced by ionophore A23187. Int Arch Allergy Appl Immunol 1978; 56:188–92.
495. Ishizaka T, Saito H, Furitsu T, Dvorak AM. Growth of human basophils and mast cells in vitro. In: Galli SJ, Austen KF, eds. Mast cell and basophil differentiation and function in health and disease. New York: Raven Press, 1989:39–47.
496. Ishizaka T, Saito H, Hatake K, Dvorak AM, Leiferman KM, Arai N, Ishizaka K. Preferential differentiation of inflammatory cells by recombinant human interleukins. Int Arch Allergy Appl Immunol 1989; 88:46–9.
497. Schrader JW. Bone marrow differentiation in vitro. CRC Crit Rev Immunol 1983; 4:197–277.
498. Yung Y-P, Moore MAS. Mast cell growth-factor. Lymphokine Res 1983; 2:127–31.
499. Ishizaka T, Adachi T, Chang T-H, Ishizaka K. Development of mast cells in vitro. II. Biologic function of cultured mast cells. J Immunol 1977; 118:211–7.
500. Dvorak AM, Furitsu T, Estrella P. Ishizaka T. Human lung-derived mature mast cells cultured alone or with mouse 3T3 fibroblasts maintain an ultrastructural phenotype different from that of human mast cells that develop from human cord blood cells cultured with 3T3 fibroblasts. Am J Pathol 1991; 139.
501. Dvorak AM, Ackerman SJ, Furitsu T, Estrella P. Letourneau L, Ishizaka T. Mature eosinophil stimulated to develop in human cord blood mononuclear clear cell cultures supplemented with recombinant human interleukin-5. II. Vesicular transport of specific granule matrix peroxidase, a mechanism for effecting piecemeal degranulation. Am J Pathol 1992; (in press).

8

Signal Mechanisms in the Activation of Basophils and Mast Cells

DONALD MACGLASHAN, JR.
Johns Hopkins University School of Medicine, Baltimore, Maryland

I. INTRODUCTION

Basophils and mast cells are central participants in allergic reactions. Both cell types secrete inflammatory mediators such as histamine in response to antigens which aggregate cell surface IgE antibody bound to a high-affinity receptor unique to these two cell types. It is generally believed that both of these cells participate in numerous other physiologic or pathophysiologic responses. For example, the basophil is known to dominate certain cell-mediated reactions such as reactions to ticks (1–3). The mast cell is generally found lining the outside of blood vessels, and it is speculated that it may act as a neuro-immuno-hormonal link in the maintenance of tissue homeostasis. However, the roles of basophils and mast cells in these situations remains unclear, and there are no good models of these reactions in which an investigation of signal transduction mechanisms would be meaningful. On the other hand, the immunologic and nonimmunologic stimulation of basophils and mast cells to produce mediators which cause allergic reactions is very amenable to study. Indeed, the IgE-mediated reaction is an excellent paradigm for cellular reactions involving the cross-linking of cell surface antibody.

While basophils and mast cells share some characteristics, the mature basophil is a mobile leukocyte which must react to events occurring in tissues and subsequently find its way through the blood vessel endothelium to participate in tissue reactions. In contrast, the mature mast cell resides in tissues throughout the body. In the airway, it is able to respond to environmental events long before the basophil. The possibility that mast cells serve both physiologic and pathophysiologic roles while basophils generally participate only in pathophysiologic reactions suggests that some of the intrinsic regulatory mechanisms will differ between these two cell types. The basophil must also possess the means to react quickly to changes in the blood vessel endothelium and presumably needs a more pronounced apparatus for movement than the mast cell. Indeed, many studies to date suggest that many characteristics of these two cell types are quite distinct, and these differences will be alluded to throughout this review. Nevertheless, at this point in time, the IgE-mediated reaction probably has a great many similarities, so that as this type of stimulation is explored, there will be significant mixing of the data to arrive at a more complete picture of this particular reaction. Time will tell if this mixing is appropriate.

This chapter will focus primarily on the reaction that is best understood in these cells, IgE-mediated degranulation. The data discussed will draw heavily upon work done in murine mast cells of various sources, but there are many interesting studies of human mast cells and basophils which help to distinguish the human cells from their rodent counterparts. For studies of human mast cells, this chapter will also primarily focus on mast cells derived from human lung parenchyma, although some differences do exist among mast cells derived from other human tissues. This chapter will also focus on mediator release from mast cells and basophils. Thus far, there have not been intensive studies of other functional endpoints. Basophils undergo extensive morphological changes during stimulation, and there are several stimuli that are known to be chemotactic. Each of these endpoints is very difficult to study in detail (only recently have quantitative morphological measurements been possible). Mast cells did not appear to have other functional endpoints until recent studies showed that mast cells secrete a variety of cytokines (4,5). While this is also a secretory reaction, it takes place on a much longer time scale (hours instead of minutes) and probably involves signaling to the nucleus and DNA transcription. Thus, the mechanisms of signal transduction may be distinctive and have certainly not been studied in detail.

II. MEDIATORS

As noted above, the functional endpoint for the basophil and mast cell reaction most commonly studied is the secretion of inflammatory mediators. Some of these mediators, e.g., histamine, are preformed and located in prominent granules. These granules carry positively charged histamine on a highly sulfated proteoglycan substrate which in many ways acts as an ion-exchange resin for histamine; when releasing the histamine in the extracellular medium, the granule contents are extruded and histamine is exchanged for other local cations. The proteoglycan substrate should not be viewed as a passive carrier for histamine. In mast cells, the predominant proteoglycan is heparin (6), which is known to enhance the activity of endothelial growth factors such as endothelial cell growth factor (7). The juxtaposition of mast cells to blood vessels walls is therefore highly suggestive of a role for mast cells in blood vessel growth. There are other preformed mediators associated with these granules whose roles are not yet clearly defined. For example, mast cells possess large quantities of tryptase (8), while basophils do not (9). The role of the enzyme remains unclear, although it has been shown that at low pH, the enzyme can generate bradykinin from kininogens (10).

In addition to the preformed mediators, basophils and mast cells secrete a number of mediators that are synthesized only during stimulation, generally products of phospholipid metabolism. The release of these mediators, relative to the release of histamine, differentiates the various stimuli which cause release in human basophils (to be discussed below). Here too, mast cells and basophils differ significantly. In basophils, arachidonic acid, which is liberated from phospholipids during activation, is metabolized primarily to leukotriene C_4 (20–200 pmoles/10^6 basophils), with small amounts of 5HETE released (11). No LTB_4 (12) or prostaglandins (11) are released in any basophil reaction studied to date. The mast cell also generates similar quantities of LTC_4, but in addition to 5HETE, LTB_4 is released in smaller quantities (1–5 pmol/10^6 cells) (13–15). In addition, prostaglandin D_2 is a major arachidonic acid metabolite from mast cells (20–200 pmol/10^6 cells) (13). It also appears that some thromboxane is released. This pattern of arachidonic acid metabolite release generally occurs in human mast cells isolated from lung, skin, intestine, and uterus (16–18).

The complete lack of prostaglandin release from basophils clearly differentiates the human basophil from the human mast cell. This difference was exploited to suggest that in experimental allergic reactions, basophils migrate into tissues several hours after the initial mast cell reaction and contribute the majority of the histamine release seen in these so-called late-phase reactions (19–22). The general pattern of mediator release in these experimental challenges following the application of antigen is an abrupt rise in histamine and prostaglandin in the tissue fluids, followed by a relative quiescent period and then a second late reaction which is thought to replicate experimentally the inflammatory reaction which characterizes asthmatic reactions. Leukocytes appear in the tissue during the late reaction; histamine is measured in the complete absence of prostaglandin D_2 (even as measured by an exquisitely sensitive GCMS technique). In addition, tryptase, another mast cell granule marker, is found only in the early reaction (23). Only the basophil and eosinophil appear to be selectively recruited in these late inflammatory reactions (24).

One additional phospholipid product, not derived from arachidonic acid, is platelet-activating factor (PAF). Mast cells appear to synthesize relatively large quantities of this mediator (25,26), while early reports suggest that the basophil does not (27). However, the basophil studies are undergoing a reexamination in light of new evidence that an acyl form of PAF can inhibit detection of PAF (alkyl form) by the standard bioassay and this acyl form may be generated in substantial quantities in basophils. As with all cells which synthesize PAF, mast cells do not appear to release this mediator. Recent studies suggest that this is an artefact of the handling procedure (28), and that a cell may release PAF if an appropriate carrier is included and also rapidly removed and replaced.

III. STIMULI

A. Non-IgE-Dependent Stimuli

While this chapter focuses primarily on IgE-mediated mediator release from human basophils and mast cells, there are other stimuli which can initiate release from these cells. Since the inflammatory reaction is not necessarily characterized by antigen-driven release, these other stimuli are important to study and may also play a role in pathophysiologic conditions not associated with type I hypersensitivity reactions.

Thus far, the human basophil responds to a broader range of stimuli than the mast cell. This statement must be qualified by noting that, in general, human mast cells from various tissues are dissociated from the tissue matrix with proteolytic enzymes. Therefore, it is possible that certain receptors are lost in the preparation of mast cells.

The basophil responds not only to the cross-linking of cell surface IgE antibody, but also to IgG antibody bound to specific receptors, probably FcγII receptors (29,30). The effects of inter-cross-linking between these two receptor types has not been explored. The bacterial peptide, formyl-methionyl-leucyl-phenylalanine (fMet), is a strong stimulus in basophils, but the magnitude of the basophil response to this stimulus and to IgE-mediated cross-linking is uncorrelated (31). A detailed comparison of the signal transduction mechanisms for these two stimuli is underway, as will be discussed below. The anaphylatoxins C5a and C3a also induce histamine release (32,33). However, while most donors' basophils respond with histamine release, very few donors possess basophils capable of releasing leukotrienes to this stimulus (11,34). Human basophils are now reported to respond to PAF (35) as well as major basic protein derived from eosinophils (36). Several polycations also induce release (37). The most recently discovered class of stimuli include the so-called histamine-releasing factors (38–42). These are proteins, derived from the culture supernatants of a wide variety of cells, which induce histamine release by mechanisms currently unknown. Several factors induce release by mechanisms unrelated to the presence of cell surface IgE (38), while others appear to be IgE dependent (41,42).

Human lung mast cells have thus far been found to secrete only in response to IgE-mediated stimulation. However, human skin mast cells respond to several univalent stimuli (43–47). Morphine, substance P, vasoactive intestinal peptide, somatostatin, and a bradykinin analog induce a rapid secretion of histamine and prostaglandins, although the amount of secreted prostaglandin D2 is less than 10% of that released in response to IgE-mediated stimulation (for equal histamine release) (46,47).

Generally, there is no relationship between the ability of basophils or mast cells to respond to one stimulus versus any other stimulus. Each stimulus appears to initiate specific biochemical events; i.e., the signal transduction pathways are distinct for each stimulus. One manifestation of these different pathways is the relative amounts of histamine and leukotriene released. Antigens and fMet peptide induce similar ratios of histamine and leukotriene release. As noted above, C5a induces histamine release only in basophils. In contrast, PAF induces more leukotriene release (per histamine release) than antigen or fMet peptide. A similar disparity exists in the skin mast cell, as noted above. These differences are useful tools toward understanding the mechanisms of signal transduction and will be expanded upon below.

B. Antigen:IgE Antibody Aggregation Reaction

Cross-linking cell surface IgE antibody with antigen is required to initiate the IgE-mediated reaction. Freely mobile IgE/receptor complexes appear to provide no signal that results in mediator release (48–50), although in RBL cells there is evidence which suggests that the univalent IgE/receptor complex might signal the cell to produce more receptor, possibly by inhibiting its endocytosis (51). With multivalent antigens possessing different epitopes and a spectrum of epitope-specific IgE antibodies on the cell surface, the aggregation reaction can be quite complex. However, it may be important to understand some of its details, since there is evidence to suggest that the form of the aggregates determines the quantitative and qualitative nature of the response.

The aggregation reaction on the surface of basophils and mast cells represents the two-dimensional analog of the classical antigen:antibody precipitin reaction in solution. In particular, the dose response curve shows suboptimal, optimal, and supraoptimal regions (see Figure 1). The concentration of antigen required for an optimal response is a complex function of the intrinsic affinity of the antibody for its antigen epitope, the valency of the antigen, the mixture of antibody specificities, and the dynamics of the cell response (since this is not an equilibrium reaction). The "avidity" of a particular

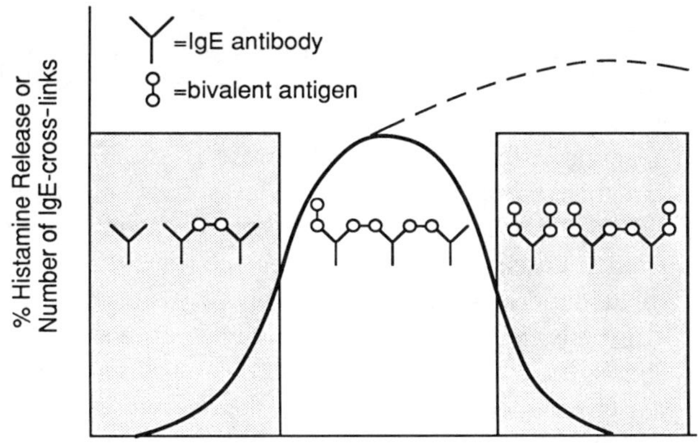

Figure 1 Characteristics of the histamine release dose response curve following challenge of basophils or mast cells with varying concentrations of bivalent antigen. The stick-and-ball drawings suggest the type of aggregation reaction occurring in different regions of the antigen dose response curve. The number of cross-linked IgE antibody molecules and the histamine release curves are essentially superimposable for simple antigens. The dashed line indicates the postulated cross-linking characteristics of anti-IgE antibody where histamine release decreases because the aggregate size becomes too large.

antibody preparation is an undefined combination of the first three factors. While the complexity of this reaction has defied mathematical solutions in analytical form, a simpler model has been studied with success. If the antigen is a hapten and bivalent forms of the hapten can be synthesized, then the dynamics of the reaction, as well as the size of aggregates formed, can be calculated (52,53). After calculations were made for the general case, the theories were tested on human basophils using the penicillin hapten and penicillin-specific IgE antibodies from penicillin-allergic patients (50,54,55). Because this hapten:antibody reaction is rapidly equilibrating, monovalent hapten could be used to dissociate the aggregates. These studies demonstrated that the cell response is a strict function of the number of cross-links (Figure 1), and that cross-links were required to maintain the release reaction (50). In other words, an ongoing reaction could be immediately stopped by the addition of monovalent hapten to dissociate cross-links. This is a powerful result because it has focused attention on signal transduction reactions which do not show transient behavior since it is clear that signal transduction events must be maintained throughout the period of the release reaction. Later studies using the mouse antidinitrophenyl (DNP) monoclonal IgE antibody demonstrated that the concentration of bivalent hapten required for optimal release was equal to $\frac{1}{2}K_a$, where K_a is the single-site affinity constant of the antibody for DNP, verifying one additional aspect of the mathematical model (56).

For some time it was accepted that dimeric aggregates were completely sufficient for activation. However, studies in RBL cells later indicated that trimeric aggregates (and larger) were 10- to 50-fold more potent stimuli of release (57). Studies in human basophils suggested that there was also a qualitative difference, since indomethacin could enhance trimeric IgE-induced release (IgE antibody covalently cross-linked and fractionated to include predominantly trimers of IgE) while having no effect or slightly inhibiting dimeric IgE-induced release (58). Later studies indicated indirectly that dimeric aggregates were generally unable to induce leukotriene release while causing only weak histamine release (59). These same studies also suggested that the ability of basophils to respond to dimeric aggregates was dependent on the donor and that basophils which could respond to dimeric aggregates were 10- to 100-fold more sensitive to antigenic stimulation than basophils which could respond only to trimeric or larger aggregates. The differential transduction of dimeric and trimeric signals may occur early in the biochemical cascade, since measurements of cytosolic calcium in human basophils indicate that dimeric signals induce only weak elevations in cytosolic calcium. Studies in RBL cells indicate that dimeric signals do not link the receptor to the underlying cytoskeleton, while trimeric signals do (60). The relevance of the cytoskeleton to general signal transduction is unclear, but the data do highlight another qualitative difference in the effects of aggregates of different sizes.

In addition to differential signal transduction at the low end of the aggregation spectrum, there are also indications that large aggregates may also be ineffective signals. For general studies of basophil histamine release, polyclonal anti-IgE (Fc-specific) antibody is employed as a nonspecific IgE antibody cross-linking reagent. However, the aggregation reaction which follows use of this antibody is complex. Suboptimal doses of anti-IgE antibody generate dimeric cross-links and therefore do not induce leukotriene release, while supraoptimal concentrations appear to generate very large aggregates. The decreased histamine release in the supraoptimal region of this dose response curve is not the result of fewer antigen:antibody aggregates, as in the case of antigens, but histamine release decreases because the aggregates are too large (61–63). Microscopic studies indicate that at high concentrations, where no histamine release occurs, patching and capping ultimately occurs (61). If monovalent Fab′ fragments of the same antibody are added to the high concentrations of the whole antibody, histamine release is increased (62). Again, this is in contrast with antigen-driven reactions where monovalent hapten further decreases the number of cross-links in the supraoptimal region and therefore decreases histamine release (53). This unusual characteristic of anti-IgE antibody appears to be related to its polyclonal nature, since monoclonal anti-IgE antibodies do not behave in the same manner (indeed, they behave more like bivalent haptens of high affinity). Circumstantial evidence suggests that overlaying multiple epitope-specific antibody dose response curves leads to the ability of the polyclonal antibody to generate these large aggregates (64). It is not yet clear whether large aggregates produce no signal for release or whether one size aggregate is equal to any other size and the overall strength of signal decreases as more antibodies are involved in the larger aggregates because of simple stochiometric considerations. This unusual characteristic of polyclonal anti-IgE antibody will resurface in the calcium studies to be discussed below.

IV. SIGNAL TRANSDUCTION

A. IgE Receptors

For many univalent receptors, the events which immediately follow the binding of ligand have become clearer in the last decade. A similar situation does not yet exist for immunoglobulin receptors that require cross-linking. Only recently has the high-affinity receptor of IgE antibody been cloned from both murine and human cells (65,66). In murine cells, such as the rat basophilic leukemia cell, this receptor is composed of three distinct subunits in a $\alpha\beta\gamma_2$ configuration. The β-subunit has not yet been cloned from human cells. It is not known whether the receptor itself possesses specific catalytic activities or whether it is immediately coupled to an intermediate similar to the GTP-binding proteins commonly employed by univalent receptor systems. The large structure of the receptor suggests that it acts in more than a ligand-binding role. The α-subunit has the high-affinity binding site for IgE (67). The γ-subunit, whose gene resides on the same chromosome as the α-subunit (68), is required for α-subunit expression in human cells while all three subunits are required in murine cells (69). The γ-subunit has homology with the ζ-subunit of the T-cell receptor and can interact with other Fc receptors (70). And while this subunit has only a cytoplasmic presentation and can be phosphorylated (71), its function is unknown. The β-subunit is intriguing. In human cells, it may be independently expressed. It has four domains which probably cross the membrane, and these regions bear homology with CD20, a protein which has recently been shown to mediate Ca^{2+} flux in B-lymphocytes. Indeed, the puzzle which must be resolved is why this receptor must be aggregated to be active. A speculative view would focus on the channel-like configuration of the β-subunit and by analogy with channel/pore proteins such as alamethicin (72,73), which might require more than one subunit (four membrane crossings) to form a complete ion channel. However, the role of these subunits in signal transduction has yet to be understood.

B. GTP-Binding Proteins

Because GTP-binding proteins mediate many univalent receptor responses, a search has begun for a GTP-binding protein which interacts with the IgE Fc receptor. At this time, the evidence remains controversial. For example, cholera toxin will increase the cytosolic calcium elevation which normally follows IgE-mediated activation of RBL cells (74). In the same cell as well as in rat peritoneal mast cells, nonhydrolyzable analogs of GTP will also up-regulate the response (75–77). In contrast, other studies have concluded that no GTP-binding protein is involved in this reaction (78). Pertussis toxin, which completely inhibits fMet peptide or C5a-induced release in human basophils, has no effect on IgE-mediated release (79). Therefore, if a GTP-binding protein regulates IgE-mediated release, it is not pertussis toxin sensitive. Because the IgE receptor bears a subunit organization similar to GTP-binding proteins, its sequence data was explored for homology but was found to be dissimilar.

C. Phospholipases

The effector enzyme for a putative GTP-binding protein also remains elusive. Phospholipases A_2, C, and D have all been implicated in the initial stages of the reaction and ultimately, each may be found to play a role. Human basophils and mast cells, as well as murine mast cells of various sources, all generate significant quantities of phospholipid metabolites. The arachidonic acid metabolites have generally been thought to be derived from the action of phospholipase A_2 on membrane phospholipids, and while some pharmacologic evidence supports this view (80–82), there has yet to be a direct demonstration of its involvement in the IgE-mediated reaction. In addition, the generation of PAF in mast cells of various types also strongly suggests the participation of a phospholipase A_2. Numerous laboratories suggest that inositol trisphosphate (83–85) is involved in the early activation cascade, and this phosphopolyol is believed to be derived from the action of a phospholipase C on the specific phosphatidylinositols. Arachidonic acid could also be derived from one of the phospholipase C byproducts, diacylglycerol (DAG), by the action of DAG-lipase (86). Diacylglycerol is a measurable metabolite in the IgE-mediated activation of rodent mast cells (87,88) and would be implicated in human basophil stimulation as well, since protein kinase C is activated in these cells (see below). However, the action of a phospholipase C on phosphatidylinositol is clearly not the only source of DAG, accounting for only 25% of the total DAG generated in rat peritoneal mast cells (87). The other likely source is phosphatidylcholine, which could be a source for DAG through the action of a phospholipase D. Recent studies have suggested that this enzyme is also active in stimulated rat peritoneal mast cells (89).

While the IgE Fc receptor may interact with a GTP-binding protein which then stimulates phospholipases, there are other pathways which might be coupled directly to receptor cross-linking. There is controversy over findings that RBL cells express a protein which can act as a calcium channel. This protein has been isolated and its addition to purified IgE Fc receptor in artificial membranes reconstitutes a calcium channel activity that depends on antigen-induced cross-linking of the receptor (90).

The role of phospholipases is almost certainly not restricted to the generation of lipid metabolites for secretion. The central paradigm of signal transduction today is the action of phospholipase C on phosphatidylinositol to generate DAG, which activates PKC, and inositol trisphosphate, which can mobilize intracellular calcium. Both of these areas are being studied intensively in mast cells and basophils.

It has been known for many years that a minimum requirement for mast cell or basophil degranulation was the presence of extracellular calcium (91). Removal of calcium at any point during the reaction immediately stopped further release. Several early studies of rat peritoneal mast cells suggested that transfer of the cells from a calcium-containing medium to a calcium-free medium simultaneously with stimulation could lead to release (92). However, it appears that the cell "shell" or "cage" calcium was acting as the source of external calcium in these reactions. Studies in RBL cells and human mast cells and basophils could not find evidence for this phenomenon. Thus, in general, the IgE-mediated reaction appears to be ultimately dependent on the mobilization of calcium from extracellular stores. Nevertheless, recent theories on cytoplasmic calcium elevations suggest that even if calcium must be replenished from the extracellular medium, the process requires the action of inositol 1,4,5-trisphosphate (IP3) on either intracellular sources of calcium or on the plasma membrane (93). Studies using RBL cells have most clearly addressed this aspect of signal transduction. IgE-mediated stimulation of these cells results in the production of IP3 and other inositol phosphates (83–85). Their generation correlates well with degranulation, and pharmacologic maneuvers that inhibit their generation also inhibit release (94,95). As will be discussed in additional detail below, there are several oscillations in cytosolic calcium levels following stimulation in calcium-free medium (96). These oscillations continue only if calcium is added to the medium. These oscillations also suggest the presence and action of IP3 on intracellular calcium stores (93). Despite this evidence, there remains some controversy over the role of IP3. The kinetics of IP3 generation is not always clearly related to the calcium elevation which follows stimulation. For example, early studies noted that IP3 generation proceeded for a period four times longer than the calcium elevation and peaked after the calcium elevation peaked. These data might suggest that

IP3 generation is a consequence of the calcium elevation, a real possibility since phospholipase C activity is sensitive to calcium (97). The primary difficulty in interpreting this data is the lack of sufficient quantitative information to draw strong conclusions. It is not known how much IP3 is required to initiate calcium mobilization, nor is it known precisely how PLC depends on calcium or other allosteric effectors, in situ.

D. Protein Kinase C

The other arm of the bifurcating pathway is the production of DAG and its activation (in cooperation with Ca^{2+}) of protein kinase C. However, the role of PKC in signal transduction is also controversial. In RBL cells, its activation appears to have little to do with degranulation (98). In the mouse PT-18 mast cell line, its activation correlates temporally and by magnitude with histamine release (86). No direct measurements have been made in human mast cells, but the available indirect evidence does not indicate a strong dependence of degranulation on its activation. Specifically, the phorbol ester, PMA, is able to down-regulate the quantity of PKC [as it does in RBL cells (97)] as assessed by the loss of mast cell inhibition by an acute treatment with PMA. Despite the apparent loss of PKC, histamine release following stimulation with anti-IgE antibody was inhibited only 30%. The kinase inhibitor, staurosporine, inhibits histamine release in mast cells, but at concentrations which leave its specificity open to question.

In contrast with human mast cells, human basophils appear to require PKC activation during IgE-mediated release (99). Several years before the phorbol esters were identified as activators of PKC, it was observed that PMA could induce significant histamine release from human basophils (100,101). In addition, pretreatment of basophils with anti-IgE antibody, while desensitizing the cells to further IgE-mediated release (see below), enhanced the basophil's response to PMA. This data (in retrospect) suggested a role for PKC in basophil degranulation. These studies have been augmented with direct measurements of PKC activity, which indicate that PKC activity correlates both temporally and in magnitude with histamine release (99). Unlike canonical PKC reactions, there was no apparent translocation of PKC from the cytosol to the membrane; the only change was found in membrane PKC activity. Furthermore, there was an increase in total PKC activity, not a simple redistribution of its activity. This distinct pattern for PKC activity raised the possibility that all stimuli induce a nonstandard form of PKC activity changes in human basophils. However, recent studies have shown that fMet peptide induces the canonical redistribution of PKC activity (102). Thus, the IgE-mediated pattern is unique to IgE-mediated release, although the significance of this pattern is unclear.

The kinase inhibitor staurosporine inhibits IgE-mediated release in basophils with a IC50 of 0.3 nM, a concentration consistent with relatively specific action of staurosporine on PKC and not other kinases (103). The IC50 of staurosporine for basophil-derived PKC, ex situ, is between 0.05 and 0.5 nM. Staurosporine has a similar IC50 for PMA-induced release in basophils (102).

These data, taken together, suggest that PKC plays a pro-degranulatory role in human basophil secretion. However, it should be noted that the actions of PMA are restricted to histamine release. PMA induces no arachidonic acid mobilization and therefore no leukotriene release (11). As in many cells, basophils stimulated with PMA show no elevation of cytosolic calcium (102). Indeed, if basophils are pretreated for 10 min with PMA, the cytosolic calcium response to antigens is nearly ablated (102). In addition, PMA can be used to stop leukotriene release at any point in the reaction, and preliminary experiments indicate that cytosolic calcium levels return rapidly to baseline following the addition of PMA to an ongoing IgE-mediated reaction. Thus, PMA stimulation is an incomplete signal. RBL cells do not respond directly to PMA, but PMA can increase the RBL cell's sensitivity to calcium ionophore (104). The combination of PMA and ionophore allows much lower cytosolic levels of calcium to induce histamine release than when using ionophore alone. However, these same studies concluded that the combination of PMA and ionophore A23187 did not entirely mimic the signals generated during IgE-mediated activation. Thus, at least three signals were felt to be necessary. Recent studies by the same group (105) conclude that modulation of cytosolic pH may be one of these additional signals.

E. Calcium

As noted above, extracellular calcium is mandatory for histamine release. Numerous studies have verified that marked elevations in cytosolic calcium follow the stimulation of mast cells and basophils with antigens or anti-IgE antibody (106–110). It is generally believed that the ultimate source of this calcium is from extracellular stores. Other than the controversial studies concerning a calcium channel protein (as noted above), the means by which calcium enters the cell remains unclear. However, the movement of calcium is not voltage dependent, nor do voltage-dependent calcium channel blockers (nifedipine, etc.) affect calcium uptake during IgE-mediated release at concentrations where their action is consistent with inhibition of a voltage-dependent channel (111,112). The kinetic curves of cytosolic calcium elevations, using fluorescent dyes such as fura-2 or quin-2, in whole-cell populations are not accurate reflections of the single-cell kinetic curves (109). In RBL cells, two events are masked by the averaging of all cell responses. First, the transition to elevated calcium levels is relatively abrupt but asynchronous among cells. The lag time between the addition of stimulus and the calcium response becomes longer in cells stimulated with suboptimal concentrations of antigen (see Figure 2). The asynchrony leads to the apparent slower average rise in whole-cell preparations. Second, the calcium levels often oscillate with a frequency of ~30 s, with oscillations superimposed on an average increase (95). These oscillations are also lost during averaging. Studies of human lung mast cells have not revealed oscillations, although similar abrupt asynchronous elevations do occur (110). Very preliminary studies in human basophils indicate that oscillations occur but that they are most easily observed during conditions of suboptimal stimulation and are almost chaotic, not periodic (see Figure 3). The significance of oscillations to the function of these cells is unclear. There are a number of cellular responses which show rhythmic oscillations in cytosolic calcium, and it is hypothesized that the signal transduction apparatus encodes the magnitude of stimulation in the frequency of the oscillations. Signal theory predicts that frequency encoding would result in better signal-to-noise ratios. However, in only one case of rhythmic oscillations has a function been correlated (113). This may soon be possible for human basophils, since these cells undergo marked morphological changes which can be quantitated and correlated, on a single-cell basis, with changes in calcium concentrations.

The abrupt nature of the transition of cytosolic calcium from resting levels to poststimulus levels suggests an all-or-nothing response by the cells. This possibility has

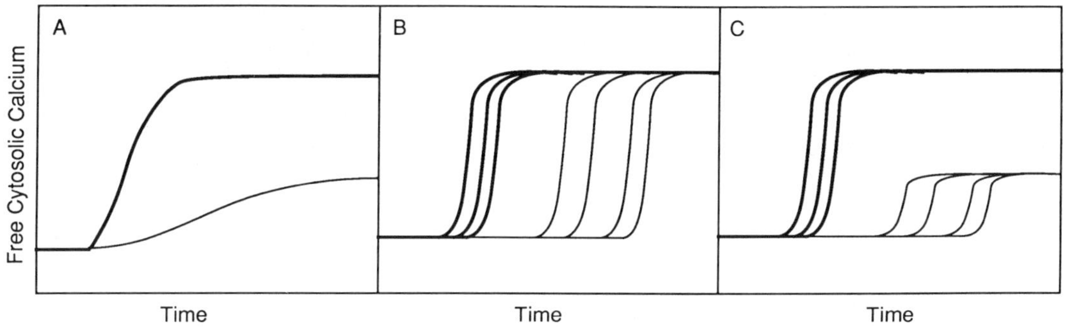

Figure 2 Idealized kinetic curves of the elevations in free cytosolic calcium which follow stimulation of mast cells (human lung mast cells or RBL cells) with anti-IgE antibody or antigen. The three panels show some possible characteristics of these curves (see text). Panel A shows the two curves obtained from average population measurements at two concentrations of stimulus (heavy and thin lines). Panel B shows the idealized form of a response which would be strictly all-or-nothing in character, variable lags in the transition times but with a constant elevation. Presumably, a smaller average response would result from fewer cells undergoing the transition. Panel C shows the idealized form as it generally appears experimentally. The lag times and the elevations are both dependent on the concentration of the stimulus resulting in a mixed all-or-nothing and graded-transition characteristic. It should be noted that individual cell responses are quite variable in form and do not always follow these idealized curves. Indeed, some transitions more closely resemble the average population response, while others show multiple small transition steps.

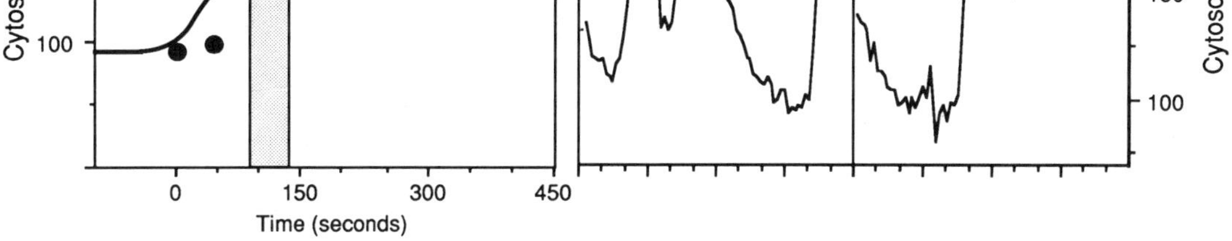

Figure 3 The elevation in free cytosolic Ca^{2+} which follows stimulation of human basophils with anti-IgE antibody at a concentration which causes less than maximal histamine release. Panel A shows the average cell population response while Panels B and C show the response of individual cells (note the change of of scale) in the time frame delimited by the stippled box in panel A. Anti-IgE was added at time zero, and the nonstimulated responses did not show these oscillations.

been debated for some time, since the release of histamine from mast cells and basophils rarely represents the total cellular stores. Thus, the question has been whether 50% histamine release implies that 50% of the cells released all their histamine, or whether all cells released 50% of their histamine. The single-cell calcium kinetics discussed above support the all-or-nothing response. However, studies in human lung mast cells suggest that the magnitude of the elevation is a graded function of the strength of stimulus (110). Thus, the calcium response has characteristics that suggest both all-or-nothing and graded responses. In the human basophil, preliminary studies have found that four measures of the cell response, at the single-cell level, show graded changes: calcium elevations (102), f-actin elevations (114), morphological changes (114), and up-regulation of specific cell surface receptors (115). Future models of the mast cell or basophil response must account for these characteristics.

F. Protein Phosphorylation

Calcium elevations, by acting through calcium/calmodulin-dependent kinases, and activation of protein kinase C, result in the phosphorylation of proteins presumably involved in degranulation and other cell functions. It is not yet clear how many steps exist between the early signals and the final act of degranulation. If the studies of nerve cell synaptic vesicle secretion were a guide (116), we could conclude that the number of steps is small since a calcium/calmodulin-dependent kinase phosphorylates a granule protein which controls granule extrusion. Unfortunately, there have been few studies of protein phosphorylation in mast cells and basophils. Several protein bands have been identified as undergoing changes in phosphorylation state during degranulation in rat mast cells or RBL cells, but their function remains obscure (117–121). However, it is interesting to note that one of the identified proteins in activated rat peritoneal mast cells is thought to participate in the desensitization (see below) of these cells (119). Several proteins have also been identified as responding to stimulation with PMA and thus may mark PKC-specific substrates (121). These studies are also important if the changes in PKC activity are to be interpreted properly, since the redistribution of PKC activity during stimulation does not necessarily imply its activation. Only substrate studies can verify its activity.

G. Comparative Studies of IgE- and fMet Peptide-Mediated Release

As noted above, human basophils respond to numerous IgE-independent stimuli. The response to fMet peptide, for example, is probably due to the fact that this cell is a leukocyte and either requires this receptor system to function as a leukocyte or has it as a vestige of its lineage. Nevertheless, the response to fMet peptide, thus far, resembles the response of neutrophils to this stimulus. Therefore, the body of knowledge acquired in neutrophil studies is applicable to basophils. This is also valuable because the signal transduction biochemistry of a univalent stimulus can be compared directly to that of IgE-mediated activation in the same cell. Comparative studies should reveal events which are specific to each type of stimulus as well as events which are common.

Detailed studies of fMet peptide- versus anti-IgE antibody-induced release have recently been described. These two stimuli, on the average, cause nearly equal levels of histamine release, produce similar arachidonic acid metabolite profiles (11), generate similar quantities of LTC4, and show similar morphological changes (114). Thus, the endpoints of the reactions are apparently identical. However, there is no correlation between the ability of a given donor's basophils to respond to fMet peptide or to anti-IgE antibody (31). Histamine release is complete within 2 min following fMet peptide stimulation while requiring 5–30 min following anti-IgE antibody. Nor do the stimuli cross-desensitize (see below). Pharmacologic studies also suggest a significant difference in the signal transduction pathways. Glucocorticosteroids (121), compounds which elevate cytosolic cAMP levels (122), and staurosporine (kinase inhibitor) (102) have no effect on fMet peptide-induced release while effectively inhibiting IgE-mediated release (especially as measured by leukotriene release). In contrast, pertussis toxin ablates mediator release following fMet peptide stimulation while having no effect on IgE-mediated release (79). Calcium elevations and PKC activity changes have also been compared. As noted above, fMet peptide induces a redistribution of PKC activity from cytosol to membrane in a manner similar to that seen with other univalent stimuli, while anti-IgE results only in an increase in membrane activity (102). Treatment of human basophils with staurosporine enhances fMet-peptide-mediated release while completely inhibiting IgE-mediated release. Staurosporine has little effect on the peak calcium response following fMet peptide while slowing the rate at which calcium returns to resting levels. PMA has opposite effects on the fMet peptide calcium response (102). Finally, a plot of the average calcium elevation versus histamine release in basophils shows that the response to fMet peptide requires a two- to three-fold higher calcium level to achieve the same histamine release, although both stimuli generate a tight correlation between the magnitude of the calcium response and histamine release. This relative sensitivity difference to calcium elevations is similar to the differences between A23187 and A23187 + PMA calcium sensitivities noted in the RBL cell (104) and suggests that IgE-mediated release is more sensitive to calcium changes because PKC plays a pro-degranulatory role. In contrast, PKC appears to play an anti-release role in fMet peptide-stimulated basophils.

The calcium response to fMet peptide and anti-IgE, at first inspection, appears qualitatively different. At anti-IgE antibody concentrations that are suboptimal to optimal for histamine release, the calcium response is slow to rise to a sustained plateau in whole-population average measurements. The fMet peptide response is characterized by a very rapid transient increase following by a slower decay to baseline. As in many cell types, the initial rapid transient response appears to be derived from intracellular stores of calcium and is somewhat resistant to pretreatment with calcium chelators. If EDTA or EGTA is added with the fMet peptide, the initial transient remains but the calcium elevations decays, within 60–120 s to baseline (123). Histamine release is only slightly inhibited, while leukotriene release is eliminated. Kinetic studies reveal that for all stimuli, LTC4 release always lags behind histamine release; for fMet peptide, LTC4 release begins after a 1- to 2-min lag (11). Thus, the initial transient is sufficient to drive degranulation while arachidonic acid metabolism, which is calcium dependent, depends on the later influx of calcium for external stores. The addition of EDTA with anti-IgE antibody at suboptimal or optimal concentrations completely eliminates the subsequent calcium response, and there is no mediator release. However, very recent studies have found that supraoptimal concentrations of anti-IgE, which cause a faster response but less histamine release, do generate a short-lived calcium transient which is insensitive to simultaneous addition of EDTA. Unlike the fMet peptide response, this transient elevation in calcium causes no mediator release. These data suggest that IgE-mediated release can mobilize intracellular calcium but, unlike fMet peptide, this calcium cannot drive degranulation. This suggests that both stimuli require the generation of an additional messenger which does not appear in basophils stimulated with supraoptimal concentrations of anti-IgE antibody in the presence of EDTA. The calcium oscillations which occur in basophils stimulated with suboptimal concentrations of anti-IgE antibody, as discussed above, provide additional circumstantial evidence for the mobilization of intracellular calcium. The data thus far appear to suggest that the asynchronous oscillations occurring at suboptimal conditions of stimulation are gradually merged into a single synchronized transient in supraoptimally stimulated cells. While the peaks of oscillations are substantial, they appear to be insufficient to drive mediator release (124).

Comparative studies of fMet peptide and C5a-induced release have also begun because these stimuli have similar characteristics (fast univalent stimuli which are inhibited by pertussis toxin) except that C5a is unable to induce leukotriene release (11,34). For reasons that are not yet clear, C5a causes a calcium transient similar to that seen with fMet peptide but without the prolonged phase of calcium elevation (123). This is a natural analog to the experiment where fMet peptide and EDTA were added simultaneously, as discussed above. Any experimental maneuver that causes C5a to generate a prolonged calcium response also causes this stimulus to generate LTC4. For example, staurosporine prolongs the slow decay phase in fMet peptide-stimulated cells and has a similar effect on the calcium response following C5a; staurosporine markedly enhances LTC4 release following C5a. In a similar fashion, overnight treatment with interleukin-3 causes a marked enhancement of the late calcium response and LTC4 release in C5a-stimulated basophils.

V. DESENSITIZATION

Aggregation of cell surface IgE generally leads to only an incomplete release of total cellular histamine. The kinetics of the release process show that a plateau of release is reached for a given concentration of stimulus, beyond which no further release may occur unless the strength of the stimulus is somehow increased. Thus, it appears that mast cells and basophils possess an intrinsic method of self-regulation. This is a general phenomenon in cell biology, and it is generally identified as desensitization or tachyphylaxis. As this is a process which is part of the full response and controls the extent of the response, studies of signal transduction must include the down-regulatory components.

Desensitization of IgE-mediated release can be demonstrated operationally by stimulating cells with antigen in the absence of extracellular calcium. For the period that the cells experience cross-linking in the absence of calcium, there is no histamine release. Upon the addition of calcium to the medium, the full degranulatory response commences. However, the longer the challenge in the absence of calcium, the smaller the subsequent histamine release (125). For human basophils this decay curve has the appearance of an exponential decay, although mathematical models suggest somewhat different forms of the decay that do not imply a proportional decay process. The $T_{1/2}$ for the rate of desensitization is approximately three times longer than the $T_{1/2}$ for histamine release in nondesensitized cells. Initially this was confusing, since it was believed that the desensitization process should be the complement of the release process. However, the mathematical models of histamine release demonstrated that this need not be true (55). In fact, the experimental protocol for desensitization studies led to the disparity in kinetic rates. Thus, it appeared that the operational method described above revealed the underlying process that controlled ongoing histamine release. Further support for a role of desensitization in controlling release in human basophils was derived from studies where diisopropylfluorophosphate (DFP) could be shown to inhibit the rate of desensitization and enhance and prolong histamine release (126). In some receptor systems, down-regulation of the response occurs because of a loss of the receptor, usually through internalization. RBL cell studies suggested that some internalization if the IgE receptor could occur during stimulation. However, only a fraction of the receptors were internalized, leaving enough cell surface IgE to maintain a strong response (127,128). Studies in human basophils have shown that no loss of cell surface IgE accompanies stimulation or desensitization (129). Thus, it appeared that the desensitization process reflected the alteration of a later signal transduction event. The DFP studies noted above did suggest that desensitization was an active event, since DFP presumably acted by inhibiting an enzyme possessing an active-site serine.

One approach to discovering the underlying mechanism of desensitization is to study the signal transduction events which occur in the absence of extracellular calcium or to examine the relationship between the kinetics of a particular event and the kinetics of histamine release. Human basophils show an increase in membrane PKC activity following antigen stimulation in the absence of extracellular calcium, conditions that are not appropriate for mediator release (99,130). There are indications in other cell types that protein kinase C plays a role in regulating the extent of the cell response. In some cases, phosphorylation of early components of the signal transduction pathway is a form of negative modulation and receptors themselves can undergo phosphorylation by protein kinase C. Unfortunately, phosphorylation studies of the high-affinity IgE receptor have been difficult, confusing, and focused primarily on the RBL cell. There has been no clear demonstration that stimulation results in any component undergoing systematic phosphorylation, although the γ-subunit is known to change phosphorylation state as well as to have a site for phosphorylation (71). It should be pointed out that a desensitization process which is directed toward the specific cross-linked receptor implies a specific form of desensitization. In human basophils and mast cells, desensitization may be either specific for the antigen causing the reaction, or it may be nonspecific, affecting all subsequent challenges with non-cross-reacting antigens (54,131). (Note: Nonspecific desensitization has no effect on IgE-independent stimulation.) The degree of nonspecificity is determined by the magnitude of the cross-linking with the first desensitizing antigen (132). It is conceivable that receptor-directed phosphorylation could become nonspecific if the kinase were to have only marginal specificity for cross-linked receptors, but it may be that a second, less specific, action by another process could account for nonspecific desensitization. Desensitization may also result from the depletion of some important intermediate and thus become nonspecific (55).

Protein kinase C may also modulate the activity of the IP3 cycle by activating a 5′-phosphomonoesterase which mediates the metabolism of IP3 to IP2 (133). This suggests that PKC may alter the calcium response. Indeed, pretreatment of human basophils or mast cells with PMA results in a significant reduction in the Ca^{2+} elevation which normally follows stimulation with anti-IgE antibody (102,134). As noted above, TPA rapidly inhibits or stops the release of LTC4 from human basophils, possibly through its action on the calcium response. However, in mast cells this observation may be deceptive. The ongoing response of mast cells shows that the calcium response persists far longer than the release of histamine (110,135). A slow decay of calcium levels back to baseline values does occur, but on a time scale far too long for it to account for the abrupt cessation of histamine release, which occurs within 5 min of stimulation. Desensitization-style experiments (treatment with anti-IgE antibody in the absence of calcium followed by the addition of calcium) also revealed that desensitization, as measured by the loss of the cell's peak calcium response, was too slow to account for the desensitization measured by the decrease in histamine release. Finally, recent studies have demonstrated indirectly that down-regulating PKC levels by long-term treatment of mast cells (human lung or skin) with PMA had no effect on the decay of calcium back to resting levels during a release experiment, nor did it alter the rate of desensitization in a desensitization-style experiment. These data indicated that whatever process controlled active release, it was not operating solely through the control of cytosolic calcium levels. Nor does PKC appear to have a role in regulating secretion under these circumstances.

Human basophils appear to use PKC in a pro-degranulatory role and, unlike the calcium response kinetics, membrane PKC activity has a kinetic profile which accounts for the kinetic profile of histamine release (see Figure 4). In other words, the PKC activity curve approximates the first derivative of the histamine-release kinetic curve. This data suggests that regulation of ongoing secretion in human basophils is handled at a point preceding the increase in membrane PKC activity, possibly through regulation of DAG levels, either its generation or its metabolism. Thus, future studies are focusing on phospholipid metabolism.

VI. RESPONSE MODULATION

A. Donor-Specific Correlates of Signal Transduction Modulation

An examination of human basophil histamine release in the general population suggests that modulation of the signal transduction apparatus may alter the sensitivity of the cells

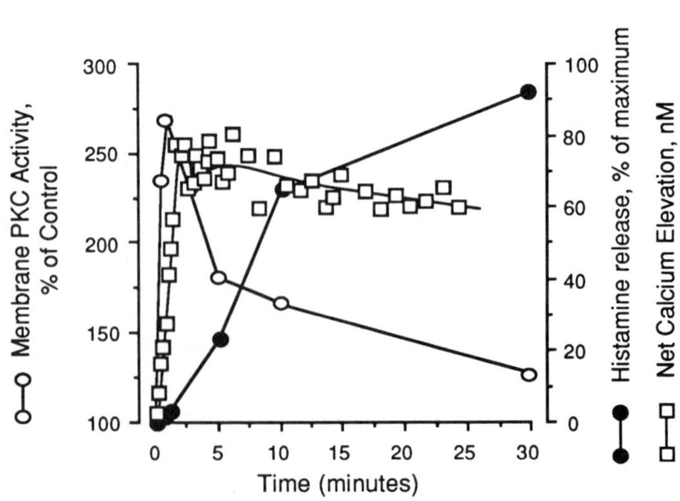

Figure 4 Kinetic curves of histamine release, membrane protein kinase C activity, and free cytosolic calcium elevations in human basophils following stimulation with anti-IgE antibody.

to stimulation. In the general population, the maximal histamine release that can be obtained following stimulation with an optimal concentration of anti-IgE antibody ranges the entire spectrum, from 0 to 100%. The population distribution of the response is bimodal, with a peak centered on 50% histamine release and a second peak at 0% (136,137). However, maximal histamine release is not necessarily a measure of the basophil's sensitivity; there is no correlation between the endogenous IgE density and the maximal response to an optimal concentration of anti-IgE antibody (138). The measurement of absolute basophil sensitivity is technically difficult but, when done, also indicates a large variation in this parameter within the general population. Some donors' basophils give a half-maximal response with as few as 500 antigen-specific IgE molecules/cell, while the others do not respond even with 1,000,000 molecules. Recent studies are focusing on the two extremes of this distribution; those cells which are exquisitely sensitive are being compared to cells which show no IgE-mediated release (nonreleasers) (137). Nonreleasing basophils possess sufficient cell surface IgE to mount a response, and it has been demonstrated that these cells generate a partial response since they also show the anti-IgE-induced increase in cell sensitivity to PMA (see above) (137). Nonreleasing cells also show normal responses to A23187, PMA, and fMet peptide, suggesting that some degranulation apparatus is intact. Measurements of PKC show that nonreleasing cells do express some PKC activity and that its kinetics resembles the PKC kinetics seen in releasing cells stimulated in the absence of extracellular calcium (99). Furthermore, there is a good correlation between the average calcium elevation and histamine release, with nonreleasing cells showing no increase in cytosolic calcium following anti-IgE antibody (102). Taken together, these data suggest that the difference between a nonreleasing and releasing basophil is the ability to elevate cytosolic calcium. Since the mechanism by which calcium levels are increased in stimulated cells remains unknown, the exact site of the difference is also unclear. One highly speculative view would suggest that a calcium transport protein or channel is missing in nonreleasing basophils. The fact that the β-subunit of the IgE receptor may function in this role (see above), and that it may be expressed independently, suggests that differences in "releasability" may be related to the relative expression of this subunit.

B. Pharmacologic Modulation and Its Role in the Control of Cellular Sensitivity

Mast cell and basophil mediator release is regulated by several external factors. Aside from the numerous drugs which are used as tools to dissect the signal transduction pathway, there are several important endogenous modulators of the response. Human basophils, in particular, are profoundly influenced by glucocorticosteroids and the interleukins and to a lesser extent by agents which increase intracellular cAMP. Any studies which examine the intrinsic control of basophil sensitivity (as above) must consider these external factors as well.

Cyclic AMP levels are controlled by compounds such as H2 agonists, β-agonists, and prostaglandins binding to specific cell surface receptors (139–141) as well as the level of phosphodiesterase activity [a cyclic GMP-insensitive PDE III appears to be the predominant PDE in basophils and mast cells (142)]. There have been reports that PDE levels in leukocytes from various atopic patients can be significantly higher than normal (144,145), leaving open the possibility that the resting levels of cAMP could be lower and basophils more sensitive to stimulation. Recent studies in mast cells suggest that cAMP could have at least two sites of action. Inhibition of histamine release requires high intracellular cAMP levels, while cAMP levels which are too low to have any effect on histamine release can completely abolish leukotriene release (143). Preliminary studies in the PT-18 murine mast cell line indicate that the site of action at low cAMP levels may be phospholipase A2.

Human basophils are inhibited by glucocorticosteroids, while mast cells are not (146,147). The inhibition requires incubations greater than several hours and presumably requires DNA transcription. The mechanism of inhibition remains unclear from human cells, but studies in murine cells [RBL cells and bone marrow-derived mast cells (BMMC)] suggest that an alteration in the early signal transduction events occurs (94,148–150). Some down-regulation of receptor number occurs in BMMC (149), but not to an extent sufficient to account for the decrease in mediator release. The RBL studies suggest that the alteration is at the level of a GTP-binding protein, which may explain earlier data demonstrating decreases in the hydrolysis of inositol phospholipids, arachidonic acid release, and elevations in cytosolic calcium. This alteration is specific for IgE-mediated release, since in both RBL cells (150) and human basophils (121), steroids have no effect on other non-IgE-dependent responses (e.g., fMet peptide in human basophils).

Most recently, cytokines have been found to have a profound influence on human basophil function (151–153). Interleukin-3 is the most potent and effacacious up-regulator of the basophil response yet found, although IL-1 and γ-interferon also cause significant up-regulation (153). There are both acute (<30 min) and long-term effects (24-h culture) of IL-3. For example, IL-3 reverses the action of glucocorticosteroids only in long-term culture. Long-term culture with 10–50 pM IL-3 leads to an average 10-fold increase in LTC4 release following IgE-mediated stimulation with a range of 3–100 fold. Preliminary studies suggest that long-term culture leads to an increased calcium response while acute treatment does not. The effects of IL-3 are global: the response to all stimuli is increased and all mediators are affected (153). Because the effects of IL-3 are significant, it is tempting to suggest that all the basophil sensitivity differences we have observed are regulated by this cytokine. Its differential effects on histamine and leukotriene release may also explain the larger distribution of leukotriene release among donors. However, the response of basophils to IgE-mediated stimuli and other univalent stimuli are not correlated, and yet IL-3 affects all stimuli to various extents, suggesting that a complete explanation of IgE-mediated basophil sensitivity may involve more than circulating IL-3 levels.

VII. SUMMARY

While several important biochemical steps have been observed to occur in basophils and mast cells, there remain some very important links to be established. Notably, it is important to understand the exact role of the IgE receptor and the need for its aggregation. The description of the GTP-binding protein involved in IgE-mediated signal transduction is necessary, as is a description of the proteins involved in calcium movement. Control mechanisms remain unclear, and the length of the signal transduction pathway has yet to be defined. Much of the data points to multiple requisite pathways, and yet only calcium elevations have a relatively well-demonstrated pro-degranulatory role. Until some of these events are understood in detail, the means by which cell sensitivity is regulated may remain a mystery. Finally, it will be important to determine if mast cells and basophils use distinctive IgE-mediated signal transduction pathways.

ABBREVIATIONS

RBL cell	Rat basophilic leukemia cell—a tumor analog of the rat mucosal *mast* cell.
HETE	Hydroxy eicosatetraenoic
LT	Leukotriene (C, D, E)
fMet peptide	Formyl-methionyl-leucyl-phenylalanine
GCMS	Gas chromatography-mass spectrometry
PL	Phospholipase (classes of A_2, C, D)
IP3	Inositol 1,4,5-trisphosphate
DAG	Diacylglycerol
PKC	Protein kinase C
PMA	Phorbol 12-myristate-13-acetate
EDTA	Ethylene diamine tetraacetic acid
IL	Interleukin

REFERENCES

1. Dvorak HJ, Mihm MC Jr, Dvorak AM, et al. Morphology of delayed type hypersensitivity reactions in man. I. Quantitative description of the inflammatory response. Lab Invest 1974; 31:111–30.
2. Dvorak AM, Mihm MC Jr, Dvorak HF. Degranulation of basophil leukocytes in allergic contact dermatitis reactions in man. J Immunol 1976; 116:687–94.
3. Brown SJ, Galli SJ, Gleich GJ, Askenase PW. Ablation of immunity to *Amblyomma americanum* by anti-basophil serum: cooperation between basophils and eosinophils in expression of immunity to ectoparasites (ticks) in guinea pigs. J Immunol 1982; 129:790–6.
4. Plaut M, Pierce JH, Watson CJ, Hanley-Hyde J, Nordan RP, Paul WE. Mast cell lines produce lymphokines in response to cross-linkage of FcϵRI or to calcium ionophores. Nature 1989; 339:64–7.
5. Wodnar-Filipowicz A, Heusser CH, Moroni C. Production of the hemopoietic growth factors GM-CSF and interleukin-3 by mast cells in response to IgE receptor-mediated activation. Nature 1989; 339:150–2.
6. Metcalfe DD, Lewis RA, Silbert JE, et al. Isolation and characterization of heparin from human lung. J Clin Invest 1979; 64:1537–43.
7. Maciag T, Mehlman T, Friesel R, Schreiber AB. Heparin binds endothelial cell growth factor, the principal endothelial cell mitogen in bovine brain. Science 1984; 225:932–5.
8. Schwartz LB, Lewis RA, Austen KF. Tryptase from human pulmonary mast cells: purification and characterization. J Biol Chem 1981; 256:11939–43.
9. Castells NC, Irani AM, Schwartz LB. Evaluation of human peripheral blood leukocytes for mast cell tryptase. J Immunol 1987; 138:2184–9.
10. Proud D, Siekierski ES, Bailey GS. Identification of human lung mast cell kininogenase as tryptase and relevance of tryptase kininogenase activity. Biochem Pharmacol 1988; 37:1473–80.
11. Warner JA, Peters SP, Lichtenstein LM, Yancey KB, Stevenson HC, Miller PJ, MacGlashan DW Jr. Differential release of mediators from human basophils: differences

in arachidonic acid metabolism following activation by unrelated stimuli. J Leuk Biol 1989; 45:558–71.

12. Warner JA, Freeland HS, MacGlashan DW Jr, Lichtenstein LM, Peters SP. Purified human basophils do not generate LTB4. Biochem Pharmacol 1987; 36:3195–9.
13. Schleimer RP, Schulman ES, MacGlashan DW Jr, Peters SP, Adams GK III, Lichtenstein LM, Adkinson NF Jr. Effects of dexamethasone on mediator release from human lung fragments and purified human lung mast cells. J Clin Invest 1983; 71:1830–5.
14. MacGlashan DW, Schleimer RP, Peters SP, Schulman ES, Adams GK III, Newball HH, Lichtenstein LM. Generation of leukotrienes by purified human lung mast cells. J Clin Invest 1982; 70:747–51.
15. Peters SP, MacGlashan DW Jr, Schulman ES, Schleimer RP, Hayes EC, Rokach J, Adkinson NF Jr, Lichtenstein LM. Arachidonic acid metabolism in purified human lung mast cells. J Immunol 1984; 132:1972–9.
16. Fox CF, Wolf EJ, Kagey-Sobotka A, Lichtenstein LM. Comparison of human lung and intestinal mast cells. J Allergy Clin Immunol 1988; 81:89–94.
17. Lawrence ID, Warner JA, Cohan VL, Hubbard WC, Kagey-Sobotka A, Lichtenstein LM. Purification and characterization of human skin mast cells: evidence for human mast cell heterogeneity. J Immunol 1987; 139:3062–9.
18. Massey W, Cohen VL, Bagavan B, Kagey-Sobotka A, Lichtenstein LM. The isolation and characterization of human uterine mast cells (UMC). J Allergy Clin Immunol 1989; 83:233.
19. Naclerio RM, Meier HL, Kagey-Sobotka A, Adkinson NF Jr, Meyers DA, Norman PS, Lichtenstein LM. Mediator release after nasal airway challenge with allergen. Am Rev Respir Dis 1983; 128:597–602.
20. Pipkorn U, Proud D, Lichtenstein LM, Kagey-Sobotka A, Norman PS, Naclerio RM. Inhibition of mediator release in allergic rhinitis by pretreatment with topical glucocorticosteroids. N Engl J Med 1987; 316:1506–10.
21. Dolovich J, Hargreave FE, Chalmers R, Shier KJ, Gauldie J, Bienenstock J. Late cutaneous allergic response in isolated IgE-dependent reactions. J Allergy Clin Immunol 1973; 52:38–46.
22. McLean J, Garkowski A, Wolomon W, Matthews K. Changes in airway resistance on antigenic challenge in allergic rhinitis. Clin Allergy 1971; 1:63–9.
23. Unpublished observations.
24. Charlesworth EN, Hoood AF, Soter NA, Kagey-Sobotka A, Norman PS, Lichtenstein LM. The cutaneous late phase response to allergen: mediator release and inflammatory cell infiltration. J Clin Invest 1989; 83:1519–26.
25. MacGlashan DW Jr, Schleimer RP, Peters SP, Schulman ES, Adams GK, Sobotka AK, Newball HH, Lichtenstein LM. Comparative studies of human basophils and mast cells. Fed Proc 1983; 42:2504–9.
26. Schleimer RP, MacGlashan DW Jr, Peters SP, Pinckard RN, Adkinson NF Jr, Lichtenstein LM. Characterization of inflammatory mediator release from purified human lung mast cells. Am Rev Respir Dis 1986; 133:614–7.
27. Betz SJ, Lotner GZ, Henson PM. Generation and release of platelet-activating factor (PAF) from enriched preparations of rabbit basophils; failure of human basophils to release PAF. J Immunol 1980; 125:2749–55.
28. Cluzel M, Undem BJ, Chilton FH. Release of platelet-activating factor and the metabolism of leukotriene B4 by the human neutrophil when studied in a cell superfusion model. J Immunol 1989; 143:3659–65.
29. Bochner BS, McKelvey AA, Schleimer RP, Hildreth JEK, Guyre PM, MacGlashan DW Jr. Flow cytometric methods for analysis of human basophil surface antigens and viability. J Immunol Meth 1989; 125:265–71.

30. Grant JA, Lichtenstein LM. Reversed in vitro anaphylaxis induced by anti-IgG: specificity of the reaction and comparison with antigen-induced histamine release. J Immunol 1972; 109:20–5.
31. Siraganian RP, Hook WA. Mechanisms of histamine release by formylmethionine containing peptides. J Immunol 1977; 119:2078–83.
32. Siraganian RP, Hook WA. Complement-induced histamine release from human basophils. II. Mechanism of the histamine release reaction. J Immunol 1976; 116:639–46.
33. Glovsky MM, Hugli TE, Ishizaka T, Lichtenstein LM, Erickson BW. Anaphylatoxin-induced histamine release with human leukocytes: studies of C3a leukocyte binding and histamine release. J Clin Invest 1979; 64:804–11.
34. Shulman ES, Post TJ, Henson PM, Giclas PC. Differential effects of the complement peptides C5a and C5a des Arg on human basophil and lung mast cell histamine release. J Clin Invest 1988; 81:918–23.
35. Okuda Y, Tsuyuguchi, Yamatodani A. Histamine release from human leukocytes by platelet-activating factor. Int Arch Appl Immunol 1988; 85:341–5.
36. O'Donnell MC, Ackerman SJ, Gleich GJ, Thomas LL. Activation of basophil and mast cell histamine release by eosinophil granule major basic protein. J Exp Med 1983; 157:1981–91.
37. Foreman JC, Lichtenstein LM. Induction of histamine secretion by polycations. Biochim Biophys Acta 1980; 629:587–603.
38. Thueson DO, Speck LS, Lett-Brown MA, Grant JA. Histamine-releasing activity (HRA). I. Production by mitogen- or antigen-stimulated human mononuclear cells. J Immunol 1979; 123:626–32.
39. Bamzai AK, Kretschmer RR. Enhancement of antigen-induced leukocyte histamine released by a mononuclear cell-derived factor. J Allergy Clin Immunol 1978; 62:137–42.
40. Kaplan AP, Haak-Frendscho M, Fauci A, Dinarello C, Halbert E. A histamine-releasing factor from activated human mononuclear cells. J Immunol 1975; 135:2027–32.
41. Liu MC, Proud D, Lichtenstein LM, MacGlashan DW Jr, Schleimer RP, Adkinson NF Jr, Kagey-Sobotka A, Schulman ES, Plaut M. Human lung macrophage-derived histamine-releasing activity is due to IgE-binding factors. J Immunol 1986; 136:2588–95.
42. MacDonald SM, Lichtenstein LM, Proud D, Plaut M, Naclerio RM, MacGlashan DW, Kagey-Sobotka A. Studies of IgE dependent histamine release factors: heterogeneity of IgE. J Immunol 1987; 139:506–12.
43. Benyon RC, Lowman MA, Church MK. Human skin mast cells: their dispersion, purification, and secretory characterization. J Immunol 1987; 138:861–7.
44. Foreman JC. Substance P and calcitonin gene-related peptide: effects on mast cells and in human skin. Int Arch Allergy Appl Immunol 1987; 82:366–71.
45. Lowman MA, Rees PH, Benyon RC, Church MK. Human mast cell heterogeneity: histamine release from mast cells dispersed from skin, lung, adenoids, tonsils and intestinal mucosa in response to IgE-dependent and non-immunological stimuli. J Allergy Clin Immunol 1988; 81:590–7.
46. Lowman MA, Benyon RC, Church MK. Characterization of neuropeptide-induced histamine release from human dispersed skin mast cells. Br J Pharmacol 1988; 95:121–30.
47. Lawrence ID, Warner JA, Cohan VL, Lichtenstein LM, Kagey-Sobotka A, Vavrek RJ, Stewart JM, Proud D. Induction of histamine release from human skin mast cells by bradykinin analogs. Biochem Pharmacol 1989; 33:227–33.
48. Segal DM, Taurog J, Metzger H. Dimeric immunoglobulin E serves as a unit signal for mast cell degranulation. Proc Natl. Acad Sci USA 1977; 74:2993–7.
49. Siraganian RP, Hook WA, Levine BB. Specific in vitro histamine release from basophils by bivalent haptens: evidence of activation by simple bridging of membrane bound antibody. Immunochemistry 1975; 12:149–57.

50. Dembo M, Goldstein B, Sobotka AK, Lichtenstein LM. Histamine release due to bivalent penicilloyl haptens: control by the number of cross-linked IgE antibodies on the basophil plasma membrane. J Immunol 1978; 121:354–8.
51. Furuichi K, Rivera J, Isersky C. The receptor for immunoglobulin E on rat basophilic leukemia cells: effect of ligand binding on receptor expression. Proc Natl Acad Sci USA 1985; 82:1522–5.
52. Dembo M, Goldstein B. A thermodynamic model of binding of flexible bivalent haptens to antibody. Immunochemistry 1978; 15:307–13.
53. Dembo M, Goldstein B. Theory of equilibrium binding of symmetric bivalent haptens to cell surface antibody: application to histamine release from basophils. J Immunol 1978; 121:345–53.
54. Sobotka AK, Dembo M, Goldstein B, Lichtenstein LM. Antigen-specific desensitization of human basophils. J Immunol 1979; 122:511–7.
55. Dembo M, Goldstein B. A model of cell activation and desensitization by surface immunoglobin: the case of histamine release from human basophils. Cell 1980; 22:59–67.
56. MacGlashan DW Jr, Dembo M, Goldstein B. Test of a theory relating to the crosslinking of IgE antibody on the surface of human basophils. J Immunol 1985; 135:4129–34.
57. Fewtrell C, Metzger H. Larger oligomers of IgE are more effective than dimers in stimulating rat basophilic leukemia cells. J Immunol 1980; 125:701–10.
58. MacGlashan DW Jr, Schleimer RP, Lichtenstein LM. Qualitative differences between dimeric and trimeric stimulation of human basophils. J Immunol 1983; 130:4–6.
59. MacGlashan DW Jr, Peters SP, Warner J, Lichtenstein LM. Characteristics of human basophil sulfidopeptide leukotriene release: releasability defined as the ability of the basophil to respond to dimeric crosslinks. J Immunol 1986; 136:2231–9.
60. Menon AK, Holowka D, Webb WW, Baird B. Cross-linking of receptor-bound IgE to aggregates larger than dimers leads to rapid immobilization. J Cell Biol 1986; 102:541–50.
61. Becker KE, Ishizaka T, Metzger H, Ishizaka K, Grimley PM. Surface IgE on human basophils during histamine release. J Exp Med 1973; 138:394.
62. Magro AM, Alexander A. Histamine release: studies of the inhibitory region of the dose-response curve. J Immunol 1974; 112:1762–5.
63. Ishizaka T, Ishizaka K. Cell surface IgE on human basophil granulocytes. Annals NY Acad Sci 1975; 254:462–75.
64. Lawson D, Fewtrell C, Gomperts B, Raff MC. Anti-immunoglobulin-induced histamine secretion by rat peritoneal mast cells studied by immunoferritin electron microscopy. J Exp Med 1975; 142:391–402.
65. Blank U, Ra C, Miller L, White K, Metzger H, Kinet JP. Complete structure and expression in transfected cells of high affinity IgE receptor. Nature 1989; 337:187–9.
66. Ra C, Jouvin MHE, Kinet JP. Complete structure of the mouse mast cell receptor for IgE (FcϵRI) and surface expression of chimeric receptors (rat-mouse-human) on transfected cells. J Biol Chem 1989; 264:15323–7.
67. Kanellopoulos JM, Liu TY, Poy G, Metzger H. Composition and subunit structure of the cell receptor for immunoglobulin E. J Biol Chem 1980; 255:9060–6.
68. Huppi K, Siwarski D, Mock BA, Kinet JP. Gene mapping of the three subunits of the high affinity Fc receptor for IgE. J Immunol 1989; 143:3787–91.
69. Miller L, Blank U, Metzger H, Kinet JP. Expression of high-affinity binding of human immunoglobulin E by transfected cells. Science 1989; 244:334–7.
70. Weissman AM, Baniyash M, Hou D, Samelson LE, Burgess WH, Klausner RD. Molecular cloning of the zeta chain of the T cell antigen receptor. Science 1988; 239:1018–21.
71. Quarto R, Metzger H. The receptor for immunoglobulin E: examination for kinase activity and as a substrate for kinases. Mol Immunol 1986; 23:1215–23.

72. Boheim G, Kolb HA. Analysis of the multi pore system of alamethicin in a lipid membrane. Part 1. Voltage jump current relaxation measurements. J Membr Biol 1978; 38:99–150.
73. Gordon LGM, Haydon DA. Kinetics and stability of alamethicin conducting channels in lipid bilayers. Biochim Biophys Act 1976; 436:541–56.
74. Narasimhan V, Holowka D, Fewtrell C, Baird B. Cholera toxin increases the rate of antigen-stimulated calcium influx in rat basophilic leukemia cells. J Biol Chem 1988; 263:19626–32.
75. Cunha-Melo JR, Beaven MA. Receptor-mediated release of inositol 1,4,5-trisphosphate and inositol 1,4-biphosphate in rat basophilic leukemia RBL-2H3 cells permeabilized with streptolysin O. Biochim Biophys Acta 1989; 1010:88–99.
76. Wilson BS, Deanin GG, Standefer JC, Vanderjaat D, Oliver JM. Depletion of guanine nucleotides with mycophenolic acid suppresses IgE receptor-mediated degranulation in rat basophilic leukemia cells. J Immunol 1989; 143:259–65.
77. Howell TW, Cockcroft S, Gomperts BD. Essential synergy between Ca^{2+} and guanine nucleotides in exocytotic secretion from permeabilized rat mast cells. J Cell Biol 1987; 105:191–7.
78. Saito H, Ishizaka K, Ishizaka T. Effect of nonhydrolyzable guanosine phosphate on IgE-mediated activation of phospholipase C and histamine release from rodent mast cells. J Immunol 1989; 143:250–8.
79. Warner JA, Yancey KB, MacGlashan DW Jr. The effect of pertussis toxin on mediator release from human basophils. J Immunol 1987; 139:161–5.
80. Marone G, Kagey-Sobotka A, Lichtenstein LM. Possible role of phospholipase A2 in triggering histamine secretion from human basophils in vitro. Clin Immunol Immunopathol 1981; 20:231–6.
81. Marone G, Kagey-Sobotka A, Lichtenstein LM. Control mechanisms of histamine release from human basophils in vitro: the role of phospholipase A2 and of lipoxygenase metabolites. Int Arch Allergy Appl Immunol 1981; 66:144–8.
82. Nakao A, Buchanan AM, Potokar DS. Possible involvement of phospholipase A2 in A23187-induced histamine release in purified rat mast cells. Int Arch Allergy Appl Immunol 1980; 63:30–5.
83. Cockroft S, Gomperts BD. Evidence for a role of phosphatidylinositol turnover in stimulus-secretion coupling. Studies with rat peritoneal mast cells. Biochem J 1979; 178:681–7.
84. Beaven MA, Moore JP, Smith GA, Hesketh TR, Metcalfe JC. The calcium signal and phosphatidylinositol breakdown in 2H3 cells. J Biol Chem 1984; 259:7137–42.
85. Cunha-Melo JR, Dean NM, Moyer JD, Maeyama K, Beaven MA. The kinetics of phosphoinositide hydrolysis in rat basophilic leukemia (RBL-2H3) cells varies with the type of IgE receptor cross-linking agent used. J Biol Chem 1987; 262:11455–63.
86. Kennerly DA, Sullivan TJ, Sylwester P, Parker CW. Diacylglycerol metabolism in mast cells: a potential role in membrane fusion and arachidonic acid release. J Exp Med 1979; 150:1039–44.
87. Kennerly DA. Diacylglycerol metabolism in mast cells. Analysis of lipid mediators pathways using molecular species analysis of intermediates. J Biol Chem 1987; 262:16305–13.
88. White JR, Pluznik DH, Ishizata K, Ishizaka T. Antigen induced increase in protein kinase C activity in the plasma membrane of mast cells. Proc Natl Acad Sci USA 1985; 82:8193–7.
89. Gruchalla RS, Dinh TT, Kennerly DA. An indirect pathway of receptor-mediated, 1,2-diacylglycerol formation in mast cells. I. IgE receptor-mediated activation of phospholipase D. J Immunol 1990; 144:2334–42.
90. Hemmerich S, Pecht I. Isolation and purification of Fc_{ϵ} receptor activation ion channel

from the rat mast cell line RBL-2H3. Biochemistry 1988; 27:7488–98.

91. Lichtenstein LM, DeBernardo R. IgE mediated histamine release: in vitro separation into two phases. Int Arch Allergy Appl Immunol 1971; 41:56–71.
92. Ennis M, Truneh A, White JR, Pearce FL. Calcium pools involved in histamine release from rat mast cells. Int Arch Allergy Appl Immunol 1980; 62:467–71.
93. Putney JW Jr. A model for receptor-regulated calcium entry. Cell Calcium 1986; 7:1–12.
94. Woldemussie E, Ali H, Takaishi T, Siraganian RP, Beaven MA. Identification of variants of the basophilic leukemia (RBL-2H3) cells that have defective phosphoinositide responses to antigen and stimulants of guanosine 5′-triphosphate-regulatory proteins. J Immunol 1987; 139:2431–8.
95. Berenstein EH, Garcia-Gil M, Siraganian RP. Dexamethasone inhibits receptor-activated phosphoinositide breakdown in rat basophilic leukemia (RBL-2H3) cells. J Immunol 1987; 138:1914–8.
96. Millard PJ, Ryan TA, Webb WW, Fewtrell C. Immunoglobulin E receptor cross-linking induces oscillations in intracellular free ionized calcium in individual tumor mast cells. J Biol Chem 1989; 264:19730–9.
97. Wilson DB, Bross TE, Hofman SL, Majerus PW. Hydrolysis of polyphosphoinositides by purified sheep seminal vesicle phospholipase C enzymes. J Biol Chem 1984; 259:11718–24.
98. White KN, Metzger H. Translocation of protein kinase C in rat basophilic leukemic cells induced by phorbol ester or aggregation of IgE receptors. J Immunol 1988; 141:942–7.
99. Warner JA, MacGlashan DW Jr. Protein kinase C (PKC) changes in human basophils: IgE-mediated activation is accompanied by an increase in total PKC activity. J Immunol 1989; 142:1669–77.
100. Schleimer RP, Gillespie E, Lichtenstein LM. Release of histamine from human leukocytes stimulated with the tumor-promoting phorbol diesters. I. Characterization of the response. J Immunol 1981; 126:570–4.
101. Schleimer RP, Gillespie E, Daiuta R, Lichtenstein LM. Release of histamine from human leukocytes stimulated with the tumor-promoting phorbol diesters. II. Interaction with other stimuli. J Immunol 1982; 128:136–40.
102. Warner JA, MacGlashan DW Jr. Signal transduction events in human basophils: a comparative study of the role of PKC in basophils activated by anti-IgE and fMet peptide. J Immunol 1990; 145:1897–1905.
103. Ruegg UT, Burgess GM. Staurosporine, K252 and UCN-01: potent but non-specific inhibitors of protein kinases. Trends Pharmacol Sci 1989; 10:218–20.
104. Beaven MA, Guthre DF, Moore JP, Smith GA, Hesketh TR, Metcalfe JC. Synergistic signals in the mechanism of antigen-induced exocytosis in 2H3 cells: evidence for an unidentified signal required for histamine release. J Cell Biol 1987; 105:1129–36.
105. Collado-Escobar DM, Beaven MA. The rise in concentration of free Ca^{2+} and of pH provides sequential, synergistic signals for secretion in antigen-stimulated rat basophilic leukemia (*RBL-2H3) cells. J Immunol 1989; 143:2626–33.
106. Foreman JC, Hallett MB, Mongar JL. The relationship between histamine secretion and ^{45}calcium uptake by mast cells. J Physiol (Lond.) 1977; 271:193–24.
107. Beaven MA, Rogers J, Moore JP, Hesketh TR, Smith GA, Metcalfe JC. The mechanism of the calcium signal and correlation with histamine release in 2H3 cells. J Biol Chem 1984; 259:7129–36.
108. Fewtrell C, Sherman E. The IgE receptor-activated calcium permeability pathway in rat basophilic leukemia (2H3) cells: measurement of the unidirectional influx of calcium using quin2-buffered cells. Biochemistry 1987; 26:6995–7003.
109. Millard PJ, Gross D, Webb WW, Fewtrell C. Imaging asynchronous changes in intracellular Ca^{2+} in individual stimulated tumor mast cells. Proc Natl Acad Sci USA 1988; 85:1854–8.

110. MacGlashan D Jr. Single cell analysis of calcium changes in human lung mast cells. I. Graded versus all-or-nothing elevations following IgE mediated stimulation. J Cell Biol 1989; 109:123–34.
111. Bindslev-Jensen C, Clementsen P, Stahl-Skov P, Svendsen UG, Thastrup O, Norn S. Comparison of the action of calcium antagonists on basophil histamine release. Allergy 1987; 42:441–6.
112. Tanizaki Y, Komagoe H, Morinaga H, Ohtani J, Nakagawa S, Maeda M, Kitani H, Takahashi K, Kimura I. The calcium antagonist, nicardipine, inhibits antigen-stimulated and anti-IgE-induced histamine release from basophilic leukocytes of atopic asthmatics. Acta Med Okayama 1985; 39:247–51.
113. Holl RW, Thorner MO, Mandell GL, Sullivan JA, Sinha YN, Leong DA. Spontaneous oscillations of intracellular calcium and growth hormone secretions. J Biol Chem 1988; 263:9682–5.
114. Warner JA, Bochner BS, MacGlashan DW Jr. Cytoskeletal rearrangement and shape change in human basophils. J Allergy Clin Immunol 1990; abstract 85:171.
115. Bochner BS, McKelvey AA, Sterbinsky SA, Hildreth JEK, Derse CP, Klunk DA, Lichtenstein LM, Schleimer RP. Interleukin-3 augments adhesiveness for endothelium and CD11b expression in human basophils but not neutrophils. J Immunol 1990; 145:1832–37.
116. Bahler M, Greengard P. Synapsin I bundles F-actin in phosphorylation-dependent manner. Nature 1987; 326:704–7.
117. Sieghart W, Theodharides TC, Alper SL, Douglas WW, Greengard P. Calcium-dependent protein phosphorylation during secretion by exocytosis in the mast cell. Nature 1978; 275:329–31.
118. Katakami Y, Kaibuchi K, Sawamura M, Takai Y, Nishizuka Y. Synergistic action of protein kinase C and calcium for histamine release from rat peritoneal mast cells. Biochem Biophys Res Commun 1984; 121:573–8.
119. Theoharides TC, Sieghart W, Greengard P, Douglas WW. Antiallergic drug cromolyn may inhibit histamine secretion by regulating phosphorylation of a mast cell protein. Science 1979:80–2.
120. Ludowyke RI, Peleg I, Beaven MA, Adelstein RS. Antigen-induced secretion of histamine and the phosphorylation of myosin by protein kinase C in rat basophilic leukemia cells. J Biol Chem 1989; 264:12492–501.
121. Sagi-Eisenburg R, Foreman JC, Raval PJ, Cockcroft S. Protein and diacylglycerol phosphorylation in the stimulus-secretion coupling of rat mast cells. Immunology 1987; 61:203–6.
122. Schleimer RP, MacGlashan DW Jr, Gillespie E, Lichtenstein LM. Inhibition of basophil histamine release by anti-inflammatory steroids. II. Studies on the mechanism of action. J Immunol 1982; 129:1632–5.
123. MacGlashan D Jr, Warner J. Stimulus-dependent leukotriene release from human basophils. A comparative study of C5a and fmet-leu-phe. J Leuk Biol 1991; 49:29–40.
124. Unpublished data.
125. Lichtenstein LM. The immediate allergic response: in vitro separation of antigen activation, decay and histamine release. J Immunol 1971; 107:1122–30.
126. Kazimierczak W, Meier HL, MacGlashan DW Jr, Lichtenstein LM. An antigen-activated DFP inhibitable enzyme controls basophil desensitization. J Immunol 1984; 132:399–405.
127. Furuichi K, Rivera J, Ishersky C. The fate of IgE bound to rat basophilic leukemia cells. III. Relationship between antigen-induced endocytosis and serotonin release. J Immunol 1984; 133:1513–20.
128. Furuichi K, Rivera J, Buonocorc LM, Isersky C. Recycling of receptor-bound IgE by rat basophilic leukemia cells. J Immunol 1986; 136:1015–22.
129. MacGlashan D Jr, Mogowski M, Lichtenstein LM. Studies of antigen binding on human basophils: II. Continued expression of antigen specific IgE during antigen induced desen-

sitization. J Immunol 1983; 130:2337–42.

130. Warner J, MacGlashan D Jr. Persistance of early crosslink-dependent signal transduction events in human basophils after desensitization. Immunol Lett 1988; 18:129–38.
131. MacGlashan DW Jr, Lichtenstein LM. Basic characteristics of human lung mast cell desensitization. J Immunol 1987; 139:501–5.
132. MacGlashan DW Jr, Lichtenstein LM. The transition from specific to nonspecific desensitization in human basophils. J Immunol 1981; 127:2410–4.
133. Connolly TM, Bross TE, Majerus PW. Isolation of a phosphomonoesterase from human platelets that specifically hydrolyzes the 5-phosphate of inositol 1, 4,5-trisphosphate. J Biol Chem 1985; 260:7868–74.
134. Sagi-Eisenberg R, Lieman H, Pecht I. Protein kinase C regulation of the receptor coupled calcium signal in histamine secreting rat basophilic leukemia cells. Nature 1985; 313:59–60.
135. MacGlashan DW Jr. Single cell analysis of free cytosolic calcium changes in human lung mast cells: II. The relationship between desensitization and the cellular regulation of calcium change. Mol Immunol 1991; 28:585–97.
136. Nguyen K, MacGlashan DW. Comparative studies of human basophils: non-releasers vs. releasers. FASEB J 1988; 2:A1251.
137. Nguyen K-L, Gillis S, MacGlashan DW Jr. A comparative study of releasing and non-releasing human basophils: Non-releasing basophils lack an early component of the signal transduction pathway which follows IgE-crosslinking. J Allergy Clin Immunol 1990; 85:1020–29.
138. Conroy MC, Adkinson NF Jr, Lichtenstein LM. Measurement of IgE on human basophils: relation to serum IgE and anti-IgE-induced histamine release. J Immunol 1977; 118:1317–21.
139. Lichtenstein LM, Margolis S. Histamine release in vitro. Inhibition by catecholamines and methylxanthines. Science 1968; 161:902–3.
140. Lichtenstein LM, Gillespie E. Inhibition of histamine release by histamine controlled by H2 receptor. Nature 1973; 244:287–8.
141. Lichtenstein LM, Gillespie E, Bourne HR, Henney CS. The effects of a series of prostaglandins on in vitro models of the allergic response and cellular immunity. Prostaglandins 1972; 2:519–28.
142. Torphy TJ, Livi GP, Balcarek JM, White JR, Chilton FH, Undem BJ. Therapeutic potential of isozyme-selective phosphodiesterase inhibitors in the treatment of asthma. Adv Cyclic Nucleotide Res (in press).
143. Undem BJ, Peachell PT, Lichtenstein LM. Isproterenol-induced inhibition of immunoglobulin E-mediated release of histamine from the human lung mast cell and arachidonic acid metabolites. J Pharmacol Exp Ther 1988; 247:209–17.
144. Grewe SR, Chan SC, Hanifin JM. Elevated leukocyte cyclic AMP-phosphodiesterase in atopic disease: a possible mechanism for cyclic AMP-agonist hyporesponsiveness. J Allergy Clin Immunol 1982: 70:452–7.
145. Butler JM, Chan SC, Stevens S, Hanifin JM. Increased leukocyte histamine release with elevated cyclic AMP-phosphodiesterase activity in atopic dermatitis. J Allergy Clin Immunol 1983; 71:490–7.
146. Schleimer RP, Lichtenstein LM, Gillespie E. Inhibition of basophil histamine release by antiinflammatory steroids. Nature 1981; 292:454–5.
147. Schleimer RP, Schulman ES, MacGlashan DM Jr, Peters SP, Adams GK III, Lichtenstein LM, Adkinson NF Jr. Effects of dexamethasone on mediator release from human lung fragments and purified human lung mast cells. J Clin Invest 1983; 71:1830–5.
148. Zor U, Her E, Talmon J, Kohen F, Harell T, Moshonov, Rivnay B. Hydrocortisone inhibits antigen-induced rise in intracellular free calcium concentration and abolishes leukotriene C4 production in leukemic basophils. Prostaglandins 1987; 34:29–40.

149. Benhamou M, Ninio E, Salem P, Hieblot C, Bessou G, Pitton C, Liu F-T, Mencia-Huerta JM. Decrease in IgE Rc receptor expression on mouse bone marrow-derived mast cells and inhibition of PAF-acether formation and of β-hexosaminidase release by dexamethasone. J Immunol 1986:1385–92.
150. Collado-Escobar D, Cunha-Melo JR, Beaven MA. Treatment with dexamethasone down-regulates IgE-receptor-mediated signals and up-regulates adenosine-receptor-mediated signals in a rat mast cell (RBL-2H3) line. J Immunol 1990; 144:244–50.
151. Hirai K, Morita Y, Misaki Y, et al. Modulation of human basophil histamine release by hemopoietic growth factors. J Immunol 1988; 141:3958–64.
152. Kurimoto Y, de Weck AL, Dhinden CA. Interleukin 3 dependent mediator release in basophils triggered by C5a. J Exp Med 1989; 170:467–79.
153. Schleimer RP, Derse CP, Friedman B, Gillis G, Plaut M, Lichtenstein LM, MacGlashan DW Jr. Regulation of human basophil mediator release by cytokines. I. Interaction with antiinflammatory steroids. J Immunol 1989; 143:1310–7.

9

Effects of Cyclic Nucleotides on Granulocytes

RONALD G. COFFEY
University of South Florida College of Medicine, Tampa, Florida

I. INTRODUCTION

The first demonstration of an effect of cyclic nucleotides on granulocytes was that of Lichtenstein and Margolis (1), who found in 1968 that agents calculated to increase intracellular levels of cAMP* caused inhibition of antigen-stimulated release of histamine from human blood leukocytes. The paper stimulated many laboratories to investigate the role of this first known "second messenger" system in a host of immune cells. A rapid accumulation of articles confirmed the inhibition by cAMP of release reactions in mast cells as well as basophils, and documented the inhibition of cAMP of nearly all differentiated functions of lymphocytes, macrophages, neutrophils, and even platelets (reviewed in 2–9).

Interest in cGMP lagged behind that of cAMP, due to technical difficulties in its assay. The development of a sensitive enzyme recycling procedure by Nelson Goldberg made feasible the measurement of cGMP in the small quantities of cells usually encountered in immune systems, resulting in the discovery in 1972 by Hadden et al. (10) that mitogenic substances increased cGMP but not cAMP in lymphocytes. Studies

---

*Abbreviations: C3 and C5, third and fifth components of complement; cAMP, adenosine 3′:5′-cyclic monophosphate; cGMP, guanosine 3′:5′-cyclic monophosphate; CHS, Chediak-Higashi syndrome; Con A, concanavalin A; DB-cAMP, N^6,2′-O-dibutyryladenosine 3′:5′-cyclic monophosphate; FMLP, N-formyl-methionyl-leucyl-phenylalanine; GM-CSF, granulocyte-macrophage colony-stimulating factor; HETE, hydroxyeisosatetraenoic acid; HPETE, hydroperoxyeicosatetraenoic acid; IBMX, 3-isobutyl-1-methylxanthine; IgG, immunoglobulin G; IP_3, inositol-1,3,4-trisphosphate; LIF, leukocyte inhibitory factor; LPS, lipopolysaccharide; LT, leukotriene, MNNG, N-methyl-N′-nitro-N-nitrosoguanidine; NECA, 5′-(N-ethylcarboxamido)-adenosine; O_2^-, superoxide; OAG, 1-octyl-2-acetyl-glycerol; PAF, platelet activating factor; PG, prostaglandin; PKC, protein kinase C; PIA, N^6-phenylisopropyladenosine; PMA, phorbol 12-myristate 13-acetate; PMSF, phenylmethylsulfonylfluoride; SRS-A, slow-reacting substance of anaphylaxis.

in granulocytes and platelets soon followed, revealing that in these cells as well, agents stimulating functions often increased cGMP levels. In several laboratories the nucleotides, or lipophilic derivatives, were added to cells. In contrast to the inhibition of responses seen by cAMP, cGMP had the opposite effect in most cases. In a few cases cGMP had no effect, and in the platelet it mimicked cAMP, inhibiting the aggregation and release reactions.

Mechanisms for the regulation of adenylate cyclase are well defined (11). Hormones, neurotransmitters, and autacoids that stimulate adenylate cyclase bind to cell surface receptors and enhance the activity of the GTP-binding protein G_s, which then mediates the activation of the enzyme. Among the agents that act in this manner on granulocytes are adenosine (A_2 receptor), histamine (H_2 receptor), prostaglandin E_2 (PGE_2), and β-adrenoceptor agonists such as epinephrine and isoproterenol. Other agents increase cAMP levels by inhibiting cAMP phosphodiesterases (methylxanthines, RO20-1724, rolipram). Some hormonal agents reduce adenylate cyclase activity by activating the G_i-protein; examples are adenosine (A_1 receptor), somatostatin, and acetylcholine (muscarinic receptor). Others reduce adenylate cyclase activity by activating phosphodiesterase (insulin). Some compounds may affect phosphodiesterase indirectly by increasing Ca^{2+} levels.

Mechanisms for the activation of guanylate cyclase are usually less direct than those for adenylate cyclase. Guanylate cyclase is activated by many oxidants, including dehydroascorbic acid and hydroperoxyeicosatetraenoic acids (HPETEs), and by substances that give rise to nitric oxide (nitroprusside, MNNG, arginine) (12,13). HPETEs are derived from lipoxygenase action on arachidonate, which in turn is produced from phospholipids by the actions of phospholipases. In addition, arachidonate can, without being metabolized, stimulate guanylate cyclase. Therefore, in leukocytes which contain phospholipases and lipoxygenases, a host of stimulants increase cGMP levels as a consequence of the more proximal phospholipase signaling systems. In some cells membrane-bound guanylate cyclase is stimulated in a direct fashion by atrial nartiuretic factor, but human leukocytes do not have receptors for this hormone (14). In certain cells, membrane and soluble forms of guanylate cyclase can be activated by phosphorylation by protein kinase C (PKC) (15,16). A membrane form of guanylate cyclase has extensive homology with protein tyrosine kinases, but it is not known whether the enzyme can phosphorylate itself or other substances (17). Activation of guanylate cyclase is therefore usually a relatively distal event in the hormone signaling sequence. Whether cGMP represents a part of the positive second message or part of a negative feedback (as in the platelet) will be discussed below.

II. BASOPHILS

The second messenger mechanisms invoked by antigen or anti-IgE in hypersensitivity reactions include a GTP-binding protein, phospholipid metabolism, Ca^{2+}, and PKC. Excellent reviews of these basophil and mast cell release mechanisms are available (18–22, and MacGlashan in Chapter 8 of this volume). The present chapter considers regulation of basophil and mast cell release reactions by the cyclic nucleotides, which may affect one or more of the above mechanisms.

A. Cyclic AMP

The observation of Lichtenstein and Margolis (1) related to basophils, since it has been abundantly demonstrated by several groups that these are the only human blood cells that release histamine. The inhibition of histamine release by β-adrenoceptor agonists and methylxanthines was thought to result from an increase of cAMP in basophils, which normally constitute less than 1% of blood granulocytes. Subsequent studies with enriched basophil populations (23–25) verified that this was indeed the case. Another important confirmation consisted in the demonstration that $N^6,O^{2'}$-dibutyryl cAMP (DB-cAMP) also inhibited release. This was the case for both direct (antigen-mediated) and "reversed anaphylaxis" (anti-IgE-mediated) histamine release (26,27). cAMP and analogs also inhibited release caused by concanavalin A (Con A) (28) and activated complement component C5a (29), but not by the tumor promoter phorbol 12-myristate 13-acetate (PMA, 30).

Lichtenstein and co-workers (31) found that allergic release of histamine from basophils can be divided into two stages: a priming stage in which cells are exposed to antigen (or anti-IgE) in the absence of Ca^{2+} and washed; followed by the release stage which is triggered by the addition of Ca^{2+} (31). Using this model, it was found that cAMP stimulants inhibited release only during the first stage (32,33). In fact, some weak cAMP stimulants such as isoproterenol were shown to inhibit release only if the reaction was "staged" (34). Marone et al. (33) showed that cAMP did not inhibit histamine release caused by the Ca^{2+} ionophore A23187, which bypasses receptors to increase Ca^{2+}. The formation and release of leukotriene (LT) C_4 was considerably more sensitive to cAMP-increasing agents than was the release of histamine (33,34).

The list of physiologically relevant hormones and other agents that activate leukocyte or basophil adenylate cyclase and also inhibit histamine release is impressive (Table 1). The effects of hormones and autacoids are receptor specific; adenosine acts on the A_2 receptor, adrenergic receptor agonists on the β_2 receptor, and histamine on the H_2 receptor to increase cAMP. Perhaps the most interesting is histamine itself, which acts in a negative-feedback manner to prevent release from cells that have not yet bound antigen (35). Histamine would not, however, interrupt an ongoing release reaction. The effects of antihistamines are interesting. All anti-H_1 drugs inhibited antigen-evoked release, the most effective being the phenothiazines (38). This inhibition was noted at less than 0.1 mM and may be related to their capacity to inhibit Ca^{2+}-calmodulin-dependent reactions. Paradoxically, anti-H_1 drugs caused histamine release at about 1 mM, coincident with a significant *fall* in cAMP levels. The most effective in causing release (cyclizine, diphenhydramine, promethazine) are considered the least specific for H_1 receptors, while the more specific H_1 antagonists (chlorpheniramine, pyrilamine) were least effective in causing release but evoked the largest drop in cAMP levels. The two actions, therefore, may not be related. H_2 receptor blockers neither caused nor inhibited release, but blocked the inhibitory effects of histamine.

The cAMP inhibitory mechanism is not well understood. Experiments in other tissues had suggested that cAMP, acting through its kinase(s), inhibits the activation of phospholipase A_2, phospholipase C, or both, thereby blocking arachidonate production. The relevance of these observations to the basophil was established by Marone and co-workers (39), who found that phospholipase inhibitors and eicosatetraynoic acid, an inhibitor of both lipoxygenase and cyclooxygenase activities, inhibited antigen-

Table 1 Agents Increasing Cyclic AMP and Inhibiting Histamine Release from Human Basophils

Agent	cAMP	References
Adenosine	nd[f]	9
β-Agonists[a]	nd	1,18,28,32,34
β-Agonists	↑	25,36,37
cAMP[b]	↑	27,28,32
Cholera toxin	nd	9
EDI[c]	↑	38
Forskolin	↑	25,33
Histamine[d]	nd	34
Histamine	↑	36,37
PDE inhibitors[e]	nd	1,26–28,32,34,36
PDE inhibitors	↑	25
$PGE_1/E_2/I_2$	nd	1,26–28,32,34,36
$PGE_1/E_2/I_2$	↑	25,37

References are cited for results with the indicated cAMP stimulants.

[a] β-Adrenoceptor agonists include epinephrine, isoproterenol, and salbutamol.

[b] cAMP analogs include DB-cAMP and 8-Br-cAMP.

[c] The eosinophil-derived inhibitor (EDI) is released by allergen or anti-IgE.

[d] Histamine H_2-receptor agonists include histamine and dimaprit.

[e] Phosphodiesterase inhibitors include the methylxanthines (caffeine, theophylline, aminophylline, and IBMX), papaverine, RO20-1724, and rolipram.

[f] nd: not done.

↑: Increased cAMP levels were measured.

provoked histamine release. By contrast, arachidonate or indomethacin and other cyclooxygenase inhibitors enhanced it. It was reasoned that the cyclooxygenase inhibitors caused the diversion of arachidonate to the lipoxygenase pathway, and that one or more products of this pathway play a key role in the release mechanism. It was then shown (40) that, among several lipoxygenase products tried, 5-HPETE and 5-HETE were able to augment antigenic histamine release. Release caused by phorbol diesters and the Ca^{2+} ionophore A23187 was also enhanced, while release caused by anti-IgE, C5a, and fMet peptides, was not.

Somewhat perplexing was the finding that the inhibition of histamine release by the adenylate cyclase stimulants isoproterenol, dimaprit (highly selective for H_2 receptors), and PGE_2 could be reversed by indomethacin (39). Since indomethacin did not prevent the generation of cAMP, it might have acted either by inhibiting cAMP-dependent protein kinase, or by stimulating the synthesis of a lipoxygenase product which possibly overcomes the step inhibited by cAMP. However, the inhibition by DB-cAMP or the cAMP phosphodiesterase inhibitor, 3-isobutyl-1-methylxantine (IBMX), could not be reversed by indomethacin. Marone et al. (39) speculated that separate pools of cAMP may exist in the cells and that only the pool generated by the hormones was affected by the drug.

Studies with highly purified basophils (from patients with basophilic leukemia) indicated that IgE itself causes a significant increase in cAMP within 30 s (18). This is followed by a decrease below basal levels at 2 min. The decrease was thought somehow to trigger the release reaction. Other studies (40) revealed that DB-cAMP can actually potentiate release when an excessive, inhibitory concentration of antigen is used. It was thought that when antigen is in excess, the drop in cAMP occurs too quickly, and addition of DB-cAMP restores the small amount of cAMP required for histamine release. This requirement apparently occurs in the second stage of the release mechanism, whereas cAMP inhibition of release occurs in the first. Several histamine-releasing agents were found to evoke a rapid rise in cAMP (peak at 45 s) in cells from a patient with basophilia [up to 70% basophils (24)]. These agents included anti-IgE, polylysine, A23187, and N-formyl-methionyl-leucyl-phenylalanine (FMLP). The increase occurred prior to histamine release in most cases, but began slowly with A23187, and did not occur with compound 48/80, a potent synthetic histamine releasor. Furthermore, adenosine and sodium fluoride caused a rapid increase in cAMP but did not stimulate histamine release. Hughes et al. (24) concluded that cAMP does not play a key role in the biochemical events leading to mediator release by human basophils. A similar conclusion was stated by Peachell et al. (25), who examined basophils purified up to 88% from human blood by Percoll density sedimentation. Anti-IgE failed to increase cAMP, and agents that did increase cAMP (IBMX > forskolin > PGE_2 > isoproterenol) caused inhibition of histamine release in proportion to the magnitude and duration of the cAMP increase. Since several sources of anti-IgE and several buffer systems were used, Hughes et al. (24) believed that, except for an undetectable increase in some cellular compartment, cAMP plays no role in the initiation of mediator release.

B. Cyclic GMP

Very few studies have involved cGMP in human basophils. Gillespie and Lichtenstein (41) found that this nucleotide modestly potentiated antigenic histamine release when medium concentrations of Ca^{2+} were low. While the cAMP-specific inhibitors rolipram (42) and RO20-1724 (43) inhibited immunologic or 48/80-induced histamine release, a cGMP-specific inhibitor (M&B 22948) did not. Thus it appears that cGMP, unlike cAMP, does not inhibit the function of basophils, and in certain circumstances cGMP may augment histamine release.

III. MAST CELLS

Mast cells are the fixed tissue counterparts of blood basophils. Mast cells are interspersed throughout the connective tissue and are especially rich in skin, respiratory epithelium, and the GI tract. Mast cells may therefore be the first cells of the immune system to respond to antigenic or injurious stimuli. In addition to histamine, mast cells release a host of other mediators of inflammation, including cytokines, enzymes such as beta-hexosaminidase, and peptide chemotactic factors for eosinophils, neutrophils, and monocytes. Nonpeptide mediators include bradykinin, heparin, and lipid-derived leukotrienes, PGD_2, and platelet-activating factor (PAF). Most of the research relevant to cyclic nucleotide regulation in mast cells, as in basophils, has involved measurement of histamine release.

A. Cyclic AMP

Cyclic nucleotide regulation has been studied extensively in rat peritoneal mast cells because they are easily purified. Older studies on chopped human and primate lung are important in demonstrating effects of cyclic nucleotides and hormones on release reactions. Procedures for purification of human lung mast cells have been developed more recently, and some very interesting experiments are reviewed here.

The diversity of agents capable of modulating cAMP and cGMP levels is indicated in Table 2. Histamine release induced by antigen or anti-IgE, the plant lectin mitogen Con A, or by a variety of noncytotoxic chemical agents such as dextran or the basic polymer 48/80 is inhibited in mast cells by cAMP (Table 3). Different results have been reported with other releasing agents. Most early studies utilized the rat peritoneal mast cell because of the ease with which it is purified; all data in Tables 2 and 3 refer to studies with these cells unless otherwise indicated.

1. Human Lung Mast Cells

In 1936, Schild (84) demonstrated the inhibition of allergic histamine release from guinea pig lung by very low (nM) levels of epinephrine. Thirty-five years later, he showed that this effect was mediated by β-adrenergic receptors, being inhibited by propranolol (85). Orange et al. (60) demonstrated that the release of slow-reacting substance of anaphylaxis (SRS-A, now known to be a mixture of LTC_4, LTD_4, and LTE_4) was similarly regulated in chopped human lung by cAMP, β-adrenergic agents, and phosphodiesterase inhibitors. The inhibition of SRS-A release was more sensitive to lower concentrations of β-adrenergic agents (60) than the release of histamine. Similarly, inhibition of both histamine and SRS-A release by β-adrenergic agents was demonstrated in monkey lung by Teruko Ishizaka et al. (89). While the two types of mediators are usually regulated in the same direction, a distinction was made with cytochalasins, which augmented the immunologic release of histamine but inhibited that of SRS-A (79). Another distinction was that carbachol prevented the inhibition by isoproterenol of the release of histamine but not of SRS-A (79). To account for these distinctions it should be noted that essentially all histamine in the lung is derived from mast cells, while SRS-A is derived from eosinophils and macrophages as well as mast cells. Therefore, different cells may respond to inhibitors to produce divergent results. On the other hand, different steps in the pathways of release of the different mediators may be regulated by cAMP. Whereas histamine is preformed and packaged in granules, SRS-A is formed after immunologic challenge. Marone et al. (33) prepared human lung mast cells to purities ranging as high as 96%. Forskolin stimulated cAMP by three- to fourfold and inhibited both LTC_4 and histamine release. With these highly purified lung mast cells, the inhibition of LTC_4 release was again more sensitive then histamine release to lower concentrations of forskolin. Similar results were obtained in purified human lung mast cells by Peachell et al. (25), who found that the elevation of cAMP by several agonists (IBMX > forskolin > PGE_2 > isoproterenol) correlated quite well with the inhibition of IgE-mediated formation of LTC_4 and histamine release. Undem et al. (83) found that the EC_{50} for inhibition by isoproterenol of immunologic histamine release was about three times higher than for the inhibition of LTC_4 or PGD_2 formation.

Using the Ca^{2+} ionophore A23187 to stimulate the release reaction, Undem et al. (83) showed that β-adrenergic stimulation completely abrogated LTC_4 release while having either no effect or potentiating histamine release from purified human lung mast

Table 2 Effects on Cyclic Nucleotides in Mast Cells

Agent	cAMP	cGMP
A23187	↓ 44–47	
ACTH	↑ 46	
Adenine	↓ 47	
Adenosine R site[a]	↑ 49	→ 49
Adenosine P site[b]	↓ 49	→ 49
α-Adrenergic	↓ Lh: 25,60,61	
β-Adrenergic[c]	↑ 44,47,56,62–64; Lh: 60,61	
Agitation	↑ 47	
Antigen challenge	↑ 46,50–52; mu: 53	↑ 50
Antigen sensitization	↓ 54	↑ 54
Anti-IgE[d]	↑ 49,50,52,55–57; ↑ Lh: 58	↑ 50,56
	↓ 59; → Lh: 25	↑ 56
Ca^{2+}	↓ 47	
Cholera toxin	↓ 65	
Cholinergic[e]	↓ 47	↑ 69
Compound 48/80	↓ 66,67; ↓ PS: 44,55,68	↑ 117; PI: 68
	→ 47,62	→ 69
Concanavalin A	↑ 52,55	→ 69
Diazoxide	↓ 47	
Disodium cromoglycate	↓ 70; ↓ PS: 55,68	↑ PI: 68
Forskolin	↑ 33; ↑ Lh: 25	
Glass exposure	↑ 47	
Glucocorticoids	↑ 71	
Histamine	↑ 47; → 64,72	
PDE inhibitors[f]	↑ 44,47,56,62–64,73	
cAMP specific[g]	↑ 74	
cGMP specific[h]		↑ 42,68
PGD_2	↑ 73, 75	
PGE_1/E_2	↑ 44,47,59,62,64; ↑ Lh: 25	
$PGF_{2\alpha}$	↑ 62,64	
Somatostatin	↓ 67	
Terfenadine	↑ 76; ↑ Lg: 76	

Reference numbers are cited for results obtained with rat mast cells unless otherwise indicated.
↑: Increase in cyclic nucleotide levels.
↓: Decrease in cyclic nucleotide levels.
→: No change in cyclic nucleotide levels.

L: Lung g: Guinea pig
PS: PDE stimulation h: Human
PI: PDE inhibition mu: mouse

[a] R-site adenosine analog: N^6-phenylisopropyl adenosine.

[b] P-site adenosine analog: Dideoxyadenosine, SQ-22536.

[c] β-Adrenergic agonists include isoproterenol and epinephrine.

[d] Anti-IgE or antibody to IgE receptor.

[e] Cholinergic compounds include acetylcholine and methacholine.

[f] Nonspecific PDE inhibitors include methylxanthines (caffeine, theophylline, IBMX), papaverine, and AA344.

[g] cAMP-specific PDE inhibitors include RO20-1724 and rolipram.

[h] cGMP-specific PDE inbhitor is M&B 22948.

Table 3 Inhibition of Mast Cell Histamine Release by Cyclic AMP Agonists

	Releasing agent					
	A23187	Antigen	Anti-IgE	Comp 48/80	Con A	PMA
β-Adrenergic agonists[a]	→ Lg: 77 → Lh: 83	↓ 78–80 ↓ Lg: 77,84,85 ↓ Lh: 60,85,88 ↓ Lmo: 89	↓ 56,81 ↓ Lh: 25,83,86	↓ 62,63,71,78,82,87 →44		→ Lg: 77
cAMP[b]	↓ 90,91 → 67,93 → Lg: 77 → mu: 94	↓ 90 ↓ Lh: 60 ↓ Lmo: 89 → 43	↓ 56,59	↓ 63,71,82	↓ 90,92,87	→ Lh: 83
Cholera toxin		→ 65				
Forskolin	→ Lg: 77	↓ 33,65,95				→ Lg: 77 → Lh: 83
Glucococorticoids				↓ 71		
Histamine[c]			↓ 75			
PDE inhibitors[d]	↓ 90,91,93	↓ 43,90	↓55,56,59, 73,81,90	↓ 43,44,63,71 82,87,96		
cAMP-specific[e]		→42				
PGD_2			→ 73			
PGE_1/E_2			↓ 59,62	↓ 44,62,82		
$PGF_{2\alpha}$				↓ 62		

Reference numbers are cited for results obtained with rat peritoneal mast cells unless otherwise indicated.
↓: Inhibition of histamine release.
→: No effect on histamine release.
L: Lung.
g: Guinea pig.
h: Human.
mo: Monkey
mu: Mouse.

[a] β-Adrenergic agonists include isoproterenol, epinephrine, and salbutamol.

[b] cAMP analogs include DB-cAMP and 8-Br-cAMP.

[c] Serotonin release was measured when histamine was added to cells.

[d] Nonspecific PDE inhibitors include methylxanthines (caffeine, theophylline, IBMX) and papaverine.

[e] cAMP-specific PDE inhibitors include RO20-1724 and rolipram.

cells. Similarly, A23187-provoked histamine release was not inhibited by cAMP, forskolin, or β-adrenergic stimulation in purified guinea pig lung mast cells (77). PMA represents another example of nonimmunologic histamine release that is not inhibited by cAMP in purified guinea pig (77) or human (83) lung mast cells. It is apparent that (a) one or more steps of phospholipid and/or arachidonate metabolism are more sensitive to cAMP inhibition than the step(s) leading to histamine release, and (b) cAMP may inhibit immunologically induced Ca^{2+} mobilization but the Ca^{2+}-dependent step of histamine release is relatively insensitive to cAMP in lung mast cells as it is in basophils.

2. *Rat Mast Cells*

Johnson and Moran (78) were the first to demonstrate β-adrenergic inhibition of antigen-induced histamine release in purified rat mast cells. Several other laboratories subsequently found that β-adrenergic agents also inhibited histamine release when stimulated by anti-IgE (81,55), dextran (97), leukocyte cationic proteins (71), or 48/80 (62,63,71,78,87). However, the rat mast cell is much less sensitive compared to human lung, and some workers (44,82) did not observe inhibition unless phosphodiesterase inhibitors were also present.

cAMP, lipophilic analogs of cAMP, and the direct adenylate cyclase stimulant forskolin inhibit rodent mast cell histamine release from rodent mast cells stimulated immunologically or with Con A, or compound 48/80 (Table 3). cAMP and its stimulants also inhibit histamine release from mast cells stimulated with dextran (97), leukocyte cationic proteins (71), and somatostatin (67). Some (90,91) but not all (67,93) workers reported inhibition of Ca^{2+} ionophore-stimulated histamine release. Several laboratories (56,70,94,95,98,99) reported that cAMP blocked immunologically induced increases in mast cell Ca^{2+}. Attempts to resolve the question of whether cAMP inhibits the mobilization of Ca^{2+} or its actions utilized permeabilized mast cells. When permeabilized by ATP, incubated with GTPγS, and resealed with Mg^{2+}, the introduction of Ca^{2+} caused histamine release (95). This release was not inhibited by cAMP or by IBMX, although antigen-stimulated release was inhibited. Antigen but not GTPγS/Ca^{2+} evoked the phospholipase C pathway, a known target of cAMP inhibition. Quite different results were obtained when mast cells were permeabilized with a nontoxic concentration of β-escin (100). These cells, which were not resealed, released histamine upon addition of Ca^{2+}, inositol 1,3,4-trisphosphate (IP_3), or GTPγS. Inhibition by cAMP (10–100 μM) was observed when Ca^{2+} or IP_3 was used. In these cells, GTPγS activated phospholipase C and released IP_3, so one may assume that cAMP would also have inhibited GTPγS-induced release.

Most workers have found that nonspecific phosphodiesterase inhibitors such as theophylline and IBMX are effective inhibitors of histamine release in rat mast cells (Table 3). However, the cAMP-specific inhibitors rolipram (42) and RO20-1724 (43) did not inhibit immunologic or 48/80-induced histamine release. Whether theophylline inhibits histamine release by increasing cAMP is unresolved. Sydbom and Fredholm (96) found that adenosine, which inhibits adenylate cyclase in rat mast cells (see below), prevents the theophylline-induced rise in cAMP but does not prevent theophylline inhibition of histamine release.

Among the most potent stimulants of mast cell cAMP are PGE_1 and PGE_2 (44,47,59,62,64). They inhibit histamine release when stimulated by anti-IgE (59,81) or by 48/80 (44,62,82). $PGF_{2\alpha}$ has a weak cAMP stimulatory effect, and is a correspondingly weak inhibitor of release (62,64). PGD_2 is of considerable interest because the mast cell is a unique source of this PG. Holgate et al. (73,75,101) showed that PGD_2 was unique in another respect: It increased cAMP, but not cAMP-dependent protein kinase. Although other cAMP-elevating agents inhibited mast cell histamine release, PGD_2 did not. One explanation for such discordant results is that PGD_2 may stimulate cAMP in an intracellular compartment that is sequestered and not accessible to protein kinase A. Another explanation is that PGD_2 provokes too small a cAMP signal. Wescott and Kaliner (75) found that histamine release could be inhibited if aminophylline were added with PGD_2. Interestingly, ^{3}H-serotonin release could be inhibited by

PGD_2 alone, suggesting that it may be packaged in granules distinct from histamine-containing granules.

The effects of histamine on rat mast cells are quite different from its effects on human basophils. Histamine, like PGD_2, has a weak effect to increase cAMP and to inhibit release (75). The receptor mediating the effect is apparently an H_1 receptor, as defined by the effective histamine analogs (75,102). These data suggest an indirect effect, since only H_2 receptors are linked directly to adenylate cyclase. Curiously, H_1 antagonists also evoked release (75).

Another argument for compartmentalization of cAMP pools was developed from data with adenosine and its analogs. Adenosine alone had no effect on histamine release from rat mast cells, but it enhanced release provoked by A23187, antigen, anti-IgE, Con A, or 48/80 (45–47,96,103–105). The effect was bimodal, with a peak at 10 μM. Austen and co-workers (49,106) found that adenosine and R-site analogs (such as N^6-phenylisopropyladenosine, modified in the purine, not the R-moiety) stimulated cAMP and promoted histamine release. By contrast, P-site analogs (such as 2′,5′-dideoxyadenosine, modified in the ribose moiety and unable to activate cell surface adenosine receptors) inhibited anti-IgE stimulation of cAMP levels, cAMP-dependent protein kinase types I and II, and histamine release. The stimulation of cAMP is probably due to the A_2 receptor (51,105), as occurs in other cells. However, several workers (47,51,104,105) proposed that the promotion of histamine release is unrelated to cAMP. Both effects are mediated by cell surface receptors, since they are prevented by inhibitors of nucleoside uptake. Of great importance is the fact that theophylline or 8-phenyltheophylline, traditional A_1 and A_2 receptor blockers, prevented adenosine stimulation of cAMP but not the effect on histamine release (47,104,105). Based on the relative actions of a series of adenosine analogs, the release potentiating receptor is in neither the A_1 nor the A_2 receptor category (51). Eposure to adenosine antagonists causes up-regulation of both cAMP-related and histamine release-related receptors, while exposure to adenosine agonists causes down-regulation of both types of receptors (107).

A final argument for compartmentalization of cAMP in mast cells derives from experiments with cholera toxin (65) and GTPγS (95). Cholera toxin ADP ribosylated the Gs GTP-binding protein of mouse mast cells. Thus it stimulated adenylate cyclase in these cells as in other cells. Cholera toxin neither enhanced nor inhibited histamine release when provoked with antigen, but enhanced release when provoked by thrombin. No effects of cholera toxin on phospholipase C, Ca^{2+}, or arachidonate release were observed. In the same cells, forskolin stimulated cAMP and inhibited all the responses.

The production of leukotrienes and PAF by rodent mast cells is much more sensitive to cAMP than the release of histamine. Undem et al. (94), working with mouse PT-18 mast cells, found that forskolin alone could inhibit the immunologic formation of the lipid mediators but had no effect on histamine release. Cytosolic Ca^{2+} was not affected. By adding forskolin with IBMX, a greater rise in cAMP and cAMP-dependent kinase activity was obtained. This combination inhibited immunologic or Ca^{2+} ionophore-stimulated histamine release as well as formation of the lipid mediators.

Mast cell cAMP levels are decreased by some agents which cause histamine release: A23187 (45,46), 48/80 (44,55,66,67,68), PMA (108), and somatostatin (67). Other agents decrease cAMP, promote histamine release caused by other agents, but by themselves do not cause histamine release: adenine, muscarinic cholinergic agents, and diazoxide (47). Still other agents stimulate histamine release but have no effect on cAMP: nerve growth factor, peptide 401, and polymyxin B (82).

The stimulation of cAMP by some histamine-releasing agents, particularly anti-IgE (46,49,50,55–57), has been the subject of considerable research. It is a rapid and brief effect, peaking at about 15 s, followed by activation of cAMP-dependent protein kinase (109). It is thought that a trypsin-like protease somehow activates adenylate cyclase (52). A secondary increase of cAMP occurs a few minutes later, and cAMP levels return to baseline before release begins. PGD_2 and PGI_2 are significantly increased by anti-IgE, and the PGs apparently account for the second cAMP increase, since indomethacin can prevent the second (20) but not the first (109) cAMP surge. Holgate et al. (49) described the parallel inhibition by the P-site adenosine analogs of anti-IgE-stimulated cAMP and histamine release. They put forth a strong argument for the essential nature of this brief cAMP surge for the sequence of events leading to histamine release. In addition to anti-IgE, Con A (55) and peptides derived from ACTH and IgE (46) also increase cAMP. However, the increase occurs during rather than prior to histamine release and may not be a necessary part of the release mechanism. It is notable that anti-IgE does not cause a change in cAMP in purified human lung mast cells (25).

Ishizaka et al. (56) observed increases in cGMP as well as cAMP within 30 s after adding anti-IgE or angi-IgE receptor antibody to rat mast cells. Phospholipid methylation occurred simultaneously, followed by Ca^{2+} uptake and histamine release. Similar events were described in mouse mast cells (110,111) and in mast cells purified from human lung by Ishizaka et al. (112). In both types of cells, the monovalent Fab′ fragment was inactive, indicating that a bridging of receptors was required for the intracellular events. The same biochemical events could be triggered in rat mast cell membranes (56). In both cells and cell membranes, 3-deaza-SIBA or 3-deaza-adenosine and homocysteine thiolactone inhibited methylation and cAMP synthesis, while theophylline or DB-cAMP inhibited methylation, suggesting that these events are mutually regulated. Interestingly, the methylation inhibitors also blocked activation of membrane adenylate cyclase by NaF, indicating a fundamental effect of the compound on adenylate cyclase or its coupling to a GTP-binding protein.

The importance of the phospholipid methylation pathway has been questioned by Holgate et al. (113), who believe the methylation inhibitors may also inhibit cAMP phosphodiesterase. However, inhibition of histamine release (as well as inhibition of desensitization) can be reversed by S-adenosyl-methionine (111), the methyl donor for methyltransferases.

3. Conclusions

To conclude this section, nearly every agent that stimulates cAMP inhibits immunologically induced mast cell degranulation. Three important exceptions are adenosine, PGD_2, and cholera toxin. It is therefore reasonable to propose that compartmentalized pools of cAMP may be formed which can inhibit, promote, or have no effect on histamine release in the isolated rat mast cell. It is possible that one subcellular compartment of cAMP is important for triggering histamine release, while another compartment functions to limit release. Kurosawa and Parker (114) described a cAMP-dependent protein kinase on the inner surface of isolated granules of rat mast cells. This kinase could mediate the effects of locally produced cAMP, thus affecting mediator release.

The mechanism of cAMP inhibition or release probably involves mobilization of Ca^{2+} and at least one other step. Release triggered by PMA is not inhibited by cAMP, while release provoked by Ca^{2+}, Ca^{2+} ionophores, or GTPγS remains controversial.

The significance or the early cAMP rise in immunologic histamine release remains unknown. Since the rise is not produced by histamine-releasing pharmacologic agents, it is not an obligatory event in the release process, but may represent a specific portion of immunologic release which is bypassed by other agents.

B. Cyclic GMP

By contrast to cAMP, cGMP does not inhibit mast cell mediator release (69), and in some tissues such as human lung, it causes a modest augmentation of release (61). In rat mast cells, however, a positive role for cGMP in promoting histamine release has not been demonstrated. In fact, the cGMP-specific phosphodiesterase inhibitor (M&B 22948) inhibited immunologic or 48/80-induced histamine release (42,43,67), while the cAMP-specific phosphodiesterase inhibitors rolipram (42) and RO20-1724 (43) did not. A role in sensitization was suggested by Sydbom et al. (54), who found that this procedure was associated with an increase in the ratio cGMP:cAMP. Other activities of mast cells may be promoted by cGMP. Kallikrein, which contributes to inflammation by catalyzing the formation of bradykinin, is released from rat mast cells activated immunologically or by other means. Rothschild (115) showed that cGMP, epinephrine, and 48/80 caused kallikrein release from a population of mast cells different from the histamine-releasing cells. The effects of each of these agents was inhibited by cAMP.

Guanylate cyclase was characterized by Taniguchi et al. (116) in rat mast cells. As in most other cells, it operates optimally at pH 8.2, with Mn^{2+}·GTP as the preferred substrate. The enzyme is entirely particulate, a characteristic not shared by guanylate cyclases of other hemopoietic cells. Anti-IgE receptor antibody increases cGMP in cell-free membranes (56). The increase of two- to three-fold occurs at 30 s, slightly after the cAMP increase, and, like cAMP, returns to baseline at 1 min. In sonicated mast cell membranes, guanylate cyclase was not stimulated by adrenergic or cholinergic agents, Con A, azide, arachidonate, or 48/80. Compound 48/80 does promote a sharp increase of cGMP in intact rat mast cells (117). Other degranulating agents that increase cGMP in mast cells are antigens (50) (Table 2). Muscarinic agonists also increase cGMP in intact cells (69). These compounds, however, do not initiate histamine release. In the human lung (61) [but not in rat mast cells (43,69)] they augment release by other agents. Several mechanisms may account for cGMP increases. The effect of 48/80 is apparently due to inhibition of cGMP phosphodiesterase (68), while that of antigen may be due to a metabolite of oxidative metabolism of arachidonate via cyclooxygenase (50). Muscarinic agonists often stimulate lipoxygenase, and products of this pathway activate guanylate cyclase in lymphocytes (118), but the mechanism has not been demonstrated in mast cells.

IV. NEUTROPHILS

The preceding chapters provide excellent overviews on the subject of neutrophil activation. The following will deal only with the effects of agents on cyclic nucleotides, and the effects of cAMP and cGMP on neutrophil function.

A. Cyclic AMP

A wide variety of agents affect cAMP in human neutrophils (Table 4). cAMP phosphodiesterase is quite active in neutrophils, and the use of phosphodiesterase inhibitors is sometimes necessary in order to be able to measure increases caused by receptor binding ligands linked to G_s, such as adenosine, histamine, isoproterenol, and PGE_2 (125,127). By contrast, it has been difficult to demonstrate the inhibitory G_i influence in neutrophils. All adenosine analogs tested to date stimulate cAMP (149). Muscarinic stimuli, usually linked to G_i-mediated decreases of cAMP, had no effect in neutrophils (134,139). Lad et al. (183) were able to measure ADP ribosylation of a 42-kD protein in neutrophil plasma membranes, but could not measure a functional G_i linked to receptors. A functional G_i linked to α-adrenergic receptors in intact cells is suggested by the findings that phentolamine augmented the stimulation of cAMP by epinephrine (135) and by isoproterenol (168). Also, combining propranolol with epinephrine to create an α-adrenergic agonist resulted in the inhibition of PGE_1 stimulation of cAMP (123). Panosian et al. (140) established the existence of α_2- (but not α_1-) adrenergic receptors by measuring the binding of specific ligands in neutrophil membranes. They noted that the α_2-specific blocker yohimbine enhanced the stimulation of cAMP by norepinephrine (acting on β-adrenergic receptors) in intact cells. Functional G_i-proteins in neutrophils are also indicated by the capacity of met-enkephalin to reduce cAMP levels (171). The reader is referred to Chapter 5 by Lad et al. for a thorough discussion of G-proteins.

Elevation of cAMP levels by hormones occurs rapidly in neutrophils, as in most systems, while stimulation by cholera toxin develops slowly (133). Colchicine and other inhibitors of microtubule formation increase cAMP levels, and greatly augment intact cell responses to all G_s-linked stimulants (137,149,154). These results suggest that microtubules restrict the association of hormones with G_s or of G_s with adenylate cyclase (138). The effect of colchicine was not observed in neutrophil homogenates (138). Glucocorticoids also augment the stimulation of cAMP by other hormones (125,126,132,151). The effect is independent of protein synthesis and phosphodiesterase inhibition. The steroids alone can increase cAMP, but the effects are small.

Sonication for more than a few seconds destroys the capacity of hormones to activate adenylate cyclase, and most workers either employ sonication for 5 s or less, or use Dounce homogenization or nitrogen cavitation to break cells (133, 143,149,158,183,185). Bourne et al. (158) stated that sonic disruption completely destroys enzyme activity. However, Stolc (119) and Galant et al. (185) measured excellent responses to histamine, isoproterenol, and PGE_1 in neutrophils sonicated for 30 s (119) or for less than 5 s (185) at a low intensity. The measurements were made with *unfractionated* sonicates immediately after sonication. In plasma membrane vesicles prepared by density-gradient centrifugation following sonication (<5 s), Lad et al. (183) measured activation by PGE_1 (sixfold) and isoproterenol (twofold) but only in the presence of GTP. Cholera toxin was able to stimulate if it was preactivated by incubation with dithiothreitol. We (149) have found that permeabilization with digitonin permits access of the enzyme to ATP, preserves responses to hormones including histamine, NECA, isoproterenol, and PGE_2, and allows good stimulation by NaF and GppNHp, which are otherwise excluded from the interior surface of the cell (119). Neutrophil adenylate cyclase is not activated by Ca^{2+}/calmodulin; indeed, it is inhibited by Ca^{2+} and stimulated by EGTA (119,149,123,183).

Table 4 Effects on Cyclic Nucleotides in Neutrophils

	cAMP	cGMP
A23187 + Ca^{2+}	↓ 119 ↑ 121,122,123,184	↑ 120
Adenosine[a]	↑ 124,125,126,127,128	
Antigen/Ab complexes	↑ 121	
Ascorbic acid	↓ 129	→ 130
α-Adrenergic agents[b]	→ 131; ↓ 123	↑ 131
β-Adrenergic agents[c]	↑ 123,124,125,126,128,131,132,133, 134,135,136,137,138,139,140,141,142 → R: 143	→ 134,135,139 ↑ 131
Chemotaxins[d]	↑ 121,122,123,144,145,146,148,184 ↓ 131	↑ 121,124,131,144,150 → 145
Cholera toxin	↑ 133,151	
Cholinergic agents	→ 120,131,134,139	↑ 120,131,134,135,139, 149,152,153
Colchicine	↑ 137,149; r: 154; → 138,155	
C-reactive protein	↑ 156	
Ethanol	↑ 157	
Fluoride[e]	↑ 149,158; R: 143	
Forskolin	↑ 149,159,160	
Glucagon	→ R: 143	
GM-CSF	↓ 124	↑ 124
GppNHp[e]	↑ 124	
Histamine[f]	↑ 125,126,138,149,161,162,163	→ 162
12-HPETE, 12-HETE	→ 164	↑ 164
Levamisole	→ 144,165,166; ↑ 139	↑ 139,144,166,167
LIF	→ 169	↑ 169
LTB_4	↑ 170	→ 170
Met-enkephalin	↓ 171	↑ 171
Muramyl dipeptide	↑ 166	↑ 166
Nitric oxide[g]		↑ 124,153
PGE_1/E_2	↑ 123,125,126,128,131,133, 136,137,138,149,158,172 ↑ R: 143	
$PGF_{2\alpha}$	↑ 172 → 131	↑ 131
PGI_2	↑ 148,173,174	
PDE inhibitors[h]	↑ 138,142 → 133,158	
cAMP specific[i]	↑ 149,173,175	
cGMP specific[j]		↑ 149,169

Table 4 Continued

	cAMP	cGMP
Phagocytic stimuli		
IgG (aggregated)	→ 134	↑ 134
Latex	↑ 176,177 → R: 143	
Zymosan (opsonized)	→ 134,152 ↑ 177,178,179	↑ 120,131,134,135,178
PMA	↓ 124; → 131	↑ 124,131,180
Tuftsin	↓ 166,181,182 → R: 143	↑ 166,181,182

Reference numbers are cited for results obtained with human neutrophils unless otherwise indicated.
↑: Stimulation of cyclic nucleotide levels.
↓: Reduction of cyclic nucleotide levels.
→: No effect on cyclic nucleotide levels.
R: Rabbit.

[a] Adenosine A_2 receptor agonists include adenosine, 2-chloro-adenosine, and NECA.

[b] α-Adrenergic agonists include norephinephrine and phenylephrine. In the presence of α_2-receptor blockade by yohimbine, norepinephrine elevated cAMP levels (140).

[c] β-Adrenergic agonists include isoproterenol, epinephrine, and salbutamol.

[d] Chemotactic agents include FMLP and other bacterially derived substances.

[e] Fluoride and GppNHp stimulate adenylate cyclase in broken or permeabilized cells.

[f] Histamine H_2-receptor agonists include histamine, 4-methylhistamine, and dimaprit.

[g] Nitric oxide-generating agents include arginine, sodium nitroprusside, and MNNG.

[h] Nonspecific phosphodiesterase inhibitors include IBMX, theophylline, and papaverine.

[i] cAMP-specific inhibitors include rolipram and RO20-1724.

[j] cGMP-specific inhibitors include M&B 22,948 and dipyridamole.

The first experiments demonstrating inhibition of human neutrophil functions by cAMP were those of May (27), who reported in 1970 that DB-cAMP inhibited zymosan-stimulated β-glucuronidase release. The following year Bourne et al. (158) published that DB-cAMP, theophylline, and PGE_1 inhibited the killing of intracellular *Candida albicans*. Subsequently, many others have reported the inhibition by cAMP of neutrophil cytotoxicity of intracellular bacteria (186,187) and antibody-dependent cytotoxicity of tumor cells (188,189). Bourne et al. (158) did not observe an effect of the drugs on phagocytosis of the *Candida albicans* fungi. Subsequently, many others have reported the inhibition by cAMP of neutrophil cytotoxicity of intracellular bacteria (186,187) and antibody-dependent cytotoxicity of tumor cells (188,189). Bourne et al. (158) did not observe an effect of the drugs on phagocytosis of the *Candida albicans* fungi. However, others (159,178,182,190) have reported inhibition by cAMP of the phagocytosis of zymosan opsonized by either IgG or $C3_{bi}$. Zymosan and other phagocytic stimuli activate several functions of neutrophils. Among these are the oxidative burst (see McPhail et al., Chapter 2), the pentose phosphate pathway (hexose monophosphate shunt), phospholipases, lipoxygenase, formation of HETEs, leukotriene B_4, and PAF, and the release of granular enzymes. All of these activities are inhibited by cAMP (Table 5). A host of phagocytic and nonphagocytic stimuli have been employed

Table 5 Effects of cAMP and cGMP on Neutrophil Function

	cAMP	cGMP
Adhesion	↑ 191	
Cytotoxicity		
Candida	↓ 133,158	
Bacteria (intracellular)	↓ 186,187	
Tumor cells (antibody dependent)	↓ 187,188	↑ 187
Enzyme release		
I. Granules[a]; stimulated by:		
A23187 + Ca^{2+}	↓ 192; ↑ G: 193	
Con A	↓ 194	
Complement C5A	↓ 192,195; ↓ G: 196	↑ 195; ↑ G: 196
FMLP	↓ 149,192,197; → 127; ↓ G: 193	
IgG (aggregated)	↓ 133,134,198,199; R: 200	↑ 134,199,204
LTB_4	↓ 192	
Platelet-activating factor	↓ 192	
Tumor cells	↓ 189	
Zymosan (opsonized)	↓ 26,133,134,135,161, 175,178,190,198,199 ↓ G: 196	↑ 134,135,178, 199 ↑ G: 196
II. Granules[b]; stimulated by:		
A23187 + Ca^{2+}	↓ 192	
FMLP	↓ 149,192; → 127	
IgG, aggregated on surface	↓ R: 200	
LTB_4	↓ 192	
Platelet-activating factor	↓ 192	
PMA	→ G: 193	
Tumor cells	↓ 189	
LTB_4 release	↓ 142,173	
Motility		
Chemotaxis	↓ 162,180,187,202,203 → 204: ↓ r: 174	↑ 144,180,202 203,204
Random movement	↑ 162	↑ 144
Oxidative burst,[c] stimulated by:		
A23187 + Ca^{2+}	↓ 141,205; → 206	
Complement C5A	↓ 145	
Con A	↓ 194	
FMLP	↓ 141,145,148,160,163,207	
Lipopolysaccharide	↓ 208	
LTB_4	↓ 141	
PMA, diacylglycerol	→ 205,206	
Zymosan (opsonized)	↓ 187,207	
Unstimulated (basal)	→ 208	↑ 208
PAF release, stimulated by antigen	↓ 178; ↓ R: 209	↑ 178

Table 5 Continued

	cAMP	cGMP
Pentose phosphate pathway (Hexose monophosphate shunt), stimulated by:		
Con A	↓ 194	
Phagocytic stimuli[d]	↓ 159,186,187,210; → 211	
Unstimulated (basal)	↓ 212	
PMA, diacylglycerol	→ 141	
Phagocytosis, stimulated by:		
Antigen	→ r: 216	
Candida	→ 158	
Zymosan (opsonized)	↓ 159,214,215; ↑ 176,216 → 133,178,190,211,217 218,219,220	↑ 178,182
Phosphatidyl inositol turnover	↓ 221,222,223	
Protein kinase C	→ 149	→ 149

Reference numbers are cited for results obtained with human neutrophils unless otherwise indicated.
↑: Stimulation by cyclic nucleotide.
↓: Inhibition by cyclic nucleotide.
→: No effect of cyclic nucleotide.
G: Guinea pig.
R: Rabbit.
r: Rat.

[a] Primary (I) granule enzymes usually measured are β-glucuronidase, myeloperoxidase, neutral protease, or N-acetyl-β-D-glucosaminidase.

[b] Secondary (II) granule enzymes usually measured are lysozyme or vitamin B_{12}-binding protein.

[c] The oxidative burst is measured by O_2^- or H_2O_2 production or by oxygen consumption; some workers have measured NADPH oxdiase in broken-cell or membrane preparations.

[d] Phagocytic stimuli include antibody- or complement-coated zymosan and bacteria.

in these studies, and in nearly all cases, cAMP or agents stimulating its synthesis proved to be inhibitory.

The effectiveness of cAMP to inhibit the various responses varies greatly. Bacterial substances such as FMLP-stimulated chemotaxis and superoxide (O_2^-) production appear to be the most sensitive. Degranulation is moderately sensitive to cAMP inhibition if the stimuli are immunologic, whereas phagocytosis and aggregation are the least. Whereas at least 10 papers documented the inhibition by cAMP of zymosan-stimulated release of primary granule enzymes, most papers showed no effect (or a weak effect) to inhibit phagocytosis (Table 5). Degranulation stimulated by FMLP was inhibited by DB-cAMP or agents increasing cAMP levels in cells in some laboratories (149,192,197), but only weak inhibition was noted by others (127). Basal or unstimulated O_2^- release was not affected by cAMP (208), and random movement was reported to be enhanced (162). Most workers have observed inhibition of degranulation by cAMP. When the stimulus was Ca^{2+} ionophore A23187, cAMP inhibited O_2^- and granule discharge in human neutrophils (141,192) but actually augmented granule release from guinea pig neutrophils (193). Release triggered by Con A, C5A, aggregated IgG, LTB_4, PAF, and by exposure to tumor cells was inhibited by cAMP (Table

5). A striking exception occurred in the case of PMA and other PKC activators (141,193,205). This is perhaps the only category of stimulant that does not act on an extracellular receptor and does not provoke an increase in intracellular Ca^{2+}.

The effects of adenosine have generated some controversy. Several laboratories (125–128) have shown that it stimulates cAMP by activating A_2 receptors. A_2 receptors also mediated the inhibition of O_2^- production by neutrophils activated by FMLP (197,224,225). Grinstein et al. (269) confirmed these observations and also found that adenosine inhibited the initial FMLP-induced acidification, but not the subsequent alkalinization. Schrier et al. (197) reported that, in addition to O_2^-, adenosine inhibited secondary granule enzyme discharge. Cronstein et al. (127), however, stated that adenosine or the more A_2 receptor-specific agonist, 5′-(N-ethylcarboxamido)-adenosine (NECA), had a trivial effect on degranulation. While all workers agree that adenosine has little or no effect on PMA-induced effects, they do not agree on effects involving Ca^{2+}. Cronstein et al. (127) stated that adenosine inhibits O_2^- and depolarization but not the increase in ionized Ca^{2+}. By contrast, Neilson and Vestal (205) reported that adenosine inhibited both O_2^- and intracellular Ca^{2+} increases in cells stimulated with either FMLP or Ca^{2+} ionophore. Whereas most workers concur that cAMP mediates the inhibition by adenosine, Cronstein et al. (127) stated that cAMP was not the second messenger for the effects of adenosine. This was due, in part, to the fact that adenosine or NECA alone did not increase neutrophil cAMP; only with the phosphodiesterase inhibitor RO20-1724 did they observe a fleeting rise in cAMP. Also, RO20-1724 synergistically enhanced the FMLP-induced increase in cAMP but not the inhibition by NECA of O_2^- production or β-glucuronidase release. Release of the secondary granule marker, vitamin B_{12}-binding protein, was not inhibited by either reagent. Since adenosine and NECA may inhibit O_2^- production in the absence of a phosphodiesterase inhibitor or demonstrable increases of cAMP, it is possible that a small pool of cAMP, localized in the plasma membrane and undetected by whole-cell measurements, is able to inhibit NADPH oxidase activation.

The effects of dopamine are interesting. In the central nervous system and a small number of peripheral tissues, it acts on β-adrenergic receptors to stimulate cAMP. In the neutrophil, however, dopamine blocked FMLP induction of O_2^- by a mechanism that was not blocked by propranolol and was associated with only a small increment in cAMP (227).

Paradoxically, FMLP and other soluble chemotactic bacterial formyl peptides increase cAMP (Table 4). Simchowitz et al. (122) found that the adenylate cyclase inhibitor SQ22536 could block the stimulation of cAMP by FMLP but did not interfere with the activation of O_2^-, β-glucuronidase release, or chemotaxis. They concluded that the increase of cAMP was not related to the biological responses of FMLP. Iannone et al. (128) determined that the increase of cAMP by endogenously produced adenosine was amplified by FMLP; incubation with SQ22536, adenosine deaminase, or with theophylline, which blocks adenosine receptors, prevented the cAMP increase by FMLP. They felt that the effects of FMLP were due to increasing adenylate cyclase rather than inhibiting phosphodiesterase. Working with isolated plasma membranes, others found that FMLP either had no effect (123,183) or had an inhibitory effect (228) on adenylate cyclase. In the latter case FMLP inhibition of forskolin stimulation was measured. Pertussis toxin prevented the inhibition by FMLP, suggesting that FMLP was linked to G_i. The possibility that FMLP may somehow cause inhibition of phosphodiesterase has been seriously considered (123). Whatever the mechanism, most workers (121–123,127,128,148,228) contend that the stimulation of cAMP by FMLP is not relevant to its biological actions.

Particulate phagocytic stimulants such as latex (176,177) and opsonized zymosan (177–179) have been reported to increase cAMP. These effects, as with FMLP, are believed by some workers to be epiphenomena. However, Przywansky et al. (179) concluded from their elegant immunocytochemical studies of cAMP distribution during phagocytosis that adenylate cyclase is activated at selective regions of the neutrophil membrane in contact with the particles and during formation of the phagosome. They suggested that ". . . the compartmentalization of cAMP at the site of particle-cell contact is probably important for initiation of phagocytosis."

Several mechanisms may account for cAMP inhibition of neutrophil functions. The first proposal was that of Weissmann et al. (196,229), who showed that cAMP interfered with the formation of microtubules. This would effectively interfere with motility and degranulation processes. cAMP has been shown to interfere with activation of phospholipases A_2 and C (159,221). However, Mueller and Sklar (206) observed cAMP inhibition of O_2^- generation in neutrophils stimulated by FMLP, but not by NaF, which is thought to act by stimulating phospholipase C. They did observe inhibition of FMLP-stimulated GTPase activation, and suggested that cAMP may inhibit signal transduction in part by blocking the interaction of the FMLP receptor with its G-protein. cAMP does not share the same inhibitory mechanism as glucocorticoids, which stimulate the synthesis of the phospholipase inhibitor lipocortin (also known as lipomodulin, macrocortin, or calpactin). This protein inhibits a least three phospholipases of the A_2 type, two of the C type, and one of the D type (231). Lipocortin is phosphorylated and inhibited by cAMP-dependent protein kinase, thus losing its ability to inhibit phospholipases (231). Several laboratories (221–223) have shown that cAMP inhibited both the breakdown and the resynthesis of inositol lipids in FMLP-stimulated neutrophils. In addition, cAMP inhibited NADPH oxidase, the first enzyme of the oxidative burst. cAMP prevented FMLP-induced increases of cytosolic Ca^{2+} (141,142,160,223), possibly as a result of inhibiting IP_3 formation. However, Kato et al. (222) found that cAMP inhibited only the second phase of Ca^{2+} increase. This is considered to result from influx rather than intracellular mobilization. Since cAMP does not affect PMA-stimulated responses, and PMA does not increase Ca^{2+} (205), it is reasonable to conclude that cAMP affects only those responses that are dependent on increased Ca^{2+}. It is therefore of great interest that inhibition by cAMP of phagocytosis was reversed by PMA and OAG (222). This suggests not only that PKC is of importance in receptor-mediated phagocytosis, but that PKC and cAMP-dependent kinase have opposing influences.

B. Cyclic GMP

Estensen, Goldberg, and co-workers (202) discovered the bidirectional control of neutrophil movement in 1973. Stimulation of directed migration toward a bacterial chemotactic factor was augmented by 8-Br-cGMP and inhibited by DB-cAMP. The peak response occurred at 10^{-8} M cGMP (180). In the same experiments, they (180,202) and others (131, Table 4) observed stimulation of chemotaxis by acetylcholine and carbamylcholine, known stimulants of cGMP in neutrophils (134,135), and by PMA, which also stimulates neutrophil cGMP (124,131). α-Adrenergic agents and $PGF_{2\alpha}$ also augmented chemotaxis. They (202) suggested that only directed movement rather than random movement is stimulated by cGMP. Levamisole, an immunopotentiator, was also found to stimulate increases in cGMP (but not cAMP) in association with enhanced chemotaxis (144).

The next observation of the opposing influences of cyclic nucleotides in neutrophils came from the laboratory of Weissmann (196). They showed that the release of lysosomal enzymes, stimulated by the activated fifth component of complement (C5A), was further augmented by cGMP and inhibited by cAMP, theophylline, and PGE_1. The enzymes measured were β-glucuronidase and myeloperoxidase, both associated with the primary granules. cGMP enhanced the release of primary granule enzymes induced by immune complexes and by serum-treated zymosan in addition to C5A (Table 5). 8-Br-cGMP was the most effective of the cGMP analogs, while the cGMP stimulants acetylcholine and carbamylcholine were equipotent, causing a doubling of immune complex-stimulated neutral protease release (201).

We are not aware of any reports testing the effects of cGMP on release of secondary granules enzymes. We have observed very minor, irreproducible effects of 8-Br-cGMP on FMLP-induced release of primary or secondary granule enzymes (149). Perhaps the cGMP-enhancable effects relate primarily to immune stimuli. Immunocytochemical techniques revealed cGMP localized in or on both primary and secondary granules, supporting the proposal that cGMP is involved in the secretion of both granules (179).

Other important immunologic responses promoted by cGMP (and inhibited by cAMP) include the antibody-dependent killing of tumor cells (187,188) and the antigen-stimulated release of PAF (178). Evidence for a role of cGMP in phagocytosis is slim (178,182).

Many of the early studies were conducted before methods of measuring very small levels of cGMP were readily available. The studies of Ignarro and co-workers (134,135) documented the stimulation of cGMP levels by opsonized zymosan, immune complexes, or aggregated IgG. These stimuli caused large increases in cGMP levels, and spectacular increases in the presence of acetylcholine, which by itself had small effects. As with so many cGMP stimulants, Ca^{2+} was required. Interestingly, the stimuli had no significant effects on cAMP levels but greatly augmented the stimulation of epinephrine.

The mechanism by which guanylate cyclase is activated varies with the stimulus, as discussed above. Opsonized zymosan stimulation of cGMP was inhibited by glucocorticoids (152), suggesting a phospholipase involvement in the activation pathway. Lad et al. (153) found that the cholinergically induced stimulation was inhibited by nordihydroguaiaretic acid, suggesting the mediation of a lipoxygenase product. Goetzl and Gorman (1964) found that 12-HPETE and, to a lesser extent, 12-HETE stimulated cGMP increases in human neutrophils. Our data with lymphocytes indicate that 5-HETE, 12-HETE, and 15-HETE can increase cGMP by a mechanism that is inhibited by NDGA, suggesting that the agents act on the cells to stimulate lipoxygenase, producing some other proximal mediator of guanylate cyclase activation (232). An HPETE is the most likely candidate, since it has oxidizing potential. LTB_4 did not stimulate cGMP in human neutrophils (170).

PMA stimulated cGMP accumulation in human neutrophils (131,180) as well as lymphocytes (233). It was shown to activate guanylate cyclase in neutrophils (124) as well as lymphocytes (16), and the stimulatory effect was demonstrated in broken cells if phosphatidylserine was added. This strongly suggests that PKC is able to phosphorylate and activate the enzyme, as shown in brain by Zwiller et al. (15).

Mechanisms by which cGMP exerts augmenting effects are largely unknown. The only relevant finding to our knowledge refers to microtubule assembly, which is promoted by cGMP, in contrast to the inhibiting effect of cAMP (144,234). Other mechanisms, less direct, could involve cGMP enhancement of a cAMP-specific phosphodiesterase.

C. Cytokines

Two cytokines have been shown to affect cyclic nucleotide levels in neutrophils: leukocyte-inhibitory factor (LIF) and granulocyte-macrophage-stimulating factor (GM-CSF). The actions of LIF are discussed by Rocklin and Borish (Chapter 12), and the biochemical effects of GM-CSF are reviewed by DiPersio (Chapter 16) and by Sullivan (Chapter 17).

In a series of articles, Bendtzen (169,235–238) described the effects of cGMP to protect LIF, an esterase, against inactivation by phenylmethylsulfonylfluoride (PMSF). cGMP apparently competes with PMSF for binding sites. The release of LIF from lymphocytes was augmented by cGMP, which had the intriguing property of reversing inhibition by cyclosporin of lymphokine secretion (239). LIF stimulated neutrophil levels of cGMP but had no effect on cAMP (169). In a curious sort of negative-feedback mechanism, the action of LIF on neutrophils was reversibly inhibited by cGMP.

We found that GM-CSF activated guanylate cyclase in a time- and dose-dependent fashion (124). This required intact cells, and was apparently not mediated by PKC, since it was not inhibited by H-7, and since PMA was able to further activate guanylate cyclase activity in homogenates prepared from cells pretreated with GM-CSF. Furthermore, GM-CSF had no effect on the activity or subcellular distribution of PKC activity. GM-CSF may stimulate other kinases, as we have observed that okadaic acid, a highly specific inhibitor of serine and threonine phosphatases, augmented the stimulation by GM-CSF (149). GM-CSF treatment reduced adenylate cyclase activity in neutrophils. The time course is somewhat different from that of guanylate cyclase activation, and pertussis toxin did not block the effect. Whether cGMP elevation is critical to the biological actions of GM-CSF has not yet been determined. The guanylate cyclase inhibitor LY83583 was able to prevent GM-CSF augmentation of FMLP-induced O_2^-, β-glucuronidase, and lysozyme release (149).

Tuftsin, a tetrapeptide cleaved from IgG, is an interesting messenger molecule. It stimulates phagocytosis, the oxidative burst, and bactericidal and tumoricidal activities of neutrophils and macrophages (181). This substance has been shown by several workers (166,181,182) to stimulate neutrophil accumulation of cGMP and to reduce cAMP levels.

V. HEMOPOIESIS

In lymphocytes and most other cell systems studied, cGMP promotes and cAMP inhibits proliferation (3,8). Kurland et al. (240) demonstrated inhibition of granulocyte-macrophage-progenitor cell proliferation by PGE_1, thus establishing the applicability of these generalizations to myeloid cell development. Imidazole, $PGF_{2\alpha}$, and carbamylcholine, three agents that increase cGMP in many cells, augmented the proliferative effects of the colony stimulating factor. In addition, Oshita et al. (241) showed that cGMP itself augmented the formation of granulocyte-macrophage colonies in the presence of colony-stimulating activity. Taetle and colleagues (242,243) confirmed these findings, showing that cGMP, $PGF_{2\alpha}$, and carbamylcholine increased the number of colony-forming units, and cAMP, PGE_1, and isoproterenol decreased them. The results are relevant to normal hemopoiesis and also have implications for the regulation of cell growth in certain types of leukemia.

VI. CONDITIONS ASSOCIATED WITH ABNORMAL CYCLIC NUCLEOTIDE RESPONSES

Several disorders of granulocytes were reviewed by Korchak et al. (244). Some of these are characterized by abnormal cAMP or cGMP levels or abnormal responses of the cyclase enzymes to stimuli.

A. Atopic Disease

In 1968, Szentivanyi (245) elaborated the hypothesis of β-adrenergic subsensitivity in atopic disease. Four years later we confirmed this hypothesis, showing that isoproterenol stimulated smaller increases of cAMP in leukocytes of asthmatic children compared to nonasthmatic children (132). Cells of steroid-treated children responded normally. Cells treated with the α-adrenergic blocker phentolamine responded much more to isoproterenol, and such treatment appeared to restore considerable β-adrenergic responsiveness in leukocytes of asthmatics (168). Our experiments involved unseparated leukocytes, which usually consist of about 65–70% neutrophils and 20–25% lymphocytes. Busse (246) later demonstrated the β-adrenergic subsensitivity to isoproterenol in isolated granulocytes of asthmatics. The response was further decreased during episodes of respiratory infection which provoked attacks of asthma. The defect is not restricted to the β-receptors, since it was shown (247) that a decreased response to histamine H_2 agonists (inhibition of opsonized zymosan-stimulated release of β-glucuronidase) also existed. Parker et al. (248,249) verified the β-adrenergic subsensitivity in leukocytes and lymphocytes of asthmatic adults, demonstrated a correlation with disease severity, and showed that the subjects responded normally to other cAMP stimuli. The essential features of the above findings have been confirmed and extended by several investigators.

β-Agonists cause a desensitization of receptor responses, which persists for about 1 week (147). The reports cited above used patients who had not taken β-agonists for at least 2, and usually for 4 weeks. Glucocorticoids not only increase the density of β-receptors (147), but attenuate the β-agonist provoked uncoupling of receptors from adenylate cyclase (250). These effects may account for the findings of normal β-receptor responses in leukocytes of steroid-treated asthmatics (132). Related to the exercise-induced asthma is Davies' intriguing discovery (251) that exercise induces a rapid decrease in the coupling of β-adrenergic receptors and adenylate cyclase activity. The effect was due to a substance in plasma. It is notable that Sano et al. (147) found no difference in β-receptor binding in granulocytes of asthmatics. Galant et al. (155) found no differences in β-receptor binding or adenylate cyclase activities in sonicates of neutrophils from asthmatics. They suggested that the defect observed in intact cells may not be in adenylate cyclase, but rather in the hormone-enzyme coupling system. Some have suggested that phosphodiesterase may be hyperactive in leukocytes of atopics; however, Busse and Anderson (175) found that the specific cAMP phosphodiesterase inhibitor RO20-1724 increased cAMP and reduced β-glucuronidase release similarly in normal and asthmatic leukocytes.

Busse and Lee (136) confirmed the reduced cAMP response to β-adrenergic agonists in both lymphocytes and granulocytes of patients with atopic dermatitis. Furthermore, they observed less inhibition by isoproterenol of β-glucuronidase release in granulocytes of atopic subjects. In both types of assays, the responses to PGE_1 were normal. Ring et al. (139) reported not only decreased cAMP responses to epinephrine, but also enhanced cGMP responses to methacholine in leukocytes of patients with atopic dermatitis.

B. Cystic Fibrosis

Cystic fibrosis represents another disease characterized by subsensitivity to β-adrenergic stimuli. Davis and co-workers (252–255) have shown that the defect is specific for the β-receptor; granulocyte and lymphocyte cAMP responses to isoproterenol are reduced, while responses to PGE_1 are normal. Adenylate cyclase activities are normal in the presence of GppNHp and PGE_1, but not isoproterenol. The defect is not due to reduced numbers of β-receptors, nor to tachyphylaxis to catecholamines. Davis et al. (255) concluded that receptor-adenylate cyclase coupling was apparently defective.

C. Affective Illness

Pandey et al. (256) discovered that patients with depressive illness had reduced granulocyte β-adrenergic stimulation of cAMP. Cells of patients with schizophrenia responded normally to isoproterenol.

D. Chediak-Higashi Syndrome and Hyper-IgE Syndrome

Granulocyte functional abnormalities in Chediak-Higashi syndrome (CHS) include giant granules, reduced microtubule formation, defective chemotaxis, and impaired degranulation and intracellular killing (165,234,245). Interestingly, the pentose phosphate pathway (hexose monophosphate shunt) and O_2^- are elevated (244). Boxer and colleagues (129,155,257) found that cGMP and cholinergic agents, added to CHS leukocytes in vitro, or ascorbate, administered to a child, corrected the impaired chemotaxis, release of β-glucuronidase, and the bactericidal capacity. The phagocytic capacity was not improved, reflecting the weak effects of cyclic nucleotides to regulate this function (Table 5). cAMP levels were elevated 10-fold in CHS leukocytes; ascorbate reduced these levels to two times normal in association with correction of chemotaxis (129). However, Wright et al. (165,167) observed a restoration of chemotaxis by cGMP or levamisole in leukocytes of hyper-IgE but not CHS patients. Furthermore, they measured no abnormalities in cAMP or cGMP in leukocytes of CHS patients, and no change upon administration of ascorbic acid (165). The vitamin was beneficial in mice but, in contrast to the results of Boxer (obtained with a child), Wright and co-workers found no benefit in adult humans. Zurier (234) reported that abnormal Con A capping was restored in human CHS neutrophils by cGMP and cGMP-raising muscarinic agents (234). Perhaps there are subtypes of CHS, only one of which is treatable with cGMP.

E. Infections

A few studies have emerged that relate increased granulocyte levels of cAMP with infections. One study (258) involved a patient with low CD4/CD8 ratio which may have represented acquired immunodeficiency syndrome. In this case the cGMP levels were normal. Another study (187) showed that *Bordetella pertussis* toxin contains a soluble, heat-stable form of adenylate cyclase that is injected into neutrophils during infection. In addition, the toxin inhibits G_i, thus permitting a greater degree of stimulation of adenylate cyclase. Sequelae include reduced chemotaxis, O_2^- production, and bacterial killing. Atkinson et al. (157) reported stimulation of cAMP levels in human neutrophils by levels of ethanol as low as 17 mM, or 0.08 g%. Methanol was ineffective; butanol and amyl alcohol were more potent than ethanol. Since ethanol is quickly metabolized, this would probably be an acute effect, but in subjects whose cells are chronically exposed to ethanol the effect might account for increased infections.

F. Aging

Interesting changes accompany leukocyte cyclic nucleotides during aging. Fulop et al. (171) have found that met-enkephalin (10^{-7}–10^{-9} M) stimulated Fcy-mediated cytotoxicity and H_2O_2 production in human granulocytes. It also decreased adenylate cyclase and increased guanylate cyclase activity. These responses were inhibited by naloxone and thus may be mediated by opiate receptors. In healthy aged (60–87 years) males, met-enkephalin failed to stimulate cGMP increases in these subjects, while it caused increases instead of decreases in cAMP. Perhaps as a consequence of these alterations in cyclic nucleotide metabolism, the capacity of met-enkephalin to stimulate H_2O_2 and cytotoxicity was greatly reduced. This laboratory obtained similar results using lymphokines to stimulate granulocytes (259).

VII. SUMMARY

The survey of agents that stimulate increases of cAMP and cGMP revealed many similarities but some differences between basophils, mast cells, and neutrophils. With procedures now available for isolation of eosinophils, it will be of great interest to learn how their cyclic nucleotides are regulated. In the granulocytes studied to date, most functions are inhibited by cAMP. In blood basophils and lung mast cells, but apparently not in rat peritoneal mast cells, cGMP can promote release reactions. Neutrophil functions are regulated by cAMP to variable degrees, O_2^- generation being the most sensitive and phagocytosis perhaps the least. cAMP controls cell surface receptor- and Ca^{2+}-dependent events but not those signaled by PKC activation. Very few cytokines have been analyzed for their effects on cyclic nucleotides. LIF and GM-CSF increase cGMP, but more studies are needed to determine whether this effect is relevant to the biological effects of the cytokines. It is conceivable that the clinical efficacy of cytokines could be enhanced by the co-administration of agents tailored to enhance the cytokines' desirable effects on cyclic nucleotides. The study of cAMP, cGMP, and other signaling systems will certainly provide material for exciting research for a considerable time.

ACKNOWLEDGMENTS

The author gratefully acknowledges the technical assistance of Christina S. Coffey. This work was supported in part by grant number CH-444 from the American Cancer Society.

REFERENCES

1. Lichtenstein LM, Margolis S. Histamine release *in vitro*: inhibition by catecholamines and methylxanthines. Science 1968; 161:902–3.
2. Bourne HR, Lichtenstein LM, Melmon KL, Henney CS, Weinstein Y, Shearer GM. Modulation of inflammation and immunity by cyclic AMP. Science 1974; 184:19–28.
3. Hadden JW. Cyclic nucleotides in lymphocyte proliferation and differentiation. In: Hadden JW, Coffey RG, Spreafico F, eds. Immunopharmacology. New York: Plenum, 1977:1–28.
4. Watson J. Involvement of cyclic nucleotides as intracellular mediators in the induction of antibody synthesis. In: Hadden JW, Coffey RG, Spreafico F, eds. Immunopharmacology. New York: Plenum, 1977:29–45.
5. Strom TB, Ludin AP II, Carpenter CB. The role of cyclic nucleotides in lymphocyte activation and function. Prog Clin Immunol 1977; 3:115–34.
6. Ignarro LJ. Regulation of polymorphonuclear leukocyte, macrophage, and platelet function. In: Hadden JW, Coffey RG, Spreafico F, eds. Immunopharmacology. New York: Plenum, 1977:61–86.
7. Coffey RG, Hadden JW. Cyclic nucleotide pharmacology of macrophage functions. In: Hadden JW, Szentivanyi A, eds. The reticuloendothelial system, vol. 8, pharmacology. New York: Plenum, 1985:27–48.
8. Coffey RG. Intracellular events during lymphocyte activation. In: Bray MA, Morley J, eds. The pharmacology of lymphocytes. New York: Springer-Verlag, 1988:83–138.
9. Plaut M, Marone G, Thomas LL, Lichtenstein LM. Cyclic nucleotides in immune responses and allergy. Adv Cyclic Nucleotide Res 1980; 12:161–72.
10. Hadden JW, Hadden EM, Haddox MK, Goldberg ND. Guanosine 3′,5′-cyclic monophosphate: a possible intracellular mediator of mitogen influences in lymphocytes. Proc Natl Acad Sci USA 1972; 69:3024–7.
11. Gilman AG. G proteins: transducers of receptor-generated signals. Ann Rev Biochem 1987; 56:615–49.
12. Goldberg ND, Graff G, Haddox MK, Stephenson JH, Glass DB, Moser ME. Redox modulation of splenic cell soluble guanylate cyclase activity: activation by hydrophilic and hydrophobic oxidants represented by ascorbic and dehydroascorbic acids, fatty acid hydroperoxides and prostaglandin endoperoxides. Adv Cyclic Nucleotide Res 1978; 9:101–30.
13. Murad F, Mittal CK, Arnold WP, Katsuki S, Kimura H. Guanylate cyclase: activation by azide, nitro compounds, nitric oxide, and hydroxyl radical and inhibition by hemoglobin and myoglobin. Adv Cyclic Nucleotide Res 1978; 9:145–58.
14. Strom TM, Weil J, Bidlingmaier F. Platelet receptors for atrial natriuretic peptide in man. Life Sci 1987; 40:769–73.
15. Zwiller J, Revel M-O, Malviya AN. Protein kinase C catalyzes phosphorylation of guanylate cyclase *in vitro*. J Biol Chem 1985; 260:1350–3.

16. Coffey RG. Phosphatidylserine and phorbol myristate acetate stimulation of human lymphocyte guanylate cyclase. Int J Biochem 1986; 18:665–70.
17. Singh S, Lowe DG, Thorpe DS, Rodriguez H, Kuang W-J, Dangott LJ, Chinkers M, Goeddel DV, Garbers DL. Membrane guanylate cyclase is a cell-surface receptor with homology to protein kinases. Nature 1988; 334:708–12.
18. Ishizaka T, Ishizaka K. Activation of mast cells for mediator release through IgE receptors. Prog Allergy 1984; 34:188–235.
19. Pearce FL. Calcium and histamine secretion from mast cells. Prog Med Chem 1982; 19:60–107.
20. Siraganian RP. Histamine secretion from mast cells and basophils. Trends Pharmacol Sci 1983; 4:432–7.
21. Beaven MA, Cunha-Melo JR. Membrane phosphoinositide-activated signals in mast cells and basophils. Prog Allergy 1988; 42:123–84.
22. Ishizaka T. Role of GTP-binding protein in histamine release from mast cells. Clin Immunol Immunopathol 1989; 50:20–9.
23. Lichtenstein LM, Sobotka AK, Malveaux FJ, Gillespie E. IgE-induced changes in human basophil cyclic AMP levels. Int Arch Allergy Appl Immunol 1978; 56:473–8.
24. Hughes PJ, Holgate ST, Roath S, Church MK. The relationship between cyclic AMP changes and histamine release from basophil-rich human leukocytes. Biochem Pharmacol 1983; 32:2557–64.
25. Peachell PT, MacGlashan DW Jr, Lichtenstein LM, Schleimer RP. Regulation of human basophil and lung mast cell function by cyclic adenosine monophosphate. J Immunol 1988; 140:571–9.
26. Lichtenstein LM, Levy DA, Ishizaka K. In vitro reversed anaphylaxis: characteristics of anti-IgE mediated histamine release. Immunology 1970; 19:831–42.
27. May CD, Levine BB, Weissman G. Effects of compounds which inhibit antigenic release of histamine and phagocytic release of lysosomal enzyme on glucose utilization by leukocytes in humans. Proc Soc Exp Biol Med 1970; 133:758–63.
28. Siraganian PA, Siraganian RP. Basophil activation by concanavalin A: characteristics of the reaction. J Immunol 1974; 112:2117–29.
29. Hook WA, Siraganian RP. Complement-induced histamine release from human basophils. 3. Effect of pharmacologic agents. J Immunol 1977; 118:679–84.
30. Schleimer RP, Gillespie E, Lichtenstein LM. Release of histamine from human leukocytes stimulated with the tumor-promoting phorbol diesters. Characterization of the response. J Immunol 1981; 126:570–4.
31. Lichtenstein LM, De Bernardo R. IgE-mediated histamine release: *in vitro* separation into two phases. Int Arch Allergy Appl Immunol 1971; 41:56–71.
32. Lichtenstein LM, De Bernardo R. The immediate allergic response: *in vitro* action of cyclic AMP-active and other drugs on the two stages of histamine release. J Immunol 1971; 107:1131–6.
33. Marone G, Columbo M, Triggiani M, Cirillo R, Genovese A, Formisano S. Inhibition of IgE-mediated release of histamine and peptide leukotriene from human basophils and mast cells by forskolin. Biochem Pharmacol 1987; 36:13–20.
34. Warner JA, MacGlashan DW Jr, Peters Sp, Kagey-Sobotka A, Lichtenstein LM. The pharmacologic modulation of mediator release from human basophils. J Allergy Clin Immunol 1988; 82:432–8.
35. Bourne HR, Melmon KL, Lichtenstein LM. Histamine augments leukocyte adenosine 3′,5′-monophosphate and blocks antigenic histamine release. Science 1971; 173:743–5.
36. Bourne HR, Lichtenstein LM, Melmon KL. Pharmacologic control of allergic histamine release *in vitro*. Evidence for an inhibitory role of 3′,5′-adenosine monophosphate in human leukocytes. J Immunol 1972; 108:695–705.

37. Hubscher T. Role of the eosinophil in the allergic reactions. I. EDI-an eosinophil-derived inhibitor of histamine release. J Immunol 1975; 114:1379–88.
38. Lichtenstein LM, Gillespie E. The effects of the H_1 and H_2 antihistamines on "allergic" histamine release and its inhibition by histamine. J Pharmacol Exp Ther 1975; 192:441–50.
39. Marone G, Kagey-Sobotka A, Lichtenstein LM. Effects of arachidonic acid and its metabolites on antigen-induced histamine release from human basophils *in vitro*. J Immunol 1979; 123:1669–77.
40. Peters SP, Kagey-Sobotka A, MacGlashan DW Jr, Siegel MI, Lichtenstein LM. The modulation of human basophil histamine release by products of the 5-lipoxygenase pathway. J Immunol 1982; 129:797–803.
41. Gillespie E, Lichtenstein LM. Histamine release from human leukocytes. Relationships between cyclic nucleotide, calcium, and antigenic concentrations. J Immunol 1975; 115:1572–6.
42. Frossard N, Landry Y, Pauli G, Ruckstuhl M. Effects of cyclic AMP- and cyclic GMP-phosphodiesterase inhibitors of immunological release of histamine and on lung contraction. Br J Pharmacol 1981; 73:933–8.
43. Sydbom A, Fredholm B, Uvnas B. Evidence against a role of cyclic nucleotides in the regulation of anaphylactic histamine release in isolated rat mast cells. Acta Physiol Scand 1981; 112:47–56.
44. Sullivan TJ, Parker KL, Eisen SA, Parker CW. Modulation of cyclic AMP in purified rat mast cells. II. Studies on the relationship between intracellular cyclic AMP concentrations and histamine release. J Immunol 1975; 114:1480–5.
45. Marquardt DL, Parker CW, Sullivan TJ. Potentiation of mast cell mediator release by adenosine. J Immunol 1978; 120:871–8.
46. Burt DS, Stanworth DR. Changes in cellular levels of cyclic AMP in rat mast cells during secretion of histamine induced by immunoglobulin E decapeptide and ACTH(1-24) peptide. Comparison with immunological and ionophore triggers. Biochim Biophys Acta 1983; 762:458–65.
47. Sullivan TJ, Parker KL, Stenson W, Parker CW. Modulation of cyclic AMP in purified rat mast cells. I Responses to pharmacologic, metabolic, and physical stimuli. J Immunol 1975; 114:1473–9.
48. Leoutsakos A, Pearce FL. The effect of adenosine and its analogues on cyclic AMP changes and histamine secretion from rat peritoneal mast cells stimulated by various ligands. Biochem Pharmacol 1986; 35:1373–80.
49. Holgate ST, Lewis RA, Austen KF. Role of adenylate cyclase in immunologic release of mediators from rat mast cells: agonist and antagonist effects of purine- and ribose-modified adenosine analogs. Proc Natl Acad Sci USA 1980; 77:6800–4.
50. Lewis RA, Holgate ST, Roberts L II, Maguire JF, Oates JA, Austen KF. Effects of indomethacin on cyclic nucleotide levels and histamine release from rat serosal mast cells. J Immunol 1979; 123:1663–8.
51. Church MK, Hughes PJ, Vardey CJ. Studies on the receptor mediating cyclic AMP-independent enhancement by adenosine of IgE-dependent mediator release from rat mast cells. Br J Pharmacol 1986; 87:233–42.
52. Takei M, Matumoto T, Itoh T, Endo K, Muramatu M. Role of cyclic AMP during histamine release. Histamine release is not directly related to increase in cyclic AMP levels in rat mast cells activated by concanavalin A, anti-IgE, antigen, prostaglandin D_2 and isoproterenol. Biol Chem Hoppe-Seyler 1988; 369:765–73.
53. White JR, Pluznik DH, Ishizaka K, Ishizaka T. Antigen-induced increase in protein kinase C activity in plasma membrane of mast cells. Proc Natl Acad Sci USA 1985; 82:8193–7.
54. Sydbom A, Fredholm BB, Uvnas B. Effect of sensitization on spontaneous and

phosphatidylserine-induced histamine release and on cyclic AMP and GMP levels in isolated rat mast cells. Acta Physiol Scand 1979; 106:473–9.
55. Sullivan TJ, Parker KL, Kulczycki A Jr, Parker CW. Modulation of cyclic AMP in purified rat mast cells. III. Studies on the effects of concanavalin A and anti-IgE on cyclic AMP concentrations during histamine release. J Immunol 1976; 117:713–6.
56. Ishizaka T, Hirata F, Sterk AR, Ishizaka K, Axelrod JA. Bridging of IgE receptors activates phospholipid methylation and adenylate cyclase in mast cell plasma membranes. Proc Natl Acad Sci USA 1981; 78:6812–6.
57. Mendoza GR, Orner FB. Adenylate cyclase, cyclic AMP and IgE-mediated desensitization in rat mast cells. Int Arch Allergy Appl Immunol 1983; 70:261–7.
58. Marquardt DL, Gruber HE, Wasserman SI. Aminophylline exposure alters mouse bone marrow-derived mast cell adenosine responsiveness. J Allergy Clin Immunol 1986; 78:462–9.
59. Kaliner M, Austen KF. Cyclic AMP, ATP, and reversed anaphylactic histamine release from rat mast cells. J Immunol 1974; 112:664–74.
60. Orange RP, Austen WG, Austen KF. Immunological release of histamine and slow-reacting substance of anaphylaxis from human lung. I. Modulation by agents influencing cellular levels of cyclic 3′,5′-adenosine monophosphate. J Exp Med 1971; 134:136s–48s.
61. Kaliner M, Orange RP, Austen KF. Immunological release of histamine and slow reacting substance of anaphylaxis from human lung. IV. Enhancement by cholinergic and alpha adrenergic stimulation. J Exp Med 1972; 136:556–67.
62. Johnson AR, Moran NC, Mayer SE. Cyclic AMP content and histamine release in rat mast cells. J Immunol 1974; 112:511–9.
63. Hayashi H, Ichikawa A, Saito T, Tomita K. Inhibitory role of cyclic adenosine 3′,5′-monophosphate in histamine release from rat peritoneal mast cells *in vitro*. Biochem Pharmacol 1976; 25:1907–14.
64. Ashida Y, Saijo T, Kuriki H, Mahi Y. Interaction of the antiallergic agent AA-344 with biogenic amines and prostaglandins in production of cyclic AMP in rat mast cells. Int Arch Allergy Appl Immunol 1980; 62:415–22.
65. Saito H, Okajima F, Molski TF, Sha'afi RI, Ul M, Ishizaka T. Effect of cholera toxin on histamine release from bone marrow-derived mouse mast cells. Proc Natl Acad Sci USA 1988; 85:2504–8.
66. Norrby K, Andersson RGG. Early changes of cyclic nucleotide levels in a mitogenic reaction in the rat mesentery. Experientia 1979; 35:1623–4.
67. Theoharides TC, Betchaku T, Douglas WW. Somatostatin-induced histamine secretion in mast cells. Characterization of the effect. Eur J Pharmacol 1981; 69:127–37.
68. Bergstrand H, Lundquist B, Schurmann A. Rat mast cell high affinity cyclic nucleotide phosphodiesterases: separation and inhibitory effects of two antiallergic agents. Mol Pharmacol 1978; 14:848–55.
69. Hanna CJ, Johnston ME, Schellenberg RR. Evaluation of the action of cholinergic agonists and cyclic guanosine monophosphate (cGMP) on histamine release from purified rat mast cells. Immunopharmacol 1981; 3:233–40.
70. Foreman JC, Garland LG. Cromoglycate and other anti-allergic drugs: a possible mechanism of action. Br Med J 1976; 1:820–2.
71. Coffey RG, Middleton E Jr. Release of histamine from rat mast cells by lysosomal cationic proteins. Possible involvement of adenylate cyclase and adenosine triphosphatase in pharmacologic regulation. Int Arch Allergy Appl Immunol 1973; 45:593–611.
72. Wescott S, Kaliner M. The effect of histamine on mast cell cyclic AMP. J Allergy Clin Immunol 1980; 65:198.
73. Holgate ST, Winslow CM, Lewis A, Austen KF. Effects of prostaglandin D_2 and theophylline on rat serosal mast cells: discordance between increased cellular levels of cyclic AMP and activation of cyclic AMP-dependent protein kinase. J Immunol 1981; 127:1530–3.

74. Kennerly DA, Secosan CJ, Parker CW, Sullivan TJ. Modulation of stimulated phospholipid metabolism in mast cells by pharmacologic agents that increase cyclic 3′,5′-adenosine monophosphate levels. J Immunol 1979; 123:1519–24.
75. Wescott S, Kaliner M. The effects of histamine and prostaglandin D_2 on rat mast-cell cyclic AMP and mediator release. J Allergy Clin Immunol 1981; 68:383–91.
76. Akagi M, Mio M, Miyoshi K, Tasaka K. Antiallergic effects of terfenadine on immediate type hypersensitivity reactions. Immunopharmacol Immunotoxicol 1987; 9:257–279.
77. Undem BJ, Graziano FM, Buckner CK. Effects of isoproterenol on histamine release induced from monodispersed guinea-pig lung cells by different secretagogues. J Pharmacol Exp Ther 1985; 233:617–22.
78. Johnson AR, Moran NC. Inhibition of the release of histamine from rat mast cells: the effect of cold and adrenergic drugs on release of histamine by compound 48/80 and antigen. J Pharmacol Exp Ther 1970; 175:632–40.
79. Austen KF, Orange RP. Bronchial asthma: the possible role of chemical mediators of immediate hypersensitivity in the pathogenesis of subacute chronic disease. Am Rev Respir Dis 1975; 112:423–36.
80. Butchers PR, Skidmore IF, Vardey CJ, Wheeldon A. Characterization of the receptor mediating the antianaphylactic effects of β-adrenoceptor agonists in human lung tissue *in vivo*. Br J Pharmacol 1980; 71:663–7.
81. Kimura Y, Inoue Y, Honda H. Further studies on rat mast cell degranulation by IgE-anti-IgE and the inhibitory effect of drugs related to cAMP. Immunology 1974; 26:983–8.
82. Loeffler LJ, Lovenberg W, Sjoerdsma A. Effects of dibutyryl-3′,5′-cyclic adenosine monophosphate, phosphodiesterase inhibitors and prostaglandin E_1 on compound 48/80-induced histamine release from rat peritoneal mast cells *in vitro*. Biochem Pharmacol 1971; 20:2287–97.
83. Undem BJ, Peachell PT, Lichtenstein LM. Isoproterenol-induced inhibition of immunoglobulin E-mediated release of histamine and arachidonic acid metabolites from the human lung mast cell. J Pharmacol Exp Ther 1988; 247:209–17.
84. Schild HO. Histamine release and anaphylactic shock in isolated lungs of guinea pigs. Quart J Exp Physiol 1936; 26:165–79.
85. Assem ESK, Schild HO. Antagonism by β-adrenoceptor blocking agents of the antianaphylactic effect of isoprenaline. Br J Pharmacol 1971; 42:620–30.
86. Peters SP, Schulman ES, Schleimer RP, MacGlashan DW Jr, Newball HH, Lichtenstein LM. Dispersed lung mast cells. Pharmacologic aspects and comparison with human lung fragments. Am Rev Respir Dis 1982; 126:1034–9.
87. Taylor WA and Sheldon D. Mast cell degranulation: a comparison of the inhibitory actions of disodium cromoglycate, drugs known to influence the level of intracellular cyclic nucleotide and diisopropylfluorophosphate (DFP). Int Arch Allergy Appl Immunol 1974; 47:696–707.
88. Hughes JM, Seale JP, Temple DM. Effect of fenoterol on immunological release of leukotrienes and histamine from human lung *in vitro*: Selective antagonism by β-adrenoceptor antagonists. Eur J Pharmacol 1983; 95:239–45.
89. Ishizaka T, Ishizaka K, Orange RP, Austen KF. Pharmacologic inhibition of the antigen-induced release of histamine and slow reacting substance of anaphylaxis (SRS-A) from monkey lung tissues mediated by human IgE. J Immunol 1971; 105:1267–73.
90. Ennis M, Truneh A, White JR, Pearce FL. Inhibition of histamine secretion from mast cells. Nature 1981; 289:186–7.
91. Truneh A, Pearce FL. Effect of cyclic AMP, disodium cromoglycate and other anti-allergic drugs on histamine secretion from rat mast cells stimulated with the calcium ionophore ionomycin. Agents Actions 1984; 14:179–84.
92. Shores AJ, Mongar JL. Modulation of histamine secretion from concanavalin A-activated rat mast cells by phosphatidylserin, calcium, cAMP, pH and metabolic inhibitors. Agents Actions 1980; 10:131–6.

93. Diamant B, Patkar SA. Stimulation and inhibition of histamine release from isolated rat mast cells. Int Arch Allergy Appl Immunol 1975; 49:183–207.
94. Undem BJ, Torphy TJ, Goldman D, Chilton FH. Inhibition by adenosine 3′,5′-monophosphate of eicosanoid and platelet-activating factor biosynthesis in the mouse PT-18 mast cell. J Biol Chem 1990; 265:6750–8.
95. Saito H, Ishizaka K, Ishizaka T. Effect of nonhydrolyzable guanosine phosphate on IgE-mediated activation of phospholipase C and histamine release from rodent mast cells. J Immunol 1989; 143:250–8.
96. Sydbom A, Fredholm BB. On the mechanism by which theophylline inhibits histamine release from rat mast cells. Acta Physiol Scand 1982; 114:243–51.
97. Baxter JH. Histamine release from rat mast cells by dextran: effects of adrenergic agents, theophylline and other drugs. Proc Soc Exp Biol Med 1972; 141:576–81.
98. Foreman JC, Hallet MB, Mongar JL. The relationship between histamine secretion and calcium uptake by mast cells. J Physiol (Lond) 1977; 271:193–214.
99. White JR, Ishizata T, Ishizata K, Sha'afi RK. Direct demonstration of increased intracellular concentration of free calcium as measured by quin-2 in stimulated rat peritoneal mast cell. Proc Natl Acad Sci USA 1984; 81:3978–82.
100. Izushi K, Tasaka K. Histamine release from β-escin-permeabilized rat peritoneal mast cells and its inhibition by intracellular Ca^{2+} blockers, calmodulin inhibitors and cAMP. Immunopharmacology 1989; 18:177–86.
101. Holgate St, Lewis RA, Maguire JF, Roberts LJ II, Oates JA, Austen KF. Effects of prostaglandin D_2 on rat serosal mast cells: discordance between immunologic mediator release and cyclic AMP levels. J Immunol 1980; 125:1367–73.
102. Wescott SL, Hunt WA, Kaliner M. Histamine H-1 receptors on rat peritoneal mast cells. Life Sci 1982; 31:1911–20.
103. Sullivan TJ, Parker CW. Pharmacologic modulation of inflammatory mediator release by rat mast cells. Am J Pathol 1976; 85:437–64.
104. Church MK, Hughes PJ. Adenosine potentiates immunological histamine release from rat mast cells by a novel cyclic AMP-independent cell-surface action. Br J Pharmacol 1985; 85:3–5.
105. Lohse MJ, Maurer K, Gensheimer HP, Schwabe U. Dual actions of adenosine on rat peritoneal mast cells. Naunyn-Schmiedebergs Arch Pharmacol 1987; 335:555–60.
106. Winslow CM, Lewis RA, Austen KF. Mast cell mediator release as a function of cyclic AMP-dependent protein kinase activation. J Exp Med 1981; 154:1125–33.
107. Marquardt DL, Walker LL. Inhibition of mast cell adenosine responsiveness by chronic exposure to adenosine receptor agonists. Biochem Pharmacol 1987; 36:4297–302.
108. Marquardt DL, Walker LL. Pretreatment with phorbol esters abrogates mast cell adenosine responsiveness. J Immunol 1989; 412:1268–73.
109. Holgate ST, Lewis RA, Austen KF. 3′,5′-cyclic adenosine monophosphate-dependent protein kinase of the rat serosal mast cell and its immunologic activation. J Immunol 1980; 124:2093–9.
110. Ishizaka T, Iwata M, Ishizaka K. Release of histamine and arachidonate from mouse mast cells induced by glycosylation-enhancing factor and bradykinin. J Immunol 1985; 134:1880–7.
111. Ishizaka T, Sterk AR, Daeron M, Becker EL, Ishizaka K. Biochemical analysis of desensitization of mouse mast cells. J Immunol 1985; 135:492–501.
112. Ishizaka T, Conrad DH, Schulman ES, Sterk AR, Ishizaka K. Biochemical analysis of intitial triggering events of IgE-mediated histamine release from human lung mast cells. J Immunol 1983; 130:2357–62.
113. Holgate ST, Benyon RC, Howart PH, Agius R, Hardy C, Robinson C, Durham SR, Kay AB, Church MK. Relationship between mediator release from human lung mast cells *in vitro* and *in vivo*. Int Arch Allergy Appl Immunol 1985; 77:47–56.

114. Kurosawa M, Parker CW. Protein phosphorylation in rat mast cell granules. Cyclic AMP dependent phosphorylation of a 44K protein associated with broken granules. Biochem Pharmacol 1987; 36:131–40.
115. Rothschild AM. Plasma kallikrein-generating activity evoked by rat peritoneal-fluid mast cells following treatment with epinephrine, 8-bromo-cyclic 3′,5′-guanosine monophosphate or compound 48/80. Biochem Pharmacol 1981; 30:481–7.
116. Taniguchi S, Nakazawa K, Fujiwara M. Characterization of adenylate and guanylate cyclases in rat peritoneal mast cells. Life Sci 1981; 29:1485–91.
117. Schinetti ML, Greco R, Bertelli A. D-penicillamine induced changes on rat mast cell cyclic GMP levels. Int J Tissue Reactions 1981; 3:83–8.
118. Coffey RG, Hadden JW. Arachidonate and metabolites in mitogen activation of lymphocyte guanylate cyclase. In: Hadden JW, Chedid L, Spreafico F, Mullen P, eds. Advances in immunopharmacology. Oxford: Pergamon, 1981:365–73.
119. Stolc V. Mechanism of regulation of adenylate cyclase activity in human polymorphonuclear leukocytes by calcium, guanosyl nucleotides, and positive effectors. J Biol Chem 1977; 252:1901–7.
120. Smith RJ, Ignarro LJ. Bioregulation of lysosomal enzyme secretion from human neutrophils: role of guanosine 3′:5′-monophosphate and calcium in stimulus-secretion coupling. Proc Natl Acad Sci USA 1975; 72:108–12.
121. Smolen JE, Korchak HM, Weissman G. Increased levels of cyclic adenosine 3′,5′-monophosphate in human polymorphonuclear leukocytes after surface stimulation. J Clin Invest 1980; 65:1077–85.
122. Simchowitz L, Spilberg I, Atkinson JP. Evidence that the functional responses of human neutrophils occur independently of transient elevations in cyclic AMP levels. J Cyclic Nucleotide Protein Phosphorylation Res 1983; 9:35–47.
123. Verghese MW, Fox K, McPhail LC, Snyderman R. Chemoattractant-elicited alterations of cAMP levels in human polymorphonuclear leukocytes require a Ca^{2+}-dependent mechanism which is independent of transmembrane activation of adenylate cyclase. J Biol Chem 1985; 260:6769–75.
124. Coffey RG, Davis JS, Djeu JY. Stimulation of guanylate cyclase activity and reduction of adenylate cyclase activity by granulocyte-macrophage colony-stimulating factor in human blood neutrophils. J Immunol 1988; 140:2695–701.
125. Marone G, Thomas LL, Lichtenstein LM. The role of agonists that activate adenylate cyclase in the control of cAMP metabolism and enzyme release by human polymorphonuclear leukocytes. J Immunol 1980; 125:2277–83.
126. Marone G, Siri L, Genovese A, Condorelli M. Betamethasone modulates the biological function of human polymorphonuclear leukocytes. Int Arch Allergy Appl Immunol 1987; 82:532–4.
127. Cronstein BN, Kramer SB, Rosenstein ED, Korchak HM, Weissman G, Hirschhorn R. Occupancy of adenosine receptors raises cyclic AMP alone and in synergy with occupancy of chemoattractant receptors and inhibits membrane depolarization. Biochem J 1988; 252:709–15.
128. Iannone MA, Wolberg G, Zimmerman TP. Chemotactic peptide induces cAMP elevation in human neutrophils by amplification of the adenylate cyclase response to endogenously produced adenosine. J Biol Chem 1989; 264:20177–80.
129. Boxer LA, Watanabe AM, Rister M, Besch HR Jr, Allen J, Baehner RL. Correction of leukocyte function in Chediak-Higashi syndrome by ascorbate. N Engl J Med 1976; 295:1041–5.
130. Atkinson JT, Weiss A, Ito M, Kelly J, Parker CW. Effects of ascorbic acid and sodium ascorbate on cyclic nucleotide metabolism in human lymphocytes. J Cyclic Nucleotide Res 1979; 5:107–123.
131. Hatch GE, Nichols WK, Hill HR. Cyclic nucleotide changes in human neutrophils induced

by chemoattractants and chemotactic modulators. J Immunol 1977; 119:450–6.
132. Logsdon PJ, Middleton E Jr, Coffey RG. Stimulation of leukocyte adenyl cyclase by hydrocortisone and isoproterenol in asthmatic and non-asthmatic subjects. J Allergy Clin Immunol 1972; 50:45–56.
133. Bourne HR, Lehrer RI, Lichtenstein LM, Weissmann G, Zurier R. Effects of cholera enterotoxin on adenosine 3′,5′-monophosphate and neutrophil function. Comparison with other compounds which stimulate leukocyte adenyl cyclase. J Clin Invest 1973; 52:698–708.
134. Ignarro LJ, George WJ. Mediation of immunologic discharge of lysosomal enzymes from human neutrophils by guanosine 3′,5′-monophosphate. Requirement of calcium, and inhibition by adenosine 3′,5′-monophosphate. J Exp Med 1974; 140:225–38.
135. Ignarro LJ, George WJ. Hormonal control of lysosomal enzyme release from human neutrophils: elevation of cyclic nucleotide levels by autonomic neurohormones. Proc Natl Acad Sci USA 1974; 71:2027–31.
136. Busse WW, Lee TP. Decreased adrenergic responses in lymphocytes and granulocytes in atopic eczema. J Allergy Clin Immunol 1976; 58:586–96.
137. Rudolph SA, Greengard P, Malawista SE. Effects of colchicine on cyclic AMP levels in human leukocytes. Proc Natl Acad Sci USA 1977; 74:3404–8.
138. Rudolph SA, Hegstrand LR, Greengard P, Malawista SE. The interaction of colchicine with hormone-sensitive adenylate cyclase in human leukocytes. Mol Pharmacol 1979; 16:805–12.
139. Ring J, Mathison DA, O'Connor R. In vitro cyclic nucleotide responsiveness of leukocytes and platelets in patients suffering from atopic dermatitis. Int Arch Allergy Appl Immunol 1981; 65:1–7.
140. Panosian JO, Marinetti GV. α-Adrenergic receptors in human polymorphonuclear leukocyte membranes. Biochem Pharmacol 1983; 32:2243–8.
141. Nielson CP. β-Adrenergic modulation of the polymorphonuclear leukocyte respiratory burst is dependent upon the mechanism of cell activation. J Immunol 1987; 139:2392–7.
142. Nielson CP, Crowley JJ, Morgan ME, Vestal RE. Polymorphonuclear leukocyte inhibition by therapeutic concentrations of theophylline is mediated by cyclic-3′,5′-adenosine monophosphate. Am Rev Respir Dis 1988; 137:25–30.
143. Constantopoulos A, Najjar VA. Adenyl cyclase of polymorphonuclear leukocytes. Nature New Biol 1973; 243:268–9.
144. Anderson R, Glover A, Koornhof HJ, Rabson AR. In vitro stimulation of neutrophil motility by levamisole: maintenance of cGMP levels in chemotactically stimulated levamisole-treated neutrophils. J Immunol 1976; 117:428–32.
145. Simchowitz L, Fischbein LC, Spilberg I, Atkinson JP. Induction of a transient elevation in intracellular levels of adenosine-3′,5′-cyclic monophosphate by chemotactic factors: an early event in human neutrophil activation. J Immunol 1980; 124:1482–91.
146. Naef A, Damerau B, Keller HU. Cytotaxin-induced cAMP peak in granulocytes: its relationship to crawling movements, chemokinesis and chemotaxis. Biochem Pharmacol 1982; 31:1573–8.
147. Sano Y, Watt G, Townley RG. Decreased mononuclear cell beta-adrenergic receptors in bronchial asthma: parallel studies of lymphocyte and granulocyte desensitization. J Allergy Clin Immunol 1983; 72:495–503.
148. Stahlberg HJ, Loschen G, Flohe L. Effects of prostacyclin analogs on cyclic adenosine monophosphate and superoxide formation in human polymorphonuclear leukocytes stimulated by formyl-methionyl-leucyl-phenylalanine. Biol Chem Hoppe-Seyler 1988; 369:329–36.
149. Coffey RG. Unpublished observations.
150. Becker EL. Chemotaxis. J Allergy Clin Immunol 1980; 66:97–105.
151. Marone G, Lichtenstein LM, Plaut M. Hydrocortisone and human lymphocytes—increases

in cyclic adenosine-3′,5′-monophosphate and potentiation of adenylate cyclase-activating agents. J Pharmacol Exp Ther 1980; 215:469–78.

152. Ignarro LJ, Cech SY. Lysosomal enzyme secretion from human neutrophils mediated by cyclic GMP: inhibition of cyclic GMP accumulation and neutrophil function by glucocorticosteroids. J Cyclic Nucleotide Res 1975; 1:283–92.
153. Lad PM, Glovsky MM, Richards JH, Smiley PA, Backstrom B. Regulation of human neutrophil guanylate cyclase by metal ions, free radicals, and the muscarinic receptor. Mol Immunol 1985; 22:731–40.
154. Deporter DA, Dunn CJ, Willoughby DA. Cyclic adenosine 3′,5′-monophosphate and the mechanism of action of three common anti-inflammatory drugs. Br J Pharmacol 1979; 65:163–5.
155. Boxer LA, Allen JM, Watanabe AM, Besch HR Jr, Baehner RL. Role of microtubules in granulocyte adherence. Blood 1978; 51:1045–50.
156. Buchta R, Fridkin M, Pontet M, Contessi E, Scaggiante B, Romeo D. Modulation of human neutrophil function by C-reactive protein. Eur J Biochem 1987; 163:141–6.
157. Atkinson JP, Sullivan TJ, Kelly JP, Parker CW. Stimulation by alcohols of cyclic nucleotide metabolism in human leukocytes—possible role of cyclic AMP in anti-inflammatory effects of ethanol. J Clin Invest 1977; 60:284–94.
158. Bourne HR, Lehrer RI, Cline MJ, Melmon KL. Cyclic 3′,5′-adenosine monophosphate in the human leukocyte: synthesis, degradation, and effects on neutrophil candidacidal activity. J Clin Invest 1971; 50:920–9.
159. Anderson T, Fallman M, Lew DP, Stendahl O. Does protein kinase C control receptor-mediated phagocytosis in human neutrophils? FEBS Lett 1988; 239:371–5.
160. Furui H, Suzuki K, Takagi K, Satake T. Effect of colforsin on human neutrophil superoxide production and intracellular calcium mobilization. Clin Exp Pharmacol Physiol 1989; 16:199–209.
161. Busse WW, Sossman J. Histamine inhibition of neutrophil lysosomal enzyme release and H_2 histamine receptor response. Science 1976; 194:737–8.
162. Anderson R, Glover A, Rabson AR. The *in vitro* effects of histamine and metiamide on neutrophil motility and their relationship to intracellular cyclic nucleotide levels. J Immunol 1977; 118:1690–6.
163. Burde R, Seifert R, Buschauer A, Schultz G. Histamine inhibits activation of human neutrophils and HL-60 leukemic cell via H_2-receptors. Nauny-Schmiedebergs Arch Pharmacol 1989; 340:671–8.
164. Goetzl EJ, Hill HR, Gorman RR. Unique aspects of the modulation of the human neutrophil function by 12-L-hydroperoxy-5,8,10,14-eicosatetraenoic acid. Prostaglandins 1980; 19:71–86.
165. Gallin JI, Elin RJ, Hubert RT, Fauci AS, Kaliner MA, Wolff SM. Efficacy of ascorbic acid in Chediak-Higashi syndrome (CHS): studies in humans and mice. Blood 1979; 53:226–34.
166. Roch-Arveiller M, Tissot M, Moachon L, Giroud JP. Effect of immunomodulating agents on leucocyte chemotaxis and cyclic nucleotides. Agents Actions 1982; 12:353–9.
167. Wright DG, Kirkpatrick CH, Gallin JI. Effects of levamisole on normal and abnormal leukocyte locomotion. J Clin Invest 1977; 59:941–50.
168. Logsdon PJ, Carnright DV, Middleton E Jr, Coffey RG. The effect of phentolamine on adenylate cyclase and on isoproterenol stimulation in leukocytes from asthmatic and non-asthmatic subjects. J Allergy Clin Immunol 1973; 52:148–57.
169. Bendtzen K, Klysner R. Increased polymorphonuclear leukocyte cGMP levels induced by the human lymphokine leukocyte migration inhibitory factor (LIF). Immunopharmacology 1979; 1:323–30.
170. Claesson HE. Leukotrienes A_4 and B_4 stimulate the formation of cyclic AMP in human leukocytes. FEBS Lett 1982; 139:305–8.

171. Fulop T Jr, Kekessy D, Foris G. Impaired coupling of naloxone sensitive opiate receptors to adenylate cyclase in PMNLs of aged male subjects. Int J Immunopharmacol 1987; 9:651–7.
172. Stolc V. Restrained adenyl cyclase in human neutrophils: stimulation of cyclic adenosine 3′:5′-monophosphate formation and adenyl cyclase activity by phagocytosis and prostaglandins. Blood 1974; 43:743–8.
173. Claesson HE, Lundberg U, Malmsten C. Serum-coated zymosan stimulates the synthesis of leukotriene B_4 in human polymorphonuclear leukocytes. Inhibition by cyclic AMP. Biochem Biophys Res Commun 1981; 99:1230–7.
174. Kainoh M, Imai R, Umetsu T, Hattori M, Nishio S. Prostacyclin and beraprost sodium as suppressors of activated rat polymorphonuclear leukocytes. Biochem Pharmacol 1990; 39:477–84.
175. Busse WW, Anderson CL. The granulocyte response to the phosphodiesterase inhibitor RO20-1724 in asthma. J Allergy Clin Immunol 1981; 67:70–4.
176. Park BH, Good RA, Beck NP, Davis BB. Concentration of cyclic adenosine 3′:5′-monophosphate in human leukocytes during phagocytosis. Nature New Biol 1971; 229:27–9.
177. Stolc V. Stimulatory effect of latex and zymosan particles on cyclic adenosine 3′,5′-monophosphate content in human granulocytes. Mol Immunol 1981; 18:773–80.
178. Alonso F, Sanchez-Crespo M, Mato JM. Modulatory role of cyclic AMP in the release of platelet-activating factor from human polymorphonuclear leucocytes. Immunol 1982; 45:493–500.
179. Pryzwansky KB, Steiner AL, Spitnagel JK, Kapoor CL. Compartmentalization of cyclic AMP during phagocytosis by human neutrophilic granulocytes. Science 1981; 211:408–10.
180. Hill HR, Estensen RD, Quie PG, Hogan NA, Goldberg ND. Modulation of human neutrophil chemotactic responses by cyclic 3′,5′-guanosine monophosphate and cyclic 3′,5′-adenosine monophosphate. Metabolism 1975; 24:447–56.
181. Najjar VA, Schmidt JJ. The chemistry and biology of tuftsin. Lymphokine Rep 1980; 1:157–79.
182. Stabinsky Y, Bar-Shavit Z, Fridkin M, Goldman R. On the mechanism of action of the phagocytosis-stimulating peptide tuftsin. Mol Cell Biochem 1980; 30:71–7.
183. Lad PM, Glovsky MM, Richards JH, Learn DB, Reisinger DM, Smiley PA. Identification of receptor regulatory proteins, membrane glycoproteins, and functional characteristics of adenylate cyclase in vesicles derived from the human neutrophil. Mol Immunol 1984; 21:627–39.
184. Naef A, Damerau B, Keller HU. Relationship between the transient cAMP increase, exocytosis from specific and azurophil granules and chemotaxis in neutrophil granulocytes. Agents Actions 1984; 14:63–71.
185. Gallant SP, Allred S, Griffiths R. Characterization of adenylate cyclase activity in asthmatic neutrophil sonicates. Am Rev Respir Dis 1980; 122:231–8.
186. Okuda K, Takahashi T, Tadokoro I, Noguchi Y. Effects of cytochalasin B and dibutyryl cyclic AMP on intraleukocytic bactericidal activity. Jap J Exp Med 1976; 46:101–10.
187. Confer DI, Eaton JW. Phagocyte impotence caused by an inverse bacterial adenylate cyclase. Science 1982; 217:948–50.
188. Gale RP and Zighelboim J. Modulation of polymorphonuclear leukocyte-mediated antibody-dependent cellular cytotoxicity. J Immunol 1974; 113:1793–800.
189. Dallegri F, Frumento G, Ballestrero A, Goretti R, Patrone F. Relationship between antibody-dependent tumour cell lysis and primary granule exocytosis by human neutrophils. Clin Exp Immunol 1987; 70:479–83.
190. Weissmann G, Dukor P, Zurier RB. Effect of cyclic AMP on release of lysosomal enzymes from phagocytes. Nature New Biol 1971; 231:131–5.

191. Pearson JD, Carleton JS, Beesley JE, Hutchings A, Gordon JL. Granulocyte adhesion to endothelium in culture. J Cell Sci 1979; 38:225–35.
192. Nourshargh S, Hoult JR. Inhibition of human neutrophil degranulation by forskolin in the presence of phosphodiesterase inhibitors. Eur J Pharmacol 1986; 122:205–12.
193. Wada Y. Cyclic AMP inhibits chemotactic-peptide-induced but not Ca^{2+}-ionophore- or tetradecanoylphorbol-acetate-induced enzyme secretion in guinea pig neutrophils. Int Arch Allergy Appl Immunol 1989; 90:194–7.
194. Romeo D, Aabucchi G, Jug M, Miani N, Soranzo MR. Concanavalin A as a probe for studying the mechanism of metabolic stimulation of leukocytes. Adv Exp Med Biol 1975; 55:273–90.
195. Goldstein I, Hoffstein S, Gallin J, Weissmann G. Mechanisms of lysosomal enzyme release from human leukocytes: microtubule assembly and membrane fusion induced by a component of complement. Proc Natl Acad Sci USA 1973; 70:2916–20.
196. Weissmann G, Goldstein I, Hoffstein S, Chauvet G, Robineaux R. Yin/yang modulation of lysosomal enzyme release from polymorphonuclear leukocytes by cyclic nucleotides. Annal NY Acad Sci 1975; 356:222–31.
197. Schrier DJ, Imre KM. The effects of adenosine agonists on human neutrophil function. J Immunol 1986; 137:3284–9.
198. Zurier RB, Hoffstein S, Weissman G. Mechanism of lysosomal enzyme release from human leukocytes. I. Effect of cyclic nucleotides and colchicine. J Cell Biol 1973; 58:27–41.
199. Ignarro LJ, Lint TF, George WJ. Hormonal control of lysosomal enzyme release from human neutrophils: effects of autonomic agents on enzyme release, phagocytosis and cyclic nucleotide levels. J Exp Med 1974; 139:1395–414.
200. Henson PM. Pathologic mechanisms in neutrophil-mediated injury. Am J Pathol 1972; 68:593–612.
201. Ignarro LJ. Stimulation of phagocytic release of neutral protease from human neutrophils by cholinergic amines and cyclic 3′,5′-guanosine monophosphate. J Immunol 1974; 122:210–21.
202. Estensen RD, Hill HR, Quie PG, Hogan N, Goldberg ND. Cyclic GMP and cell movement. Nature 1973; 245:258–60.
203. Pham HT. Chemotaxis of human leucocytes: II. Effects of lectins, colchicine, cytochalasin B, cyclic nucleotides and immuno-stimulatory products. Biomedicine 1979; 30:121–4.
204. Bendtzen L, Palit J. In vitro modulation of human leucocyte migration and migration inhibitory factor (LIF) activity by cyclic 3′,5′-AMP and cyclic 3′,5′-GMP. Acta Pathol Microbiol Scand 1977; 85C:78–80.
205. Nielson CP, Vestal RE. Effects of adenosine on polymorphonuclear leukocyte function, cyclic 3′:5′-adenosine monophosphate, and intracellular calcium. Br J Pharmacol 1989; 97:882–8.
206. Mueller H, Sklar LA. Coupling of antagonistic signalling pathways in modulation of neutrophil function. J Cell Biochem 1989; 40:287–94.
207. Gryglewski RJ, Szczelic A, Wandzilak M. The effect of six prostaglandins, prostacyclin and iloprost on generation of superoxide anions by human polymorphonuclear leukocytes stimulated by zymosan or formyl-methionyl-leucyl-phenylalanine. Biochem Pharmacol 1987; 24:4209–13.
208. Spirer Z, Zakuth V, Golander A, Bogair N. The influence of cyclic nucleotides (c-AMP and c-GMP) on the nitrous blue tetrazolium reduction by human polymorphonuclear leucocytes. Experientia 1975; 31:118–20.
209. Bussolino F, Benveniste J. Pharmacological modulation of platelet-activating factor (PAF) release from rabbit leucocytes. I. Role of cAMP. Immunology 1980; 40:367–76.
210. Flyer RH, Finch SC. The effects of prostaglandin E_1 on human granulocyte metabolism during phagocytosis. J Reticuloendothel Soc 1973; 14:325–31.

211. Schell-Frederick E, Van Sande J. Evidence that cyclic AMP is not the chemical mediator of the metabolic changes accompanying phagocytosis. J Reticuloendothel Soc 1974; 15:139–48.
212. Qualliotone D, De Chatelet LR, McCall CE, Cooper MR. Stimulation of oxidative metabolism in polymorphonuclear leukocytes by catecholamines. J Reticuloendothel Soc 1972; 11:263–76.
213. Deporter DA, Dieppe PA, Glatt M, Willoughby DA. The relation of cyclic AMP levels to phagocytosis and enzyme release in acute inflammation in vivo. J Pathol 1977; 121:129–39.
214. Stossel TP, Mason RJ, Hartwig J, Vaughan M. Quantitative studies of phagocytosis by polymorphonuclear leukocytes: use of emulsions to measure the initial rate of phagocytosis. J Clin Invest 1972; 51:615–24.
215. Cox JP, Karnovsky ML. The depression of phagocytosis by exogenous cyclic nucleotides, prostaglandins, and theophylline. J Cell Biol 1973; 59:480–90.
216. Muschel RJ, Rosen N, Rosen OM, Bloom BR. Modulation of Fc-mediated phagocytosis by cyclic AMP and insulin in a macrophage-like cell line. J Immunol 1977; 119:1813–20.
217. Stossel TP, Murad F, Mason RJ, Vaughan M. Regulation of glycogen metabolism in polymorphonuclear leukocytes. J Biol Chem 1970; 245:6228–34.
218. Manganiello V, Evans WH, Stossel TP, Mason RJ, Vaughan M. The effect of polystyrene beads on cyclic 3′,5′-adenosine monophosphate concentration in leukocytes. J Clin Invest 1971; 50:2741–4.
219. Seyberth HW, Schmidt-Gayk H, Jakobs KH, Hackenthal E. Cyclic adenosine monophosphate in phagocytizing granulocytes and alveolar macrophages. J Cell Biol 1973; 57:567–71.
220. Deporter DA. Cyclic AMP and the mechanism of leucocyte lysosomal enzyme release during an immediate hypersensitivity reaction in vivo. J Pathol 1977; 123:129–34.
221. Della Bianca V, De Togni P, Grzeskowiak M, Vicentini LM, DiVirgilio F. Cyclic AMP inhibition of phosphoinositide turnover in human neutrophils. Biochim Biophys Acta 1986; 886:441–7.
222. Kato H, Ishitoya J, Takenawa T. Inhibition of inositol phospholipids metabolism and calcium mobilization by cyclic AMP-increasing agents and phorbol ester in neutrophils. Biochem Biophys Res Commun 1986; 139:1272–8.
223. Tecoma ES, Motulsky HJ, Traynor AE, Omann GM, Muller H, Sklar LA. Transient catecholamine modulation of neutrophil activation: kinetic and intracellular aspects of isoproterenol action. J Leuk Biol 1986; 40:629–44.
224. Cronstein BN, Rosenstein ED, Kramer SB, Weissman G, Hirschhorn R. Adenosine: a physiologic modulator of superoxide anion generation by human neutrophils. Adenosine acts via an A_2 receptor on human neutrophils. J Immunol 1985; 135:1366–71.
225. Roberts PA, Newby AC, Hallett MB, Campbell AK. Inhibition by adenosine of reactive oxygen metabolite production by human polymorphonuclear leucocytes. Biochem J 1985; 227:669–74.
226. Grinstein S, Furuya W. Cytoplasmic pH regulation in activated human neutrophils: effects of adenosine and pertussis toxin on Na^+/K^+ exchange and metabolic acidification. Biochim Biophys Acta 1986; 889:301–9.
227. Yamazaki M, Matsuoka T, Yasui K, Komiyama A, Akabane T. Dopamine inhibition of superoxide anion production by polymorphonuclear leukocytes. J Allergy Clin Immunol 1989; 83:967–72.
228. Lad PM, Olson CV, Smiley PA. Association of the N-formyl-met-leu-phe receptor in human neutrophils with a GTP-binding protein sensitive to pertussis toxin. Proc Natl Acad Sci USA 1985; 82:869–73.
229. Weissmann G, Zurier RB, Hoffstein S. Leukocyte proteases and the immunologic release of lysosomal enzymes. Am J Pathol 1972; 68:539–60.

230. Lapetina EG, Schmitges CJ, Chandrabose K, Cuatrecasas P. Regulation of phospholipase activity in platelets. Adv Prostaglandin Thromboxane Res 1978; 3:89–95.
231. Hirata F. The regulation of lipomodulin, a phospholipase inhibitory protein, in rabbit neutrophils by phosphorylation. J Biol Chem 1981; 256:7730–3.
232. Coffey RG, Hadden JW. Arachidonate and metabolites in mitogen activation of lymphocyte guanylate cyclase. In: Hadden J, Chedid L, Spreafico F, Mullen P, eds. Oxford: Pergamon, 1981:365–73.
233. Coffey RG, Hadden JW. Phorbol myristate acetate stimulation of lymphocyte guanylate cyclase and cyclic GMP phosphodiesterase and reduction of adenylate cyclase. Cancer Res 1983; 43:150–8.
234. Zurier RB. Cyclic nucleotides and the Chedia-Higashi syndrome. Adv Cyclic Nucleotide Res 1980; 12:173–9.
235. Bendtzen K. Human leukocyte migration inhibitory factor (LIF). IV. 3′,5′-cGMP protects LIF against inactivation by the esterase inhibitor phenylmethylsulfonylfluoride. Scand J Immunol 1977; 6:1357–61.
236. Bendtzen K. Human leucocyte migration inhibitor factor (LIF). V. Specific regulation of the lymphokine serine protease activity by 3′,5′-cGMP and, possibly, 2′,3′-cCMP. Scand J Immunol 1978; 8:53–61.
237. Bendtzen K. Leukocyte migration inhibitory factor. A serine esterase release by stimulated human lymphocytes. Kinetic analysis and inhibition by cyclic GMP. Biochim Biophys Acta 1979; 566:183–91.
238. Bendtzen K. Evidence for the esterase and protease nature of human leukocyte migration inhibitory factor (LIF) and its modulation by cGMP. Lymphokine Rep. 1980; 1:41–62.
239. Svenson M, Bendtzen K. Effects of cyclic GMP agonists on ciclosporin-induced suppression of human lymphokine production. Allergy 1985; 40:529–34.
240. Kurland JI, Hadden JW, Moore MAS. Role of cyclic nucleotides in the proliferation of committed granulocyte-macrophage progenitor cells. Cancer Res 1977; 37:4534–8.
241. Oshita AK, Rothstein G, Lonngi G. cGMP stimulation of stem cell proliferation. Blood 1977; 49:585–91.
242. Taetle R, Koessler A. Effects of cyclic nucleotides and prostaglandins on normal and abnormal human myeloid progenitor proliferation. Cancer Res 1980; 40:1223–9.
243. Taetle R, Mendelsohn J. Modulation of normal and abnormal myeloid progenitor proliferation by cyclic nucleotides and PGE_1. Blood Cells 1980; 6:701–18.
244. Korchak HM, Hoffstein ST, Weissmann G. The neutrophil granules. In: Poisner AM, Trifao JM, eds. The secretory granule—the secretory process, vol. 1. Amsterdam: Elsevier, 1982:317–56.
245. Szentivanyi A. The beta-adrenergic theory of the atopic abnormality in bronchial asthma. J Allergy 1968; 42:203–32.
246. Busse WW. Decreased granulocyte response to isoproterenol in asthma during upper respiratory infections. Am Rev Respir Dis 1977; 115:783–91.
247. Busse WW and Sosman J. Decreased H_2 histamine response of granulocytes of asthmatic patients. J Clin Invest 1977:1080–7.
248. Parker CW, Smith JW. Alterations in cyclic adenosine monophosphate metabolism in human bronchial asthma. I. Leukocyte responsiveness to β-adrenergic agents. J Clin Invest 1973; 52:48–59.
249. Parker CW, Baumann ML, Huber MG. Alterations in cyclic AMP metabolism in human bronchial asthma. II. Leukocyte and lymphocyte responses to prostaglandins. J Clin Invest 1973; 52:1336–41.
250. Davies AO, Lefkowitz RJ. In vitro desensitization of beta-adrenergic receptors in human neutrophils—attenuation by corticosteroids. J Clin Invest 1983; 71:565–71.
251. Davies AO. Exercise-induced fall in coupling of human β-adrenergic receptors. Metabolism Clin Exp 1988; 37:916–8.

252. Davis PB, Braunstein M, Jay C. Decreased adenosine 3′,5′-monophosphate response to isoproterenol in cystic fibrosis leukocytes. Pediatr Res 1978; 12:703–7.
253. Davis PB. Plasma factors do not account for the leukocyte beta-adrenergic defect in cystic fibrosis. IRCS Med Sci—Biochem 1980; 8:413.
254. Davis PB, Laundon SC. Adenylate cyclase in leukocytes from patients with cystic fibrosis. J Lab Clin Med 1980; 96:75–84.
255. Davis PB, Dieckman L, Boat TF, Stern RC, Doershuk CF. Beta adrenergic receptors in lymphocytes and granulocytes from patients with cystic fibrosis. J Clin Invest 1983; 71:1787–95.
256. Pandey GN, Dysken MW, Garver DL, Davis JM. Beta-adrenergic receptor function in affective illness. Am J Psychiatr 1979; 136:675–8.
257. Boxer LA, Rister M, Allen JM, Baehner RL. Improvement of Chediak-Higashi leukocyte function by cyclic guanosine monophosphate. Blood 1977; 49:9–17.
258. Soligo D, Lambertenghi-Deliliers G, Capsoni F, Villa M, Neri A, Peracchi M, Benazzi E, Valenti F, Polli E. Defective granulocyte chemotaxis and natural killer activity in a patient with recurrent infections. J Clin Lab Immunol 1986; 21:49–53.
259. Hauck M, Fulop T Jr, Foris G, Leovey A. Divergent effects of human lymphokine derived oligopeptides on PMNLs function of young and aged healthy subjects. Int J Immunopharmacol 1987; 9:3–8.

B

Effects of Cytokines: Basic Research

10

Regulatory Effects of Cytokines on Myelopoiesis

F. HERRMANN and R. MERTELSMANN
University of Freiburg, Freiburg, Germany

I. INTRODUCTION

Recombinant DNA technology has been central in answering some of the most relevant questions in the research of regulation of the functional status of hematopoietic stem/progenitor cells and their progeny. This chapter will focus on recent results that have emerged from studies utilizing recombinant human cytokines that control myelopoietic blood cell development. The following features will be detailed: the biological characteristics and biochemistry of hematopoietic growth factors, synergizing factors and growth factor-releasing factors, their role in the regulation of myelopoiesis, their cellular sources, and regulation of production.

A number of distinct biological regulators termed cytokines have been identified, and many of them have been purified to homogeneity and molecularly cloned. These cytokines may stimulate or inhibit stem/progenitor cell growth either by acting directly or by modifying the production or action of other regulatory molecules. Table 1 lists the molecularly cloned cytokines involved in the regulation of myelopoiesis, along with their synonyms, chromosomal localization of their genes, transcript size, protein size, mode of secretion, and primary cellular source. Included are the hematopoietic growth factors, also referred to as colony-stimulating factors (CSF): granulocyte-macrophage (GM)-CSF, G-CSF, M-CSF, multi-CSF (IL-3), eosinophil-CSF (IL-5), erythropoietin (Epo), as well as other cytokines that do not appear to exert direct CSF activity but can up- and down-modulate CSF action or production and encompass IL-1, IL-2, IL-4 to IL-5, possibly IL-7 to IL-9, tumor necrosis factor (TNF)-α, lymphotoxin (LT), the interferons (IFN) (α, β_1, -γ), transforming growth factor (TGF)-β, leukemia inhibitory factor (LIF), monocyte chemotactic and activating factor (MCAF), activin, inhibin, oncostatin M, and the macrophage inflammatory proteins (MIP) 1 and 2. Other molecules not belonging to the class of cytokines may also act as hematopoietic regulators and involve lactoferrin, acidic isoferritin, transferrin, and E-type prostaglandins.

Table 1 Cytokines Involved in the Regulation of Hematopoiesis

Molecule	Synonym	Chromosome Localization	mRNA (kb)	MW (kD)	Secretion[a]	Main Source[b]
1. Hematopoietic growth factors						
Multi-CSF	IL-3	5q	1	14–28	p	T
GM-CSF	CSF-alpha	5q21-32	1	14–35	e; p	T,E,F
G-CSF	CSF-beta	17q11-22	1.6	18–22	e; p	M,G,E,F
M-CSF	CSF-1	5q33	1.8–4.0	36–90	e; a	M,G,E,F
Erythropoietin		7q21	2.0	32–35	p	Kidney
2. Non-CSF interleukins						
IL-1-alpha	Hemopoietin-1	2q14	2.2	17–31	e; p; a	M,G,E,F
IL-1-beta		2q14	1.6	17–31	e; p; a	M,G,E,F
IL-2	TCGF	4p	0.9	15	e; p; a	T
IL-4	BSF-1	5q	0.9	15–20	e; p; a	T
IL-5	BCGF-II, TRF	5q	1.7	12–18	e; p	T
IL-6	IFN-beta2, BSF2	7p21	1.3–1.6	24	p	T,M,F,E,G
IL-7		8q12–13	1.8–2.4	17	a; p	T
IL-9	p40	nd[c]	0.8	40	p	T
3. Growth factor-inducing factors						
TNF-alpha	Cachectin	6p23	1.6	17	e; p; a	M,T,G,E,F
Lymphotoxin	TNF-beta	6p23	1.7		e; p	T
IL-6	see above					
IFN-gamma	type-II IFN	12	1.7	15–45	p	T
4. Chemotactic factors						
IL-8	NCF/NAP, TCF	nd	1.8	10	p	M,F,E
MCAF	E, MCP-1	17q11-12	0.7	32	p	M,F,E
MIP-1		nd	nd	8–10	p	M
MIP-2		nd	nd	8	p	M
5. Others						
LIF	HILDA	22q12	4.0	24	p	T,E,F,
Activin		nd	nd		e	Sertoli, granulosa cells
Inhibin		nd	nd	32	e	Sertoli, granulosa cells
Oncostatin M		nd	2.0	28	nd	M
TGF-beta		nd	2.5	25	p	Plt
6. Iron-binding proteins (No Cytokines)						
Lactoferrin						
Acidic isoferritin						
Transferrin						

[a] e; endocrine p; paracrine a; autocrine

[b] T, T-lymphocytes; M, monocytes; G, granulocytes; E, endothelial cells; F, fibroblasts; Plt, platelets; T (B)CGF, T (B)-cell growth factor; BSF, B-cell stimulating factor; TGF, transforming growth factor; TRF, T-cell replacing factor; NCF/NAP, neutrophil chemotactic factor/neutrophil activating protein; MCP-1, Monocyte chemoattractant protein-1; LIF, leukemia inhibitory factor; HILDA, human interleukin for DA cells; MCAF, monocyte chemotactic and activating factor; MIP, macrophage inflammatory protein.

[c] nd; not determined

Cytokines are produced and secreted by accessory cells upon appropriate stimulation (Figure 1). While these cytokines and CSF have a well-established role in the activation of the functional repertoire of mature end cells, their action on hematopoietic stem/progenitor cells is less completely understood. In the present chapter the in-vitro activities of cytokines in regulating white blood cell development will be briefly reviewed.

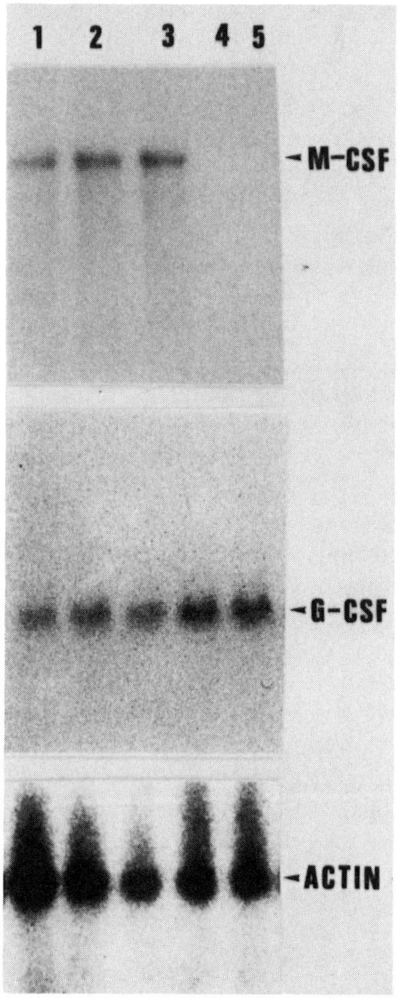

Figure 1 Expression of G-CSF and M-CSF transcripts in various types of human cells. Lane 1; peripheral blood neutrophils activated for 12 h with recombinant human (rh) GM-CSF (25 ng/ml). Lane 2; peripheral blood monocytes activated for 4 h with rh TNF-α (20 ng/ml). Lane 3; embryonic lung fibroblasts activated for 12 h with rh IL-1β (10 U/ml). Lane 4; cells of the squamous cell carcinoma line CHU-2. Lane 5; blasts obtained from a patient with acute myelogenous leukemia. Filters were reprobed with an α-actin cDNA to control for RNA loading in single lanes.

II. HEMATOPOIETIC CELLS

After entering the circulation, nucleated bone marrow-derived myeloid cells are extremely short-lived, with a half-life ranging from a few hours to a few days. To provide the necessary supply of functional competent end-stage cells required for maintenance of steady-state hematopoiesis, the process of blood cell formation must be tightly regulated. Cellular elements of the blood-forming system encompass hematopoietic stem and progenitor cells, which while present in the bone marrow in low frequency, generate the mature cell population circulating in the blood. Proliferation and differentiation of the stem and progenitor cell pool are controlled by accessory cells such as T- and B-lymphocytes, natural killer cells, monocytes/macrophages, endothelial cells, and fibroblasts (Figure 1). Stem/progenitor cells and accessory cells cooperate in a complex network of stimulatory and inhibitory loops, which may be established by direct cellular interactions or through an accessory cell-derived soluble regulator (1–3). Extracellular matrix molecules may have a role in this scenario as well, by compartmentalizing these regulators (4,5). Stem cells can self-renew to generate more stem cells or can differentiate to produce progeny (i.e., progenitor cells), which are unable to self-renew but will undergo deterministic divisions and terminal maturation.

Stem cells can be quantitated by their ability to reconstitute hematopoiesis in potentially lethally irradiated recipients (6); clonogenic multipotent cells with self-renewal ability can also be assayed by their ability to generate hematopoietic foci (colony-forming units-S, CFU-S) on the spleen of irradiated mice (7) or by their ability to form colonies in semisolid media containing mature cells of several hematopoietic lineages (8) (CFU-Mix). Lineage-committed progenitor cells are also able to produce clones containing mature cells. These include the granulocyte/macrophage colony-forming cells (CFU-GM), which develop into mature neutrophils, eosinophils, and macrophages; erythroid progenitor cells (BFU-E and CFU-E), which produce mature erythrocytes; and megakaryocyte progenitor cells (CFU-mega), which produce megakaryocytes. The survival, proliferation, and development of these cell populations in vitro is independent on exogenous growth factors (Figure 2). In vivo, the situation seems to be less clear. On a speculative basis, it might be possible that nonproliferative cells are in an equilibrium maintained by counteracting stimulatory and inhibitory regulators and that activation into the proliferative state would occur if there were either an increase in stimulatory signals, a decrease of inhibitory signals, or a combination of both (9).

III. HEMATOPOIETIC COLONY-STIMULATING FACTORS AND THEIR ACTION ON HEMATOPOIETIC STEM AND PROGENITOR CELLS

Experimental evidence using purified populations suggest that CSF can act directly at the level of stem/progenitor cells but may also act indirectly by inducing or enhancing the release of other hematopoietic regulators by accessory cells (Figure 1). The CSF exert their effect by binding to their specific receptors (10) but may also have their effects mediated through other cell surface components. One such component, the protein encoded by the FES protooncogene, has been shown to mediate some activities of GM-CSF (11). Also, the CD 45 surface structure has been implicated in the action of CSF (12). Some of the CSF have growth-promoting effects on more than one cell population: the earliest-acting factor, IL-3, can induce development of CFU-Mix-type

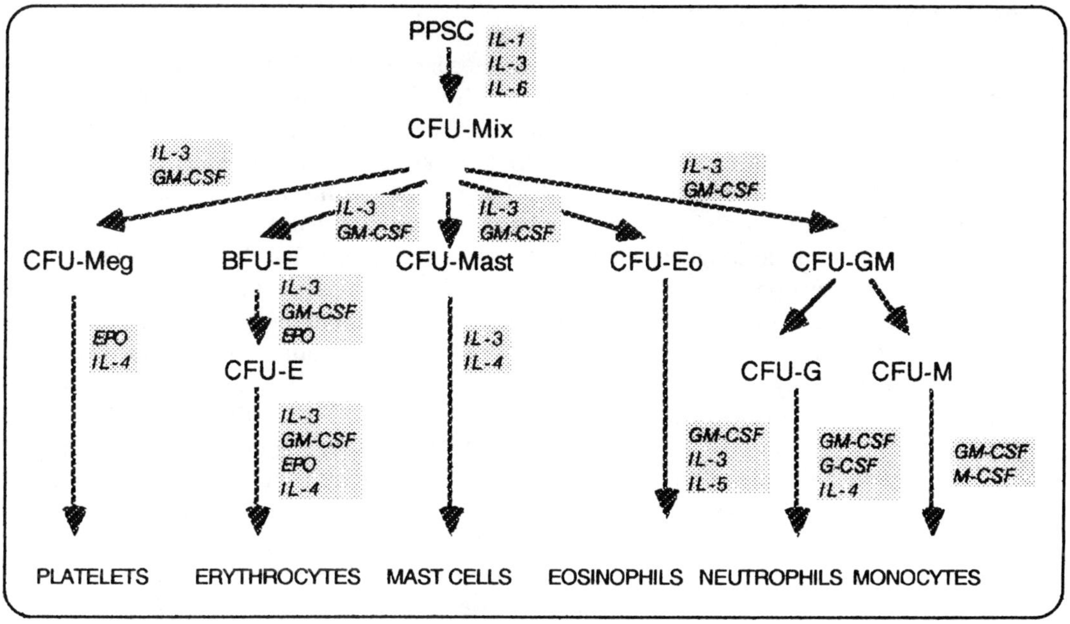

Figure 2 Interaction of the hematopoietic growth factors and non-CSF interleukins with hematopoietic cells. See text for abbreviations.

colonies and can recruit clonal growth of BFU-E, CFU-GM, and CFU-Eo (13,14); G-CSF acts on CFU-G (15), while M-CSF stimulates CFU-GM and CFU-M to undergo growth into monocytes/macrophages (16) (Figure 3). Of perhaps greater significance regarding stem/progenitor cell regulation is that synergies were seen when various CSFs were combined in culture: G-CSF synergizes with GM-CSF and M-CSF (17). Synergy was also seen when M-CSF was combined with GM-CSF or IL-3 (18,19) or when a combination of IL-1 with M-CSF or GM-CSF was analyzed (20).

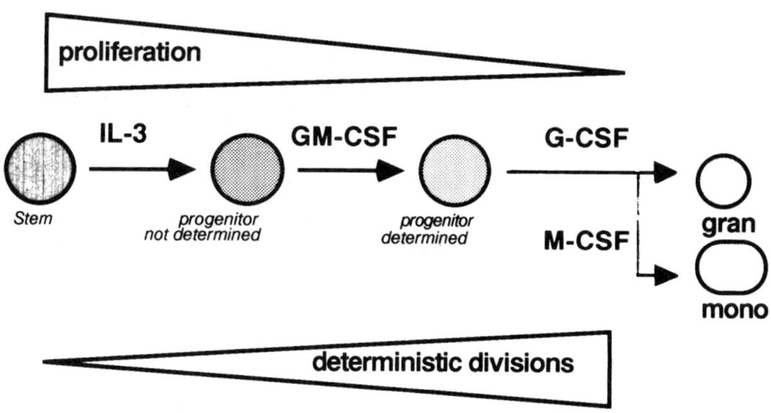

Figure 3 Sequential action of hematopoietic growth factors on hematopoietic stem/progenitor cells to stimulate their proliferation and differentiation into mature end cells. See text for abbreviations.

IV. NON-CSF INTERLEUKINS

The interleukins IL-1, IL-2, IL-4 to IL-6 do not appear to act as CSF. It is not yet clear whether the lymphoid growth factors IL-7 and IL-9 have intrinsic CSF activity. IL-1 exists in two forms, IL-1α and IL-1β. Both IL-1 species are able to induce release of CSF from antigen-activated T-cells (21), monocytes (16), and mesenchymal cells (22). Through its hemopoietin-1 activity (23), IL-1 enhances the hematopoietic activity of IL-3 (24). The use of purified progenitor populations suggests that this effect may relate to a direct action on the progenitor cells rather than being mediated through the induction of CSF production or release. IL-2 is a T-cell growth factor that either directly down-modulates CSF-stimulated colony growth (25) or inhibits hematopoietic colony growth via induction of release of γ-IFN by T-cells (26). Depending on the culture system applied, IL-2 may also trigger T-cell release of GM-CSF and IL-3 (27). IL-4, first described as B-cell growth factor-1 (BCGF-1), enhances G-CSF-stimulated CFU-G growth and Epo-stimulated colony formation by BFU-E (28) and is an essential growth factor for connective tissue-type mast cells (29). Whereas no synergism of IL-4 and GM-CSF exists, M-CSF-stimulated colony formation by CFU-M (30) and IL-3-stimulated BFU-E growth (31) is inhibited by IL-4. On the other hand, IL-4 can also enhance the release of CSF activity from mitogen-activated T-cells (32) and monocytes (33) and synergizes with IL-1 to stimulate release of M-CSF by fibroblasts (34). IL-6 can also induce the release of hematopoietic cytokines by accessory cells (Table 2) and acts in synergy with IL-3 to stimulate blast-cell-colony growth (46). It also synergizes with M-CSF and GM-CSF in the formation of monocyte and granulocyte colonies (47,48).

V. CHEMOTACTIC FACTORS

IL-8 is a cytokine with numerous synonyms reflecting its pleiotropic functions (49 for review). It has been termed neutrophil chemotactic factor (NCF), neutrophil activating protein (NAP), monocyte derived neutrophil activating protein (MONAP), and T-cell chemotactic factor (TCF). The major IL-8-producing cells were identified to be peripheral blood monocytes, keratinocytes, dermal fibroblasts, and endothelial cells. Endotoxin, IL-1 and TNF-α have been identified as IL-8 inducers in these cells, whereas glucocorticoids inhibit expression. Intravenous injection of human IL-8 into rabbits causes rapid neutrophilia (50). However, IL-8 does not stimulate colony formation by CFU-GM or CFU-G but may rather cause neutrophilia by increasing vascular permeability through enzyme release by the exocytosis of neutrophil granule contents. Injection of IL-8 into lymphocyte drainage areas of lymph nodes in rats results in an acceleration of immigration of T-cells into high endothelial venules of the draining lymph node. IL-8 is also able to stimulate antifungal activities of neutrophils but not of monocytes. It does not augment neutrophil cytostatic activity against tumor cells; its role in inducing superoxide anion generation by granulocytes is not yet clear. IL-8 is also chemotactic for human basophils (but not for eosinophils) and stimulates histamine release.

IL-8 shares 21% amino acid homology with another monocyte-derived chemotactic factor termed MCAF (49). MCAF mRNA expression is also augmented by endotoxin, IL-1, and TNF. MCAF has no effect on granulocytes but exerts its effect on mononuclear phagocytes. It is not only chemotactic for these cells but also activates them to

Table 2 Cytokine-Accessory Cell Interactions in the Production of Hematopoietic Growth Factors

Cytokine-producing cell	Inducing cytokine	Induced cytokine	Reference
Endothelial cells	IL-1	GM-CSF	35
		G-CSF	35
		M-CSF	35
	TNF-α	GM-CSF	35
		G-CSF	35
		M-CSF	35
	IL-6	M-CSF	36
Fibroblasts	IL-1	GM-CSF	22
		M-CSF	34
		IL-6	37
	TNF-α	GM-CSF	38
		G-CSF	39
		M-CSF	39
		IL-6	40
Monocytes	γ-IFN	G-CSF	41
		M-CSF	42
		IL-1	43
	TNF-α	G-CSF	44
		M-CSF	44
		IL-6	45
	IL-4	M-CSF	33
		G-CSF	33
T-cells	IL-1	GM-CSF	21
	IL-2	GM-CSF	27
		IL-3	27

augment their cytostatic activity against tumor tissues. MCAF also causes superoxide anion production and release of lysosomal enzymes by monocytes but has no detectable effect on the development of their progenitor cells. MCAF shows a 55% homology with MIP-1 at the amino acid level (51). The MIP (MIP-1 and MIP-2) are members of two families of heparin-binding chemotactic cytokines whose cDNA have been cloned from activated fibroblasts, T-cells and monocytes (52 for review). When injected into the footpads of C3H/HeJ mice, MIP-1 induces a localized inflammatory reaction with invading granulocytes followed by a monocyte infiltrate. It also causes granulocytes to degranulate, inducing the release of lysozyme. In contrast to MIP-1, MIP-2 also causes a localized inflammatory reaction upon injection. In contrast to IL-8 and M-CAF, MIP-1 and MIP-2 exhibit synergy with GM-CSF and M-CSF to enhance colony growth of CFU-GM (53).

VI. INHIBIN AND ACTIVIN

Inhibin is a cytokine produced by Sertoli cells of the testis and granulosa cells of the ovary (54 for review). It inhibits secretion of follicle-stimulating hormone (FSH) of the pituitary gland. In addition to its endocrine effects, inhibin has been found to suppress growth of CFU-Mix, BFU-E, and erythroid colony-forming cells (55) (CFU-E), but only when these progenitor cells are stimulated by the FSH-releasing factor activin (56). Inhibin has no effect on growth of CFU-GM, CFU-G, or CFU-M. The stimulatory effects of activin on CFU-Mix, BFU-E, and CFU-E growth seem to be mediated through T-lymphocytes, since some of the hematopoietic enhancing activities of activin could be inactivated by preincubation of T-lymphocyte-conditioned medium with antibodies against GM-CSF, IL-3, or erythroid potentiating activity (EPA). There is also evidence to suggest that activin may be able to synergize with EPA, IL-3, GM-CSF, and G-CSF on the stem/progenitor cell level (57).

VII. ONCOSTATIN M

Oncostatin M is produced by activated human monocytes and T-cells as a 252-amino acid polypeptide (58). Oncostatin M was originally identified by its ability to inhibit in synergy with TGF-β the replication of some human tumor cell lines but not normal diploid fibroblasts. Oncostatin M also shares limited homology with several hematopoietic growth factors which have an N-terminal consensus sequence in common of Ala-Ser-Xaa-Ser or Ala-Pro-Xaa-Arg (59).

VIII. TRANSFORMING GROWTH FACTOR β

TGF-β is a negative regulator of hematopoiesis and acts directly at the level of stem/progenitor cells (9 for review). Platelets are the prime cellular source of TGF-β. Multipotential and bipotential progenitor cells appear to be sensitive to the inhibitory action of TGF-β, whereas unipotential, more mature progenitor cells are insensitive (60).

IX. TUMOR NECROSIS FACTORS

TNF-α and lymphotoxin (LT; also termed TNF-β) are myelosuppressive, have synergistic suppressive activities with interferons, have direct-acting effects on hematopoietic stem/progenitor cells (61), but are also able to induce or augment the release of CSF and other hematopoietic regulators from accessory cells (Table 2). Although both TNF species share the same receptor, TNF-α is believed to be a stronger cytokine inducer than LT (44). Interestingly, TNF-α has been reported to stimulate the growth of myeloid leukemia cells when used in combination with GM-CSF, contrasting the results obtained with normal cells (62).

X. INTERFERONS

α-, β_1-, and γ- have direct-acting suppressive effects on hematopoietic stem/progenitor cells in vitro (63). γ-INF also has a differentiating capacity on myeloid leukemia cells. In addition to direct-acting suppressive effects on progenitors, IFN can also induce or enhance release of CSF and other cytokines from accessory cells (Table 2). Depending on the costimulus, γ-IFN can also down-regulate accessory cell expression of hematopoietic regulators such as IL-1 and G-CSF (64,65).

XI. LEUKEMIA INHIBITORY FACTOR

LIF does not directly influence the growth of normal hematopoietic progenitor cells but does suppress the differentiation of normal pluripotent embryonic stem cells (66). LIF was originally identified by its ability to induce differentiation and inhibit proliferation of mouse M1 leukemic cells (67).

XII. E-TYPE PROSTAGLANDINS

The E-type prostaglandins PGE 1 and PGE 2 have inhibitory activities on granulocyte-macrophage progenitor cells, with CFU-M being the most sensitive cells for their suppressive activity (68). PGE has, however, no activity on CFU-G but can enhance growth of BFU-E by effects mediated through T-cells (69).

XIII. IRON-BINDING HEMATOPOIETIC REGULATORS

Lactoferrin (LF), acidic isoferritin (AIF), and transferrin (TF) are iron-binding proteins that have been implicated as regulators of hematopoiesis. Although iron is necessary for the action of these molecules, the role in its effect on hematopoiesis is presently unknown. It might well be that the iron molecule causes a conformational change of the binding proteins and thus allows them to bind to their receptors. LF is produced and stored in cells of the granulocyte lineage. LF decreases release of CSF from monocytes and also decreases IL-1 production which could then spur other cells to secrete CSF (70,71). TNF-α has been shown to control the expression of LF. Leukemia cells seem to be less responsive than normal progenitor cells to its suppressive effects (72). Like LF, TF has been found to inhibit release of CSF from accessory cells (73). AIF has direct-acting myelosuppressive effects on hematopoietic progenitor cells (74). As with LF, decreased responsiveness of leukemia cells to the effects of AIF have been reported (72).

REFERENCES

1. Cline MJ, Golde DW. Nature 1979;277:177.
2. Broxmeyer HE. Int J Cell Clon 1986;4:378.
3. Clark SC, Kamen R. Science 1987; 236:1229.
4. Roberts RA, Gallagher J, Spooncer E et al. Nature 1988; 332:376.
5. Gordon MY, Riley GP, Clarke D. Leukemia 1988; 2:804.
6. Harrison DE, Astle CM. J Exp Med 1982; 156:1767.
7. Till JE, McCulloch E. Biochem Biophys Acta 1980; 605:431.
8. Fauser AA, Messner HA. Blood 1978; 52:1243.
9. Axelrad AA. Exp Hematol 1990; 18:143.
10. Nicola NA. Immunol Today 1987; 8:134.
11. Weber SC, Lalik PH, Farley BA et al. Blood 1989; 74:192 (abstr).
12. Broxmeyer HE, Hangoc G, Cooper S, Shen F. Blood 1989; 74:111 (abstr).
13. Leary AG, Yang YC, Clark SC et al. Blood 1987; 70:1343.
14. Sieff CA, Niemeyer CM, Natahn DG et al. J Clin Invest 1987; 79:48.

15. Platzer E, Welte K, Gabrilove J et al. J Exp Med 1985; 162:1788.
16. Ralph P, Warren MK, Nakoinz I et al. Immunobiology 1986; 172:194.
17. Sieff CA, Neimeyer CM. Behring Inst Mitt 1988; 83:97.
18. Carraciolo D, Shirsat N, Wong GG et al. J Exp Med 1987; 166:1851.
19. Breen FN, Hume DA, Weidemann MJ. Br J Haematol 1990; 74:138.
20. Schaafsma RM, Falkenburg JHF, Duinkerken N et al. Blood 1989; 74:2398.
21. Herrmann F, Oster W, Meuer SC et al. J Clin Invest 1988; 81:1415.
22. Zucali JR, Dinarello CA, Oblon DJ et al. J Clin Invest 1986; 77:1837.
23. Stanley ER, Bartocci A, Patinkin A et al. Cell 1986; 45:667.
24. Hangoc G, Williams DE, Falkenburg JHF et al. J Immunol 1989; 142:4329.
25. Naldini A, Fleischmann WR, Ballas ZK et al. J Immunol 1987; 139:1880.
26. Burdach SEG, Levitt L. Blood 1987; 69:1368.
27. Oster W, Lindemann A, Mertelsmann R, Herrmann F. Eur J Immunol 1989; 19:543.
28. Peschel C, Paul W, Ohara J, Green I. Blood 1987; 70:254.
29. Tsuji K, Nakahata T, Takagi M et al. Blood 1990; 75:421.
30. Jansen JH, Wientjens GJHM, Fibbe WE et al. J Exp Med 1989; 170:577.
31. De Wolf JTM, Beentjes JAM, Esselink MT. Br J Haematol 1990; 74:246.
32. Broxmeyer HE, Lu L, Cooper S et al. J Immunol 1988; 141:3852.
33. Wieser M, Bonifer R, Oster W et al. Blood 1989; 73:1105.
34. Henschler R, Mantovani L, Oster W et al. Br J Haematol 1990 (in press).
35. Seelentag WK, Mermod JJ, Montesano R, Vasalli P. EMBO J 1987; 6:2261.
36. Mantovani L, Henschler R, Brach MA. Eur J Biochem 1990 (in press).
37. Van Damme J, Opdenakker G, Simpson RJ et al. J Exp Med 1987; 165:914.
38. Munker R, Gasson J, Ogawa M, Koeffler HP. Nature 1986; 323:79.
39. Koeffler HP, Gasson J, Tobler A. Mol Cell Biol 1988; 8:3423.
40. Akashi M, Louissararian AH, Adelman DC et al. J Clin Invest 1990; 85:121.
41. Klein H, Becher R, Lübbert W et al. J Exp Med 1990 (in press).
42. Rambaldi A, Young DC, Griffin JD. Blood 1987; 69:1409.
43. Herrmann F, Cannistra SA, Lindemann A et al. J Immunol 1989; 142:138.
44. Oster W, Lindemann A, Horn S et al. Blood 1987; 70:1700.
45. Brach MA, Henschler R, Hirano T et al. FEBS Lett 1990 (in press).
46. Ikebuchi K, Wong GG, Clark SC et al. Proc Natl Acad Sci USA 1987; 84:9035.
47. Bot F, van Eijk L, Broeders L et al. Blood 1989; 73:435.
48. Carraciolo D, Clark SC, Rovera G. Blood 1989; 73:666.
49. Matsushima K, Oppenheim JJ, Cytokine 1989; 1:2.
50. Van Damme J, van Beeumen J, Opdenakker G, Billiau A. J Exp Med 1988; 167:1364.
51. Davatelis, G, Tekamp-Olson P, Wolpe SD et al. J Exp Med 1988; 167:1939.
52. Wolpe SD, Cerami A. FASEB J 1989; 3:2565.
53. Broxmeyer HE. In: Mertelsman R, Hermann F, eds. Hematopoietic growth factors in clinical applications. New York: Marcel Dekker, 1990 (in press).
54. Val W, Hsueh A, Rivier C, Yu Y. In: Sporn MB, Roberts AB, eds. Peptide growth factors and their receptors. New York: Springer Verlag, 1990 (in press).
55. Yu Y, Shao LE, Lemas V et al. Nature 1987; 330:765.
56. Yu J, Shao LE, Vaughan J et al. Blood 1989; 73:952.
57. Lu L, Lin ZH, Shen RN et al. Blood 1989; 74:74 (abstr).
58. Malik N, Kallestad JC, Gunderson N et al. Mol Cell Biol 1989; 9:2847.
59. Schrader JW, Ziltner JH, Leslie KB. Proc Natl Acad Sci USA 1986; 74:2458.
60. Keller JR, Mantel C, Sing GK et al. J Exp Med 1988; 168:737.
61. Broxmeyer HE, Williama DE, Lu L et al. J Immunol 1986; 136:4487.
62. Hoang T, Levy B, Onetto N et al. J Exp Med 1989; 170:15.
63. Broxmeyer HE, Lu L, Platzer E et al. J Immunol 131:1300.
64. Ghezzi P, Dinarello CA. J Immunol 140:4238.

65. Riedel D, Lindemann A, Otto J et al. Cancer Res (submitted).
66. Williams RL, Hilton DJ, Pease S et al. Nature 1988; 336:684.
67. Gough NM, Gearing DP, King JA et al. Proc Natl Acad Sci USA 1988; 85:2632.
68. Pelus LM, Broxmeyer HE, Kurland JI, Moore MAS. J Exp Med 1979; 150:277.
69. Lu L, Broxmeyer HE. Exp Hematol 1985; 13:989.
70. Broxmeyer HE, Smithyman A, Eger RR et al. J Exp Med 1978; 148:1052.
71. Babgy GC, Mcall E, Bergstrom KA et al. J Clin Invest 1981; 68:156.
72. Broxmeyer HE. In: de Souza M, Brock JH, eds. Iron in immunity and inflammation. New York: John Wiley, 1978:199.
73. Broxmeyer HE, Lu L, Bognacki J. Blood 1983; 62:37.
74. Williams, DE, Cooper S, Broxmeyer HE. Cancer Res 1988; 48:1548.

11

Cytokine-Stimulated Emigration of Granulocytes in Vivo

DENNIS E. VAN EPPS
Baxter Healthcare Corporation, Round Lake, Illinois

I. INTRODUCTION

Chemotactic factors released at sites of inflammation or antigenic challenge play a major role in the recruitment of leukocytes from the circulation to these sites. The nature of this cellular response differs dramatically depending on the stimulus and can range from a predominantly neutrophil infiltrate as observed with IgG antibody-antigen complex mediated responses to a mononuclear cell infiltrate associated with T-cell-mediated reactions. The basis for the selective appearance of different cell types in association with these different inflammatory reactions is thought to be due to the production and release of unique chemoattractants at the site of inflammation as well as to the presence of the specific receptors for these individual chemoattractants on selected cell types. One of the best examples of this selectivity is the classic Arthus response associated with an antibody-antigen-mediated complement activation and leading to a cellular infiltrate consisting predominantly of neutrophils (PMN). The preferential emigration of PMN in this type of response can be attributed to a large extent to the release of the complement-derived chemoattractant C5a, which selectively attracts these cells. In this case, the nature of the reaction (immune complex-stimulated complement activation) and the restricted expression of C5a receptors on neutrophils and monocytes (1) governs the types of cells that respond. In addition, the predominance of PMN in this reaction reflects their great number in the peripheral circulation as well as their ability to migrate rapidly from the vasculature into the tissues. This preferential recruitment of specific cell types has also been postulated for reactions associated with T-lymphocytic infiltrates, where antigen-driven production of T-cell chemotactic factors such as IL-2 or other lymphocyte chemoattractants (2–6) may be produced. Likewise, selective stimuli for monocyte chemotaxis (7) and eosinophil chemotaxis (8) have also been described and may account for an accumulation of these cells in reactions associated with

T-cell-mediated immune responses (lymphocyte-derived monocyte chemotactic factors) or allergic reactions (eosinophil chemotactic factors).

Although it is tempting to associate the in-vitro chemotactic activity of cytokines for a specific cell type with their ability to stimulate the influx of particular cell types in vivo, it is important to note that other factors may influence the mobilization of leukocytes to an inflammatory site and that, generally, it is not just a single chemoattractant that is produced at that site. Figure 1 summarizes some of the major factors and responses that may influence both the nature and the magnitude of the leukocyte response in vivo. These include vascular responses, which can potentially alter blood flow and cell delivery; the responsiveness and numbers of circulating cells themselves; changes in endothelial cells, which can influence vasopermeability; adherence of leukocytes to vessel walls; and the generation and regulation of inflammatory mediators and cytokines at the inflammatory site, which may stimulate or suppress the emigration of leukocytes. As shown in Figure 1, the mobilization of leukocytes to an inflammatory site involves a complex set of events subject to positive and negative regulation at a number of different steps. It is the cumulative effect of all of these events that dictates the nature and amplitude of the cellular response at a site of inflammation.

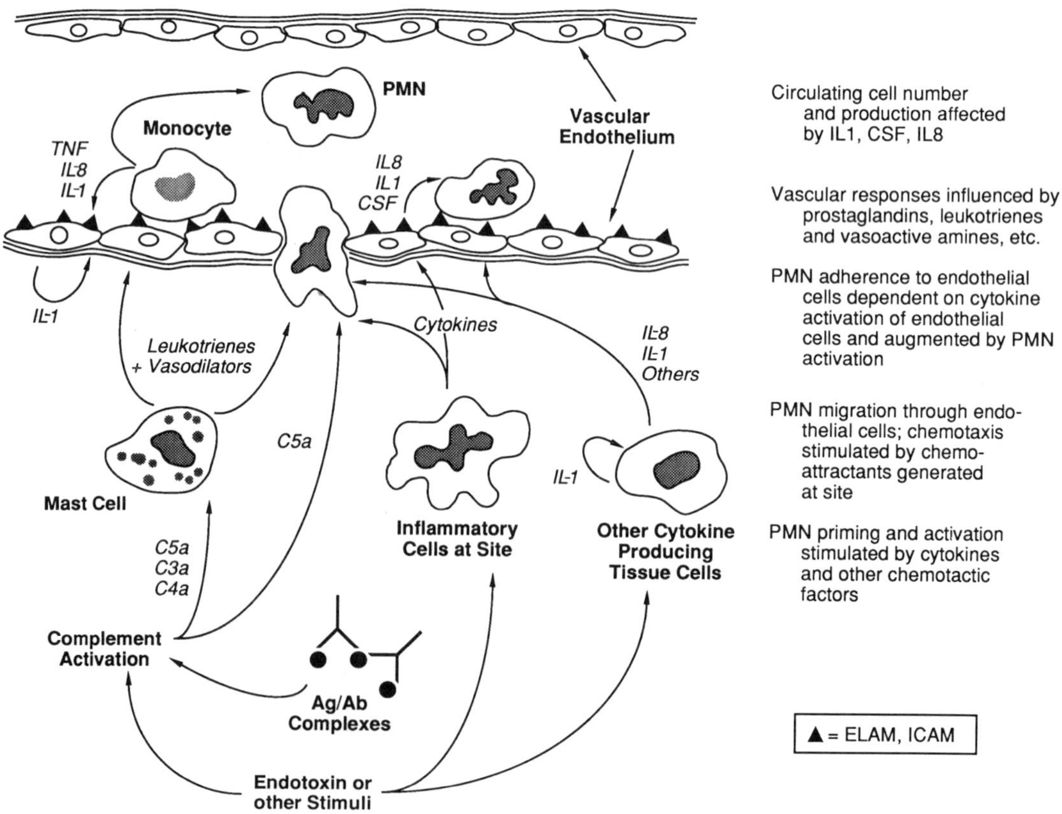

Figure 1 Model of the interactions of cytokines and regulators that influence PMN mobilization in vivo.

Over the past several years it has become apparent that several cytokines play an important role in the in-vivo mobilization of leukocytes to an inflammatory site. Many of the advances made in our understanding of these events have resulted from the production of recombinant cytokines, which have provided a means to efficiently evaluate and compare the actions and interactions of these bioactive polypeptides both in vitro and in vivo. Until this occurred, most of our knowledge of the role of these cytokines in the inflammatory response resulted from in-vitro studies using individual cytokines and single-cell populations in classic assays of leukocyte chemotaxis such as the Boyden chamber (9) or agarose methods (10). However, it has become apparent that these cytokines and other chemotactic factors do not act alone, but rather in concert with one another, both in vitro and in vivo. In many cases, such as with interleukin-1 (IL-1) and tumor necrosis factor α (TNF_α), it is clear that one cytokine not only acts collaboratively with another, but can induce the production of other cytokines or the same cytokine itself in an autocrine fashion, thereby amplifying the inflammatory process. Furthermore, it is apparent that there is not a single target cell, but multiple targets for many of these cytokines, which greatly adds to the complexity of the in-vivo inflammatory reaction. It is the purpose of this review to focus on the role of those cytokines in the stimulation of neutrophil migration in vivo and to discuss the interrelationships of these agents in the development of the inflammatory response. Table 1 lists the major cytokines that have been found to stimulate neutrophil function in vitro or to elicit a neutrophil response in vivo.

I. INTERLEUKIN-1 AS A STIMULUS FOR PMN EMIGRATION

One of the most extensively studied cytokines with the potential to stimulate PMN function and emigration in vivo is the 16- to 18-kDa protein, IL-1. IL-1 exists in at least two forms, α and β, which are the products of two different genes. Although the two proteins have only 28% sequence homology, they have similar biological activities. They have been shown to compete for the same receptors, although recent studies have indicated that IL-1 receptors may be of more than one type (11,12). IL-1 is produced by a variety of different cell types and has a broad spectrum of physiological functions and target cells (reviewed in Ref. 13). The most important sources of this cytokine with respect to PMN emigration in vivo are monocytes, endothelial cells (13–15), tissue macrophages (16–20), keratinocytes and Langerhans cells (21,22), T-cells (23), PMN (24), and fibroblasts (25). These cells may serve as either an initial source of IL-1 following an inflammatory stimulus or as amplifier cells providing additional IL-1 at a site where other cytokines or mediators trigger IL-1 production. Examples of agents that may trigger IL-1 production include bacteria, viruses, silica, asbestos and urate crystals (reviewed in Ref. 13), and exposure to ultraviolet irradiation (26). IL-1 can also be produced as a result of antigen recognition and processing by antigen-presenting cells and T-cells (27–32). This in turn can result in an autocrine response by the T-cell or macrophage, leading to additional IL-1 production (33–35) or to the generation of other cytokines that can in turn trigger IL-1 production. Some of the cytokines that have been shown to stimulate IL-1 production include GM-CSF, TNF_α (36), TGF_β (37), and α- and β-interferon (38). C5a has also been shown to stimulate IL-1 mRNA transcription and IL-1 and TNF production by human monocytes (39) and murine macrophages (40), indicating an additional link between complement-induced inflammation and IL-1 production.

Table 1 Cytokines That Stimulate Neutrophil Function and/or Emigration

Cytokine	Source	Activity on PMN Response	References
Interleukin-1	Monocytes, endothelial cells, keratinocytes, epithelial cells, fibroblasts	• Increases PMN adhesion to endothelial cells • Priming • Stimulates Il-1, TNF, and NAP-1 production by other cells • Stimulates in-vivo emigration • Increases circulating number	88,92,111,146
Tumor necrosis factors alpha and beta	Macrophages, T-cells	• Immigration in vivo • Chemotaxis • Priming • Superoxide production • Adherence to endothelial cells • Degranulation • Increases circulating number	86,88,91,92,96, 111,147–149
Interleukin-8 NAP-1 LCF MONAP-1 GCP NAF NCF TCF LDCF	Monocytes, T-cells, endothelial cells, fibroblasts, keratinocytes, chondrocytes	• Chemotaxis • Priming • Inhibition of endothelial cell-PMN adherence • In-vivo accumulation of PMN and plasma leakage • Increases CR1 expression • Degranulation • Increases circulating number	42,90,111,115, 119,122,150,151
GM-CSF G-CSF	T-cells, fibroblasts	• Priming • Degranulation • Increases surface receptors (CR1, CR3), FCR III	44–47,130,147
γ-Interferon	T-cells	• Increases in FCRI and FCR III • Synergy with TNF	96,130

IL-1 itself also initiates the release of a variety of other cytokines, which in turn play an active role in augmenting PMN emigration. For example, it has been shown that IL-1 stimulates the production of TNF (41) and neutrophil-activating peptide (NAP-1), also known as IL-8 (42,43). IL-1 has also been shown to stimulate the release of GM-CSF and G-CSF from fibroblasts, endothelial cells, and T-lymphocytes (44–48). Release of these colony-stimulating factors in turn enhances the production of PMN by the bone marrow, activates circulating PMN, and primes PMN so that they become hyperresponsive to a second stimulus, thereby enhancing their function (49–56). The complexity of these interrelationships makes it difficult to define a direct or indirect role for IL-1 in controlling the in-vivo mobilization of PMN. It is likely that IL-1 acts both ways to trigger PMN emigration in vivo, with the amplitude and regulation of an IL-1-induced PMN response depending on the type of stimulus, the site of inflammation, and the synergy between it and other cytokines.

Early studies with mononuclear cell-derived IL-1 suggested that IL-1 had chemotactic activity for human granulocytes (57), but these studies have not been confirmed with recombinant IL-1 (58), and it is felt that there is only minimal, if any, direct chemotactic activity associated with IL-1 alone. It is clear, however, that even though r-IL1 does not stimulate a strong PMN emigration in vitro, it is a major stimulus for PMN emigration in vivo (59–61), thus emphasizing the point that in-vivo and in-vitro responses with respect to leukocyte chemotaxis do not always agree.

The evaluation of PMN emigration in vivo has been studied using many different model systems, ranging from skin windows (62) to direct injection of the synovium, peritoneal cavity, footpad, or skin, to sponge-implantation models where responding cells can be extracted and quantitated (59–61). Although a variety of stimuli have been studied using these techniques, this review will focus on only those where in-vivo PMN emigration in response to cytokines has been evaluated. In the case of IL-1, Cybulski et al. (63) have described a rabbit model system using ^{51}Cr-neutrophils to evaluate the PMN influx in response to intradermal injection of IL-1 into skin. In this model a marked influx of PMN was observed within hours of injection. By comparison with TNF_{α}, IL-1α was a superior stimulus (61), showing a threshold response at 10^{-14} M for IL-1 as compared to 10^{-11} M for TNF. In other studies, both IL-1α and -β were found to be effective stimuli for PMN emigration, with IL-1α being the more potent of the two (64). The timing of the response was similar with IL-1 and TNF, showing a peak neutrophil influx in 1 to 2 h with clearance of the majority of ^{51}Cr label from the tissue by 3 h. Similar results were also obtained with murine macrophage IL-1, with a peak response occurring at 3 h. Histological studies of PMN emigration in response to IL-1 were performed by Granstein et al. using epidermal cell-derived thymocyte-activating factor (ETAF) produced by keratinocytes and biochemically equivalent to IL-1 (65). In their studies using mouse-footpad injection of IL-1, PMN were found to emigrate into injected regions with a peak response occurring at approximately 4 h. This was preceded by margination of PMN in blood vessels, which was observed 1 h after injection. Although these studies demonstrate that PMN respond to IL-1 in vivo, they did not provide quantitative data on the comparative immigration of PMN, monocytes/macrophages, or lymphocytes, so it is difficult to draw any conclusions as to the selective recruitment of a particular cell type by IL-1.

In other studies (59), a model system was developed to evaluate and quantitate the influx of PMN, lymphocytes, and monocytes in response to IL-1. In this system, collagen sponges were implanted subcutaneously in mice. After a 48-h recovery time, these sponges were injected with rIL-1α or control buffer. At various times after injection, sponges were removed and digested with collagenase, resulting in a suspension of the emigrating cells. As shown in Figure 2, cell counts and differentials showed an influx of PMN which peaked at 6 h, followed by resolution of the response by 14 h. It is apparent that the predominant cell type responding to IL-1 under these conditions is the PMN (59), with no significant increase in the emigration of macrophages or lymphocytes. As compared to other studies, the peak emigration of PMN in response to IL-1 is somewhat slower in this model, which may reflect the necessity for cells to migrate a greater distance into the sponge rather than into the tissue as in previous studies. Because IL-1 shows little chemotactic activity in vitro, the mechanism of PMN immigration in response to IL-1 must be dependent on other IL-1 mediated events.

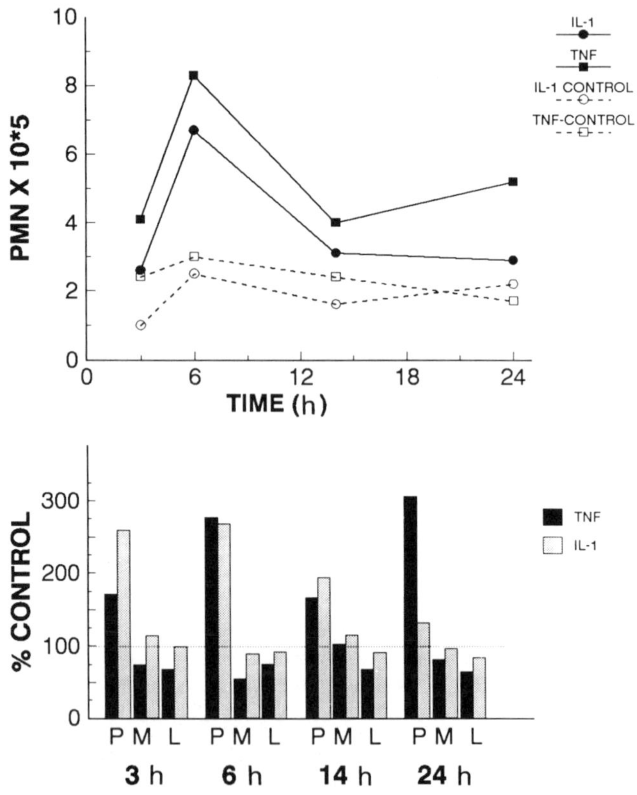

Figure 2 Emigration of leukocytes into subcutaneous collagen sponge implants in response to the injection of 5U of IL-1 over 0.2 μg of TNF$_{\alpha}$. The emigration of PMN into sponges over time as compared to control-media injections is shown in the upper panel. Each point represents the mean of at least three injected sponges. Significant ($p < 0.03$) increases as compared to the control populations were observed with IL-1 at 6 and 14 h and with TNF at 6 and 24 h. The distributions of cell types (P = PMN, M = macrophage, L = lymphocytes) in the harvested populations are shown in the lower panel. Data on cell distribution are expressed as a percent of the number of similar cell types in the control population. Details of this methodology using this murine model can be found in Ref. 60.

In considering the action of IL-1, it is apparent that it can potentially affect the emigration of PMN in three ways. First, as has been shown by several investigators, IL-1 stimulates the expression of endothelial leukocyte adherence molecule (ELAM) and intracellular adherence molecules 1 and 2 (ICAM-1 and -2) (66–70) on endothelial cells. These proteins, which are recognized by PMN, adhere to the endothelium and subsequently traverse this cellular lining into the tissue. This response is dependent not only on the expression of adherence proteins on the endothelium, but also on the expression of complementary adhesion proteins such as LFA-1 (CD11a) and CR3 (CD11b) on the PMN. This interaction represents a primary step in mobilizing PMN to the inflammatory site. However, it does not convey the cell specificity observed after IL-1 injection, because T-lymphocytes can also bind to IL-1-stimulated endothelial cells (71).

Second, IL-1 affects PMN emigration by stimulating the release of PMN from the bone marrow (reviewed in Refs. 13, 72, and 73), thereby increasing the numbers of PMN in the circulation that are able to respond to inflammatory stimuli. This may explain the slightly increased number of PMN found even in control sites in the murine sponge model of PMN emigration following distal injection of IL-1 (Figure 2). In addition, IL-1 can trigger the release of colony-stimulating factors such as G or GM-CSF, which in turn stimulate the production of PMN by the bone marrow. This action, however, may not effect the immediate influx of PMN, since the response time for production of PMN would be relatively slow by comparison to the influx of PMN.

Third, IL-1 can modulate PMN emigration by serving as a potent stimulus for the release of vasoactive agents such as PGI_2 (74) or PGE_2 (75) and chemoattractants such as NAP-1/IL-8, and CSF, which in turn can specifically attract PMN to the inflammatory site (76–78). This action of IL-1 may explain why it is a particularly potent stimulus for PMN emigration, since it may serve to amplify the local production of multiple PMN chemoattractants. In addition to stimulating the release of other cytokine chemoattractants, IL-1 can also stimulate endothelial cells to release platelet-activating factor (PAF), which is a potent in-vitro PMN chemoattractant (79,80) and an in-vivo chemoattractant for PMN when tested in rats with the skin window method (62).

Thus it is clear that IL-1, although lacking in-vitro chemotactic activity for PMN, is a potent stimulus for PMN emigration in vivo. Its ability to alter endothelial cells, to mobilize circulating PMN, and to induce the production of a variety of PMN chemoattractants indicates that this cytokine plays a major role in the inflammatory process. The importance of IL-1 in triggering the inflammatory process in vivo is further emphasized by its broad presence in cells throughout the host and its induction by many exogenous stimuli. This action, coupled with its multitude of physiological effects, including acute-phase reactant release and induction of fever (81) corticosteroid (82) and prostaglandin (83) release, demonstrate that IL-1 is a major mediator of the local inflammatory reaction as well as the systemic response associated with an excessive inflammatory reaction.

III. TUMOR NECROSIS FACTOR AS A STIMULUS FOR PMN EMIGRATION

TNF_α, also known as cachectin, is a macrophage-derived, 18-kDa cytokine which shares many of the functional properties of IL-1. Early in-vitro studies of partially purified TNF_α showed that it was a potent chemoattractant for PMN (84), but like IL-1, later studies with recombinant TNF_α indicated that it lacked in-vitro chemotactic activity (58). There has, however, been some controversy with respect to the chemotactic activity of TNF_α in vitro, with some investigators actually reporting that TNF_α (85) inhibited PMN migration. More recent studies by Newman and Wilkinson (86) show that both TNF_α and TNF_β (lymphotoxin) stimulate morphological polarization of PMN, locomotion into micropore filters, and orientation in a TNF gradient. This response, however, is much lower than that observed with the classic chemoattractants such as formylated peptides. These latter data indicate that TNF is indeed a PMN chemoattractant by multiple criteria, although its potency may be less than that of other well-defined chemotactic factors. In spite of the controversy about in-vitro chemotactic activity, most studies have shown that TNF_α is a very potent in-vivo stimulus of PMN emigration (59,60,72,87,88).

TNF, like IL-1, stimulates mononuclear cells, fibroblasts, and keratinocytes to produce the well-characterized PMN chemoattractant NAP-1/IL-8 in vitro (42,89). Similarly, TNF has been shown to induce the production of NAP-1/IL-8 by endothelial cells (43,90), keratinocytes, and fibroblasts (42), and also to stimulate the emigration of PMN in vivo in rabbits, mice, and baboons (59,63,91). This cellular infiltrate is predominantly PMN, with little indication of a monocyte or lymphocyte response, as shown in Figure 2 using the subcutaneous murine-sponge-implant model described previously (59).

Like IL-1, TNF can influence the PMN emigration response in multiple ways. It can induce expression of adherence molecules such as ELAM and ICAM on endothelial cells (67–70), as well as augment the circulating PMN count (72). As mentioned previously, this activation of endothelial cells by TNF or IL-1 may be particularly important in the ability of PMN to bind to and migrate through endothelial cells into the tissues (92). This binding to endothelial cells is dependent on the expression of PMN adherence proteins (CD11b, CD11a) that are capable of recognizing activation/adherence proteins on endothelial cells (93).

Interestingly, neutrophilia induced by high doses of TNF is biphasic, with an initial peak occurring approximately 1.5 h after intravenous injection followed by a second peak 6 h later (72). Studies using indomethacin, which blocks IL-1-induced neutrophilia, show that only the second peak of TNF-induced neutrophilia is inhibited. This supports the hypothesis that TNF can induce IL-1 in vivo, with IL-1-induced PG then being responsible for the second-phase response. The induction of IL-1 release from endothelial cells and mononuclear cells in vitro also supports this concept (94,95). Not only can TNF act in concert with IL-1 by inducing its release, it also acts synergistically with IL-1 in both the stimulation of neutrophilia (72) and in-vivo emigration of PMN (59), providing a further augmentation of the inflammatory reaction. A similar synergy has been demonstrated with γ-interferon in vitro in assays of PMN superoxide production, receptor up-regulation, and phagocytosis (96). Thus, mobilization of PMN to an inflammatory site may be quickly amplified through the generation of multiple cytokines at that site.

Although a variety of chemotactic factors have been shown to induce PMN emigration in vivo, including C5a (59,88,97), leukotriene B_4, and formylated peptide (88), recent in-vivo studies by Cybulsky et al. (88) and by Rampart and Williams (87) indicate that the mechanisms of induction with different factors are quite independent. Specifically, PMN emigration in response to TNF and IL-1 appears to be highly dependent on protein synthesis and is inhibited by local injections of actinomycin D, cycloheximide, or puromycin, whereas C5a des arg (activated plasma) and formyl peptide-induced emigration of PMN in the rabbit is unaffected by these protein synthesis inhibitors. These studies imply that IL-1 and TNF effects in vivo may depend more on the induction and synthesis of other peptide chemoattractants, which in turn are responsible for the attraction of PMN to the site of inflammation.

IV. ROLE OF NAP-1/IL-8 IN THE EMIGRATION OF PMN IN VIVO

More recently, a cytokine that stimulates human PMN migration in vivo and in vitro, and now commonly referred to as NAP-1 or IL-8, has been described. This cytokine was discovered several years ago, and its final identification and function were approached from two directions due to its action on both human T-cell and PMN migration.

From the T-cell source, several investigators described a chemotactic factor produced in the mixed lymphocyte reaction (4) or by mitogen or antigen-stimulated mononuclear cells or T-cells (2,3,5,6) which stimulated the in-vitro chemotaxis of T-cells. It was later found that these supernatants contained at least two T-cell chemoattractants, one of which was IL-2 (2) and the other of which was a 10- to 18-KDa protein distinct from IL-2, IL-1, and other cytokines known at the time (2,3,5,6,98). This second chemoattractant was found to be produced by T-cells and to specifically stimulate CD4 but not CD8 T-cell migration in vitro (3). Evaluation of PMN chemotactic activity showed that at the concentrations found in concanavalin A-stimulated mononuclear and isolated T-cell supernatants there was little activity on other cell types including PMN. This T-cell chemotactic factor has been referred to as lymphocyte chemotactic factor (LCF), lymphocyte-derived chemotactic factor (LDCF), or T-cell chemotactic factor (TCF). With purification of the native material to homogeneity, it was discovered that this cytokine also had chemotactic activity for PMN, although dose-response curves showed that the in-vitro chemotactic activity for T-cells was greater than that for PMN (ED_{50} of approximately 1 nM for T-cells versus approximately 50 nM for PMN (Van Epps and Potter, unpublished data). Similar factors with T-lymphocyte chemotactic activity have since been described by Leonard et al. for NAP-1 (99) and by Larson et al. and Van Damme et al. for IL-8 (98,100). These latter studies defined a cytokine which was first discovered based on its PMN chemotactic activity, and was later found to also have chemotactic activity for T-cells.

NAP-1/IL-8 was first described in the supernatants of LPS-stimulated mononuclear cells (58), and was found to be produced by monocytes (101). This cytokine has now been cloned and well characterized (102) and is described in more detail elsewhere in this book (see Chapter 13). Subsequent sequence analysis of the T-lymphocyte chemotactic factor (LCF) harvested from concanavalin A-stimulated human mononuclear cells (2) shows that the sequence of the N-terminal 19 amino acids (Van Epps and Potter, unpublished data) is comparable to NAP-1/IL-8 (101), indicating that the T-cell chemotactic factor described in previous studies (2,3) and NAP-1/IL-8 are closely related, if not identical. LyNAP, described by Schroeder et al., has similar sequence homology (103).

Several investigators have now characterized multiple factors that compare closely in their primary amino acid sequence (58,89,100,101,104–108), which represent a "supergene" family of closely related cytokines with both T-cell and/or PMN chemotactic activity (109–111). This supergene family includes NAP-1/IL-8, platelet factor 4 (112), macrophage inflammatory protein-2 (110), and melanoma growth-stimulating activity [MGSA (113,114)]. NAP-1/IL-8 has been most extensively studied and has also been found to be produced by IL-1, TNF, and LPS but not by IL-6-stimulated endothelial cells (43,111), as well as by IL-1 and TNF-stimulated fibroblasts (90,115), keratinocytes (42), hepatocytes (116), and chondrocytes (117). Indeed, it may be that NAP-1/IL-8 represents the chemoattractant that is produced as a result of IL-1 or TNF injection in vivo, which in turn leads to the emigration of PMN. In vitro, NAP-1/IL-8 has been reported to stimulate a variety of PMN functions, including chemotaxis, superoxide anion production, and degranulation (105,118), although the production of superoxide anion has not been observed in other laboratories (111) including this one.

Some in-vivo studies with NAP-1/IL-8 have shown that it induces plasma leakage and neutrophil accumulation when injected into rabbit skin in picomole quantities (119). This response, however, required the co-injection of prostaglandin E, suggesting a synergism between this vasodilatory agent and the chemotactic peptide. In these studies the half-time to PMN immigration (72 min) and plasma leakage (56 min) were similar to that observed with formyl peptide (64 and 52 min, respectively). The rapid time course of the response to NAP-1/IL-8 as compared to the responses observed in other studies with IL-1 and TNF again suggests that IL-8 may be the effector substance triggered by IL-1 or TNF injection. In other studies, the intraperitoneal injection of NAP-1/IL-8 into mice resulted in a rapid increase in the number of PMN in the peripheral circulation as well as a selective increase in the number of PMN in the peritoneal cavity (111) over a period of hours. Subcutaneous injection of NAP-1/IL-8 induced the margination and emigration of lymphocytes as well as PMN in these studies, consistent with the dual activity of NAP-1/IL-8 as both a PMN and a T-cell chemoattractant.

Studies where NAP-1/IL-8 was injected into lymph nodes of Fisher rats resulted in an immigration of only lymphocytes, while intradermal injection resulted in both PMN and lymphocytes depending of dosage (78). Preliminary studies by Leonard et al. (120) indicate that intradermal injection of NAP-1/IL-8 in humans also stimulates a PMN infiltration.

Similarly, in-vivo PMN emigration was observed with the NAP-1/IL-8-related peptide MSGA in a rat model where 10^{-9} M MSGA was injected intradermally. The mechanism of this PMN mobilization is likely the same as that shown with NAP-1/IL-8, since studies indicate that these two peptides bind to the same receptor on PMN (111). This receptor has now been defined as a 58-KDa protein with a density of approximately 75,000 sites per PMN (121).

NAP-1/IL-8 has also been shown to induce the expression of CR1 (122) and CR3 (CD11b) on PMN, indicating that it, like other chemotactic factors such as C5a and FMLP, can induce the expression of cell surface proteins which enhance the functional activity and adherence of PMN to endothelial cells. The latter is particularly important in the mobilization of PMN to an inflammatory site in vivo, since the adherence to endothelial cells is highly dependent on CD11b (123). In contrast, however, to studies with IL-1, there is evidence that NAP-1/IL-8 may actually inhibit the binding of PMN to endothelial cells (124). Thus this cytokine may serve dual purposes in the mobilization of PMN to inflammatory sites in vivo. Still other studies by Carveth et al. (125) showed that NAP-1/IL-8 stimulated PMN adherence to endothelial cells via a mechanism that involved CD11/CD18 glycoproteins. The relationship between PMN stimulation and inhibition of binding to endothelial cells is not fully understood and will require further study to resolve what appears to be antagonist and agonistic activities of NAP-1/IL-8.

V. ACTIVITY OF COLONY-STIMULATING FACTORS AND γ-INTERFERON

Colony-stimulating factors, in particular G-CSF and GM-CSF, have been shown to activate PMN in vitro, increasing phagocytosis, superoxide anion production, and expression of CD11a, CD11b, and formyl peptide receptors (49,54,55,126,127). Although the specific role of CSFs in the emigration of PMN to an inflammatory site in vivo is not fully understood, their ability to stimulate the production of granulocytes by the bone marrow, to increase the circulating neutrophil counts, and to activate mature PMN implies that these cytokines can play an active role in the inflammatory process and neutrophil function. This role is further supported by the fact that endothelial cells are a source of colony-stimulating factors and can be triggered to produce these cytokines in response to IL-1, TNF, and lipopolysaccharide (LPS) (79). Thus these cytokines can be produced locally in response to a stimulus, and act both locally to activate PMN and systemically to stimulate the production of PMN by the bone marrow. More recent studies (53,128) have shown that intraperitoneal injection of GM-CSF as well as local production of GM-CSF in transgenic mice carrying an extra GM-CSF gene copy results in the presence of large numbers of macrophages and some neutrophils in the peritoneal cavity. This, however, appears to be due to the local production of cells in response to GM-CSF production and not totally to the influx of cells in response of GM-CSF.

γ-Interferon, although not an active stimulus for PMN migration, can also affect the mobilization and function of PMN through its synergistic activity with other cytokines as well as its ability to induce ICAM-1 expression on endothelial cells (79) and CR3 and high-affinity Fc receptors on PMN (129,130). As discussed previously, ICAM-1 serves as a receptor for LFA-1 and can enhance the binding of inflammatory cells to endothelial cells, thus providing the initial steps of the mobilization of PMN to an inflammatory site. It may also suppress myelopoiesis (131–133) and thus has the potential to influence PMN mobilization by direct action on the circulating cell number.

VI. REGULATION OF THE MIGRATION OF PMN IN VIVO

Regulation of the migration of PMN to an inflammatory site can occur at several levels. These include inhibition of cytokine production or function, alteration of the PMN ability to respond to the inflammatory stimulus, or changes in vascular permeability or the endothelial cell surface. Although a variety of substances and factors have been shown to inhibit cytokine production or the response of neutrophils to these cytokines in vitro, there is much less information available on the specific role of inhibitory substances on neutrophil emigration in vivo.

Inhibition of cytokine activity or production has probably been best studied with IL-1. Natural inhibitors of IL-1 synthesis and/or function include PGE_2, corticosteroids, uromodulin, TGF-β, and a variety of other less well characterized materials (reviewed in Ref. 134). PGE_2 is a particularly interesting regulator, since it both increases vascular leakage (119) when used in conjunction with NAP-1/IL-8 and inhibits the production of NAP-1/IL-8 (LCF) by stimulated T-cells (135) in vitro. It also plays an inhibitory role in the production of PMN by the bone marrow by suppressing hematopoietic cell proliferation (136) and the synthesis of colony-stimulating factors. These inhibitors can be produced by monocytes, the adrenals, virus-infected macrophages, granulocytes, keratinocytes, and lymphocytes. It is not difficult to imagine how such inhibitors might act in vivo to suppress IL-1 production or its function following the induction of an inflammatory reaction. More recently, a specific IL-1 receptor antagonist that appears to be a competitive inhibitor of IL-1 binding has been described (137,138). This protein has 26% homology with IL-1β and 19% homology with IL-1α but lacks IL-1 activity. This molecule may represent a unique mechanism for regulating IL-1 responses and consequently the in-vivo production of chemotactic factors and endothelial cell responses.

A naturally occurring neuropeptide, α-MSH, has also been studied in vivo by several investigators and found to be a potent inhibitor of IL-1 and TNF-mediated responses (73,139), including neutrophil emigration (60). This peptide has a broad spectrum of activity and has been shown to inhibit IL-1, endotoxin, and TNF-induced fever, leukocytosis, and acute-phase reactant release (73,139) in mice and rabbits. In addition, MSH has been shown to inhibit histamine-induced vasopermeability in rabbits, suggesting that it may act at the level of the vasculature (140). Figure 3 summarizes the inhibitory action of a single 0.1-ml intraperitoneal injection of 5×10^{-5} M

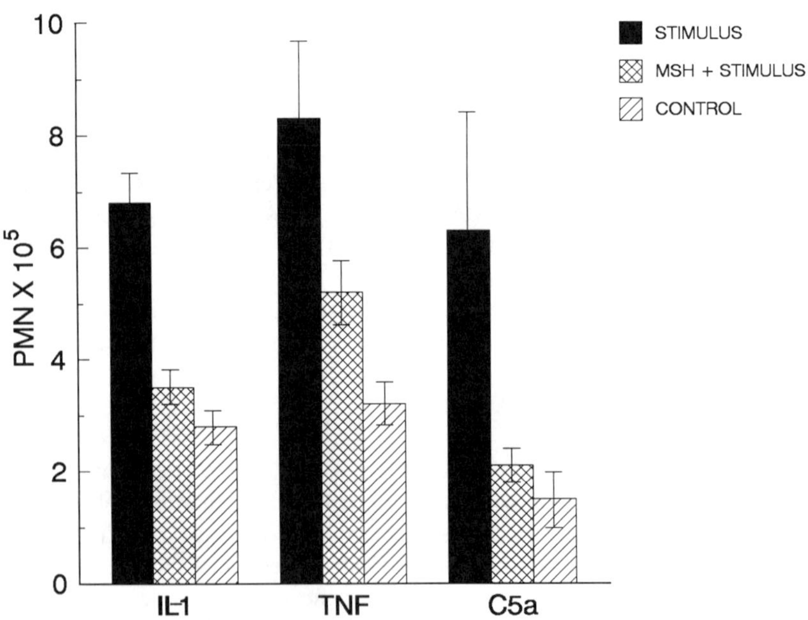

Figure 3 Inhibitory effect of intraperitoneal injection of α-MSH on the emigration of PMN into subcutaneous collagen sponges in response to 5U of IL-1, 0.2 μg of TNF_{α}, or 0.1 ml of 10^{-7} M human C5a. Each bar represents the mean of a minimum of six sponges, with the standard deviations indicated. In each case, the stimulus or control medium was injected into the subcutaneous sponge simultaneously with the intraperitoneal injection of 0.1 ml of 5×10^{-5} M α-MSH. All sponges were harvested 6 h postinjection. Details of this study can be found in Ref. 60.

MSH on the 6-h emigration of PMN into a site of TNF, IL-1, or C5a injection in the murine subcutaneous-sponge-implantation model (60). As shown, this peptide is highly effective at suppressing PMN emigration in vivo and is stimulus nonspecific, indicating that it does not interfere with the binding of TNF or IL-1 to their specific receptors. Previous studies have also shown (60) that, as with most good regulatory molecules, the inhibitory activity is short-lived; if MSH is injected more than 30 min prior to, or 60 min following, the injection of the inflammatory stimulus (IL-1), little inhibition of PMN emigration is observed. Of particular interest with respect to the action of this peptide in regulating the in-vivo migration of PMN is that MSH is released from the pituitary under conditions of stress (141,142), which provides a mechanism for rapid release and responsiveness to peripheral stimuli. The amino acid sequence of this peptide shows that it is homologous to the first 13 N-terminal amino acids of adrenocorticotropic hormone (ACTH), which is also released from the pituitary in response to IL-1 (82,143) and serves to stimulate the subsequent release of immunosuppressive corticosteroids from the adrenals. Although the mechanism through which MSH inhibits PMN emigration in vivo is not fully understood, its broad spectrum of activity, its regulated presence in the peripheral circulation (82,143), its reversible activity, and its limited duration of activity are consistent with a regulatory function.

A second mechanism of regulating the mobilization of PMN to an inflammatory site in vivo has been demonstrated by Cybulsky et al. (64), who showed that a primary injection of IL-1 or TNF into the skin of rabbits results in a cytokine-specific tachyphylaxis when tested 6 h later. In most cases, this primary injection of cytokine resulted in >75% reduction in the mobilization of PMN into inflammatory sites. Of importance in these experiments was that IL-1, but not TNF, induced a tachyphylaxis to LPS injection; and conversely, a primary LPS injection induced tachyphylaxis to IL-1, but not to TNF or other chemoattractants. These data indicate that receptor modulation within the tissue site may be involved in the regulation of PMN emigration to particular stimuli. Indeed, a similar type of cytokine-specific tachyphylaxis has been observed by Pober et al. (144) with endothelial cell expression of surface antigen in response to IL-1 or TNF. This inferred loss of cytokine receptor may provide a means of selectively modulating the inflammatory process to different stimuli. Without such regulation, infections or chronic production of an inflammatory mediator could result in the overproduction of cytokines through autocrine mechanisms, leading to an excessive and adverse inflammatory reaction.

Receptor modulation may play a major role in regulating the response of PMN to cytokines or other chemoattractants. It is clear from the literature that receptors for chemotactic factors capable of stimulating PMN emigration in vivo can be down-regulated following exposure to ligand. This is apparent from in-vitro studies with fluorescent C5a, where the ligand-receptor complex has been shown to be rapidly and specifically internalized within minutes (145). This internalization results in a loss of functional responsiveness (H_2O_2 production) to C5a after approximately 50% of the receptors have been internalized (Van Epps et al., manuscript submitted). The disappearance of these receptors is temporary, with reexpression occurring within 2 h in vitro through a protein synthesis-independent process (145). Full functional responsiveness also returns once these receptors return to at least 50% of their original level. Although functional responsiveness has not been correlated with a loss of cytokine receptors on PMN, recent data with NAP-1/IL-8 demonstrate that the receptor for this cytokine is down-regulated on PMN much like the receptor for C5a (111). In addition, similar to the PMN C5a receptor, IL-8 receptors are down-regulated and reexpressed within 10 min in a protein synthesis-independent manner, with this reexpression inhibited by the carboxylic ionophore for Na^+, monensin. This latter effect of monensin, which prevents lysosomal acidification, suggests that ligand-receptor dissociation is required for receptor recycling. It is thought that this process of receptor internalization and reexpression is essential to the directional migration of PMN in response to chemoattractants.

Although NAP-1/IL-8 has been shown to stimulate PMN function, it may also function as a regulator of the inflammatory process. Studies by Gimbrone et al. (124) have shown that cultured endothelial cells produce an inhibitor of neutrophil adhesion to cytokine-activated endothelial cells and protect these cells from PMN-mediated damage. This inhibitor was determined to be endothelial cell-derived IL-8, which is an extended amino-terminal variant of IL-8. This same phenomenon was also observed with recombinant NAP-1/IL-8. These observations demonstrate the complexity of the inflammatory reaction and the consequent influx of PMN in response to cytokine mediators.

VII. CONCLUSION

As summarized in this chapter, it is clear that cytokines play a major role in the mobilization of PMN to inflammatory sites in vivo. It is also apparent that these peptides do not act alone, but in synergy with one another. As with many other critical systems in the host, the inflammatory response can be triggered through a variety of mediators derived from the fixed tissue cells, infiltrating leukocytes, vascular endothelium, the complement and coagulation systems, as well as the neuroendocrine system. This apparent duplication of function provides an efficient host defense mechanism which cannot be easily subverted by the loss or inactivation of a single cytokine or inflammatory mediator. This makes it much more difficult for an invading microorganism to circumvent the host defenses and also provides a rapid means for the host to amplify the inflammatory response through the local generation of a multitude of stimuli. The major advances in the role of cytokines to date have been focused primarily on how the peptides trigger an inflammatory response and the consequent emigration of PMN. It would appear that the next step in understanding this response will be to determine how it is controlled in vivo and which cytokines and/or other agents regulate this response.

REFERENCES

1. Van Epps DE, Chenoweth DE. Analysis of the binding of fluorescent C5a and C3a to human peripheral blood leukocytes. J Immunol 1984; 132:2862–7.
2. Potter JW, Van Epps DE. Human T-lymphocyte chemotactic activity: nature and production in response to antigen. Cell Immunol 1986; 97:59–66.
3. Van Epps DE, Durant DA, Potter JW. Migration of human helper/inducer T cells in response to supernatants from Con A-stimulated suppressor/cytotoxic T cells. J Immunol 1983; 131:697–700.
4. El-Naggar AL, Van Epps DE, Williams RC. A human lymphocyte chemotactic factor produced by the mixed lymphocyte reaction. J Lab Clin Med 1982; 100:558–65.

5. Center DM, Cruikshank W. Modulation of lymphocyte migration by human lymphokines. I. Identification and characterization of chemoattractant activity for lymphocytes from mitogen-stimulated mononuclear cells. J Immunol 1982; 128:2563–8.
6. Cruikshank W, Center DM. Modulation of lymphocyte migration by human lymphokines. II. Purification of a lymphotactic factor (LCF). J Immunol 1982; 128:2569–74.
7. Leonard EJ, Yoshimura T. Human monocyte chemoattractant protein-1 (MCP-1). Immunol Today 1990; 11:97–101.
8. Kay AB, Stechschulte DJ, Austen KF. An eosinophil leukocyte chemotactic factor of analphylaxis. J Exp Med 1971; 133:602–19.
9. Boyden S. The chemotactic effect of mixtures of antibody and antigen on polymorphonuclear leukocytes. J Exp Med 1962; 135:453–66.
10. Nelson RD, Fiegel VD, Simmons RL. Chemotaxis of human polymorphonuclear neutrophils under agarose: morphologic changes associated with the chemotactic response. J Immunol 1976; 117:1676–83.
11. Lowenthal JW, MacDonald HR. Binding and internalization of Interkeukin 1 by T Cells. J Exp Med 1986; 164:1060–74.
12. Savage N, Puren AJ, Orencole SF, Ikejima T, Clark BD, Dinarello CA. Studies on IL-1 receptors on D10S T-helper cells: demonstration of two molecularly and antigenically distinct IL-1 binding proteins. Cytokine 1989; 1:23–35.
13. di Giovine FS, Duff GW. Interleukin 1: the first interleukin. Immunol Today 1990; 11:13–20.
14. Libby P, Ordovas JM, Birinyi KR, Auger KR, Dinarello CA. Inducible interleukin-1 gene expression in human vascular smooth muscle cells. J Clin Invest 1986; 78:1432–8.
15. Wagner CR, Vetto RM, Burger DR. Expression of I-region-associated antigen (Ia) and interleukin 1 by subcultured human endothelial cells. Cell Immunol 1985; 93:91–104.
16. Simon PL, Willoughby WF. The role of subcellular factors in pulmonary immune function: physicochemical characterization of two distinct species of lymphocyte-activating factor produced by rabbit alveolar macrophages. J Immunol 1981; 126:1534–41.
17. Dinarello CA, Bodel PT, Atkins E. The role of the liver in the production of fever and in pyrogenic tolerance. Trans Assoc Am Physicians 1968; 81:334–44.
18. Wood DD, Ihrie EJ, Hamerman D. Release of interleukin-1 from human synovial tissue *in vitro*. Arthr Rheum 1985; 28:853–62.
19. Murphy PA, Simon PL, Willoughby WF. Endogenous pyrogens made by rabbit peritoneal exudate cells are identical with lymphocyte-activating factors made by rabbit alveolar macrophages. J Immunol 1980; 124:2498–501.
20. Di Giovine FS, Malawista SE, Nuki G, Duff GW. Interleukin 1 (IL 1) as a mediator of crystal arthritis stimulation of T cell and synovial fibroblast mitogenesis by urate crystal-induced IL 1. J Immunol 1987; 138:3213–8.
21. Luger TA, Stadler BM, Luger BM, Mathieson BJ, Mage M, Schmidt JA, Oppenheim JJ. Murine epidermal cell-derived thymocyte-activating factor resembles murine interleukin 1. J Immunol 1982; 128:2147–52.
22. Sauder DN, Dinarello CA, Morhenn VB. Langerhans cell production of interleukin-1. J Invest Dermatol 1984; 82:605–7.
23. Tartakovsky B, Kovacs EJ, Takacs L, Durum SK. T cell clone producing an IL-1-like activity after stimulation by antigen-presenting B cells. J Immunol 1986; 137:160–6.
24. Goto K, Nakamura S, Goto F, Yoshinaga M. Generation of an interleukin-1-like lymphocyte-stimulating factor at inflammatory sites: correlation with the infiltration of polymorphonuclear leukocytes. Br J Exp Pathol 1984; 65:521–32.
25. Iribe H, Koga T, Kotani S, Kusumoto S, Shiba T. Stimulating effect of MDP and its adjuvant-active analogues on guinea pig fibroblasts for the production of thymocyte-activating factor. J Exp Med 1983; 157:2190–5.

26. Araneo BA, Dowell T, Moon HB, Daynes RA. Regulation of murine lymphokine production *in vivo*. Ultraviolet radiation exposure depresses IL-2 and enhances IL-4 production by T cells through an IL-1-dependent mechanism. J Immunol 1989; 143:1737–44.
27. Mizel SB. The interleukins. FASEB J 1989; 3:2379–88.
28. Durum SK, Gershon RK. Interleukin 1 can replace the requirement for I-A-positive cells in the proliferation of antigen-primed T cells. Proc Natl Acad Sci USA 1982; 79:4747–50.
29. Smith KA, Lachman LB, Oppenheim JJ, Favata MF. The functional relationship of the interleukins. J Exp Med 1980; 151:1551–6.
30. Scala G, Oppenheim JJ. Antigen presentation by human monocytes: evidence for stimulant processing and requirement for interleukin 1. J Immunol 1983; 131:1160–6.
31. DeFreitas EC, Chesnut RW, Grey HM, Chiller JM. Macrophage-dependent activation of antigen-specific T cells requires antigen and a soluble monokine. J Immunol 1983; 131:23–9.
32. Weaver CT, Unanue ER. T cell induction of membrane IL 1 on macrophages. J Immunol 1986; 137:3868–73.
33. Durum SK, Schmidt JA, Oppenheim JJ. Interleukin 1: an immunological perspective. Ann Rev Immunol 1985; 3:263–87.
34. Warner SJC, Auger KR, Libby P. Human interleukin 1 induces interleukin 1 gene expression in human vascular smooth muscle cells. J Exp Med 1987; 165:1316–31.
35. Manson JC, Symons JA, Di Giovine FS, Poole S, Duff GW. Autoregulation of interleukin 1 production. Eur J Immunol 1989; 19:261–5.
36. Dinarello CA, Cannon JG, Wolff SM, Bernheim HA, Beutler B, Cerami A, Figari IS, Palladino MA Jr, O'Connor JV. Tumor necrosis factor (cachectin) is an endogenous pyrogen and induces production of interleukin 1. J Exp Med 1986; 163:1433–50.
37. Wahl SM, Hunt DA, Wakefield LM, McCartney-Francis N, Wahl LM, Roberts AB, Sporn MB. Transforming growth factor type beta induces monocyte chemotaxis and growth factor production. Proc Natl Acad Sci USA 1987; 84:5788–92.
38. Candler RV, Rouse BT, Moore RN. Regulation of interleukin 1 production by alpha and beta interferons: evidence for both direct and indirect enhancement. J Interferon Res 1985; 5:179–89.
39. Okusawa S, Yancey KB, Van der Meer JWM, Endres S, Lonnemann G, Hefter K, Frank MM, Burke JF, Dinarello, CA, Gelfand JA. C5a stimulates secretion of tumor necrosis factor from human mononuclear cells *in vitro*. Comparison with secretion of interleukin 1 beta and interleukin 1 alpha. J Exp Med 1988; 168:443–8.
40. Goodman MG, Chenoweth DE, Weigle WO. Induction of interleukin 1 secretion and enhancement of humoral immunity by binding of human C5a to macrophage surface C5a receptors. J Exp Med 1982; 156:912–7.
41. Philip R, Epstein LB. Tumour necrosis factor as immunomodulator and mediator of monocyte cytotoxicity induced by itself, alpha-interferon and interleukin-1. Nature 1986; 323:86–9.
42. Larsen CG, Anderson AO, Oppenheim JJ, Matsushima K. Production of interleukin-8 by human dermal fibroblasts and keratinocytes in response to interleukin-1 or tumour necrosis factor. Immunology 1989; 68:31–6.
43. Strieter RM, Kunkel SL, Showell HJ, Remick DG, Phan SH, Ward PA, Marks RM. Endothelial cell gene expression of a neutrophil chemotactic factor by TNF-alpha, LPS, and IL-1 beta. Science 1989; 243:1467–9.
44. Zucali JR, Dinarello CA, Oblon DJ, Gross MA, Anderson L, Weiner RS. Interleukin 1 stimulates fibroblasts to produce granulocyte-macrophage colony-stimulating activity and prostaglandin E2. J Clin Invest 1986; 77:1857–63.
45. Sieff CA, Schickwann T, Faller DV. Interleukin 1 induces cultured human endothelial cell production of granulocyte-macrophage colony-stimulating factor. J Clin Invest 1987; 79:48–51.

46. Bagby GC Jr, Dinarello CA, Wallace P, Wagner C, Hefeneider S, McCall E. Interleukin 1 stimulates granulocyte macrophage colony-stimulating activity release by vascular endothelial cells. J Clin Invest 1986; 78:1316–23.
47. Segal GM, McCall E, Stueve T, Bagby GC Jr. Interleukin 1 stimulates endothelial cells to release multilineage human colony-stimulating activity. J Immunol 1987; 138:1772–8.
48. Herrmann F, Oster W, Meuer SC, Lindemann A, Mertelsmann RH. Interleukin 1 stimulates T lymphocytes to produce granulocyte-monocyte colony-stimulating factor. J Clin Invest 1988; 81:1415–8.
49. Kitagawa S, Yuo A, Souza LM, Saito M, Miura Y, Takaku F. Recombinant human granulocyte colony-stimulating factor enhances superoxide release in human granulocytes stimulated by the chemotactic peptide. Biochem Biophys Res Commun 1987; 144:1143–6.
50. Platzer E, Welte K, Gabrilove JL, Lu L, Harris P, Mertelsmann R, Moore MAS. Biological activities of a human pluripotent hemopoietic colony stimulating factor on normal and leukemic cells. J Exp Med 1985; 162:1788–801.
51. Lopez AF, Williamson DJ, Gamble JR, Begley CG, Harlan JM, Klebanoff SJ, Waltersdorph A, Wong G, Clark, SC, Vadas MA. Recombinant human granulocyte-macrophage colony-stimulating factor stimulates *in vitro* mature human neutrophil and eosinophil function, surface receptor expression, and survival. J Clin Invest 1986; 78:1220–8.
52. Gasson JC, Weisbart RH, Kaufman SE, Clark SC, Hewick RM, Wong GG, Golde DW. Purified human granulocyte-macrophage colony-stimulating factor: direct action on neutrophils. Science 1984; 226:1339–42.
53. Metcalf D, Begley CG, Johnson GR, Nicola NA, Vadas MA, Lopez AF, Williamson DJ, Wong GG, Clark SC, Wang EA. Biologic properties *in vitro* of a recombinant human granulocyte-macrophage colony-stimulating factor. Blood 1986; 67:37–45.
54. Shirafuji N, Matsuda S, Ogura H, Tani K, Kodo H, Ozawa K, Nagata S, Asano S, Takaku F. Granulocyte colony-stimulating factor stimulates human mature neurophilic granulocytes to produce interferon-alpha. Blood 1990; 75:17–9.
55. Cairo MS, Vende Ven C, Toy C, Mauss D, Sheikh K, Kommareddy S, Modanlou H. Lymphokines: enhancement by granulocyte-macrophage and granulocyte colony-stimulating factors of neonatal myeloid kinetics and functional activation of polymorphonuclear leukocytes. Rev Infect Dis 1990; 12:S492–7.
56. Kondo S, Okamura S, Ohhara N, Niho Y. Direct action of human granulocyte colony-stimulating factor on mature human neutrophils: flow-cytometric analysis. Res Commun Chem Pathol Pharmacol 1990; 67:249–57.
57. Sauder DN, Mounessa NL, Katz SI, Dinarello CA, Gallin JI. Chemotactic cytokines: the role of leukocytic pyrogen and epidermal cell thymocyte-activating factor in neutrophil chemotaxis. J Immunol 1984; 132:828–32.
58. Yoshimura T, Matsushima K, Oppenheim JJ, Leonard EJ. Neutrophil chemotactic factor produced by lipopolysaccharide (LPS)-stimulated human blood mononuclear leukocytes: partial characterization and separation from interleukin 1 (IL 1). J Immunol 1987; 139:788–93.
59. Mason MJ, Van Epps DE. *In vivo* neutrophil emigration in response to interleukin-1 and tumor necrosis factor-alpha. J Leuk Biol 1989; 45:62–8.
60. Mason MJ, Van Epps DE. Modulation of IL-1, tumor necrosis factor, and C5a-mediated murine neutrophil migration by alpha-melanocyte-stimulating hormone. J Immunol 1989; 142:1646–51.
61. Movat HZ, Cybulsky MI. Neutrophil emigration and microvascular injury role of chemotaxins, endotoxin, interleukin-1 and tumor necrosis factor-alpha. Inflammation 1987; 6:153–76.
62. Humphrey DM. Inflammatory exudates in skin windows induced by 1-O-alkyl-2-acetyl-sn-glyceryl-3-phosphorylcholine. Am J Pathol 1990; 136:467–77.

63. Cybulsky MI, Colditz IG, Movat HZ. The role of interleukin-1 in neutrophil leukocyte emigration induced by endotoxin. Am J Pathol 1986; 124:367–72.
64. Cybulsky MI, McComb DJ, Movat HZ. Neutrophil leukocyte emigration induced by endotoxin mediator roles of interleukin 1 and tumor necrosis factor alpha. J Immunol 1988; 140:3144–9.
65. Granstein RD, Margolis R, Mizel SB, Sauder DN. *In vivo* inflammatory activity of epidermal cell-derived thymocyte activating factor and recombinant Interleukin 1 in the mouse. J Clin Invest 1986; 77:1020–7.
66. Bevilacqua MP, Stengelin S, Gimbrone, MA Jr, Seed B. Endothelial leukocyte adhesion molecule 1: an inducible receptor for neutrophils related to complement regulatory proteins and lectins. Science 1989; 243:1160–5.
67. Bevilacqua MP, Pober JS, Mendrick DL, Cotran RS, Gimbrone MA Jr. Identification of an inducible endothelial-leukocyte adhesion molecule. Proc Natl Acad Sci USA 1987; 84:9238–42.
68. Pober JS, Gimbrone MA Jr, Lapierre LA, Mendrick DL, Fiers W, Rothlein R, Springer TA. Overlapping patterns of activation of human endothelial cells by interleukin 1, tumor necrosis factor, and immune interferon. J Immunol 1986; 137:1893–6.
69. Cotran RS, Gimbrone MA Jr, Bevilacqua MP, Mendrick DL, Pober JS. Induction and detection of a human endothelial activation antigen *in vivo.* J Exp Med 1986; 164:661–6.
70. Dustin ML, Rothlein R, Bhan AK, Dinarello CA, Springer TA. Induction by IL 1 and interferon-gamma: tissue distribution, biochemistry, and function of a natural adherence molecule (ICAM-1). J Immunol 1986; 137:245–54.
71. Van Epps DE, Potter J, Vachula M, Smith CW, Anderson DC. Suppression of human lymphocyte chemotaxis and transendothelial migration by anti-LFA-1 antibody. J Immunol 1989; 143:3207–10.
72. Ulich TR, del Castillo J, Keys M, Granger GA, Ni RX. Kinetics and mechanisms of recombinant human interleukin 1 and tumor necrosis factor-alpha-induced changes in circulating numbers of neutrophils and lymphocytes. J Immunol 1987; 139:3406–15.
73. Daynes RA, Robertson BA, Cho BH, Burnham DK, Newton R. Alpha-melanocyte-stimulating hormone exhibits target cell selectivity in its capacity to affect interleukin 1-inducible responses *in vivo* and *in vitro.* J Immunol 1987; 139:103–9.
74. Rossi V, Breviario F, Ghezzi P, Dejana E, Mantovani A. Prostacyclin synthesis induced in vascular cells by interleukin-1. Science 1985; 229:174–6.
75. Balavoine JF, deRochemonteix B, Williamson K, Seckinger K, Cruchaud A, Dayer JM. Prostaglandin E2 and collagenase production by fibroblasts and synovial cells is regulated by urine-derived human interleukin 1 and inhibitor(s). J Clin Invest 1986; 78:1120–4.
76. Broudy VC, Kaushansky K, Harlan JM, Adamson JW. Interleukin 1 stimulates human endothelial cells to produce granulocyte-macrophage colony-stimulating factor and granulocyte colony-stimulating factor. J Immunol 1987; 139:464–8.
77. Sieff CA, Neimeyer CM, Mentzer SJ, Faller DV. Interleukin-1, tumor necrosis factor, and the production of colony-stimulating factors by cultured mesenchymal cells. Blood 1988; 72:1316–23.
78. Wang JM, Chen ZG, Cianciolo GJ, Snyderman R, Breviario F, Dejana E, Mantovani A. Production of a retroviral P15E-related chemotaxis inhibitor by IL-1-treated endothelial cells. A possible negative feedback in the regulation of the vascular response to monokines. J Immunol 1989; 142:2012–7.
79. Mantovani A, Dejana E. Cytokines as communication signals between leukocytes and endothelial cells. Immunol Today 1989; 10:370–5.
80. Bussolino F, Breviario F, Aglietta M, Sanavio F, Bosia A, Dejana E. Studies on the mechanism of interleukin 1 stimulation of platelet activating factor synthesis in human endothelial cells in culture. Biochem Biophys Acta 1987; 927:43–5.

81. Dinarello CA. Interleukin-1 and the pathogenesis of the acute-phase response. N Engl J Med 1984; 311:1413–8.
82. Besedovsky H, DelRey A, Sorkin E, Dinarello CA. Immunoregulatory feedback between interleukin-1 and glucocorticoid hormones. Science 1986; 233:652–4.
83. Dayer JM, deRochemonteix B, Burrus B, Demczuk S, Dinarello CA. Human recombinant IL-1 stimulates collagenase and prostoglandin E production by human synovial cells. J Clin Invest 1986; 77:645–8.
84. Ming WJ, Bersani L, Mantovani A. Tumor necrosis factor is chemotactic for monocytes and polymorphonuclear leukocytes. J Immunol 1987; 138:1469–74.
85. Atkinson YH, Marasco WA, Lopez AF, Vadas MA. Recombinant human tumor necrosis factor-alpha regulation of N-formyl-methionyl-leucyl-phenylalanine receptor affinity and function on human neutrophils. J Clin Invest 1988; 81:759–65.
86. Newman I, Wilkinson PC. Chemotactic activity of lymphotoxin and tumour necrosis factor alpha for human neutrophils. Immunology 1989; 66:318–20.
87. Rampart M, Williams TJ. Evidence that neutrophil accumulation induced by interleukin-1 requires both local protein biosynthesis and neutrophil CD18 antigen expression *in vivo.* Br J Pharmacol 1988; 94:1143–8.
88. Cybulsky MI, McComb DJ, Movat HZ. Protein synthesis dependent and independent mechanisms of neutrophil emigration. Different mechanisms of inflammation in rabbits induced by interleukin-1, tumor necrosis factor alpha or endotoxin versus leukocyte chemoattractants. Am J Pathol 1989; 135:227–37.
89. Matsushima K, Morishita K, Yoshimura T, Lavu S, Kobayashi Y, Lew W, Appella E, Kung HF, Leonard EJ, Oppenheim JJ. Molecular cloning of a human monocyte-derived neutrophil chemotactic factor (MDNCF) and the induction of MDNCF mRNA by interleukin 1 and tumor necrosis factor. J Exp Med 1988; 167;1883–93.
90. Schroder JM, Sticherling M, Henneicke HH, Preissner WC, Christophers E. IL-1 alpha or tumor necrosis factor-alpha stimulate release of three NAP-1/IL-8-related neutrophil chemotactic proteins in human dermal fibroblasts. J Immunol 1990; 144:2223–32.
91. Munro JM, Pober JS, Cotran RS. Tumor necrosis factor and interferon-gamma induce distinct patterns of endothelial activation and associated leukocyte accumulation in skin of *Papio anubis.* Am J Pathol 1989; 135:121–33.
92. Furie MB, McHugh DD. Migration of neutrophils across endothelial monolayers is stimulated by treatment of the monolayers with interleukin-1 or tumor necrosis factor-alpha. J Immunol 1989; 143:3309–17.
93. Tonnesen MG. Neutrophil-endothelial cell interactions: mechanisms of neutrophil adherence to vascular endothelium. J Invest Dermatol 1989; 93:53S-8S.
94. Bachwich PR, Chensue SW, Larrick JW, Kunkel SL. Tumor necrosis factor stimulates interleukin-1 and prostaglandin E2 production in resting macrophages. Biochem Biophys Res Commun 1986; 136:94–101.
95. Nawroth PP, Bank I, Handley D, Cassimeris J, Chess L, Stern D. Tumor necrosis factor/cachectin interacts with endothelial cell receptors to induce release of interleukin 1. J Exp Med 1986; 163:1363–75.
96. Livingston DH, Appel SH, Sonnenfeld G, Malangoni MA. The effect of tumor necrosis factor-alpha and interferon-gamma on neutrophil function. J Surg Res 1989; 46:322–6.
97. Yancey KB, Swerlick RA, Lawley TJ. C5a as a mediator of cutaneous inflammation. Am J Dematopathol 1987; 9(2):138–43.
98. Larsen CG, Anderson AO, Appella E, Oppenheim JJ, Matsushima K. The neutrophil-activating protein (NAP-1) is also chemotactic for T lymphocytes. Science 1989; 243:1464–6.
99. Leonard EJ, Skeel A, Yoshimura T, Noer K, Kutvirt S, Van Epps DE. Leukocyte specificity and binding of human neutrophil attractant/activation protein-1. J Immunol 1990; 144:1323–30.

100. Van Damme J, Van Beeumen J, Opdenakker G, Billiau A. A novel, NH_2-terminal sequence-characterized human monokine possessing neutrophil chemotactic, skin-reactive, and granulocytosis-promoting activity. J Exp Med 1988; 167:1364–76.
101. Yoshimura T, Matsushima K, Tanaka S, Robinson E, Appella E, Oppenheim JJ, Leonard EJ. Purification of a human monocyte-derived neutrophil chemotactic factor that has peptide sequence similarity to other host defense cytokines. Proc Natl Acad Sci USA 1987; 84:9233–7.
102. Furuta R, Yamagishi J, Kotani H, Sakamoto F, Fukui T, Matsui Y, Sohmura Y, Yamada M, Yoshimura T, Larsen CG, Oppenheim JJ, Matsushima K. Production and characterization of recombinant human neutrophil chemotactic factor. J Biochem 1989; 106:436–41.
103. Gregory H, Young J, Schroder JM, Mrowietz U, Christophers E. Structure determination of a human lymphocyte derived neutrophil activating peptide (LYNAP). Biochem Biophys Res Commun 1988; 151:883–90.
104. Walz A, Peveri P, Aschauer H, Baggiolini M. Purification and amino acid sequencing of NAF, a novel neutrophil-activating factor produced by monocytes. Biochem Biophys Res Commun 1987; 149:755–61.
105. Schroder JM, Mrowietz U, Morita E, Christophers E. Purification and partial biochemical characterization of a human monocyte-derived, neutrophil-activating peptide that lacks interleukin 1 activity. J Immunol 1987; 139:3474–83.
106. Schroder JM, Mrowietz U, Christophers E. Identification of different charged species of a human monocyte derived neutrophil activating peptide (MONAP). Biochem Biophys Res Commun 1988; 152:277–84.
107. Peveri P, Walz A, Dewald B, Baggiolini M. A novel neutrophil-activating factor produced by human mononuclear phagocytes. J Exp Med 1988; 167:1547–59.
108. Lindley I, Aschauer H, Seifert JM, Lam C, Brunowsky W, Kownatzki E, Thelen M, Peveri P, Dewald B, Von Tscharner V, Walz A, Baggiolini M. Synthesis and expression in *Escherichia coli* of the gene encoding monocyte-derived neutrophil-activating factor: biological equivalence between natural and recombinant neutrophil-activating factor. Proc Natl Acad Sci USA 1988; 85:9199–203.
109. Westwick J, Li SW, Camp RD. Novel neutrophil-stimulating peptides. Immunol Today 1989; 10:146–7.
110. Wolpe SD, Cerami A. Macrophage inflammatory proteins 1 and 2: members of a novel superfamily of cytokines. FASEB J 1989; 3:2565–73.
111. Matsushima K, Oppenheim JJ. Interleukin 8 and MCAF: novel inflammatory cytokines inducible by IL 1 and TNF. Cytokine 1989; 1:2–13.
112. Deuel TF, Keim PS, Farmer M, Heinrikson RL. Amino acid sequence of human platelet factor 4. Proc Natl Acad Sci USA 1977; 74:2256–8.
113. Moser B, Clark-Lewis I, Zwahlen R, Baggiolini M. Neutrophil-activating properties of the melanoma growth-stimulatory activity. J Exp Med 1990; 171:1797–802.
114. Schroder JM, Persoon NLM, Christophers E. Lipopolysaccharide-stimulated human monocytes secrete, apart from neutrophil-activating peptide 1/interleukin 8, a second neutrophil-activating protein NH2-terminal amino acid sequence identity with melanoma growth stimulatory activity. J Exp Med 1990; 171:1091–100.
115. Mielke V, Bauman JGJ, Sticherling M, Ibs T, Zomershoe AG, Seligmann K, Henneicke HH, Schroder JM, Sterry W, Christophers E. Detection of neutrophil-activating peptide mRNA in human recombinant IL-1 alpha- and human necrosis factor-alpha-stimulated human dermal fibroblasts An immunocytochemical and fluorescent in situ hybridization study. J Immunol 1990; 144:153–61.
116. Thornton AJ, Strieter RM, Lindley I, Baggiolini M, Kunkel SL. Cytokine-induced gene expression of a neutrophil chemotactic factor/IL-8 in human hepatocytes. J Immunol 1990; 144:2609–13.

117. Van Damme J, Bunning RAD, Conings R, Graham R, Russell G, Opdenakker G. Characterization of granulocyte chemotactic activity from human cytokine-stimulated chondrocytes as interleukin 8. Cytokine 1990; 2:106–11.
118. Peveri P, Walz A, Dewald B, Baggiolini M. A novel neutrophil-activating factor produced by human mononuclear phagocytes. J Exp Med 1988; 167:1547–59.
119. Rampart M, Van Damme J, Zonnekeyn L, Herman AG. Granulocyte chemotactic protein/interleukin-8 induces plasma leakage and neutrophil accumulation in rabbit skin. Am J Pathol 1989; 135:21–5.
120. Leonard E. NAP-1(IL-8). Immunol Today 1990; 11:223–4.
121. Grob PM, David E, Warren TC, DeLeon RP, Farina PR, Homon CA. Characterization of a receptor for human monocyte-derived neutrophil chemotactic factor/interleukin-8. J Biol Chem 1990; 265:8311–6.
122. Paccaud JP, Schifferli JA, Baggiolini M. NAP-1/IL-8 induces up-regulation of CR1 receptors in human neutrophil leukocytes. Biochem Biophys Res Commun 1990; 166:187–92.
123. Smith CW, Rothlein R, Hughes BJ, Mariscalco MM, Rudloff HE, Schmalstieg FC, Anderson DC. Recognition of an endothelial determinant for CD18-dependent human neutrophil adherence and transendothelial migration. J Clin Invest 1988; 82:1746–56.
124. Gimbrone MA, Obin MS, Brock AF, Luis EA, Hass PE, Hebert CA, Yip YK, Leung DW. Endothelial interleukin-8: a novel inhibitor of leukocyte-endothelial interactions. Science 1989; 246:1601–3.
125. Carveth HJ, Bohnsack JF, McIntyre TM, Baggiolini M, Prescott SM, Zimmerman GA. Neutrophil activating factor (NAF) induces polymorphonuclear leukocyte adherence to endothelial cells and to subendothelial matrix proteins. Biochem Biophys Res Commun 1989; 162:387–93.
126. Coffey RG. Mechanism of GM-CSF stimulation of neutrophils. Immunol Res 1989; 8:236–48.
127. Weisbart RH, Golde DW, Clark SC, Wong GC, Gasson JC. Human granulocyte-macrophage colony-stimulating factor is a neutrophil activator. Nature 1985; 314:361–3.
128. Metcalf D, Moore JG. Divergent disease patterns in granulocyte-macrophage colony-stimulating factor transgenic mice associated with different transgene insertion sites. Proc Natl Acad Sci USA 1988; 85:7767–71.
129. Perussia B, Kobayashi M, Rossi ME, Anegon I, Trinchieri G. Immune interferon enhances functional properties of human granulocytes: role of Fc receptors and effect of lymphotoxin, tumor necrosis factor, and granulocyte-macrophage colony-stimulating factor. J Immunol 1987; 138:765–74.
130. Buckle AM, Hogg N. The effect of IFN-gamma and colony-stimulating factors of the expression of neutrophil cell membrane receptors. J Immunol 1989; 143:2295–301.
131. Gajewski TF, Goldwasser E, Fitch FW. Anti-proliferative effect on IFN-gamma in immune regulation. J Immunol 1988; 141:2635–42.
132. Barber KE, Crosier PS, Watson JD. The differential inhibition of hemopoietic growth factor activity by cytotoxins and interferon-gamma. J Immunol 1987; 139:1108–12.
133. Lu L, Welte K, Gabrilove JL, Hangoc G, Bruno E, Hoffman R, Broxmeyer HE. Effects of recombinant human tumor necrosis factor A, recombinant human gamma-interferon and prostaglandin E on colony formation of human hematopoietic progenitor cells stimulated by natural human pluripotent colony-stimulating factor, pluripoietin A, and recom. Cancer Res 1986; 46:4357–61.
134. Larrick JW. Native interleukin 1 inhibitors. Immunol Today 1989; 10:61–6.
135. Brown SL, Van Epps DE. Suppression of T lymphocyte chemotactic factor production by the opioid peptides beta-endorphin and met-enkephalin. J Immunol 1985; 134:3384–90.
136. Kurland JI, Bockman RS, Broxmeyer HE, Moore MAS. Limitation of excessive myelopoiesis by the intrinsic modulation of macrophage-derived prostaglandin E. Science 1977; 199:552–5.

137. Hannum CH, Wilcox CJ, Arend WP, Josln FG, Dripps DJ, Heimdal PL, Armes LG, Sommer A. Interleukin-1 receptor antagonist activity of a human interleukin-1 inhibitor. Nature 1990; 343:336–40.
138. Eisenberg SP, Evans RJ, Arend WP, Verderber E, Brewer MT, Hannum CH, Thompson RC. Primary structure and functional expression from complementary DNA of a human interleukin 1 receptor antagonist. Nature 1990; 343:341–6.
139. Murphy MT, Richards DB, Lipton JM. Antipyretic potency of centrally administered alpha-melanocyte stimulating hormone. Science 1983; 221:192–3.
140. Hiltz ME, Lipton JM. Anti-inflammatory activity of a COOH-terminal fragment of the neuropeptide alpha-MSH. FASEB J 1989; 3:2282–4.
141. Kastin AJ, Schally AV, Viosca S, Miller MC. MSH activity in plasma and pituitaries of rats after various treatments. Endocrinology 1969; 84:20–7.
142. Khorram O, Bedran de Castro JC, McCann SM. Stress-induced secretion of alpha-melanocyte-stimulating hormone and its physiological role in modulating the secretion of prolactin and luteinizing hormone in the female rat. Endocrinology 1985; 117:2483–9.
143. Woloski BM, Smith EM, Meyer WJ, Fuller GM, Blalock JE. Corticotropin-releasing activity of monokines. Science 1985; 230:1035–7.
144. Pober JS, Lapierre LA, Stolpen AH, Brock TA, Springer TA, Fiers W, Bevilacqua MP, Mendrick DL, Gimbrone MA Jr. Activation of cultured human endothelial cells by recombinant lymphotoxin: comparison with tumor necrosis factor and interleukin 1 species. J Immunol 1987; 138:3319–24.
145. Van Epps DE, Simpson S, Bender JG, Chenoweth DE. Regulation of C5a and formyl peptide receptor expression on human polymorphonuclear leukocytes. J Immunol 1990; 144:1062–8.
146. Beck G, Habicht GS, Benach JL, Miller F. Interleukin 1: a common endogenous mediator of inflammation and the local Shwartzman reaction. J Immunol 1986; 136:3025–31.
147. Richter J, Andersson T, Olsson I. Effect of tumor necrosis factor and granulocyte/macrophage colony-stimulating factor on neutrophil degranulation. J Immunol 1989; 142:3199–205.
148. Figari IS, Mori NA, Palladino MA Jr. Regulation of neutrophil migration and superoxide production by recombinant tumor necrosis factors-alpha and -beta: comparison to recombinant interferon-gamma and interleukin-1 alpha. Blood 1987; 70:979–84.
149. Ferrante A, Nandoskar M, Walz A, Goh DHB, Kowanko IC. Effects of tumour necrosis factor-alpha and interleukin-1-alpha and beta on human neutrophil migration, respiratory burst and degranulation. Int Arch Allergy Appl Immunol 1988; 86:82–91.
150. Djeu JY, Matsushima K, Oppenheim JJ, Shiotsuki K, Blanchard DK. Functional activation of human neutrophils by recombinant monocyte-derived neutrophil chemotactic factor/IL-8. J Immunol 1990; 144:2205–10.
151. Yoshimura T, Leonard EJ. Secretion by human fibroblasts of monocyte chemoattractant protein-1, the product of gene JE. J Immunol 1990; 144:2377–83.

12

Physiological Studies with Human Leukocyte Inhibitory Factor

LARRY BORISH
National Jewish Center for Immunology and Respiratory Diseases, University of Colorado Health Sciences Center, Denver, Colorado

ROSS ROCKLIN
Boehringer Ingelheim Pharma, Inc., Ridgefield, Connecticut

I. PHYSIOCHEMICAL PROPERTIES OF LIF

A. Introduction

Human leukocyte inhibitory factor (LIF) has been partially characterized by a variety of physiochemical techniques; these findings are shown in Table 1 (1). LIF has been shown to be heat stable to 80°C for 30 min and is stable between pH 4 and 10. Its properties have been shown to be generally those of a protein through studies in which LIF activity was destroyed by treatment with chymotrypsin and by the demonstration of its buoyant density in cesium chloride gradients similar to that of a reference protein. Sialic acid does not appear to be important for the expression of biological activity of LIF, as has been demonstrated by the inability of neuraminidase to inactivate it. The molecular weight of LIF has been estimated to be approximately 60,000 Da by gel filtration using Sephadex G-100 chromatography. At pH 9.1, LIF has a charge similar to that of albumin when subjected to electrophoresis on polyacrylamide gels. It has also been reported that LIF activity is abolished following incubation with L-cysteine and 2-mercaptoethanol, suggesting the presence of disulfide linkages. Attempts to purify LIF by isoelectric focusing in sucrose gradients has led to the demonstration of two peaks of activity with differing fractions having pH ranges of 5.0–5.5 and 8.0–8.5. Furthermore, when each activity was rechromatographed on Sephadex G-75 gels, both preparations were found to be sensitive to diisopropylphosphofluoridate (DFP), suggesting the presence of active serine sites on the molecule.

B. Esterase Nature of LIF

LIF is an intriguing molecule because, as mentioned above, it has been found to have some of the characteristics of an esterase (2). A variety of esterase inhibitors in addition to DFP, including a benzamidine derivative, phenylmethylsulfonylfluoride

Table 1 Physiochemical Properties of Human LIF

Heat	Stable 56°C, 30 min; diminished 80°C, 30 min
pH stability	4–10
MW	60,000 Da
Buoant density	Protein
Gel electrophoresis (pH 9.1)	Albumin
Chymotrypsin	Sensitive
Neuraminidase	Resistant
L-Cysteine	Sensitive
2-Mercaptoethanol	Sensitive
Isoelectric point	5.0–5.5; 8.0–8.5
DFP	Sensitive

(PMSF), and eserine, have been shown to abolish LIF activity. These inhibitors bind irreversibly to serine groups at the active site of known esterases and presumably, therefore, in LIF molecules also. To determine if DFP was serving as a substrate for LIF, experiments were carried out in which the kinetics of inactivation were measured. The inactivation of LIF by DFP appeared to follow standard enzyme-substrate kinetics in that the reaction was time, temperature, pH, and concentration dependent. However, since there may have been other esterases present in the preparation, the K_m values could not be determined.

On the basis of indirect evidence that an amide of the oligopeptide benzoyl-phenylalanyl-valyl-arginine might have high and selective affinity for LIF, an ester of this oligopeptide was prepared. Benzoyl-phenylalanyl-valyl-arginine (^{3}H) methyl ester (^{3}H-BPVAME) was employed for the direct measurement of LIF activity in a double-phase radioenzyme assay. The hydrolysis of ^{3}H-BPVAME followed enzyme-substrate kinetics in that the reaction was time, temperature, pH, and concentration dependent. ^{3}H-BPVAME proved to be more selective and approximately 20 times more sensitive as a substrate for LIF than previously used radiolabeled substrates such as ^{3}H-BAEE and ^{3}H-TAME. Moreover, hydrolysis of ^{3}H-BPVAME by partially purified LIF preparations was significantly inhibited by 10^{-8} M to 10^{-5} M guanosine 3′,5′-cyclic monophosphate (cGMP), suggesting that cGMP acts as a regulator of LIF activity. Inhibition of LIF-induced esterolysis also occurred by dibutyryl cGMP, but only at concentrations of 10^{-7} to 10^{-5} M; 8-bromo cGMP and adenosine 3′,5′-cyclic monophosphate were both ineffective. These results provide support for the use of ^{3}H-BPVAME as a more selective substrate to detect esterase activity in LIF preparations than heretofore described and suggest the possible development of a biochemical assay for the measurement of this lymphokine.

C. Biochemical Effects of LIF on PMN

We investigated the role of calcium in the activation of PMN by LIF (3). Using the fluorescent probe fura-2, we demonstrated that LIF induced a small but significant dose-dependent increase in intracellular calcium in the presence of both calcium-containing (71 nM to 158 nM) and calcium-free (53 nM to 144 nM) buffer solutions. Thus, LIF releases calcium from both membrane channels and from intracellular stores. In contrast to the signals generated by formyl-methionyl-leucyl-phenylalanine (fMLP), maximal calcium fluxes were of a much lower magnitude and not observed until 10–15 min after its application (Figure 1). The importance of calcium to the metabolic effects of LIF was demonstrated by the abilities of the calmodulin inhibitor trifluoroperazine, the calcium chelator EGTA, and the intracellular calcium chelator fura 2 to significantly inhibit LIF-mediated degranulation. Contrariwise, TMB-8, which inhibits the release of calcium from intracellular stores, had no effect on LIF-mediated PMN activation. These data suggest that the activation of PMN by LIF is calcium dependent and that this calcium is primarily derived from the slow influx of calcium from the extracellular pool.

II. PURIFICATION OF LEUKOCYTE INHIBITORY FACTOR

Leukocyte inhibitory factor (LIF) was originally named an inhibitory factor secondary to its capacity to inhibit the random migration of neutrophils (PMN). We were eager, however, to determine whether this reflected its immunoregulatory role in vivo. A putative role for LIF could be proposed by ascertaining the spectrum of effects of LIF on neutrophil functions. The performance of these studies obviously necessitated the

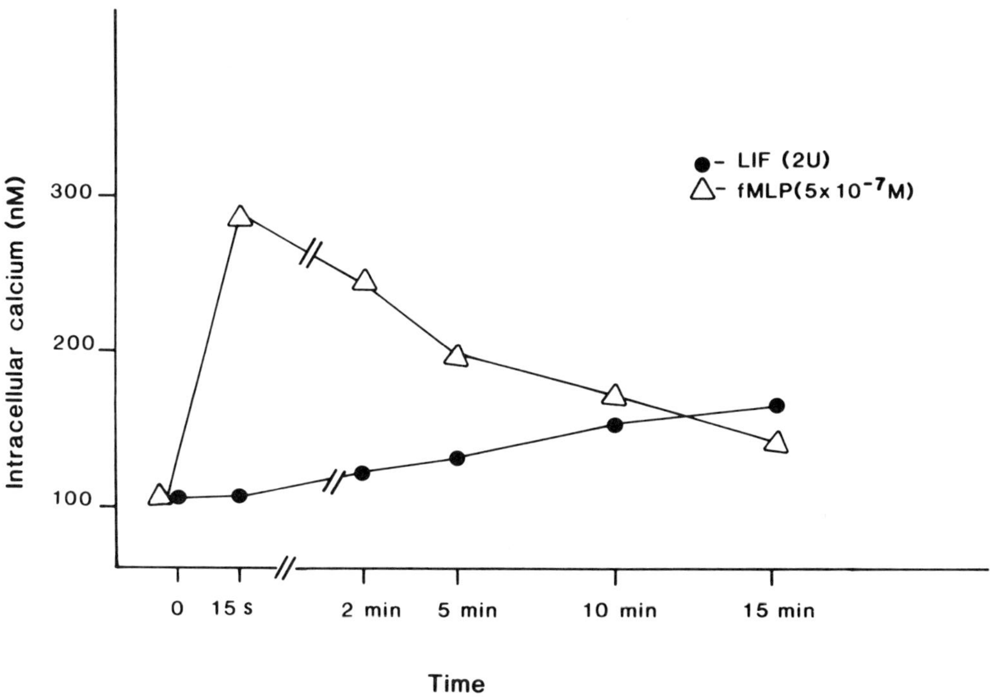

Figure 1 PMN were loaded with the calcium probe Fura 2am. PMN were stimulated with LIF or fMLP (5×10^{-7} M). Fluorescence was measured for 15 min with the fluorometer set to measure emission at 510 nM and with the excitation wavelength scanning from 340 to 380 nM. Intracellular calcium concentrations were derived from standard formulas.

availability of purified LIF. The initial, analytical, purification scheme for LIF was established using LIF bioactivity obtained from a human non-T, non-B leukemia cell line (REH) (4). LIF was known to be a glycoprotein, and the initial purification step was performed via affinity binding to Con A-Sepharose and elution with α-methyl mannoside. Subsequent purification utilized hydrophobic interaction chromatography (HIC) and established that while LIF bound to all types of hydrophobic agarose, hexylagarose produced the highest recovery of LIF activity. Fractions obtained from HIC were subjected to gel filtration on Sephadex G-100 and the bioactive fraction (MW = 58 kDa) obtained. The combination of these three separation techniques produced a preparation that was 80–90% pure, and an apparently homogeneous product was subsequently identified via electrofocusing (Figure 2). From 10 L of serum-free supernatant, 1.3 μg

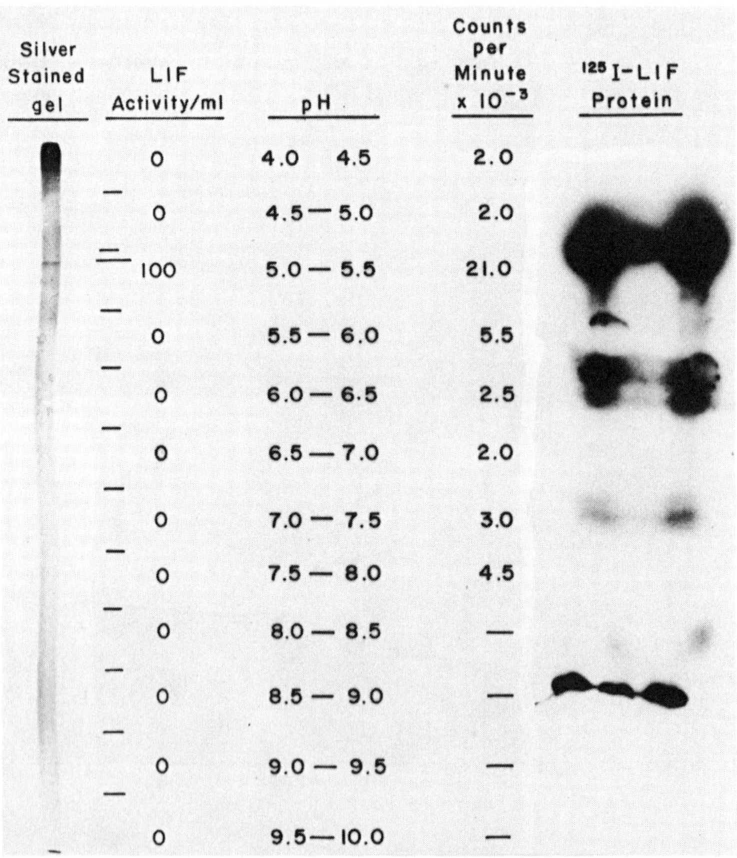

Figure 2 Purification of REH-derived LIF. Part of the LIF obtained after affinity chromatography, hydrophobic chromatography, and gel filtration was iodinated and both unlabeled and ^{125}I-labeled samples were separated on slab gels via isoelectric focusing. One stainable band (pH 5.0–5.5) was detected, and biologic LIF activity was recovered in this same region of the gel. The major radiolabeled band had the same pI (5.1), consonant with this representing a homogenous preparation.

of protein with LIF activity could be obtained, which represented an 80,000-fold purification over the initial crude supernatants. To perform physiological studies with LIF, subsequent experiments substituted preparative isoelectrofocusing in an agarose gel matrix for analytical IEF in acrylamide (5).

III. EFFECTS OF LIF ON NEUTROPHIL PHYSIOLOGICAL FUNCTIONS

A. Chemotaxis

The most important question to be answered in order to propose a putative in-vivo role for LIF was to determine the effect of LIF on chemotactic stimuli. These studies would determine whether LIF did, in fact, function as an *inhibitory factor* by inhibiting the directed migration and preventing neutrophil accumulation at inflammatory sites or, alternatively, whether it was pro-inflammatory by promoting the passive accumulation of neutrophils. Preliminary studies demonstrated that LIF by itself was neither chemotactic nor chemokinetic toward PMN (6). When subjected to increasing concentrations of LIF, as would be predicted, inhibition of random migration into the nitrocellulose filters was observed. To our great surprise, when PMN were pretreated with low concentrations of LIF (1/4 to 2 units) and then subjected to a chemotactic gradient of formyl-methionyl-leucyl-phenylalanine (fMLP), not only did LIF not inhibit directed migration, a potentiation of chemotaxis was observed (Figure 3). Only when exposed to

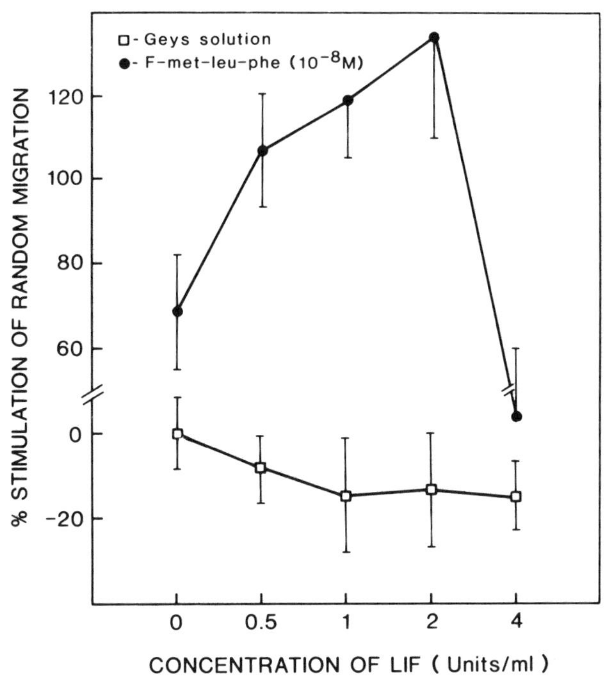

Figure 3 Neutrophils were preincubated with either control supernatant or varying concentrations of LIF. PMN were placed in modified Boyden chambers containing Gey's solution alone or with the additional presence of fMLP (10^{-8} M). Chemotaxis was measured as the distance of migration along the leading front. Data are expressed as the percent stimulation of migration observed by untreated PMN in the absence of the chemoattractant.

higher concentrations (≥4 U) was incubation with LIF associated with inhibition of fMLP-directed chemotaxis. Together, these observations suggest that at low concentrations of LIF, such as would be seen distant to inflammatory reactions, neutrophils would have enhanced responsiveness toward a chemotactic agent. At the site of inflammation, the higher concentrations of LIF present would promote the accumulation of neutrophils.

B. Respiratory Burst

Subsequent experiments were performed to investigate the effects of LIF on an array of PMN physiological functions associated with microbicidal function (6). At no concentration was LIF able to induce a respiratory burst, even when PMN were primed with cytochalasin B or endotoxin, or stimulated for as long as 16 h. However, as with chemotaxis, exposure to low concentrations of LIF (1/4 to 1 U) enhanced by as much as 151.6 ±77.0% the concentration of superoxide, and by 54.9 ±15.5% the concentration of hydrogen peroxide by fMLP (10^{-7} M)-stimulated PMN.

C. Degranulation

PMN were subsequently exposed to a range of concentrations of purified LIF and supernatants assayed for degranulation products (6,7). LIF was shown to induce secretory (secondary) granule secretion, as demonstrated by the release of both lysozyme (28.1% secreted) and lactoferrin (8.2%) in the absence of β-glucuronidase (2.0%). LIF was not toxic toward neutrophils, as shown by the absence of lactate dehydrogenase (LDH) release.

IV. EFFECTS OF LIF ON NEUTROPHIL RECEPTOR EXPRESSION AND FUNCTION

A. Formyl Peptide Receptor Expression

Neutrophil-specific granules are known to contain an intracellular pool of receptors for fMLP, and upon degranulation provide the surface membrane with a fresh source of receptors (8,9). Our data that LIF induced secondary granule secretion suggested that LIF potentiation of fMLP-mediated chemotaxis and respiratory burst might be mediated, at least in part, by increasing the number of available membrane receptors for fMLP. Radioligand receptor analysis using f-met-leu-[^{3}H]phe (Figure 4) showed that LIF exposure was associated with an average increase in fMLP receptors from 18,600 to 27,000 (6). Binding coefficients declined from an average of 0.046 nM^{-1} to an average of 0.030 nM^{-1} after treatment. LIF does, however, have a more generalized effect on the transduction of neutrophil activation stimuli, as it also mediated a 35.8% increase in superoxide production after exposure to the receptor-independent stimulus calcium ionophore A23187 (6).

B. Complement Receptor Expression

Our observations that LIF induced both secretory granule release and increased formyl peptide receptor expression led us to investigate the effects of LIF on neutrophil complement receptors. In addition to receptors for C5a, PMN contain receptors for the

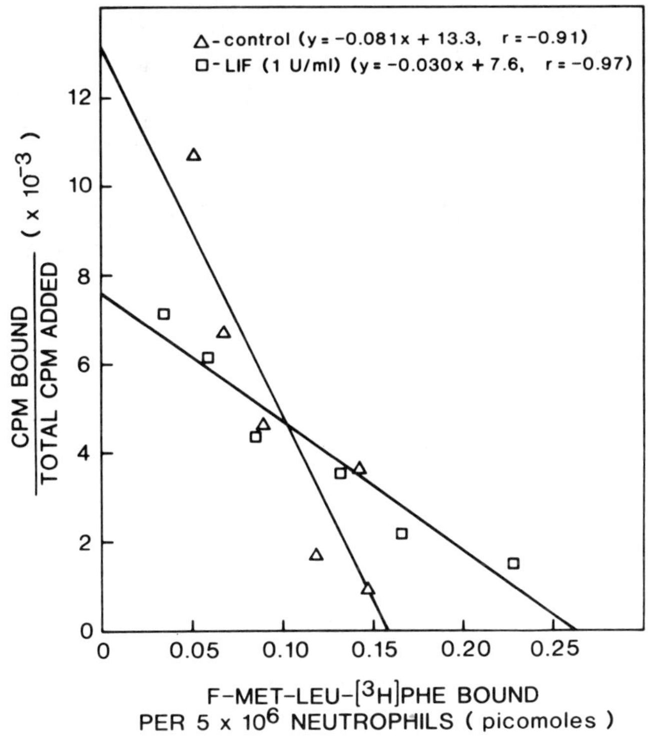

Figure 4 Scatchard analysis of a representative f-met-leu-phe radioligand receptor-binding assay. PMN were exposed to a range of concentrations of f-met-leu-[^{3}H] phe with or without pretreatment with LIF (1 U/ml).

complement components C3b (complement receptor, type 1 or CR1) and C3bi (CR3) (10–13). These latter receptors were of particular interest to us because, as with the fMLP receptor, these have an intracellular pool which, in the presence of PMN-activating stimuli, produce increased surface expression (14–17). Furthermore, in the case of CR3 this intracellular pool has been localized to the secretory granule (14). Utilizing indirect immunofluorescence analysis, LIF was shown to induce a 38.2% increase in CR1 and a 96.1% increase in CR3 expression (18). These receptors mediate the respiratory burst and adherence to appropriately opsonized targets (C3b- and C3bi-coated, respectively) and, in the presence of an additional signal (e.g., phorbol esters, fibronectin, serum amyloid P component, or IgG) induce phagocytosis (19–23). In this regard, it was significant that LIF increased by 97.1% superoxide production by opsonized zymosan, and adhesion to EAC3b and EAC3bi by 137.4% and 59.4%, respectively (Figure 5). However, LIF did not serve as a signal for complement receptor-mediated phagocytosis (18).

C. Adhesion and Aggregation

The type 3 complement receptor has recently been shown to have physiological activities beyond its capacities as a ligand for complement products. CR3 is a heterodimer

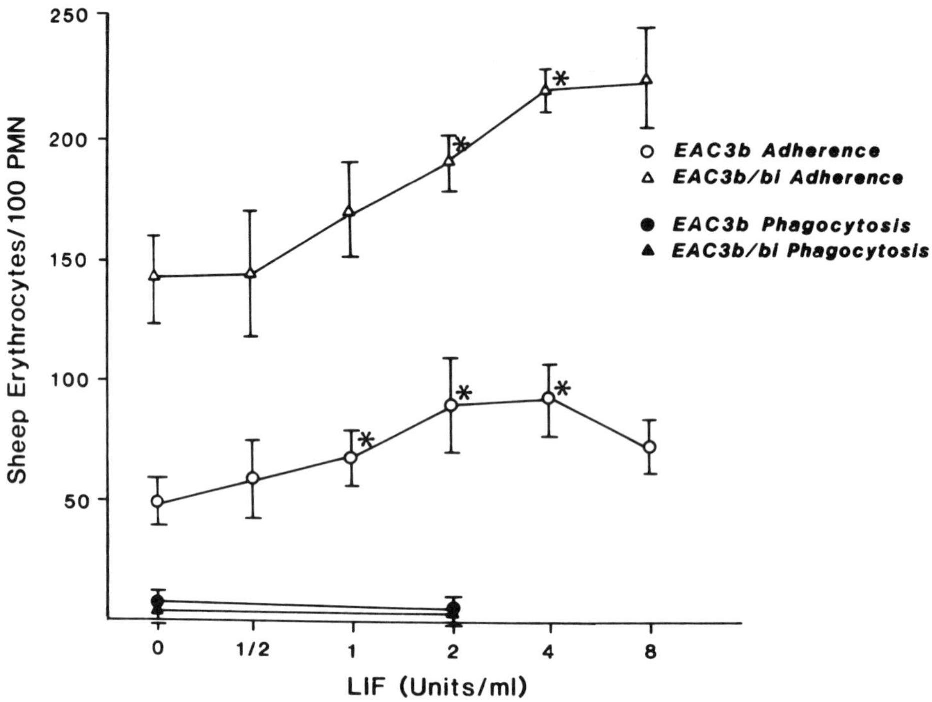

Figure 5 PMN were pretreated with a range in concentrations of LIF and then exposed to sheep erythrocytes (E) opsonized with C3b or C3bi. Phagocytosis was assayed after extracellular and adherent E were lysed with NH_4Cl. Data are expressed as the mean number of E associated with 100 consecutive PMN. * Differences were significant ($p < 0.05$).

which shares a common 95-KDa β-chain with lymphocyte functional antigen type 1 (LFA-1) and complement receptor type 4 (gp 95,150) (24–27). Together these three surface proteins have been shown to be critically important in cellular adhesive processes. Thus, PMN exposed to anti-beta-chain antibodies or obtained from patients congenitally lacking in these receptors cannot be stimulated to demonstrate aggregation (neutrophil-to-neutrophil adherence) or adherence to endothelial cells (EC), and they have defective chemotaxis (i.e., neutrophil to ground substance adherence) (24–27). Our observation that LIF stimulated CR3 expression therefore led us to speculate that LIF might thereby enhance PMN aggregation and EC adherence. We found that exposure to up to 16 U of LIF was not able to directly induce PMN clumping (28). However, preincubation with LIF for 10 min produced a dose-dependent augmentation of aggregation with fLMP (up to 94.5 ±3.1% increase), leukotriene B_4 (183.1 ±8.2%), and 100 μg of serum-opsonized zymosan (29.8 ±8.6%).

Unlike aggregation, LIF was shown to directly stimulate PMN to adhere to EC (68.6% adherence at 4 U LIF) (29). The effect of LIF on the PMN was blocked through co-exposure to anti-CR3 antibodies. This observation is consistent with a role for the LIF-stimulated expression of CR3 in inducing increased adherence. LIF was also shown to stimulate isolated EC to bind more PMN. LIF (4 U)-treated EC bound up to 91.1% of applied neutrophils, as compared to 28.8 ±3.1% for untreated EC (Figure 6) (29). Modulation of EC function required new protein synthesis. LIF-treated

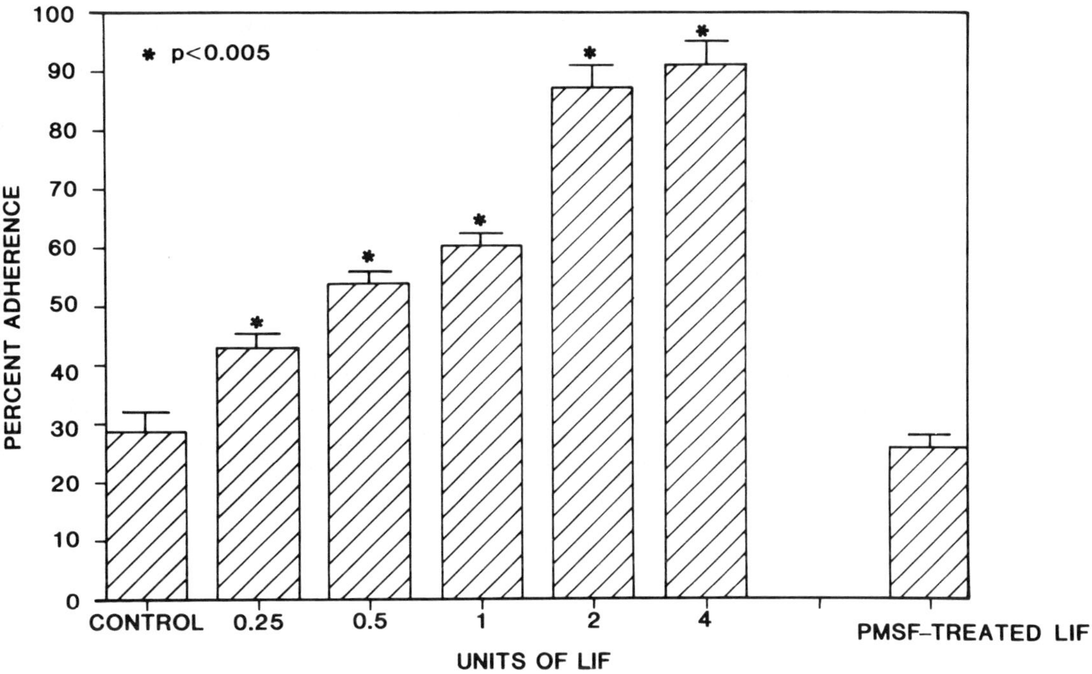

Figure 6 Endothelial cells were pretreated (4 h) with HBSS or a range of concentrations of LIF and then washed extensively. PMN were ^{51}Cr-labeled and applied to the EC monolayers. After 45 min the nonadherent PMN were carefully aspirated and remaining cells were lysed. The percent adherence was determined.

EC were stimulated to secrete interleukin-1 (IL-1). IL-1 produced by LIF-treated EC may thereby function in an autocrine fashion as a second messenger for adherence (30,31). With Jordan Pober (unpublished data), it was shown that LIF up-regulated their expression of intracellular adhesion molecule 1 (ICAM-1). ICAM-1 is the EC ligand for LFA-1, and its induction by LIF is an alternative mechanism by which LIF may stimulate EC to bind PMN (32).

D. Fcγ Receptor Expression and Function

Unlike complement receptors, the PMN Fcγ receptors do mediate phagocytosis directly. However, using opsonized ^{14}C-labeled, heat-killed *staphylococcus aureus,* LIF was shown to potentiate Fcγ-mediated phagocytosis by up to 57.2% (33). Similarly, LIF enhanced the phagocytosis of IgG-opsonized sheep erythrocytes (EA) by up to 124.4%. Unlike the complement receptor-dependent effects, LIF did not up-regulate type 3 Fcγ receptor expression. An effect on type 1 Fcγ receptor expression might still be a mechanism for these observations; however, this has yet to be studied. Our data that exposure to anti-FcγIII receptor antibodies abrogated the LIF-mediated enhancement of phagocytosis of EA suggests that this is probably not the case. Furthermore, the stimulation of phagocytosis was produced, at least in part, through a receptor-independent mechanism, as LIF was shown to enhance the phagocytosis of unopsonized latex particles (59.9%).

V. PRO-INFLAMMATORY ACTIVITIES OF LIF ON OTHER CELL TYPES

The studies on the interaction of LIF with endothelial cells represent the first observations to extend the activities of LIF beyond the neutrophil (29). With Stephanie Pincus, however, we have obtained preliminary data that LIF also interacts with eosinophils to stimulate secretion of eosinophil granule peptides and to stimulate a respiratory burst (unpublished observations).

VI. EFFECTS OF LIF ON NEUTROPHIL KILLING

A. Microbicidal Activity

Our next series of experiments were to confirm that LIF could potentially function as a pro-inflammatory peptide in vivo by assessing its influence on both intracellular and extracellular killing by the neutrophil. LIF potentiated the killing of opsonized *Staphylococcus aureus* by up to 51.6%, consonant with its capacities to enhance phagocytosis, the respiratory burst, and degranulation (33).

B. Antibody-Dependent Cellular Cytotoxicity

Extracellular killing (antibody-dependent cellular cytotoxicity; ADCC) was assayed using ^{51}chromium-labeled K562 targets opsonized with heterologous rabbit antisera (34). Highly purified LIF induced a dose-dependent potentiation of neutrophil ADCC by up to 54.9% (Figure 7). The degree of cytotoxicity was found to correlate (r =

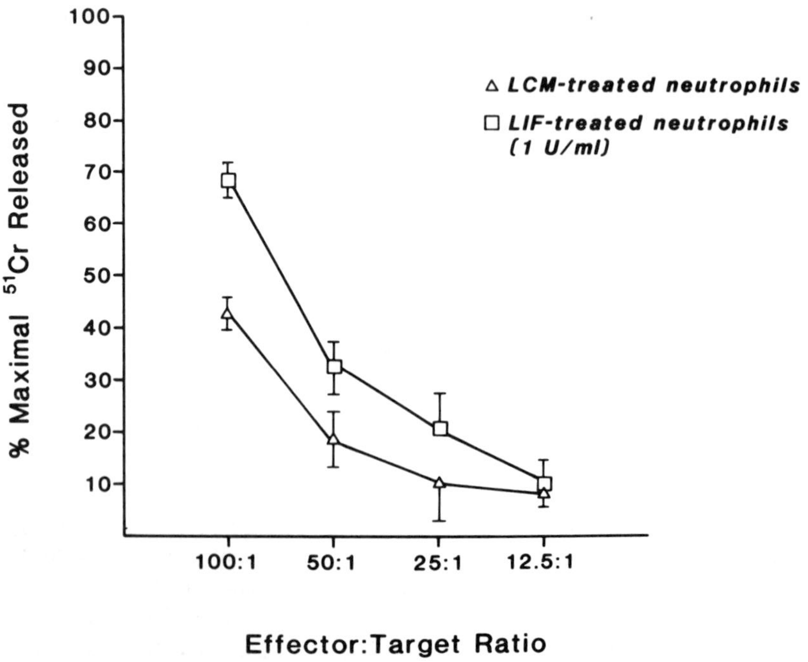

Figure 7 PMN were pretreated with LIF and exposed to ^{51}Cr-labeled antibody-coated K562 targets at varying effector:target ratios. Released ^{51}Cr was determined, and data are expressed as the percent of maximal release.

0.99) with increased secretion of superoxide into the assay media. Furthermore, our observation that anaerobic conditions inhibited cytotoxicity lends support to the concept that enhanced ADCC by LIF was mediated through increased superoxide production and not, for example, via increased degranulation. Enhanced ADCC was also associated with increased adherence of PMN to opsonized targets (average 3.3:1 effector:target ratio in untreated cells and 4.8:1 after treatment with LIF).

VII. SUMMARY

LIF has been shown to be a potentially important activator of neutrophil function. By means of its dose-dependent dichotomous effects on chemotaxis, LIF can be predicted to both enhance the potency of chemotactic stimuli and promote the passive accumulation of PMN at inflammatory loci. Furthermore, LIF's stimulatory effects on both PMN- and endothelial cell-mediated adherence will promote the migration of neutrophils from the circulation to the inflammatory site. We have demonstrated LIF stimulation of fMLP, CR1, and CR3 expression and function, as well a stimulated FcγRIII function. Through both receptor-dependent and -independent effects, LIF produces increased target cell attachment, phagocytosis, respiratory burst activity, and degranulation. Together, these effects result in a significant increase in killing of both phagocytosed targets and extracellular targets.

REFERENCES

1. Rocklin R. Properties and mechanisms of action of human leukocyte migration inhibitory factor (LIF). In: Lymphokines, vol. 2. New York: Academic Press, 1981:163–77.
2. Rocklin RE, Bendtzen K. Lymphokines that affect the migration of polymorphonuclear leukocytes. In: Hadden JW, Stewart WE II, eds. The Lymphokines. Humana Press, 1981:33–54.
3. Borish L, Rosenbaum R, Rocklin R. Role of calcium in the activation of neutrophils by leukocyte inhibitory factor (LIF). Lymphokine Res 1987; 6:341–9.
4. Meshulam DH, Blair HE, Wong BL, Charm S, Minowada J, Rocklin RE. Purification of a lymphoid cell product with leukocyte inhibitory factor activity. Proc Natl Acad Sci USA 1982; 79:601–5.
5. Borish L, O'Reilly D, Rocklin RE. Purification of human leukocyte inhibitory factor. J Allergy Clin Immunol 1984; 73:185A.
6. Borish L, O'Reilly D, Klempner MS, Rocklin RE. Leukocyte inhibitory factor (LIF) potentiates neutrophil responses to formyl-methionyl-leucyl-phenylalanine. J Immunol 1986; 137:1897–903.
7. Klempner MS, Rocklin RE. Effects of leukocyte inhibitory factor (LIF) on human neutrophil function. Inflammation 1985; 7:145–53.
8. Fletcher MP, Gallin JI. Degranulating stimuli increase the availability of receptors on human neutrophils for the chemoattractant f-met-leu-phe. J Immunol 1980; 124:1585–8.
9. Fletcher MP, Gallin JI. Human neutrophils contain an intracellular pool of putative receptors for the chemoattractant N-formyl-methionyl-leucyl-phenylalanine. Blood 1983; 62:792–9.
10. Fearon DT. Identification of the membrane glycoprotein that is the C3b receptor of the human erythrocyte, polymorphonuclear leukocyte, B lymphocyte and monocyte. J Exp Med 1980; 152:20–30.
11. Stossel TP, Field RJ, Gitlin JD, Alper CA, Rosen FS. The opsonic fragment of the third component of human complement. J Exp Med 1975; 141:1329–47.

12. Wright SD, Rao PE, VanVoorhis WC, Craigmyle LS, Iida K, Talle MA, Westberg EF, Goldstein G, Silverstein SC. Identification of the C3bi receptor of human monocytes and macrophages using monoclonal antibodies. Proc Natl. Acad Sci USA 1983; 80:5699–703.
13. Huey R, Hugli TE. Characterization of a C5a receptor on human polymorphonuclear leukocytes (PMN). J Immunol 1985; 135:2063–8.
14. O'Shea JJ, Brown EJ, Seligmann BE, Metcalf JA, Frank MM, Gallin JI. Evidence for distinct intracellular pools of receptors for C3b and C3bi in human neutrophils. J Immunol 1985; 134:2580–7.
15. Berger M, O'Shea J, Cross AS, Folks TM, Chused TM, Brown EJ, Frank MM. Human neutrophils increase expression of C3bi as well as C3b receptors upon activation. J Clin Invest 1984; 74:1566–71.
16. Berger M, Cross AS. Lymphoblastoid cell supernatants increase expression of C3b receptors on human polymorphonuclear leukocytes: direct binding studies with ^{125}I-C3b. Immunology 1984; 51:431–9.
17. Esparza I, Fox RI, Schreiber RD. Interferon-γ-dependent modulation of C3b receptors (CR1) on human peripheral blood monocytes. J Immunol 1986; 136:1360–5.
18. Borish L, Audera C, Rosenbaum R, Rocklin RE. Enhancement of the function of neutrophil type-1 and type-3 complement receptors by human leukocyte inhibitory factor (LIF). Cell Immunol 1988; 113:320–8.
19. Pommier CG, Inada S, Fries LF, Takashi T, Frank MM, Brown EJ. Plasma fibronectin enhances phagocytosis of opsonized particles by human peripheral blood monocytes. J Exp Med 1983; 157:1844–54.
20. Wright SD, Craigmyle LS, Silverstein SC. Fibronectin and serum amyloid P component stimulate C3b- and C3bi-mediated phagocytosis in cultured human monocytes. J Exp Med 1983; 158:1338–43.
21. Wright SD, Silverstein SC. Tumor-promoting phorbol esters stimulate C3b and C3b′ receptor-mediated phagocytosis in cultured human monocytes. J Exp Med 1982; 156:1149–64.
22. O'Shea JJ, Siwik SA, Gaither TA, Frank MM. Activation of the C3b receptor: effect of diacylglycerols and calcium mobilization. J Immunol 1985; 135:3381–7.
23. O'Shea JJ, Brown EJ, Gaither TA, Takahashi T, Frank MM. Tumor-promoting phorbol esters induce rapid internalization of the C3b receptor via a cytoskeletal-dependent mechanism. J Immunol 1985; 135:1325–30.
24. Anderson DC, Schmalstieg, FC, Arnaout MA, Kohyl S, Tosi MF, Dana N, Buffone GJ, Hughes BJ, Brinkley BR, Dickey WD, Abramson JS, Springer T, Boxer LA, Hollers JM, Wayne Smith C. Abnormalities of polymorphonuclear leukocyte function associated with a heritable deficiency of high molecular weight surface glycoproteins (GP138): common relationship to diminished cell adherence. J Clin Invest 1984; 74:536–51.
25. Harlan JM, Kilen PD, Senecal FM, Schwartz BR, Yee EK, Taylor RF, Beatty PG, Price TH, Ochs HD. The role of neutrophil membrane glycoprotein GP-150 in neutrophil adherence to endothelium in vitro. Blood 1985; 66:167–78.
26. Fischer A, Seger R, Durandy A, Grospierre B, Virelizier JL, LeDeist F, Griscelli C, Fischer E, Kazatchkine M, Bohler M-C, Descapms-Latscha B, Trung PH, Springer TA, Olive D, Mawas C. Deficiency of the adhesive protein complex lymphocyte function antigen 1, complement receptor type 3, glycoprotein p150,95 in a girl with recurrent bacterial infections: effects on phagocytic cells and lymphocyte functions. J Clin Invest 1985; 76:2385–92.
27. Schwartz BR, Ochs HD, Beatty PG, Harlan JM. A monoclonal antibody-defined membrane antigen complex is required for neutrophil-neutrophil aggregation. Blood 1985; 65:1553–6.
28. Schainberg H, Borish L, Rocklin RE. Potentiation of neutrophil aggregation by human leukocyte inhibitory factor. Inflammation 1988; 12:203–11.

29. Schainberg H, Borish L, King M, Rocklin R, Rosenwasser LJ. Leukocyte inhibitory factor (LIF) stimulates neutrophil endothelial cell adhesion. J Immunol 1988; 141:3055–60.
30. Furie MB, McHugh DD. Migration of neutrophils across endothelial monolayers is stimulated by treatment of the monolayers with interleukin-1 or tumor necrosis factor-α. J Immunol 1989; 143:3309–17.
31. Schleimer RP, Rutledge BK. Cultured human vascular endothelial cells acquire adhesiveness for neutrophils after stimulation with interleukin 1, endotoxin, and tumor-promoting phorbol diesters. J Immunol 1986; 136:649–54.
32. Makgoba MW, Sanders ME, Ginther Luce GE, Dustin ML, Springer TA, Clark EA, Mannoni P, Shaw S. ICAM-1 a ligand for LFA-1-dependent adhesion of B, T, and myeloid cells. Nature 1988; 331:86–8.
33. Borish L, Rocklin RE. Effects of leukocyte inhibitory factor (LIF) on neutrophil phagocytosis and bacterial killing. J Immunol 1986; 138:1475–9.
34. Borish L, Rocklin RE. Effects of leukocyte inhibitory factor (LIF) on neutrophil-mediated antibody-dependent cellular cytotoxicity. J Immunol 1986; 138:1480–4.

13

The Biology of NAP-1/IL-8, a Neutrophil-Activating Cytokine

JENS-M. SCHRÖDER and ENNO CHRISTOPHERS
University of Kiel, Kiel, Germany

I. INTRODUCTION

Inflammatory diseases besides cancer and vascular occlusion disorders are among the major health hazards of humans. In these conditions tissue destruction following inflammation is a common consequence, and in these events the neutrophil is being implicated with increasing frequency as the principal mediator cell. Disorders ranging from chronic obstructive lung diseases, respiratory distress syndromes, rheumatoid arthritis, and myocardial reperfusion injury to thrombotic occlusion syndromes or ulcerative colitis are known to be associated with activated neutrophils as well as their constituents, e.g., toxins, enzymes, and pro-inflammatory mediators (1).

Neutrophil-related disorders are frequent in human skin and include pustule-forming disorders, diseases with generalized blistering, vasculitis syndromes, as well as a group of disorders showing psoriatic tissue alterations (2,3). In these conditions intraepidermal accumulation of neutrophils is associated with augmented keratinocyte growth, leading to chronic relapsing inflammation and scaling.

Whereas the neutrophil, when activated for function, is unable to recognize differences between foreign and host tissue, the specificity of neutrophil responses resides in the nature of the stimuli and the corresponding membrane receptors.

A number of stimuli eliciting strong functional activities in human neutrophils have been defined in recent years. With the exception of the bacterial chemotactic formylated tripeptide N-formyl-methionyl-leucyl-phenylalanine (fMLP) (4), known PMN (polymorphonuclear leukocytes, neutrophils) stimuli are derived from mammalian cells or tissues and include $C5a/C5a_{des\,arg}$ (5), leukotriene B_4 (LTB_4) (6), as well as platelet-activating factor (PAF) (7). For each of these endogenous stimuli, appropriate receptors have been isolated on the PMN membrane eliciting the cell's spectrum of functions.

Recently, when working with lesional scale material from patients with psoriasis, we noted fractions exhibiting powerful neutrophil-stimulating activities. This observation led to the isolation of an apparently novel type of endogenous chemoattractant for neutrophils. A new neutrophil-activating protein was first detected in diseased skin (8) and thereupon has shown to be produced by a number of cells intimately associated with cutaneous inflammation.

II. STIMULATED MONOCYTES SECRETE A NOVEL PMN CHEMOATTRACTANT

When extracts of psoriatic scales were separated by Sephadex G-75 gel chromatography, the existence of a second neutrophil attractant apart from $C5a_{des\,arg}$ was observed (8). We tentatively termed this factor "*a*nionic *n*eutrophil-*a*ctivating *p*eptide" (ANAP). Partially purified psoriasis-derived ANAP was able to desensitize degranulation of PMN, which were preincubated with supernatants of lipopolysaccharide (LPS)-stimulated monocytes (8). Moreover, when psoriasis scale extracts were separated by G-75 gel chromatography and PMN were preincubated with supernatants of LPS-stimulated monocytes, the peak of PMN function-stimulating activity eluting in fractions 21–26 disappeared (Figure 1). Therefore we concluded that the PMN-activating protein present in psoriatic scale extracts as well as supernatants of LPS-stimulated monocytes binds to the same (postulated) receptor on PMN and, also, both factors could represent structurally related or homologous chemoattractants.

Initially it was suggested that PMN-stimulating activities present in the supernatants of LPS-stimulated monocytes as well as keratinocytes derive from interleukin-1 (IL-1) (9,10). However, when recombinant IL-1 was available and biochemical separation of PMN-stimulating activity from IL-1 activity was achieved, it became evident that IL-1 was not a PMN chemotactic and activating factor (11). These findings prompted us to purify and further characterize the *m*onocyte-derived *n*eutrophil-*a*ctivating *p*eptide (MONAP).

As known from recent attempts to characterize monocyte-derived neutrophil chemotactic activity, the molecular mass appeared to be 10,000–15,000 Da (12,13). For purification of MONAP we first applied supernatants to a G-75 gel column. PMN-stimulating activity eluted in fractions corresponding to $M_r = 12{,}000$ (14). A second peak eluting with a corresponding M_r of 50,000 appeared to consist of aggregated or complexed forms of the same chemotaxin, because both chemotaxin preparations showed cross-desensitization with each other (14). MONAP binds to a cation-exchange HPLC column (14) and could be eluted by increasing the ionic strength. Although this method separated large amounts of impurities, recovery of biological activity was low. Nevertheless, by subsequently performed size-exclusion HPLC followed by reversed-phase HPLC (Figure 2), we were able to obtain essentially pure MONAP material which upon SDS-PAGE analysis showed a single line corresponding to an M_r near 10,000 (14).

When MONAP was analyzed for its aminoterminal amino acid sequence, there was evidence for a pure preparation giving the sequence SAKELRXQXIKTYSKPFHPK . . . (15).

At the time we obtained amino acid sequence data for MONAP, a thorough computer search revealed MONAP as a unique polypeptide. Interestingly, in the same year it became clear that Schmid and Weissmann (1987) had isolated a cDNA from mitogen-stimulated mononuclear cells which they termed 3-10C (16). For the deduced

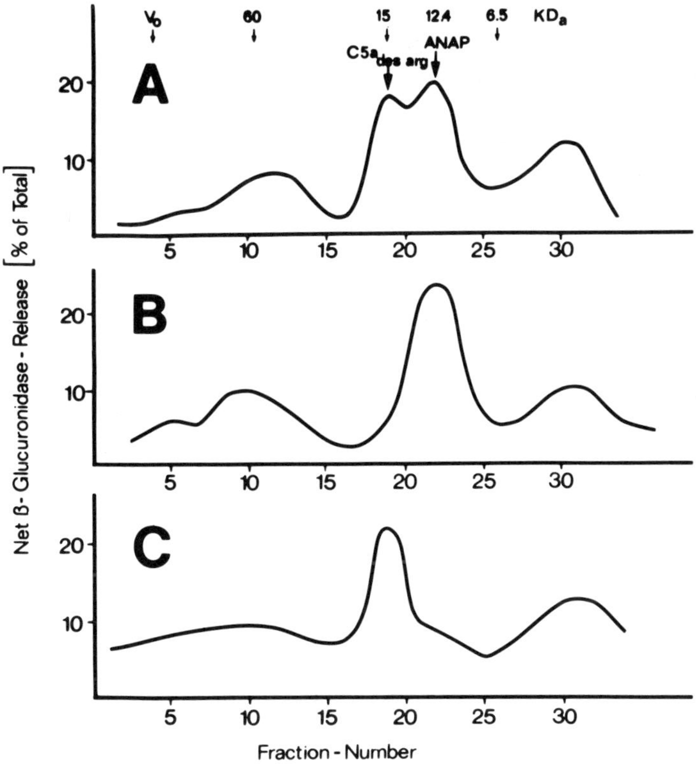

Figure 1 Sephadex G-75 gel chromatography of a psoriatic scale extract. An acidic extract of psoriatic scales was chromatographed on a Sephadex G-75-gel column. Fractions were tested for degranulating activity in PMN, pretreated with cytochalasin B. (A) Profile when normal PMN were used. (B) Profile when PMN were treated with 10^{-8} M C5a prior to cytochalasin B treatment. (C) Same experiment as (B), but using concentrated supernatants of LPS-stimulated human mononuclear cells instead of C5a. Note the reduction of peak I ($C5a_{des\ arg}$), when test PMN were pretreated with C5a as well as reduction of peak II (ANAP) when test PMN were treated with supernatants of LPS-stimulated mononuclear cells.

protein this gave the same amino acid sequence as we obtained from MONAP (16). Obviously, MONAP is the gene product of 3-10C.

Nevertheless, at the time when we isolated and characterized MONAP we became aware that in independent work three other groups had characterized the same cytokine, termed "monocyte-derived neutrophil chemotactic factor" (MDNCF) (17,18), "neutrophil-activating factor" (NAF) (19,20), as well as "granulocyte chemotactic protein" (GCP) (21). To avoid confusion about different names for the same cytokine, at a meeting in Vienna (with three of the groups involved) the name NAP-1 (which stands for "*n*eutrophil-*a*ctivating/*a*ttracting *p*rotein") was agreed. Because NAP-1 also attracts lymphocytes, the term "Interleukin-8" (IL-8) was suggested (22,23). Therefore in this report this novel cytokine will be termed "NAP-1/IL-8."

The production of a neutrophil-attracting protein by activated monocytes or macrophages was recognized 10 years ago. Merrill et al. (12), as well as Tono-Oka et al.

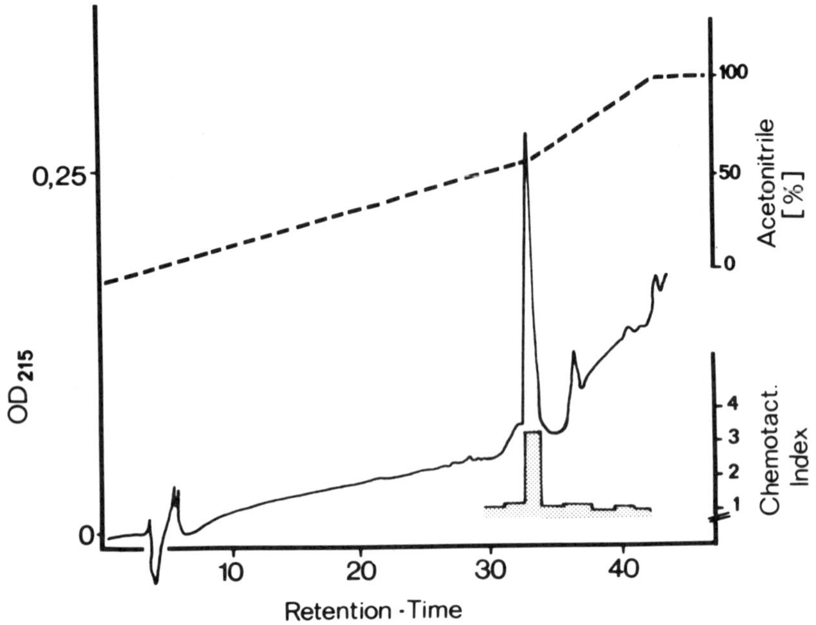

Figure 2 Final purification of MONAP by reversed-phase HPLC. MONAP, partially purified by cation-exchange HPLC followed by size-exclusion HPLC, was chromatographed on a RP-18 HPLC column. Proteins (———) were eluted using a gradient of increasing concentrations of acetonitrile. Note the presence of a single peak, absorbing at 215 nm, which contained most of the PMN chemotactic activity.

(24), identified neutrophil chemotactic activity of proteinaceous nature, which was partially purified. Interestingly, in Merrill's report, charge heterogeneity of neutrophil chemotactic proteins corresponding to pI's near 4 and 5.5 was described (12). Isoelectrofocusing of crude leukocytic pyrogen revealed two chemotactic activity peaks which eluted at pH 4–5.5 as well as the second peak near pH 6.8 (9). These findings were supported by our own experiments. We isolated neutrophil chemotactic NAP-1/IL-8 from LPS-stimulated monocytes by reversed-phase HPLC, a procedure which avoids separation of different charged types of the cytokine. Although a single line could be detected upon SDS-PAGE, analytical IEF analysis revealed the presence of differently charged types of NAP-1/IL-8 with pI's near 4.7, 4.9, 6.4, and 6.9 (25) (Figure 3).

A. Biochemical Properties of NAP-1/IL-8

Aminoterminal amino acid sequence characterization of NAP-1/IL-8 revealed this peptide to be a novel cytokine with no structural homologies to known cytokines such as IL-1 or tumor necrosis factor (TNF). By sequencing of tryptic and chymotryptic fragments of reduced and alkylated NAP-1/IL-8, this cytokine was found to consist of 72 residues (MW: 8386) containing four half-cysteines and 14 basic amino acids (15,26). The primary structure of NAP-1/IL-8 was supported by solid-phase synthesis: A synthesized peptide with identical sequence found for natural NAP-1/IL-8 showed the same biological behavior (27). Although the secondary and tertiary structure is currently being studied by X-ray cristallography (K. Matsushima, personal communica-

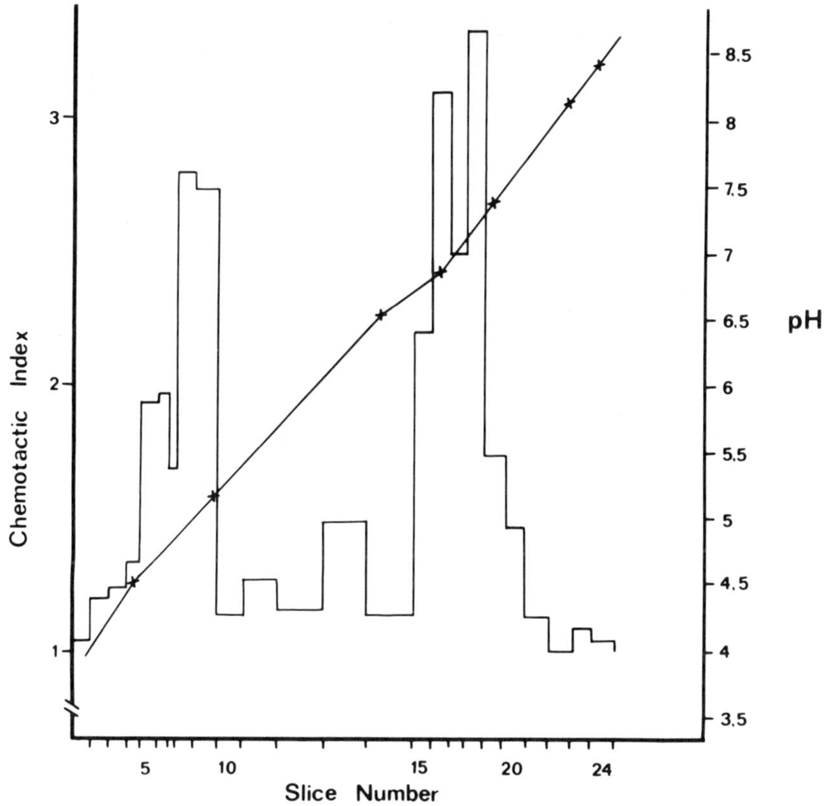

Figure 3 Analytical IEF of purified MONAP. MONAP purified by reversed-phase HPLC was analyzed for charge heterogeneity by analytical IEF. After focusing, lanes bearing MONAP were fixed and stained with silver (lower part of the figure). A second gel slice bearing MONAP was extracted and the extract assayed for chemotactic activity. Note the presence of different protein bands containing PMN chemotactic activity. (From Ref. 25.)

tion) and nuclear magnetic resonance spectroscopy (28,29), it appears that the NAP-1/IL-8 monomer contains a triple standard antiparallel β-sheet with a long carboxyterminal α-helix and that IL-8 forms dimers in solution (28).

Disulfide bridges most likely occur from cysteine-7 to cysteine-34 and from cysteine-9 to cysteine-50, giving a two-loop configuration (Figure 4). The secondary structure appears to be closely related to that of platelet factor 4 as well β-thromboglobulin, both platelet α-granule-derived polypeptides, which belong to the same superfamily of cytokines as NAP-1/IL-8 does (15,18,26,30,31). In addition, the structure of NAP-1/IL-8 was supported by production of recombinant material (32). NAP-1/IL-8 expressed in *E. coli* has been found to be fully biologically active (26,32). These findings suggest that formation of disulfide bridges may occur spontaneously in the correct manner, because upon storage reduced NAP-1/IL-8 as well as recombinant NAP-1/IL-8 are able to recover full biological activity (26,27). Apart from the 72-residue form of NAP-1/IL-8, several extended as well as NH_2-terminally truncated forms (Table 1) have been isolated from mononuclear cell supernatants (33,34). These findings point toward the presence of different peptidase activities in cell supernatants.

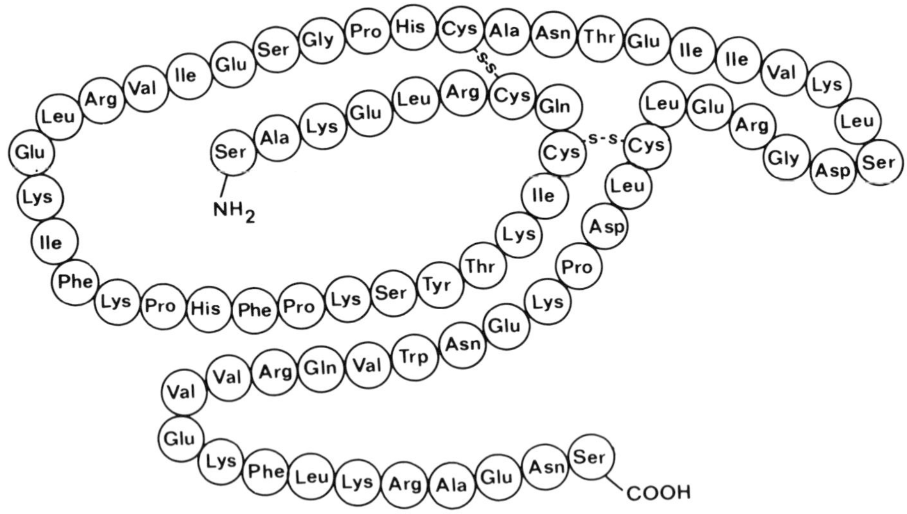

Figure 4 Primary structure of NAP-1/IL-8.

However, cleavage of extended forms may also occur spontaneously, which makes it difficult to isolate all these different forms of NAP-1/IL-8 (33).

When we isolated NAP-1/IL-8 from supernatants of LPS-stimulated monocytes by affinity chromatography using our monoclonal antibodies against NAP-1/IL-8, a polypeptide could be isolated apart from NAP-1/IL-8, which obviously is a COOH-terminal cleavage product of NAP-1/IL-8 (35). Therefore it appears that next to NH_2-terminal extended forms COOH-terminal-truncated products also exist.

B. NAP-1/IL-8 Is a Member of a Novel Supergene Family

NAP-1/IL-8 has strong sequence homology with some platelet α-granule products such as β-thromboglobulin (β-TG) (Figure 5), which is known to be a cleavage product of the platelet basic protein (PBP). PBP is the precursor form of connective tissue activating peptide III (CTAP III) (36). None of these peptides expresses any significant PMN chemotactic activity (34,37).

Table 1 Different NH_2-Terminal Variants of NAP-1/IL-8[a]

NH_2-terminal sequence	Percent	Reference
EGAVLPRSAKELRCQCI . . .	0–10	33
AVLPRSAKELRCQCI . . .	10–20	15,26,33,34
SAKELRCQCI . . .	>70	15,26,33,34
AKELRCQCI . . .	0–8	26,33,34
KELRCQCI . . .	45[b]	34
ELRCQCI . . .	3–13	26,33,34

[a] The single-letter code for amino acids is used.

[b] A single observation.

```
                         1        10        20        30        40        50        60        70        80        90
hβ-TG                  ...GKEESLDSDLYAELRCMCIKTTSG-IHP-KNIQSLEVIGK-GTHCNQV-EVIATL-KDGRKICLDPDAPRIKK-IVQKKLAGDESAD
hNAP-1/IL-8                   AVLPRSAKELRCQCIKTYSKPFHP-KFIKELRVIES-GPHCANT-EIIVKL-SDGRELCLDPKENWVQR-VVEKFLKRAENS
ch9E3                 ...ALSQGRTLVKMGNELRCQCISTHSKFIHP-KSIQDVKLTPS-GPHCKNV-EIIATL-KDGREVCLDPTAPWVQL-IV-KALMAKAQLNSDAPL
hMGSA/GRO                        ASVATELRCQCLQTLQG-IHP-KNIQSVMVKSP-GPHCAQT-EVIATL-KNGRKACLNPASPIVKK-IIEKMLNSDKSN
mKC/N51                         GAPIANELRCQCLQTMAG-IHL-KNIQSLKVLPS-GPHCTQT-EVIATL-KNGREACLDPEAPLVQK-IVQKMLKGVPK
haGRO                            APVANELRCQCLQTMTG-VHL-KNIESLKVTPP-GPHCTQT-EVIATL-KNGQEACLNPEAPMVQK-IVQKMLKSGIRK
mMIP-2                           AVVASELRCQCLKTLPR-VDF-KNIQSLSVTPP-G...
hPF-4                           EAEEDGDLQCLCVKTTSQ-VRP-RHITSLEVIKA-GPHCPTA-QLIATL-KDGRKICLDLQAPLYKK-II-KKLLES
hIP-10                           VPLSRTVRCTCISISNQPVNP-RSLEKLEIIPA-SQFCPRV-EIIATMKKKGEKRCLNPESKAIKN-LL-KAVSKEMSKRSP
mm3                           ...IPLARTV-CMCIDDGPVRMRA---IGKLEIIPA-SLSCPRV-EIIATMKKNDEQRCLNPESKTIKN-LM-KAFSQKRSKRAP

mMIP-1α/SiSα                   APYGADTPTAC-CFSY-SRKI-PRQFIVD-Y-FETSSL-CSQP-GVIF-LTKRNRQICADSKETWVQRYI--TDLELNA
hLD78/SiShβ/pAT464                 ADTPTAC-CFSYTSRQI-PQNFIAD-Y-FETSSQ-CSKP-GVIF-LTKRSRQVCADPSEEWVQKYV--SDLELSA
mMIP1β/SiSh                    APMGSDPPTSC-CFSYTSRQL-HRSFVMD-Y-YETSSL-CSKP-AVVF-LTKRGRQICANPSEPWVTEYM--SDLELN
hACT-2                      ...APMGSDPPTSC-CFSYTARKL-PRNFVVD-Y-YETSSL-CSQP-AVVF-QTKRSKQVCADPSESWVQEYV--YDLELN
hPAT744/SiSh                   APMGSDPPTAC-CFSYT-REA-SSNFVVD-Y-YETSSL-CSQP-AVVF-QTKRSKQVCADPSESWVQEYV--YDLELN
hRANTES/SiS                     SPYSSDTTPC-CFAYIARPL-PRAHIKE-Y-FYTSGK-CSNP-AVVF-VTRKNRQVCANPEKKWVREYI--NSLEMS
mJE                                  APLTC-CYSFTSKMI-PMSRLES-YKRITSSR-CPKE-AVVF-VTKLKREVCADPKKEWVQTYI--KNLDRNQMRSE
hMCAF                          QPDAINAPVTC-CYNFTNRKI-SVQRLAS-YRRITSSK-CPKE-AVIF-KTIVAKEICADPKQKWVQDSM--DHLDKQTQTPKT
```

Figure 5 The β-thromboglobulin superfamilies containing the C-X-C- as well as C-C structural elements. Sequences of human β-thromboglobulin (hβ-TG) (39), human NAP-1/IL-8 (15,18,26), 9E3 from chicken fibroblasts (ch 9E3) (45,46), human melanoma growth-stimulatory activity, product of the growth-regulated oncogene gro (hMGSA/gro) (50,53), murine KC/N51 (mKC/N51) (47,48), murine macrophage inflammatory protein-2 (mMIP-2) (49), human platelet factor 4 (hPF-4) (46), human γ-interferon-inducible protein 10 (h-IP-10) (41), and the murine equivalent of IP 10 (mm3) (44) are listed in the upper part of the figure. Note that all of these polypeptides contain a C-X-C- structural element. The second group of β-thromboglobulin-like proteins contains two adjacent cysteines (C-C) as major structural elements. Members of this superfamily are murine macrophage inflammatory protein-1 (mMIP-1α and β) (61), human LD78 (hLD78) (63), human ACT-2 (hACT-2), (64), human PAT 744 (hPAT 744) (65), human RANTES (hRANTES) (64), murine JE (mJE) (60), and human monocyte chemotactic and activating factor, now termed human monocyte chemotactic protein 1 (hMCAF/MCP-1) (57,59). Conserved common structural elements (cysteines) are shaded. The single-letter code for amino acids is used. Gaps are indicated by (—).

Another α-granule product, platelet factor 4 (PF-4), belongs to the same family of cytokines and appears to have a similar secondary structure (38) as found for β-TG (39) as well as NAP-1/IL-8 (28). PF-4 has been described as a PMN chemotactic factor (40). However, its potency appears to be rather low, giving an ED_{50} near 1 μg/ml, which is approximately 1000-fold higher than that found for NAP-1/IL-8 (14,26). A number of additional members of this family have recently been identified which are mainly secretory products from mononuclear cells.

Inflammatory protein 10 (IP-10) is a cytokine secreted by γ-interferon-activated mononuclear cells (41,42). Similar to NAP-1/IL-8, the IP-10 gene is expressed in macrophages, endothelial cells, and fibroblasts, as well as keratinocytes. Its biological function is yet unknown. IP-10 immunoreactivity could be identified in pathological conditions such as type IV immune reaction (43), indicating a possible role of IP-10 in special types of inflammation. The murine equivalent of IP-10 has recently been identified and is termed m3 (44). In transformed chicken fibroblasts, a gene termed 9E3/pCEF has been detected, whereby the deduced protein sequence shows 60%

homology to human NAP-1/IL-8 (Figure 5) (45,46). It appears that 9E3/pCEF is the avian equivalent of NAP-1/IL-8, although biological studies have not been done so far.

Recently two genes have been detected in the murine system which were termed KC/N51 (47,48) and macrophage inflammatory protein 2 (MIP-2) (49). The deduced proteins, both of which are chemotactic for PMN (49), show 20–30% homology to human NAP-1/IL-8. The human analog of KC/N51, which shows more than 50% homology with NAP-1/IL-8, is termed melanoma growth-stimulatory activity (MGSA) (50). MGSA is a protein which, apart from β-thromboglobulin, so far shows the closest structural homology to human NAP-1/IL-8 (Figure 5). MGSA was originally identified in melanomas as well-growing melanocytes and appears to be a mitogen for transformed fibroblasts (51,52). MGSA is the product of the oncogene gro (growth-stimulating gene product), which is known to be expressed in tumorigenic fibroblast cell lines (53). Expression of the MGSA/gro gene has been shown to occur apart from melanoma cells in fibroblasts (54,55) as well as endothelial cells (56).

A typical feature of all of these members of the β-TG family is the presence of four cysteine residues with an identical relative positioning, forming a two-looped molecule (Figure 4). In contrast to the family of β-TG-related polypeptides, which as a common characteristic bear the presence of a single residue between the first and the second cysteine with the sequence C-X-C, a second subfamily does exist, demonstrating four cysteines at identical positions. A second feature in common with all members of this subfamily is the lack of a residue between the first and the second cysteines, giving the sequence C-C (Figure 5). Most of the genes of these members are expressed in macrophages or lymphocytes. Although the biological role of most of these gene products is unknown, some of these were characterized via their biological activity.

One of these members is the monocyte chemotactic/activating protein 1 (MCAF, MCP-1) (57–59), which is known to be a monocyte-specific chemotaxin (58,59). The murine equivalent appears to be the product of the gene JE (60).

Another member of the subfamily, termed macrophage inflammatory protein 1α (MIP 1α), which is a murine cytokine, is known to be a weak PMN chemotaxin (61). Recently, however, MIP 1α has been identified as a potent inhibitor of hemopoietic stem cell proliferation (52). The human equivalent of MIP 1α is the gene product of a cDNA termed LD 78 (63), Sishβ (64), or pAT 646 (65). Although final evidence has not been given so far, this could represent a human inhibitor of hemopoietic stem cell proliferation.

The genes for IP-10 and PF-4 as well as NAP-1/IL-8 have been identified on chromosome 4 (66). Moreover, the gene for MGSA/gro has been localized on chromosome 4Q21 (50). These findings, together with the close structural similarities of the cytokines described above, make it likely that all these are members derived from an ancestral gene and are formed by gene duplication and divergence.

C. Biological Properties of NAP-1/IL-8

1. Migration-Stimulating Activity of NAP-1/IL-8 in PMN

Originally, NAP-1/IL-8 was identified, but not characterized, as a neutrophil chemotactic factor (12,13,24). Purification allowed specific characterization of its activity. NAP-1/IL-8 now is known to be an extremely potent in-vitro chemotactic factor with an ED_{50} near 0.1–0.8 nM depending on the method used (Figure 6) (14,26). The

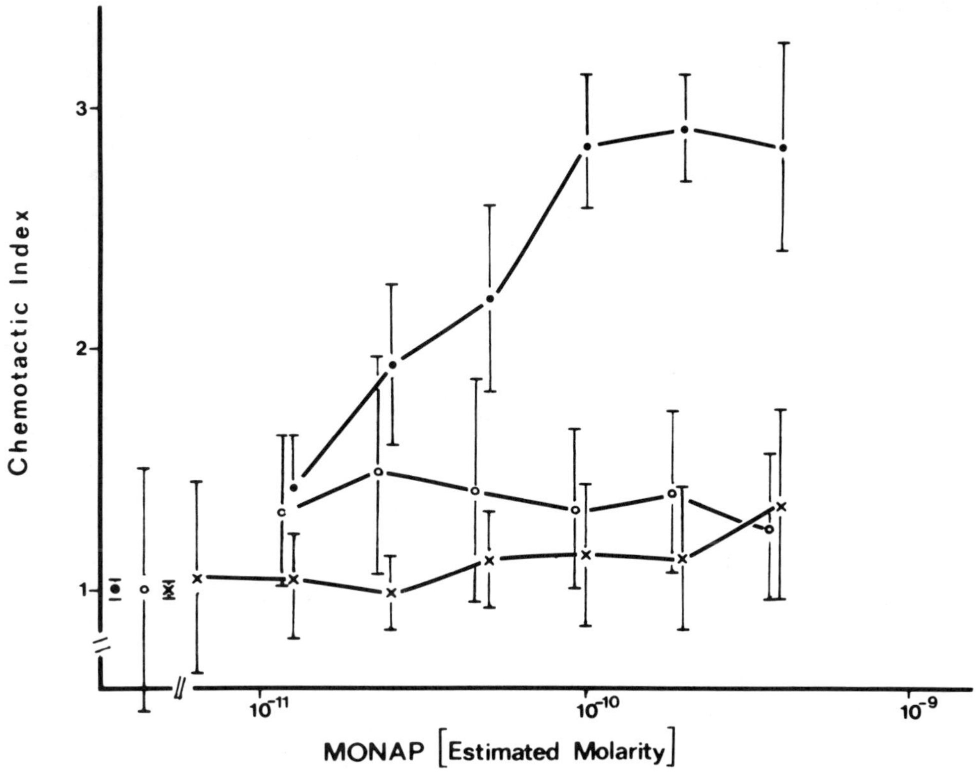

Figure 6 Investigations of chemotactic activity for leukocytes by purified NAP-1/IL-8. Chemotactic activity was investigated for different types of leukocytes (-●-) indicates chemotactic activity for PMN, whereas chemotaxis for human monocytes is shown by (-×-). Chemotactic responses of human eosinophils are given in (-○-). (From Ref. 14.)

numbers of PMN migrating at optimal doses are similar to those seen with the most potent known PMN chemotaxins, C5a and LTB_4 (14). Also, apart from chemotactic migration, NAP-1/IL-8 is chemokinetically active (14). In contrast to other well-characterized chemotactic factors, NAP-1/IL-8 apparently is not a chemotactic factor for either human monocytes or eosinophils (Figure 6) (14,18), indicating some specificity of NAP-1/IL-8 for neutrophils.

2. *Secretory Responses*

PMN chemotactic factors are known to elicit the release of primary granule contents when cells are preincubated with the microfilament-binding agent cytochalasin B (67). Also, NAP-1/IL-8 could be identified as eliciting the release of either β-glucuronidase (14), elastase (19,20), or myeloperoxidase (14) (Figure 7).

The release of cellular elastase has been used to characterize NAP-1/IL-8 (19). Apart from degranulation of primary (azurophilic) PMN granules, release of vitamin B_{12}-binding protein or lactoferrin from secondary (specific) granules could be elicited by NAP-1/IL-8. This was achieved in a dose-dependent fashion (20,68), even in the absence of any pretreatment of PMN (68).

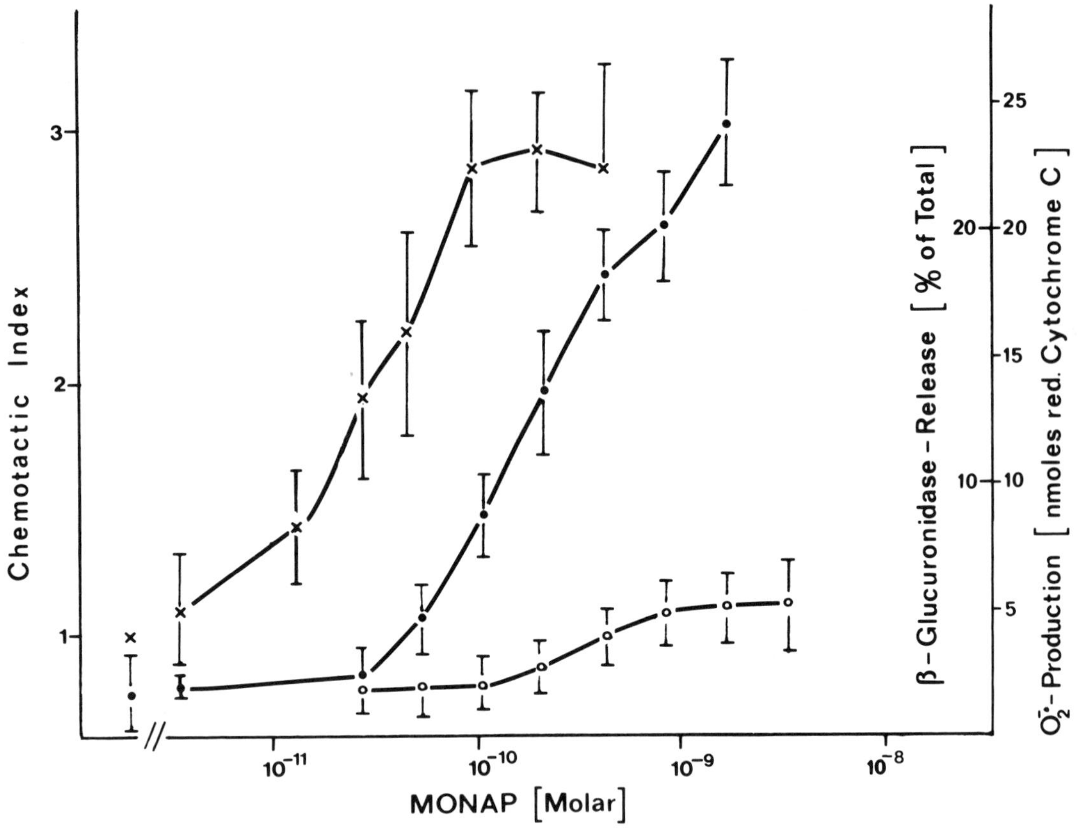

Figure 7 Activation of secretory responses by NAP-1/IL-8. Human PMN were pretreated with cytochalasin B and subsequently challenged with variable doses of NAP-1/IL-8. Either the release of β-glucuronidase (-●-) or the superoxide dismutase-inhibitable cytochrome C reduction O_2^- production (-○-) are indicated. Note the very weak, O_2^- release after NAP-1/IL-8 stimulation, when PMN were pretreated with cytochalasin B. (From Ref. 14.)

NAP-1/IL-8 therefore could be responsible for the lactoferrin-releasing activity of the partially purified "leukocytic pyrogen" (69), which is now known to be identical with IL-1. This cytokine, however, lacks any neutrophil-stimulating activity (11).

3. Activation of the Respiratory Burst

Partially purified leukocyte pyrogen has been described as activating the respiratory burst of human neutrophils [shown by increased tetrazolium blue precipitate (70)]. However, this biological activity is not elicitable by IL-1 because hrIL-1 did not activate the respiratory burst of PMN (11). The most likely explanation would be that NAP-1/IL-8, present in the leukocyte pyrogen preparation, was responsible for activation of the PMN respiratory burst. Indeed, we (14) as well as other investigators (20) found NAP-1/IL-8-induced activation of membrane NADPH-oxidase as measured either by cytochrome C reduction (14) or by chemiluminescence (20). Nevertheless, NAP-1/IL-8 is a very weak activator of the respiratory burst. Similar to stimulation by LTB_4, O_2^- production (measured via cytochrome C reduction) was detectable only when

when PMN were used at high cell numbers and when preincubated with cytochalasin B (14). This may explain why some investigators were unable to detect any respiratory burst induction (27) and supports the suggestion that NAP-1/IL-8 is similar to LTB_4 in its biological behavior. LTB_4 is known to be a highly potent PMN chemotactic factor, a weaker inducer of enzyme release, and a very weak activator of the respiratory burst (71).

4. *Induction of LTB_4 Synthesis by NAP-1/IL-8*

A number of well-characterized PMN chemotactic factors such as C5a, fMLP, or PAF have been reported to activate the PMN 5-lipoxygenase, an enzyme leading to the formation of LTB_4 (72).

In a recent investigation it has been shown that monocyte-derived IL-1 preparations are able to elicit LTB_4 release in the absence of arachidonic acid as a substrate (73). Although it was initially suggested that IL-1 is the activator of cellular 5-lipoxygenase (73), it was concluded that a different neutrophil-activating factor might be responsible for this observation (74).

In a study conducted in our laboratory, the ability of human monocytes to secrete a cytokine which stimulates the formation of LTB_4 was investigated (75). Interestingly, when supernatants of LPS-stimulated monocytes were separated by reversed-phase HPLC and fractions were analyzed for induction of LTB_4 production, no such activity could be detected, despite the fact that the crude supernatant revealed such activity. Therefore the experiment was repeated by adding exogenous arachidonic acid to the cells. Now a single peak of LTB_4-forming activity could be detected in fractions which were shown to contain NAP-1/IL-8 (75). Indeed, purification of the 5-lipoxygenase-stimulating activity revealed a polypeptide with identical biochemical as well as biological properties as found for NAP-1/IL-8 (Figure 8) (75). The failure of HPLC column fractions to induce LTB_4 production in PMN directly might be the result of a two-step event of LTB_4 production: One step is the liberation of arachidonic acid (i.e., by activation of cellular phospholipases/diacylglycerol lipases) and the other consists of the activation of the PMN 5-lipoxygenase.

Furthermore, it is intriguing to speculate that both processes may be activated by different cytokines, which could be separated by reversed-phase HPLC. This suggestion is supported by our own findings: NAP-1/IL-8 is not able to elicit LTB_4 production in the absence of exogenous arachidonic acid, even at nonphysiological concentrations (75). This fits well with other findings, that after prelabeling of PMN with ^3H-arachidonic acid NAP-1/IL-8 did not activate the release of cellular ^3H-arachidonic acid or metabolites (75).

Interestingly, another cytokine, GMCSF, is known to prime for the activation of cellular phospholipases and diacylglycerol lipases, and—as shown for C5a or fMLP (76)—pretreatment of PMN with this cytokine may induce the release of LTB_4 when cells are stimulated with NAP-1/IL-8. Alternatively, the LPS-activated monocytes may have released sufficient arachidonic acid to serve as substrate for neutrophil 5-lipoxygenase.

5. *Effects of NAP-1/IL-8 on Adherence or Expression of Adherence Proteins*

Chemotactic factors such as fMLP or LTB_4 have been shown to increase adherence of PMN to cultured human endothelial cell monolayers (77,78). This effect appeared to be PMN dependent rather than endothelium dependent. Recently conducted studies using NAP-1/IL-8 revealed that this cytokine was able to stimulate PMN to adhere to cul-

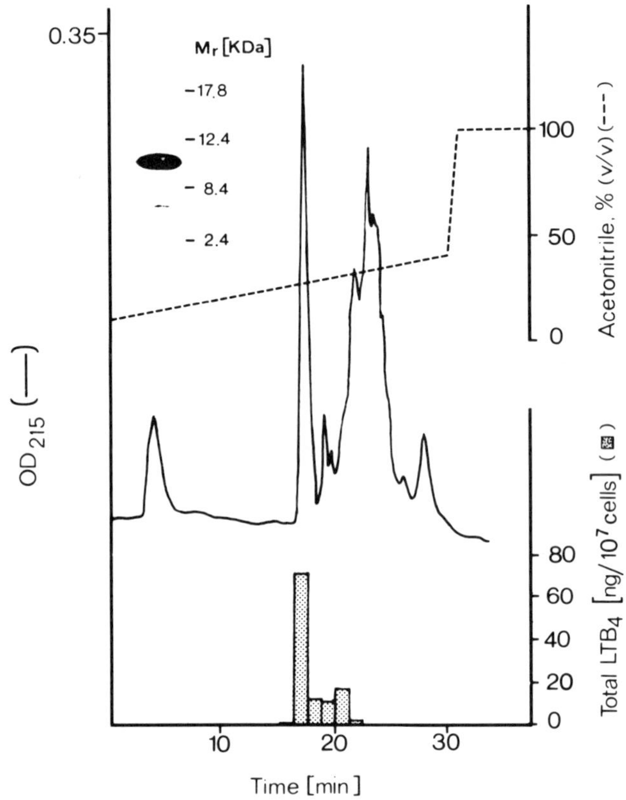

Figure 8 Purification of an LTB_4 synthesis-inducing cytokine. RP-8 HPLC-purified LTB_4 synthesis-inducing activity in supernatants of LPS-stimulated monocytes was finally purified by CN-propyl HPLC. The major peak of LTB_4 synthesis-inducing activity eluted in a single peak absorbing at 215 nm, showing a single line near 10 kDa upon SDS-PAGE (inset). (From Ref. 75.)

tured human endothelial cell monolayers (79). NAP-1/IL-8-induced PMN adhesion to EC has been found to be concentration dependent with a threshold at 10^{-9}–10^{-8} M and a maximum at 10^{-6} M (79). Interestingly, adhesion to EC layers was rapid, with a peak at 10 min, but binding was rapidly reversed, with a return to control values by 30 min (79). Adherence of NAP-1/IL-8-stimulated PMN is found to be associated with increased expression of the leukocyte CD_{11}/CD_{18} integrins (80); the latter could be inhibited by a monoclonal antibody against CD_{18}. It appears that NAP-1/IL-8 may promote the adhesion of activated PMN to the endothelium.

Interestingly, biochemical characterization of an endothelial cell-derived leukocyte adhesion inhibitor (LAI) revealed identity with the five-amino acid extended form of NAP-1/IL-8 (81). It appears that LAI shows the opposite effect as found for NAP-1/IL-8. Surprisingly, recombinant NAP-1/IL-8 showed the same inhibitory effect. In contrast to studies using untreated endothelial layers (79), in these investigations EC were pretreated with IL-1. Therefore it appears likely that, depending on pretreatment of EC layers, NAP-1/IL-8 may function as either an adherence promotor or inhibitor.

6. *Detection of NAP-1/IL-8-Specific Receptors on PMN*

Preincubation of PMN with NAP-1/IL-8 diminished the enzyme release following a second challenge with NAP-1/IL-8. In similar experiments, responses to other chemotaxins such as C5a, fMLP, PAF, or LTB_4 were not affected (14). Specific desensitization was also obtained when the respiratory burst was studied: Preincubation of PMN with NAP-1/IL-8 resulted in a diminished chemiluminescence when cells were restimulated with the same stimulus, but not with other stimuli (20).

These results led to the suggestion that NAP-1/IL-8 binds to a specific receptor on PMN. Indeed, as shown by incubation of PMN with ^{125}I-NAP-1/IL-8, saturable binding of radioactivity to the PMN membrane could be observed (82), and this binding of radioactivity could be prevented by adding nonradioactive NAP-1/IL-8 (82). Furthermore, Scatchard analysis revealed the presence of 20,000 receptors per cell with a K_D near 8×10^{-10} M (82). After chemical cross-linking of ^{125}I-NAP-1/IL-8 and the receptor complex, two distinct polypeptides could be detected upon SDS-PAGE followed by autoradiography (82). The M_r of the NAP-1/IL-8-binding proteins were estimated to be 67 and 59 kDa; reasons for the heterogeneity are so far unknown (82).

Studies of Besemer et al. (83) supported the existence of an NAP-1/IL-8-specific receptor on PMN. Interestingly, these investigators observed two receptor types, one with high (K_D = 11–35 pM) and the other with lower (K_D = 640–830 pM) affinity. The numbers of the low-affinity binding sites were approximately 34,000, and those with high affinity were 5,200 per cell (83). These findings are similar to those found for fMLP (84) and LTB_4 (85).

Comparison of receptor binding activities in various inflammatory cell types revealed that NAP-1/IL-8 receptor expression was observed mainly in PMN. Blood monocytes, monocytic cell lines, as well as lymphocyte preparations also bound NAP-1/IL-8 to a limited extent (82,83). Platelets and erythrocytes did not bind significant amounts of NAP-1/IL-8 (82,83).

Interestingly, binding of NAP-1/IL-8 to its receptor is characterized by two steps: One consists of binding to the receptor in an acid-sensitive form (at 4°C); the other consists of rapid formation of an acid-resistant form which occurs at 37°C (66). Addition of lysosomotropic agents such as ammonium chloride, although not inhibiting binding of the ligand or ligand internalization, partially inhibited reappearance/recycling of the NAP-1/IL-8 receptors (66). It appeared that NAP-1/IL-8 receptor expression is dynamically regulated by NAP-1/IL-8 itself, and rapid recycling of NAP-1/IL-8 receptors may be essential for chemotaxis of PMN (86).

7. *Mechanisms of PMN Activation by NAP-1/IL-8*

Well-characterized PMN-activating factors such as fMLP, C5a, PAF, or LTB_4 are known to bind to distinct receptors eliciting several biological responses, i.e., chemotactic migration, exocytosis, or activation of the respiratory burst. Signal transduction through the chemotaxin receptors seems to be similar or identical. Therefore it became interesting to know if similar mechanisms may occur with NAP-1/IL-8.

Thelen et al. (87) have shown that NAP-1/IL-8 causes a rapid (<3 s) rise in cytosolic free Ca^{2+} concentration, which could be inhibited by Bortedella pertussin toxin. In addition, superoxide production by NAP-1/IL-8 was blocked when cells were pretreated with either 17-hydroxywortmannin or staurosporine. Based on these data it has been suggested that GTP-binding proteins may be associated with the NAP-1/IL-8-receptor and protein kinase C activation may be essential for activation by NAP-1/IL-8

(87). Moreover, it has been mentioned that NAP-1/IL-8 rapidly phosphorylates a cytosolic 48-kDa protein. This has been reported to be phosphorylated when PMN were activated with other chemoattractants and is claimed to be involved in the superoxide anion production (87).

8. *NAP-1/IL-8 Also Activates Other Cells*

Purification of lipopolysaccharide/phytohemagglutinin (LPS/PHA)-stimulated human mononuclear cell supernatants for lymphocyte chemotactic activity led to a polypeptide with the same aminoterminal amino acid sequence as found for NAP-1/IL-8 (22).

Chemotactic activity of NAP-1/IL-8 for human lymphocytes was confirmed by the use of recombinant material. This has been found to be active at concentrations below 10^{-12} M (88). The number of lymphocytes migrating when stimulated with NAP-1/IL-8, however, appears to be low, which supports the suggestion that NAP-1/IL-8 represents primarily a chemotaxin with relatively high specificity for PMN (89). Apart from these findings, it was recently shown that NAP-1/IL-8 also attracts basophils (90).

In addition, recent studies on basophils revealed that NAP-1/IL-8, either as natural or recombinant material, is able to cause histamine release. However, this occurred at a concentration found to be two orders of magnitude higher ($\sim 10^{-6}$ M) than the optimal NAP-1/IL-8 concentration required for basophil chemotaxis (90). The net histamine release by NAP-1/IL-8 was nearly half of that observed with the potent inducer anti-IgE (90). NAP-1/IL-8 at concentrations $< 10^{-7}$ M did not elicit a significant release of histamine by basophils (90). Interestingly, pretreatment (priming) of basophils with 20 ng/ml of interleukin-3 (IL-3) resulted in an enhancement of responsiveness to NAP-1/IL-8 (90). IL-3-pretreated basophils showed a similar dose-response curve either in the NAP-1/IL-8-induced release of histamine or sulfido-leukotrienes, when compared with the secretion of azurophilic granule enzymes (ED_{50}: 10 nM).

Thus, not only can NAP-1/IL-8 induce infiltration of neutrophils and possibly lymphocytes, it could also be involved in the pathogenesis of type I hypersensitivity reactions.

A summary of known biological properties in vitro is given in Table 2.

Table 2 Biological Properties of NAP-1/IL-8 in Vitro

	References
Stimulation of PMN chemotaxis	14,18,21,27
Stimulation of PMN chemokinesis	14
Activation of the respiratory burst in PMN	14,20
Exocytosis of (a) azurophilic granule constituents	14,20,27
(b) specific granule constituents	20,68
Induction of PMN adherence	79
Activation of PMN 5-lipoxygenase	75
Inhibition of PMN adherence to endothelial cells	81
Increased expression of CD_{11}/CD_{18} integrins in PMN	80
Stimulation of T-lymphocyte chemotaxis	22
Attraction of basophils	90
Release of histamine in basophils	90,91

III. EFFECTS OF NAP-1/IL-8 IN VIVO

A. Investigations in Animals

Intravenous injection of NAP-1/IL-8 into the rabbit was rapidly followed by a profound granulocytosis, which peaked at 1/2 to 2 h after injection. The effects were found to be dose dependent (21). IL-1β, known to elicit granulocytosis of later onset, was suggested to promote its effect via induction of NAP-1/IL-8 synthesis and release (21).

Intradermal injection of NAP-1/IL-8—either as natural compound or as recombinant material—into rabbits led to a mild infiltration predominantly by PMN (92–94). When the vasodilator PGE_2 was injected together with NAP-1/IL-8, a profound neutrophil accumulation could be detected in rabbit ear skin, which occurred at lower doses of NAP-1/IL-8 than those seen for fMLP (92,93). Indeed, 10^{-14} mol per site were found to be sufficient to detect significant PMN influx (94). In addition to infiltration by PMN, NAP-1/IL-8 led to plasma exudation into the skin at a dose response similar to that seen for PMN infiltration (92,93). The kinetics of the NAP-1/IL-8-induced inflammatory responses resembled those of other established chemotactic factors such as the complement fragment C5a and the bacterial tripeptide fMLP (92–94). Because NAP-1/IL-8 could be produced endogenously (e.g., by tissue macrophages, fibroblasts, or endothelial cells), it may be involved in the acute phase of an inflammatory response to microbial stimuli.

Injection of rNAP-1/IL-8 into lymphatic drainage areas of lymph nodes in rats caused an increase of lymph node weight as well as increase in lymphocyte traffic (22). The effective dose has been found between 0.01 and 1 μg of NAP-1/IL-8 (22). When rNAP-1/IL-8 was injected into ear skin of rats, a dose-related accumulation of PMN as well as lymphocytes, but not monocytes, was observed in the edematous sites of injection (22). Low doses of rNAP-1 (1 ng/ml) selectively attracted lymphocytes, whereas at higher doses predominantly PMN were attracted (22).

B. Investigations in Humans

1. *In-Vivo Effects in Human Skin*

When human NAP-1/IL-8—either as a natural product or as recombinant material—was injected intracutaneously at various doses ranging from 1 ng to 1 μg per injection, no clinical symptoms were observed except for the transient bleb caused by injection of a 40–100 μL volume (95,96). Because of the absence of a wheal and flare reaction as well as pruritus, it was suggested that NAP-1/IL-8 does not induce mast cells to release histamine (95,96). This hypothesis was supported by electron micrographs of NAP-1/IL-8-injected skin areas showing that cutaneous mast cells failed to show signs of degranulation (95). Moreover, there was a moderate swelling of capillary endothelial cells and an inflammatory cell infiltrate which consisted predominantly of neutrophils. Only a few mononuclear cells were observed, mainly in or around the vessels of the superficial and mid dermis (95,96). Interestingly, no significant migration into the surrounding dermis was observed. These findings are totally different from those seen with C5a as a chemoattractant, where a massive dermal PMN infiltrate could be observed (97,98).

The failure to detect signs of a dermal neutrophil infiltrate following NAP-1/IL-8 injection was further ascertained by a newly developed skin blister assay in which subepidermal bullae raised by suction are filled with known chemotaxins for various lengths of time. Again, in contrast to C5a and LTB_4, which are potent in-vivo PMN chemotaxins in human skin (97,98), no migratory PMN response could be elicited with NAP-1/IL-8 (our unpublished results).

Our results were quite unexpected, not only because of the well-documented in-vitro effectiveness of NAP-1/IL-8 in stimulating neutrophils, but also because this cytokine proved to be a powerful pro-inflammatory agent in several laboratory animals. As pointed out above, injection of NAP-1/IL-8 in rabbit ear skin (together with PGE_2) resulted in plasma exudation and perivascular accumulation of neutrophils (92,93). Massive neutrophil infiltration following intradermal injections was also observed in rats, mice, guinea pigs, and dogs (99).

Reasons for this failure to exert signs of massive inflammation in human skin could be manifold and include the need for a second stimulus acting as cofactor together with NAP-1/IL-8. On the other hand, rapid inactivation by human skin proteases appears possible, although at present the fate of this cytokine after production is unknown.

IV. NAP-1/IL-8 IS A CYTOKINE OF MULTICELLULAR ORIGIN

Originally, monocytes were identified as a source of NAP-1/IL-8. These cells were shown to express the NAP-1/IL-8 gene or release the mature cytokine, when stimulated with various stimuli such as LPS, IL-1α, IL-1β, or TNF_α (30,66,100). The dose of these stimuli has been found to be in the namomolar range, indicating a very high sensitivity of the NAP-1/IL-8 gene expression (101). Activated monocytes are by far the most potent producers of NAP-1/IL-8. For example, by the use of affinity chromatography we were able to obtain 50 μg of pure NAP-1/IL-8 from 100 mL of supernatant, corresponding to a ratio of 0.1 pg per cell, which is in a similar order as found by other investigators.

Apart from monocytes, lung macrophages were similarly found to secrete PMN chemotactic material with some biochemical similarities to NAP-1/IL-8 (12). Although this chemotactic peptide has not yet been fully characterized, a recent reinvestigation showed by NH_2-terminal amino acid sequence analysis that the major NAP produced by lung-lavage macrophages is indeed identical with NAP-1/IL-8 (102).

A. Lymphocytes as a Source of NAP-1/IL-8

Whereas the production of NAP-1/IL-8 by mononuclear phagocytes has been observed by several laboratories, formation of NAP-1/IL-8-related PMN chemotaxins by lymphocytes remained a point of discussion. Using purified lymphocyte preparations, we could show that purified T-lymphocyte preparations indeed are able to produce NAP-1/IL-8 (103). The lymphocyte-derived NAP preparation (LYNAP) contained 70% NAP-1/IL-8 and 30% of the five-amino-acid extended form of NAP-1/IL-8 (15). This latter finding contrasts to results obtained from monocyte preparations, where we did not find any extended forms of NAP-1/IL-8 (six experiments). However, we reproducibly detected extended forms of NAP-1/IL-8 in supernatants of PHA or concanavalin A (Con A)-stimulated lymphocyte preparations or supernatants of mononuclear cell mixtures.

The failure to detect any PMN chemotactic activity in stimulated lymphocyte preparations may derive from the presence of mitogens or lymphocyte-derived leukocyte migration-inhibiting substances (LIFs), which can affect the assay system, or the use of LPS, which is not a stimulus for T-lymphocytes (103).

Production of NAP-1/IL-8 by lymphocytes could be further proven by the use of cell lines: HUT-78 cells (from lymphoma) apparently constitutively secrete low amounts of NAP-1/IL-8 (data not shown).

In comparison to monocytes, highly purified T-lymphocyte preparations produce only low amounts of NAP-1/IL-8. Reasons for these differences are not clear but could be the result of too low numbers of contaminating macrophages, which are known to be necessary for secretion of large amounts of lymphokines. At the moment the in-vivo relevance of the production of NAP-1/IL-8 by lymphocytes cannot be elucidated. It appears that activation of T-cells to produce NAP-1/IL-8 needs more complicated activation kinetics. Moreover, it cannot be excluded that only subpopulations are able to produce sufficient amounts of NAP-1/IL-8. These findings suggest that a lymphokine chemotactic for PMN initially reported in the 1970s (104) may actually have been NAP-1/IL-8.

B. Endothelial Cells Secrete NAP-1/IL-8-Related Polypeptides

Among the earliest responses of PMN to an inflammatory stimulus (e.g., infection) is adherence to the endothelial lining of postcapillary vessels. Investigations of Mercandetti et al. (105) have shown that cultivated human umbilical vein endothelia cells (HUVEC) secrete a biochemically undefined protein which is chemotactic for PMN. Recently it was shown that LPS or IL-1 treatment of HUVEC enhances adherence of PMN (106,107) as well as transendothelial migration (108). Moreover, intradermal injection of these factors resulted in enhanced adherence of PMN to capillary vessels, with the subsequent appearance of a perivascular infiltrate (109).

Therefore we were interested to know whether HUVEC upon LPS stimulation are able to secrete a PMN chemotactic protein. As a result we demonstrated that HUVEC indeed produces two proteinaceous PMN attractants, tentatively termed α- and β-endothelial cell-derived neutrophil-activating peptide (ENAP) (110).

The most potent form of these two attractants appeared biochemically as well as biologically similar to NAP-1/IL-8 (110). Furthermore, upon SDS-PAGE this chemotaxin migrated with slightly enhanced molibility, which points toward an M_r smaller than that of NAP-1/IL-8 (110).

Finally, aminoterminal sequence analysis revealed β-ENAP to be identical with an aminoterminally truncated product of NAP-1/IL-8 starting with glutamic acid (unpublished results).

These findings were supported by Strieter et al., who showed that HUVEC express the NAP-1/IL-8 gene when stimulated with either TNFα, LPS, or IL-1β (111,112). These authors were also able to confirm the presence of PMN chemotactic proteins with an M_r similar to NAP-1/IL-8 in stimulated HUVEC. As much as 0.5 ng of TNFα or IL-1β were found to be sufficient to induce significant NAP-1/IL-8 gene expression. As mentioned above (Section II.C.5), secretion of NAP-1/IL-8 by stimulated endothelial cells was further confirmed by Gimbrone et al. (81), who detected a "leukocyte adherence inhibiting protein" (LAIP), shown to be identical with the 77-residue form of NAP-1/IL-8, whereas our group detected the 69-residue form in supernatants of LPS-stimulated HUVEC. Gimbrone et al. isolated the 77-residue form of NAP-1/IL-8 as a major product when endothelial cells were stimulated with IL-1. Reasons for these differences are presently unknown and need further investigation. Nevertheless, it appears that vascular endothelial cells, by their strategic position, may regulate interactions of circulating leukocytes and the tissue either by facilitating or inhibiting adherence and diapedesis.

B. Fibroblasts Secrete a Pro-Protein Form of NAP-1/IL-8

As has been pointed out, tissue infiltration with PMN following injections of hrIL-1 (113) or hrTNFα (114) was supposed to be related to IL-1 or TNF, both considered as chemoattractants for PMN in vitro (115). There is now ample evidence that neither cytokine activates migratory responses of PMN in vitro (11,116–118), indicating that tissue cells, upon IL-1 or TNF stimulation, may secrete PMN chemotactic factors. Evidence that these could be secreted by fibroblasts was first provided by Matsushima et al. (100), who have shown by Northern blot experiments that dermal fibroblasts, upon stimulation with IL-1 or TNFα, express the NAP-1/IL-8 gene. These findings were confirmed by studies of Golds et al. (54), who were able to isolate the 77-residue form of NAP-1/IL-8 as one of the major low-molecular-mass proteins, when fibroblasts were stimulated with IL-1 or TNF.

The same 77-residue form of NAP-1/IL-8 could be isolated from virus-infected dermal fibroblasts or fibroblasts incubated with double-stranded RNA (119). Studies on gene expression revealed that IL-1β is the most potent inducer of its NAP-1/IL-8 gene expression, indicating that a dose of 0.02 ng of IL-1β/ml proved to be sufficient to give a high response (120,121). Interestingly, LPS—even at concentrations as high as 10 μg/mL—did not induce any significant NAP-1/IL-8 gene expression (119–121).

These findings were confirmed by our own experiments investigating PMN chemotactic proteins in human dermal fibroblasts (55). When supernatants of IL-1α or TNFα-stimulated dermal fibroblasts were analyzed for PMN chemotactic proteins, three PMN chemotaxins could be separated by HPLC techniques. The major chemotaxin was identified as a 77-residue form of NAP-1/IL-8 containing 15% of the 79-residue form (55). Interestingly, the fibroblast-derived 77-residue form was found to be of lower potency in chemotaxis when compared to the 72-residue form of NAP-1/IL-8 (55).

Reasons for these differences are unknown. However, similarities to the β-thromboglobulin/NAP-2 system are apparent (37). Whereas the structurally related β-thromboglobulin is devoid of any PMN chemotactic activity, cleavage of 11 aminoterminal amino acids results in formation of a highly potent PMN-activating protein termed NAP-2 (37,122).

Apart from dermal fibroblasts, other connective tissue cells were noted to be able to secrete NAP-1/IL-8. Recently it has been shown that synovial cells, upon IL-1 stimulation, secrete NAP-1/IL-8-related proteins (123). Interestingly, such cells apparently did not respond to TNFα (124).

C. Secretion of NAP-1/IL-8 or NAP-1/IL-8 Gene Expression by Other Cells

The pro-protein form of NAP-1/IL-8 has been detected in the culture fluid of the human lung giant carcinoma cell line LU 65C (125). Production of this cytokine did not need any stimulus. The relevance of this finding is unknown. Secretion of NAP-1/IL-8 by tumor cells might be important as the first step of immunosurveillance by PMN in their host defense function.

Epithelial cells including hepatocytes were recently found to express NAP-1/IL-8 mRNA in response to IL-1α, IL-1β, or TNFα (126). Using human keratinocytes, the amounts of NAP-1/IL-8-related proteins secreted after stimulation were very low (our unpublished results). It appears that cells of different origin are able to express the NAP-1/IL-8 gene and secrete NAP-1/IL-8 at a cell-specific rate. In addition, each cell type appears to respond to a different set of stimuli (Table 3); i.e., the most potent producers of NAP-1/IL-8 are monocytes/macrophages, followed by fibroblasts and endothelial cells. Low amounts of NAP-1/IL-8 can be obtained from purified and stimulated T-lymphocytes or keratinocytes (Table 3). It cannot be excluded that cells which apparently produce only low amounts of NAP-1/IL-8 need different activation kinetics or stimuli for maximal secretion of NAP-1/IL-8. Nevertheless, it is interesting to know that there do exist several stimuli, such as IL-1, TNFα or LPS, PHA, Con A, or PMA that activate production of NAP-1/IL-8. On the other hand, cytokines such as α-, β-, and γ-interferon, IL-2, or IL-6 apparently do not directly activate any one of these cell types for NAP-1/IL-8 gene expression or secretion of NAP-1/IL-8 (30), although pretreatment of keratinocytes with γ-interferon apparently primes keratinocytes for TNFα-dependent NAP-1/IL-8 gene expression (127).

Cellular sources of NAP-1/IL-8 are summarized in Table 3.

V. DETECTION OF OTHER STRUCTURALLY RELATED NEUTROPHIL CHEMOATTRACTANTS

A. NAP-2

Investigation of platelet-containing cultures of stimulated human blood mononuclear cells for PMN-activating polypeptides led to the detection of a novel neutrophil-activating peptide termed NAP-2 (122,128). Amino acid sequence analysis of purified NAP-2 revealed identity with a 70-residue fragment (see Figure 9) of platelet basic protein (PBP) as well as connective tissue-activating peptide III (CTAP III), which is also known as "low-affinity platelet factor 4" (36). The absence of NAP-2 activity in cultures of purified stimulated human monocytes has led to the hypothesis that NAP-2 is possibly a product of mononuclear cell/platelet interaction. Indeed, it was recently shown that mononcyte-derived proteases are able to cleave PBP or CTAP III between Tyr and Ala, giving mature NAP-2 (128). NAP-2 behaves like a typical chemotactic factor receptor agonist, inducing cytosolic free calcium changes, chemotaxis, and exo-

```
                      1       10        20        30
NAP-1 (IL-8)            SAKELRCQCIKTYSKPFHPKFIKELRVIESGPHCA

NAP-2                     AELRCMCIKTTSG-IHPKNIQSLEVIGKGTHCN

NAP-3 (MGSA/GRO)      ASVATELRCQCLQTLQG-IHPKNIQSVMVKSPGPHCA

                        40        50        60        70
NAP-1 (IL-8)          NTEIIVKLSDGRELCLDPKENWVQRVVEKFLKRAENS

NAP-2                 QVEVIATLKDGRKICLDPDAPRIKKIVQKKLAGDESAD

NAP-3 (MGSA/GRO)      QTEVIATLKNGRKACLNPASPIVKKIIEKMLNSDKSN
```

Figure 9 Amino acid sequences of different neutrophil-activating proteins. The sequences are aligned according to the compared cysteine residues. The single-letter code for amino acids is used.

Table 3 Cellular Source and Stimuli for NAP-1/IL-8 Gene Expression/Secretion

Source	Stimuli	Gene expression/ secretion	References
Blood monocytes	LPS/TNF/IL-1	+ + + + +	14,16,18,19,21,59,101
Alveolar macrophages	LPS	+ + + + +	102
T-cell preparations	PHA/Con A	+	15,103
Endothelial cells	LPS/IL-1/TNF	+ + + +	110,111,112
Fibroblasts	IL-1/double-stranded RNA/virus infection, TNFα	+ + + +	54,55,59,119,120,121
Synovial cells	IL-1	+ + + +	123
Epithelial cells	TNF/IL-1	+	126
Keratinocytes	IL-1/TNFα	+	121
	after pretretment with γ-interferon	+ + +	127
Hepatoma cells	IL-1	+ +	126
Lung giant carcinoma cells	None	+ + +	125
Chondrocytes	IL-1	+ + +	124
Neutrophils	LPS	+	101

cytosis (37). Although the relative potency (ED_{50}) of NAP-2 for chemotaxis as well as degranulation is similar to that observed for NAP-1/IL-8, the efficiency (percentage of elastase release at optimal concentration of the agonist) is lower (37). It appears that neutrophils found in association with platelet aggregates are presumably attracted by the release of chemotaxins following platelet activation. Therefore, it has been suggested that formation of platelet-derived chemotaxins may constitute a mechanism for degranulation of thrombotic deposits and recanalization of obstructed vessels (128). Interestingly, three precursors of NAP-2—namely, PBP, CTAP III, as well as β-TG—apparently are completely inactive as neutrophil activators (up to 100 nM) (37). Although it is not yet clear whether similar precursor forms of NAP-1/IL-8 lack neutrophil-activating activity, we saw some evidence that preparations of the 77-residue form of NAP-1/IL-8, which contained only traces of the highly active 72-residue form, show lower specific activity than the mature protein (55).

B. MGSA/gro Is a Neutrophil Activator

When we studied PMN-activating polypeptides in supernatants of endotoxin-stimulated human monocytes upon reversed-phase HPLC, we reproducibly observed a second peak of PMN chemotactic activity apart from NAP-1/IL-8 eluting at a lower acetonitrile concentration (129). Purification of this factor led to the detection of a polypeptide eluting from a size-exclusion HPLC column as a protein with an apparent M_r near 9 kDa (130). Aminoterminal amino acid sequence analysis of the purified peptide, tentatively termed NAP-3, revealed a sequence identical to the published sequence of so-called melanoma growth-stimulating activity (MGSA) (129), which is identical with the gene product of the oncogene gro (129).

Similar to NAP-2, NAP-3 (MGSA/gro) was found to be of equivalent potency (ED_{50}) in eliciting neutrophil responses such as chemotaxis or degranulation when compared with NAP-1/IL-8 (129). Interestingly, PMN chemotaxis showed a strongly bell-shaped dose-response curve; at concentrations higher than 200 ng/ml (corresponding to 2.5×10^{-8} M), no significant chemotactic activity could be detected (129,130).

Cross-desensitization studies with NAP-3 and NAP-1/IL-8 revealed cross-desensitization of each other, but not with other chemotaxins such as C5a, fMLP, or the lipid-like factors (129). These results indicate that NAP-3 binds to a similar—or identical—receptor on PMN. This suggestion was recently confirmed by receptor studies (66). The role of MGSA/gro as a PMN activator was supported by recent findings in our laboratory: When we investigated neutrophil attractants released by dermal fibroblasts stimulated with IL-1 or TNFα, a PMN chemoattractant could be identified which showed the same aminoterminal amino acid sequence as was found for MGSA/gro (55). In addition, biological behavior of this fibroblast-derived MGSA/gro was identical to that obtained from monocytes. Further support for PMN-activating activity of MGSA/gro was obtained when authentic MGSA or recombinant gro were tested for PMN chemotactic properties (K. Matsushima, personal communication; R. Sager, personal communication). Both preparations were found to contain potent PMN chemotactic activity. Furthermore, a synthetic polypeptide with the amino acid sequence predicted for MGSA/gro has been found to be a potent neutrophil activator (M. Baggiolini, personal communication). The role of MGSA/gro as a signal for leukocyte accumulation in vivo is yet not clear. It is possible that MGSA/gro is the ancestral form of NAP-1/IL-8. In the human system, NAP-1/IL-8 could be of importance for leuko-

of NAP-1/IL-8. In the human system, NAP-1/IL-8 could be of importance for leukocyte accumulation in vivo, whereas in rodents it appears that only MGSA/gro-related peptides such as KC/N51 or MIP-2 exist (47–49).

VI. NAP-1/IL-8 AND RELATED PMN ATTRACTANTS IN DISEASE

The apparent neutrophil specificity of NAP-1/IL-8 raises the question of whether, in diseases showing predominantly PMN as infiltrate cells, this novel cytokine may be responsible for the PMN infiltration.

In psoriasis neutrophils are typically present in the upper epidermal layer of diseased skin. Only a few lymphocytes or macrophages and no eosinophils can be detected (131). Indeed, by far the most abundant PMN attractant in psoriatic lesions, termed ANAP, showed closed biochemical as well as biological similarities to NAP-1/IL-8 (8). Whereas ANAP was not fully characterized at that time, we were later able to purify ANAP to homogeneity. The most surprising observation was the finding that ANAP consists of nine biochemically different chemoattractants, all of which bind to the same PMN receptor and are therefore chemotaxin homologs.

The three major ANAPs could be characterized by aminoterminal amino acid sequence analysis and were identified as NAP-1/IL-8, the 69-residue form of NAP-1/IL-8, and—most interestingly—melanoma growth-stimulatory activity, MGSA (gro) (132 and our unpublished observation). The levels of NAP-1/IL-8-related PMN chemoattractants were found up to 150 times the amounts seen in normal heel callus, where NAP-1/IL-8-related peptides were found to be nearly absent (132). Similar amounts of MGSA were detected in psoriatic scale material (132). Preliminary data recently observed in human keratinocyte cultures revealed an apparently specific mitogenic effect of NAP-1/IL-8 for keratinocytes, but not fibroblasts (133). This appears to be a most interesting finding and may partly explain epidermal hyperproliferation in diseased psoriatic skin.

NAP-1/IL-8 could also be involved in other diseases, such as rheumatoid arthritis, since it has been shown that IL-1-stimulated synovial cells produce NAP-1/IL-8-like activity (123). Moreover, idiopathic pulmonary fibrosis and asbestosis are characterized predominantly by PMN infiltrates in the alveolar space. The major inflammatory cell in adult respiratory distress syndrome, where tissue damage is attributed to neutral proteinases such as elastase, is the neutrophil. Therefore, search for NAP-1/IL-8 and related attractants in these diseases may lead to a better understanding of the pathophysiology of PMN infiltration in diseased tissue.

VII. CONCLUSIONS

In this brief review, rapidly accumulating knowledge on NAP-1/IL-8 has been presented. This cytokine proved to be a highly stable polypeptide with apparent specificity for neutrophils. The fact that large amounts of NAP-1/IL-8 could be recovered from inflamed skin surfaces despite the presence of various degrading enzymes supports the stability of this molecule.

Of interest is the observation that a variety of cells are able to produce and secrete the cytokine in response to specific stimuli, e.g., IL-1 and TNF acting on endothelial cells, fibroblasts, monocyte/macrophages, and lipopolysaccharide as additional stimulus in endothelial cells and macrophages. This points toward a high survival value of NAP-1/IL-8.

The induction of this cytokine, except in T-cells, depends on cytokines secreted by other cells, which indicates that a hierarchy of regulatory signals can be envisioned. The exact role that NAP-1/IL-8 may play in this hierarchy is not exactly clear at this moment. The fact that, as recently shown (75), NAP-1/IL-8 is able to stimulate LTB_4 production in PMN, indicates that NAP-1/IL-8, in addition to being a potent chemotaxin, may also act as an amplifier of other cell functions.

In this respect, it is important to remember that in-vitro experiments testing one effect of a single cytokine are unlikely to reflect the in-vivo situation. As pointed out by DiGione and Duff (134), cells in vivo probably never see a sudden change in concentration of a single cytokine. Also, interaction of cytokines forming a regulatory network reflect normal conditions rather than the exception.

In summary, NAP-1/IL-8 has proven to be a member of a newly detected peptide family with potent pro-inflammatory and/or growth-stimulating activities. In skin this cytokine is produced by resident cells (e.g., endothelial cells, fibroblasts) as well as immune-competent cells (monocyte/macrophages, T-cells). This may indicate a major need for this peptide in cutaneous pathology, especially in host defense. With its outstanding role as a protective organ, skin may indeed play an important role in the production of NAP-1/IL-8. This could be especially important in the cutaneous response to injury, the most common pathological event in skin. In this case the peptide could play a role as a critical cytokine in wound repair.

ACKNOWLEDGMENT

We thank I. Brandt for expert secretarial assistance in preparing the manuscript and Deutsche Forschungsgemeinschaft (grant Schr 305/1-2) for financial support.

REFERENCES

1. Weiss SJ. Tissue destruction by neutrophils. N Engl J Med 1989; 320:365–76.
2. Christophers E. Neutrophile Dermatosen. In: Braun-Falco O, Schill WB, eds. Fortschritte der praktischen Dermatologie und Venerologie. Berlin-Heidelberg-New York, London, Paris, Tokyo: Springer Verlag, 1987:195–202.
3. Jorizzo JL. Neutrophilic dermatoses: Sweet's syndrome and pyoderma gangrenosum. In: Gallin JI, Goldstein IM, Snyderman R, eds. Inflammation. New York: Raven Press, 1988:785–802.
4. Schiffman E, Corcoran BA, Wahl SM. N-formylmethionyl peptides as chemoattractants for leukocytes. Proc Natl Acad Sci USA 1975; 72:1059–62.
5. Fernandez HN, Henson PM, Otani H, Hugli TE. Chemotactic response to human C3a and C5a anaphylatoxins. I. Evaluations of C3a and C5a leukotaxis in vivo and in vitro. J Immunol 1978; 120:109–15.
6. Ford-Hutchinson AW, Bray MA, Doig MV, Shipley ME, and Smith MJH. Leukotriene B_4, a potent chemokinetic and aggregating substance released from polymorphonuclear leucotyes. Nature 1980; 286:264–8.
7. Braquet P, Touqui L, Shen TY, Vargaftig BB. Perspectives in platelet-activating factor research. Pharmacol Rev 1987; 39:97–145.
8. Schröder J-M, Christophers E. Identification of $C5a_{des\ arg}$ and an anionic neutrophil-activating peptide (ANAP) in psoriatic scales. J Invest Dermatol 1986; 87:53–8.

9. Sauder DN, Mounessa NL, Katz SI, Dinarello CA, Gallin JI. Chemotactic cytokines: the role of leukotactic pyrogen and epidermal cell thymocyte activating factor in neutrophil chemotaxis. J Immunol 1984; 132:828–32.
10. Luger TA, Charon JA, Colot M, Micksche M, Oppenheim JJ. Chemotactic properties of partially purified human epidermal cell-derived thymocyte-activating factor (ETAF) for polymorphonuclear and mononuclear cells. J Immunol 1983; 131:816–20.
11. Georgilis K, Schäfer C, Dinarello CA, Klempner MS. Human recombinant interleukin 1β has no effect on intracellular calcium or on functional responses of human neutrophils. J Immunol 1987; 139:3403–7.
12. Merril WW, Naegel GA, Matthay RA, Reynolds HY. Alveolar macrophage-derived chemotactic factor: kinetics of in vitro production and partial characterization. J Clin Invest 1980; 65:268–76.
13. Kownatzki E, Kapp A, Uhrich S. Novel neutrophil chemotactic factor derived from human peripheral blood mononuclear leucocytes. Clin Exp Imunol 1986; 64:214–22.
14. Schröder J-M, Mrowietz U, Morita E, Christophers E. Purification and partial biochemical characterization of a human monocyte-derived neutrophil-activating peptide that lacks interleukin 1 activity. J Immunol 1987; 139:3474–83.
15. Gregory H, Young J, Schröder J-M, Mrowietz U, Christophers E. Structure determination of a human lymphocyte derived neutrophil activating peptide (LYNAP). Biochem Biophys Res Commun 1988; 151:883–90.
16. Schmid J, Weissmann C. Induction of mRNA for a serine protease and a β-thromboglobulin-like protein in mitogen-stimulated human leukocytes. J Immunol 1987; 139:250–6.
17. Yoshimura T, Matsushima K, Oppenheim JJ, Leonard EJ. Neutrophil chemotactic factor produced by lipopolysaccharide (LPS)-stimulated human blood mononuclear leucocytes: partial characterization and separation from interleukin 1 (IL 1). J Immunol 1987; 139:788–93.
18. Yoshimura T, Matsushima K, Tanaka S, Robinson EA, Apella E, Oppenheim JJ, Leonard EJ. Purification of a human mononcyte-derived neutrophil chemotactic factor that shares sequence homology with other host defense cytokines. Proc Natl Acad Sci USA 1987; 84:9233–7.
19. Walz A, Peveri P, Aschauer H, Baggiolini M. Purification and amino acid sequencing of NAF, a novel neutrophil-activating factor produced by monocytes. Biochem Biophys Res Commun 1987; 149:755–61.
20. Peveri P, Walz A, Dewald B, Baggiolini M. A novel neutrophil-activating factor produced by human mononuclear phagocytes. J Exp Med 1988; 167:1547–59.
21. Van Damme J, Van Beeumen J, Opdenakker G, Billiau A. A novel, NH_2-terminal sequence-characterized human monokine possessing neutrophil chemotactic, skin-reactive and granulocytosis-promoting activity. J Exp Med 1988; 167:1364–76.
22. Gronhoj-Larsen C, Anderson AO, Apella E, Oppenheim JJ, Matsushima K. The neutrophil-activating protein (NAP-1) is also chemotactic for T lymphocytes. Science 1989; 243:1464–6.
23. Westwick J, Li SW, Camp RD. Novel neutrophil stimulating peptides. Immunol Today 1989; 10:146–7.
24. Tono-Oka T, Nakayama M, Matsumoto S. Human monocyte-derived chemotactic factor for granulocytes. Immunology 1980; 39:607–13.
25. Schröder J-M, Mrowietz U, Christophers E. Identification of different charged species of a monocyte derived neutrophil activating peptide (MONAP). Biochem Biophys Res Commun 1988; 152:277–84.
26. Lindley I, Aschauer H, Seifert J-M, Lam C, Brunowsky W, Kownatzki E, Thelen M, Peveri P, Dewald B, von Tscharner V, Walz A, Baggiolini M. Synthesis and expression in *Escherichia coli* of the gene encoding monocyte-derived neutrophil-activating factor: bio-

logical equivalence between natural and recombinant neutrophil-activating actor. Proc Natl Acad Sci USA 1988; 85:9199–203.

27. Tanaka S, Robinson EA, Yoshimura T, Matsushima K, Leonard EJ, Appella E. Chemical synthesis and biological characterization of a monocyte-derived neutrophil chemotactic factor (MDNCF). FEBS Lett 1988; 236:467–70.
28. Clore CM, Appella E, Yamada M, Matsushima K, Gronenborn AM. Determination of the secondary structure of interleukin 8 by nuclear magnetic resonance spectroscopy. J Biol Chem 1990; 264:18907–11.
29. Clore GM, Appella E, Yamada M, Matsushima K, Gronenborn AM. Three-dimensional structure of interleukin 8 in solution. Biochemistry 1990; 29:1689–96.
30. Baggiolini M, Walz A, Kunkel SL. Neutrophil-activating peptide-1/interleukin 8, a novel cytokine that activates neutrophils. J Clin Invest 1989; 84:1045–9.
31. Wolpe SD, Cerami A. Macrophage inflammatory proteins 1 and 2: members of a novel superfamily of cytokines. FASEB J 1989; 3:2565–73.
32. Furuta R, Yamagishi J, Kotani H, Sakamoto F, Fukui T, Matsui Y, Sohmura Y, Yamada M, Yoshimura T, Larsen CG, Oppenheim JJ, Matsushima K. Production and characterization of recombinant human neutrophil chemotactic factor. J Biochem 1989; 106:436–41.
33. Yoshimura T, Robinson EA, Apella E, Matsushima K, Showalter SD, Skeel A, Leonard EJ. Three forms of monocyte-derived neutrophil chemotactic factor (MDNCF) distinct by different lengths of the aminoterminal sequence. Mol Immunol 1989; 26:87–93.
34. Van Damme J, Van Beeumen JV, Conings R, Decock B, Billiau A. Purification of granulocyte chemotactic peptide interleukin-8 reveals N-terminal sequence heterogeneity similar to that of β-thromboglobulin. Eur J Biochem 1989; 181:337–44.
35. Sticherling M, Schröder J-M, Christophers E. Production and characterization of monoclonal antibodies against the novel neutrophil activating peptide NAP-1/interleukin-8. J Immunol 1989; 143:1628–34.
36. Castor CW, Miller JW, Walz DA. Structural and biological characteristics of connective tissue activating peptide (CTAP-III), a major human platelet-derived growth factor. Proc Natl Acad Sci USA 1983; 80:765–9.
37. Walz A, Dewald B, von Tscharner V, Baggiolini M. Effects of the neutrophil-activating peptide NAP-2, platelet basic protein, connective tissue-activating peptide III, and platelet factor 4 on human neutrophils. J Exp Med 1989; 170:1745–50.
38. St Charles R, Walz DR, Edwards BFP. The three-dimensional structure of bovine platelet factor 4 at 2.0-A resolution. J Biol Chem 1989; 264:2092–8.
39. Begg GS, Pepper DS, Chesterman CN, Morgan FJ. Complete covalent structure of human β-thromboglobulin. Biochemistry 1978; 17:1739–44.
40. Deuel TF, Senior RM, Chang D, Griffin DL, Heinrikson RL, Kaiser ET. Platelet factor 4 is chemotactic for neutrophils and monocytes. Proc Natl Acad Sci USA 1981; 78:4584–7.
41. Luster AD, Unkeless JC, Ravetch JV. Interferon transcriptionally regulates an early-response gene containing homology to platelet proteins. Nature 1985; 315:672–6.
42. Luster AD, Ravetch JV. Biochemical characterisation of a γ-interferon-inducible cytokine (IP-10). J Exp Med 1987; 166:1084–97.
43. Kaplan G, Luster AD, Hancock G, Cohn ZA. The expression of an interferon-induced protein (IP-10) in delayed immune responses in human skin. J Exp Med 1987; 166:1098–108.
44. Vanguri P, Farber J. Cloning of the mouse homolog of IP-10 from lymphokine-activated RAW264.7 cells. Cytokine 1989; 1:147 (abstr).
45. Sugano S, Stoeckle MY, Hanafusa H. Transformation by Rous sarcoma virus induces a novel gene with homology to a mitogenic platelet protein. Cell 1987; 49:321–8.
46. Bedard PA, Alcorta D, Simmons DL, Luck K-C, Erikson RL. Constitutive expression of a gene encoding a polypeptide homologous to biologically active human platelet protein in Rous sarcoma virus-transformed fibroblasts. Proc Natl Acad Sci USA 1987; 84:6715–9.

47. Oquendo P, Alberta J, Wen D, Graycar JL, Derynck R, Stiles CD. The platelet-derived growth factor inducible KC gene encodes a secretory protein related to platelet α-granule proteins. J Biochem 1989; 264:4133–7.
48. Ryseck RP, MacDonald-Bravo H, Mattel MG, Bravo R. Cloning and sequencing of a secretory protein induced by growth factors in mouse fibroblasts. Exp Cell Res 1989; 180:266–75.
49. Wolpe SD, Sherry B, Juers D, Davatelis G, Yurt RW, Cerami A. Identification and characterization of macrophage inflammatory protein 2. Proc Natl Acad Sci USA 1989; 86:612–6.
50. Richmond A, Balentien E, Thomas HG, Flaggs G, Barton DE, Spiess J, Bardoni R, Francke U, Derynck R. Molecular characterization and chromosomal mapping of melanoma growth stimulatory activity, a growth factor structurally related to β-thromboglobulin. EMBO J 1988; 7:2025–33.
51. Richmond A, Thomas HG. Melanoma growth stimulatory activity: isolation from human melanoma tumors and characterization of tissue distribution. J Cell Biochem 1988; 36:185–98.
52. Lawson DH, Thomas HG, Roy RGB, Gordon DS, Chawla RK, Nixon DW, Richmond A. Preparation of a monoclonal antibody to a melanoma growth-stimulatory activity released into serum-free culture medium by Hs 0294 malignant melanoma cells. J Cell Biochem 1987; 34:169–85.
53. Anisowicz A, Bardwell L, Sager R. Constitutive overexpression of a growth-regulated gene in transformed Chinese hamster and human cells. Proc Natl Acad Sci USA 1987; 84:7188–92.
54. Golds EE, Mason PP, Nyirkos P. Inflammatory cytokines induce synthesis and secretion of gro protein and a neutrophil chemotactic factor but not β_2-microglobulin in human synovial cells and fibroblasts. Biochem J 1989; 259:585–8.
55. Schröder J-M, Sticherling M, Henneicke H-H, Preissner WC, Christophers E. IL-1α or TNFα stimulate release of three IL-8-related neutrophil chemotactic proteins in human dermal fibroblasts. J Immunol 1990; 144:2223–32.
56. Wen D, Rowland A, Derynck R. Expression and secretion of gro/MGSA by stimulated human endothelial cells. EMBO J 1989; 8:1761–6.
57. Yoshimura T, Yuhki N, Moore SK, Appella E, Lerman MI, Leonard EJ. Human monocyte chemoattractant protein-1 (MCP-1): full-length cDNA cloning, expression in mitogen-stimulated blood mononuclear leukocytes, and sequence similarity to mouse competence gene JE. FEBS Lett 1989; 244:487–93.
58. Yoshimura T, Robinson EA, Tanaka S, Appella E, Leonard EJ. Purification and amino acid analysis of two human monocyte chemoattractants produced by phytohemagglutinin-stimulated human blood mononuclear leukocytes. J Immunol 1989; 142:1956–64.
59. Matsushima K, Larsen CG, DuBois G, Oppenheim JJ. Purification and characterization of a novel monocyte chemotactic and activating factor produced by human myelomonocytic cell line. J Exp Med 1989; 169:1485–90.
60. Rollins BJ, Morrison EE, Stiles CD. Cloning and expression of JE, a gene inducible by platelet-derived growth factor and whose product has cytokine-like properties. Proc Natl Acad Sci USA 1988; 85:3738–42.
61. Wolpe SD, Davatelis G, Sherry B, Beutler B, Hesse DG, Nguyen HT, Moldawer LL, Nathan CF, Lowry SF, Cerami A. Macrophages secrete a novel heparin-binding protein with inflammatory and neutrophil chemokinetic properties. J Exp Med 1988; 167:570–81.
62. Graham GJ, Wright EG, Hewick R, Wolpe SD, Wilkie NM, Donaldson D, Lorimore S, Pragnell IB. Identification and characterization of an inhibitor of haemopoietic stem cell proliferation. Nature 1990; 344:442–6.
63. Obaru K, Fukuda M, Maeda S, Shimara K. A cDNA clone used to study mRNA inducible

in human tonsillar lymphocytes by a tumor promotor. J Biochem (Tokyo) 1986; 99:885–94.

64. Brown KD, Zurawski SM, Mosmann TR, Zurawski G. A family of small inducible proteins secreted by leukocytes are members of a new superfamily that includes leukocyte and fibroblast-derived inflammatory agents, growth factors and indicators of various activation processes. J Immunol 1989; 142:679–87.
65. Zipfel PF, Balke J, Irwing SG, Kelly K, Siebenlist U. Mitogenic activation of human T cells induces two closely related genes which share structural similarities with a new family of secreted factors. J Immunol 1989; 142:1582–90.
66. Matsushima K, Oppenheim JJ. Interleukin 8 and MCAF: novel inflammatory cytokines inducible by IL 1 and TNF. Cytokine 1989; 1:2–13.
67. Hartwig JH, Stossel TP. Interactions of actin, myosin, and an actin-binding protein of rabbit pulmonary macrophages. III. Effects of cytochalasin B. J Cell Biol 1976; 71:295–303.
68. Willems J, Joniau M, Cinque S, van Damme J. Human granulocyte chemotactic peptide (IL-8) as a specific neutrophil degranulator: comparison with other monokines. Immunology 1989; 67:540–3.
69. Klempner MS, Dinarello CA, Gallin JI. Human leukocytic pyrogen induces release of specific granule contents from human neutrophils. J Clin Invest 1978; 61:1330–6.
70. Klempner MS, Dinarello CA, Henderson WR, Gallin JI. Stimulation of neutrophil oxygen-dependent metabolism by human leukocyte pyrogen. J Clin Invest 1979; 64:996–1002.
71. Palmblad J, Gyllenhammar H, Lindgren JA, Malmsten CL. Effects of leukotrienes and f-met-leu-phe on oxidative metabolism of neutrophils and eosinophils. J Immunol 1984; 132:3041–5.
72. Samuelsson B. Leukotrienes: mediators of immediate hypersensitivity reactions and inflammation. Science 1983; 220:568–72.
73. Smith RJ, Epps DE, Justen JM, Sam LM, Wynalda MA, Fitzpatrick FA, Yein FS. Human neutrophil activation with interleukin 1. A role for intracellular calcium and arachidonic acid lipoxygenation. Biochem Pharmacol 1987; 36:3851–8.
74. Smith RJ, Sam LM, Justen JM, Bundy GL, Fitzpatrick FA, Wynalda MA. Archidonic acid and 15(S)-hydroxyl-5,8,11-cis-13-trans-eicosatetraenoic acid modulate human polymorphonuclear neutrophil activation by monocyte derived neutrophil activating factor. Biochem Biophys Res Commun 1987; 148:636–45.
75. Schröder J-M. The monocyte-derived neutrophil activating peptide (NAP/interleukin 8) stimulates human neutrophil arachidonate 5-lipoxygenase but not the release of cellular arachidonate. J Exp Med 1989; 170:847–63.
76. Dahinden CA, Zingg J, Maly FE, de Weck AL. Leukotriene production in human neutrophils primed by recombinant human granulocyte/macrophage colony stimulating factor and complement component C5a and FMLP as second signals. J Exp Med 1988; 167:1281–93.
77. Hoover J, Briggs R, Karnovsky M. The adhesive interaction between polymorphonuclear leukocytes and endothelial cells in vitro. Cell 1978; 14:423–8.
78. Smith R, Lackie J, Wilkinson P. The effect of chemotactic factors on thc adhesiveness of rabbit neutrophil granulocytes. Exp Cell Res 1979; 122:169–74.
79. Carveth JH, Bohnsack JF, McIntyre TM, Baggiolini M, Prescott SM, Zimmerman CA. Neutrophil activating factor (NAF) induces polymorphonuclear leukocyte adherence to endothelial cells and to subendothelial matrix proteins. Biochem Biophys Res Commun 1989; 162:387–93.
80. Detmers PA, Olsen-Egbert E, Peveri P, Walz A, Baggiolini M, Cohn ZA. Neutrophil activating factor (NAF) enhances the binding activity of CD11b/CD18. FASEB J 1989; 3:A1087.

81. Gimbrone MA, Obins MS, Brock AF, Luis EA, Hass PE, Hèbert CA, Yip YK, Leung DW, Lowe DG, Kohr WJ, Dabonne WC, Bechtal KB, Baker JB. Endothelial interleukin-8: a novel inhibitor of leukocyte-endothelial interactions. Science 1989; 246:1601–3.
82. Samanta AK, Oppenheim JJ, Matsushima K. Identification and characterization of specific receptors for monocyte-derived neutrophil chemotactic factor (MDNCF) on human neutrophils. J Exp Med 1989; 169:1185–9.
83. Besemer J, Hujber A, Kuhn B. Specific binding, internalization, and degradation of human neutrophil activating factor by human polymorphonuclear leukocytes. J Biol Chem 1989; 264:17409–15.
84. Goetzl EJ, Foster DW, Goldman DW. Isolation and partial characterization of membrane protein constituents of human neutrophil receptors for chemotactic F-Met-peptides. Biochemistry 1981; 20:5717–22.
85. Goldman DW, Goetzl EJ. Selective transduction of human polymorphonuclear leucocyte functions by subsets of receptors for leukotriene B_4. J Allergy Clin Immunol 1984; 74:373–7.
86. Samanta AK, Oppenheim JJ, Matsushima K. Interleukin 8 (MDNCF) dynamically regulates its own receptor expression on human neutrophils. J Biol Chem 1990; in press.
87. Thelen M, Peveri P, Kernen P, von Tscharner V, Walz A, Baggiolini M. Mechanism of neutrophil activation by NAF, a novel monocyte-derived peptide agonist. FASEB J 1988; 2:2702–6.
88. Bacon KB, Westwick J, Camp RDR. Potent and specific inhibition of IL-8, IL-1α- and IL-1β-induced in vitro human lymphocyte migration by calcium channel antagonists. Biochem Biophys Res Commun 1989; 165:349–54.
89. Leonard EJ, Skeel A, Yoshimura T, Noer K, Kutvird S, Van Epps DE. Leukocyte specificity and binding of human neutrophil attractant/activation protein-1. J Immunol 1990; 144:1323–31.
90. White MV, Yoshimura T, Hook W, Kaliner MA, Leonard EJ. Neutrophil attractant/activation protein-1 (NAP-1) causes human basophil histamine release. Immunol Lett 1989; 22:151–4.
91. Dahinden CA, Kurimoto Y, De Weck AL, Lindley I, Dewald B, Baggiolini M. The neutrophil-activating peptide NAF/NAP-1 induces histamine and leukotriene release by interleukin 3-primed basophils. J Exp Med 1989; 170:1787–92.
92. Foster SJ, Aked DM, Schröder J-M, Christophers E. Acute inflammatory effects of a monocyte-derived neutrophil-activating peptide in rabbit skin. Immunology 1989; 67:181–4.
93. Rampart M, van Damme J, Zonnekeyn L, Herman AG. Granulocyte chemotactic protein/interleukin-8 induces plasma leakage and neutrophil accumulation in rabbit skin. Am J Pathol 1989; 135:635–42.
94. Colditz I, Zwahlen R, Dewald B, Baggioloni M. In vivo inflammatory activity of neutrophil-activating factor, a novel chemotactic peptide derived from human monocytes. Am J Pathol 1989; 134:755–60.
95. Schubert C, Schröder J-M, Isai T, Swensson O, Christophers E. Morphological patterns of endothelial cell activation after intracutaneous injection of MONAP and $C5a_{des\ arg}$. J Invest Dermatol 1988; 91:399.
96. Leonard EJ, Yoshimura T, Tanaka S, Raffeld M. Neutrophil infiltration caused by intradermal injection of neutrophil attractant protein-1 (NAP-1/IL-8) into human skin. Cytokine 1989; 1:151 (abstr).
97. Yancey KB, Hammer CH, Harvath L, Renfer L, Frank MM, Lawley TJ. Studies of human C5a as a mediator of inflammation in normal human skin. J Clin Invest 1985; 75:485–95.
98. Michel L, Mencia-Huerta J-M, Benveniste J, Dubertret L. Biologic properties of LTB_4 and Paf-acether in vivo in human skin. J Invest Dermatol 1978; 88:675–81.

99. Rot A, Lam C, Lindley IJD. Recombinant human NAP-1/IL-8 shows differing chemotactic and stimulatory activity on cells from different species. Cytokine 1989; 1:147 (abstr).
100. Matsushima K, Larsen CG, Dubois G, Oppenheim JJ. Purification and characterization of a novel monocyte chemotactic and activating factor produced by human myelomonocytic cell line. J Exp Med 1989; 169:1485–90.
101. Strieter RM, Chensue SW, Standiford TJ, Basha MA, Showell HJ, Kunkel SL. Disparate gene expression of chemotactic cytokines by human mononuclear phagocytes. Biochem Biophys Res Commun 1990; 166:886–91.
102. Sylvester I, Rankin JA, Yoshimura T, Tanaka S, Leonard EJ. Secretion of neutrophil attractant/activation protein (NAP-1) by lipopolysaccharide-stimulated lung macrophages, determined by both enzyme-linked immunosorbent assay and N-terminal sequence analysis. Am Rev Respir Dis 1990; 141:683–8.
103. Schröder J-M, Mrowietz U, Christophers E. Purification and partial biologic characterization of a human lymphocyte-derived peptide with potent neutrophil-stimulating activity. J Immunol 1988; 140:3534–40.
104. Verghese MW, Snyderman R. Role of chemotactic and inflammatory cytokines. In: Oppenheim JJ and Shevach E, eds. Textbook of immunophysiology. New York: Oxford University Press, 1989:274–305.
105. Mercandetti AJ, Lane TA, Colmerauer EM. Cultured human endothelial cells elaborate neutrophil chemoattractants. J Lab Clin Med 1984; 104:370–80.
106. Tonnesen MG, Anderson DC, Springer TA, Knedler A, Audi N, Henson PM. Endotoxin directly enhances neutrophil adherence to endothelial cells by a MAC-1 glycoprotein-dependent mechanism. J Invest Dermatol 1987; 88:521 (abstr).
107. Schleimer RP, Rutledge BK. Cultured human vascular endothelial cells acquire adhesiveness for neutrophils after stimulation with interleukin 1, endotoxin, and tumor-promoting phorbol-diesters. J Immunol 1986; 136:649–54.
108. Furie MB, McHugh DD. Migration of neutrophils across endothelial monolayers is stimulated by treatment of the monolayers with interleukin-1 or tumor necrosis factor-α. J Immunol 1989; 143:3309–17.
109. Sayers TJ, Wiltrout TA, Bull CA, Denn AC, Polaro AM, Lokesh B. Effect of cytokines on polymorphonuclear neutrophil infiltration in the mouse. J Immunol 1988; 141:1670–7.
110. Schröder J-M, Christophers E. Secretion of novel and homologous neutrophil activating peptides by LPS-stimulated human endothelial cells. J Immunol 1989; 142:244–51.
111. Strieter RM, Kunkel SL, Showell HJ, Marks RM. Monokine-induced gene expression of a human endothelial cell-derived neutrophil-chemotactic factor. Biochem Biophys Res Commun 1989; 156:1340–5.
112. Strieter RM, Kunkel SL, Showell HJ, Remick GD, Phan SH, Ward PA, Marks PM. Endothelial cell gene expression of a neutrophil chemotactic factor by TNF, IL-1 and LPS. Science 1989; 243:1467–9.
113. Dowd PM, Camp RDR, Greaves MW. Human recombinant interleukin-1α is proinflammatory in normal human skin. Skin Pharmacol 1989; 1:30–7.
114. Movat HZ, Cybulsky MI. Neutrophil emigration and microvascular injury. Role of chemotaxins, endotoxin, interleukin 1 and tumor necrosis factor alpha. Pathol Immunopathol Res 1987; 6:153–76.
115. Ming WJ, Bersani L, Mantovani A. Tumor necrosis factor is chemotactic for mononcytes and polymorphonuclear leukocytes. J Immunol 1987; 138:1469–78.
116. Mrowietz U, Schröder J-M, Christophers E. Recombinant human tumor necrosis factor α lacks chemotactic activity for human peripheral blood neutrophils and mononcytes. Biochem Biophys Res Commun 1988; 153:1223–8.
117. Ferrante A, Nandoskar M, Walz A, Goh DHB, Kowanko IC. Effects of tumour necrosis factor alpha and interleukin-1 alpha and beta on human neutrophil migration, respiratory burst and degranulation. Int Arch Allergy Appl Immunol 1989; 86:82–91.

118. Yonemaru M, Stephens KE, Ishizaka A, Zheng H, Hogue RS, Crowley JJ, Hatherill JR, Raffin TA. Effects of tumor necrosis factor on PMN chemotaxis, chemiluminescence, and elastase activity. J Lab Clin Med 1989; 114:674–81.
119. Van Damme J, Decock B, Conings R, Lenaerts J-P, Opdenakker G, Billiau A. The chemotactic activity for granulocytes produced by virally infected fibroblasts is identical to monocyte-derived interleukin 8. Eur J Immunol 1989; 19:1189–94.
120. Strieter R, Phan SH, Showell HJ, Remick DG, Lynchz JP, Genord M, Raiford C, Eskandari M, Marks RM, Kunkel SL. Monokine-induced neutrophil chemotactic factor gene expression in human fibroblasts. J Biol Chem 1989; 264:10621–6.
121. Larsen CG, Anderson AO, Oppenheim JJ, Matsushima K. Production of interleukin 8 by human dermal fibroblasts and keratinoctes in response to interleukin 1 or tumor necrosis factor. Immunology 1989; 68:31–8.
122. Walz A, Baggiolini M. A novel cleavage product of β-thromboglobulin formed in cultures of stimulated mononuclear cells activates human neutrophils. Biochem Biophys Res Commun 1989; 159:969–75.
123. Watson ML, Lewis GP, Westwick, J. Neutrophil stimulation by recombinant cytokines and a factor produced by IL-1 treated human synovial cell cultures. Immunology 1988; 65:567–72.
124. Van Damme J, Bunning RAD, Conings R, Graham R, Russel G, Opdenakker G. Characterization of granulocyte chemotactic activity from human cytokine-stimulated chondrocytes as interleukin-8. Cytokine 1990; 2:106–111.
125. Suzuki K, Miyasaka H, Ota H, Yamakawa Y, Tagawa M, Kuramoto A, Mizuno S. Purification and partial primary sequence of a chemotactic protein for polymorphonuclear leukocytes derived from human lung giant cell carcinoma LU65C cells. J Exp Med 1989; 169:1895–902.
126. Kunkel SL, Strieter RM, Chensue SW, Remick DG. Regulation of tumor necrosis factor-alpha and neutrophil activating protein-1 gene expression: potential role of cytokine directed cell communication during multiple organ injury. In: Bringham K, Stahlmann M, eds. Respiratory distress syndrome: molecular to man. Nashville, TN: Vanderbilt University Press, 1990: in press.
127. Barker JNWN, Sama V, Mitra RS, Dixit VM, Nickoloff BJ. Marked synergism between tumor necrosis factor α and interferon-γ in regulation of keratinocyte-derived adhesion molecules and chemotactic factors. J Clin Invest 1990; 85:605–8.
128. Walz A, Baggiolini M. Generation of the neutrophil-activating peptide NAP-2 from platelet basic protein or connective tissue-activating peptide III through monocyte proteases. J Exp Med 1990; 171:449–54.
129. Schröder J-M, Persoon N, Christophers E. Lipopolysaccharide-stimulated human monocytes secrete apart from NAP-1/IL-8 a second neutrophil-activating protein: NH_2-terminal aminoacid sequence-identity with melanoma growth stimulatory activity (MGSA/gro). J Exp Med 1990; 171:1091–100.
130. Schröder J-M, Christophers E. Human melanoma growth stimulating activity (MGSA/gro) is a neutrophil activator. In: Powanda MC, Oppenheim JJ, Kluger MJ, Dinarello CA, eds. Molecular and cellular biology of cytokines. New York: Alan Riss, 1990: 351–6.
131. Christophers E, Krueger G. Psoriasis. In: Fitzpatrick TB, Eisen AZ, Wolff K, Freedberg IM, Austen KF, eds. Dermatology in general medicine, vol 1, 3d ed. New York: McGraw-Hill, 1986:461–91.
132. Schröder J-M, Young J, Gregory H, Christophers E. Amino acid sequence characterization of two strukturally related neutrophil activating peptides obtained from lesional psoriatic scales. J Invest Dermatol 1989; 92:515 (abstr).
133. Krueger G, Jörgensen C, Miller C, Schröder J-M, Sticherling M, Christophers E. Effects of IL-8 on epidermal proliferation. J Invest Dermatol 1990; 94:545 (abstr.)
134. Di Gione FS, Duff GW. Interleukin 1 the first interleukin. Immunol Today 1990; 11:13–20.

14

Activation of Neutrophils by Interleukins-1 and -2 and Tumor Necrosis Factors

ANTONIO FERRANTE
University of Adelaide and Adelaide Children's Hospital, Adelaide, South Australia

I. INTRODUCTION

Tumor necrosis factors (TNFs), interleukin-1 (IL-1), and interleukin-2 (IL-2) are among a number of polypeptide cytokines which have been shown to modulate neutrophil functions. Others include interleukin-4, interleukin-6, interleukin-8, granulocyte macrophage colony-stimulating factor, and γ-interferon. Some of these may be released following interaction of mononuclear leukocytes with microbial components of bacterial, viral, or parasite origin (particularly in relation to TNF_{α}). In other cases the release may be slower and more persistent, involving antigen- or mitogen-stimulated T-lymphocytes. By the release of these factors, neutrophils may be educated in their search for microorganisms in body tissues as well as destruction of the organisms. It is important to realize, however, that the effects of these polypeptide cytokines may not be unique. That is, their effects are also common to other mediators such as the complement peptide C5a and lipids such as LTB_4, arachidonic acid, and tissue breakdown products.

Cytokines such as IL-1 and TNF_{α} are released by a range of cell types including local tissue cells. Microbial perturbation of cells can lead to the release of these cytokines and the pathophysiology which accompanies infections. On the other hand, a highly regulated inflammatory response leading to controlled release of cytokines by macrophages and lymphocytes in proximity to neutrophils can be of major benefit to the host. Both T-cells and neutrophils have been found in the same cellular infiltrate in vivo. It has also been shown that T-cells, through a cell-mediated immune response, regulate the migration and function of neutrophils (1–5). To date, presumably because of technical problems, very little work has been conducted to assess the importance of polypeptide cytokines on neutrophil-mediated antimicrobial activity in vivo. Therefore the role of these in defense against infection derives primarily from in-vitro studies.

II. RECEPTORS FOR TNFs ON NEUTROPHILS

TNF_α is a neutrophil modulator. The action of TNF_α is most likely mediated via receptors to this cytokine present on the neutrophil surface. Receptors of TNF_α have been demonstrated (6,7). Neutrophils contain a single class of high-affinity receptors. Approximately 6000 TNF_α receptor sites per cell were suggested by Scatchard analysis of competitive binding studies in one investigation, and 2200 receptors per cell in another (6,7). From these studies the dissociation constant was of the order of 10^{-9} to 10^{-10} M. Of biological significance was the finding that a linear relationship existed between neutrophil TNF_α binding and cell adherence to plastic surfaces (7). It is interesting that although lymphocytes, macrophages, and neutrophils respond to TNF_α, the neutrophils have a greater number of receptors (6). This may explain our previous results, which showed that the neutrophil-stimulating activity of TNF_α-rich medium could be readily absorbed with neutrophils but only poorly with mononuclear cells (8). There is a strong amino acid homology between TNF_α and TNF_β, and this is consistent with the finding that TNF_α and TNF_β share the same receptor on neutrophils (6). The cell's capacity to respond to TNF_α and TNF_β is likely to depend on the state and number of these receptors on the cell. Recently it was demonstrated that challenging human macrophages with bacterial lipopolysaccharide (LPS) modulated (down-regulated) the number of TNF_α receptors (9). Similar results were obtained when neutrophils were treated with stimulators such as fMLP, C5a, PAF, LTB_4, and PMA (10,11).

III. EFFECTS OF IL-1, IL-2, AND TNFs ON NEUTROPHIL ADHERENCE

Recent studies by Seow et al. (12) have shown that treatment of human neutrophils with recombinant human IL-1α decreases their adherence to dacron fiber while TNF_α enhanced neutrophil adherence. Only a few minutes' treatment of leukocytes with these cytokines was adequate to achieve optimal depression (with IL-1) or optimal enhancement (with TNF_α) of adherence. Treatment of neutrophils with TNF_α also increases their adherence to cultured human umbilical vein endothelial cells (13). Both the chemotactic peptide N-formyl-L-methionyl-L-leucyl-L-phenylalanine (fMLP) and phorbol myristate acetate (PMA) enhance neutrophil adherence to dacron fiber. Pretreatment of neutrophils with IL-1α depressed the enhancement induced by both stimulators (12), while treatment of neutrophils with TNF_α enhanced the fMLP- and PMA-induced adherence (12). The addition of both IL-1α and TNF_α to neutrophils resulted in no change in adherence (12).

The findings that TNF_α enhances not only the adherence response induced by a surface receptor-acting stimulus, fMLP, but also the response to an activator of protein kinase C (PMA), shows that this phenomenon is also relevant to stimuli which "bypass" the surface receptor. This suggests that the adherence response induced by other stimuli, including the types generated during the inflammatory response which act on cell surface receptors, can be augmented by exposure of neutrophils to TNF_α. The opposite effects would be expected if the cells are exposed to IL-1. Macrophages thus release two cytokines, IL-1 and TNF_α, which appear to have different effects on neutrophil adherence: one up-regulates and the other down-regulates this response. While IL-1 and TNF_α share many biological properties such as thermoregulation, cytocidal activity for tumor cells, osteoclast-activating factor activity, and stimulation of synovial cell production of prostaglandin E2 and collagenase, IL-1 lacks the cachectic activity of TNF_α and TNF_α lacks the lymphocyte-activating activity of IL-1 (14–17).

The T-lymphocyte product TNF_β showed similar enhancement of neutrophil adherence as TNF_α (18). TNF_β-treated human neutrophils showed increased adherence to dacron fibers. As with TNF_α, only a few minutes' pretreatment were adequate to achieve these modifications. TNF_β-pretreated neutrophils showed enhancement of the fMLP- and PMA-induced response. In contrast to the effects of TNF_β, IL-2 depressed basal neutrophil adherence (18). Furthermore, pretreatment of cells with IL-2 decreased the fMLP- and PMA-induced adherence response (18). Treatment of cells with a combination of IL-2 and TNF_β resulted in no modulation of adherence property of the cell. This demonstrates that T-cells, upon antigenic or mitogenic stimulation, release cytokines which can have opposite effects on neutrophil adherence. Preferential expression of one or the other by T-lymphocytes may dictate the type of effect on neutrophils.

IV. EFFECT OF IL-1, IL-2, AND TNFs ON NEUTROPHIL MIGRATION AND CHEMOTAXIS

A number of investigators have attempted to establish a chemotactic property for TNFs (5,19–24). In all these cases rHu TNFs were used. Ming et al. (19) reported the chemotactic property of both TNF_α and TNF_β for human neutrophils and monocytes. Using a filter microchamber technique, TNF_α was chemotactic for neutrophils and monocytes at a concentration range of 1 to 10^4 U/ml and 0.01 to 10^4 U/ml, respectively. Maximal responses were observed between 10 and 10^3 U/ml. The level of chemotaxis induced by TNF_α was comparable to that elicited by standard chemotactic agents, fMLP and C5a. The studies also demonstrated that both TNFs were not chemokinetic. The TNFs were not chemotactic for large granular lymphocytes nor for endothelial cells, although both of these express receptors for TNF. The chemotactic properties of TNF_α and TNF_β were demonstrated also by Figari et al. (21) using polycarbonate filters. However, these were found to be chemokinetic as well as chemotactic. In these studies it was found that TNF_α was more active on a molar basis than was TNF_β. In contrast, Ferrante et al. (5,20), using a migration-under-agarose assay, showed that both TNF_α and TNF_β lacked chemotactic activity. Similar findings have been obtained by Mrowietz et al. (22) using Boyden chambers. Using a recently developed improved method of measuring chemotaxis of neutrophils, employing a "sparse-pore" polycarbonate membrane in a Boyden chamber, we have found no evidence to show that either TNF_α or TNF_β is chemotactic for neutrophils (24). The reasons for the differences observed in the chemotactic properties of TNFs is difficult to appreciate. All the different investigator groups used at least one preparation of TNF_α/TNF_β from the same supplier. Ferrante et al. (5,20) demonstrated that while the TNF_α and TNF_β preparations were not chemotactic, these induced a respiratory response in the same cell preparations. It would seem reasonable to assume at this stage that the question of whether TNFs are chemotactic or not remains to be resolved.

The studies of Ferrante et al. (5,20) showed that TNF_α and TNF_β were migration inhibitory for human neutrophils. These were demonstrated in a migration-under-agarose method. Migration-inhibitory effects were shown for both random and chemotactic migration, using fMLP. The migration inhibition-inducing properties of TNFs were found to be created within a short pretreatment period of 30 min with the cytokines. The effects of TNF_α on migration were also evidenced by the studies of Shalaby et al. (6). The migration-inhibitory properties of TNF_α and TNF_β were confirmed using a recently described improved chemotaxis method based on a Boyden chamber but using a "sparse-pore" polycarbonate membrane (24).

Although initial studies using leukocyte-derived purified IL-1 showed it to be chemotactic (25,26), recent studies with recombinant human IL-1α showed these not to be chemotactic using the migration-under-agarose method (20) and modified Boyden chambers using a polycarbonate membrane (21). Using the sparse-pore polycarbonate membrane, we found IL-1α and IL-1β to be chemotactic for neutrophils. However, these were nowhere near as active as fMLP (24).

Some reports have shown that IL-2 is a neutrophil modulator (27). Studies examining the chemotactic activity of IL-2 in migration under agarose failed to demonstrate activity using both a leukocyte-purified human IL-2 and recombinant IL-2 (27). However, IL-2-treated neutrophils showed inhibited migration–randomly and toward fMLP (27).

V. ENHANCEMENT OF ANTIBODY-DEPENDENT CELLULAR CYTOTOXICITY

Both TNF_α and TNF_β have been shown to augment antibody-dependent neutrophil cytotoxicity (28,29). Using antibody-coated chicken erythrocytes, Shalaby et al. (28) showed that human TNF_α and TNF_β increased the neutrophil-mediated cytotoxicity against this target. These findings were confirmed by Perussia et al. (29) using a different target, antibody-sensitized mouse mastocytoma P815y. The augmentation of neutrophil antibody-dependent cellular cytotoxicity developed rapidly in the presence of TNF_α and TNF_β compared to 18 h with γ-interferon. The effects of TNFs were, however, short-lived and probably independent of protein synthesis. It is unlikely that either TNF_α or TNF_β enhances antibody-independent neutrophil cytotoxicity. For example, we have found that (PHA) phytohaemagglutinin-activated mononuclear leukocyte-conditioned medium containing both TNF_α and TNF_β (Figure 1) increased the damage against amebae and tumor cells when the targets were sensitized with antibody but not in the absence of sensitization (30,31). These results indicate synergism between TNF receptor activation and Fc receptor action. The inability of TNF to stimulate cytotoxicity in an antibody-independent system could be partly explained by the incubation periods of the cytotoxicity assays. Shau (32) found that TNF_α could modestly stimulate this type of cytotoxicity reaction if the incubation periods were extended to over 24 h. The studies of Shou (32), however, did show that TNF_α-primed neutrophils had markedly increased cytostatic properties toward tumor targets.

VI. TNFs AND NEUTROPHIL ANTIMICROBIAL ACTIVITY

It has been observed that a leukocyte-conditioned medium of cells stimulated with mitogens such as PHA or formalin-fixed *S. aureus* primes human neutrophils for increased amebicidal, fungicidal, and bactericidal activity (30,31,33). Recently these media have been shown to be rich in TNF_α and TNF_β (34–36) (Figure 1). Some initial studies have also shown that the recombinant human TNFs increase antimicrobial activity of neutrophils.

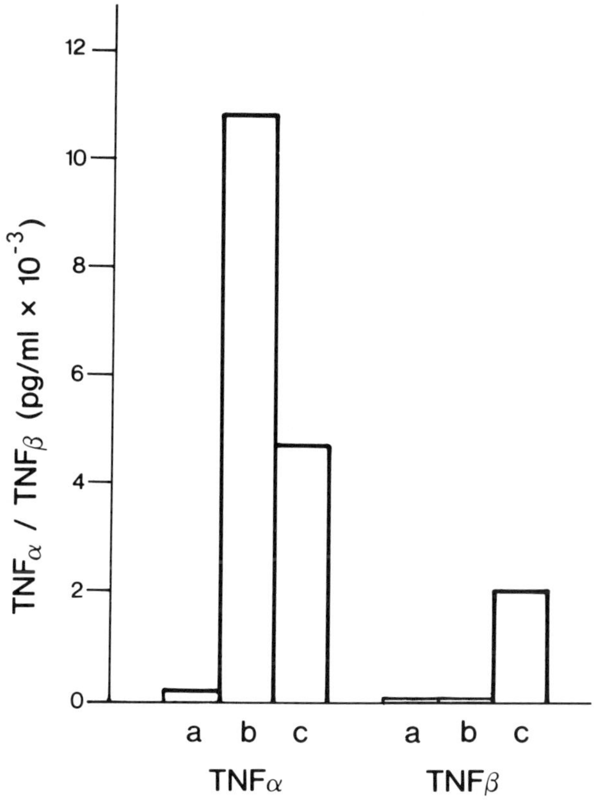

Figure 1 Production of TNF_α and TNF_β by human MNL stimulated by either *S. aureus* or PHA. Key: (a) no mitogen; (b) *S. aureus;* (c) PHA. MNL were cultured for 3 days and then the supernatants harvested for TNF determination. The concentration of TNF_α and TNF_β was measured by enzyme-linked immunosorbent assay essentially as described previously (32). Results are the means from 34 different individuals.

The ability of TNF_α to alter neutrophil antifungal activity was examined by Djeu et al. (37). Human neutrophils treated with TNF_α showed significantly increased growth inhibition of *Candida albicans.* This activity occurred in the absence of serum opsonic factors. These findings were extended by the work of Ferrante (38), which showed that the killing of both *C. albicans* and *Torulopsis glabrata* by human neutrophils was augmented by pretreating the leukocytes with TNF_α, in suspension assays and in the presence of serum opsonins (Table 1). A similar stimulation of neutrophil bactericidal activity by TNF_α was found (Table 1). The results, presented in Table 2, show that TNF_α fails to stimulate killing of *T. glabrata* by neutrophils in the absence of serum opsonins. If human serum used as a source of opsonin were heated to inactivate complement and absorbed with the fungus to remove antibodies, TNF_α was unable to increase the fungicidal activity of neutrophils (Table 2). Using these suspension assays, it has been found that TNF_β also increases the fungicidal and bactericidal activity of neutrophils (Figure 2). However, TNF_α always caused greater augmentation of the fungicidal activity than did TNF_β.

Table 1 Effects of TNF_α on Neutrophil Fungicidal and Bactericidal Activity[a]

Neutrophil treatment	Percent survival[b]	
	Fungi	Bacteria
Diluent	49.6 ± 6.3	16.3 ± 5.4
TNF_α	19.4 ± 4.0	2.7 ± 0.9

[a] Human neutrophils were pretreated with 50 U/10^6 cells of $rHuTNF_\alpha$ for 30 min at 37°C and then challenged with *T. glabrata* and *S. aureus* as previously described.

[b] Shows survival of fungi and bacteria at 3 h and 1 h, respectively. Viable count was made by assessing the ability of the organisms to form colonies. The results represent the mean ±SD of five (fungi) or three (bacteria) experiments.

Examination of kinetics of fungal killing by TNF_α-treated neutrophils showed that enhancement by this cytokine was evident in the first few minutes of the incubation. That is, there was an increase in initial rate of killing, but after 1 h the rates of killing by TNF_α-treated and nontreated neutrophils were essentially the same (38). The difference between the two cell populations was evident even after overnight incubation. It is interesting that the amount of killing by nontreated cells did not eventually reach that of the TNF_α-primed cells. In the same study it was established that the degree of enhancement by TNF_α was dependent on the preincubation time. Preincubation times of 60 min and 30 min were highly effective, while if TNF_α was added at 0 time (just prior to the fungi), very little effect occurred. If it was added after the fungi had been added, then no effect was observed. This may be related to either a requirement for TNF_α to modulate surface receptor expression or a fungal-induced change in TNF_α receptors (10,11).

Killing of *Legionella pneumophila* by neutrophils could also be augmented by treating leukocyte with TNF_α (39). Studies with the protozoa *Entamoeba histolytica* showed that while γ-interferon-activated neutrophils were stimulated to kill these amebae, TNF_α was ineffective (40). However TNF_α and γ-interferon were synergistic in this system. Kumaratilake et al. (41) have demonstrated that TNF_α stimulates the neutrophil-mediated killing of *P. falciparum*-infected erythrocytes. The cytokine

Table 2 Effects of Serum Opsonins on TNF_α Enhancement of Neutrophil Fungicidal Activity[a]

Addition	Percent survival[b]	
	Diluent	TNF_α
1% BSA	93.4 ± 7.5	97.6 ± 14.8
1% PHS	40.4 ± 10.1	25.2 ± 3.8
1% adsorbed-heated PHS	69.8 ± 8.3	86.8 ± 10.8

[a] Human neutrophils were treated with 100U $rHuTNF_\alpha/10^6$ cells for 30 min prior to challenge with *T. glabrata*. The fungicidal reaction was carried out in the presence of bovine serum albumin (BSA), pooled human group AB serum (PHS), or fungi absorbed heat-inactivated (56°C/20 min) PHS.

[b] The results are present as mean ±SD of five experiments.

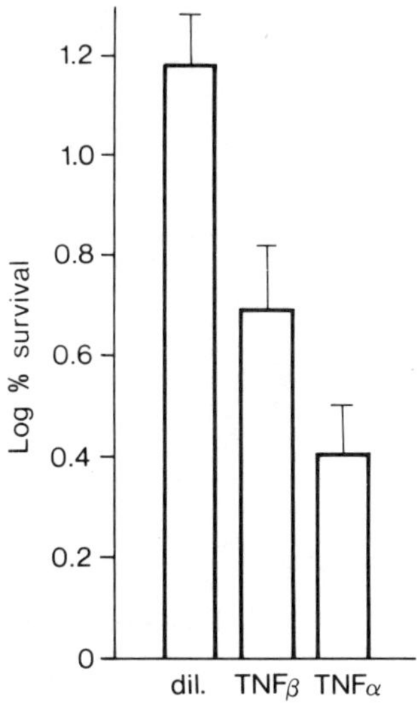

Figure 2 The effects of rHuTNF$_\beta$ on neutrophil bactericidal (*S. aureus*) activity. The bactericidal assays were conducted as described previously (31). Human neutrophils were pretreated with 500 U rHuTNF$_\beta$ for 30 min at 37°C and then challenged with bacteria. This was compared with the optimal concentration of rHuTNF$_\alpha$ (100 U). The results are the mean ±SEM of three experiments.

enhanced the killing in the absence of serum opsonin, in the presence of complement, and in the presence of antimalarial antibodies. The greatest killing occurred in the presence of antibody and TNF$_\alpha$-treated neutrophils. The results also showed that killing occurred by engulfment of the parasites by neutrophils (41). Recent studies with TNF$_\beta$ have shown comparable results to TNF$_\alpha$ in the *P. falciparum* system (42).

VII. CHANGES IN THE OXYGEN-DEPENDENT RESPIRATORY ACTIVITY

NADPH oxidase has been recognised as the key enzyme responsible for the respiratory burst. Stimulation of neutrophils with a range of stimuli leads to the activation of the NADPH oxidase and the consumption and reduction of oxygen by the cell. This process leads to the formation and release of oxygen-derived reactive species, which are very important in the microbicidal activity of the cell.

TNFs have been shown to augment the size of the respiratory burst induced by a range of neutrophil stimuli. Figure 3 demonstrates the lucigenin-dependent chemiluminescence response (a measure of superoxide formation) in neutrophils primed with TNF$_\alpha$ and then stimulated with fMLP. Similar findings can be seen when measuring superoxide by the cytochrome c reduction assay (Table 3). Pretreatment of neutrophils with TNF$_\alpha$ augments their response to fMLP. There is now overwhelming evidence that TNF$_\alpha$ increases the neutrophil response to a range of cell stimuli (5,6, 20,21,34,38,43–46).

TNF$_\alpha$ binds and induces a respiratory burst in neutrophils in a concentration, related manner (Figure 4). This is a consistent finding by many investigators. However, this type of result may be difficult to interpret, a fact brought out clearly in the work of

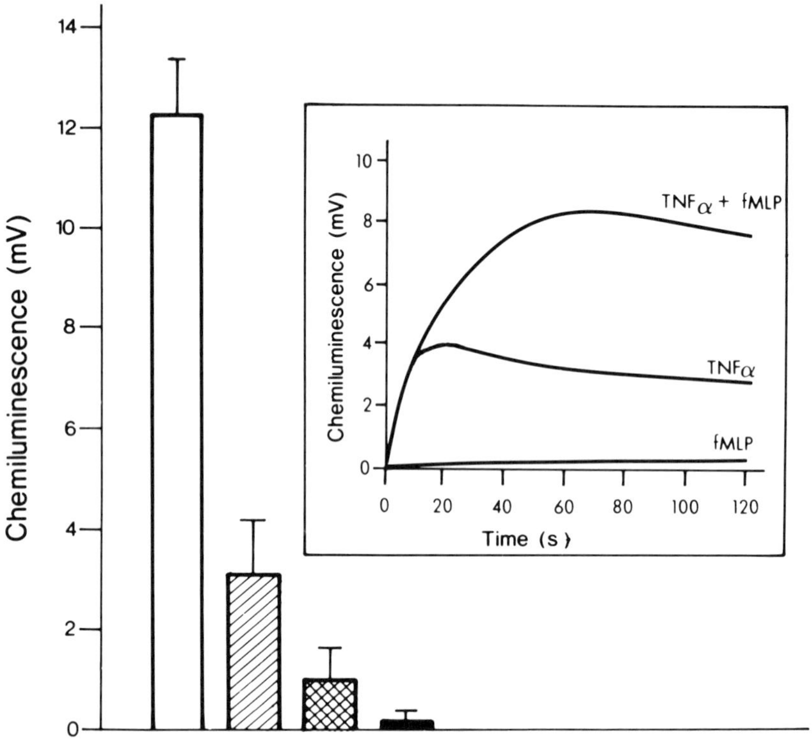

Figure 3 The effects of rHuTNF$_\alpha$ on the fMLP-induced human neutrophil lucigenin-dependent chemiluminescence response. Bars represent mean ±SD of eight separate experiments. Insert shows the time-related changes in rate of chemiluminescence production by neutrophils. The bars indicate (□) TNF$_\alpha$ primed and fMLP challenged, (▨) TNF$_\alpha$ primed diluent challenged, (▩) diluent primed and fMLP challenged, and (■) diluent primed and challenged.

Table 3 Enhancement of fMLP-Induced Superoxide Production by TNF$_\alpha$[a]

Priming agent	$O_2^{\bar{\cdot}}$ (nmol/10^6 cells) Diluent	fMLP
Diluent	1.25 ± 0.77	7.41 ± 1.41
TNF$_\alpha$	6.17 ± 2.79	17.13 ± 2.56

[a] Human neutrophils were pretreated with 100 U of rHuTNF$_\alpha$/10^6 cells for 30 min at 37°C and then challenged with fMLP. The superoxide response was measured as the difference in absorption of the reduction of cytochrome C in the presence or absence of superoxide dismutase. Assays were terminated 5 min after the addition of fMLP. Results are the mean ±SD of three experiments.

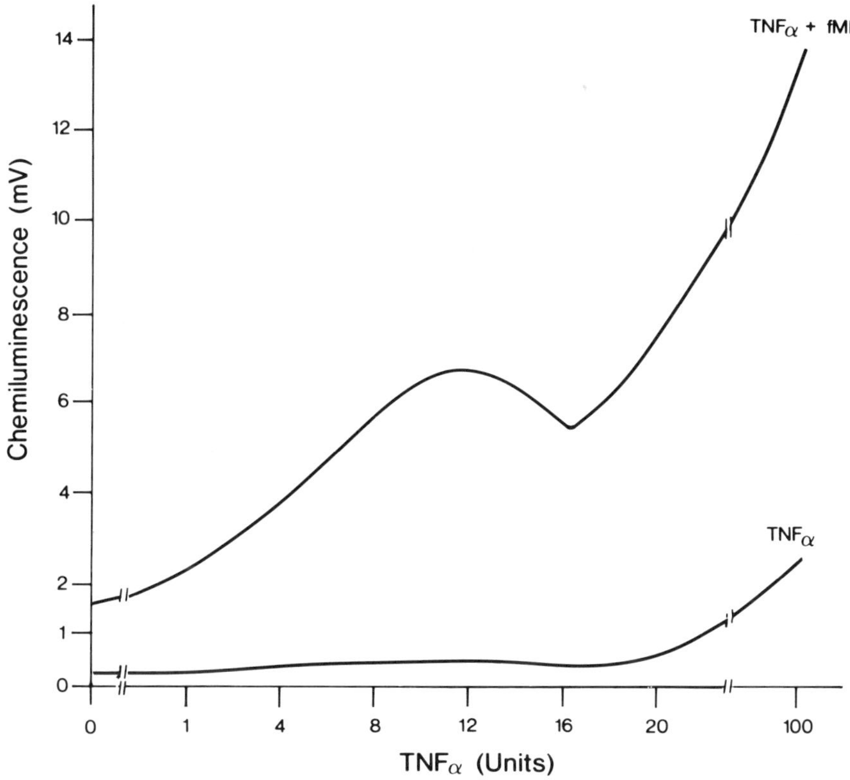

Figure 4 The effects of different rHuTNF$_\alpha$ concentrations on the fMLP-induced lucigenin-dependent chemiluminescence response. For each concentration, the maximal rate of chemiluminescence production is recorded.

Nathan (45). In these studies both TNF$_\alpha$ and TNF$_\beta$ did not induce a respiratory burst if the neutrophils were incubated in suspension and in low cell concentrations. The data suggest that the observed reported rapid respiratory burst induced by TNFs is due to a second stimulus through cell-cell adhesion and/or adherence to the culture vessel. Under conditions where the response due to binding to polystyrene surface was prevented (i.e., coated plates with fetal bovine serum, fibronectin, or other), TNFs did induce a respiratory burst, but this was quite delayed (lag of 30 min). This result was interpreted to suggest that, upon adherence of neutrophil to intra- or extravascular surface, they undergo a massive and prolonged respiratory burst in rsponse to TNFs released by macrophages and lymphocytes.

TNF$_\alpha$- and TNF$_\beta$-pretreated neutrophils show an augmented response to a range of soluble and particle stimuli. fMLP, which binds to a surface receptor on neutrophils, induces a rapid and modest response in neutrophils. Pretreatment of neutrophils with TNF$_\alpha$ or TNF$_\beta$ for 30 min primes the cells for an augmented response (5,20,21,46–48). Responses to other surface receptor-binding simuli have been reported to be modified by priming with TNFs. The production of H_2O_2 by human neutrophils in response to nonopsonized zymosan was increased by pretreating with TNF$_\alpha$ (43). TNF$_\alpha$-containing stimulated conditioned medium has been shown to prime neutrophils for increased superoxide production in response to opsonized *Staphylococcus aureus* (8,33,49). Further studies of effects of TNF_α on neutrophil-fungal interactions showed that the lucigenin-dependent chemiluminescence and superoxide production in response to opsonized *C. albicans* and *T. glabrata* was augmented by TNF_α pretreatment (38). TNF_β has also the ability to enhance the chemiluminescence response to opsonized fungi. The neutrophil oxidative response against other organisms such as bacteria (45) and pathogenic free-living amebae (34,50) was also enhanced by TNF_α priming. However, the effects of TNF are not restricted to surface-acting stimuli. It has been shown that TNF_α and TNF_β enhance the superoxide response to PMA, which acts on an intracellular-receptor, protein kinase C (5,20).

Both IL-1α and IL-1β have been shown to increase the neutrophil chemiluminescence response and H_2O_2 production by neutrophils challenged with fMLP (20). IL-2, a T-lymphocyte growth factor, was also shown to increase the chemiluminescence and H_2O_2 production by neutrophils in response to fMLP or PMA (27). The ability of TNFs, IL-1, and IL-2 to prime neutrophils was highly time dependent (5,20,27). It was essential to add the cytokines prior to the addition of a stimulus.

VIII. EFFECTS ON LYSOSOMAL ENZYME RELEASE

The ability of TNF_α to modulate neutrophil lysosomal enzyme release was highlighted by the work of Klebanoff et al. (43). These investigations reported that TNF_α was a weak direct stimulus for degranulation but augmented neutrophil degranulation in response to nonopsonized zymosan, particularly in relation to the specific granule release. Interpretation of these results were complicated by the finding that TNF_α was toxic to the neutrophils. It is not clear why this should be so, as we have found that concentrations up to 10,000 U/10^6 cells is not toxic to neutrophils. Extensive studies on direct effects on degranulation have given rise to the conclusion that TNF_α causes release primarily from the specific granules of the neutrophil (Table 4) (20,34,38). In addition, the cytokine augments quite markedly the response of neutrophil degranulation to fMLP, opsonized fungi, and opsonized amebae. Release from both granule components was augmented. TNF_β was similarly shown to enhance the quantity of enzymes released from specific and azurophilic granules, in response to cytochalasin B-fMLP (5).

Table 4 Differential Effects of TNF_α on Neutrophil Specific and Azurophilic Granule[a]

	Granule marker (percentage release)	
Stimulant	Specific granule (vitamin B_{12} binding protein)	Azurophilic granule (β-glucuronidase)
Diluent	11.2 ± 1.8	8.0 ± 2.8
TNF_α	18.9 ± 4.2	8.9 ± 2.0

[a] Human neutrophils were stimulated with 100 U rHuTNF_α/10^6 cells and the supernatants collected after 15 min incubation at 37°C. The granule constituents vitamin B_{12} binding protein and β-glucuronidase were measured as described previously (35). Results are the mean ±SD of three experiments.

IL-1 (rHu IL-1α) pretreatment of human neutrophils also resulted in augmented degranulation responses to cytochalasin B-fMLP stimulation (20). The results demonstrated that IL-1 enhanced release from azurophilic granules, but it was not clear whether it increased release from specific granules. IL-2 was also found to modulate the granule release response of neutrophils. Kowanko and Ferrante (27) showed that IL-2-treated neutrophils were induced to release constituents of specific but not azurophilic granules. However, the cytokine enhanced release from both granules in response to opsonized zymosan.

IX. CYTOKINE SYNERGISM

Since polypeptide cytokines most likely occur as a mixture in body fluids, it may be more relevant to study their combined addition to cells. To date, however, very little has been done to address this question. Studies on antibody-dependent neutrophil cytotoxicity showed that γ-interferon and TNF_β were synergistic in this system and also in neutrophil phagocytosis (28). Djeu et al. (37) showed that γ-interferon and TNF_α were synergistic in activating neutrophils for increased anti-*C. albicans* activity. Similarly, the killing of *E. histolytica* by human neutrophils was augmented by the combined treatment of the leukocytes with γ-interferon and TNF_α (40). Addition of two cytokines, GM-CSF and TNF_α, which act on distinct receptors on neutrophils, did not result in a synergistic effect (Table 5).

X. IN-VIVO EVIDENCE FOR A ROLE OF CYTOKINES IN NEUTROPHIL ACTIVATION

To date it is still difficult to appreciate the role of IL-1, TNF_α, and IL-2 in neutrophil activation. The levels of cytokines found to be required to activate neutrophils in vitro are present in body fluids and in supernatants of stimulated macrophages and lymphocytes. The results in Table 6 show that TNF_α was a more powerful primer of the fMLP response in the presence of serum, suggesting that the observed in-vitro effects are pertinent to the in-vivo environment. Averbook et al. (51) showed that TNF_β injected into normal rabbit skin induced a local inflammatory reaction in which neutro-

Table 5 Effect of Combined Treatment of Neutrophils with TNF_α and GM-CSF on the fMLP Response[a]

	$O_2^{\cdot}$ (nmol/10^6 cells)	
Pretreatment	Diluent	fMLP
Diluent	0.56 ± 0.30	5.16 ± 2.19
GM-CSF	0.64 ± 0.79	13.19 ± 3.41
TNF_α	3.65 ± 1.62	17.44 ± 4.07
GM-CSF + TNF_α	4.07 ± 2.05	16.62 ± 5.40

[a] Human neutrophils were pretreated with 50 U of recombinant human cytokine/10^6 for 30 min and then stimulated with fMLP. Superoxide was measured by the cytochrome C reduction assay. The results represent mean ± SD of five experiments.

Table 6 Effects of Human Serum Addition on TNF_{α} Priming of the fMLP-Induced Respiratory Activity of Neutrophils[a]

Serum concentration (%)	Challenge stimulus: Diluent — Diluent	Diluent — TNF_{α}	fMLP — Diluent	fMLP — TNF_{α}
0	0.01 ± 0.10	2.45 ± 2.1	0.45 ± 0.28	5.87 ± 3.56
0.1	0.03 ± 0.08	4.19 ± 3.46	0.80 ± 0.44	11.38 ± 5.80
1	0.11 ± 0.11	3.81 ± 2.02	3.37 ± 3.95	13.82 ± 1.87
5	0.09 ± 0.02	7.12 ± 4.53	4.92 ± 3.68	27.77 ± 2.13
10	0.09 ± 0.05	11.95 ± 7.20	6.71 ± 4.70	36.26 ± 3.55

[a] Human neutrophils were pretreated for 30 min with 100 U $rHuTNF_{\alpha}/10^6$ cells in the presence of the indicated concentrations of human serum, and then challenged with fMLP. The results are the maximal rate of lucigenin-dependent chemiluminescence production, and are presented as mean ±SD of three experiments.

quite prominent. However, in-vivo studies of this type are difficult to interpret because of the multitudinal effects of cytokines.

XI. MECHANISM OF PRIMING AND ENHANCEMENT

The mechanisms which lead to increased neutrophil responsiveness following TNF_{α}, and IL-1 and IL-2 treatment remain essentially undefined. Very few studies have been conducted on IL-2 and neutrophil function. We were unable to demonstrate IL-2 receptors on neutrophils (Kowanko and Ferrante, unpublished). Activation of lymphocyte proliferation by IL-2 has been shown to be inhibited by the protein kinase C inhibitor H-7 (52). It is possible that IL-2 may mediate its activation of neutrophils via the protein kinase C system.

IL-1α and IL-1β bind with similar affinities to the same receptor on neutrophils (53), and their mechanism of priming may be similar to TNF_{α} and TNF_{β}, both of which bind to the same class of surface receptor on neutrophils. The binding of TNFs to receptors triggers an oxidative burst of respiratory activity, priming the cell to display an increased response to various agonists. The relationship between priming and cell activation by TNFs is not understood. However, it is necessary to realize that priming for an increased response is not restricted just to cytokines. fMLP interaction with neutrophil surface receptors leads to enhancement of the bactericidal activity of the cell (Figure 5). fMLP also directly activates a weak respiratory burst (Figure 3). The data presented in Table 7 are against the requirement for an associated respiratory activity in the TNF_{α}-induced priming. Pretreatment of neutrophils with cytochalasin-B severely decreased the cell's response to TNF_{α} without affecting the priming for an fMLP response by TNF_{α}. This finding reinforces the view derived from the studies of Nathan (45) which showed that priming of neutrophils by TNF_{α}, under conditions which prevented adhesion and a TNF_{α}-induced respiratory activity, still occurred.

Further support for a nonrequirement of a respiratory burst is shown by making comparisons between the effects of γ-interferon and TNF_{α} on the NADPH oxidase activity and the killing of *E. histolytica.* The killing of this organism by neutrophils is

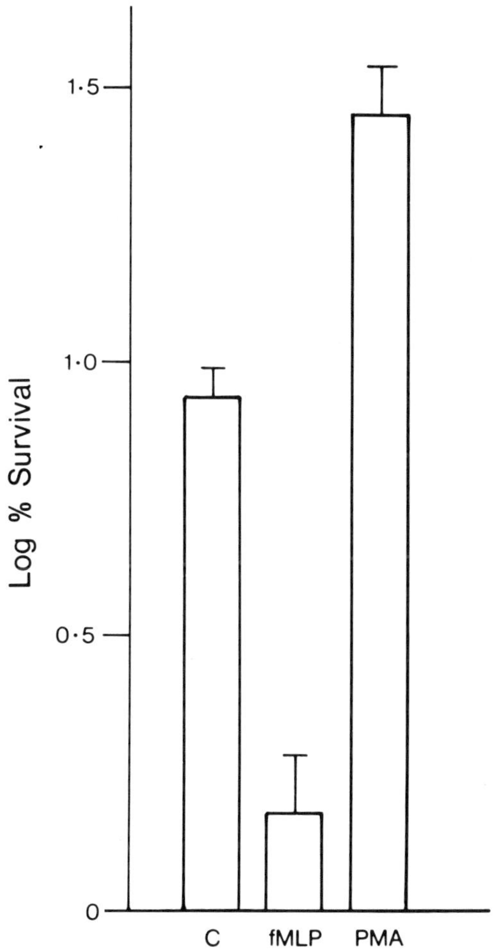

Figure 5 The effect of fMLP and PMA on neutrophil bactericidal (*S. aureus*) activity. Human neutrophils were pretreated for 30 min at 37°C with fMLP or PMA and then challenged with bacteria. The results are the mean ±SD of three experiments. C = diluent-treated cells.

Table 7 Effects of Cytochalasin B on TNF_α-Neutrophil Priming[a]

	Chemiluminescence (mV)	
Pretreatment	Diluent	fMLP
Diluent	0.37 ± 0.08	3.07 ± 0.80
Cyt B-diluent	0.09 ± 0.02	5.20 ± 1.09
TNF_α	5.45 ± 1.16	11.41 ± 0.80
Cyt B-TNF_α	0.16 ± 0.03	19.21 ± 3.10

[a] Human neutrophils were pretreated with cytochalasin B (Cyt B) for 10 min and followed by 100 U of $rHuTNF_\alpha/10^6$ cells for 20 min and then challenged with fMLP. The results represent mean ±SD of three experiments.

stimulated by γ-interferon but not TNF_α, although the two cytokines show a synergistic effect (40). The killing is highly dependent on H_2O_2. However, an examination of data in Table 8 shows that γ-interferon shows a very weak stimulation of respiratory activity compared with TNF_α.

Besides the stimulation of the cell's NADPH oxidase by TNFs, the neutrophils show depressed locomotion. This effect could be related to TNF-induced increased adhesiveness of the neutrophils to the substrate. Although there is still some controversy, TNFs appear not to be chemotactic but do cause an inhibition of migration of cells in a chemotactic gradient generated with fMLP. This could be related to changes in fMLP receptor affinity induced by TNFs (45). Changes in the expression of surface receptors are induced by TNFs and include the CR3 (13) and CR1 complement receptors (54). TNFs may induce these changes in surface receptor expression by causing release of these receptors from neutrophil-specific granules. In support of this is the finding that TNFs cause release of constituents from these granules. Following modulation of either the number or affinity of surface receptors, the cells may respond to other stimuli, such as fMLP or complement/antibody opsonized particles, more effectively. The effects of cytokines on neutrophils appear to be transient. Studies on the fungicidal activity of TNF treated neutrophils showed that only the initial rate of killing is increased (38). Promotion of the translocation of components of the NADPH oxidase, presumably contained in the specific (or specific-like) granules by TNF_α may also be a factor in cell priming. It is unlikely that this event is itself responsible for increased microbicidal activity of the cell by pregenerating ODRS and release of lysosomal enzymes. Instead it is envisaged that the increased response of the primed cells to the second challenge is the major cause of the enhanced microbicidal or tumoricidal activity. Evidence in support of this belief is derived from our studies in which neutrophils were pretreated with cytochalasin B and then examined to see if these could be primed by TNF_α. The results showed that although cytochalasin B markedly depressed the neutrophil response to TNF_α, it augmented the TNF_α priming for an fMLP response (Table 7). The cell is primed for a more effective release of ODRS and granule constituents from specific and azurophilic granules.

It is difficult to develop concepts which began with the binding of TNF to its receptor and actual modulation of receptors. It has been found that TNF_α priming of neutrophils is independent of a pertussis toxin-sensitive guanine nucleotide regulatory protein

Table 8 Comparison of Effects of rHu γ-Interferon and rHu TNF_α on Neutrophil Chemiluminescence[a]

	Chemiluminescence (mV)	
Priming agent	Diluent	fMLP
Diluent	0.07 ± 0.02	2.0 ± 0.52
γ-Interferon	0.11 ± 0.06	3.83 ± 0.89
TNF_α	2.37 ± 0.78	26.16 ± 2.32

[a] Human neutrophils pretreated for 30 min at 37°C with the cytokines (100 U/10^6 cells) and then challenged with fMLP. The results represent the mean ±SE of six experiments of the lucigenin-dependent chemiluminescence response.

(47,55). In support of this finding is our data which showed that TNF_α and TNF_β prime neutrophils to a stimulus which bypasses the surfaces receptor and acts directly on protein kinase C (i.e., PMA). The cytokines also do not induce translocation of the calcium and phospholipid-dependent protein kinase C. Evidence is in fact against the role for protein kinase C activation in signal transduction by TNF_α. Pretreatment of neutrophils with a protein kinase C inhibitor H-7 failed to inhibit the TNF_α-augmented fMLP response (Figure 6). However, this response was inhibited by an inhibitor, W-7, of the calmodulin-dependent pathway of activation (Figure 6). This suggests that the mechanism of TNF_α-induced priming of neutrophils is independent of protein kinase C.

The possibility that TNF_α induces the release of other mediators such as AA, LTB_4, and PAF which may be involved in a cascade of events leading to maximal cell priming needs to be studied. Although some investigators have been unable to show TNF_α induction of LTB_4 (56) and AA (47) production, others have demonstrated LTB_4, AA, and PAF release upon stimulation with TNF_α (57). All of these neutrophil inflammatory mediators have the capacity to prime neutrophil functions (Figure 7). It is even of major interest that these mediators act synergistically with TNF_α (Figure 7).

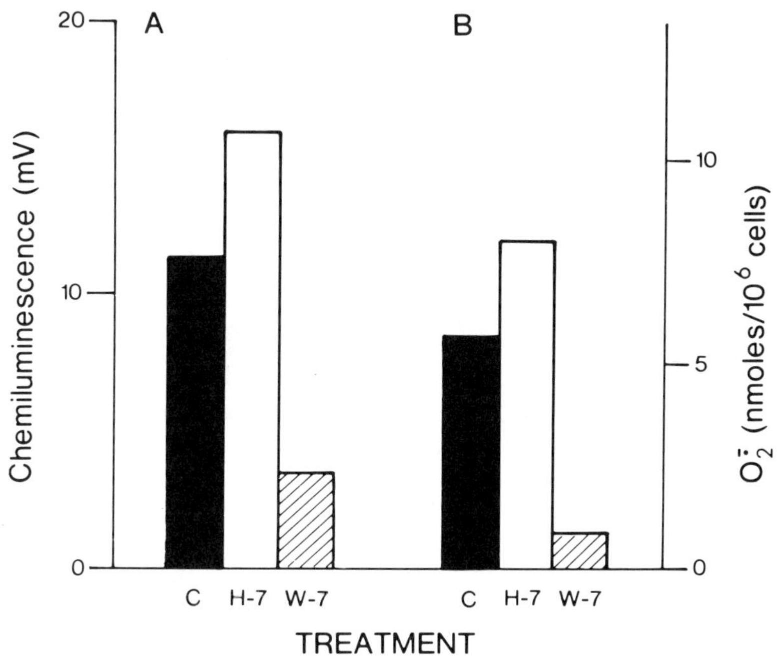

Figure 6 The effect of 1-(5-isoquinolinylsulfonyl)-2 methylpiperazine (H-7) and N-(6-aminohexyl)-5-chloro-1-naphthalenesulfonamide (W-7) on rHuTNF_α-primed fMLP-induced respiratory burst examined by the lucigenin-dependent chemiluminescence assay and the SOD-inhibitable cytochrome C reduction assay. The neutrophils were pretreated with 100 μM of either H-7 or W-7 10 min prior to priming with TNF_α. The results are the mean of three experiments.

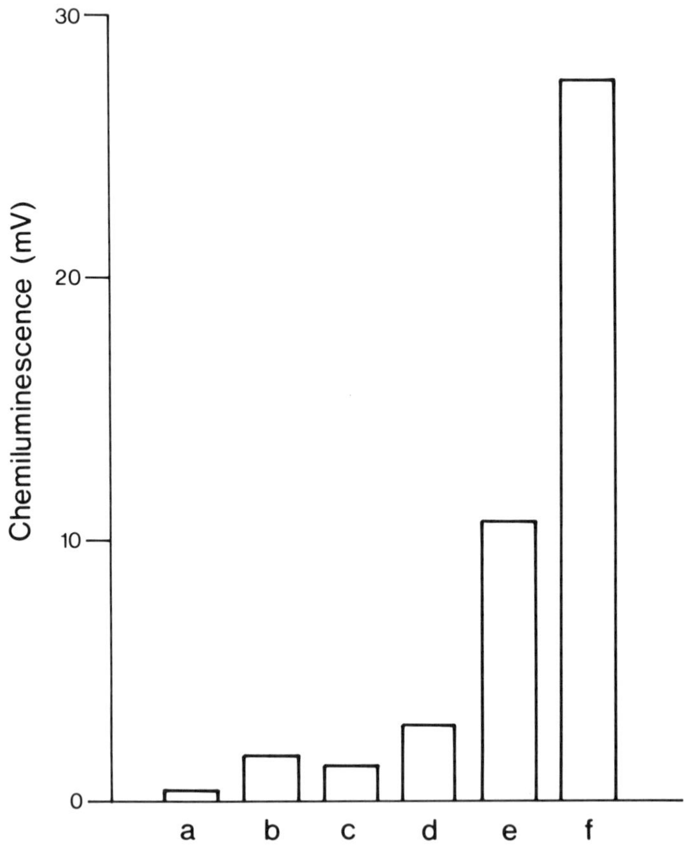

Figure 7 The effects of platelet-activating factor (PAF) on the neutrophil respiratory burst. Human neutrophils were pretreated with either diluent (a), (b); PAF, (c), (d); or TNF_α (e), (f) and then challenged with either diluent a, c, e, or fMLP b, d, and f.

XII. SUMMARY

This review outlines evidence that IL-1, IL-2, and TNFs modulate neutrophil functions. These cytokines affect some or all of the following functions of the neutrophil: adherence, cell migration, respiratory burst, lysosomal enzyme release, and cell surface receptor expression. TNFs, especially TNF_α, remains one of the most highly studied cytokine with respect to regulation of neutrophil function. TNFs are a direct stimuli for the neutrophil respiratory burst and weak stimuli of lysosomal enzyme release. The cytokines enhance cell adhesion and inhibit neutrophil migration. The TNFs augment the oxidative burst and lysosomal enzyme release response to a wide range of soluble and particulate cell stimuli. These changes in the cell seem to be closely correlated with the increased fungicidal, bactericidal, tumoricidal, and protozoacidal activity of the TNF-primed neutrophils. In contrast to TNFs, IL-1 and IL-2 inhibit neutrophil adherence, and this provides evidence that the cytokine family represents a regulatory system. Another form of regulation of TNF_α and IL-1 neutrophil-activating activity is by the release of inhibitors to these cytokines (58). We have evidence which shows that the soluble TNF_α inhibitor (a cleaved product of the TNF_α receptor) (59) binds and inhibits TNF from activating and priming neutrophils (60). Priming of neutrophils by TNFs involves surface receptor binding but is independent of protein kinase C system, pertussis toxin-sensitive guanine nucleotide regulatory protein, and direct burst of respiratory activity. The translocation of cell surface receptors and constituents of the NADPH oxidase from stored vesicles may be the major mechanism of TNF-induced cell priming.

ACKNOWLEDGMENTS

I am indebted to my departmental colleagues Edna J. Bates, Inge Kowanko, and Laki Kumaratilake and to Jean-Michel Dayer of the Division of Immunology and Allergy, Hospital Cantonal University of Geneva, for stimulating discussions, Trish Harvey and Kathy Carman for excellent technical assistance, and Pru Russell-Taylor for secretarial assistance. I am grateful to A. Adolf from the Ernst-Boehringer Institut, Vienna, for providing the $rHuTNF_\alpha$, $rHuTNF_\beta$, and rHuIFN-γ, and to P. Lomedico, Hoffmann-La Roche, Inc., Nutley, NJ, for the gift of rHuIL-1α which were used in the author's work. The work of the author has been supported by grants from the National Health and Medical Research Council, UNDP/WORLD BANK/WHO Special Programme for Research and Training in Tropical Diseases, Channel 7 Children's Medical Research Foundation, Adelaide Children's Hospital Research Foundation, and University of Adelaide Research Grants.

REFERENCES

1. Pelletier M, Cirre C, Giroud JP. Induction of macrophage DNA synthesis in vitro, by non-immunological inflammatory sera: effect of irradiation and thymus or bone marrow cell reconstitution. J Pathol 1979; 131:157–63.
2. Czuprynski CJ, Henson PM, Campbell PA. Enhanced accumulation of inflammatory neutrophils and macrophages mediated by transfer of T cells from mice immunized with *Listeria monocytogenes.* J Immunol 1985; 134:3449–54.
3. Palmer DG, Hogg N, Revell PA. Lymphocytes, polymorphonuclear leukocytes, macrophages and plates in synovium involved by rheumatoid arthritis. A study with monoclonal antibodies. Pathology 1986; 18:431–7.
4. Felice GA, Niewoehner DE. Contribution of neutrophils and cell-mediated immunity to control of *Nocardia asteroids* in murine lungs. J Infect Dis 1987; 156:113–21.
5. Ferrante A, Nandoskar M, Bates EJ, Goh, DHB, Beard LJ. Tumour necrosis factor-beta (lymphotoxin) inhibits locomotion and stimulates respiratory burst and degranulation of neutrophils. Immunology 1988; 63:507–12.
6. Shalaby MR, Palladin MA Jr, Hirabayashi SE, Eessalu TE, Lewis GD, Shepard HM, Aggarwal BB. Receptor binding and activation of polymorphonuclear neutrophils by tumour necrosis factor-alpha. J Leukocyte Biol 1987; 41:196–204.
7. Pichyangkul S, Schick D, Jia F, Berent S, Bollon A, Kahn A. Binding of tumour necrosis factor alpha (TNFα) to high-affinity receptors on polymorphonuclear cells. Exp Hematol (New York) 1987; 15:1055–9.
8. Ferrante A, Bates EJ, Nandoskar M. Neutrophil stimulating activity released by Staphylococcus-stimulated mononuclear leukocyte conditioned medium: further characterization and partial purification. J Chromatogr 1988; 440:105–18.

9. Ding AH, Sanchez E, Srimal S, Nathan CF. Macrophages rapidly internalize their tumor necrosis factor receptors in response to bacterial lipopolysaccharide. J Biol Chem 1989; 3924–9.
10. Porteu F, Nathan C. Shedding of tumor necrosis factor receptors by activated human neutrophils. J Exp Med 1990; 172:599–607.
11. Schieiffenbaum B, Fehr J. The tumor necrosis factor receptor and human neutrophil function: deactivation and cross-deactivation of tumor necrosis factor-induced neutrophil responses by receptor down-regulation. J Clin Invest 1990; 86:184–95.
12. Seow WK, Thong YH, Ferrante A. Macrophage-neutrophil interactions: contrasting effects of the monokine interleukin-1 and tumour necrosis factor (chachectin) on human neutrophil adherence. Immunology 1988; 82:357–61.
13. Gamble JR, Harlan JM, Klebanoff SJ, Vadas MA. Stimulation of the adherence of neutrophils to umbilical vein endothelium by human recombinant tumour necrosis factor. Proc Natl Acad Sci USA 1985; 82:8667–71.
14. Onozaki K, Matsushima K, Aggarwal BB, Oppenheim JJ. Human interleukin-1 is a cytocidal factor for several tumor cell-lines. J Immunol 1985; 135:3962–8.
15. Dinarello CA, Mier JW. Interleukins. Ann Rev Med 1986; 37:173–8.
16. Mannel DN. Biological aspects of tumor necrosis factor. Immunobiology 1986; 172:283–90.
17. Beutler B, Cerami A. Cachectin: more than a tumour necrosis factor. N Engl J Med 1987; 317:379–85.
18. Seow WK, Thong YH, McCormack JG, Ferrante A. Lymphocyte-neutrophil interactions: Opposite effects of interleukin-2 and tumour necrosis factor-beta (lymphotoxin) on human neutrophil adherence. Int Arch Allergy Appl Immunol 1988; 85:63–8.
19. Ming WJ, Bersani L, Mantovani A. Tumor necrosis factor is chemotactic for monocytes and polymorphonuclear leukocytes. J Immunol 1987; 138:1469–74.
20. Ferrante A, Nandoskar M, Walz A, Goh DHB, Kowanko IC. Effects of tumour necrosis factor alpha and interleukin-1 alpha and beta human on neutrophil migration, respiratory burst and degranulation. Int Arch Allergy Appl Immunol 1988; 86:82–91.
21. Figari IS, Mori NA, Palladino MA Jr. Regulation of neutrophil migration and superoxide production by recombinant tumour necrosis factors-α and β: comparison to recombinant interferon-γ and interleukin-1α. Blood 1987; 70:979–84.
22. Mrowietz U, Schroder J-M, Christophers E. Recombinant human tumor necrosis factor a lacks chemotactic activity for human peripheral blood neutrophils and monocytes. Biochem Biophys Res Commun 1988; 153:1223–8.
23. Newman I, Wilkinson PC. Chemotactic activity of lymphotoxin and tumour necrosis factor alpha for human neutrophils. Immunology 1989; 66:318–20.
24. Bignold LP, Ferrante A, Haynes DR. Studies of chemotactic, chemotactic movement-inhibiting and random movement-inhibiting effects of interleukin-1 alpha and beta, tumour necrosis factors alpha and beta and interferon gamma on human neutrophils in assays using "sparse-pore" polycarbonate (nuclepore) membrane in the Boyden chamber. Int Arch Allergy Appl Immunol 1990; 91:1–7.
25. Luger TA, Stadler BM, Luger BM, Sztein MB, Schmidt JA, Hawley-Nelson P, Grabner G, Oppenheim JJ. Characteristics of an epidermal cell thymocyte-activating factor (ETAF) produced by human epidermal cells and a human squamous cell carcinoma cell line. J Invest Dermatol 1983; 81:187–93.
26. Sauder DN, Mousnessa NL, Katz SI, Dinarello CA, Galin JI. Chemotactic cytokines: the role of leukocytic pyrogen and epidermal cell thymocyte-activating factor in neutrophil chemotaxis. J Immunol 1984; 132:828–32.
27. Kowanko IC, Ferrante A. Interleukin-2 inhibits migration and stimulates the respiratory burst and degranulation of human neutrophils in vitro. Immunol Lett 1987; 15:285–9.

28. Shalaby MR, Aggarwal BB, Rinderknecht E, Svedersky LP, Finkle BS, Palladino MA Jr. Activation of human polymorphonuclear neutrophil functions by interferon-γ and tumour necrosis factors. J Immunol 1985; 135:2069–73.
29. Perussia B, Kobayashi M, Rossi ME, Angeon I, Trinchieri G. Immune interferon enhances functional properties of human granulocyte: role of Fc receptors and effect of lymphotoxin, tumour necrosis factor, and granulocyte-macrophage colony stimulating factor. J Immunol 1987; 138:765–74.
30. Ferrante A, Mocatta T. Human neutrophils require activation by mononuclear leucocyte-conditioned medium to kill the pathogenic free-living amoeba, *Naegleria fowleri*. Clin Exp Immunol 1984; 56:559–66.
31. Ferrante A, Abell TJ. Conditioned medium from stimulated mononuclear leukocytes augments human neutrophil mediated-killing of a virulent Acanthaemoeba. Infect Immun 1986; 51:607–17.
32. Shau H. Cytostatic and tumoricidal activities of tumor necrosis factor-a treated neutrophils. Immunol Lett 1988; 88:47–51.
33. Ferrante A, Harvey D, Bates EJ. *Staphylococcus aureus* stimulated MNL conditioned medium increases the neutrophil bactericidal activity, and augments the oxygen radical production and degranulation in response to the bacteria. Clin Exp Immunol 1989; 78:366–71.
34. Ferrante A. Augmentation of neutrophil responses to *Naegleria fowleri* by tumour necrosis factor alpha. Infect Immun 1989; 57:3110–5.
35. Ferrante A, Seow WK, Rowan-Kelly B, Thong YH. Tetrandrine, a plant alkaloid, inhibits the production of tumour necrosis factor alpha (cachectin) by human monocytes. Clin Exp Immun 1990; 80:232–5.
36. Ferrante A, Staugas REM, Rowan-Kelly B, Bresatz S, Kumaratilake LM, Rzepczyk CM, Adolf GR. Production of tumour necrosis factor alpha and beta by human mononuclear leukocytes stimulated with mitogens and microbial components. Infect Immun 1990; 58:3996–4003.
37. Djeu JY, Blanchard DK, Halkias H, Friedman H. Growth inhibition of *Candida albicans* by human polymorphonuclear neutrophils: activation by interferon-γ and tumour necrosis factor. J Immunol 1986; 137:2980–4.
38. Ferrante A. Tumour necrosis factor alpha potentiates neutrophil antimicrobial activity: increased fungicidal activity against *Torulopsis glabrata/Candida albicans* and associated increases in oxygen radical production and lysosomal enzyme release. Infect Immun 1989; 57:2115–22.
39. Blanchard DK, Friedman H, Klein TW, Djeu JY. Induction of interferon-gamma and tumor necrosis factor by *Legionella pneumophilia:* augmentation of human neutrophil bactericidal activity. J Leuk Biol 1989; 45:538–45.
40. Denis M, Chadee K. Human neutrophils activated by interferon-γ and tumour necrosis factor-α kill *Entamoeba histolytica* trophozoites in vitro. J Leuk Biol 1989; 46:270–4.
41. Kumaratilake L, Ferrante A, Rzepczyk CM. Tumour necrosis factor enhances the neutrophil mediated killing of *Plasmodium falciparum.* Infect Immun 1990; 58:788–93.
42. Kumaratilake L, Ferrante A, Rzepczyk CM. The role of T lymphocytes in immunity to *Plasmodium falciparum:* enhancement of neutrophil-mediated parasite killing by lymphotoxin and interferon gamma and comparisons with tumour necrosis factor effects. J Immunol 1991; 146:762–7.
43. Klebanoff SJ, Vadas MA, Harlan JM, Sparks LH, Gamble JR, Agosti JM, Waltersdorph AM. Stimulation of neutrophils by tumour necrosis factor. J Immunol 1986; 136:4220–5.
44. Tsujimoto M, Yokota S, Vilvek J, Weissman G. Tumour necrosis factor provokes superoxide anion generation from neutrophils. Biochem Biophys Res Commun 1986; 137:1094–100.

45. Nathan CF. Neutrophil activation on biological surfaces: massive secretion of hydrogen peroxide in response to products of macrophages and lymphocytes. J Clin Invest 1987; 80:1550–60.
46. Atkinson YH, Marasco WA, Lopez AF, Vadas MA. Recombinant human tumour necrosis factor-α: regulation of N-formylmethionyl/leucylphenylalanine receptor affinity and function on human neutrophils. J Clin Invest 1988; 81:759–65.
47. Berkow RL, Dodson MR. Biochemical mechanisms involved in the priming of neutrophils by tumour necrosis factor. J Leuk Biol 1988; 44:345–52.
48. Knownatzki E, Kapp A, Uhrich S. Modulation of human neutrophilic granulocyte functions by recombinant human tumor necrosis factor and recombinant human lymphotoxin. Promotion of adherence, inhibition of chemotactic migration and superoxide anion release from adherence cells. Clin Exp Immunol 1988; 74:143–8.
49. Ferrante A, Nandoskar M, Bates EJ, Goh DHB. *Staphylococcus aureus* stimulated human mononuclear leucocytes conditioned medium augments the basal and stimuli-induced neutrophil respiratory burst and degranulation. Immunology 1987; 60:431–8.
50. Ferrante A. Immunity to Acanthamoeba. Rev Infect Dis 1991; 13 (suppl 5):403–9.
51. Averbook BJ, Yamamoto RS, Ulich TR, Jeffes EWB, Masunaka I, Granger GA. Purified native and recombinant human alpha lymphotoxin [tumor necrosis factor (TNF)-beta] induces inflammatory reactions in normal skin. J Clin Immunol 1987; 7:333–40.
52. Mukaida N, Yagisawa H, Kawai T, Kasahara T. The role of protein kinase C activation in signal transmission by interleukin 2. Biochem Biophys Res Commun 1988; 154:187–93.
53. Dower SK, Kronheim SR, Hopp TP, Cantrell M, Deeley M, Gillis S, Henney CS, Urdal DL. The cell surface receptors for interleukin-1 alpha and interleukin-1 beta are identical (letter). Nature 1986; 324:266–7.
54. Berger M, Wetzler EM, Wallis RS. Tumor necrosis factor is the major monocyte product that increases complement receptor expression on mature human neutrophils. Blood 1988; 71:151–8.
55. Meurer R, McIntyre DE. Lack of effect of pertussis toxin on the TNFα-induced formation of reaction oxygen intermediates by human neutrophils. Biochem Biophys Res Commun 1989; 159:763–9.
56. Roubin R, Elsas PP, Fiers W, Dessein AJ. Recombinant human tumour necrosis factor (rTNF)^2 enhances leukotriene biosynthesis in neutrophils and eosinophils stimulated with the Ca^{++} ionophore A23187. Clin Exp Immunol 1987; 70:484–90.
57. Camussi G, Tetta G, Bussolino F, Baglioni C. Tumor necrosis factor stimulates human neutrophils to release leukotriene B_4 and platelet-activating factor. Eur J Biochem 1989; 182:661–6.
58. Ferrante A, Kumaratilake L, Rzepczyk CM, Dayer J-M. Killing of *Plasmodium falciparum* by cytokine activated effector cells (neutrophils and macrophages). Immunol Lett 1990; 25:179–88.
59. Seckinger P, Zhang JH, Hauptmann B, Dayer J-M. Characterization of a tumor necrosis factor α (TNF-α) inhibitor: evidence of immunological cross-reactivity with the TNF receptor. Proc Natl Acad Sci USA 1990; 20:1167–74.
60. Ferrante A, Hauptmann B, Seckinger P, Dayer J-M. Inhibition of tumour necrosis factor alpha (TNF-α) induced neutrophil respiratory burst by a TNF inhibitor. Immunology 1991; 72:440–2.

15

Modulation of Neutrophil Functions by γ-Interferon

GIORGIO BERTON and MARCO A. CASSATELLA
Institute of General Pathology,
University of Verona, Verona, Italy

I. INTRODUCTION

γ-Interferon (γ-IFN) is a cytokine produced by T-lymphocytes and natural killer cells whose multiple actions on cells of different lineage have been extensively characterized in the last few years.

In its natural form, γ-IFN is secreted as a single polypeptide showing heterogeneity in its molecular weight due to different extents of glycosylation. Human γ-IFN is encoded by a unique gene located on chromosome 12 (reviewed in Ref. 1), while the gene encoding its high-affinity cell surface receptor is located on chromosome 6 (1–4).

Studies initiated in the early 1980s permitted identification of γ-IFN as the major cytokine having the capability to activate macrophage microbicidal and cytotoxic functions (reviewed in Refs. 5–9). Studies on a possible effect of γ-IFN on neutrophils were delayed, probably owing to the assumption that these are terminally differentiated cells fully capable of exerting their effector functions. More recently, it has been appreciated that several cytokines affect neutrophils behavior (this volume and Ref. 10).

In this chapter we review the evidence demonstrating that γ-IFN is indeed a "neutrophil-activating factor." It must be anticipated that this conclusion does not rely only on phenomenological studies demonstrating that γ-IFN modulates several selective neutrophil functions. In fact, observations are emerging which permit the understanding of the molecular basis of γ-IFN actions. In this respect, the research on neutrophil-γ-IFN interaction is entering a new phase which will potentially shed light on full understanding of neutrophil behavior in the inflammatory site.

II. ALTERATIONS OF EXPRESSION OF NEUTROPHIL PLASMA MEMBRANE MOLECULES INDUCED BY γ-IFN

A. Identification of γ-IFN as a Neutrophil-Activating Factor Able to Increase Surface Expression of the High-Affinity Receptor for IgG

The first evidence that γ-IFN is able to modulate neutrophil functions was obtained by Perussia et al. in 1983 (11). These investigators demonstrated that while neutrophils cultivated for 18 h in serum-containing medium do not show specific high-affinity binding for monomeric human IgG1, neutrophils cultivated in the presence of γ-IFN bind IgG1 with high affinity. Scatchard plots of IgG1 binding revealed that γ-IFN induces the appearance of approximately 13,600 binding sites per cell with an average affinity of 13 nM. The calculated number of IgG1 binding sites on γ-IFN treated neutrophils was even higher than that on untreated monocytes, which showed a constitutive expression of about 10,000 binding sites. Treatment of monocytes for 18 h with γ-IFN increased the number of IgG1 binding sites about threefold, with an affinity of about 16 nM, comparable to that of γ-IFN-treated neutrophils.

These observations established that the neutrophil expression of the high-affinity receptor for the Fc portion of IgG—now referred to as FcγRI (see Ref. 12 for a review)—is strictly dependent on γ-IFN treatment.

The same (13) and other (14–17) investigators extended the studies on this topic by investigating the binding of the monomeric mouse monoclonal antibody (Mab) B137.17 (13) and of Mabs directed against FcγRI. Mabs used for this purpose were those designated 32.2 (14–16), 10.1 (17), and 44.1 (16).

B137.17 was shown to bind to a highly variable proportion (10–40%) of freshly isolated neutrophils although at a very low density (13). Less than 5% or an undetectable number of freshly isolated neutrophils were bound by 32.2 (14) or 10.1 (17), respectively. Some discrepancy exists about the effect of cultivation on the expression of FcγRI by neutrophils. Maintenance of neutrophils for 18–24 h in serum-containing medium caused a decrease of B137.17 (13) and 32.2 binding (14). In similar culture conditions, the proportion of neutrophils which bound Mab 10.1 increased to a highly variable but, in a few cases, very high extent (5–70%) after 12 h of cultivation (17).

Despite these discrepancies in the effect of cultivation on the constitutive expression of FcγRI, all the studies mentioned above demonstrated that cultivation of neutrophils in the presence of γ-IFN clearly enhances the expression of FcγRI. After 18 h of cultivation with γ-IFN, the proportion of neutrophils expressing FcγRI approximated, on average, 70% and 85% as revealed by binding of Mabs B137.17 (13) and 32.2 (14), respectively. The proportion of neutrophils of 13 different donors which, after cultivation in the presence of γ-IFN for 12 h, were bound by the anti-FcγRI Mab 10.1 was more variable but consistently higher than that of control neutrophils (17). All these investigations reported that γ-IFN treatment enhances not only the proportion of FcγRI-positive neutrophils but also the level of FcγRI expression.

Quantitative binding studies with the anti-FcγRI Mab 32.2 confirmed the results obtained with IgG1 binding (see above), showing that γ-IFN treated neutrophils express about 17,000 receptor molecules per cell while there are about 1,300 in control neutrophils (15).

The enhancement of FcγRI expression by γ-IFN requires that neutrophils are cultivated with the cytokine for several hours. Incubation of neutrophils with γ-IFN for 1 h does not enhance FcγRI expression (17). This can be observed, however, after 12 h of incubation and increases up to 48 h (15), that is, at the limit of the neutrophils' lifespan in culture. As detailed in the following sections, the modulation of other neutrophil functions by γ-IFN, i.e., the activation of the capability to generate toxic oxygen molecules, requires only a few hours of incubation. It must be emphasized, however, that the mRNA encoding FcγRI starts to accumulate within 1 h of γ-IFN treatment (see Section II.B), thus indicating that the long times required to detect enhanced expression of FcγRI on the surface are related mainly to the processes of synthesis of the protein and its targeting to the plasma membrane.

In terms of enhanced expression of FcγRI, neutrophils are very sensitive to the action of γ-IFN. Doses of 0.5 U/ml of γ-IFN were shown to have a maximal effect (17). This type of response of neutrophils is also very selective for γ-IFN, since other cytokines known to modulate neutrophil functions, such as granulocyte-macrophage colony-stimulating factor (13,17), granulocyte colony-stimulating factor (17), and tumor necrosis factors α and β (13) do not enhance FcγRI receptor expression.

B. Molecular Basis of Enhanced Expression of FcγRI in Neutrophils Exposed to γ-IFN

Studies have been done on expression of mRNA encoding FcγRI (18,19). These have shown that, while mRNA encoding FcγRI is below the limit of detection in freshly isolated neutrophils and does not increase upon cultivation up to 18 h, γ-IFN induces FcγRI mRNA. The induction of FcγRI mRNA is evident within 1 h of exposure to γ-IFN, plateaus in a few hours, and remains stable up to 18 h of incubation; as shown with expression of the FcγRI protein (see Ref. 19), induction of the message can be observed with very low doses (1 U/ml) of γ-IFN.

These observations establish that enhanced expression of FcγRI at the neutrophil surface caused by γ-IFN is due to an increase of the mRNA encoding the protein and contributes to the notion that in neutrophils γ-IFN is also able to increase steady-state levels of mRNA (see Section VI).

C. Effect of γ-IFN on the Expression of FcγRII, FcγRIII and Other Plasma Membrane Molecules

Although expression of FcγRI on the neutrophil surface appears to be strictly dependent on exposure to γ-IFN, neutrophils constitutively express the other two types of receptors for IgG designated FcγRII and FcγRIII (12).

Studies performed in different laboratories showed that γ-IFN does not change expression of FcγRII (14,17). Some effect has been reported, however, on expression of FcγRIII.

Early studies (13,15) showed that at doses of 200–300 U/ml, γ-IFN causes a slight enhancement (20–30%) of binding of 3G8, a Mab directed to FcγRIII. A more recent study performed on neutrophils of 22 different donors showed that γ-IFN can increase, decrease, or have no effect on FcγRIIII expression (17). These different effects were shown to depend on the constitutive level of FcγRIII expression by the neutrophil population studied which, although more than 90% of neutrophils were positive for 3G8 binding, was highly variable. Excluding five samples in which the expression of FcγRIII was particularly high and decreased after treatment with γ-IFN, γ-IFN had a clear effect on the level of FcγRIII expression, causing an average increase of about threefold.

The modulation of FcγRIII expression by γ-IFN described by Buckle and Hogg (17) differs from that of FcγRI in some aspects: (a) It is not γ-IFN-specific in the sense that GM-CSF and G-CSF also affect FcγRIII expression, causing the same pattern of modulation (increase, decrease, no change) in dependence on the levels of constitutive expression by the neutrophil population studied; and (b) it requires much higher doses of γ-IFN (100–1000 U/ml). Analogously to FcγRI, expression of FcγRIII is also enhanced after 12 h of incubation with γ-IFN.

The mechanism(s) of enhanced expression of FcγRIII in response to γ-IFN have not yet been investigated. Preliminary studies indicate that neutrophils express high levels of FcγRIII mRNA and that γ-IFN does not enhance its steady-state level (M. A. Cassatella, R. M. Flynn, and G. Trinchieri, unpublished observation). Since evidence has been presented that FcγRIII is shed from the plasma membrane during cultivation of neutrophils (20), it would be worth testing whether γ-IFN and GM- and G-CSF decrease shedding.

Some effect of γ-IFN has also been reported on expression of members of the leukocyte integrins. A 20–40% enhancement of binding of the anti-CR3 (CD11b/CD18) Mab OKM1 to γ-IFN-treated neutrophils has been observed (13,15). Measurement of the expression of the common beta chain (CD18) of the three integrins present on the neutrophil surface (LFA-1, CR3, gp150/95) gave indications of a more consistent increase of expression which, in nine independent experiments, averaged 60% (17). It is of interest that γ-IFN was shown to increase steady-state levels of beta-chain mRNA in EBV-transformed B-cells derived from both normal subjects and a patient affected by leukocyte adhesion deficiency (LAD) (21).

III. ENHANCEMENT OF THE NEUTROPHIL CAPABILITY TO KILL EUKARYOTIC CELLS BY γ-IFN

The identification of γ-IFN as a cytokine able to enhance expression of FcγRI in neutrophils was soon followed by the observation that γ-IFN enhances neutrophil antibody-dependent cell-mediated cytotoxicity (ADCC) to different target cells.

Incubation of neutrophils in serum-containing medium with 100 U/ml γ-IFN for 1 h followed by co-cultivation for 4 h with antibody-coated chicken erythrocytes was shown to cause a consistent enhancement of target lysis (22). This observation was confirmed by subsequent investigations done by using the same target (14,23,24) or the P815y tumor cell line (13) and with both human (13,14,22,23) and bovine (24) neutrophils.

Although the production of heteroantibodies consisting of Fab of an anti-FcγRI Mab (32.2) linked to Fab anti-target Ab proved that FcγRI can mediate cytotoxicity (14), several observations substantiate the notion that the enhancement of neutrophil ADCC by γ-IFN is not due simply to the enhancement of FcγRI expression. A significant enhancement of ADCC was observed after 5 h (22), 6 h (23), and 7 h (24) of exposure of neutrophils to γ-IFN, while enhancement of FcγRI expression can be appreciated after 12 h of treatment and increases markedly after longer times (15). When, after incubation with γ-IFN, neutrophils were sorted in populations expressing FcγRI at high or low density, no correlation was found between expression of FcγRI and ADCC (13). Finally, γ-IFN was shown to enhance antibody-independent cytotoxicity (24).

Contrary to the expression of FcγRI, which shows an absolute selectivity of response to γ-IFN (see Section II), neutrophil ADCC is also enhanced by other cytokines such as GM-CSF, TNF_{α}, and TNF_{β} (13, and this volume). However, while the enhancement of ADCC is maximal after 3 h of incubation with GM-CSF, TNF_{α}, and TNF_{β} and declines after 18 h, the potentiation of ADCC by γ-IFN is evident after 18 h (13). Together with the evidence that these cytokines act in synergism with γ-IFN in enhancing ADCC (13, see Section VI) these observations suggest that the mechanism of activation of neutrophil ADCC by γ-IFN is unique.

The available data indicate that γ-IFN, GM-CSF, and TNF are all able to enhance the neutrophil capability to release cytotoxic molecules. The potentiation induced by γ-IFN is prolonged, and we will discuss in Section IV that this has been established at least for the activation of the capability to produce toxic oxygen molecules. The state of "prolonged activation" induced by γ-IFN eventually synergizes with the enhanced expression of FcγRI, which, as discussed above, requires relatively long times to be optimal.

IV. MODULATION OF NEUTROPHIL OXYGEN METABOLISM BY γ-IFN

A. Identification of γ-IFN as a Cytokine Able to Enhance the Generation of Toxic Oxygen Molecules by Neutrophils in Response to Different Stimuli

As discussed in the previous section, studies on cell cytotoxicity indicate that the enhanced capability of neutrophils to kill eukaryotic cells after exposure to γ-IFN may well be dependent on an enhanced production of cytotoxic molecules. One of the mechanisms responsible for the role played by phagocytes as effector cells of cytotoxic reactions is the activation of a multicomponent system, universally referred to as NADPH oxidase, which catalizes the monovalent transfer of electrons from NADPH to oxygen with formation of superoxide anion (O_2^-), hydrogen peroxide (H_2O_2), and hydroxyl radical ($OH\cdot$) (reviewed in Ref. 25).

The results of studies performed in our laboratory were the first to demonstrate that γ-IFN is able to modulate the generation of toxic oxygen molecules by neutrophils (26). We demonstrated that incubation of neutrophils in serum-containing medium with γ-IFN for a few hours causes a doubling of their capability to generate O_2^- in response to formyl-methionyl-leucyl-phenylalanine (fMLP) and concanavalin A (Con A), and a 50% enhancement of the response to low, submaximal stimulatory doses of phorbol myristate acetate (PMA). Similar results were obtained by measuring the total, cyanide-insensitive oxygen consumption.

These results were confirmed by studies on the PMA-stimulated chemiluminescence (13) or H_2O_2 generation (27), the fMLP-stimulated oxygen consumption (28), chemiluminescence (29) and O_2^- generation (30), and the chemiluminescence generated during phagocytosis of *Staphilococcus aureus* (29). We also extended our previous studies to show that γ-IFN treatment enhances the neutrophil capability to generate H_2O_2 in response to fMLP, Con A, immune complexes, and PMA (31).

These in-vitro studies were substantiated by investigations on neutrophils isolated both from children affected by chronic granulomatous disease (CGD) or mice after in-vivo treatment with γ-IFN. Neutrophils isolated from the peritoneal cavity of mice, injected i.m. with γ-IFN 5 h before cell harvesting, were shown to generate 10-fold more O_2^- in response to PMA than neutrophils from control animals (32). As we will discuss in detail in Section IV.C, γ-IFN treatment caused a partial correction of the defect of NADPH oxidase activity which characterizes CGD neutrophils (33,34).

In-vitro studies defined several aspects of the modulation of neutrophil oxygen metabolism by γ-IFN. The effect of γ-IFN was observed after 1 to 4 h of incubation (26–28) and lasted up to 18–24 h (13,31). For example, we showed that the enhancement of H_2O_2 generation in response to Con A required times of incubation longer than 30 min and was optimal after 90–240 min (31). γ-IFN acts at relatively low doses, and we calculated a half-maximal effect at 2 U/ml (31), a concentration close to that effective on the induction of FcγRI expression (see Section II.A).

As shown in Figure 1, another important aspect of modulation of neutrophil oxygen metabolism by γ-IFN is its dependence on de-novo RNA and protein synthesis. This same dependence was demonstrated in studies of modulation of ADCC in human (13) and of antibody-independent cytotoxicity and random migration in bovine neutrophils (35).

The general significance of these observations will be discussed in Section VI. In relation to the modulation of oxygen metabolism, the data described in the next section suggest, however, that RNA and protein synthesis are required to enhance the expression of at least one of the components of NADPH oxidase.

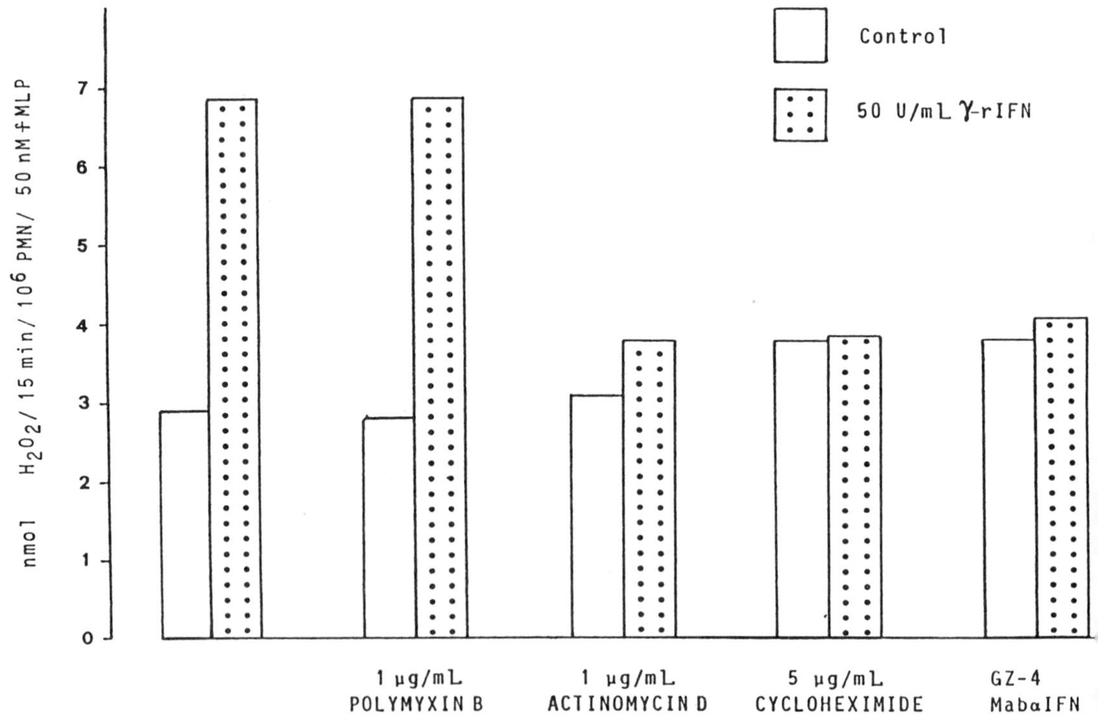

Figure 1 Effect of different inhibitors on the capability of γ-IFN to enhance the H_2O_2 production by neutrophils in response to fMLP. The indicated inhibitors were added together with 50 U/mL of γ-IFN at the beginning of the incubation period. Neutrophils were incubated in serum-containing medium for 4 h before the assay (see Ref. 31). Reproduced from Immunology 1988; 63:499–506 with the permission of Blackwell Scientific Publication Limited.

B. Molecular Basis of Modulation of Neutrophil Oxygen Metabolism by γ-IFN

Activation of NADPH oxidase is thought to depend on three distinct steps (see Ref. 25 and Chapter 2, this volume, for a review): (a) binding of an appropriate stimulus to specific cell surface receptors; (b) generation of second messengers acting intracellularly; (c) the actual shift of the NADPH oxidase from a dormant to an activated state, which catalyzes the transfer of electrons from NADPH to oxygen and which can possibly be conceived as the assembly of discrete components.

Theoretically, the capability of γ-IFN to enhance neutrophil oxygen metabolism could depend on actions exerted at the level of any of these three steps.

Both indirect and direct evidence indicate that enhanced expression of receptors for agonists of NADPH oxidase activation does not play a major role in modulation of neutrophil oxygen metabolism by γ-IFN. In fact, γ-IFN-treated neutrophils generate higher amounts of toxic oxygen molecules in response to different, unrelated stimuli, including PMA, which acts through a receptor-independent, direct activation of protein kinase C. We have shown that the higher Con A-stimulated oxygen consumption by γ-IFN-treated neutrophils is not accompanied by an enhanced binding of the lectin to the cell surface (31).

The possible influence of γ-IFN on the transmembrane signaling which ensues from ligand-receptors interaction has not been thoroughly investigated. We performed studies on the basal and stimulated levels of cytoplasmic free calcium and the formation of inositol phosphates in γ-IFN-treated neutrophils in response to different stimuli (31). The basal levels of cytosolic calcium after cultivation of neutrophils for 4 h in serum-containing medium were about 90 nM and did not change if γ-IFN was included in the incubation medium. Stimulation of neutrophils with fMLP or Con A caused an elevation of cytosolic calcium which was comparable in control and γ-IFN-treated cells. Formation of inositol phosphates in response to Con A was also unaffected by treatment with γ-IFN. These results exclude the possibility that γ-IFN modulates phosphoinositides turnover, altering, for example, the activity of phosphatidylinositol-specific phospholipase C. However, they do not discourage further investigations on a possible effect of γ-IFN on the generation of other putative messengers derived, for example, by the hydrolysis of other membrane phospholipids such as phosphatidylcholine. It has been in fact appreciated in the last few years that activation of NADPH oxidase in neutrophils does not necessarily involve turnover of phosphoinositides (see Ref. 36 and the literature quoted therein). Recently, interest has been focused on a possible role of phosphatidic acid (37) and diacylglycerol (38) generated by phospholipases D or C acting on phosphatidylcholine, although there is no direct proof that these messengers are involved in NADPH oxidase activation. Nonetheless, these recent findings justify the investigation of the possible effect of γ-IFN on neutrophil phospholipid metabolism and turnover.

As anticipated at the end of Section VI.A, there are grounds to conclude that one of the mechanisms by which γ-IFN modulates the capability of neutrophils to metabolize oxygen can be the enhanced expression of one of the NADPH oxidase components.

NADPH oxidase activity has been recognized as depending on different polypeptides, some of which have been definitively identified. The first component of NADPH oxidase whose biochemical and molecular nature has been characterized is a phagocyte-specific, low-potential cytochrome b, also referred to as cytochrome b_{558} or cytochrome b_{-245} according to its spectroscopic or potentiometric properties, respectively (reviewed in Ref. 39). Cytochrome b_{-245} is composed of a high-molecular-weight subunit, which in its glycosylated natural form has a molecular weight of 91 kDa, and of a low-molecular-weight, nonglycosylated subunit of 22 kDa. The high-molecular-weight subunit is also referred to as X-CGD protein, owing to the recognition that its mRNA is missing in patients affected by the X-linked form of chronic granulomatous disease (39). cDNAs encoding both subunits have been cloned (39).

Other proteins certainly involved in the NADPH oxidase activity are at least two cytosolic components, referred to as p47phox and p67 (40). The cDNAs encoding these proteins have been cloned (41–43). There is a general consensus that a flavoprotein which has not yet been identified also participates in NADPH oxidase activity (reviewed in Ref. 44).

Newburger et al. (45) were the first to show that exposure of neutrophils to γ-IFN causes an enhancement of the steady-state levels of mRNA encoding the high-molecular-weight subunit of cytochrome b_{-245}, the X-CGD protein. Treatment of neutrophils for 90 min with γ-IFN increased X-CGD mRNA about threefold (45). Studies performed in our laboratory showed that the increase of steady-state levels of X-CGD mRNA is accompanied by an increase of the relative protein (46). This was evident after times of treatment with γ-IFN at which an enhancement of the neutrophil capability to metabolize oxygen was observed. As we will discuss in Section IV.C, previous studies by Ezekowitz et al. (33) and Sechler et al. (34) on CGD neutrophils demonstrated an enhancing effect of γ-IFN on the X-CGD protein. Furthermore, induction of differentiation of myelomonocytic leukemic cell lines with γ-IFN and TNF_{α} established a link between the acquisition of the NADPH oxidase activity and expression of the X-CGD mRNA (47).

No evidence of a significant enhancement of the light-chain mRNA expression in γ-IFN-treated neutrophils has been obtained (45,46). Studies on a possible effect of γ-IFN on the expression of the p47phox mRNA, one of the two well-characterized cytosolic NADPH oxidase components, showed that γ-IFN decreases p47 mRNA in neutrophils (46) after times of incubation at which X-CGD mRNA is enhanced.

Figure 2 summarizes the data obtained in studies on the effect of γ-IFN on neutrophil expression of mRNAs encoding the high- and low-molecular-weight subunits of cytochrome b_{-245}, and the p47phox (46).

There is no study on the effect of γ-IFN on the expression of a 45-kDa protein which has been proposed as the FAD-binding component of NADPH oxidase and can be probed by diphenylene iodonium binding (48). However, induction of U937 differentiation with γ-IFN is accompanied by up-regulation of this protein (49).

The data so far obtained indicate that expression of the X-CGD protein could be the limiting factor for enhancing NADPH oxidase activity and that the capability of γ-IFN to modulate neutrophil oxygen metabolism depends on the enhancement of X-CGD mRNA and protein expression.

Why an enhanced expression of the X-CGD protein following γ-IFN treatment causes a potentiation of the NADPH oxidase is not clear. In fact, the function of the X-CGD protein is known only in part. Although lack of expression of the X-CGD mRNA and protein causes the total absence of the typical cytochrome b spectrum and the deficit of NADPH oxidase activity which characterizes the classic X-linked form of CGD, evidence has been presented that the actual heme-binding subunit of cytochrome b_{-245} is the 22-kDa light chain (50).

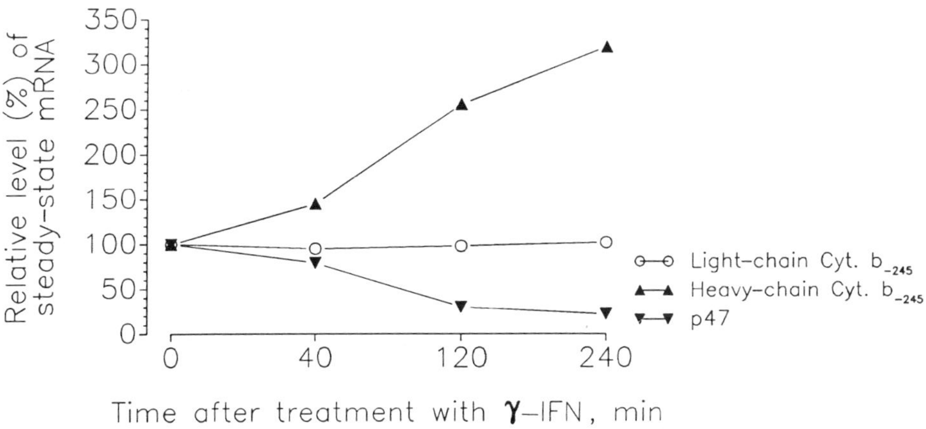

Figure 2 Neutrophils were cultivated in serum-containing medium in the presence of 100 U/mL of γ-IFN for the indicated times. RNA was recovered from γ-IFN-treated neutrophils and from control neutrophils cultivated for 2 h. Autoradiograms were scanned densitometrically and the values normalized on the basis of phosphoglycerate kinase mRNA expression.

It has not been possible to establish a linear correlation between the cell content of cytochrome b_{-245}, the expression of the X-CGD protein, and the capability of phagocytes to produce toxic oxygen molecules. We showed that γ-IFN treatment does not increase the apparent amount of the spectrophotometrically determinable cytochrome b_{-245} in neutrophils (31). In-vitro studies on neutrophils of CGD patients showed that the partial correction of their capability to generate O_2^- by γ-IFN occurs in the complete absence of any spectrophotometric detectability of cytochrome b (51). However, later investigations demonstrated that in-vivo treatment of some CGD patients with γ-IFN enhances neutrophil content of cytochrome b_{-245} (33). Indications that generation of toxic oxygen molecules does not depend linearly on the content of cytochrome b_{-245} also derived from the evidence that in-vivo activation of mouse macrophages, by means which presumably involve release of cytokines by T-lymphocytes, is not accompanied by an enhancement of cytochrome b_{-245} (52).

The available data do not allow us to draw any conclusion about the role of the X-CGD protein except to suggest that this protein might play a role in regulating the assembly of cytochrome b_{-245} subunits (53) and possibly of other NADPH oxidase components. Useful indications could derive from the extension of studies which indicate that the X-CGD protein may bind cytosolic components of NADPH oxidase (54).

Another intriguing aspect of modulation of NADPH oxidase activity by γ-IFN concerns the differences observed in studies performed with macrophages and neutrophils. We showed that the NADPH oxidase assayed in detergent lysates of human monocyte-derived macrophages treated for 48 h with γ-IFN displays a higher affinity for NADPH, evident as a decrease of about 10-fold of the apparent K_m measured in untreated macrophage cultures (55). However, we could not observe any alteration of the K_m of NADPH oxidase of γ-IFN-treated neutrophils (31). Ezekowitz et al. also reported that the partial correction of the O_2^--generating capacity of CGD neutrophils upon treatment in vitro with γ-IFN is not accompanied by alterations of K_m of the oxidase (51).

One way to interpret the different effects of γ-IFN on neutrophil and macrophage NADPH oxidase is to assume that in neutrophils all the NADPH oxidase components are fully expressed and some of these are implicated in the regulation of the oxidase activity for its substrate. On the contrary, differentiation of monocytes to macrophages could be accompanied by down-modulation of the expression of some NADPH oxidase components, and their reinduction by γ-IFN also cause an increase of the oxidase affinity for NADPH. Some support for this hypothesis derives from our observation that, in monocyte-derived macrophages treated with γ-IFN, the K_m of NADPH oxidase is about 30 μM, a value comparable to that of about 20 μM characterizing the NADPH oxidase of monocytes cultivated for 1 day (55). Concordant with this interpretation is the observation that, in monocytes cultured for 3 days, whose NADPH oxidase displays a K_m of about 30 μM, γ-IFN does not cause any alteration of the K_m (56).

C. γ-IFN Enhances the Capability of Neutrophils of CGD Patients to Metabolize Oxygen

An outstanding contribution to the establishment of the notion that γ-IFN is able to modulate neutrophil functions derived from studies on CGD patients (Table 1).

Starting from its description in 1959 (57), a great deal has been learned about the molecular basis of CGD, which is recognized as a defect of activation by different stimuli of the NADPH oxidase of phagocytes. CGD is a heterogeneous disorder, and both X-linked and autosomal recessive patterns of inheritance have been described (reviewed in Ref. 58). In most of the X-linked cases, a defective expression of cytochrome b_{-245} has been documented. Autosomal recessive cases are mainly cytochrome b_{-245} positive but lack cytosolic components involved in NADPH oxidase activity.

Ezekowitz, Orkin, and Newburger were the first to show that in-vitro treatment of neutrophils of some CGD patients with γ-IFN enhances their capability to produce toxic oxygen molecules (51). Neutrophils which responded to in-vitro treatment with γ-IFN were those obtained from patients affected by the "variant" form of X-linked CGD. Neutrophils of these patients contain trace amounts of cytochrome b_{-245} (33), produce very low amounts of toxic oxygen molecules, and show an altered NADPH

Table 1 Effect of γ-IFN on X-CGD Neutrophils[a]

	In-vitro effects	In-vivo effects
Enhancement of O_2^- generation in response to phorbol myristate acetate	Positive effects with X-linked "variants" (51); no effect with "classic" X-linked forms (51)	Positive effects on patients with X-linked "classic" and "variant" forms (33) and autosomal recessive forms (34)
Enhancement of the expression of NADPH oxidase components	ND	Enhanced expression of the X-CGD protein (33,34)

[a] References are indicated in parentheses. ND, not determined. A clear in-vitro effect of γ-IFN on O_2^- generation by monocytes of patients affected by different forms of CGD has been reported (34).

oxidase kinetic, which consists of an elevated K_m. Incubation of neutrophils of three out of four of these patients with γ-IFN caused more than a doubling of their capability to produce O_2^- in response to PMA. However, neutrophils of patients affected by the "classic" form of CGD or by the autosomal recessive one did not respond to γ-IFN. Subsequent studies by Sechler et al. on a larger number of patients showed that monocytes of patients affected by all the forms of CGD can acquire the capability to produce greater amounts of O_2^- after 3 days of treatment with γ-IFN, although the enhancement induced by γ-IFN in monocytes of different patients was highly variable and only monocytes of four out of 13 patients affected by the X-linked form responded to γ-IFN (34).

The capability of γ-IFN to augment the oxygen metabolism of CGD neutrophils was further established by in-vivo studies. Subcutaneous injection of 0.1 mg of γ-IFN/m^2 on two consecutive (33) or of 0.1 mg/m^2 on five consecutive (34) days was shown to ameliorate the neutrophil defect to produce O_2^- of three "variant" and one "classic" CGD patients (33) and one autosomal recessive patient (34). The amelioration of the neutrophil defect was observed after a few days from the injection of γ-IFN and lasted for a few weeks. These in-vivo studies also demonstrated that the capability of neutrophils to kill *Staphylococcus aureus* increased in parallel with their capability to metabolize oxygen.

As anticipated in the previous section, studies on CGD neutrophils indicate that an enhanced expression of the high-molecular-weight subunit of cytochrome b_{-245}, the X-CGD protein, may underlie the amelioration of the capability of CGD neutrophils to metabolize oxygen by γ-IFN. Western blot analysis showed that after in-vivo administration of γ-IFN, the X-CGD protein increases in neutrophils of patients with both the X-linked variant (33) and the autosomal recessive (34) form of CGD. It is not known if this increase of the X-CGD protein in CGD neutrophils after treatment with γ-IFN is also accompanied by an enhanced expression of the X-CGD mRNA, although this was shown to occur in CGD monocytes after in-vitro (51) and in-vivo (33) administration of γ-IFN. In neutrophils of a cytochrome b-negative CGD patient, the possible relation between the γ-IFN dependent enhancement of the X-CGD protein and the capability to metabolize oxygen is understandable in the light of results of in-vivo studies which showed that γ-IFN treatment increase the cell content of cytochrome b_{-245} (33). More difficult is to establish a causal relation between the amelioration of the defect of neutrophils of an autosomal recessive cytochrome b-positive patient and the enhanced expression of the X-CGD protein after γ-IFN treatment (34). It may be that γ-IFN also enhances the expression of cytosolic component(s) of the NADPH oxidase which are lacking in this form of the disease. Alternatively, as discussed in Section IV.B, an enhancement of the X-CGD protein could favor the proper assembly of different components, albeit these are expressed at a low level.

V. MODULATION OF NEUTROPHIL MICROBICIDAL ACTIVITY BY γ-IFN

Detailed investigations performed over the last 7 years established the notion that γ-IFN is the major endogenous "macrophage-activating factor," on the basis of the evidence that this cytokine induces alterations of macrophage functions which had been previously recognized to accompany the acquirement of cell-mediated immunity (reviewed in Refs. 59–61). To be considered "activated," macrophages must have the capacity to kill eukaryotic targets, to generate high amounts of O_2^- and H_2O_2, and to kill facultative intracellular parasites.

As discussed in the previous sections, γ-IFN enhances both cytotoxic activity and oxygen metabolism in neutrophils. Several studies demonstrated that this cytokine also augments the capability of neutrophils to kill bacteria, fungi, and protozoa. These observations add further ground to the conclusion that γ-IFN is also a "neutrophil-activating factor."

An enhancement of neutrophil microbicidal activity by γ-IFN has been demonstrated with *Candida albicans* (13,62), *Blastomyces dermatitidis* (63), *Staphylococcus aureus* (29), *Legionella pneumophila* (64), and *Entamoeba histolytica* (65). With the exception of *Staph. aureus,* whose rate of killing is enhanced after only 10 min of neutrophil preincubation with γ-IFN (29), the enhancement of microbicidal activity requires a few hours of preincubation followed by co-cultivation of the cells with the parasite in the presence of γ-IFN for different times.

The enhancement of neutrophil microbicidal activity by γ-IFN has been also demonstrated with in-vivo studies. Neutrophils isolated from mice injected i.m. with γ-IFN kill *Blastomyces dermatitidis* more efficiently (63). Treatment of CGD patients with γ-IFN ameliorates their capability to kill *Staph. aureus* (33,34).

Evidence has been obtained that the enhanced killing ability of neutrophils treated with γ-IFN is due, at least in part, to an enhanced generation of toxic oxygen molecules. Phagocytosis of *Staph. aureus* stimulates a higher chemiluminescence in γ-IFN-treated neutrophils (29). The ability of γ-IFN-treated neutrophils to kill *Blastomyces dermatitidis* is inhibited by superoxide dismutase and catalase (63) and that to kill *Entamoeba histolytica* by catalase (65).

It is likely, however, that besides the enhanced generation of toxic oxygen molecules, other mechanisms are responsible for the enhancement of neutrophil microbicidal activity by γ-IFN. In fact, in-vivo studies with some CGD patients have shown that, after γ-IFN treatment, the amelioration of the neutrophil microbicidal activity is more substantial than the enhancement of O_2^- production. In one "variant" and one "classic" CGD patient, treatment with γ-IFN augmented the neutrophil killing of *Staph. aureus* up to 40% of that of normal neutrophils, while the capability to generate of O_2^- was below 20% of control (33). Furthermore, in two patients with autosomally inherited, cytochrome b_{-245}-positive CGD, a substantial enhancement of *Staph. aureus* killing by neutrophils was observed in the absence of any increase in the cell capability to produce O_2^- (34).

The oxygen-independent mechanisms of killing possibly enhanced by γ-IFN have not been identified. Although there is no evidence that γ-IFN affects lysosome-phagosome fusion, it has been shown that γ-IFN does enhance secretion of granule constituents. A dose-dependent enhancement of both the basal and the opsonized zymosan-stimulated lysozyme release has been reported to occur in neutrophils after 1 h of incubation with γ-IFN (27). We also reported that, after incubation with γ-IFN for 4 h, neutrophils secrete two- to threefold more vitamin B_{12}-binding protein in response to PMA, Con A, and fMLP (31). The issue of the potentiation of oxygen-independent mechanisms of killing by γ-IFN deserves to be investigated further in the light of the observation that this cytokine has been shown to enhance the microbicidal or microbistatic activity of endothelial, epithelial, and parenchymal cells which do not metabolize oxygen with production of toxic molecules (reviewed in Refs. 7 and 8).

VI. NEUTROPHIL-γ-IFN INTERACTION: RECEPTORS, SIGNALS, AND MECHANISMS OF ACTION

Receptors for γ-IFN on human neutrophils have been recently characterized by studies with ^{125}I-labeled recombinant γ-IFN (66). Scatchard analysis of γ-IFN binding at 4°C revealed only one class of high-affinity receptors with a K_a of about 6.0×10^{-11} M and in number about 1100 per cell. At 4°C, the binding of γ-IFN was maximal after 30 min and reached saturation with doses of 300–500 U of γ-IFN/mL; half-maximal binding was observed at 50 U of γ-IFN/mL. With saturating concentrations of γ-IFN, the rate of binding at 37°C was faster and saturation was observed within 6 min. Studies performed at 37°C indicated that about 50% of bound γ-IFN is internalized within 30 min and that the ligand is in part degraded. As expected from studies on other cells, α- and β-interferons did not compete for binding of γ-IFN.

Interestingly, it was observed that incubation of neutrophils in Krebs-Ringer's phosphate buffer at 37°C causes a loss of 80% of binding sites for γ-IFN, and this was in part prevented by IL-1. This observation prompts studies to define factors possibly involved in expression and turnover of γ-IFN receptors. For example, we observed that the potentiation of the neutrophil capability to generate toxic oxygen molecules by γ-IFN is optimal when serum is included in the incubation medium (26), and it could be that some serum components affects γ-IFN receptor expression. Furthermore, the described effect of IL-1 encourages studies on a possible synergism of the two cytokines in modulating neutrophil function. To our knowledge there is no study of a possible synergistic effect of γ-IFN and IL-1 on neutrophils. In fact, as we will discuss in Section VII, the ability of γ-IFN to act in synergism with other cytokines has been investigated, almost exclusively, in relation to tumor necrosis factors. Since the study of Hansen and Finbloom (66) showed that TNF does not prevent the loss of γ-IFN binding sites which occurs during maintenance of neutrophils at 37°C, it can be anticipated that the capability of TNF to synergize with γ-IFN in modulating neutrophil functions does not likely depend on an action at the receptor level.

Whether interaction of γ-IFN with specific receptors on the neutrophil surface is accompanied by generation of secondary messengers acting intracellularly is absolutely unknown. This lack of knowledge reflects the paucity of data on the mechanisms of transmembrane signals involved in cytokine, and especially γ-IFN, actions. In fact, the only direct evidence that γ-IFN receptors trigger the generation of secondary messengers was obtained with human diploid fibroblasts which were shown to generate diaclyglycerol and inositol tris-phosphate in response to γ-IFN (67). Studies with macrophages also provided indications, albeit indirect, that elevation of cytoplasmic free calcium and activation of protein kinase C might be involved in modulation of cell functions by γ-IFN (reviewed in Ref. 68).

Whatever are the early events following γ-IFN-receptor interaction, there is ground to conclude that the main mechanism responsible for the modulation of neutrophil functions by this cytokine is an enhanced transcription of different genes and/or an enhanced synthesis of proteins involved in selective functions.

Indirect evidence supporting this conclusion has derived from studies with inhibitors of RNA and protein synthesis. In fact, these were shown to prevent the modulation by γ-IFN of the neutrophil capability to generate toxic oxygen molecules and to secrete vitamin B_{12}-binding protein (26,31), to undergo random migration (35), and to exert both antibody-dependent (13) and -independent (35) cytotoxicity.

As discussed in Sections II and IV, direct evidence that γ-IFN enhances mRNA steady-state levels was obtained with the FcγRI and the X-CGD protein transcripts. The observation that cycloheximide does not induce these mRNAs in neutrophils (Cassatella, unpublished observation) does indeed suggest that this might be due to a true enhancement of gene transcription.

De-novo protein synthesis in γ-IFN-treated neutrophils has been investigated by different means. As detailed in Sections II and IV, antibodies have been used to detect enhanced expression of known polypeptides, indicating that γ-IFN treatment causes an enhanced synthesis of FCγRI, FcγRIII, CD18, and the X-CGD protein. Other proteins whose synthesis is enhanced by γ-IFN have been identified by ^{35}S-methionine labeling of neutrophils followed by electrophoresis and autoradiographic analysis of total cell extracts or of immunoprecipitates done with antibodies against previously recognized proteins.

When human neutrophils were incubated for 1 h in medium supplemented with ^{35}S-methionine with or without γ-IFN, the cytokine was shown to increase incorporation of label into trichloroacetic acid-precipitable material (30,69). Two-dimensional polyacrylamide gel electrophoresis analysis of labeled proteins showed that, although it was impossible to identify polypeptides whose expression was detectable only in γ-IFN-treated neutrophils, γ-IFN caused an increase of several proteins. ^{35}S-methionine-labeled proteins of apparent molecular weight of 45, 34, 25, and 14 kDa increased 2.7-, 5.5-, 20.2-, and 2.1-fold, respectively, when neutrophils were incubated in the presence of γ-IFN (69). Studies done using the same approach with bovine neutrophils reported a consistent increase in the synthesis of a 60- and 94- to 95-kDa protein (35). At present, the nature of these proteins is unknown. Steinbeck and colleagues speculated that the 94- to 95-kDa polypeptide, whose synthesis is enhanced by γ-IFN, might be the β-chain of the leukocyte integrins (35). It would be of interest to obtain a direct proof of that. In fact, as discussed in Section II.C, the β-chain of leukocyte integrins is up-modulated by γ-IFN treatment. Furthermore, normal neutrophils have been shown to express the β-chain transcript constitutively but to be unable to synthesize the protein (70). These observations indicate that γ-IFN might increase protein synthesis acting at post-transcriptional levels.

An interesting approach to identifying polypeptides whose synthesis is enhanced by γ-IFN in neutrophils has been recently exploited by Rubin and colleagues (71). These investigators made use of antibodies previously raised against proteins whose synthesis is increased in interferon-treated fibroblasts (72–74). Neutrophils were incubated with ^{35}S-methionine in either the presence or the absence of α-IFN or γ-IFN and cell extracts immunoprecipitated with different antibodies. This approach demonstrated that, in neutrophils, α-IFN enhances the synthesis of a 67-kDa protein and induces de-novo synthesis of a 56-kDa protein. γ-IFN had the same effect on the 67-kDa protein and a much greater effect on the 56-kDa one. Moreover, γ-IFN induced selectively the de-novo synthesis of a 42-kDa protein. The evidence that actinomycin D prevented the effect of both types of interferons on the synthesis of these polypeptides indicates that RNA synthesis was necessary for their action.

The immunoprecipitated 42-kDa protein has been clearly identified as indoleamine 2,3-dioxygenase (74), thus further supporting a possible role of γ-IFN-activated neutrophils in tumor cell destruction. The identities of the γ-IFN-induced 67- and 56-kDa proteins are still unclear. These authors suggested that the 67-kDa protein could be related to a guanylate-binding protein which is induced by γ-IFN in human diploid fibroblasts (75). The cytosolic localization of this protein and its affinity for guanine nucleotides favors the speculation that it could be related to the 67-kDa cytosolic component of NADPH oxidase (see Section IV.B) which has been purified by GTP-agarose affinity chromatography (40). However, the protein described by Cheng et al. (75) showed an exquisite specificity for guanine nucleotides, while the 67-kDa cytosolic NADPH oxidase component appears also to bind adenine nucleotides (40).

Concerning the nature of the 56-kDa protein, Rubin and colleagues proposed that it could be a protein of similar molecular weight identified by Ulker and colleagues as a component of intermediate filaments and which is induced by γ-IFN in amnion U cells and fibroblasts (76,77).

Taken together, these data indicate that the ability of γ-IFN to modulate neutrophil function is definitely due to the induction of the synthesis of different polypeptides whose identity has been clarified only in part. Table 2 summarizes the data available up to now on proteins whose synthesis is modulated by γ-IFN. As discussed above and in previous sections, a correlation has been demonstrated between the enhanced expression of some proteins and an increase in steady-state levels of the specific mRNA. Additional mechanisms acting at the level of protein synthesis cannot be excluded, however.

Table 2 Proteins Whose Expression Is Enhanced or Induced in γ-IFN-Treated Neutrophils[a]

Protein	Method of detection	Function
FcγRI	Antibodies and binding of monomeric IgG (11,13–17)	Binding of monomeric IgG
FcγRIII	Antibodies (13,15,17)	Binding of immune complexes
CR3 (CD11b/CD18)	Antibodies (13,15,17)	Homotypic and heterotypic adhesion
CD18	Antibodies (17) ^{35}S-methionine labeling (?,35)	
X-CGD	Antibodies (33,34,46)	Component of the NADPH oxidase
94–95 kDa	^{35}S-methionine labeling (35)	CD18 (35)
60 kDa	^{35}S-methionine labeling (35)	Precursor of 94–95 (35)
45 kDa 34 kDa 25 kDa 14 kDa	^{35}S-methionine labeling (69)	Unknown
42 kDa	^{35}S-methionine labeling and immunoprecipitation with specific antibodies (71)	Indoleamine 2,3-dioxygenase
56 kDa	^{35}S-methionine labeling and (71) immunoprecipitation with specific antibodies	Component of intermediate filaments (?)
67 kDa	^{35}S-methionine labeling (71) and immunoprecipitation with specific antibodies	Guanylate binding protein (?)

[a] References are indicated in parentheses.

VII. SYNERGISM OF γ-IFN AND OTHER CYTOKINES IN MODULATING NEUTROPHIL FUNCTIONS

Several observations suggest that, in sites of inflammation, other cytokines can synergize with γ-IFN in enhancing neutrophil effector functions.

The first evidence in line with this conclusion derived from studies by Shalaby and colleagues, who showed that the enhancement of neutrophil ADCC induced by low doses of TNF_{β} (0.1–1 U/mL) in combination with 1 U/mL of γ-IFN exceeded the enhancement caused by similar doses of either cytokine alone (23). This observation was extended by studies on the enhancement of neutrophil ADCC caused by GM-CSF, TNF_{α}, and TNF_{β}, where it was shown that the cytokine-induced killing was higher in neutrophils which had been pretreated with γ-IFN (13). A clear synergistic effect of both TNF_{β} and TNF_{α} with γ-IFN was demonstrated in studies of killing of *Candida albicans* and *Entamoeba histolytica,* respectively (62,65). Finally, TNF_{α} and γ-IFN were shown to synergize in enhancing both the chemiluminescence response and phagocytosis of *Staph. aureus* (78). A clear synergistic effect of TNF_{α} and γ-IFN has been demonstrated in inducing myeloid cell lines to express NADPH oxidase activity and NADPH oxidase components (47).

The molecular basis of the capability of TNFs to act in synergism with γ-IFN are presently unknown. Studies on this topic and also on the ability of other cytokines to synergize with γ-IFN in enhancing neutrophil functions would provide important clues to understand how factors present in the inflammatory site drive this cell to a state of activation whose possible relevance began to be appreciated only a few years ago.

ACKNOWLEDGMENTS

The authors wish to thank Filippo Rossi for his contribution to our studies mentioned in this review and for his critical reading of the manuscript. We also acknowledge the financial support of the Italian Association for Cancer Research (A.I.R.C.) for the studies we are currently performing on this topic.

REFERENCES

1. Pestka S, Langer JA, Zoon KC, Samuel CE. Interferons and their actions. Ann Rev Biochem 1987; 56:727–77.
2. Rashidbaigi A, Langer JA, Jung V, Jones C, Morse HG, Tischfield JA, Trill JJ, Kung HF, Petska S. The gene for the human immune interferon receptor is located on chromosome 6. Proc Natl Acad Sci USA 1986; 83:384–8.
3. Pfizenmaier K, Wiegman K, Scheurich P, Kronke M, Merlin G, Aguet M, Knowles BB, Ucer U. High affinity human IFN-γ binding capacity is encoded by a single receptor gene located in proximity to c-ros on human chromsome region 6q16 to 6q22. J Immunol 1988; 141:856–60.
4. Aguet M, Dembic Z, Merlin G. Molecular cloning and expression of the human interferon-γ receptor. Cell 1988; 55:273–80.
5. Schreiber RD. Identification of gamma-interferon as a murine macrophage-activating factor for tumor cytotoxicity. In: Adams DO, Hanna MG, eds. Contemporary topics in immunobiology, vol. 13, Macrophage activation. New York: Plenum Press, 1984:171–98.
6. Trinchieri G, Perussia B. Immune interferon: a pleiotropic lymphokine with multiple effects. Immunol Today 1985; 4:131–6.

7. Murray HW. Interferon-gamma, the activated macrophage, and host defence against microbial challenge. Ann Intern Med 1988; 108:595–608.
8. Nathan C, Yoshida R. Cytokines: interferon-γ. In: Gallin JI, Goldstein M, Snyderman R, eds. Inflammation: basic principles and clinical correlates. New York: Raven Press, 1988:229–51.
9. Dijkmans R, Billiau A. Interferon-γ: a master key in the immune system. Curr Opinion Immunol 1988; 1:269–74.
10. Steinbeck MJ, Roth JA. Neutrophil activation by recombinant cytokines. Rev Infect Dis 1989; 11:549–68.
11. Perussia B, Dayton ET, Lazarus S, Fanning V, Trinchieri G. Immune interferon induces the receptor for monomeric IgGI on human monocytic and myeloid cells. J Exp Med 1983; 158:1092–113.
12. Unkeless JC. Human Fcγ receptors. Curr Opinion Immunol 1989; 2:63–7.
13. Perussia B, Kobayashi M, Rossi ME, Anegon I, Trinchieri G. Immune interferon enhances functional properties of human granulocytes: role of Fc receptors and effect of lymphotoxin, tumor necrosis factor, and granulocyte-macrophage colony-stimulating factor. J Immunol 1987; 138:765–74.
14. Shen L, Guyre PM, Fanger MW. Polimorphonuclear leukocyte function triggered through the high affinity Fc receptor for monomeric IgG[1]. J Immunol 1987; 139:534–8.
15. Petroni KC, Shen L, Guyre PM. Modulation of human polymorphonuclear leukocyte IgG Fc receptors and Fc receptor-mediated functions by IFN-γ and glucocorticoids. J Immunol 1988; 140:3467–72.
16. Ceuppens JL, Baroja ML, Van Vaek F, Anderson CL. Defect in the membrane expression of high affinity 72-KD Fc γ receptors on phagocytic cells in four healthy subjects. J Clin Invest 1988; 82:571–8.
17. Buckle AM, Hogg N. The effect of IFN-γ and colony-stimulating factors on the expression of neutrophil cell membrane receptors. J Immunol 1989; 143:2295–301.
18. Pan L, Mendel DB, Zurlo J, Guyre PM. Regulation of the steady state level of FcγRI mRNA by IFN-γ and dexamethasone in human monocytes, neutrophils, and U-937 cells. J Immunol 1990; 145:267–75.
19. Cassatella MA, Flynn RM, Aste Amezaga M, Bazzoni F, Vicentini F, Trinchieri G. Interferon γ induces in human neutrophils and macrophages expression of the mRNA for the high affinity receptor for monomeric IgG (FcγR-I or CD64). Biochem Biophys Res Commun 1990; 170:582–8.
20. Huizinga TWJ, Van Der Schoot CE, Jost C, Klaassen R, Kleijer M, Von Dem Borne AEG, Roos D, Tetteroo PAT. The PI-linked receptor FcRIII is released on stimulation of neutrophils. Nature 1988; 333:667–8.
21. Dimanche-Boitrel MT, Le Deist F, Quillet A, Fischer A, Griscelli C, Lisowska-Grospierre BL. Effects of interferon-γ (IFN-γ) and tumor necrosis factor-α (TNF-α) on the expression of LFA-1 in the moderate phenotype of leukocyte adhesion deficiency (LAD). J Clin Immunol 1989; 9:200–7.
22. Basham TY, Smith WK, Mcrigan TC. Interferon enhances antibody-dependent cellular cytotoxicity when suboptimal concentrations of antibody are used. Cell Immunol 1984; 88:393–400.
23. Shalaby MR, Aggarwal BB, Rinderknecht E, Svedersky LP, Finkle BS, Palladino MA Jr. Activation of human polimorphonuclear neutrophil functions by interferon-γ and tumor necrosis factors. J Immunol 1985; 135:2069–73.
24. Steinbeck MJ, Roth JA, Kaeberle ML. Activation of bovine neutrophils by recombinant interferon-γ. Cell Immunol 1986; 98:137–44.
25. Rossi F. The O_2^--forming NADPH oxidase of the phagocytes: nature, mechanisms of activation and function. Biochim Biophys Acta 1986; 853:65–89.

26. Berton G, Zeni L, Cassatella MA, Rossi F. Gamma interferon is able to enhance the oxidative metabolism of human neutrophils. Biochem Biophys Res Commun 1986; 138:1276–82.
27. Kowanko IC, Ferrante A. Stimulation of neutrophil respiratory burst and lysosomal enzyme release by human interferon-gamma. Immunology 1987; 62:149–51.
28. Lappegard KT, Benestad HB, Rollag H. Interferons affect oxygen metabolism in human neutrophil granulocytes. J Interferon Res 1988; 8:665–77.
29. Edwards SW, Say JE, Hughes V. Gamma interferon enhances the killing of *Staphylococcus aureus* by human neutrophils. J Gen Microbiol 1988; 134:37–42.
30. Edwards SW, Holden CS, Humphreys JM, Hart A. Granulocyte-macrophage colony-stimulating factor (GM-CSF) primes the respiratory burst and stimulates protein biosynthesis in human neutrophils. FEBS Lett 1989; 256:62–6.
31. Cassatella MA, Cappelli R, Della Bianca V, Grzeskowiak M, Dusi S, Berton G. Interferon-gamma activates human neutrophil oxygen metabolism and exocytosis. Immunology 1988; 63:499–506.
32. Morrison CJ, Brummer E, Isenberg MA, Stevens DA. Activation of murine polymorphonuclear neutrophils for fungicidal activity by recombinant gamma interferon. J Leuk Biol 1987; 41:434–40.
33. Ezekowitz RAB, Dinauer MC, Jaffe HS, Orkin SH, Newburger PE. Partial correction of the phagocyte defect in patients with X-linked chronic granulomatous disease by subcutaneous interferon gamma. New Engl J Med 1988; 319:146–51.
34. Sechler, JMG, Malech HL, White J, Gallin JI. Recombinant human interferon-γ reconstitutes defective phagocyte function in patients with chronic granulomatous disease. Proc Natl Acad Sci USA 1988; 85:4874–8.
35. Steinbeck MJ, Webb DSA, Roth JA. Role of arachidonic acid metabolism and protein synthesis in recombinant bovine interferon-γ-induced activation of bovine neutrophils. J Leuk Biol 1989; 46:450–60.
36. Della Bianca V, Grzeskowiak M, Rossi F. Studies on molecular regulation of phagocytosis and activation of the NADPH oxidase in neutrophils: IgG- and C3b-mediated ingestion and associated respiratory burst independent of phospholipid turnover and Ca^{2+} transients. J Immunol 1990; 144:1411–7.
37. Rossi F, Grzeskowiak M, Della Bianca V, Calzetti F, Gandini G. Phosphatidic acid and not diacylglycerol generated by phospholipase D is functionally linked to the activation of the NADPH oxidase by fMLP in human neutrophils. Biochem Biophys Res Commun 1990; 168:320–7.
38. Besterman JM, Duronio V, Cuatrecasas P. Rapid formation of diacylglycerol from phosphatidylcholine: a pathway for generation of second messenger. Proc Natl Acad Sci USA 1986; 83:6785–9.
39. Orkin SH. Molecular genetics of chronic granulomatous disease. Ann Rev Immunol 1989; 7:277–307.
40. Volpp BD, Nauseef WM, Clark RA. Two cytosolic components absent in autosomal chronic granulomatous disease. Science 1988; 242:1295–7.
41. Lomax KJ, Leto TL, Nunoi H, Gallin JI, Malech HL. Recombinant 47-kilodalton cytosol factor restores NADPH oxidase in chronic granulomatous disease. Science 1989; 245:409–11.
42. Volpp BD, Nauseef WM, Donelson JE, Moser DR, Clark RA. Cloning of the cDNA and functional expression of the 47-kilodalton cytosolic component of human neutrophil respiratory burst oxidase. Proc Natl Acad Sci USA 1989; 86:7195–9.
43. Leto TL, Lomax KJ, Volpp BD, Sechler JMG, Nunoi H, Nauseef WM, Clark RA, Gallin JI, Malech HL. Neutrophil oxidase components share homology with regulatory domains of the arc related tyrosine kinase family. J Cell Biol 1989; 109:49A.
44. Bellavite P. The superoxide forming enzymatic system of phagocytes. Free Rad Biol Med 1988; 4:225–61.

45. Newburger PE, Ezekowitz RAB, Whitney C, Wright J, Orkin SH. Induction of phagocyte cytocrome b heavy chain gene expression by interferon γ. Proc Natl Acad Sci USA 1988; 85:5215–9.
46. Cassatella MA, Bazzoni F, Flynn RM, Dusi S, Trinchieri G, Rossi F. Molecular basis of interferon gamma and lypolysaccharide enhancement of phagocyte respiratory burst capability. Studies on the gene expression of several NADPH oxidase components. J Biol Chem 1990; 265:20241–6.
47. Cassatella MA, Hartman L, Perussia B, Trinchieri G. Tumor necrosis factor and immune interferon synergistically induce cytochrome b_{-245} heavy-chain gene expression and nicotinamide-adenine dinucleotide phosphate oxidase in human leukemic myeloid cells. J Clin Invest 1989; 83:1570–9.
48. Yea CM, Cross AR, Jones OTG. Purification and some properties of the 45 kDa diphenylene iodonium-binding flavoprotein of neutrophil NADPH oxidase. Biochem J 1990; 265:95–100.
49. Andrew PW, Robertson AK, Lowrie DB, Cross AR, Jones OTG. Induction of synthesis of components of the hydrogen peroxide-generating oxidase during activation of the human monocytic cell line U937 by interferon-γ. Biochem J 1987; 248:281–3.
50. Yamaguchi T, Hayakawa T, Kaneda M, Kakinuma K, Yoshikawa A. Purification and some properties of the small subunit of cytochrome b558 from human neutrophils. J Biol Chem 1989; 264:112–8.
51. Ezekowitz RAB, Orkin SH, Newburger PE. Recombinant interferon gamma augments phagocyte superoxide production and X-chronic granulomatous disease gene expression in X-linked variant chronic granulomatous disease. J Clin Invest 1987; 80:1009–16.
52. Berton G, Cassatella MA, Bellavite P, Rossi F. Molecular basis of macrophage activation. Expression of the low potential cytochrome b and its reduction upon cell stimulation in activated macrophages. J Immunol 1986; 136:1393–9.
53. Parkos CA, Dinauer MC, Walker LE, Allen RA, Jesaitis AJ, Orkin SH. Primary structure and unique expression of the 22-kilodalton light chain of human neutrophil cytochrome b. Proc Natl Acad Sci USA 1988; 85:3319–23.
54. Rotrosen D, Nunoi H, Gallin JG, Malech HL. Evidence for interaction of neutrophil 47 kD phosphoprotein with cytochrome b558 during activation of the respiratory burst. Clin Res 1989; 37:438A.
55. Cassatella MA, Della Bianca V, Berton G, Rossi F. Activation by gamma interferon of human macrophage capability to produce toxic oxygen molecules is accompanied by decreased Km of the superoxide-generating NADPH oxidase. Biochem Biophys Res Commun 1985; 132:908–14.
56. Thelen M, Wolf M, Baggiolini M. Activation of monocytes by interferon-gamma has no effect on the level or affinity of the nicotinamide adenine dinucleotide-oxidase and on agonist-dependent superoxide formation. J Clin Invest 1988; 81:1889–95.
57. Bridges RA, Berendes H, Good RA. A fatal granulomatous disease of childhood. The clinical, and laboratory features of a new syndrome. J Dis Child 1959; 97:387–408.
58. Curnutte JT. Classification of chronic granulomatous disease. Hematol Oncol Clin North Am 1988; 2:241–52.
59. North RJ. The concept of activated macrophage. J Immunol 1978; 121:806–9.
60. Karnovsky ML, Lazdins JK. Biochemical criteria for activated macrophages. J Immunol 1978; 121:809–13.
61. Cohn ZA. The activation of mononuclear phagocytes: facts, fancy and future. J Immunol 1978; 121:813–6.
62. Djeu JY, Blanchard DK, Halkias D, Friedman H. Growth inhibition of *Candida albicans* by human polymorphonuclear neutrophils: activation by interferon-γ and tumor necrosis factor. J Immunol 1986; 137:2980–4.
63. Morrison CJ, Brummer E, Stevens DA. In vivo activation of peripheral blood polymor-

phonuclear neutrophils by gamma interferon results in enhanced fungal killing. Infect Immun 1989; 57:2953–8.
64. Blanchard DK, Friedman H, Klein TW, Djeu JY. Induction of interferon-gamma and tumor necrosis factor by *Legionella phneumophila:* augmentation of human neutrophil bactericidal activity. J Leuk Biol 1989; 45:538–45.
65. Denis M, Chadee K. Human neutrophils activated by interferon-γ and tumor necrosis factor-α kill *Entamoeba histolytica* triphozoites in vitro. J Leuk Biol 1989; 46:270–4.
66. Hansen BD, Finbloom DS. Characterization of the interaction between recombinant interferon-γ and its receptor on human polymorphonuclear leukocytes. J Leuk Biol 1990; 47:64–9.
67. Yap WH, Teo TS, Tan YH. An early event in the interferon-induced transmembrane signalling process. Science 1986; 234:355–8.
68. Hamilton TA, Adams DO. Molecular mechanisms of signal transduction in macrophages. Immunol Today 1987; 8:151–8.
69. Humphreys JM, Hughes V, Edwards SW. Stimulation of protein synthesis in human neutrophils by γ-interferon. Biochem Pharmacol 1989; 38:1241–6.
70. Jack RM, Fearon DT. Selective synthesis of mRNA and proteins by human peripheral blood neutrophils. J Immunol 1988; 140:4286–93.
71. Rubin BY, Anderson SL, Lunn RM, Smith LY. Induction of proteins in interferon-α- and interferon-γ-treated polymorphonuclear leukocytes. J Leuk Biol 1989; 45:396–400.
72. Rubin BY, Anderson SL, Lunn RM, Hellermann GR, Richardson NK, Smith LJ. Production of a monoclonal antibody directed against an interferon-induced 56,000-dalton protein and its use in the study of this protein. J Virol 1988; 62:1875–80.
73. Rubin BY, Anderson SL, Lunn RM, Richardson NK, Hellermann GR, Smith LJ, Old LJ. Tumor necrosis factor and IFN induce a common set of proteins. J Immunol 1988; 141:1180–4.
74. Rubin BY, Anderson SL, Hellermann GR, Richardson NK, Lunn RM, Yalinsky JE. The development of antibody to the interferon-induced indoleamine 2,3-dioxygenase and the study of the regulation of its synthesis. J Interferon Res 1988, 8:691–702.
75. Cheng YSE, Becker-Manley MF, Chow TP, Horan DC. Affinity purification of an interferon-induced human guanylate-binding protein and its characterization. J Biol Chem 1985; 260:15834–9.
76. Ulker N, Zhang X, Samuel CE. Mechanism of interferon action. I. Characterization of a 54-kDa protein induced by γ interferon with properties similar to a cytoskeletal component. J Biol Chem 1987; 262:16798–803.
77. Ulker N, Samuel CE. Mechanism of interferon action. II. Induction and decay kinetics of the antiviral state and protein p54 in human amnion U cells treated with γ interferon. J Biol Chem 1987; 262:16804–7.
78. Livingston DH, Appel SH, Sonnenfeld G, Malangoni MA. The effect of tumor necrosis factor-α and interferon-γ on neutrophil function. J Surg Res 1989; 46:322–6.

16

Activation of Neutrophils by Granulocyte-Macrophage Colony-Stimulating Factor

JOHN F. DiPERSIO and CAMILLE N. ABBOUD
University of Rochester School of Medicine and Dentistry, Rochester, New York

I. INTRODUCTION

Hematopoietic growth factors both stimulate the growth and maturation of marrow precursor cells and enhance the functional activities of mature myelomonocytic effector cells. These biological effects are consistent with the expression of functional high-affinity cytokine receptors on both granulocytes and monocytes. Granulocyte-macrophage colony-stimulatory activity (GM-CSF) is a 22,000-Da glycoprotein produced by activated T-cells, endothelial cells, fibroblasts, and macrophages (Clark and Kamen, 1987). Recently, several reports suggest that GM-CSF is also made by acute myeloid blast cells (Herrmann and Vellenga, 1990; Young et al., 1987). This glycoprotein hormone stimulates the production of granulocytes and monocytes both in vivo and in vitro (Metcalf, 1986). The cDNA encoding this CSF has been cloned and expressed in *Escherichia coli,* yeast, and eukaryotic cells, allowing the production of large amounts of purified material necessary for in-vitro studies and in-vivo clinical trials (Gough, 1990; Broxmeyer and Vadhan-Raj, 1989; Groopman et al., 1986; Appelbaum, 1989).

The expression of GM-CSF is regulated by both 5′- and 3′ flanking regions of the genomic coding sequences (Shaw and Kamen, 1986; Chan et al., 1986; Nimer et al., 1988). GM-CSF is produced only by activated and not resting T-cells in a fashion similar to the expression of two other important T-cell-specific cytokines, IL-5 and IL-3 (Takatsu and Tominaga, 1990; Oster et al., 1991). It is of interest that all three of these cytokines promote the growth of eosinophilic precursors and increase the survival of eosinophils in vitro (Sanderson et al., 1985; Lopez et al., 1986; Owen et al., 1987). In addition, all three of these eosinophilopoietins possess simlar exon-intron structures, and all map to the long arm of chromosome 5 (Yang et al., 1988; Le Beau et al., 1989). Whether the deletion of one or more of these genes in patients with the 5q-syndrome contribute to the hematological abnormalities seen in these patients is currently still unknown (Nimer and Golde, 1987).

The expression of GM-CSF in endothelial cells, fibroblasts, and macrophages as well as acute myelogenous leukemia cells is regulated differently (Zsebo et al., 1988; Ernst et al., 1989; Nimer et al., 1989). Unlike in T-cells, where activation results primarily in increased GM-CSF mRNA transcription (Nimer et al., 1988), activation of fibroblasts, endothelial cells, and macrophages with lipopolysaccharide (LPS), tumor necrosis factor (TNF), or interleukin 1 (IL-1) results in increased GM-CSF mRNA stability and thus increased protein synthesis (Koeffler et al., 1987, 1988; Munker et al., 1986). It has been shown that specific "AUUUA"-rich sequences in the 3′ flanking region of the GM-CSF mRNA are important in allowing rapid degradation of the GM-CSF mRNA (Shaw and Kamen, 1986).

II. EFFECT OF GM-CSF ON THE ACTIVATION STATE OF HUMAN NEUTROPHILS

GM-CSF has been shown to directly activate or indirectly "prime" mature effector cells for enhanced response to secondary stimuli such as parasites, bacteria, immune serum, and chemotactic factors (Fleischman et al., 1986; Lopez et al., 1986; Silberstein et al., 1986; Weisbart et al., 1987). We and others have shown that GM-CSF receptors exist on human neutrophils (Gasson et al., 1986; DiPersio et al., 1988c; Park et al., 1986). There appears to be a single class of high-affinity receptors (kDa 50–100 pM) expressed in low levels (200–800 receptors/cell) on normal human neutrophils (DiPersio et al., 1988c). We have looked extensively at many patients with chronic neutropenia, myelodysplasia, and active and chronic myeloid leukemias but have been unable to identify patients whose neutrophils express dramatically altered numbers or affinities of GM-CSF receptors (unpublished observations). There is some evidence that the expression of high-affinity GM-CSF receptors is developmentally regulated in a human myeloid leukemia cell line, HL-60 (DiPersio et al., 1988c). When these cells are induced to differentiate to mature neutrophils using dibutryl cAMP, dimethyl sulfoxide, or retinoic acid, high-affinity GM-CSF receptor expression increases coincident with the increased expression of other receptors such as the IgA receptor, the f-Met-Leu-Phe (fMLP) receptor, and the leukotriene B_4 (LTB_4) receptor as well as with obvious morphologic neutrophilic differentiation (unpublished observations).

In spite of the multitude of studies showing effects of GM-CSF on neutrophil function (see Table 1), it has been very difficult to demonstrate direct activation of neutrophils by GM-CSF and other CSFs. Early studies demonstrated that GM-CSF had no direct effect on neutrophils but enhanced the response of neutrophils to secondary stimuli such as ionophore or chemotactic factors: Measurable responses included superoxide generation (Weisbart et al., 1987; Corey and Rosoff, 1989); killing of bacteria (Fleischmann et al., 1986; Djeu and Blanchard, 1987a), parasite (Silberstein et al., 1986; Villalta and Kierszenbaum, 1986), or tumor cells (Grabstein et al., 1986; Lopez et al., 1986; Djeu et al., 1987b; Fabian et al., 1987); calcium flux (Naccache et al., 1988; Mege et al., 1989); arachidonic acid release (DiPersio et al., 1988c; Sullivan et al., 1987); leukotriene synthesis (DiPersio et al., 1988b, 1988c; Dahinden et al., 1988); and platelet-activating factor (PAF) synthesis (Wirthmueller et al., 1989; DiPersio et al., 1990b).

Table 1 Biological Effects of Recombinant GM-CSF on Neutrophils

Effect	Reference
Neutrophils—direct:	
Increased cell survival	Begley et al., 1986; Lopez et al., 1986
Increased stimulation of superoxide generation	Yuo et al., 1989
Inhibition of random migration	Gasson et al., 1984; Weisbart et al., 1985
Increase forward light scatter/ruffing	Fletcher and Gasson, 1988; Abboud et al., 1990
Increase F-actin polymerization, and cell polarity	Abboud et al., 1990
Induction of early response genes: c-fos, c-myc, TIS-8 (Egr-1)	Colotta et al., 198; Tsai-Morris et al., 1988; Varnum et al., 1989
Stimulation of guanylate-cyclase	Coffey et al., 1988
Decrease of adenylate cyclase	Coffey et al., 1988
Induction of IL-1	Lindemann et al., 1988
Cellular alkalinization	Gomez-Cambronero et al., 1989
Altered tyrosine phosphorylation	Gomez-Cambronero et al., 1989; DiPersio et al., 1990a
Activation of a pertussis toxin-sensitive G-protein	Corey and Rosoff, 1989; Gomez-Cambronero et al., 1989; McColl et al., 1989
Increase fMLP receptor expression	Weisbart et al., 1986
Increase Mo-1 expression	Arnaout et al., 1986; Socinski et al., 1988; Devereux et al., 1989
Increased CD35 and Class I MHC expression	Neuman et al., 1990
Increase IgA Fc receptor expression	Weisbart et al., 1989
Decrease LTB_4 receptor expression	DiPersio et al., 1991a
Decrease LAM-1 adhesion protein expression	Griffin et al., 1990
Synthesis and release of LTB_4 and PAF	DiPersio et al., 1991a, 1990c
Synthesis and release of a 23-kDa protein	McColl et al., 1990
Neutrophils—indirect:	
Enhanced antibody-dependent tumor cell killing	Lopez et al., 1986; Djeu et al., 1987b
Enhanced killing of organisms	Villalta and Kierszenbaum, 1986; Baldwin et al., 1988
Enhanced degranulation	Kaufman et al., 1989; Richter et al., 1989; Devereux et al., 1990[a]
Enhanced chemotaxis	Weisbart et al., 1986
Enhanced phagocytosis	Fleischmann et al., 1986; Djeu and Blanchard, 1987a
Enhanced superoxide generation	Weisbart et al., 1986[a]
Blunted intracellular alkalinization	Sullivan et al., 1987; Naccache et al., 1988; Mege et al., 1989[a]
Enhanced intracellular acidification	Naccache et al., 1988
Enhanced arachidonic acid release	Sullivan et al., 1988; DiPersio et al., 1988b; Corey and Rosoff, 1989[a]
Enhanced LTB_4 and lipoxin synthesis	DiPersio et al., 1988a, 1988b; Dahinden et al., 1988; Fiore and Serhan, 1990[a]
Enhanced PAF synthesis	Wirthmueller et al., 1989; DiPersio et al., 1990b, 1990c[a]
Enhanced phosphatidic acid release and phospholipid D activation	Bougoin et al., 1990

[a] May also be a direct effect.

Not all secondary stimuli such as phorbol esters were enhanced by GM-CSF (Weisbart et al., 1986; Mege et al., 1989), suggesting that priming by GM-CSF may proceed through separate and distinct pathways. In addition, "priming" of neutrophils is not a property limited to GM-CSF or other CSFs, since other agents such as phorbol esters

(Dewald et al., 1984), PAF (Shalit et al., 1987; Vercelotti et al., 1988), LTB_4 (Gay et al., 1988), LPS (Guthrie et al., 1984), and fMLP (Karnard et al., 1989) can all effectively "prime" neutrophils when used at low concentrations (10^{-12}–10^{-9} M), concentrations which do not usually result in the direct activation of human neutrophils.

Pathways of "priming" by GM-CSF and other neutrophil-activating agents will be discussed below but are generally poorly understood. Recent data suggest that pathways of direct activation in neutrophils by 10^{-7} M fMLP utilizing pertussis toxin-sensitive G-proteins may not operate when neutrophils are "primed" by 10^{-10} M fMLP. In this case, fMLP appears to prime neutrophils through a calcium-independent pertussis toxin-insensitive pathway (Karnad et al., 1989).

The process of "priming" by GM-CSF may be physiologically advantageous to the host. If one considers GM-CSF and other cytokines as circulating hormones, one would not want the increased blood levels of these hormones during stress to result in direct activation of neutrophils (i.e., superoxide generation, or degranulation) at inappropriate times or distances from offending stimuli. Instead, GM-CSF may arm neutrophil effectors for enhanced response to physiologically relevant agents (chemotactic factors, leukotrienes, PAF, interleukin-8), all of which may be released locally at sites of inflammation (König et al., 1990; Matsushima and Oppenheim, 1989). These secondary stimuli can directly activate chemotaxis, the respiratory burst, arachidonic acid metabolism, calcium fluxes, phagocytosis, and degranulation, but their effects would be dramatically potentiated by preexposure of the neutrophils to GM-CSF (Cairo et al., 1990).

III. DIRECT EFFECTS OF GM-CSF ON NEUTROPHIL FUNCTION

Recent studies by our laboratory and others, using very sensitive assays of neutrophil function, have suggested that GM-CSF directly activates multiple biological effects in neutrophils, eosinophils, and normal human monocytes. These effects include release of free arachidonic acid (Sullivan et al., 1988; DiPersio et al., 1988a; Corey and Rosoff, 1989), LTB_4 and its 20-omega metabolites (DiPersio et al., 1988a, 1988b; Dahinden et al., 1988), lipoxins (Fiore and Serhan, 1990), and PAF (Wirthmueller et al., 1989; DiPersio et al., 1990b). All of these inflammatory products of neutrophil arachidonic acid metabolism can both "prime" and directly activate neutrophil effector function; this effect will be discussed at greater length later in this chapter.

In addition to directly activating subtle changes in the arachidonic acid cascade, GM-CSF has been shown by our laboratory and others to acutely inhibit the chemotactic factor and phorbol ester-induced cellular alkalinization as well as directly inducing, over longer periods of time (10–60 min), increasing intracellular pH in both neutrophils and monocytes, presumably by activation of the Na^+/H^+ antiport (Naccache et al., 1988; Sullivan et al., 1987; Mege et al., 1989; Gomez-Cambronero et al., 1989; Vallance et al., 1990). Similar results have been reported by Bussolino et al. (1989a) using GM-CSF-treated endothelial cells. To date no studies have demonstrated any direct effects of GM-CSF or neutrophil Na^+/H^+ antiport gene expression, protein synthesis, post-translational modification (i.e., phosphorylation), or cellular translocation.

Since the time course of GM-CSF on a multiplicity of neutrophil-signaling events is quite slow (i.e., superoxide generation, PAF synthesis, cellular alkalinization, etc.), it is conceivable that these effects may not be a direct effect of GM-CSF but due to the accumulation and release of inflammatory intermediates such as PAF or LTB_4 by GM-CSF-treated neutrophils. It is also conceivable that "priming" of neutrophils in response to GM-CSF may reflect the accumulation of these intermediates, which have been shown when used in low concentrations (10^{-11}–10^{-9} M) to "prime" and not directly activate human neutrophils.

A. Effect of GM-CSF on Chemotaxis and Neutrophil Migration

Weisbart et al. (1987) first demonstrated that GM-CSF has a biphasic effect on neutrophil motility. Chemotaxis along a chemical gradient to fMLP was enhanced immediately (5–15 min) after incubation with GM-CSF. Longer incubations with GM-CSF (30–120 min) resulted in a significant decrease in "random migration" of neutrophils, a result also reported by Atkinson et al. (1988) in vitro and Addison et al. in vivo (1989). It has been very difficult to study the very early effects of GM-CSF in reproducible chemotactic assays; however, significant evidence both in vitro and in vivo suggests that GM-CSF decreases the random migration of human neutrophils, increases the surface expression of the Mo-1 adhesion molecule, and increases leukocyte aggregation (Arnaout et al., 1986; Socinski et al., 1988). A number of investigators have described a profound and reproducible drop in the absolute neutrophil count after intravenous boluses of GM-CSF and G-CSF (Peters et al., 1988; Lindemann et al., 1989a; Lieschke et al., 1989). Indium-labeled neutrophil studies suggest that neutrophils are transiently sequestered in the lungs (Devereux et al., 1987). This transient decrease in absolute numbers of circulating neutrophils, eosinophils, and monocytes is reversible after 6 h and correlates with a dramatic decrease in random migration of neutrophils in vitro (Kownatzki et al., 1990; Kharazmi et al., 1988; Wang et al., 1988).

Decreased neutrophil migration was also demonstrated in vivo by measuring random migration of neutrophils into skin windows of patients before and after the administration of GM-CSF (Peters et al., 1988). Several studies have suggested that this may be due to the increased expression of neutrophil adhesion molecules, whose increased surface expression by GM-CSF may be due to the ability of GM-CSF to directly promote degranulation of neutrophils (Socinski et al., 1988). We and others have demonstrated that other proteins stored in neutrophil secondary specific granules such as the fMLP receptor (Weisbart et al., 1986), B_{12}-binding protein (Kaufman et al., 1989; Richter et al., 1989; Smith et al., 1990), plasminogen activator in monocytes (Hart et al., 1990), and CR1 and CR3 are released or expressed in higher levels on the neutrophil cell surface (Neuman et al., 1990).

GM-CSF has profound effects on other neutrophil surface receptors. GM-CSF has been shown to increase the number and affinity of neutrophil IgA Fc receptors (Weisbart et al., 1989), and down-regulate the expression of human LTB_4 receptors (DiPersio et al., 1991a), interleukin-8 receptors (DiPersio et al., 1990a), and LAM-1, another important adhesion molecule (Griffin et al., 1990). These rapid and direct effects on surface adhesion molecule/receptor expression by GM-CSF may result in a more efficient migration of mature and "primed" effector neutrophils to areas of inflammation. They may also promote or facilitate appropriate neutrophil and monocyte aggregation, margination, and egress from the vascular space to potential sites of tissue injury.

B. Direct Effects of GM-CSF on Neutrophil Actin Polymerization

There are other explanations for the drop in neutrophil count after in-vivo administration of GM-CSF. Recent studies have suggested that antibodies to Mo-1 do not block the GM-CSF-induced drop in random migration and GM-CSF-induced neutropenia in vivo (Lundberg and Wright, 1990; Yong et al., 1990). Recent data by our laboratory suggests that GM-CSF has a direct but slow (10–30 min at room temperature) effect on neutrophil F-actin polymerization. It is likely that increased F-actin polymerization may contribute to increased mechanical stiffness and increased neutrophil trapping in the microvasculature of the lungs (Yong et al., 1990; Worthen et al., 1989). Indeed, in one patient described by Yong et al. (1990) with partial leukocyte adhesion deficiency, GM-CSF administration in vivo was still associated with neutrophil margination despite no detectable up-regulation of CD11b on his neutrophils, clearly implying other mechanisms in this process.

Our interest in the role of cytokines in the egress of mature neutrophils from the marrow led us to investigate the role of GM-CSF on F-actin polymerization in vitro, using NBD-phallacidin staining and analysis by flow cytometry (Packman and Lichtman, 1990). When compared to active chemoattractants such as fMLP or platelet-derived growth factor (PDGF), the action of GM-CSF on F-actin polymerization in blood-derived neutrophils is delayed and requires 10–20 min to reach its maximum at room temperature. Figure 1 shows the direct effects of recombinant human granulocyte-macrophage colony-stimulating factor on human neutrophil F-actin at 30 min. Both 40 and 200 pg/mL of GM-CSF were able to increase relative F-actin by 1.4 times over control buffer. One nanomolar fMLP (positive control) causes, in contrast, a twofold increase in PMN-relative F-actin that peaks at 1 min (data not shown).

In view of our earlier findings that GM-CSF is able to prime neutrophils to a variety of second stimuli including fMLP and C5A, we investigated its action on fMLP-

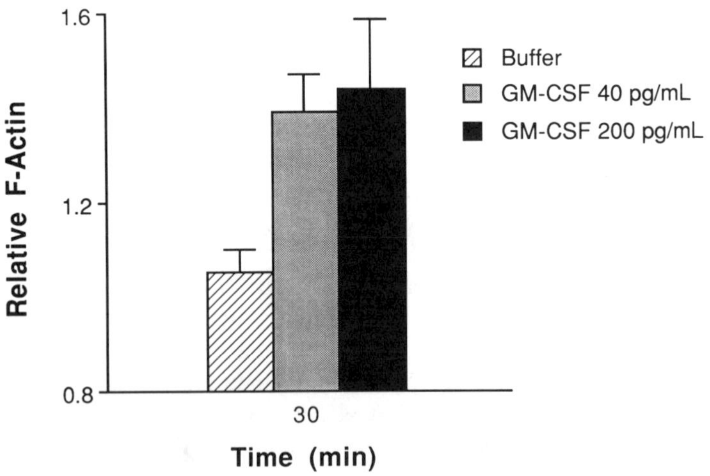

Figure 1 Direct effects of recombinant GM-CSF (40 and 200 pg/mL [Genzyme, Cambridge, MA]) on F-actin polymerization in human neutrophil, using NBD-phallacidin staining and flow cytometry. Data represent mean and SEM of five experiments. Note the increase in relative F-actin at 30 min above control, in cells exposed to GM-CSF.

induced F-actin polymerization in human neutrophils. Neutrophils preincubated with GM-CSF [16 pg/mL (0.7 pM), for 20 min at room temperature] were "primed" for enhanced F-actin polymerization when compared with neutrophils incubated with diluent control (Figure 2); similar results were observed with incubations at 37°C. These changes in F-actin conformation may help explain some of the previously reported changes in receptor expression and degranulation effects (Kapp et al., 1988), since most agonists that are associated with degranulation are also ones that cause F-actin polymerization in PMNs, such as LTB_4, PAF, fMLP, TNF. In addition to being able to migrate effectively toward their targets, CSF-activated neutrophils display increased adhesiveness and increased cytotoxicity toward opsonized targets (Socinski et al., 1988; Yuo et al., 1989; Devereux et al., 1989). Detailed examination of such cells by scanning electron microscopy allows one to depict the membrane ruffling that clearly occurs in these activated cells, as indicated in Figure 3 [A, control untreated PMN; B, PMN + 1 nM fMLP at 1 min; C, PMN + GM-CSF 2 ng/mL (1 nM) for 20 min]. The delayed effects of GM-CSF on cell shape and polarity (Abboud et al., 1990) suggest perhaps that these changes may be secondary to the generation of other agonists such as LTB_4 and PAF. Studies are currently aimed at addressing those questions.

C. Effects of GM-CSF on Arachidonic Acid/Leukotriene B_4 (LTB_4) Production

Arachidonic acid (AA) and its metabolites are at the center of neutrophil activation. Membrane and cytosol-associated AA is generated through the activation of the calcium-dependent enzyme phospholipase A2 (PLA2). Free AA may then be metabolized along multiple pathways. Calcium-dependent PLA2 stimulates the cleavage of AA from the 2(R)-position of the phospholipid 1-alkyl-2-acyl-glycerophosphocholine as well as other substrates. PLA2 generates not only free AA, which can be metabolized

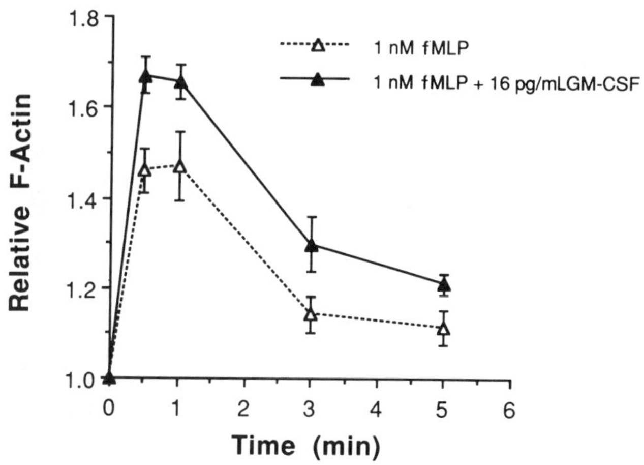

Figure 2 Priming effect of low-dose GM-CSF on fMLP-induced neutrophil F-actin polymerization. Cells were incubated with 16 pg/mL GM-CSF for 20 min at room temperature, prior to the addition of 1 nM fMLP at time 0. Note the increase in relative F-actin at 0.5–5 min in neutrophils exposed to GM-CSF (solid line) as compared to control cells (dashed line) after treatment with 1 nM fMLP. Data represent the mean and SEM of three experiments.

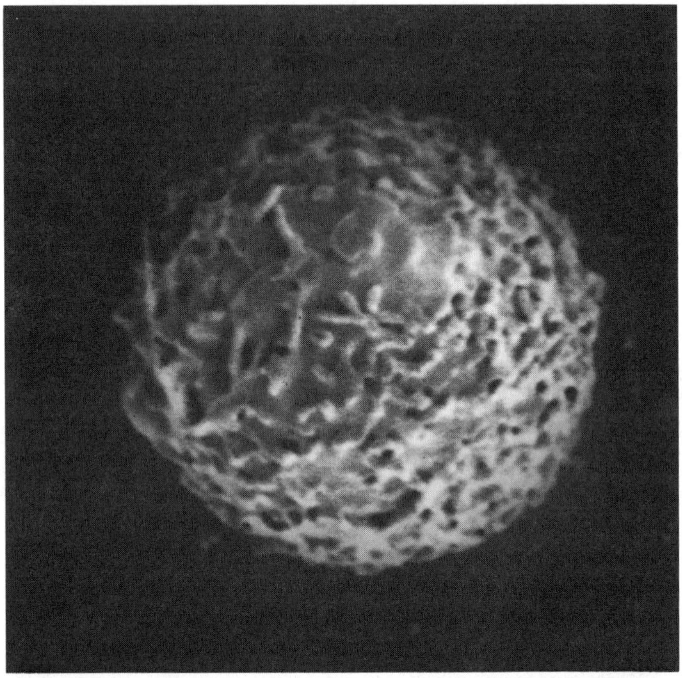

(A)

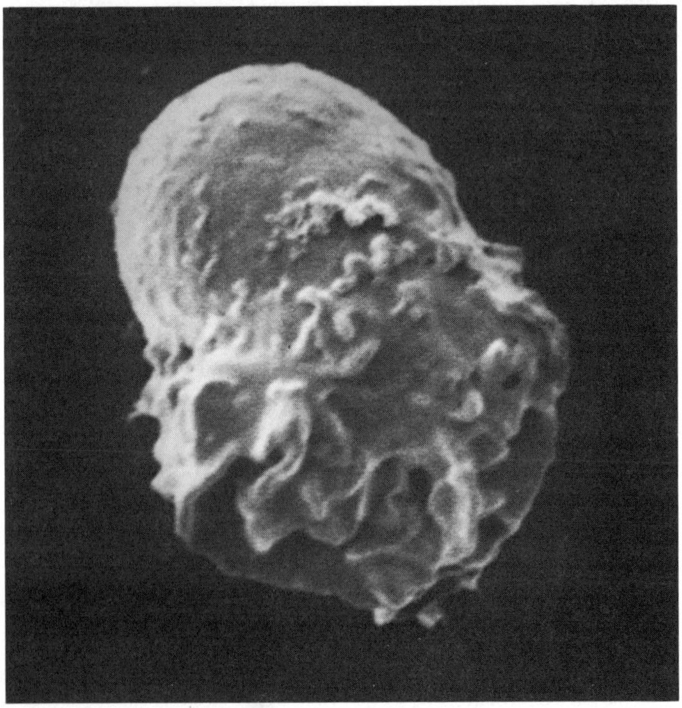

(B)

Figure 3 Scanning electron microscopy of human neutrophil (10,575× magnification). A: untreated neutrophil; B: neutrophil treated with 1 nM fMLP at 1 min; C: neutrophil treated with GM-CSF (2 ng/ml G-enzyme, for 20 min at room temperature).

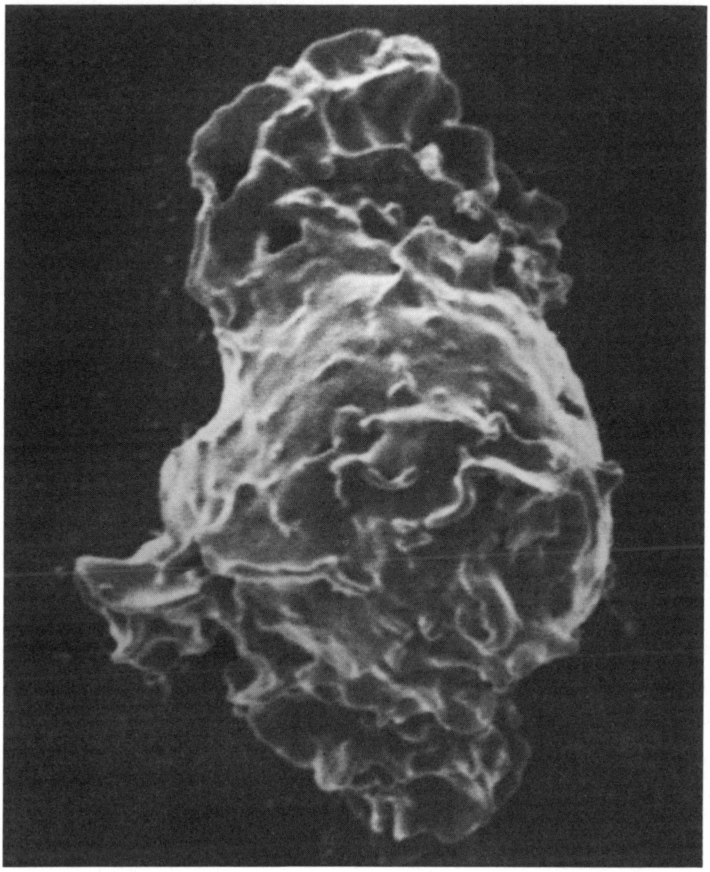

(C)

by cyclooxygenases to prostaglandins (PG) and prostacyclin and by lipoxygenases to leukotrienes (LT), but also results in the generation of lyso-PAF, the precursor of PAF (Figure 4). Prostaglandins, LTs, and PAF are all potent mediators of inflammation. Mature effector cells such as neutrophils and monocytes can not only synthesize these inflammatory intermediates but also express receptors for LTs and PAF which can be activated in an autocrine or paracrine fashion by these same intermediates (Goldman and Goetzl, 1984; Valone and Goetzl, 1983; O'Flaherty et al., 1986a, 1986b). LTB_4 and PAF directly activate neutrophils (superoxide generation, etc.) and are potent chemotactic factors for neutrophils and eosinophils (Sanjar et al., 1990; Czarnetzki et al., 1989). Bomalaski et al. (1989) demonstrated that LTB_4 may promote neutrophil chemotaxis by modulating phospholipid methylation. Enhanced phospholipid methylation has been observed in human neutrophil membranes following stimulation with other chemotactic agents, specifically opsonized zymosan, mitogenic lectins (Hirata et al., 1979), and the formylated peptide fMLP (Niwa et al., 1984).

Leukotrienes and PAF modulate the synthesis of each other. Lipoxygenase products of AA metabolism modulate the synthesis of PAF in human neutrophils via activation of PLA2 (Billah et al., 1985). Likewise, PAF stimulates neutrophil LTB_4 synthesis. Recent data suggest that platelets cooperate with neutrophils for both LTB_4 (Fiore and

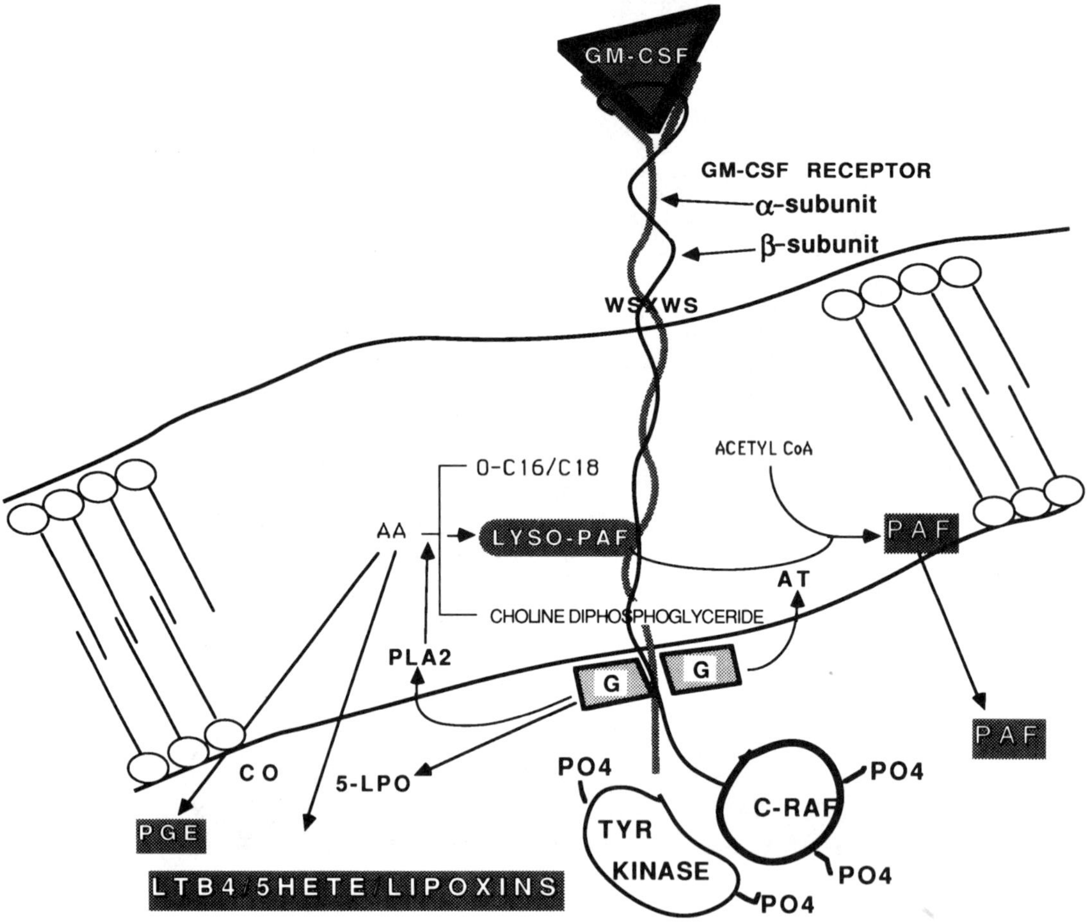

Figure 4 Model of GM-CSF signaling in normal human neutrophils. GM-CSF binds to a heterodimeric high-affinity receptor consisting of a low-affinity ligand-binding subunit (α-subunit) and an associated signal-transducing subunit (β-subunit). Both subunits contain the WSXWS consensus sequence in the extracellular domain. Engagement of the GM-CSF ligand induces receptor conformational changes resulting in the activation of both pertussis toxin-sensitive and -insensitive G-proteins (G), receptor-associated tyrosine kinases, and the c-raf serine/threonine kinase. Phospholipase A2 (PLA2) is activated through unclear mechanisms, resulting in the release of free arachidonic acid (AA) and the generation of lyso-PAF from its precusor 1-O-alkyl(C16 or C18)-2(R)-acyl-glycero-3-phosphorylcholine. This provides substrates for activated 5-lipoxygenase (5-LPO), lyso-PAF acetyltransferase (AT), and cyclooxygenase. These activated neutrophil enzymes utilize both neutrophil as well as platelet substrates to generate potent autocrine/paracrine mediators, platelet-activating factor (PAF), leukotriene B_4 (LTB_4), lipoxins, 5-HETE, and prostaglandins (PGE).

Serhan, 1990) and PAF (Coeffier et al., 1990) synthesis. The interrelationship of these intermediates underscores the ability of separate neutrophil agonists to amplify the inflammatory response by simulating neutrophils to synthesize either LTB_4 or PAF.

We and others have studied the effects of GM-CSF on neutrophil AA release and metabolism (Sullivan et al., 1987; DiPersio et al., 1988a; Corey and Rosoff, 1989). GM-CSF, and to a lesser extent tumor necrosis factor (TNF) and G-CSF, prime neutrophils for enhanced synthesis and release of AA in response to secondary stimuli such as chemotactic factors and calcium ionophore (DiPersio et al., 1988a). Although very subtle, GM-CSF could directly induce the release of very low levels of free AA. Neither direct or priming effects could be inhibited by protein kinase C (PKC) inhibitors such as staurosporine or H-7, or by pertussis toxin (PT) or inhibitors of protein and RNA synthesis (Figure 5). Hannigan et al. (1991) demonstrated that 5,8,11,14-eicosatetraynoic acid (ETYA), an inhibitor of AA epoxygenation, blocks the biological effects of α-interferon on a mouse fibroblast cell line. Similar events may be responsible for neutrophil activation or priming in response to GM-CSF.

The products of AA released by GM-CSF-primed neutrophils in response to fMLP and A23187 were examined by both reverse-phase HPLC and by LTB_4 radioimmunoassay (RIA). In addition to small amounts of free AA, significantly increased amounts of LTB_4 and its 20-omega metabolites were synthesized and released by GM-

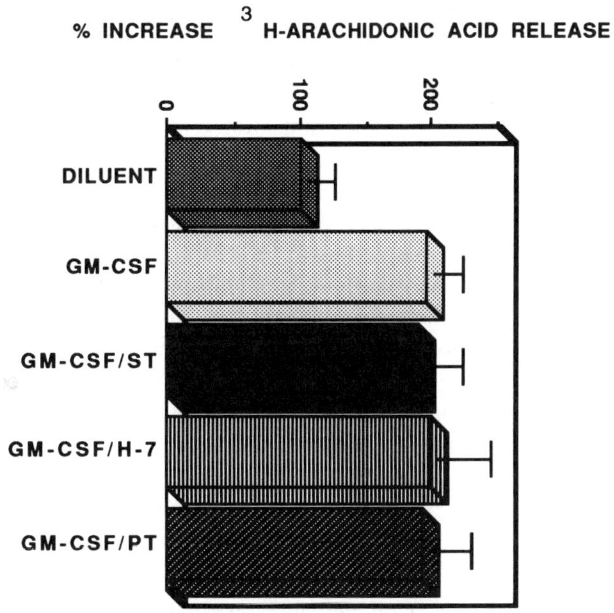

Figure 5 Effect of GM-CSF on arachidonic acid release by normal human neutrophils. Neutrophils were loaded with ^{3}H-arachidonic acid for 1 h at 23°C. After washing these cells and preincubating the cells for 30 min with diluent control, staurosporin (ST), H-7, or pertussin toxin (PT), the cells were stimulated for 30 min at 37°C with either diluent control or 1 nM GM-CSF. After removing the neutrophils, the supernatants were extracted and counted in a liquid scintillation counter. GM-CSF directly induces the release of small but detectable amounts of free arachidonic acid. This effect was not inhibited by staurosporin, H-7, or pertussin toxin. Data represents the mean and SEM of six experiments.

CSF-primed neutrophils (DiPersio et al., 1988b). Similar results were recently obtained by Dahinden et al. (1989). By developing a very sensitive $^{3}H-LTB_4$ radioreceptor binding assay and a very sensitive LTB_4 RIA, we observed that GM-CSF directly induced a dramatic decrease in the surface expression of high-affinity LTB_4 receptors coincident with a direct stimulation of very low but easily measured levels of LTB_4 (DiPersio et al., 1991a; Figure 6). These effects could be consistently inhibited by NDGA (5-lipoxygenase inhibitor) and two inhibitors of tyrosine kinases (erbstatin and genistein) (DiPersio et al., 1990a).

These results suggest that GM-CSF may directly activate both PLA2 and 5-LPO, resulting in the synthesis of small amounts of LTB_4 which may in turn bind and down-regulate the neutrophil high-affinity LTB_4 receptor. It is of interest that Gay et al. (1984) have shown that low concentrations of LTB_4, lower concentrations than can directly activate neutrophils, are able to prime neutrophils for enhanced response to fMLP in a fashion similar to that of GM-CSF. Low concentrations of other neutrophil agonists such as PAF (Ingraham et al., 1987; Shalit et al., 1987; Vercellotti et al., 1988), phorbol esters (Dewald et al., 1984; Bass et al., 1987; Bauldry et al., 1988), and fMLP (Karnad et al., 1989) can prime neutrophils for enhanced effector function in response to secondary stimuli as well. Although fMLP, PAF, and LTB_4 appear to directly activate neutrophils through pertussis toxin-sensitive pathways involving G-proteins and phospholipase C, low concentrations of at least one of these agonists, fMLP, "prime" neutrophils through an entirely different mechanism (Karnad et al., 1989). Although the direct effect of GM-CSF on LTB_4 synthesis is small, it is significant and reproducible. It is conceivable that the direct effects of GM-CSF on PLA2, 5-lipoxygenase, and PAF acetyltransferase (the rate-limiting enzyme for PAF synthesis) may generate "priming" concentrations of LTB_4 or PAF sufficient to enhance the response of neutrophils to secondary stimuli such as calcium ionophore or chemotactic factors. It is also possible that synthesis of LTB_4, PAF, and down-regulation of the LTB_4 receptor may be late, secondary, and irrelevant events occurring as a consequence of more immediate effects of GM-CSF on neutrophil signaling, such as tyrosine phosphorylation or phospholipid methylation. It is of interest that many of the direct effects of GM-CSF on neutrophils (LTB_4 synthesis, LTB_4 receptor down-regulation, cellular alkalinization, degranulation, AA release, PAF synthesis) take at least 10–30 min. That is a distinctly slower time course than that seen when fMLP, LTB_4, PAF, C5a, A23187, or PMA are used to directly stimulate neutrophils.

In our hands, pertussis toxin (PT) does not selectively inhibit GM-CSF's effects on AA, LTB_4, and PAF synthesis. It is possible that some of the PT-sensitive effects that have been described for GM-CSF may be due to the production of low concentrations of potent autocrine/paracrine PT-inhibitable activators such as LTB_4 or PAF. We have recently shown that GM-CSF and IL-3 prime a human GM-CSF/IL-3-dependent cell line, MO7E (Avanzi et al., 1988), for enhanced LTB_4 synthesis and PAF synthesis in response to stimulation with the calcium ionophore A23187 (unpublished results). Recently, Shibata et al. (1990) have demonstrated that IL-3 and GM-CSF both prime bone marrow precursors for enhanced LT synthesis. These results may shed some light on why patients who have myeloid leukemias appear to have more systemic toxicities when given GM-CSF in vivo. Indeed, timely studies by Denzlinger et al. (1990) have shown that patients with myelodysplasia treated in vivo with GM-CSF excreted increased urinary cysteinyl leukotrienes when compared to untreated cohorts. The

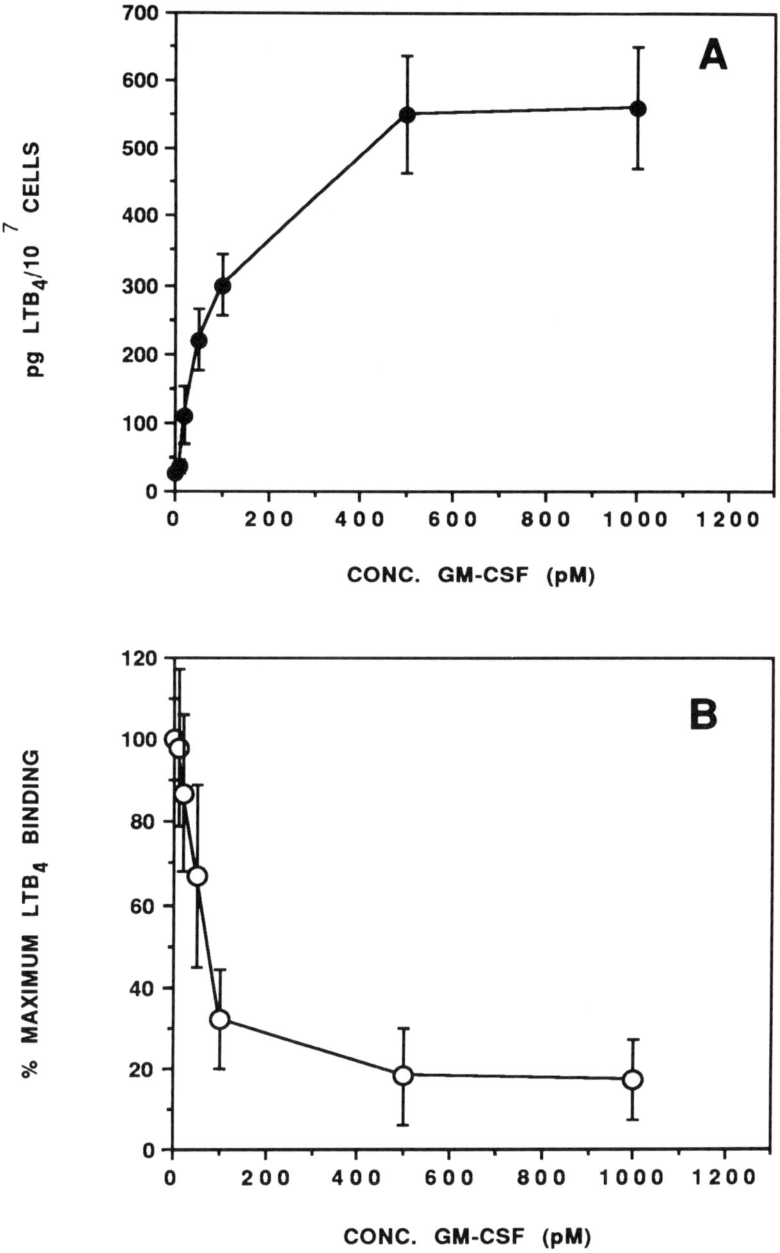

Figure 6 Effect of GM-CSF on LTB_4 receptor expression (A) and neutrophil LTB_4 synthesis. Neutrophils were incubated for 30 min at 37°C with increasing concentrations of human GM-CSF. ^3H-LTB_4 radioreceptor binding assay was performed as previously described (A), and total LTB_4 was measured by a sensitive radioimmunoassay (B), (Goldman and Goetzl, 1984; DiPersio et al., 1988). GM-CSF induces a rapid decrease in the surface expression of the high-affinity LTB_4 receptor coincident with the production of increasing amounts of LTB_4. The data represent the mean and SEM of eight separate experiments.

increased urinary excretion of these LT derivatives correlated with an expansion of the white blood cell count. Again, both in-vitro and in-vivo studies suggest that GM-CSF directly stimulates both mature effector cells as well as marrow precursors to synthesize and secrete a wide array of eicosanoids.

D. Effect of GM-CSF on Platelet-Activating Factor (PAF) Production by Human Neutrophils

As mentioned previously, GM-CSF "primes" neutrophils for enhanced PAF synthesis in response to secondary stimuli (Wirthmueller et al., 1989; Gomez-Cambronero et al., 1989; DiPersio et al., 1990b). We have studied the effects of GM-CSF on neutrophil PAF synthesis by developing a very sensitive RIA for PAF. This RIA can detect as little as 20–500 pg of PAF. GM-CSF directly stimulates the production of PAF by human neutrophils in a time (max. 30–60 min) and concentration (max. 50 pM–1 nM) fashion (Figure 7). Of interest is that comparable levels of PAF were stimulated by 10^{-7} M LTB_4 and that 90% ±5% of the PAF synthesized in response to GM-CSF and LTB_4 remained cell associated and very little (<10%) could be detected in the supernatant. The importance of cell-associated PAF remains controversial. Some data suggest that the enhanced binding of neutrophils to TNF or IL-1α-treated endothelial cells as well as release of icosanoids and superoxide anions from neutrophils may be blocked by PAF receptor antagonists (Zimmerman et al., 1990; Toothill et al., 1990; Vercellotti et al., 1988; Stewart et al., 1990; Dubois et al., 1989; Yue et al., 1990; Häkansson and Venge, 1990). We have found that low concentrations of NDGA (5–10 μM) block GM-CSF-induces LT synthesis without blocking GM-CSF-induced PAF synthesis, suggesting that LT synthesis is not required for PAF synthesis. We are currently using both PAF antagonists as well as metabolic inhibitors of both PLA2 and PAF synthesis to determine if PAF synthesis is essential for GM-CSF-induced priming of neutrophils. The mechanism by which GM-CSF induced increased PAF accumulation in neutrophils remains unclear. Recent evidence from our laboratory suggests that GM-CSF directly stimulates increased activity of the rate-limiting microsomal-associated enzyme for PAF synthesis, the lyso-PAF acetyltransferase (AT). Figure 7 demonstrates that maximum GM-CSF-induced acetyltransferase activity occur after approximately 5–10 min. This enhanced enzyme activity precedes by 10–15 min the maximum accumulation of GM-CSF-induced PAF.

It is presently not understood how PLA2, 5-LPO, or the lyso-PAF AT enzymes are activated by GM-CSF or other agonists. Previous studies by Rouzer et al. (1990) suggest that A23187 may activate the 5-LPO by inducing the translocation of the cytosolic enzyme to the plasma membrane and a specific membrane-associated protein called the 5-LPO-activating protein ("FLAP") (Miller et al., 1990; Dixon et al., 1990). Tumor necrosis factor, TNF_{α}, has been shown to increase levels of PLA2 activating protein ("PLAP") in endothelial cells (Clark et al., 1988). This protein is antigenically and functionally related to melittin, a bee venom peptide which has been shown to stimulate PLA2 activity (Bomalaski et al., 1989). PLAP has been shown to stimulate neutrophil PLA2, leukotriene synthesis, neutrophil aggregation, and superoxide generation. It is possible that GM-CSF stimulates PLAP in a way similar to TNF, resulting in increased neutrophil AA, LTB_4, and PAF synthesis.

Platelets cooperate with neutrophils for PAF synthesis (Coeffier et al., 1990), similar to that noted for LTB_4. In addition, recent in-vivo studies in both guinea pigs (Sanjar et

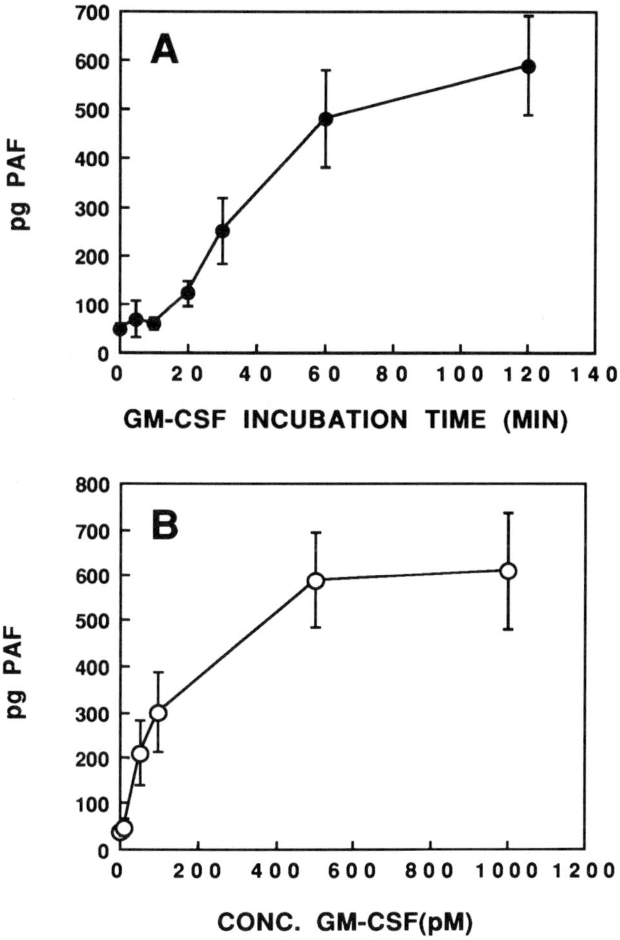

Figure 7 Effect of GM-CSF on neutrophil platelet-activating factor (PAF) synthesis. Neutrophils were treated for varying times (A) and with varying concentrations of GM-CSF (B) prior to cellular extraction and measurement of total cell-associated PAF by RIA. GM-CSF induces a time- and concentration-dependent production of PAF in human neutrophils. The data represent the mean and SEM of seven experiments.

al., 1990) and humans (Aglietta et al., 1990) suggest that GM-CSF both enhances PAF-induced eosinophil accumulation in guinea pig airways and primes human neutrophils in vivo for enhanced PAF synthesis in response to secondary stimuli. Again, in-vivo studies support the effect of GM-CSF on granulocyte PAF synthesis in addition to LTB_4 synthesis.

IV. CLINICAL CORRELATES OF GM-CSF-INDUCED PMN ACTIVATION

It is well known that in-vivo administration of GM-CSF in both primates and humans induces a leukocytosis and monocytosis. GM-CSF in high enough doses can induce significant toxicities, such as fever, myalgias, rash, capillary leak syndrome, bone pain, and pericardial and pleural effusions (Brandt et al., 1988; Champlin et al., 1989). These toxicities may be due in part to the effects of GM-CSF on mature effector cells (Devereux et al., 1990). A number of investigators have described a reproducible and profound drop in the absolute neutrophil and monocyte count after intravenous boluses of both GM-CSF and G-CSF. It was determined that GM-CSF induced a rapid sequestration of neutrophils in the lung coincident with increased surface expression of Mo-1 and dramatic decreases in random neutrophil migration through skin windows (Peters et al., 1988). These effects may be due to TNF_α synthesis and release or to the induction and release of autocrine regulators such as LTB_4 and PAF, both of which can prime or directly activate neutrophils. Our work demonstrating direct induction of shape changes and F-actin polymerization by GM-CSF suggests another explanation of the observed leukopenia seen after CSF administration in vivo. Specifically, changes in mechanical deformability induced by GM-CSF may render them stiffer and thereby increase their entrapment in the capillary networks. This hypothesis was advanced previously for fMLP by others (Worthen et al., 1989). Recent work by Lundberg and Wright (1990), showing that the chemoattractant-induced leukopenia is not reversed by Mo-1 antibody administration in vivo, seems to provide additional indirect proof that this effect may not depend on specific adhesive receptor/endothelial interactions. We are currently investigating the effects of GM-CSF on the mechanical properties of neutrophils and correlating F-actin changes with filtration properties of these cells.

V. OTHER POTENTIAL GM-CSF SIGNALING PATHWAYS

A. Association with G-Proteins

GM-CSF indirectly primes neutrophils and monocytes for enhanced effector function in response to secondary stimuli such as chemotactic factors and immune serum. A number of laboratories have attempted to define pathways of GM-CSF signal transduction in neutrophils. These studies have been complicated by several factors, including the potential self-activation of neutrophils during the isolation process and subsequent incubation at 37°C. This process is gradual over time and may overshadow the direct effects of GM-CSF on neutrophils, which are subtle and frequently detectable only after the addition of secondary stimuli such as chemotactic factors. Many secondary activating factors are chemotactic agents whose effects on neutrophils are mediated through pertussis toxin (PT)-sensitive G-proteins. Therefore, using PT in an attempt to block the priming effect of GM-CSF could potentially be misinterpreted, since any inhibition by PT might be due to its effect on the secondary stimulus and not to the priming effect of GM-CSF. Some investigators have suggested that this priming effect of GM-CSF in vitro is simply to hasten activation events set in motion by the isolation and incubation of PMNs at 37°C (English et al., 1988). It should be noted in this regard that treatment with PT requires a prolonged incubation a 37°C (60–120 min) to achieve maximal ADP ribosylation and inhibition of the signal-transducing G-proteins. Furthermore, unless very purified populations of target cells (neutrophils) are used, one cannot eliminate the possibility that GM-CSF might directly stimulate the release of chemotactic factors or neutrophil-activating molecules such as LTB_4, PAF, or IL-8 from contaminating cells (i.e., monocytes), or perhaps, in an autocrine fashion, from neutrophils themselves. These activating molecules could then bind to their respective receptors on neutrophils and directly activate the cell. Since these activating molecules all transduce their signals through PT-sensitive G-proteins, the priming effect of GM-CSF might be falsely attributed to a direct association of the GM-CSF receptor with PT-sensitive G-proteins.

Nevertheless, several groups including our own have suggested that GM-CSF transduces selected signals via PT-sensitive G-proteins (Corey and Rosoff, 1989; Gomez-Cambronero et al., 1989; McColl et al., 1989; Mege et al., 1989; Richter et al., 1989). Indeed, because of these problems, the association of GM-CSF with neutrophil G-proteins has yet to be demonstrated conclusively. Such an association has been more clearly demonstrated in HL-60 cells and monocytes for both TNF and CSF-1 (Imamura et al., 1988a). In spite of these results, many effects of these cytokines are not inhibited by PT.

The ability of GM-CSF to directly activate a PT-inhibitable GTPase in purified neutrophil membranes, to increase the binding of ^{35}S-GTPγS to purified plasma membranes, to promote the co-purification of a GTP-binding protein with the human GM-CSF receptor (Polakis et al., 1988), or the demonstration that the GM-CSF receptor has multiple membrane-spanning domains similar to the muscarinic receptor, would, individually or together, lend strong support to such an association. The muscarinic receptor provides an example where binding of ligand results in the stimulation of a membrane-associated GTPase and activation of a G-protein. Recently, Matsuda et al. (1989) have underscored this finding by showing direct activation of a membrane-associated-GTPase by G-CSF in a murine myeloblastic cell line, NFS-60.

B. Association with the Phospholipase C and D Cascades

There has been no evidence thus far that GM-CSF activates the phospholipase C cascade. We and others have not shown any direct effect on calcium fluxes, protein kinase C activity or distribution, or generation of inositol phosphates or diacylglycerol (Sullivan et al., 1987; Coffey et al., 1988; Naccache et al., 1988; Corey and Rosoff, 1989; DiPersio et al., 1990b). Our laboratory demonstrated that GM-CSF, although without direct effect, could significantly enhance the ability of chemotactic factors to increase intracellular concentrations of free calcium in normal human neutrophils (Naccache et al., 1988). It is not clear if this enhanced calcium flux came from release of intracellular stores or from influx of calcium from the extracellular medium. Recent studies by Buorgoin et al. (1990) suggest that, in contrast to phospholipase C (PLC), GM-CSF can prime neutrophils in vitro for enhanced phosphatidic acid and diacylglycerol production via activation of neutrophil phospholipase D. Indeed, studies in other systems have indicated that intracellular alkalinization secondary to Na^+/H^+ exchange regulates hormone-associated DAG accumulation (Grinstein et al., 1989). The relationship of this pathway to GM-CSF signaling is discussed below.

C. Activation of Na^+ and K^+ Influx

Two independent reports suggest that both CSF-1 (Imamura and Kufe, 1988b) and TNF (Imamura et al., 1988a) directly stimulate Na^+ influx in mature monocytes and HL-60 cells, respectively. This effect could be inhibited by pertussis toxin, ouabain, and amiloride, suggesting the activation of a G-protein-induced Na^+/K^+ ATPase. GM-CSF has been shown to induce similar events in both human neutrophils (Gomez-Cambronero et al., 1989; DiPersio et al., 1990b) and human endothelial cells (Bussolino et al., 1989b).

These events are delayed and occur within 10 min of its addition to target cells. They therefore may not be the earliest signaling events after GM-CSF binding. The observed increase of intracellular pH seen after stimulation of neutrophils with chemotactic factors and phorbol esters (Simchowitz and Cragoe, 1988; Grinstein and Furuya, 1986) is paradoxically blocked by GM-CSF (Sullivan et al., 1987; Naccache et al., 1988; Gomez-Cambronero et al., 1989). This is not due to a direct inhibition of the Na^+/H^+ antiport. Although this seems contrary to the experiments mentioned above, a subtle activation of the Na^+/H^+ exchange mechanism by GM-CSF may inhibit further stimulation of this system with chemotactic agents or phorbol esters. This may also explain the increased chemotactic factor and phorbol ester-induced intracellular acidification when neutrophils are primed with GM-CSF. There are many other effects of GM-CSF which are resistant to pertussis toxin, suggesting alternative pathways of signaling. In addition, many of these inhibitors, such as ouabain, PT, and amiloride, have nonspecific inhibitory effects on cell function and viability, making interpretation of these results problematic.

D. Association with Cellular Tyrosine Kinases

A number of reports using murine and human myeloid leukemia cell lines suggest that GM-CSF and IL-3 induce the rapid phosphorylation of specific substrates (Farrar et al., 1990; Linnekin and Farrar, 1990; Evans et al., 1986; Evans et al., 1987; Sorenson et al., 1989; Ferris et al., 1988; Carroll et al., 1990; Kanakura et al., 1990, 1991). Recently, Gomez-Combronero et al. (1989) demonstrated that GM-CSF induced the rapid phosphorylation of a series of substrates in human neutrophils. We have found similar results, using antiphosphotyrosine immunoblotting—namely, that GM-CSF induces a rapid phosphorylation of at least 6 neutrophil substrates (150,000, 120,000, 95,000, 70,000, 54,000, and 40,000 Da). We have shown that two inhibitors of tryosine kinases (erbstatin and genistein) inhibit certain biological effects of GM-CSF coincident with their abilities to inhibit tyrosine phosphorylation induced by GM-CSF (DiPersio et al., 1990a). The effects of tyrosine phosphorylation in both neutrophils and leukemic cell lines occurs within minutes after GM-CSF-receptor engagement.

Of interest is that neither the α- nor β-subunits of the human GM-CSF receptor contain consensus sequences for classic tyrosine kinases. Therefore, the GM-CSF receptor-associated tyrosine kinase remains elusive. Recent data suggest that c-raf (a cellular threonine/serine kinase) is phosphorylated on both serine and tyrosine, resulting in activation of the c-raf kinase activity by both GM-CSF and IL-3 in IL-3/GM-CSF-dependent mouse and human myeloid leukemia cell lines (Carroll et al., 1990; Kanakura et al., 1991). Cellular proto-oncogenes are critical elements for signaling in many growth-factor target cell systems (Kahn and Graf, 1986). Again, the tyrosine kinases activated by GM-CSF which are required for c-raf phosphorylation remain a mystery. There are presently no data to suggest that c-raf is phosphorylated in neutrophils by GM-CSF. However, we and others have shown that 70,000-Da neutrophil substrate is phosphorylated on tyrosine by GM-CSF. The identity of this as c-raf awaits confirmation.

VI. GM-CSF RECEPTOR

Recent studies by Gearing et al. (1989) and Hayashida et al. (1990) suggest that the GM-CSF receptor is composed of at least two subunits (Figure 4). Both subunits are members of a novel superfamily of cytokine receptors (review: Cosman et al., 1990). The α-subunit, which is an 84,000-Da glycoprotein, is expressed in both hematopoietic and nonhematopoietic cells (Gasson et al., 1986; DiPersio et al., 1988c, 1991b). When expressed transiently in COS cells, this cDNA encodes a protein which binds GM-CSF with markedly decreased affinity ($K_d \approx$1-10 nM) compared to the endogenous high-affinity GM-CSF receptor. The β-subunit has significant homology with the murine IL-3 receptor cDNA, and when it is co-expressed with the α-subunit it converts low-affinity GM-CSF receptors ($k_d \approx$1-10 nM) to high-affinity receptors ($k_d \approx$10-50 pM). Neutrophils appear to express only the high-affinity recrptors (K_d 20–100 pM) composed of probable α/β-heterodimers. As noted, neither subunit is a tyrosine kinase and neither has multiple membrane-spanning domains similar to G-protein-associated receptors such as the PAF receptor (Honda et al., 1991), the fMLP receptor (Boulay et al., 1990), and rhodopsin-type receptors (Dohlman et al., 1987). How GM-CSF activates cellular tyrosine and serine/threonine kinases and stimulates the production of AA, PAF, and LTB_4 in neutrophils remains an active area of investigation, epecially if common receptor-signaling cascades operate in other cytokine-driven triggering systems such as interleukin-2-mediated T-cell mitogenesis (Farrar et al., 1990).

VII. SUMMARY

A hypothetical pathway of GM-CSF-induced signaling in human neutrophils is presented in Figure 4. The earliest postreceptor events leading to activation of cellular kinases and phosphorylation of c-raf on tyrosine and serine remain a mystery. It is conceivable that downstream events such as the production of LTB_4 and PAF as well as other autocrine or paracrine activators of neutrophil-activation function may be involved in neutrophil activation and priming, or they may be downstream events irrelevant in the signaling cascade. The association of GM-CSF signaling and G-proteins, PLD, c-raf, tyrosine kinases, and the Na^+/H^+ antiport remain poorly understood.

ACKNOWLEDGMENTS

This work was supported in part by grants from the American Cancer Society, number 4-444930-58633 and number 4-444930-58554; PHS grant HL 18208-15; and BRSG grant S7RR05403-27.

REFERENCES

1. Abboud CN, Kempski MC, Brennan JK. Neutrophil activation by colony-stimulating factors and interleukins: effects on cell shape and polarity. Blood 1990; 76(suppl):175a (abstr 690).
2. Addison IE, Johnson B, Devereux S, Goldstone AH, Linch DC. Granulocyte-macrophage colony-stimulating factor may inhibit neutrophil migration *in vivo.* Clin Exp Immunol 1989; 76:149–53.
3. Aglietta M, Monzeglio C, Apra F, Mossetti C, Stern AC, Giribaldi G, Bussolino F. In vivo priming of human neutrophils by granulocyte-macrophage colony-stimulating factor: effect on the production of platelet activating factor. Br J Haematol 1990; 75:333–9.
4. Appelbaum FR. The clinical use of hemopoietic growth factors. Sem Hematol 1989; 26(3, suppl 3):7–14.

5. Arnaout MA, Wang EA, Clark SC, Sieff CA. Human recombinant granulocyte-macrophage colony-stimulating factor increases cell-cell adhesion and surface expression of adhesion-promoting surface glycoproteins on mature granulocytes. J Clin Invest 1986; 78:597–601.
6. Atkinson YH, Lopez AF, Marasco WA, Lucas CM, Wong GG, Burns GF, Vadas MA. Recombinant human granulocyte-macrophage colony-stimulating factor (rH GM-CSF) regulates f Met-Leu-Phe receptors on human neutrophils. Immunology 1988; 64:519–25.
7. Avanzi GC, Lista P, Giovinazzo G, Miniero R, Saglio G, Benetton G, Coda R, Cattoretti G, Pegoraro L. Selective growth response to IL-3 of a human leukaemic cell line with megakaryoblastic features. Br J Haematol 1988; 69:359–66.
8. Baldwin GC, Gasson JC, Quan SG, Fleischmann J, Weisbart R, Oette D, Mitsuyasu RT, Golde DW. Granulocyte-macrophage colony-stimulating factor enhances neutrophil function in acquired immunodeficiency syndrome patients. Proc Natl Acad Sci USA 1988; 85:2763–6.
9. Bass DA, Gerard C, Olbrantz P, Wilson J, McCall CE, McPhail LC. Priming of the respiratory burst of neutrophils by diacyglycerol. Independence from activation or translocation of protein kinase C. J Biol Chem 1987; 262:6643–9.
10. Bauldry SA, Wykle RL, Bass DA. Phospholipase A2 activation in human neutrophils. Differential actions of diacylglycerols and aklylacyglycerols in priming cells for stimulation by N-formyl-Met-Leu-Phe. J Biol Chem 1988; 263:16787–95.
11. Begley CG, Lopez AF, Nicola NA, Warren DJ, Vadas MA, Sanderson CJ, Metcalf D. Purified colony-stimulating factors enhance the survival of human neutrophils and eosinophils in vitro: a rapid and sensitive microassay for colony-stimulating factors. Blood 1986; 68:162–6.
12. Billah MM, Bryant RW, Siegel MI. Lipoxygenase products of arachidonic acid modulate biosynthesis of platelet-activating factor (1-O-alkyl-2-acetyl-sn-glycero-3-phosphocholine) by human neutrophil via phospholipase A2. J Biol Chem 1985; 260:6899–906.
13. Bomalaski JS, Baker DG, Brophy L, Spilberg RNV I, Muniain M, Clark MA. A phospholipase A2-activity protein (PLAP) stimulates human neutrophil aggregation and release of lysomal enzymes, superoxine and eicosanoids. J Immunol 1989; 142:3957–62.
14. Boulay F, Tardif M, Bruchon L, Vignais P. Synthesis and use of a novel N-formyl peptide derivative to isolate a human N-fotmyl peptide receptor cDNA. Biochem Biophys Res Commun 1990; 168:1103–9.
15. Bourgoin S, Plante E, Gaudry M, Naccache PH, Borgeat P, Poubelle PE. Involvement of a phospholipase D in the mechanism of action of granulocyte-macrophage colony-stimulating factor (GM-CSF): priming of human neutrophils in vitro with GM-CSF is associated with accumulation of phosphatidic acid and diradylglycerol. J Exp Med 1990; 172:767–77.
16. Brandt ST, Peters WP, Atwater SK, Kuerzberg J, Borowitz MJ, Jones RB, Shpall EJ, Bast RC, Gilbert CJ, Oette DH. Effect of recombinant human granulocyte-macrophage colony stimulating factor on hematopoietic reconstitution after high dose chemotherapy and autologous bone marrow transplantation. N Engl J Med 1988; 318:869–876.
17. Broxmeyer HE, Vadhan RS. Preclinical and clinical studies with the hematopoietic colony-stimulating factors and related interleukins. Immunol Res 1989; 8:185–201.
18. Bussolino F, Wang JM, Turrini F, Alessi D, Ghigo D, Costamagna C, Pescarmona G, Mantovani A, Bosia A. Stimulation of the Na^+/H^+ exchanger in human endothelial cells activated by granulocyte- and granulocyte-macrophage-colony-stimulating factor. J Biol Chem 1989a; 264:18284–7.
19. Bussolino F, Wang JM, DiFilippi P, Turrini F, Sanavio F, Edgell CJ, Aglietta M, Arese P, Mantovani A. Granulocyte and granulocyte-macrophage colony stimulating factors induce endothelial cells to migrate and proliferate. Nature 1989b; 337:471–3.

20. Cairo MS, VandeVen C, Toy C, Mauss D, Sheikh K, Kommareddy S, Modanlou H. Lymphokines: enhancement by granulocyte-macrophage and granulocyte colony-stimulating factors of neonatal myeloid kinetics and functional activation of polymorphonuclear leucocytes. Rev Infect Dis 1990; 12(suppl 4):492–7.
21. Carroll M, Clark-Lewis I, Rapp U, May WS. Interleukin 3 and granulocyte-macrophage colony-stimulating factor mediate rapid phosphorylation and activation of cytosolic c-raf. J Biol Chem 1990; 265:19812–7.
22. Champlin RE, Nimer SD, Ireland P, Oette DH, Golde DW. Treatment of refractory aplastic anemia with recombinant human granulocyte-macrophage-colony-stimulating factor. Blood 1989; 73:694–9.
23. Chan JY, Slamon DJ, Nimer SD, Golde DW, Gasson JC. Regulation of expression of human granulocyte-macrophage colony-stimulating factor. Proc Natl Acad Sci USA 1986; 83:8669-73.
24. Clark SC, Kamen R. The human hematopoietic colony-stimulating factors. Science 1987; 236:1229–37.
25. Clark MA, Chen MJ, Crooke ST, Bomalaski JS. Tumor necrosis factor (Cachectin) induces phospholipase A2 activity and the synthesis of a phospholipase A2 activating protein (PLAP) in endothelial cells. Biochem J 1988; 250:125–32.
26. Coëffier E, Delautier D, Le Couedic J-P, Chignard M, Denizot Y, Benveniste J. Cooperation between platelets and neutrophils for Paf-Aceter (platelet-activating factor) formation. J Leukocyte Biol 1990; 47:234–43.
27. Coffey RG, Davis JS, Djeu JY. Stimulation of guanylate cyclase activity and reduction of adenylate cyclase activity by granulocyte-macrophage colony-stimulating factor in human blood neutrophils. J Immunol 1988; 140:2695–701.
28. Colotta F, Wang JM, Polentarutti N, Mantovani A. Expression of c-fos protooncogene in normal human peripheral blood granulocytes. J Exp Med 1987; 165:1224–9.
29. Corey SJ, Rosoff PM. Granulocyte-macrophage colony-stimulating factor primes neutrophils by activating a pertussis toxin-sensitive G protein not associated with phosphatidylinositol turnover. J Biol Chem 1989; 264:14165–71.
30. Cosman D, Lyman SD, Idzerda RL, Beckmann MP, Park LS, Goodwin RG, March CJ. A new cytokine receptor superfamily. TIBS 1990; 15:265–70.
31. Czarnetzki BM, Csato M. Comparative studies of human eosinophil migration towards platelet-activating factor and leukotriene B4. Int Arch Allergy Appl Immunol 1989; 88:191–3.
32. Dahinden CA, Zingg J, Maly FE, De Weck AL. Leukotriene production in human neutrophils primed by recombinant human granulocyte-macrophage colony-stimulating factor and stimulated with complement component C5A and FMLP as second signals. J Exp Med 1988; 167:1281–95.
33. Denzlinger C, Kapp A, Grimberg M, Gerhartz HH, Wilmanns W. Enhanced endogenous leukotriene biosynthesis in patients treated with granulocyte-macrophage colony-stimulating factor. Blood 1990; 76:1765–70.
34. Devereux S, Linch DC, Campos CD, Spittle MF, Jelliffe AM. Transient leucopenia induced by granulocyte-macrophage colony-stimulating factor (letter). Lancet 1987; 2:1523–4.
35. Devereux S, Bull HA, Campos-Costa D, Saib R, Linch DC. Granulocyte-macrophage colony-stimulating factor induced changes in cellular adhesion molecule expression and adhesion to endothelium: in vivo and in vitro studies in man. Br J Haematol 1989; 71:323–30.
36. Devereux S, Porter JB, Hoyes KP, Abeysinghe RD, Saib R, Linch DC. Secretion of neutrophil secondary granules occurs during granulocyte-macrophage colony stimulating factor induced margination. Br J Haematol 1990; 74:17–23.

37. Dewald B, Payne TG, Baggiolini M. Activation of NADPH oxidase of human neutrophils. Potentiation of chemotactic peptide by a diacylglycerol. Biochem Biophys Res Commun 1984; 125:367–73.
38. DiPersio JF, Billing P, Williams R, Gasson JC. Human granulocyte-macrophage colony-stimulating factor and other cytokines prime human neutrophils for enhanced arachidonic acid release and leukotriene B_4 synthesis. J Immunol 1988a; 140:4315–22.
39. DiPersio JF, Naccache PH, Borgeat P, Gasson JC, Nguyen M, McColl SR. Characterization of the priming effects of human granulocyte-macrophage colony-stimulating factor on human leukotriene synthesis. Prostaglandins 1988b; 36:673–91.
40. DiPersio JF, Billing P, Kaufman S, Eghtesady P, William RE, Gasson JC. Characterization of the human granulocyte-macrophage colony-stimulating factor receptor. J Biol Chem 1988c; 263:1834–41.
41. DiPersio JF, Aggarwal S, Naccache PH, Umizawa K, McColl S. Effect of GM-CSF on neutrophil LTB4 and IL-8 receptor expression: association with a cellular tyrosine kinase. Blood 1990a; 76(suppl 1):179a (abs 708).
42. DiPersio JF, Golde DW, Gasson JC. GM-CSF:receptor structure and transmembrane signaling. Int J Cell Cloning 1990b 8(suppl 1):63–74.
43. DiPersio JF, Aggarwal S, Golde DW. GM-CSF induces neutrophil platelet activating factor (PAF) synthesis: activation of lyso-PAF acetyltransferase. Blood 1990c; 76(suppl 1):179a (abst 707).
44. DiPersio JF, Hedvat C, Gasson JC. GM-CSF activates neutrophils via distinct autocrine pathways: direct effect on LTB_4 synthesis and LTB_4 receptor down regulation. Submitted 1991a.
45. DiPersio JF, Hedvat C, Ford CF, Golde DW, Gasson JC. Characterization of the soluble human GM-CSF receptor complex. J Biol Chem 1991b; 266:279–86.
46. Dixon RA, Diehl RE, Opas E, Rands E, Vickers PJ, Evans JF, Gillard JW, Miller DK. Requirements of a 5-lipoxygenase-activating protein for leukotriene synthesis. Nature 1990; 343:282–4.
47. Djeu JY, Blanchard DK. Regulation of human polymorphonuclear neutrophil (PMN) activity against *Candida albicans* by large granular lymphocytes via release of a PMN-activating factor. J Immunol 1987a; 139:2761–7.
48. Djeu JY, Serboursek D, Smith-Joyner M, Blanchard DK. Enhancement of anti-tumor activity in human polymorphonuclear neutrophils (PMN) and monocytes by granulocyte-macrophage colony-stimulating (GM-CSF). Fed Proc 1987b; 46:1511 (abst 6972).
49. Dohlman HG, Carron MG, Lefkowitz RJ. A family of receptors coupled to guanine nucleotide regulatory proteins. Biochemistry 1987; 26:2657–64.
50. Dubois C, Bissonnette E, Rola-Pleszczynski M. Platelet-activating factor (PAF) enhances tumor necrosis factor production by alveolar macrophages: prevention by PAF receptor antagonists and lipoxygenase inhibitors. J Immunol 1989; 143:964–70.
51. English D, Broxmeyer HE, Gabig TG, Akard LP, Williams DE, Hoffman R. Temporal adaptation of neutrophil oxidative responsiveness to n-formyl-methionyl-leucyl-phenylalanine. Acceleration by granulocyte-macrophage colony stimulating factor. J Immunol 1988; 141:2400–6.
52. Ernst TJ, Ritchie AR, O'Rourke R, Griffin JD. Colony-stimulating factor gene expression in human acute myeloblastic leukemia cells is posttranscriptionally regulated. Leukemia 1989; 3:620–5.
53. Evans SW, Rennick D, Farrar WL. Multilineage hematopoietic growth factor IL-3 and direct activators of protein kinase C stimulate phosphorylation of common substrates. Blood 1986; 68:906–13.
54. Evans SW, Rennick D, Farrar WL. Identification of a signal-transduction pathway shared by haemopoietic growth factors with diverse biological specificity. Biochem J 1987; 244:683–91.

55. Fabian I, Baldwin GC, Golde DW. Biosynthetic granulocyte-macrophage colony-stimulating factor enhances neutrophil cytotoxicity toward human leukemia cells. Leukemia 1987; 1:613–7.
56. Farrar WL, Linnekin D. Lymphohematopoietic factors and biological control mechanisms. Prog Clin Biol Res 1990; 352:269–76.
57. Farrar WL, Garcia G-G, Evans G, Michiel D, Linnekin D. Cytokine regulation of protein phosphorylation. Cytokine 1990; 2:77–91.
58. Ferris DK, Willete-Brown J, Martensen T, Farrar WL. IL-3 stimulation of tyrosine kinase activity in FDCP-P1 cells. Biochem Biophys Res Commun 1988; 154:991–6.
59. Fiore S, Serhan CN. Formation of lipoxins and leukotrienes during receptor-mediated interactions of human platelets and recombinant human granulocyte/macrophage colony-stimulating factor-primed neutrophils. J Exp Med 1990; 172:1451–7.
60. Fleischmann J, Golde DW, Weisbart RH, Gasson JC. Granulocyte-macrophage colony-stimulating factor enhances phagocytosis of bacteria by human neutrophils. Blood 1986; 68:708–11.
61. Fletcher MP, Gasson JC. Enhancement of neutrophil functions by granulocyte-macrophage colony-stimulating factor involves recruitment of a less responsive subpopulation. Blood 1988; 71:652–8.
62. Garcia JGN, Azghani A, Callahan KS, Johnson AR. Effect of platelet activating factor on leukocyte-endothelial cell interactions. Thrombosis Res 1988; 51:83–96.
63. Gasson JC, Weisdorf RH, Kaufman SE, Clark SC, Hewick RM, Wong GC, Golde DW. Purified granulocyte-macrophage colony-stimulating factor: direct action on neutrophils. Science 1984; 226:1339–42.
64. Gasson JC, Kaufman SE, Weisbart RH, Tomonaga M, Golde DW. High-affinity binding of granulocyte-macrophage colony-stimulating factor to normal and leukemic human myeloid cells. Proc Natl Acad Sci USA 1986; 83:669–73.
65. Gay JC, Beckman, JK, Brash AR, Oates JA, Lukens JN. Enhancement of chemotactic factor-stimulated neutrophil oxidase metabolism by leukotriene B4. Blood 1984; 64:780–5.
66. Gearing D, King JA, Gough NA, Nicola NA. Expression cloning of a receptor for human granulocyte-macrophage colony-stimulating factor. EMBO J 1989; 8:3667–76.
67. Goldman DW, Goetzl EJ. Heterogeneity of human polymorphonuclear leukocyte receptors for leukotriene B4. Identification of a subset of high affinity receptors that transduce the chemotactic response. J Exp Med 1984; 159:1027–41.
68. Gomez-Chambronero J, Yamazaki M, Metwally F, Molski TF, Bonak VA, Huang C, Becker EL, Sha'afi RI. Granulocyte-macrophage colony-stimulating factor and human neutrophils: roles of guanine nucleotide regulatory proteins. Proc Natl Acad Sci USA 1989; 86:3569–73.
69. Gough NM. The hemopoietic growth factor, granulocyte-macrophage colony stimulating factor. In: Habenicht A, ed. Growth factors, differentiation factors and cytokines. Berlin Heidelberg: Springer-Verlag 1990:177–87.
70. Grabstein KH, Urdal DL, Tushinski RJ, Mochizuki EY, Price VL, Cantrell MA, Gillis S, Conlon PJ. Induction of macrophage tumoricidal activity by granulocyte-macrophage colony-stimulating factor. Science 1988; 232:506–8.
71. Griffin JD, Spertini O, Ernst TJ, Belvin MP, Levine HB, Kanakura Y, Tedder TF. Granulocyte-macrophage colony-stimulating factor and other cytokines regulate surface expression of the leukocyte adhesion molecule-1 on human neutrophils, monocytes, and their precursors. J Immunol 1990; 145:576–84.
72. Grinstein S, Furuya W. Characterization of the amiloride-sensitive Na^+/H^+ antiport of human neutrophils. Am J Physiol 1986; C283–91.
73. Grinstein S, Rotin D, Mason MJ. Na^+/H^+ exchange and growth factor-induced cytosolic pH changes. Role in cellular proliferation. Biochim Biophys Acta 1989; 988:73–97.

74. Groopman JE, Mitsuyasu RT, DeLeo MJ, Oette DH, Golde DW. Effect of recombinant human granulocyte-macrophage colony-stimulating factor on myelopoiesis in the acquired immunodeficiency syndrome. N Engl J Med 1987; 317:593–8.
75. Guthrie LA, McPhail LC, Henson PM, Johnston RJ. Priming of neutrophils for enhanced release of oxygen metabolites by bacterial lipopolysaccharide. Evidence for increased activity of the superoxide-producing enzyme. J Exp Med 1984; 160:1656–71.
76. Häkansson L, Venge P. Inhibition of neutrophil and eosinophil chemotactic responses to PAF by the PAF-antagonists WEB-2086, L-652,731, and SRI-63441. J Leukocyte Biol 1990; 47:449–56.
77. Hannigan G, Williams R. Signal transduction by interferon alpha through arachidonic acid metabolism. Science 1991; 251:204–7.
78. Hart PH, Vitti GF, Burgess DR, Whitty GA, Royston K, Hamilton JA. Activation of human monocytes by granulocyte-macrophage colony-stimulating factor: increased urokinase-type plasminogen activator activity. Blood 1991; 77:841–8.
79. Hayashida K, Kitamura T, Gorman DM, Arai KI, Yokota T, Miyajima A. Molecular cloning of a second subunit of the receptor for human granulocyte-macrophage colony-stimulating factor (GM-CSF): reconstitution of a high affinity GM-CSF receptor. Proc Natl Acad Sci USA 1990; 87:9655–9.
80. Herrmann F, Vellenga E. The role of colony-stimulating factors in acute leukemia. J Cancer Res Clin Oncol 1990; 116:275–82.
81. Hirata F, Axelrod J, Crews FT. Concanavalin A stimulates phospholipid methylation and phosphatidylserine decarboxylation in rat mast cells. Proc Natl Acad Sci USA 1979; 76:4813–6.
82. Honda Z-I, Nakamura M, Miki I, Minami M, Watanabe T, Seyama Y, Okado H, Toh H, Ito K, Miyamoto T, Shimizu T. Cloning by functional expression of platelet-activating factor receptor from guinea-pig lung. Nature 1991; 349:342–50.
83. Imamura K, Sherman ML, Spriggs D, Kufe D. Effect of tumor necrosis factor on GTP binding and GTPase activity in HL-60 and L929 cells. J Biol Chem 1988a; 263:10247–53.
84. Imamura K, Kufe D. Colony-stimulating factor 1-induced Na^+ influx into human monocytes involves activation of a pertussis toxin-sensitive GTP-binding protein. J Biol Chem 1988b; 263:14093–8.
85. Ingraham LM, Lafuze JE, Boxer LA, Baehner RL. In vitro and in vivo effects of treatment by platelet-activating factor on N-formyl-met-leu-phe-mediated responses of polymorphonuclear leukocytes. Br J Haematol 1987; 66:219–25.
86. Kahn P, Graf T. Oncogenes and growth control. Berlin Heidelberg: Springer Verlag, 1986:138–146, 253–258.
87. Kanakura Y, Druke B, Cannistra SA, Furukawa Y, Torimoto Y, Griffin JD. Signal transduction of the human granulocyte-macrophage colony-stimulating factor and interleukin-3 receptors involves tyrosine phosphorylation of a common set of cytoplasmic proteins. Blood 1990; 76:706–15.
88. Kanakura Y, Drucker B, Wood KW, Mamon HJ, Okuda K, Roberts TM, Griffin JD. Granulocyte-macrophage colony-stimulating factor and interleukin-3 induce a rapid phosphorylation and activation of the proto-oncogene Raf-1 in human factor dependent myeloid cell line. Blood 1991; 77:243–8.
89. Kapp A, Zeck-Kapp G, Danner M, Luger TA. Human granulocyte-macrophage colony-stimulating factor: an effective direct activator of human polymorpho-nuclear neutrophilic granulocytes. J Invest Dermatol 1988; 91:49–55.
90. Karnad AB, Hartshorn KL, Wright J, Myers JB, Schwartz JB, Tauber AI. Priming of human neutrophils with N-Formyl-Methionyl-Leucyl-Phenylalanine by a calcium-independent, pertussis toxin-insensitive pathway. Blood 1989; 74:2519–26.
91. Kauffman SE, DiPersio JF, Gasson JC. Effects of human GM-CSF on neutrophil degranulation in vitro. Exp Hematol 1989; 17:800–4.

92. Kharazmi A, Nielsen H, Bendtzen K. Modulation of human neutrophil and monocyte chemotaxis and superoxide responses by recombinant TNF-alpha and GM-CSF. Immunobiology 1988; 177:363–70.
93. Koeffler HP, Gasson JC, Ranyard J, Souza L, Shepard M, Munker R. Recombinant human TNF alpha stimulate production of granulocyte colony-stimulating factor. Blood 1987; 70:55–9.
94. Koeffler HP, Gasson J, Tobler A. Transcriptional and posttranscriptional modulation of myeloid growth factor expression by tumor necrosis factor and other agents. Mol Cell Biol 1988; 8:3432–8.
95. König W, Schönfeld W, Raulf M, Köller M, Knöller J, Scheffer J, Brom J. The neutrophil and leukotrienes—role in health and disease. Eicosanoids 1990; 3:1–22.
96. Kownatzki E, Liehl E, Aschauer H, Uhrich S. Inhibition of chemotactic migration of human neutrophilic granulocytes by recombinant human granulocyte-macrophage colony-stimulating factor. Immunopharmacology 1990; 19:139–43.
97. Le Beau MM, Lemons RS, Espinosa R III, Larson RA, Arai N, Rowley JD. Interleukin-4 and interleukin-5 map to the human chromosome 5 in a region encoding growth factors and receptors and are deleted in myeloid leukemias with a del(5q). Blood 1989; 73:647–50.
98. Lieschke GJ, Cebum J, Morstyn G. Characterization of the clinical effects after the first dose of bacterially synthesized recombinant human granulocyte-macrophage colony-stimulating factor. Blood 1989; 74:2634–43.
99. Lindemann A, Riedel D, Oster W, Meuer SC, Blohm RH, Mertelsmann RH, Hermann F. Granulocyte/macrophage colony-stimulating factor induces interleukin 1 production by human polymorphonuclear neutrophils. J Immunol 1988; 140:837–9.
100. Lopez AF, Williamson DJ, Gamble JR, Begley CG, Harlan JM, Klebanoff SJ, Waltersdorph A, Wong GC, Clark SC, Vadas MA. Recombinant human granulocyte-macrophage colony-stimulating factor stimulates in vitro mature human neutrophils and eosinophil function, surface receptor expression, and survival. J Clin Invest 1986; 78:1220–8.
101. Lundberg C, Wright SD. Relation of the CD11/CD18 family of leucocyte antigens to the transient neutropenia caused by chemoattractants. Blood 1990; 76:1240–5.
102. Matsuda S, Shirafuji N, Asano S. Human granulocyte colony-stimulating factor specifically binds to murine myeloblastic NFS-60 cells and activates their guanosine triphosphate binding proteins/adenylate cyclase system. Blood 1989; 74:2343–8.
103. Matsushima K, Oppenheim JJ. Interleukin 8 and MCAF: novel inflammatory cytokines inducible by IL 1 and TNF. Cytokine 1989; 1:2–13.
104. McColl SR, Kreis C, DiPersio JF, Borgeat P, Nacchache PH. Involvement of guanine nucleotide binding proteins in neutrophil activation and priming by GM-CSF. Blood 1989; 73:588–91.
105. McColl SR, Paquin R, Beaulieu AD. Selective synthesis and secretion of a 23 kd protein by neutrophils following stimulation with granulocyte-macrophage colony-stimulating factor and tumor necrosis factor-alpha. Biochem Biophys Res Commun 1990; 172:1209–16.
106. Mege J, Gomez-Cambronero J, Molski TFP, Becker EL, Sha'afi RI. Effect of granulocyte-macrophage colony-stimulating factor on superoxide production in cytoplasts and intact human neutrophils: role of protein kinase and G-proteins. J Leukocyte Biol 1989; 46:161–8.
107. Metcalf D. The molecular biology and functions of the granulocyte-macrophage colony-stimulating factors. Blood 1986; 67:257–67.
108. Miller DK, Gillard JW, Vickers PJ, Sadowski S, Leveille C, Mancini JA, Charleson P, Dixon RA, Ford-Hutchinson AW, Fortin R, Gauthier JY, Rodkey J, Rosen R, Rouzer C, Sigal IS, Strader CD, Evans JF. Identification and isolation of a membrane protein necessary for leukotriene production. Nature 1990; 343:278–81.
109. Munker R, Gasson JC, Ogawa M, Koeffler HP. Recombinant human TNF induces production of granulocyte-macrophage colony-stimulating factor. Nature 1986; 323:79–82.

110. Naccache PH, Faucher N, Borgeat P, Gasson JC, DiPersio JF. Granulocyte-macrophage colony-stimulating factor modulates the excitation coupling sequence in human neutrophils. J Immunol 1988; 140:3541–6.
111. Neuman E, Huleatt JW, Jack RM. Granulocyte-macrophage colony-stimulating factor increases synthesis and expression of CR1 and CR3 by human peripheral blood neutrophils. J Immunol 1990; 145:3325–32.
112. Nimer SD, Morrita EA, Martis MJ, Waschman W, Gasson JC. Characterization of the human granulocyte-macrophage colony-stimulating factor promoter region by genetic analysis: correlation with DNase I footprinting. Mol Cell Biol 1988; 8:1979–84.
113. Nimer SD, Gates MJ, Koeffler HP, Gasson JC. Multiple mechanisms control the expression of granulocyte-macrophage colony-stimulating factor by human fibroblasts. J Immunol 1989; 143:2374–7.
114. Niwa Y, Sakane T, Taniguchi S. Phospholipid transmethylation in the membrane of human neutrophils and lymphocytes. Arch Biochem Biophys 1984; 234:7–14.
115. O'Flaherty JT, Surles JR, Redman J, Jacobson JD, Piantadosi C, Wylke RL. Binding and metabolism of platelet-activating factor by human neutrophils. J Clin Invest 1986a; 78:381–8.
116. O'Flaherty JT, Kosfeld S, Nishihira J. Binding and metabolism of leukotriene B4 by neutrophils and their subcellular organelles. J Cell Physiol 1986b; 126:359–70.
117. Oster W, Schulz G. Interleukin 3: biological and clinical effects. Int J Cell Cloning 1991; 9:5–23.
118. Owen WJ, Rothenberg ME, Silberstein DS, Gasson JC, Stevens RL, Austen KF, Soberman RJ. Regulation of human eosinophil viability, density, and function by granulocyte/macrophage colony-stimulating factor in the presence of 3T3 fibroblasts. J Exp Med 1987; 166:129–41.
119. Packman CH, Lichtman MA. Activation of neutrophils: measurement of actin conformational changes by flow cytometry. Blood Cells 1990; 16:193–207.
120. Park LS, Friend D, Gillis S, Urdal DL. Characterization of the cell surface receptor for granulocyte-macrophage colony-stimulating factor. J Biol Chem 1986; 261:4177–83.
121. Peters W, Stuart A, Affronti M, Kim C, Coleman R. Neutrophil migration is defective during recombinant human granulocyte-macrophage colony-stimulating factor infusion after autologous bone marrow transplantation in humans. Blood 1988; 72:1310–5.
122. Polakis PG, Uhing RJ, Snyderman R. The formylpeptide chemoattractant receptor copurifies with a GTP-binding proten containing a distinct 40-kDa pertussis toxin substrate. J Biol Chem 1988; 263:4969–76.
123. Richter J, Andersson T, Olsson I. Effect of tumor necrosis factor and granulocyte/macrophage colony-stimulating factor on neutrophil degranulation. J Immunol 1989; 42:3199–205.
124. Rouzer CA, Ford-Hutchinson AW, Morton HE, Gillard JW. MK886, a potent and specific leukotriene biosynthesis inhibitor blocks and reverses the membrane association of 5-lipoxygenase in ionophore-challenged leukocytes. J Biol Chem 1990; 265:1436–42.
125. Sanderson CJ, Warren DJ, Strath M. Identification of a lymphokine that stimulates eosinophil differentiation in vitro. Its relationship to interleukin 3, and functional properties of eosinophils produced in cultures. J Exp Med 1985; 162:60–74.
126. Sanjar S, Smith D, Kings MA, Morley J. Pretreatment with rh-GMCSF, but not IL-3 enhances PAF-induced eosinophil accumulation in guinea-pig airways. Br J Pharmacol 1990; 100:399–400.
127. Shalit M, Dabiri GA, Southwick FS. Platelet-activating factor both stimulates and "primes" human polymorphonuclear leukocyte actin filament assembly. Blood 1987; 70:1921–7.
128. Shaw G, Kamen R. A conserved AU sequence from the 3′ untranslated region of GM-CSF

mRNA mediates selective mRNA degradation. Cell 1986; 46:659–67.

129. Shibata Y, McCaffrey PG, Sato H, Oghiso Y. Calcium ionophore but not phorbol ester promotes eicosanoids release by proliferating interleukine-3-dependent bone marrow cells. Blood 1990; 76:1586–92.

130. Silberstein DS, Owen WF, Gasson JC, DiPersio JF, Golde DW, Bina JC, Soberman R, Austen KF, David JR. Enhancement of eosinophil cytotoxicity and leukotriene synthesis by biosynthetic (recombinant) granulocyte-macrophage colony-stimulating factor. J Immunol 1986; 137:3290–4.

131. Simchowitz L, Cragoe EJ. Na^{+}-Ca^{2+} exchange in human neutrophils. Am J Physiol 1988; 254:C150–64.

132. Smith RJ, Justen JM, Sam LM. Recombinant human granulocyte-macrophage colony-stimulating factor induces granule exocytosis from human polymorphonuclear neutrophils. Inflammation 1990; 14:83–92.

133. Socinski MA, Cannistra SA, Sullivan R, Elias A, Antman K, Schnipper L, Griffin JD. Granulocyte-macrophage colony-stimulating factor induces the expression of the CD11b surface adhesion molecule on human granulocytes in vivo. Blood 1988; 72:691–7.

134. Sorenson PHB, Mui A, Murthy S, Krystal G. IL-3, GM-CSF, and TPA induce distinct phosphorylation events in an IL-3 dependent multipotential cell line. Blood 1989; 13:406–18.

135. Stewart AG, Dubbin PN, Harris T, Dusting GJ. Platelet-activating factor may act as a second messenger in the release of icosanoids and superoxide anions from leukocytes and endothelial cells. Proc Natl Acad Sci USA 1990; 87:3215–9.

136. Sullivan R, Griffin JD, Simons ER, Schafer AI, Meshulam T, Fredette JP, Maas AK, Gadenne AS, Leavitt JL, Melnick DA. Effects of recombinant human granulocyte and granulocyte-macrophage colony-stimulating factors on signal transduction pathways in human granulocytes. J Immunol 1987; 139:3422–30.

137. Sullivan R, Griffin JD, Wright J, Melnick DA, Leavitt JL, Fredette JP, Horne JH, Lyman CA, Lazzari KG, Simons ER. Effects of recombinant human granulocyte-macrophage colony-stimulating factor on intracellular pH in mature granulocytes. Blood 1988; 72:1665–73.

138. Takatsu K, Tominaga A. Interleukin 5 as a hematopoietic and differentiation factor. In: Habenicht A, ed. Growth factors, differentiation factors and cytokines. Berlin Heidelberg: Springer Verlag, 1990:147–62.

139. Toothill VJ, Van-Mourik JA, Niewenhuis HK, Metzelaar MJ, Pearson JD. Characterization of the enhanced adhesion of neutrophil leucocytes to thrombin-stimulated endothelial cells. J Immunol 1990; 145:283–91.

140. Tsai-Morris CH, Cao X, Sukhatme VP. 5′ Flanking sequence and genomic structure of egr-1, a murine mitogen inducing zinc finger. Nucleic Acid Res 1988; 16:8835–45.

141. Vallance SJ, Downes P, Cragoe EJ, Whetton AD. Granulocyte-macrophage colony-stimulating factor can stimulate macrophage proliferation via persistent activation of the Na^{+}/H^{+} antiport. Biochem J 1990; 265:359–64.

142. Valone FJ, Goetzl EJ. Specific binding by human polymorphonuclear leucocytes of the immunological mediator 1-O-hexadecyl/octadecyl-2-acetyl-sn-glycero-3-phosphorylcholine. Immunology 1983; 48:141–9.

143. Varnum BC, Lim RW, Kujubu DA, Luner SJ, Kaufman SE, Greenberger JS, Gasson JC, Herschman HR. Granulocyte-macrophage colony-stimulating factor and tetradecanoyl phorbol acetate induce a distinct, restricted subset of primary response TIS genes in both proliferating and terminally differentiated myeloid cells. Mol Cell Biol 1989; 9:3580–3.

144. Vercellotti GM, Yin HQ, Gustafson KS, Nelson RD, Jacob HS. Platelet-activating factor primes neutrophil responses to agonists: role in promoting neutrophil-mediated endothelial damage. Blood 1988; 71:1100–7.

145. Villalta F, Kierszenbau MF. Effects of human colony stimulating factor on the uptake and destruction of a pathogenic parasite (*Trypanozoma cruzi*) by human neutrophils. J Immunol 1986; 137:1703–7.
146. Wang JM, Collela S, Allavena P, Mantovani A. Chemotactic activity of human recombinant granulocyte-macrophage colony-stimulating factor. Immunoloy 1987; 60:439–44.
147. Weisbart RH, Golde DW, Clark SC, Wong GC, Gasson JC. Human granulocyte-macrophage colony-stimulating factor is a neutrophil activator. Nature 1985; 314:361–3.
148. Weisbart RH, Golde DW, Gasson JW. Biosynthetic human GM-CSF modulates the number and affinity of neutrophil f-Met-Leu-Phe receptors. J Immunol 1986; 137:3584–7.
149. Weisbart RH, Kwan L, Golde DW, Gasson JC. Human GM-CSF primes neutrophils for enhanced oxidative metabolism in response to the major physiological chemoattractants. Blood 1987; 69:18–21.
150. Weisbart RH, Kacena H, Schuh A, Golde DW. GM-CSF induces human neutrophil IgA-mediated phagocytosis by an IgA Fc receptor activation mechanism. Nature 1988; 332:647–8.
151. Wirthmueller U, De Weck AL, Dahinden CA. Platelet-activating factor production in human neutrophils by sequential stimulation with granulocyte-macrophage colony-stimulating factor and the chemotactic factors C5A and formyl-methionyl-leucyl-phenylalanine. J Immunol 1989; 142:3213–8.
152. Worthen GS, Schwab B III, Elson EL, Downey GP. Mechanisms of stimulated neutrophils: cell stiffening induces retention in capillaries. Science 1989; 245:183–6.
153. Yang YC, Kovaciacs S, Kris R, Wolf S, Clark SC, Wellems TE, Neinhuis A, Epstein N. The human genes for GM-CSF and IL-3 are closely linked in tandem on chromosome 5. Blood 1988; 71:958–68.
154. Yong K, Rowles P, Webster ADB, Linch DC. GM-CSF-mediated neutrophil adhesion to endothelium. Blood 1990; 76(suppl 1):199a (abs 786).
155. Young DC, Wagner K, Griffin JD. Constitutive expression of the GM-CSF gene in acute myeloblastic leukemia. J Clin Invest 1987; 79:100–6.
156. Yue TL, Rabinovici R, Farhat M, Feurstein G. Pharmacologic profile of BN 50739 a new PAF antagonist in vitro and in vivo. Prostaglandins 1990; 39:469–80.
157. Yuo A, Kitagawa S, Ohsaka A, Ohta M, Miyazono K, Okabe T, Urabe A, Saito M, Takaku F. Recombinant human granulocyte-macrophage colony-stimulating factor as an activator of human granulocytes: potentiation of responses triggered by receptor-mediated agonists and stimulation of C3bi receptor expression and adherence. Blood 1989; 74:2144–9.
158. Zimmerman GA, McIntyre TM, Mehra M, Prescott SM. Endothelial cell-associated platelet-activating factor: a novel mechanism for signaling intercellular adhesion. J Cell Biol 1990; 110:529–40.
159. Zsebo KM, Yuschenkoff VN, Schiffer S, Chang D, McCall E, Dinarello CA, Brown MA, Altrock B, Bagby GJ. Vascular endothelial cells and granulopoiesis: interleukin-1 stimulates release of G-CSF and GM-CSF. Blood 1988; 71:99–103.

17

Biochemical Effects of Human Granulocyte-Macrophage Colony-Stimulating Factor (GM-CSF) on the Human Neutrophil

RICHARD SULLIVAN
Baylor College of Medicine,
Houston, Texas

I. INTRODUCTION

Granulocyte-macrophage colony-stimulating factor (GM-CSF) is a hematopoietic hormone which, in addition to its ability to stimulate the production of neutrophils, eosinophils, and monocytes within the bone marrow, greatly augments the function of these phagocytes, once they become fully mature, through a process known as priming (1). While GM-CSF does not by itself activate these cells to produce large quantities of toxic oxygen species or to undergo substantial degranulation, these functions are significantly enhanced when cells that have first been exposed to GM-CSF are then stimulated by strong chemoattractants (2–4). Since GM-CSF receptors have been identified by human neutrophils (5,6), and since these cells are relatively simple to isolate in large numbers and exhibit functional responses to GM-CSF that are easy to quantitate, considerable work has been carried out on the stimulus-response coupling of the GM-CSF receptor in the neutrophil. The purpose of this review is to summarize information gained to date, through use of this model, which pertains to the signal transduction of the GM-CSF receptor.

II. HUMORAL REGULATION OF HEMATOPOIESIS

The proliferation and terminal differentiation of blood cells are regulated by a family of glycoprotein cytokines referred to as hematopoietic colony-stimulating factors (CSFs) (7), of which GM-CSF is a prominent member. These cytokines are produced by a variety of mesenchymal cells in the body and exert their effects both individually and synergistically at various ontogenetic stages of hematopoiesis (1). While the trophic activities of CSFs have primarily been defined using in-vitro cultures of hematopoietic progenitor cells (8), these growth factors are widely considered to represent true hormones which regulate blood cell production physiologically. Within recent years, the genes for many murine and human CSFs have been identified, cloned, and expressed in recombinant tissue culture systems, and, as a result, a number of highly purified synthetic CSFs have been made available for study (9–18). As a consequence, and owing to the work of many laboratories, our understanding of the endocrine control of blood cell production has broadened considerably in a relatively brief period of time.

GM-CSF is a member of this family of cytokines that has been studied particularly extensively. Produced by a variety of types of mesenchymal cells in response to lymphokines and monokines elaborated during the immune response, GM-CSF stimulates the proliferation of virtually all classes of progenitor cells in the bone marrow (1). However, its most pronounced and apparent effects are clearly exerted upon cells of the phagocyte lineage. GM-CSF not only stimulates the proliferation of immature phagocyte precursor cells but also facilitates the release of mature phagocytes from the bone marrow and enhances the microbicidal and cytotoxic functions of mature neutrophils (2–5,19–30), eosinophils (3,31), basophils (32,33), and macrophages (34–39).

The observation that GM-CSF exerts different effects at separate stages of phagocytic maturation has led to the concept that receptors for this cytokine, which appear during early hematopoiesis, may be retained throughout the entire ontogeny of granulocytes and monocytes and subserve quite different functions in proliferating cells than in their mature progeny. The notion that a single hormone may exert both proliferative and functional effects on receptor-bearing cells at different maturational stages is not new to endocrinology (40–43). However, the possibility remains that more than one type of receptor may exist for GM-CSF and that separate functions attributed to this glycoprotein may be mediated through structurally different receptors.

III. PRIMING OF NEUTROPHILS BY GM-CSF

In 1985, shortly after the gene for human GM-CSF was cloned, Weisbart et al. (2) noted that recombinant human GM-CSF (GM-CSFrh) was incapable of directly activating the respiratory burst of neutrophils. When these cells were preincubated with GM-CSFrh for 15–120 min, however, they became "primed" in such a way that they subsequently produced about twice the amount of superoxide anion (O_2^-) that they ordinarily would in response to cellular activation by the chemotactic peptide N-formyl-Met-Leu-Phe (fMLP). Subsequent studies have shown that GM-CSFrh-primed neutrophils generate more O_2^- in response to most chemoattractant stimuli (e.g., the complement component C5a, leukotriene B_4, and opsonized microbes) (4,28) and that many other chemoattractant-stimulated microbicidal and cytotoxic functions of the neutrophil [e.g. phagocytosis (3), cellular adhesion (29), and antibody-dependent cell-mediated cytotoxicity (3)] are also enhanced when the cells have been preexposed to GM-CSFrh. More recently, it has been reported that GM-CSF may directly induce the release of a very small fraction of the contents of neutrophilic specific granules (44) and stimulate the generation of small quantities of toxic oxygen radicals (21,26), particularly when the cells have been allowed to adhere to surfaces; however, there is little doubt that the major effect of the cytokine lies in its capacity to enhance, or "prime," the neutrophil's response to more potent agonists. As discussed below, it is likely that much of the priming effect which GM-CSFrh exerts on the cytotoxic and microbicidal functions of the activated neutrophil can be accounted for by the ability of this cytokine to upregulate, through a poorly understood mechanism, the surface expression of several classes of proteins important in cell function, such as the C3bi receptor CD11b (29) which plays a major role in cell adhesion, IgA receptors (45), and formyl peptide receptors (27,30,46). However, other direct effects of GM-CSFrh on the metabolism of the neutrophil have now been described, and a number of them have provided important clues to the stimulus-response network through which GM-CSF preactivates these cells.

In order to gain insight into the stimulus-response coupling of GM-CSF in the neutrophil, several laboratories have carried out systematic studies aimed toward discerning whether the signal transduction of the GM-CSF receptor in the neutrophil may be similar to that of other growth factors. Other studies have been designed to determine whether this cytokine activates metabolic pathways of known important in ligand-mediated neutrophil activation. A brief overview of cytokine receptor signal transduction and of stimulus-response coupling in the neutrophil, on which the majority of the studies described in this view have been based, is summarized below.

IV. GROWTH FACTOR RECEPTOR STRUCTURE AND FUNCTION

From studies of other growth factor receptors that have been identified and studied in detail, at least four categories of receptors may be considered: (a) large receptors with a single membrane-spanning region which exhibit intrinsic tyrosine kinase activity (47), (b) receptors which are directly coupled to G-proteins (48), (c) receptors which share homologous domains with the immunoglobulin superfamily (49), and (d) smaller receptors (~45–50 kDa) which comprise the newly described hematopoietic cytokine receptor superfamily (50,51). Very little is known about the early events in signal transduction by receptors in this last group, which includes the GM-CSF receptor. However, the biochemical class of its receptor has so far proven to be of only limited value in predicting the stimulus-response coupling of any given growth factor, since considerable transcommunication appears to take place commonly between early signal transduction pathways.

Activation of membrane Na^+/H^+ antiporters frequently occurs in response to growth factors, regardless of their receptor type, giving rise to elevation of the cytosolic pH by 0.15–0.25 pH units (52). Although the alkalinization may enhance DNA synthesis and other aspects of cell growth, the exact role of the antiporter's activation is unclear. One such antiporter has recently been cloned and expressed as a recombinant protein (53). Through studies carried out using this synthetic plasma membrane protein, Sardet et al. have recently shown that activation of the Na^+/H^+ antiporter in response to certain growth factors may be mediated by serine phosphorylation, which might give rise to an increased affinity for H^+ ions at the internal proton-binding site of the molecule (54).

Gearing et al. (55) have recently cloned the gene for a 45-kDa GM-CSF receptor in the human neutrophil which shares structural similarities with other members of the hematopoietic cytokine receptor superfamily (51). Whether other classes of GM-CSF receptors are present in the mature neutrophil or in proliferative myeloid cells remains to be established.

V. STIMULUS-RESPONSE COUPLING IN THE NEUTROPHIL

Several laboratories have carried out studies designed to determine whether GM-CSF activates signal transduction pathways of known importance in ligand-mediated neutrophil activation. While there is considerable "cross-talk" among these pathways, they may be conveniently divided as follows: (a) the phospholipase C-inositol phosphate pathway, through which a transient rise in the concentration of intracellular calcium ions ($[Ca^{2+}]_i$) is mediated (48); (b) the protein kinase C pathway, which plays a central role in the activation of the neutrophil's oxidative burst (56); and (c) the arachidonate cascade, which results in the formation of eicosanoid derivatives such as leukotriene B_4 (LTB_4), which facilitate activation of several aspects of the cell's microbicidal functions (57). A very brief description of these pathways and of the metabolic signals which they generate follows.

The phospholipase C-inositol phosphate pathway, which couples the formyl chemotactic peptide receptor to cellular activation, plays a pivotal role in the microbicidal function of the mature neutrophil. When the formyl peptide receptor, which is coupled to a *Bordetella pertussis* toxin-inhibitable GTP-binding protein, is occupied, phospholipases C are activated, giving rise to the liberation of inositol trisphosphates (IP3) and diacylglycerols from membrane-associated phosphoinositol bisphosphate (PIP2). One particular isomer of IP3, inositol 1,4,5 trisphosphate, is especially active in inducing the liberation of Ca^{2+} ions from bound stores, an event which effects a transient elevation of $[Ca^{2+}]_i$ (58). A rise in $[Ca^{2+}]_i$ is an important signal in cellular activation owing to diverse effects which include facilitation of the activation of a variety of phospholipases and protein kinases (59). Diacylglycerols derived from PIP2 directly activate protein kinases C, setting into motion the respiratory burst, through as yet unknown processes (56).

Two ionic epiphenomena of protein kinase C activation accompany the generation of toxic oxygen radicals during this sequence: (a) membrane depolarization, which may result from the influx of Na^+ (60) but which also is accompanied by alterations in intracellular concentrations of K^+ (61) and H^+ (62); and (b) acidification of the cell's interior, which is due largely to the liberation of H^+ ions generated by the hexose monophosphate shunt (63), which supplies reduced NADPH as a cofactor for the oxidase that reduces molecular O_2 to O_2^-. Like an elevation of $[Ca^{2+}]_i$, both of these ionic "events" have been implicated as transduction signals which may play direct roles in stimulus-response coupling in the neutrophil. While the function of depolarization is not entirely clear, it may facilitate cellular activation by opening voltage-gated ion channels in organellar or plasma membranes (64). The role of acidification of the cell's interior, on the other hand, is much more clearly established. An acidic pH within organelles such as endosomes, lysosomes, and receptosomes is crucial for the separation of internalized ligands from their receptors, for the fusion of membranes, and for the action of a number of lysosomal enzymes (65).

The release of arachidonic acid via hydrolysis of membrane phospholipids represents another pathway of cellular activation in the neutrophil. While phospholipases A2, which are facilitated by an elevation of $[Ca^{2+}]_i$, are well recognized to induce arachidonate release, other pathways exist through which hydrolytic cleavage of this fatty acid from its phospholipid storage sites can be initiated. For example, diacylglycerols released through the action of phospholipases C may serve as a source of arachidonate through the subsequent action of diacylglycerol lipases (59). Arachidonic acid is then free to be converted via cyclooxygenases to prostaglandins and thromboxanes or via lipoxygenases to leukotrienes. The most potent derivative of the latter pathway in the neutrophil is LTB_4, which causes adhesion and chemotactic movement of neutrophils and stimulates aggregation, enzyme release, and generation of O_2^- anion (57).

With this information as background, several laboratories have undertaken systematic studies aimed toward elucidating the stimulus-response coupling of GM-CSF in the neutrophil. Based on this approach, certain clues to the signal transduction of GM-CSF receptors in the neutrophil have emerged. The following paragraphs summarize these recent studies.

VI. SURFACE RECEPTOR UP-REGULATION BY GM-CSF

In 1986, Arnaout et al. reported that a 15-min exposure of neutrophils to GM-CSFrh gave rise to a two- to threefold increase in the plasma membrane expression of two species of leukocyte adhesion molecules, Mol and LeuM5 (P150,95) (29). The optimal concentration of GM-CSF in their study was 500 pM, at which concentration neutrophil migration was inhibited. They proposed that GM-CSF promoted neutrophil adhesion through this mechanism. In the same year, Weisbart et al. (27) observed that GM-CSF induced up-regulation of formyl peptide receptors on the neutrophil's surface. The kinetics of receptor up-regulation which they observed were similar to those reported for leukocyte adhesion molecules in that the concentration of GM-CSF required, the length of time before up-regulation occurred, and the quantitative degree of increased expression were similar. More recently, GM-CSF has been found to increase the surface expression of IgA receptors as well (45). The mechanisms through which up-regulation of these particular plasma membrane proteins is induced by GM-CSF is unclear.

English et al. (46) have found that when neutrophils are incubated at 37°C in physiologic buffer, the surface expression of formyl peptide receptors increases slowly over approximately a 1-hr period. In the presence of GM-CSF, they found that the increase in the expression of these receptors was quantitatively greater and extended over a longer period. They proposed the interesting hypothesis that up-regulation of surface receptors important in neutrophil activation, such as formyl peptide receptors, may be a normal consequence of cell aging, and that priming agents such as GM-CSF may accelerate that process. Regardless of the mechanisms through which such up-regulation of surface receptors in response to GM-CSF takes place, it seems clear that remodeling of the plasma membrane induced by this cytokine is likely to account for many of the cellular alterations which characterize GM-CSF priming.

VII. EFFECTS OF GM-CSF ON THE PHOSPHOLIPASE C-INOSITOL PHOSPHATE PATHWAY

Considerable evidence indicates that while direct activation of the phospholipase C-inositol phosphate pathway in the neutrophil by GM-CSF is not likely to play a significant role in the signal transduction of this cytokine, most of the signals generated when this pathway is activated by formyl peptides appear to be accentuated in GM-CSF-primed cells.

GM-CSF has been reported to have no direct effect on the cellular content of inositol trisphosphates (19,66) and to induce either no or very little release of intracellular diacylglycerols (24). Consistent with these observations, GM-CSF has furthermore been found to exert no direct effect on $[Ca^{2+}]_i$ (19,20,22) or resting transmembrane electrical potentials (ψ) (22,67) in the neutrophil.

In contrast to these findings, when neutrophils are preincubated with GM-CSF and then stimulated with fMLP, most of the effects of phospholipase C activation are augmented. Corey and Rosoff (66) found that in GM-CSF-primed cells, there was no difference in the amount of IP3 or DAG released in response to fMLP. However, their data are in disagreement with those of Tyagi et al. (24), who reported large increases in fMLP-induced DAG generation in neutrophils that had been primed with GM-CSF. Furthermore, in GM-CSF-primed cells, fMLP-induced increases in $[Ca^{2+}]_i$ (20) and in the rate and degree of membrane depolarization (67) have been reported to be augmented. Enhancement of the metabolic signals produced through occupancy of formyl peptide receptors were predictable in view of the well-established observation that the rates of O_2^- generation following fMLP are substantially increased in GM-CSF-pretreated neutrophils.

Whether the augmentation in the metabolic signals generated in response to fMLP in GM-CSF-primed neutrophils can be entirely accounted for by increases in the number of formyl peptide receptors on the plasma membrane induced by this cytokine is unclear.

VIII. EFFECTS OF GM-CSF ON ARACHIDONATE RELEASE

In 1987, we reported that when neutrophils that had been preincubated with ^3H-labeled arachidonic acid were exposed to GM-CSF for 5 min, small quantities of the radiolabeled arachidonate were released by the cells directly in response to the cytokine (22). Others have found that in GM-CSF-primed neutrophils, fMLP-stimulated arachidonic acid release is substantially increased (68). Furthermore, in GM-CSF-primed neutrophils, the conversion of liberated arachidonic acid to eicosanoid derivatives such as leukotriene B_4 may be increased (25,68). In a similar manner, the production of leukotriene C_4 has been reported to be increased in eosinophils that have been preincubated with GM-CSF before activation with fMLP (31).

Dahinden et al. (25) noted that when neutrophils were stimulated with fMLP or the complement component C5a, the cells elaborated no measurable leukotriene B_4 unless exogenous arachidonic acid had been added to the cell suspension. In contrast, when the cells had first been primed with GM-CSF, they generated large quantities of eicosanoid conversion products, including LTB_4, in response to fMLP and C5a even in the absence of added arachidonic acid. Similar results were reported by DiPersio et al. (68). These interesting observations raised the possibility that, as a consequence of GM-CSF priming, arachidonic acid may be released more freely from the plasma membrane of the neutrophil, thereby providing increased quantities of substrate for conversion via the lipoxygenase pathway. Such an increase in arachidonic acid availability could result either from the activation of enzymes which hydrolyze arachidonate from membrane phospholipids (phospholipases A2) or from diacylglycerols (diacylglycerol lipases) or from enhanced synthesis of membrane phospholipids which contain arachidonic acid.

In addition to these findings, Bourgoin et al. have reported that phosphilipase D activity is increased in GM-CSF primed neutrophils, following fMLP stimulation (69), resulting in the liberation of increased quantities of phosphatidic acid and diradylglycerol, both of which are potential sources of free arachidonic acid. Furthermore, phosphatidic acid itself may play a direct role in cell signaling, since it has been reported to activate the hydrolysis of inositol phospholipids in other cell systems (70).

IX. EFFECTS OF GM-CSF ON TRANSMEMBRANE Na^+/H^+ EXCHANGE

When the neutrophil's respiratory burst is activated with agonists such as fMLP or phorbol myristate acetate (PMA), acidification of the cytosol takes place which has been shown to be due primarily to the release of H^+ ions by the hexose monophosphate shunt (63). The fall in cytosolic pH ceases after 30–45 s, and realkalinization of the cytoplasm occurs due to Na^+/H^+ exchange via plasma membrane antiporters (71). Often, the cytosolic pH achieved after reequilibration is higher than the initial resting pH; therefore, ligands such as PMA or fMLP may effect changes in the antiporter which result in a higher affinity of proton-binding sites and consequent reestablishment of a slightly higher resting cytosolic pH.

The effects of GM-CSF priming on the kinetics of cytosolic pH change following fMLP or PMA are pronounced. When neutrophils are preincubated with GM-CSF and then stimulated with either fMLP or PMA, the initial fall in cytosolic pH is greater than in unprimed cells, and realkalinization is delayed (20,72). We found that these changes are partially but not entirely due to increased H^+ liberation coupled to the increased amount of O_2^- generated in primed neutrophils, since they were shown to be diminished but not ablated entirely in neutrophils from patients with chronic granulomatous disease (72).

Gomez-Cambronero et al. (73) have recently reported that GM-CSF directly induces a low and subtle alkalinization of the neutrophil's cytoplasm which begins as soon as 5 min after the cytokine is added to neutrophils in suspension and which results in an increase in the cytosolic pH of as much as 0.25 pH unit. They further observed that GM-CSF-induced cytoplasmic alkalinization was inhibited by amiloride and *B. pertussis* toxin, findings which indicated that alkalinization resulted in activation by GM-CSF of Na^+/H^+ antiporters in the plasma membrane through a pathway that contained GTP-binding proteins (73).

X. ROLE OF G-PROTEINS IN GM-CSF PRIMING

Guanine nucleotide-binding proteins (G-proteins) have been implicated in the stimulus-response coupling of GM-CSF in the neutrophil by several groups of investigators (see this volume, Chapter 5). It now appears that a number of distinct metabolic events stimulated by GM-CSF depend on activation of *B. pertussis* toxin-sensitive G-proteins. McColl et al. (74) found that exposure to GM-CSF gave rise to increases in measurable levels of c-fos mRNA in human neutrophils, and that this response was inhibited by *B. pertussis* toxin. They further observed that when neutrophils were primed with GM-CSF, elevations in $[Ca^{2+}]_i$ induced by platelet-activating factor were enhanced, and, in addition, the stimulation of leukotriene synthesis by the calcium ionophore A23187 was augmented. Both of these responses to GM-CSF were blocked by treatment of the cells with *B. pertussis* toxin. Corey and Rosoff (66) reported that when GM-CSF-primed neutrophils were stimulated with either arachidonic acid or the nonhydrolyzable guanosine triphosphate (GTP) analog GTPγS, they released significantly more O_2^- than unprimed cells; both of these enhanced responses were inhibited by *B. pertussis* toxin. Finally, Gomez-Cambronero et al. (73) found that plasma membranes isolated from GM-CSF-pretreated neutrophils had higher than normal basal and stimulated GTPase activities. Furthermore, they observed that GM-CSF activated Na^+/H^+ exchange through plasma membrane antiporters, and that this event was significantly diminished by *B. pertussis* toxin.

These reports provide strong evidence that G-proteins participate in the stimulus-response coupling of GM-CSF in the neutrophil. That so many separate metabolic responses to GM-CSF are blocked by *B. pertussis* toxin suggests that it may have a proximal role in the signal transduction of GM-CSF in these cells. However, direct coupling of GM-CSF receptors to G-proteins has not been established and would seem unlikely based on the size and biochemical properties of GM-CSF receptors which have been characterized to date.

XI. EFFECTS OF GM-CSF ON CYCLIC NUCLEOTIDE GENERATION

Coffey et al. (19) observed that GM-CSF directly increased the concentration of cyclic guanosine monophosphate (cGMP) in human neutrophils. They found that guanylate cyclase activities in both membrane and cytosol fractions were increased after brief exposures of cells to the cytokine. Adenylate cyclase activity was inhibited by GM-CSF by approximately 50%. Their findings are of considerable interest in view of prior studies that indicate that many of the microbicidal functions of the neutrophil are enhanced in the presence of high cytosolic concentrations of cyclic GMP (75) and conversely dampened when cytosolic concentrations of cyclic AMP are increased (76,77). Furthermore, a number of studies have indicated that agents which stimulate adenylate cyclase activity may impede granulocyte production by inhibiting the proliferative response of precursor cells to colony-stimulating factors (78) or by suppressing the production of some of these cytokines (79). The precise role that alterations in cellular concentrations of cyclic GMP and AMP play in the signal transduction of GM-CSF is presently unknown but is likely to be multifactorial, since many pathways are recognized to be affected by levels of these metabolites.

XII. EFFECTS OF GM-CSF ON PROTEIN KINASES

Gomez-Cambronero et al. (1989) reported that when human neutrophils are incubated with GM-CSF, five separate cellular proteins are phosphorylated on tyrosine residues (73). These proteins range in size from 40 to 118 kDa, and their functions are to date unclear. These findings indicate that one or more tyrosine kinases are activated when GM-CSF receptors are occupied on the neutrophil's surface. On the other hand, GM-CSF has been found to exert no direct effect on plasma membrane (80) or cytosolic (19,22) concentrations of active protein kinase C. It is of interest that Lopez et al. found in parallel studies that protein kinase C levels in the plasma membranes of cells of the progranulocytic leukemia cell line HL-60 were enhanced by GM-CSF (80). The discrepancy between the effects of GM-CSF on this class of enzymes in HL-60 cells and in mature neutrophils has as yet not been explained.

XIII. SUMMARY

Through studies of the stimulus-response coupling of GM-CSF in the neutrophils, important clues to the nature of the signal transduction of GM-CSF receptors are starting to emerge. GM-CSF receptors which have to date been identified and characterized biochemically appear to be too small to contain internal tyrosine kinase domains. Nonetheless, tyrosine phosphorylation of five separate proteins results when neutrophils are incubated with GM-CSF (73). The most appealing explanation for this interesting observation is that one or more tyrosine kinases lie distal to GM-CSF receptors in their signal transduction pathway. While less likely, the possibility exists that another class of GM-CSF receptors which exhibit intrinsic tyrosine kinase activity remains to be identified. Characterization of the specific proteins which are phosphorylated on tyrosine residues ought to provide important insights into the signal transduction of this cytokine. On the other hand, direct activation of protein kinases C has not been observed following exposure of neutrophils to GM-CSF (19,22,80).

GM-CSF induces the release of small quantities of arachidonic acid from the plasma membrane of the neutrophil (22). Arachidonic acid is primarily released directly through the effects of phospholipases A2 on membrane phospholipids or indirectly through activation of phospholipases C or D, which release compounds that can serve as a source of arachidonic acid when hydrolyzed by specific enzymes. Direct activation of phospholipases C in the neutrophil by GM-CSF appears most unlikely, since GM-CSF does not elevate $[Ca^{2+}]_i$ or induce the release of detectible quantities of inositol trisphosphates or diacylglycerols in these cells. Therefore, the possibility that GM-CSF may directly activate phospholipases A2 is quite plausible.

GM-CSF directly activates Na^+/H^+ antiporters in the plasma membrane of the neutrophil, resulting in alkalinization of the cytoplasm of approximately 0.1–0.25 pH unit (73). The function of cytoplasmic alkalinization in the priming of mature neutrophils is unclear. However, evidence exists in other cell systems that cytoplasmic alkalinization may be important in inducing cell proliferation, since the pH optima of several enzymes necessary for DNA synthesis are slightly more alkaline than the resting pH of the cytosol. Many types of growth factors which initiate cell division through occupancy of surface receptors give rise to cytoplasmic alkalinization through just such a mechanism (52). Therefore, it seems likely that GM-CSF may activate Na^+/H^+ antiporters in the plasma membranes of hemic progenitor cells which bear GM-CSF receptors and which proliferate in response to this cytokine.

In the brief period of time since recombinant human GM-CSF was first synthesized in 1985, considerable progress has been made in elucidating the subcellular effects that this important cytokine exerts on hemic cells which bear its receptors. As these studies continue over the next several years, considerable clarification of the precise signal transduction pathway which couples GM-CSF receptors to activation of cell proliferation in hematopoietic progenitor cells and to priming of the neutrophil's cytotoxic and microbicidal functions ought to be forthcoming.

REFERENCES

1. Cannistra SA, Griffin JD. Regulation of the production and function of granulocytes and monocytes. Sem Hematol 1988; 25:173–88.
2. Weisbart RH, Golde DW, Clark SC, Wong GC, Gasson JC. Human granulocyte-macrophage colony-stimulating factor is a neutrophil activator. Nature 1985; 314:361–3.
3. Lopez AF, Williamson DJ, Gamble JR, Begley CG, Harlan JM, Klebanoff SJ, Waltersdorph A, Wong G, Clark SC, Vadas MA. Recombinant human granulocyte-macrophage colony-stimulating factor stimulates in vitro mature human neutrophil and eosinophil function, surface receptor expression, and survival. J Clin Invest 1986; 78:1220–8.

4. Weisbart RH, Kwan L, Golde DW, Gasson JC. Human GM-CSF primes neutrophils for enhanced oxidative metabolism in response to the major physiological chemoattractants. Blood 1987; 69:18–21.
5. DiPersio J, Billing P, Kaufman S, Eghtesady P, Williams RE, Gasson JC. Characterization of the human granulocyte-macrophage colony-stimulating factor receptor. J Biol Chem 1988; 263:1834–41.
6. Gasson JC, Kaufman SE, Weisbart RH, Tomonaga M, Golde DW. High-affinity binding of granulocyte-macrophage colony-stimulating factor (GM-CSF) to normal and leukemic human myeloid cells. Proc Natl Acad Sci USA 1986; 83:669–73.
7. Metcalf D. The colony-stimulating factors: discovery, development, and clinical applications. Cancer 1990; 65:2185–95.
8. Nicola NA, Vadas M. Hemopoietic colony-stimulating factors. Immunol Today 1984; 5:76–80.
9. Souza LM, Boone TC, Gabrilove J, Lai PH, Zsebo KM, Murdock, DC, Chazin VR, Bruszewski J, Lu H, Chen KK, Barendt J, Platzer E, Moore MAS, Mertelsmann R, Welte K. Recombinant human granulocyte colony-stimulating factor: effects on normal and leukemic myeloid cells. Science 1986; 232:61–5.
10. Gabrilove JL, Welte K, Harris P, Platzer E, Lu L, Levi E, Mertelsmann R, Moore MAS. Pluripoietin α: a second human hematopoietic colony-stimulating factor produced by the human bladder carcinoma cell line 5637. Proc Natl Acad Sci USA 1986; 83:2478–82.
11. Kawasaki ES, Ladner MB, Wang AM, Van Arsdell J, Warren MK, Coyne MY, Schweickart VL, Lee M-T, Wilson KJ, Boosman A, Stanley ER, Ralph P, Mark DF. Molecular cloning of a complementary DNA encoding human macrophage-specific colony-stimulating factor (CSF-1). Science 1985; 230:291–6.
12. Wong GG, Witek JS, Temple PA, Wilkens KM, Leary AC, Luxenberg DP, Jones SS, Brown EL, Kay RM, Orr EC, Shoemaker C, Golde DW, Kaufman RJ, Hewick RM, Wang EA, Clark SC. Human GM-CSF: molecular cloning of the complementary DNA and purification of the natural and recombinant proteins. Science 1985; 228:810–5.
13. Yang Y-C, Ciarletta AB, Temple PA, Chung MP, Kovacic S, Witek-Giannotti JS, Leary AC, Kriz R, Donahue RE, Wong GG, Clark SC. Human IL-3 (multi-CSF): identification by expression cloning of a novel hematopoietic growth factor related to murine IL-3. Cell 1986; 47:3–10.
14. Rajavashisth TB, Eng R, Shadduck RK, Waheed A, Ben-Avram CM, Shively JE, Lusis AJ. Cloning and tissue-specific expression of mouse macrophage colony-stimulating factor mRNA. Proc Natl Acad Sci USA 1987; 84:1157–61.
15. Gough NM, Gough J, Metcalf D, Kelso A, Grail D, Nicola NA, Burgess AW, Dunn AR. Molecular cloning of cDNA encoding a murine haematopoietic growth regulator, granulocyte-macrophage colony-stimulating factor. Nature 1984; 309:763–7.
16. Tsuchiya M, Asano S, Kaziro Y, Nagata S. Isolation and characterization of the cDNA for murine granulocyte colony-stimulating factor. Proc Natl Acad Sci USA 1986; 83:7633–7.
17. Miyatake S, Yokota T, Lee F, Arai K-I. Structure of the chromosomal gene for murine interleukin 3. Proc Natl Acad Sci USA 1985; 82:316–20.
18. Fung MC, Hapel AJ, Ymer S, Cohen DR, Johnson RM, Campbell HD, Young IG. Molecular cloning of cDNA for murine interleukin-3. Nature 1984; 307:233–7.
19. Coffey RG, Davis JS, Djeu JY. Stimulation of guanylate cyclase activity and reduction of adenylate cyclase activity by granulocyte-macrophage colony-stimulating factor in human blood neutrophils. J Immunol 1988; 140:2695–701.
20. Naccache PH, Faucher N, Borgeat P, Gasson JC, DiPersio JF. Granulocyte-macrophage colony-stimulating factor modulates the excitation-response coupling sequence in human neutrophils. J Immunol 1988; 140:3541–6.
21. Nathan CF. Respiratory burst in adherent human neutrophils: triggering by colony-stimulating factors CSF-GM and CSF-G. Blood 1989; 73:301–6.

21. Nathan CF. Respiratory burst in adherent human neutrophils: triggering by colony-stimulating factors CSF-GM and CSF-G. Blood 1989; 73:301–6.
22. Sullivan R, Griffin JD, Simons ER, Schafer AI, Meshulam T, Fredette JP, Maas AK, Gadenne A-S, Leavitt JL, Melnick DA. Effects of recombinant human granulocyte and macrophage colony-stimulating factors on signal transduction pathways in human granulocytes. J Immunol 1987; 139:3422–30.
23. Kharazmi A, Nielsen H, Bendtzen K. Modulation of human neutrophil and monocyte chemotaxis and superoxide responses by recombinant TNF-alpha and GM-CSF. Immunobiology 1988; 177:363–70.
24. Tyagi SR, Winton EF, Lambeth JD. Granulocyte/macrophage colony-stimulating factor primes human neutrophils for increased diacylglycerol generation in response to chemoattractant. FEBS Lett 1989; 257:188–90.
25. Dahinden CA, Zingg J, Maly FE, De Weck AL. Leukotriene production in human neutrophils primed by recombinant human granulocyte/macrophage colony-stimulating factor and stimulated with the complement component C5a and fMLP as second signals. J Exp Med 1988; 167:1281–95.
26. Kapp A, Zeck-Kapp G, Danner M, Luger TA. Human granulocyte-macrophage colony stimulating factor: an effective direct activator of human polymorphonuclear neutrophilic granulocytes. J Invest Dermatol 1988; 91:49–55.
27. Weisbart RH, Golde DW, Gasson JC. Biosynthetic human GM-CSF modulates the number and affinity of neutrophil f-met-leu-phe receptors. J Immunol 1986; 137:3584–7.
28. Fleischmann J, Golde DW, Weisbart RH, Gasson JC. Granulocyte-macrophage colony-stimulating factor enhances phagocytosis of bacteria by human neutrophils. Blood 1986; 68:708–11.
29. Arnaout MA, Wang EA, Clark SC, Sieff CA. Human recombinant granulocyte-macrophage colony-stimulating factor increases cell-to-cell adhesion and surface expression of adhesion-promoting surface glycoproteins on mature granulocytes. J Clin Invest 1986; 78:597–601.
30. Atkinson YH, Lopez AF, Marasco WA, Lucas CM, Wong GG, Burns GF, Vadas MA. Recombinant human granulocyte-macrophage colony-stimulating factor (rH GM-CSF) regulates f-met leu phe receptors on human neutrophils. Immunology 1988; 64:519–25.
31. Silberstein DS, Owen WF, Gasson JC, DiPersio JF, Golde DW, Bina JC, Soberman R, Austen KF, David JR. Enhancement of human eosinophil cytotoxicity and leukotriene synthesis by biosynthetic (recombinant) granulocyte-macrophage colony-stimulating factor. J Immunol 1986; 137:3290–4.
32. Haak-Frendscho M, Arai N, Arai K, Baeza ML, Finn A, Kaplan AP. Human recombinant granulocyte-macrophage colony-stimulating factor and interleukin 3 cause basophil histamine release. J Clin Invest 1988; 82:17–20.
33. Hirai K, Morita Y, Misaki Y, Ohta K, Takaishi T, Suzuki S, Motoyoshi K, Miyamoto T. Modulation of human basophil histamine release by hemopoietic growth factors. J Immunol 1988; 141:3958–64.
34. Fischer H-G, Frosch S, Reske K, Reske-Kunz AB. Granulocyte-macrophage colony-stimulating factors activates macrophages derived from bone marrow cultures to synthesis of MHC class II molecules and to augmented antigen presentation function. J Immunol 1988; 141:3882–8.
35. Belosevic M, Davis CE, Meltzer MS, Nacy CA. Regulation of activated macrophage antimicrobial activities. Identification of lymphokines that cooperate with IFN-gamma for induction of resistance to infection. J Immunol 1988; 141:890–6.
36. Reed SG, Nathan CF, Pihl DL, Rodricks P, Shanebeck K, Conlon PJ, Grabstein KH. Recombinant granulocyte-macrophage colony-stimulating factor activates macrophages to

inhibit trypanozoma cruzi and release hydrogen peroxide. Comparison with interferon gamma. J Exp Med 1987; 166:1734–46.
37. Coleman DL, Chodakewitz JA, Bartiss AH, Mellors JW. Granulocyte-macrophage colony-stimulating factor enhances selective effector functions of tissue-derived macrophages. Blood 1988; 72:573–8.
38. Weiser WY, Van Niel A, Clark SC, David JR, Remold HG. Recombinant human granulocyte/macrophage colony-stimulating factor activates intracellular killing of *Leishmania donovani* by human monocyte-derived macrophages. J Exp Med 1987; 166:1436–46.
39. Grabstein KH, Urdal DL, Tushinski RJ, Mochizuki DY, Price VL, Cantrell MA, Gillis S, Conlon PJ. Induction of macrophage tumoricidal activity by granulocyte-macrophage colony-stimulating factor. Science 1986; 232:506–8.
40. Collip JB, Anderson EM, Thompson DL. The adrenotropic hormone of the anterior pituitary lobe. Lancet 1933; 225:347–8.
41. Evans HM. Present position of our knowledge of anterior pituitary function. JAMA 1933; 101:425–32.
42. Aschner B. Ueber die Funktion der Hypophyse. Pfleugers Archiv Ges Physiol 1912; 146:1–146.
43. Liddle GW, Island D, Meador CK. Normal and abnormal regulation of corticotropin secretion in man. Rec Prog Hormone Res 1962; 18:125–66.
44. Richter J, Andersson T, Olsson I. Effect of tumor necrosis factor and granulocyte/macrophage colony-stimulating factor on neutrophil degranulation. J Immunol 1989; 142:3199–205.
45. Weisbart RH, Kacena A, Schuh A, Golde DW. GM-CSF induces human neutrophil IgA-mediated phagocytosis by an IgA Fc receptor activation mechanism. Nature 1988; 332:647–8.
46. English D, Broxmeyer HE, Gabig TG, Akard LP, Williams DE, Hoffman R. Temporal adaptation of neutrophil oxidative responsiveness to n-formyl-methionyl-leucyl-phenylalanine. J Immunol 1988; 141:2400–6.
47. Yarden Y, Ullrich A. Growth factor receptor tyrosine kinases. Ann Rev Biochem 1988; 57:443–78.
48. Hokin LE. Receptors and phosphoinositide-generated second messengers. Ann Rev Biochem 1985; 54:205–35.
49. Williams AF, Barclay AN. The immunoglobulin superfamily—domains for cell surface recognition. Ann Rev Immunol 1988; 6:381–405.
50. Nicola NA. Hemopoietic cell growth factors and their receptors. Ann Rev Biochem 1989; 58:45–77.
51. Cosman D, Lyman SD, Idzerda RL, Beckmann MP, Park LS, Goodwin RG, March CJ. A new cytokine receptor superfamily. TIBS 1990; 15:265–70.
52. Moolenaar WH. Effects of growth factors on intracellular pH regulation. Ann Rev Physiol 1986; 48:363–76.
53. Sardet C, Franchi A, Pouyssegur J. Molecular cloning, priming structure, and expression of the human growth factor-activatable Na^+/H^+ antiporter. Cell 1989; 56:271–80.
54. Sardet C, Counillon L, Franchi A, Pouyssegur J. Growth factors induce phosphorylation of the Na^+/H^+ antiporter, glycoprotein of 110 kD. Science 1990; 247:723–6.
55. Gearing DP, King JA, Gough NM, Nicola NA. Expression cloning of a receptor for human granulocyte-macrophage colony-stimulating factor. EMBO J 1989; 12:3667–76.
56. Tauber AI. Protein kinase C and the activation of the human neutrophil NADPH-oxidase. Blood 1987; 69:711–20.
57. Needleman P, Turk J, Jakschik BA, Morrison AR, Lefkowith JB. Arachidonic acid metabolism. Ann Rev Biochem 1986; 55:69–102.

58. Berridge MJ, Irvine RF. Inositol phosphates and cell signalling. Nature 1989; 341:197–205.
59. Berridge MJ. Inositol trisphosphate and diacylglycerol: two interacting second messengers. Ann Rev Biochem 1987; 56:159–93.
60. Korchak HM, Weissman G. Stimulus-response coupling in the human neutrophil: transmembrane potential and the role of extracellular Na^+. Biochim Biophys Acta 1980; 601:180–94.
61. Naccache PH, Showell HJ, Becker EL, Sha'afi RI. Transport of sodium, potassium, and calcium across rabbit polymorphonuclear leukocyte membranes: effect of chemotactic factor. J Cell Biol 1977; 73:428–44.
62. Grinstein S, Furuya W. Amiloride-sensitive Na^+/H^+ exchange in human neutrophils: mechanism of activation by chemotactic factors. Biochem Biophys Res Commun 1984; 122:755–62.
63. Borregaard N, Schwartz JH, Tauber AI. Proton secretion by stimulated neutrophils. Significance of hexose monophosphate shunt activity as source of electrons and protons for the respiratory burst. J Clin Invest 1984; 74:455–9.
64. Sullivan R, Fredette JP, Griffin JD, Leavitt JL, Simons ER, Melnick DA. An elevation in the concentration of free cytosolic calcium is sufficient to activate the oxidative burst of granulocytes primed with recombinant human granulocyte-macrophage colony-stimulating factor. J Biol Chem 1989; 264:6302–9.
65. Mellman I, Fuchs R, Helenius A. Acidification of the endocytic and exocytic pathways. Ann Rev Biochem 1986; 55:663–700.
66. Corey SJ, Rosoff PM. Granulocyte-macrophage colony-stimulating factor primes neutrophils by activating a pertussis toxin-sensitive G protein not associated with phosphatidylinositol turnover. J Biol Chem 1989; 264:14165–71.
67. Sullivan R, Fredette JP, Leavitt JL, Gadenne A-S, Griffin JD, Simons ER. Effects of recombinant human granulocyte-macrophage colony-stimulating factor (GM-CSFrh) on transmembrane electrical potentials in granulocytes: relationship between enhancement of ligand-mediated depolarization and augmentation of superoxide anion (O_2^-) production. J Cell Physiol 1989; 139:361–9.
68. DiPersio JF, Billing P, Williams R, Gasson JC. Human granulocyte-macrophage colony-stimulating factor and other cytokines prime human neutrophils for enhanced arachidonic acid release and leukotriene B4 synthesis. J Immunol 1988; 140:4315–22.
69. Bourgoin S, Plante E, Gaudry M, Naccache PH, Borgeat P, Poubelle PE. Involvement of a phospholipase D in the mechanism of action of granulocyte-macrophage colony-stimulating factor (GM-CSF): priming of human neutrophils in vitro with GM-CSF is associated with accumulation of phosphatidic acid and diradylglycerol. J Exp Med 1990; 172:767–77.
70. Kroll MH, Zavoico GB, Schafer AI. Second messenger function of phosphatidic acid in platelet activation. J Cell Physiol 1989; 139:558–64.
71. Wright J, Schwartz JH, Olson R, Kosowsky JM, Tauber AI. Proton secretion by the sodium/hydrogen ion antiporter in the human neutrophil. J Clin Invest 1986; 77:782–8.
72. Sullivan R, Griffin JD, Wright J, Melnick DA, Leavitt JL, Fredette JP, Horne JH Jr, Lyman CA, Lazzari KG, Simons ER. Effects of recombinant human granulocyte-macrophage colony-stimulating factor on intracellular pH in mature granulocytes. Blood 1988; 72:1665–73.
73. Gomez-Cambronero J, Yamazaki M, Metwally F, Molski TFP, Bonak VA, Huang C-K, Becker EL, Sha'afi RI. Granulocyte-macrophage colony-stimulating factor and human neutrophils: role of guanine nucleotide regulatory proteins. Proc Natl Acad Sci USA 1989; 86:3569–73.
74. McColl SR, Kries C, DiPersio JF, Borgeat P, Naccache PH. Involvement of guanine

nucleotide binding proteins in neutrophil activation and priming by GM-CSF. Blood 1989; 73:588–91.
75. Ignarro LJ, Cech SY. Bidirectional regulation of lysosomal enzyme secretion and phagocytosis in human neutrophils by guanosine 3′,5′-monophosphate and adenosine 3′,5′-monophosphate. Proc Soc Exp Biol Med 1976; 151:448–52.
76. Bourne HR, Lehrer RI, Cline MJ, Melmon KL. Cyclic 3′,5′-adenosine monophosphate in the human leukocyte: synthesis, degradation, and effects on neutrophil candidacidal activity. J Clin Invest 1971; 50:920–9.
77. Weissman G, Dukor P, Zurier RB. Effect of cyclic AMP on release of lysosomal enzymes from phagocytes. Nature New Biol 1971; 231:131–5.
78. Morley A, Quesenberry P, Garrity M, Stohlman F Jr. Inhibition of marrow growth by cyclic AMP. Proc Soc Exp Biol Med 1971; 138:57–9.
79. Ramsey R, Hays EF. Factors promoting colony stimulating activity (CSA) production in macrophages and epithelial cells. Exp Hematol 1979; 7:245–54.
80. Lopez AF, Hardy SJ, Eglinton J, Gamble J, To LB, Dyson P, Wong G, Clark S, Murray AW, Vadas MA. Recombinant human granulocyte-macrophage colony-stimulating factor (rh GM-CSF) induces different intracellular signals in mature and immature myeloid cells. In: Powanda MC, Oppenheim JJ, Kluger MJ, Dinarello CA, eds. Monokines and other nonlymphocytic cytokines. New York: Alan R. Liss, 1988:235–42.

18

Mechanisms of Host Tissue Damage by Cytokine-Activated Neutrophils

ANTONIO FERRANTE, INGE C. KOWANKO, and EDNA J. BATES
University of Adelaide and Adelaide Children's Hospital, Adelaide, South Australia

I. INTRODUCTION

The inflammatory response is a highly coordinated and regulated process consisting of a network of interactions among a wide variety of tissue cells and infiltrating leukocytes usually involving cell adhesion and cell-derived mediators. The characteristic of the inflammatory response is highly dependent on the inducing agent. The cellular infiltrate is made up of lymphocytes, mononuclear phagocytes, and neutrophils in proportions characteristic of the type of inflammation and its phase. A number of classical mediators have been examined exhaustively for their role in the initiation, development, and resolution of the inflammatory reaction. In the last few years we have seen the identification, characterization, and preparation of a range of polypeptide cytokines released by lymphocytes, macrophages, and tissue cells. Consequently, new dimensions have been opened in efforts to clarify the network of interactions which occur in the inflammatory process. Although polypeptide cytokines have been regarded as possible therapeutic agents, it is unlikely that they will be used in this capacity. By far the most rewarding aspect of research in this field will be the contribution it will make toward the understanding of mechanisms of inflammatory processes. This review is concerned with the role of polypeptide cytokine regulation of the neutrophil, a major cell involved in defense against infection but which also contributes significantly to tissue damage during inflammation.

A variety of polypeptide cytokines with multifaceted effects have been described recently. Some are produced by a wide variety of body cells, while others may be highly restricted to specific cell types such as T-lymphocytes. Among the varied properties of these cytokines is their ability to alter phagocytic cell function (1–12). This is considered to be relevant to tissue damage which occurs in many different types of inflammatory diseases.

The effects of various cytokines on neutrophil functions are shown in Table 1. Cytokines are capable of altering a wide range of functions of neutrophils which are essential in the evolution of the inflammatory response and in the tissue damage that accompanies this response. These include adherence and chemotaxis, which promote cellular infiltration in tissues, increased oxygen-dependent respiratory activity leading to the production of reactive oxygen intermediates, and release of lysosomal enzymes and proteins.

Interaction of neutrophils with appropriate particulate or soluble stimuli results in a respiratory burst characterized by an increase in oxygen consumption and generation of oxygen-derived reactive species (ODRS). Enzymes and other proteins stored in lysosomal granules are released together with a variety of bioactive lipids such as platelet-activating factor (PAF), leukotrienes, and prostaglandins (for reviews see Refs. 13–15). The involvement of these released substances in leukocyte-induced tissue injury has been addressed frequently (13,16,17).

Table 1 Effects of Polypeptide Cytokines on Neutrophil Functions[a]

	Cytokine								
Function	IL-1	IL-2	IL-4	IL-6	IL-8	γ-IFN	TNF_{α}	TNF_{β}	GM-CSF
Adherence	Dec.	Dec.				Inc.	Inc.	Inc.	Inc.
Chemotactic				None	Yes		?	?	?
Migration							Dec.	Dec.	Dec.
Expression of surface receptors							Inc.		Inc.
Respiratory burst:									
Direct	Inc.	Inc.	None		None		Inc.	Inc.	None
fMLP	Inc.	Inc.	Inc.		Inc.		Inc.	Inc.	Inc.
PMA			None		Inc.		Inc.	Inc.	None
Bacteria							Inc.		
Fungi							Inc.		Inc.
Amebas							Inc.	Inc.	
Degranulation:									
Specific granules									
Direct	None		Inc.				Inc.		None
fMLP	Inc.		Inc.				Inc.	Inc.	Inc.
Fungi							Inc.		Inc.
Amebas							Inc.		
Azurophilic granules									
Direct	None		None		Inc.				None
fMLP	Inc.		Inc.				Inc.	Inc.	Inc.
Fungi							Inc.		Inc.
Amebas							Inc.		Inc.

[a] Dec. = decreased; Inc. = increased; ? = controversial; None = no activity; Yes = activity present.

II. THE NEUTROPHIL OXIDATIVE RESPIRATORY BURST AND TISSUE INJURY

A. Oxygen-Derived Reactive Species

During the respiratory burst, superoxide anion ($O_2^{\bar{\cdot}}$) is formed via the univalent reduction of oxygen (18) and can be converted into H_2O_2, through either spontaneous or superoxide dismutase (SOD)-catalyzed dismutation. The H_2O_2 formed is thought to react via the metal-catalyzed Haber-Weiss reaction to produce the highly reactive hydroxyl radical ($OH^{\cdot}$). In this reaction $O_2^{\bar{\cdot}}$ reduces the oxidized transition metal ion and H_2O_2 then reacts with the reduced metal ion (19):

$$O_2^{\bar{\cdot}} + Fe^{3+} \rightarrow O_2 + Fe^{2+}$$

$$Fe^{2+} + H_2O_2 \rightarrow Fe^{3+} + OH^{\cdot} + OH^-$$

Most stimuli that induce $O_2^{\bar{\cdot}}$ production by neutrophils also cause the release of the azurophilic granule enzyme myeloperoxidase (MPO) (14), and in the presence of this enzyme, H_2O_2 can react with Cl^- to form hypochlorous acid (HOCl). Reaction of MPO-generated HOCl with amines forms long-lived chloramines which have been implicated in an amplification of the oxidizing potential of the peroxidase system (20).

In aqueous solution, $O_2^{\bar{\cdot}}$ is poorly reactive, rapidly dismutating to H_2O_2, which is more reactive and can cross biological membranes with the possibility of giving rise to more reactive species within cells. The $OH^{\cdot}$ is highly reactive, and in vivo it will react at or close to its site of formation.

B. The Importance of ODRS in Tissue Injury in Vivo

The potential involvement of $O_2^{\bar{\cdot}}$, H_2O_2, and $OH^{\cdot}$ in tissue damage in various biological systems has been well studied (13,16,17,19). A role for $OH^{\cdot}$ in tissue injury associated with rheumatoid arthritis has been suggested based on in-vitro experimentation, and indirect evidence also suggests an in-vivo role for this oxygen radical. There are reports that rheumatoid synovial fluid contains more iron than normal fluid (21). More recently, Fe^{3+} in a form suitable for catalysis has been found in only 40% of rheumatoid arthritis synovial fluids (22). Lactoferrin (an iron-binding protein present in specific granules of neutrophils) can increase $OH^{\cdot}$ production in vitro, presumably by its ability to provide iron as a catalyst for the reduction of H_2O_2 by $O_2^{\bar{\cdot}}$ (23). $OH^{\cdot}$ has also been proposed to be important in an experimental model of inflammation by the inhibitory effect of an iron chelator (24).

Recently the hypothesis of $OH^{\cdot}$ generation by neutrophils in vivo has been challenged by Winterbourne (25), who found that the production of $OH^{\cdot}$ by the iron-catalyzed Haber-Weiss reaction was not favored in the presence of active MPO; she concluded that under conditions where neutrophils release MPO as well as $O_2^{\bar{\cdot}}$ and H_2O_2, breakdown of H_2O_2 by MPO would make conditions unfavorable for $OH^{\cdot}$ production.

Cationic derivatives of catalase (CAT) and peroxidase (but not superoxide dismutase) with a strong affinity for negatively charged articular cartilage have been shown to be effective in suppressing two different types of experimental arthritis (26), suggesting a role for peroxides (H_2O_2, lipid peroxides) in the inflammatory response. Free radical oxidation products have been found in the synovial fluid of patients with rheumatoid arthritis (27).

C. Effects of ODRS on Cartilage

Enzymatically generated ODRS (using xanthine oxidase and hypoxanthine, XO/HX) have been found to inhibit the synthesis of proteoglycan by bovine articular cartilage (28). Protein synthesis was also inhibited. The active species involved was found to be H_2O_2 (29). When H_2O_2 was added directly or generated with a glucose oxidase/glucose system, a similar inhibition of synthesis was observed (29). Hyaluronic acid synthesis was inhibited in parallel with that of proteoglycan (30). These results have been confirmed by others (31,32), with the added observation that DNA synthesis was also impaired (32). Chondrocyte viability was maintained (29,32) in the presence of ODRS.

Other studies have shown that added HOCl was also inhibitory to proteoglycan synthesis and caused degradation of proteoglycan (33). H_2O_2 itself was found to have no effect on the degradation of proteoglycan (33). Other workers have found that prolonged incubation of cartilage with a XO/HX system for 12 h with replacement of the XO/HX every 2 h resulted in a release of proteoglycan (uronic acid) and collagen fragments (hydroxyproline) from cartilage (34). Exposure of cartilage slices prelabeled with [^{35}S] sulfate to $O_2^{\cdot-}$ and $OH^{\cdot}$ resulted in the release of products which chromatographed similarly to free chondroitin-sulfate chains (35).

D. Effects of ODRS on Macromolecules Relevant to Cartilage Injury and the Inflammatory Response

Hyaluronic acid is the major macromolecular component of synovial fluid, and synovial fluid loses viscosity in rheumatoid arthritis (36). Depolymerization of the hyaluronic acid molecule has been suggested as the cause (37). Hyaluronic acid is thought to be degraded by $OH^{\cdot}$ (36–38). However, more recently it has been shown that both purified hyaluronic acid and bovine synovial fluid react with HOCl, resulting in a decrease in their specific viscosities (39). Other workers have also provided evidence in support of the hypothesis that peroxidase activity controls the effect of $O_2^{\cdot-}$ generation on hyaluronic acid (40).

Proteoglycan-hyaluronate aggregate in solution is susceptible to degradation by ODRS (41,42), although the proteoglycan monomer is relatively insensitive (42). The active species is thought to be $OH^{\cdot}$ (42), in agreement with effects of ODRS on hyaluronic acid in solution (36–38).

The inability of collagen solutions to gel normally after exposure to a XO/HX system has been known for some years (43). More recently the same system was found to degrade the collagen-liberating peptides smaller than the α-chains of collagen (44). The $OH^{\cdot}$ is suggested to be important in the degradation of collagen (45), and the molecule can become more susceptible to proteolytic degradation.

The MPO/halide/H_2O_2 system results in the oxidation of lysine side chains of elastin (46). This also occurred with normal neutrophils, but not with MPO-deficient neutrophils unless exogenous MPO was added (46), suggesting that MPO-mediated reactions may affect cross-linking of elastin at sites of injury.

Tissue damage in inflammatory diseases is due in part to α_1-proteinase activity, which is normally controlled by α_1-proteinase inhibitor. Oxidation of methionine at the active site of α_1-proteinase inhibitor (α_1-PI) by the MPO/H_2O_2/halide system results in suppression of inhibitory activity (47). Human neutrophils are found to suppress α_1-PI activity, although cells from a patient with chronic granulomatous disease (CGD) are unable to suppress activity (48). The MPO system is again implicated in these whole-cell systems. Neutrophils are able to suppress the antielastase activity of bronchial antileucoprotease by a MPO system (49), which may play a role in pulmonary disease.

When human IgG is exposed to ODRS-generating systems such as ultraviolet radiation, perioxidizing lipids, or activated neutrophils, characteristic fluorescent monomeric and polymeric IgG is formed (50). These complexes can stimulate O_2^- production by neutrophils, and identical complexes have been found in fresh rheumatoid sera and synovial fluids (50). It is suggested that the formation of these complexes may be self-perpetuating within the inflamed joint. It has also been found that incubation of human IgG with a MPO/H_2O_2/halide system results in the generation of large amounts of covalently cross-linked IgG aggregates that behave as typical immune complexes (51). More recently, human neutrophils incubated over immune complexes attached to a solid phase have been found to mediate covalent cross-linking of a significant proportion of these molecules by a process requiring the MPO/halide/H_2O_2 system and the generation of HOCl (52). Thus nonspecific aggregation and cross-linking of immune complexes to themselves and connective-tissue macromolecules may play an important pathogenic role in establishing and maintaining inflammation.

E. Intracellular Changes Occurring as a Result of ODRS Tissue Injury

H_2O_2, when incubated with articular cartilage, causes an immediate decrease in ATP levels. This has been shown to be due to the oxidative inactivation of glyceraldehyde-3-phosphate dehydrogenase (32). The authors suggest that intrachondrocyte oxidant damage occurs through the oxidation of the sensitive thiol residue at the active center of the enzyme with subsequent reduction in the rate of glycolytic ATP synthesis and the intracellular concentration of ATP, which is required for DNA, protein, proteoglycan, and hyaluronic acid synthesis. H_2O_2 has also been shown to reduce ATP levels in endothelial cells (53).

Other workers have presented evidence that one of the early targets of H_2O_2-induced cell injury may be the cytoskeleton. This was assessed by examining the distribution of actin and cytokeratin filaments in A_{549} cells derived from human lung carcinoma. These changes occurred earlier than ^{51}Cr release or trypan blue uptake (54). Shasby et al. (55), using a XO-xanthine system, have demonstrated that ODRS-mediated increase in endothelial permeability to macromolecules is associated with reversible changes in endothelial cell shape and actin filaments, which in turn are related to changes in endothelial calcium homeostasis (55). Potassium efflux and the release of cytoplasmic purines have also been shown to result from H_2O_2 damage to endothelial cells (56).

H_2O_2 caused single-strand breaks in DNA of fibroblasts in the same concentration range in which it produced cell killing (57). This was mediated through the generation of $OH^{\cdot}$, with iron complexed to chromatin functioning as the catalyst.

There is much experimental evidence suggesting that lipid peroxidation reactions on the cell membrane may play an important role in ODRS-mediated cell injury (19). There was no evidence of lipid peroxidation products after treatment of cartilage with the XO/HX system (29). Other workers have obtained evidence for both lipid peroxidation-dependent and -independent pathways of hepatocyte killing by H_2O_2 (58). It has been suggested that the H_2O_2-induced increase in endothelial calcium permeability and PAF synthesis results from the generation of lipid peroxides (59), which can act as Ca^{2+} ionophores (60). The synthesis of PAF is temporally dissociated from lytic cell injury.

III. LYSOSOMAL GRANULE RELEASE AND TISSUE INJURY

In addition to releasing ODRS, neutrophils can release lysosomal granules (14) in response to appropriate stimuli. There are at least two distinct types of lysosomal granules. The azurophilic or primary granules contain potential tissue-destructive enzymes and proteins such as MPO, cationic proteins, and neutral proteases (elastase and cathepsin G), whereas the specific or secondary granules contain enzymes such as lysozyme, collagenase, and plasminogen activator. A third, less well characterized granule contains gelatinase activity.

A. Elastase

Of the lysosomal enzymes released by neutrophils, elastase has received much attention with regard to its involvement in tissue damage. Elastase is known to degrade a wide range of connective tissue proteins (61–64). Both elastase and cathepsin G have been demonstrated in articular cartilage in rheumatoid arthritis (65). Others have found that leukocyte elastase in the synovial fluid of rheumatoid arthritis patients is complexed with α_1-PI and that no free elastase is detectable (66). However, incubation of elastase and α_1-PI in equimolar concentrations or even with α_1-PI in excess resulted in significant tissue destruction as assessed by histological staining for proteoglycan, release of uronic acid, and loss of mechanical stability. Immunofluorescent staining indicated elastase penetration into the matrix (66).

Bartholomew et al. (67) have shown that a purified low-molecular-weight elastase from rabbit neutrophils can degrade proteoglycan in bovine cartilage in culture as well as elicit a prolonged, severe inhibition of proteoglycan biosynthesis by cartilage. Neutrophil granule extract (at a concentration equivalent to 10^7 neutrophils) also caused proteoglycan degradation and inhibited its synthesis, the effects being partially reversed by the specific elastase inhibitor MAAPV-CMK (33).

More recently (68), it has been demonstrated that chondrocytes in culture have a specific cell surface receptor for leukocyte elastase and that endocytosis of elastase occurs as a secondary event after cell binding.

Elastase, while removing proteoglycans from cartilage, also demasks collagen fibers, thus giving collagenase access to them (69). It also solubilizes collagen at a sizable rate (69). Neutrophil collagenase is not able to initiate degradation of native human articular cartilage unless the cartilage is first treated with leukocyte elastase (69). Others have shown that cartilage subjected to elastase treatment was more susceptible to ODRS attack (34), with resultant proteoglycan degradation.

B. Plasminogen Activator

Evidence has been presented that most of the plasminogen activator in resting neutrophils is associated with the specific granule membranes; upon activation, plasminogen activator translocates to the plasma membrane, thus equipping the neutrophil with surface-associated proteolytic activity (70). Plasminogen activator is then released. Its substrate plasminogen is derived from plasma or synovial fluid, and is converted to the active plasmin.

Plasmin can cause degradation of proteoglycan in cartilage (71,72) as well as activate latent collagenases and proteoglycanases (73,74), which have been isolated from connective tissue or cell cultures of chondrocytes. However, an in-vivo role for plasmin in cartilage degradation has been questioned on the grounds that plasmin might be too large to enter normal cartilage in appreciable amounts and also because of the presence of α_2-antiplasmin in synovial fluid. However, plasmin could act first at the surface of cartilage and then, as proteoglycans are lost, the increased permeability of cartilage (75) would facilitate the entry of plasmin. Close apposition to its substrate and/or excess of enzyme in the disease tissue could allow plasmin to escape its primary inhibitor, α_2-antiplasmin. Chondrocytes have been shown to produce plasminogen activator themselves (76).

C. Cationic Proteins (Defensins)

Defensins are a family of low-molecular-weight (<3500 Da) cationic proteins found in the azurophilic granules (77). There are three human defensins, which are antibacterial, antifungal, and antiviral in vitro. Other, larger bactericidal proteins (15–60 kDa) have also been isolated from human neutrophils (78). Neutrophils contain 4–5 μg of defensins/10^6 cells and release 3–8% of this extracellularly when stimulated with opsonized zymosan or phorbol 12-myristate-13-acetate (PMA). The defensins adsorb to neutrophils, and high concentrations could develop in intercellular clefts between neutrophils and tissues. Defensins have been shown to be cytotoxic to a range of mammalian cells in vitro (79). These defensins were synergistic with H_2O_2 in this activity.

IV. NEUTROPHILS AND TISSUE INJURY

A. Involvement of Neutrophils in Tissue Damage

Human neutrophils degrade proteoglycan and inhibit proteoglycan synthesis when incubated with cultures of either human or bovine articular cartilage coated with heat-aggregated IgG (33,80–82). Preincubation of the cartilage with the specific elastase inhibitor MAAPC-CMK partially reversed these damaging effects of neutrophils (33). The degradation of proteoglycan by neutrophils was a direct effect of the neutrophils and was not mediated by the chondrocytes, as similar results were obtained with both living and dead cartilage (81,82). Others have shown that exposure of murine patellar cartilage to neutrophils stimulated with N-formyl-met-leu-phe (fMLP) or A23187 resulted in an inhibition of proteoglycan synthesis and breakdown of proteoglycan (83). This was prevented by a serine protease inhibitor and a specific elastase inhibitor. The authors also showed that close contact between neutrophils and cartilage by pelleting the cells onto the tissue prevented some of the effect of α_1-PI (83). Our studies with human neutrophils have shown that PMA activates these cells to degrade proteoglycan and inhibit its synthesis, using bovine articular cartilage (Figures 1 and 2).

Complement-stimulated neutrophils damage endothelial cells as measured by ^{51}Cr release (84), and the inclusion of SOD and CAT partially reduced the damage. Cells treated with cytochalasin B were more effective in damaging the tissue (84). Weiss et al. (85) have presented evidence using PMA-stimulated neutrophils and umbilical vein

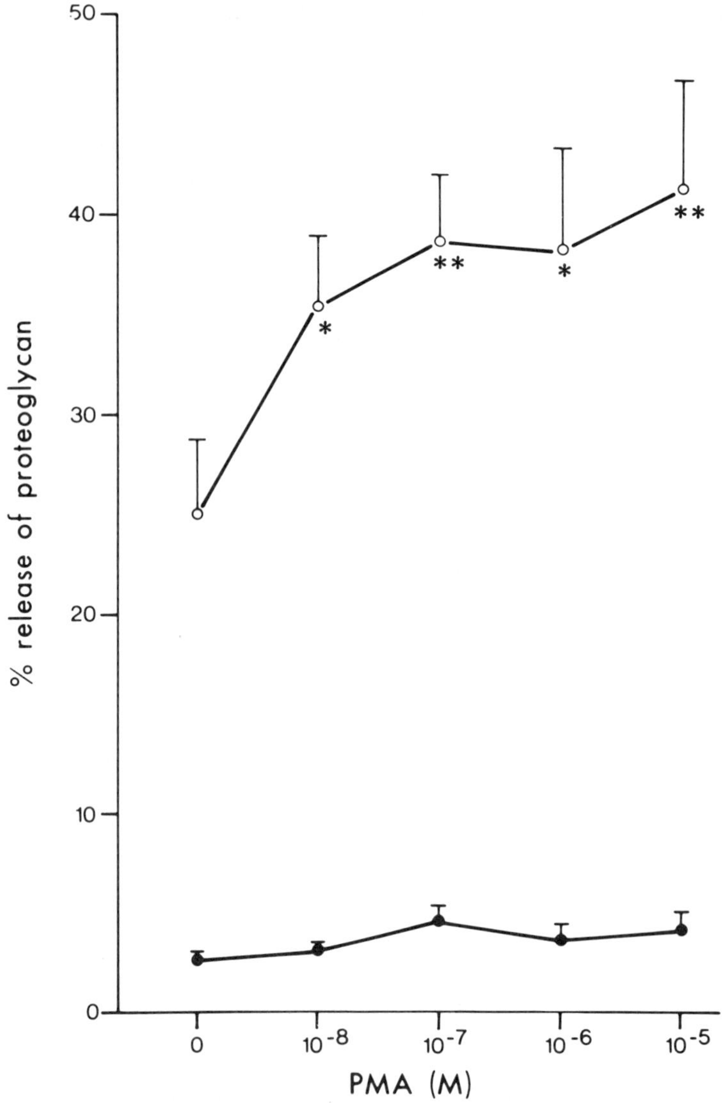

Figure 1 Effect of phorbol myristate acetate (PMA) on neutrophil-mediated cartilage degradation. Bovine cartilage was incubated with (○) or without (●) human neutrophils for 2.5 h in the absence or presence of the indicated concentrations of PMA. Cartilage degradation is expressed as percent release of proteoglycan into the medium during the incubation. Results are means ±SD of three to four replicate cultures. *, ** indicate $p < 0.01$, $p < 0.005$, respectively, for the effect of PMA on neutrophils.

endothelial cells that cytotoxicity is a result of H_2O_2 generation and not HOCl. This conclusion was based on data that neutrophils from a chronic granulomatous disease (CGD) patient did not destroy targets, whereas those from a MPO-deficient patient did. They also found that a cell-free MPO-glucose oxidase system did destroy endothelial cells, and this was prevented by scavengers of HOCl. This suggests that the neutrophil

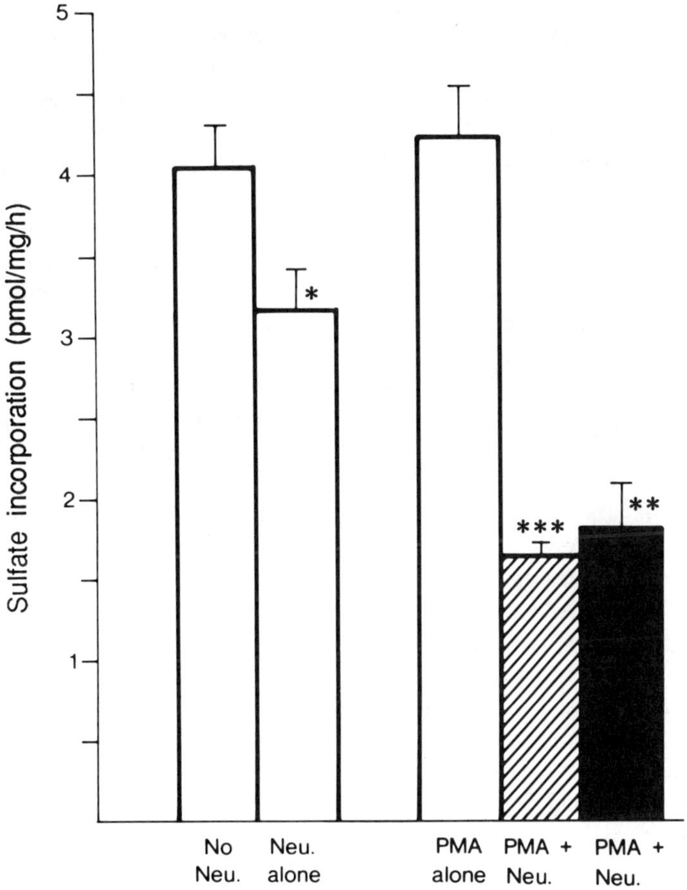

Figure 2 Effect of phorbol myristate acetate (PMA) on neutrophil-mediated inhibition of proteoglycan synthesis. Bovine cartilage was incubated in the absence and presence of human neutrophils for 2.5 h. Neutrophils were either untreated or pretreated with PMA (10^{-6} M) for 30 min and washed before addition to heat-aggregated gamma globulin (HAGG)-coated cartilage (solid bar). In some incubations, untreated neutrophils were incubated with cartilage in the presence of PMA (10^{-6} M; hatched bar). The incorporation of ^{35}S-sulfate into cartilage proteoglycans was subsequently determined. Results are mean ± SD of three or four replicate cultures. * indicates $P < 0.01$ for the effect of neutrophils alone; ** indicates $p < 0.005$ for the effect of preincubation of neutrophils with PMA; *** indicates $p < 0.001$ for the effect of PMA in the presence of neutrophils.

does not require the MPO-H_2O_2-halide system to destroy endothelial cells. Similar cytotoxic neutrophil effects have been shown using immune complexes and aggregated IgG as stimulus, with CAT reducing the cytotoxicity (86). Smedly et al. (87) have found that chemotactic factor-stimulated neutrophil injury to microvascular endothelial cells (^{111}In release) is enhanced by lipopolysaccharide and is largely mediated by neutrophil elastase, as injury occurred with neutrophils from a CGD patient and the elastase inhibitor reversed 63% of the neutrophil-mediated injury.

Endothelial cell detachment has been shown to occur as a result of neutrophils activated by zymosan (88). No cell lysis resulted, and the detachment was inhibited by neutral protease inhibitors but not CAT or SOD. Neutrophils from a CGD patient also caused endothelial cell detachment (88). Using endothelial monolayers on polycarbonate filters, Harlan et al. (89) have shown that fMLP-stimulated neutrophils produced a marked increase in the passage of ^{125}I-albumin across bovine aortic or pulmonary-artery endothelial monolayers. There was, however, no ^{51}Cr- release or detachment of cells. Neutrophils from a CGD patient produced a similar disruption of the endothelium. CAT was unable to reverse the increased passage of albumin. Cell-free postsecretory supernatants of neutrophils stimulated by fMLP, leukotrieneC_4 (LTC_4), and PAF also had no effect on the passage of ^{125}I-albumin. However, neutrophils from a patient with a congenital abnormality of neutrophil adhesion and chemotaxis did not increase the passage of ^{125}I-albumin (89). They conclude that activated neutrophils mediate nonlytic disruption of endothelial monolayer integrity by an ODRS-independent mechanism that requires neutrophil-endothelial contact.

Neutrophils are known to adhere to glomerular basement membrane (GBM) in glomerulonephritis. Using a model consisting of isolated GBM impregnated with IgG aggregates (90), it has been shown that neutrophil damage to the membrane is through the action of serine proteases with the solubilization of type IV collagen. This model has also been used to demonstrate that H_2O_2 is generated in the contact area between neutrophils and GBM (91). Electron microscopy demonstrated deposits of cerium chloride (use to detect H_2O_2) only in the contact area; but when PMA was used as the neutrophil stimulus instead of impregnated IgG, cerium deposits were seen over the whole surface of the neutrophil (91). These authors also indicated that the neutrophil respiratory burst has little effect on GBM degradation. Other workers have demonstrated that the MPO/H_2O_2/halide system causes glomerular injury in a model where MPO followed by H_2O_2 was infused in a chloride-containing solution into the renal artery of rats (92). Iodination of glomeruli in a neutrophil-mediated model of experimental glomerulonephritis also suggests a role for MPO/H_2O_2/halide system in vivo (93). Cationic proteins may also cause changes in physiology of the glomeruli (94). Evidence has also been presented that in-vivo transient hepatic parenchymal cell injury with postoperative sepsis may be mediated by the margination of activated neutrophils in the liver (95).

As described above, neutrophils may damage tissues directly, by releasing damaging molecules such as ODRS and lysosomal enzymes, without active participation of the tissue. This has been shown using heat-aggregated gamma globulin (HAGG)-coated cartilage, where neutrophil degradation of the tissue is the same for both living and dead tissue (33,80–82). The ability of tumor necrosis factors TNF_α, TNF_β, or conditioned medium to enhance neutrophil-mediated degradation of cartilage was observed with both living and dead cartilage (80–82).

Alternatively, neutrophils cause damage by an indirect action involving the tissue itself. Latent collagenase and proteoglycanase of cartilage may be activated by neutrophil release of mediators such as plasminogen activator (73,74). It is also known that latent collagenase of neutrophils is activated by HOCl (96), and this may also be true of cartilage collagenase. This type of mechanism may be operative to "turn on" tissue destruction.

In addition, endogenous tissue inhibitors may be inhibited by neutrophils. For example, a tissue inhibitor of metalloproteinases from cultured bovine dental pulp can be inhibited by human neutrophil elastase (97). This might allow the uncontrolled destruction of proteoglycans, type IV collagen, laminin, and fibronectin in the tissue.

Finally, neutrophil products may stimulate the tissue to produce other active mediators, and these may be involved in damage to the tissue. Cathepsin G stimulates prostglandin I_2 (PGI_2) production by porcine aortic endothelial cells (98). Neutrophil elastase had little effect but inhibited PGI_2 production in response to other stimuli, especially ATP. Other workers have shown that both human leukocyte elastase and H_2O_2 can stimulate endothelial cells to release PAF (59,99).

Neutrophils are known to release both TNF_α and interleukin-1 (IL-1) (100,101). These cytokines may turn on tissue destructive processes. For example, both IL-1 and TNF_α cause proteoglycan degradation and inhibit proteoglycan synthesis in cartilage cultures (82,102–104).

B. Cytokine Modulation of Neutrophil-Mediated Tissue Injury

The ability of cytokines to modulate tissue injury by neutrophils has only recently been addressed. Cytokines such as IL-1, IL-2, TNF_α, TNF_β, γ-interferon (γ-INF), and granulocyte-macrophage colony-stimulating factor (GM-CSF) are known to have many effects on neutrophil function (Table 1). Both TNF_α and TNF_β have been shown to enhance neutrophil-mediated proteoglycan degradation in cartilage (81,82) (Figure 3). However, TNF_α had no effect on the neutrophil inhibition of proteoglycan synthesis (82), and indeed TNF_β abrogated the inhibition of synthesis induced by neutrophils (81) (Figure 4). Mononuclear leukocyte-conditioned medium augmented both neutrophil-mediated degradation and inhibition of proteoglycan synthesis (80). We have established that this medium contains high concentrations of TNF_α and IL-1 (105,106), but no TNF_β (107). Therefore these results suggest that there must be factors in the conditioned medium other than TNF_α which prime neutrophils for enhanced inhibition of proteoglycan synthesis. Although we suspected IL-1, our recent studies have shown that recombinant human IL-1α is not responsible (unpublished).

While some evidence suggests that TNF_α fails to prime neutrophils for enhanced release of azurophilic granule constituents (108), other studies have shown that enhanced release is induced by TNF_α in relation to exposure to a stimulus of "frustrated phagocytosis" (8,9,109–111) such as cytochalasin B/fMLP, cytochalasin B/fungi, or large organisms such as amebae.

It is not clear to us why TNF_α-primed neutrophils do not show enhanced inhibition of proteoglycan synthesis in culture, since the cytokine augments release of enzymes such as elastase and also the production of ODRS. Both elastase and ODRS such as H_2O_2 cause inhibition of proteoglycan synthesis (28,29,33). Other neutrophil agonists (e.g., PMA) which enhance ODRS production augment neutrophil-mediated inhibition of proteoglycan synthesis (Figure 2). Even more intriguing is the finding that TNF_β suppresses the inhibition of proteoglycan synthesis induced by neutrophils (81) (Figure 4). These results show that two cytokines which bind to the same receptor on neutrophils (109) and have almost identical effects on cells show major differences in their effects on neutrophil-mediated inhibition of proteoglycan synthesis.

The capacity of TNF_α and TNF_β to increase neutrophil-mediated proteoglycan degradation is consistent with the finding that both cytokines prime for the release of ODRS and of enzymes from specific and azurophilic granules. While ODRS alone do not induce degradation of proteoglycan, the product H_2O_2 in combination with MPO

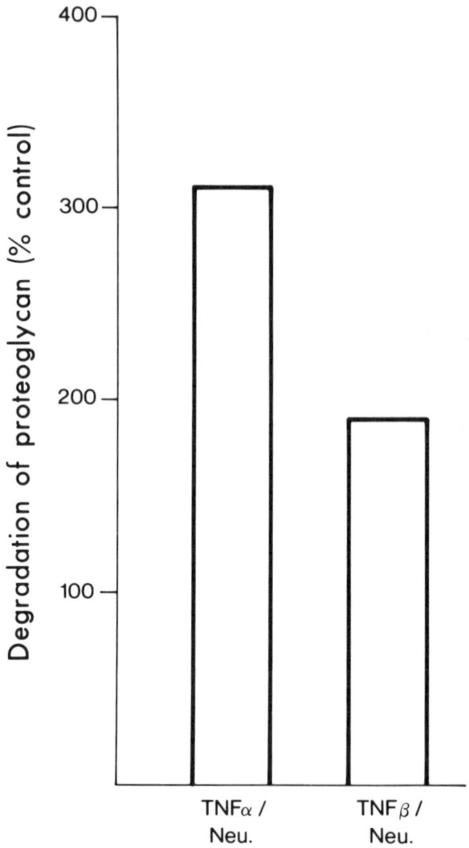

Figure 3 Effect of neutrophils preincubated with TNF_{α} or TNF_{β} on cartilage proteoglycan degradation. Human neutrophils were preincubated for 30 min with TNF_{α} (10^5 units/10^7 cells) or TNF_{β} (5×10^4 units/10^7 cells). After washing, the neutrophils were incubated for 2.5 h with HAGG-coated human cartilage prelabeled with ^{35}S-sulfate. Proteoglycan degradation was determined (release of ^{35}S-labeled glucosaminoglycans) during the 2.5-h incubation. Results are expressed as percentage of control (100%; neutrophils preincubated in the absence of TNFs).

and a halide (leading to formation of HOCl) causes proteoglycan degradation (33). This is another method by which TNF_{α} and TNF_{β} may augment neutrophil proteoglycan degradation.

Studies in our laboratory have shown that PAF causes a marked decrease in proteoglycan synthesis in bovine articular cartilage (Figure 5). While TNF_{α} induces PAF release from human neutrophils (see later), TNF_{α}-treated neutrophils do not show increased inhibition of proteoglycan synthesis.

Other mechanisms by which TNFs increase proteoglycan degradation by neutrophils are related to their ability to increase expression of cell surface receptors (110,111). These changes promote increased adherence to targets (2,3,110) and thereby promote the effective delivery of neutrophil mediators on the tissue surface. Neutrophils display increased adherence to endothelial cells in culture when either the neutrophils or the endothelial cells are treated with TNF_{α} (110,112). Similarly, neutrophils treated with

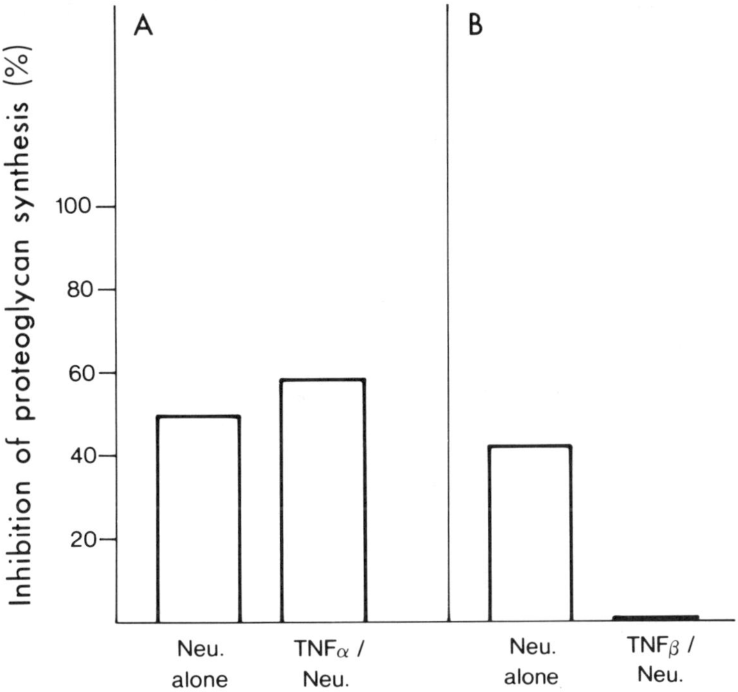

Figure 4 Effect of neutrophils preincubated with TNF_α or TNF_β on cartilage proteoglycan synthesis. Human neutrophils were preincubated for 30 min the absence and in the presence of TNF_α (10^5 units/10^7 cells; panel A) or TNF_β (5×10^4 units/10^7 cells; panel B). After washing, the neutrophils were incubated for 2.5 h with HAGG-coated human cartilage. The incorporation of ^{35}S-sulfate into cartilage proteoglycans was subsequently determined.

TNF_α-rich conditioned medium showed increased adherence to human articular cartilage tissue (80).

Although the discussion has centered mainly on TNFs, the ability of other polypeptide cytokines to regulate neutrophil function (Table 1) implies that cytokines in general may promote the neutrophil-mediated tissue injury. For example, our recent observations suggest that GM-CSF and γ-interferon augment the damage to cartilage mediated by human neutrophils (128,129).

Evidence suggests that cartilage damage by neutrophils involves a combination of lysosomal enzymes and also products of the oxygen-dependent respiratory burst. Our initial studies, data shown in Figure 6, show that TNF_α primes human neutrophils for a potentiated oxygen-dependent respiratory response to challenge with cartilage.

C. Involvement of Platelet-Activating Factor

As outlined above, both elastase and H_2O_2 can cause increased synthesis of platelet-activating factor (PAF) by endothelial cells (59,99). PAF is 1000-fold more potent than histamine in increasing vascular permeability (113). PAF has been shown to cause cultured human endothelial cells to change shape (114) as well as induce ^{125}I-albumin diffusion with a concentration dependence similar to that for PAF-induced cytoskeletal

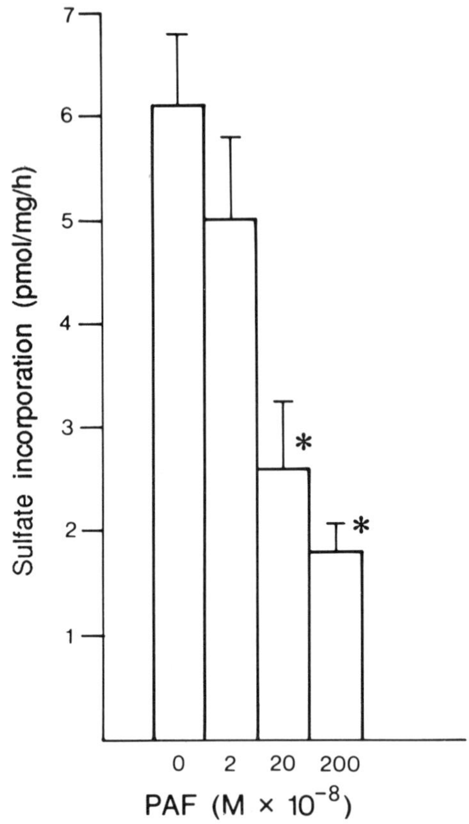

Figure 5 Effect of platelet-activating factor on cartilage proteoglycan synthesis. Bovine cartilage was incubated in the absence or presence of the indicated concentrations of PAF for 2.5 h, washed, and recultured overnight in DMEM supplemented with 20% newborn calf serum. ^{35}S-sulfate incorporation into proteoglycan was then measured. Results are means ± SD of triplicate cultures. * indicates $p < 0.001$ for incubations in the absence of PAF compared with incubations in its presence.

changes (114). TNF_α causes PAF synthesis by both endothelial cells (115,116) and neutrophils (117), and PAF enhances neutrophil responses to subsequent activation by agonists such as fMLP and PMA (118), with increased respiratory burst, degranulation, and adhesion to endothelium. PAF-primed neutrophils are extremely damaging to cultured endothelium (118) and cartilage (manuscript submitted). In addition, neutrophils can be stimulated directly by PAF with an increased respiratory burst and degranulation (15). When neutrophils are preincubated with TNF_α, a synergism exists between PAF and TNF_α that results in increased superoxide production (119). Thus interactions among TNF_α, PAF, neutrophils, and tissues (such as endothelium) may amplify the resultant tissue damage. Similar interactions involving other cytokines such as IL-1 may also be operative (120,121).

PAF has also been shown to release plasminogen activator from vessel walls (122). This may also be relevant in neutrophil-mediated damage.

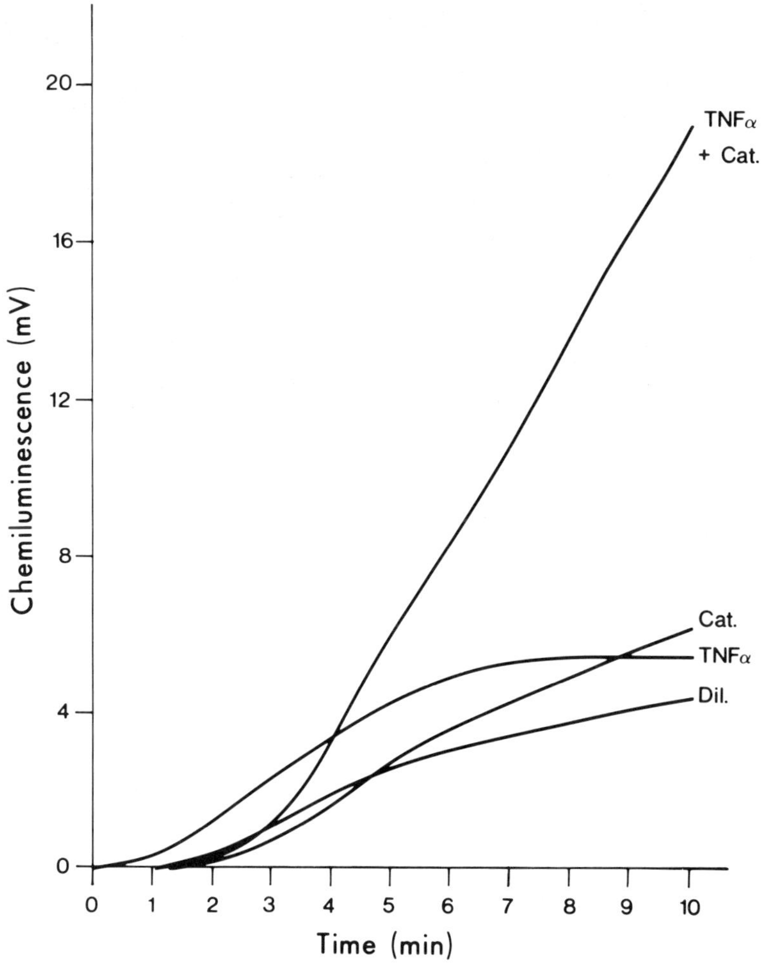

Figure 6 Production of chemiluminescence by neutrophils using cartilage as a stimulus. Bovine cartilage was killed by repeated freeze/thawing before coating with HAGG. Neutrophils were preincubated for 30 min the absence and presence of TNF_α (10^2 units/10^6 cells) before addition to cartilage (Cat). Lucigenin-enhanced chemiluminescence was measured at 10-s intervals over 10 min. Dil. indicates chemiluminescence of neutrophils preincubated in the absence of TNF_α with no added cartilage.

D. Cell-Substrate Contact

It has been suggested that neutrophils might degrade the extracellular matrix in the presence of plasma inhibitors by oxidatively inactivating the elastase-inhibitory capacity of α_1-PI (48). However, Campbell et al. (123) have found, using a model system in which PMA or opsonized zymosan-stimulated neutrophils are held in close proximity to a proteinase-sensitive connective-tissue substrate (^{125}I-labeled fibronectin), that the neutrophils quickly spread on the substrate and rapidly degrade it using predominantly elastase. There was no evidence of oxidative inactivation of proteinase inhibitors α_1-PI or α_2-macroglobulin. Close contact between neutrophils and substrate results in proteolysis, even in the presence of an excess of proteinase inhibitors (123). More recently (124), it has been shown using opsonized fibronectin as substrate that spreading of neutrophils on the surface is enhanced and the penetration of α_1-PI is reduced into zones of contact between neutrophils and substrate as a result of opsonization.

Other workers (125) have provided data concluding that neutrophils can use cooperatively an oxidant (thought to be HOCl) and the lysosomal enzyme elastase to negate the protective effects of α_1-PI in order to attack the subendothelial matrix. More recently, these authors (126) have suggested that nonoxidatively linked proteolysis can occur in the presence of a large excess of α_1-PI. They found that CGD neutrophils degrade the subendothelial matrix at apparently normal rates in the absence of α_1-PI. In its presence, CGD neutrophils had a reduced ability to degrade, and the levels seen were equivalent to those of normal neutrophils in the presence of azide or CAT (126). Neutrophils migrating on a fibrinogen-coated surface in response to fMLP form zones of close contact with fibrinogen, and only 81–85% of the resultant fibrinogenolysis can be blocked by undiluted serum or plasma, whereas 99% can be blocked by a specific low-molecular-weight elastase inhibitor (127).

In a cartilage model, it has been demonstrated that α_1-PI is not as effective in reversing the effects of neutrophils on cartilage when the cells are pelleted onto the cartilage rather than in suspension (83).

Of interest is the finding that low concentrations of plasma antiproteinase can inhibit PAF synthesis in neutrophils induced by TNF_α or stimulated by phagocytosis (99). Addition of elastase or cathepsin G stimulates PAF release much faster than TNF_α. A proteinase activated on the surface of TNF_a-treated neutrophils or secreted by these cells may be involved in promoting PAF synthesis. These findings suggest that PAF production may be limited to zones of close contact between cells which exclude antiproteinase (124,127).

V. SUMMARY

Although extensive investigations into the role of neutrophils and their products in tissue injury have been conducted, very little work has been carried out on the role of polypeptide cytokines in the regulation of neutrophil-mediated tissue damage. A range of cytokines are known to promote a wide variety of functions of the neutrophil, including neutrophil adhesion, surface receptor expression, ODRS production, and release of lysosomal constituents. Evidence has been presented to show that these products, either singly or in combination, cause tissue injury. At this stage, TNF_α and TNF_β are cytokines which have been shown to regulate neutrophil tissue injury. From this work it is suggested that TNFs promote neutrophil-mediated tissue damage.

ACKNOWLEDGMENTS

We are grateful to Gina Clemente for her skillful technical assistance and to Pru Russell-Taylor for her dedicated secretarial assistance. This work was supported by grants from the National Health and Medical Research Council the National Heart Foundation of Australia and the Arthritis Foundation.

REFERENCES

1. Steinbeck MJ, Roth JA. Neutrophil activation by recombinant cytokines. Rev Infect Dis 1989; 11:549–68.
2. Seow WK, Thong YH, Ferrante A. Macrophage neutrophil interactions: contrasting effects of the monokines interleukin-1 and tumour necrosis factor (cachetin) on human neutrophil adherence. Immunology 1987; 62:357–61.
3. Seow WK, Thong YH, McCormack JG, Ferrante A. Lymphocyte-neutrophil interactions: opposite effect of interleukin-2 and tumour necrosis factor beta (lymphotoxin) on human neutrophil adherence. Int Arch Allergy Appl Immunol 85:63–8.
4. Ferrante A, Nandoskar M, Watz A, Goh, DHB, Kowanko IC. Effects of tumour necrosis factor alpha and interleukin-1 alpha and beta on human neutrophil migration, respiratory burst and degranulation. Int Arch Allergy Appl Immunol 1988; 86:82–91.
5. Ferrante A, Nandoskar M, Bates EJ, Goh, DHB, Beard LJ. Tumour necrosis factor beta (lymphotoxin) inhibits locomotion and stimulates the respiratory burst and degranulation of neutrophils. Immunology 1988; 63:507–12.
6. Newman I, Wilkinson PC. Chemotactic activity of lymphotoxin and tumour necrosis factor alpha for human neutrophils. Immunology 1989; 66:318–20.
7. Sauder DN, Mousnessa NL, Katz SI, Dinarello CA, Galin JI. Chemotactic cytokines: the role of leukocytic pyrogen and epidermal cell thymocyte-activating factor in neutrophil chemotaxis. J Immunol 1984; 132:828–32.
8. Ferrante A, Harvey D, Bates EJ. *Staphylococcus aureus* stimulated MNL conditioned medium increases the neutrophil bactericidal activity, and augments the oxygen radical production and degranulation in response to the bacteria. Clin Exp Immunol; 1989; 78:366–71.
9. Djeu HY, Blanchard DK, Halkias H, Friedman H. Growth inhibition of *Candida albicans* by human polymorphonuclear neutrophils: activation by interferon-γ and tumour necrosis factor. J Immunol 1986; 137:2980–4.
10. Boey H, Rosenbaum R, Castracane J, Borish L. Interleukin-4 is a neutrophil activator. J Allergy Clin Immunol 1989; 83:978–84.
11. Kharazmi A, Nielsen H, Rechnitzer C, Bendtzen K. Interleukin-6 primes human neutrophil and monocyte oxidative burst response. Immunol Lett 1989; 21:177–84.
12. Peveri P, Walz A, Dewald B, Baggiolini M. A novel neutrophil-activating factor produced by human mononuclear phagocytes. J Exp Med 1988; 167:1547–60.
13. Fantone JC, Ward PA. Role of oxygen derived free radicals and metabolites in leukocyte dependent inflammatory reactions. Am J Pathol 1982; 107:396–418.
14. Baggioli M, Dewald B. Exocytosis by neutrophils. In: Snyderman R, ed. Regulation of leukocyte function; Contemporary topics in immunology, Vol. 14. New York and London: Plenum Press, 1984:221–46.
15. Baggioli M, Dewald B, Thelen M. Effects of PAF on neutrophils and mononuclear phagocytes. Prog Biochem Pharmacol 1988; 22:90–105.
16. Jackson JH, Cochrane CG. Leukocyte-induced tissue injury. Haematol/Oncol Clin N Am 1988; 2:317–34.
17. Henson PM, Johnston RB. Tissue injury in inflammation. Oxidants, proteinases and cationic proteins. J Clin Invest 1987; 79:669–74.
18. Babior BM, Kipnes RS, Curnutte JT. Biological defense mechanism. The production by leukocytes of superoxide, a potent bactericial agent. J Clin Invest 1973; 52:571–744.
19. Halliwell B. Free radicals, oxygen toxicity and aging. In: Sohal RS, ed. Age pigments. Amsterdam: Elsevier/North Holland Biomedical Press, 1981:1–62.
20. Weiss SJ, Lampert MB, Test ST. Long-lived oxidants generated by human neutrophils: characterization and bioactivity. Science 1983; 222:625–8.
21. Wong SF, Halliwell B, Richmond R, Skowroneck WR. The role of superoxide and

hydroxyl radicals in the degradation of hyaluronic acid induced by metal ions and by ascorbic acid. J Inorganic Biochem 1981; 14:127–34.
22. Gutteridge JMC. Bleomycin—detectable iron in knee-joint synovial fluid from arthritis patients and its relationship to the extracellular antioxidant activities of caeruloplasmin, transferrin and lactoferrin. Biochem J 1987; 245:415–21.
23. Ambruso DR, Johnston RB. Lactoferrin enhances hydroxyl radical production by human neutrophils, neutrophil particulate fractions, and an ezymatic generating system. J Clin Invest 1981; 67:352–60.
24. Blake DR, Hall ND, Bacon PA, Dieppe PA, Halliwell B, Gutteridge JMC. Effect of a specific chelating agent on animal models of inflammation. Ann Rheum Dis 1983; 42:89–93.
25. Winterbourn CC. Myeloperoxidase as an effective inhibitor of hydroxyl radical production. Implications for the oxidative reactions of neutrophil. J Clin Invest 1986; 78:545–50.
26. Schalkwijk J, van den Berg WB, van de Putte LBA, Joosten LAB, van den Bersselaar L. Cationization of catalase, peroxidase and superoxide dismutase. Effect of improved intraarticular retention on experimenter arthritis in mice. J Clin Invest 1985; 76:198–205.
27. Lunec J, Halloran SP, White AG, Dormandy TL. Free radical oridation (peroxidation) products in serum and synovial fluid in rheumatoid arthritis. J Rheumatol 1981; 8:233–45.
28. Bates EJ, Lowther DA, Handley CJ. Oxygen free radicals mediate an inhibition of proteoglycan synthesis in cultured articular cartilage. Ann Rheum Dis 1984; 43:462–9.
29. Bates EJ, Johnson CC, Lowther DA. Inhibition of proteoglycan synthesis by hydrogen peroxide in cultured bovine articular cartilage. Biochim Biophys Acta 1985; 838:221–8.
30. Bates EJ, Lowther DA, Johnson CC. Hyaluronic acid synthesis in articular cartilage: an inhibition by hydrogen peroxide. Biochem Biophys Res Commun 1985; 132:714–20.
31. Schalkwijk J, van den Berg WB, Levinus BA, van de Putte LBA, Joosten LAB. Hydrogen peroxide suppresses the proteoglycan synthesis of intact articular cartilage. J Rheumatol 1985; 12:205–10.
32. Baker MS, Feigan J, Lowther DA. The mechanisms of chondrocyte hydrogen peroxide damage. Depletion of intracellular ATP due to suppression of glycolysis caused by oxidation of glyceraldehyde-3-phosphate dehydrogenase. J Rheumatol 1989; 16:7–14.
33. Kowanko IC, Bates EJ, Ferrante A. Mechanisms of human neutrophil-mediated cartilage damage in vitro: the role of lysosomal enzymes, hydrogen peroxide and hypochlorous acid. Immunol Cell Biol 1989; 67:321–9.
34. Burkhardt H, Schwingel M, Menninger H, McCartney HW, Tschesche H. Oxygen radicals as effectors of cartilage destruction. Direct degradative effect on matrix components and indirect action via activation of latent collagenase from polymorphonuclear leukocytes. Arthritis Rheum 1986; 29:379–87.
35. Dean RT, Roberts CR, Forni L. Oxygen centered free radicals can efficiently degrade the polypeptide of proteoglycans in whole cartilage. Biosci Rep 1984; 4:1017–26.
36. Greenwald RA, Moy WW. Effect of oxygen derived free radicals on hyaluronic acid. Arthritis Rheum 1980; 23:455–63.
37. Greenwald RA, Moak SA. Degradation of hyaluronic acid by polymorphonuclear leukocytes. Inflammation 1986; 10:15–30.
38. Betts WH, Cleland LG. Effect of metal chelators and anti-inflammatory drugs on the degradation of hyaluronic acid. Arthritis Rheum 1982; 25:1469–76.
39. Baker MS, Green SP, Lowther DA. Changes in the viscosity of hyaluronic acid after exposure to a myeloperoxide derived oxidant. Arthritis Rheum 1989; 32:461–7.
40. Weitz Z, Moak SA, Greenwald RA. Degradation of hyaluronic acid by neutrophil derived oxygen radicals is stimulus dependent. J Rheumatol 1988; 15:1250–3.
41. Greenwald RA, Moy WW, Lazarus D. Degradation of cartilage proteogylcans and collagen by superoxide radicals. Arthritis Rheum 1976; 19:799 (abstr).
42. Bates EJ, Harper GS, Lowther DA, Preston BN. Effect of oxygen-derived reactive species on cartilage proteoglycan hyaluronate aggregates. Biochem Int 1984; 8:629–37.

43. Greenwald RA, Moy WW. Inhibition of collagen gelation by action of the superoxide radical. Arthritis Rheum 1979; 22:251–9.
44. Monboisse JC, Braquet P, Randoux A, Borel JP. Non-enzymatic degradation of acid soluble calf skin collagen by superoxide ion: protective effect of flavenoids. Biochem Pharmacol 1983; 32:53–8.
45. Curran SF, Amoruso MA, Goldstein BD, Berg RA. Degradation of soluble collagen by ozone or hydroxyl radicals. FEBS Lett 1984; 176:155–60.
46. Clark RA, Szot Z, Williams MA, Kagan HM. Oxidation of lysine side-chains of elastin by the myeloperoxidase system and by stimulated human neutrophils. Biochem Biophys Res Commun 1986; 135:451–7.
47. Johnson D, Travis J. The oxidative inactivation of human alpha-1-proteinase inhibitor: further evidence for methionine at the active centre. J Biol Chem 1979; 254:4022–6.
48. Carp H, Janoff A. Potential mediator of inflammation. Phagocyte-derived oxidants suppress the elastase inhibitory capacity of alpha 1-proteinase inhibitor *in-vitro*. J Clin Invest 1980; 66:987–95.
49. Kramps JA, Twisk CU, Klasen EC, Dijkman JH. Interactions among stimulated human polymorphonuclear leukocytes, released elastase and bronchial antileucoprotease. Clin Sci 1988; 75:53–62.
50. Lunec J, Blake DR, McCleary SJ, Brailsford S, Bacon PA. Self-perpetuating mechanisms of immunoglobulin G aggregation in rheumatoid arthritis. J Clin Invest 1985; 76:2084–90.
51. Jasin HE. Generation of IgG aggregates by the myeloperoxidase-hydrogen peroxide system. J Immunol 1983; 130:1918–23.
52. Jasin HE. Oxidative cross-linking of immune complexes by human polymorphonuclear leukocytes. J Clin Invest 1988; 81:6–15.
53. Spragg RG, Hinshaw DB, Hyslop PA, Schraufstattler IU, Cochrane CG. Alterations in adenosine triphosphate and energy charge in cultured endothelial cells and P388D_1 cells after oxidant injury. J Clin Invest 1985; 78:462–71.
54. Raghu G, Striker L, Harlan J, Gown A, Striker G. Cytoskeletal changes as an early event in hydrogen peroxide induced cell injury: a study in A549 cells. Br J Exp Pathol 1986; 67:105–12.
55. Shasby DM, Lind SE, Shasky SS, Goldsmith JC, Hunninghake GW. Reversible oxidant induced increases in albumin transfer across cultured endothelium: alterations in cell shape and calcium homeostasis. Blood 1985; 65:605–14.
56. Ager A, Gordon JL. Differential effects of hydrogen peroxide on indices of endothelial cell function. J Exp Med 1984; 159:592–603.
57. Mello Filho AC, Meneghini R. *In vivo* formation of single strand breaks in DNA by hydrogen peroxide is mediated by the Haber-Weiss reaction. Biochem Biophys Acta 1984; 781:56–63.
58. Rubin R, Farber JL. Mechanisms of the killing of cultured hepatocytes by H_2O_2. Arch Biochem Biophys 1984; 228:450–9.
59. Lewis MS, Whatley RE, Cain P, McIntyre T, Prescott S, Zimmerman GA. Hydrogen peroxide stimulates the synthesis of platelet activating factor by endothelium and induces endothelial cell-dependent neutrophil adhesion. J Clin Invest 1988; 82:2045–55.
60. Serhan C, Anderson P, Goodman E, Dunham P, Weissman G. Phosphatidate and oxidised fatty acid are calcium ionophores. Studies employing arsenazo III in liposomes. J Biol Chem 1981; 256:2736–41.
61. Gadek JE, Fells GA, Wright DG, Crystal RG. Human neutrophil elastase functions as a type III collagen "collagenese." Biochim Biophys Res Commun 1980; 95:1815–22.
62. Mainardi CL, Dixit SN, Kang AH. Degradation of type IV (basement membrane) collagen by a proteinase isolated from human polymorphonuclear leukocyte granules. J Biol Chem 1980; 255:5435–41.
63. Roughly PJ. The degradation of proteoglycan by leukocyte elastase. Biochem Soc Trans 1977; 5:443–5.

64. Janoff A. Elastase in tissue injury. Annu Rev Med 1985; 36:207–216.
65. Velvart M, Fehr K. Degradation *in vivo* of articular cartilage in rheumatoid arthritis and juvenile chronic arthritis by cathepsin G and elastase from polymorphonuclear leukocytes. Rheumatol Int 1987; 7:195–202.
66. Burkhardt H, Kasten M, Rauls S, Rehkopf E. Interference of cartilage surface with interaction of granulocyte elastase with α_1 proteinase inhibitor. Rheumatol Int 1987; 7:133–8.
67. Bartholomew JS, Lowther DA, Handley CJ. Changes in proteoglycan biosynthesis following leukocyte elastase treatment of bovine articular cartilage in culture. Arthritis Rheum 1984; 27:905–12.
68. Bartholomew JS, Lowther DA. Receptor-mediated binding of leukocyte elastase by chondrocytes. Arthritis Rheum 1987; 30:431–8.
69. Baici A, Salgam P, Cohen G, Fehr K, Boni A. Action of collagenase and elastase from human polymorphonuclear leukocytes on human articular cartilage. Rhematol Int 1982; 2:11–6.
70. Heiple JM, Ossowski L. Human neutrophil plasminogen activator is localised in specific granules and is translocated to the cell surface by exocytosis. J Exp Med 1986; 164:826–40.
71. Lack CH, Rogers HJ. Action of plasmin on cartilage. Nature 1958; 182:948–9.
72. Machan E, Keler T. Plasmin degradation of cartilage proteoglycan. Biochem Biophys Acta 1984; 800:312–5.
73. Wert Z, Mainardi CL, Vater CA, Harris ED. Endogenous activation of latent collagenase by rheumatoid synovial cells—evidence for the role of plasminogen activator. N Engl J Med 1977; 296:1017–23.
74. Collier SA, Ghosh P. The role of plasminogen in IL-1 mediated cartilage degradation. J Rhematol 1988; 15:1129–37.
75. Maroudas A. Transport of solutes through cartilage: permeability to large molecules. J Anat 1976; 122:335–47.
76. Meats JE, McGuire MB, Russell RGG. Human synovium releases a factor which stimulates chondrocyte production of PGE and plasminogen activator. Nature 1980; 286:891–2.
77. Ganz T, Selsted ME, Szklarek D, Harwig SSL, Daher K, Bainton DF, Lehrer RI. Defensins. Natural peptide antibiotics of human neutrophils. J Clin Invest 1985; 76:1427–35.
78. Elsbach P, Weiss J. A re-evaluation of the roles of the O_2 dependent and O_2 independent microbicidal systems of phagocytes. Rev Infest Dis 1983; 5:843–53.
79. Lichtenstein A, Ganz T, Selsted ME, Lehrer RI. *In vitro* tumour cell cytolysis mediated by peptide defensins of human and rabbit granulocytes. Blood 1986; 69:1407–10.
80. Bates EJ, Kowanko IC, Ferrante A. Conditioned medium from stimulated mononuclear leucocytes potentiates the ability of human neutrophils to damage human articular cartilage. Ann Rheum Dis 1988; 47:1–9.
81. Kowanko IC, Bates EJ, Ferrante A. Tumour necrosis factor-β modulates human neutrophil-mediated cartilage damage. Scand J Immunol 1988; 28:591–8.
82. Kowanko IC, Bates EJ, Ferrante A. Neutrophil-mediated cartilage injury *in vitro* is enhanced by tumour necrosis factor alpha. Rheumatol Int 1990; 10: 85–90.
83. Schalkwijk J, van den Berg WB, van de Putte LBA, Joosten LAB. Elastase secreted by activated polymorphonuclear leuocytes causes chondrocyte damage and matric degradation in intact articular cartilage—escape from inactivation by alpha-1-proteinase inhibitor. Br J Exp Pathol 1987; 68:81–8.
84. Sacks T, Moldow CF, Craddock PR, Bowers TK, Jacob HS. Oxygen radicals mediate endothelial cell damage by complement-stimulated granulocytes. J Clin Invest 1978; 61:1161–7.
85. Weiss SJ, Young J, Lobuglio AF, Slivka A, Nimeh NF. Role of H_2O_2 in neutrophil mediated destruction of cultured endothelial cells. J Clin Invest 1981; 68:714–21.

86. Hashimoto Y, Tanimoto K, Yoshinoya S, Miyamoto T. Destruction of cultured vascular endothelial cells and red blood cells by immune-activated polymorphonuclear leukocytes. Inflammation 1987; 11:201–10.
87. Smedly LA, Tonnesen MG, Sandhaus RA, Haslett C, Guthrie LA, Johnston RB, Henson PM, Worthen CS. Neutrophil-mediated injury to endothelial cells. Enhancement by endotoxin and essential role of neutrophil elastase. J Clin Invest 1986; 77:1233–43.
88. Harlan JM, Killen PO, Harker LA, Striker GE, Wright DC. Neutrophil mediated endothelial injury *in vitro*. Mechanisms of cell detachment. J Clin Invest 1981; 68:1394–403.
89. Harlan JM, Schwartz BR, Reidy MA, Schwartz SM, Ochs HD, Harker LA. Activated neutrophils disrupt endothelial monolayer integrity by an oxygen radical independent mechanism. Lab Invest 1985; 52:141–50.
90. Vissers MCM, Winterbourn CC, Hunt JS. Degradation of glomerular basement membrane by human neutrophils *in vitro*. Biochim Biophys Acta 1984; 804:154–60.
91. Vissers MCM, Day WA, Winterbourn CC. Neutrophils adherent to a non-phagocytosable surface (glomerular basement membrane) produce oxidants only at the site of attachment. Blood 1985; 66:161–6.
92. Johnston RJ, Couser WG, Chi EY, Adler S, Klebanoff SJ. New mechanism for glomerular injury. Myeloperoxide-hydrogen peroxide system. J Clin Invest 1987; 79:1379–87.
93. Couser WG, Johnson RJ, Adler S, Ochi RF, Klebanoff SJ. The myeloperoxidase-hydrogen peroxide-halide system: evidence for participation in neutrophil-mediated glomerulonephritis. Kidney Int 1986; 29:271 (abstr).
94. Camussi G, Tetta C, Segoloni G, Coda R, Vercellone A. Localization of neutrophil cationic proteins and loss of anionic charges in glomeruli of patients with systemic lupus erythematosis glomerulonephritis. Clin Immunol Immunopathol 1982; 24:299–314.
95. Holman JM, Saba TM. Hepatocyte injury during post-operative sepsis: activated neutrophils as potential mediators. J Leukocyte Biol 1988; 43:193–203.
96. Weiss SJ, Peppin G, Ortiz X, Ragsdale C, Test ST. Oxidative autoactivation of latent collagenase by human neutrophils. Science 1985; 227:747–9.
97. Okado Y, Watanabe S, Nankanishi I, Kishi J, Hayakawa T, Watorek W, Travis J, Nagase H. Inactivation of tissue inhibitor of metalloproteinases by neutrophil elastase and other serine proteases. FEBS Lett 1988; 229;157–60.
98. LeRoy EC, Ager A, Gordon JL. Effects of neutrophil elastase and other proteases on porcine aortic endothelial prostaglandin I_2 production, adenine nucleotide release and responses to vasoactive agents. J Clin Invest 1984; 74:1003–10.
99. Camussi G, Tetta C, Bussolino F, Baglioni C. Synthesis and release of platelet activating factor is inhibited by plasma α_1 proteinase inhibitor or α_1 antichymotrypsin and is stimulated by proteinases. J Exp Med 1988; 168:1293–306.
100. Lindemann A, Riedel D, Oster W, Ziegler-Heitbrock HWL, Mertelsmann R, Herrmann F. Granulocyte-macrophage colony-stimulating factor induces cytokines secretion by human polymorphonuclear leukocytes. J Clin Invest 1989; 83:1308–12.
101. Lindemann A, Riedel D, Oster W, Meuer SC, Blohm D, Mertelsmann RH, Herrmann F. Granulocyte-macrophage colony-stimulating factor induces interleukin-1 production by human polymorphonuclear neutrophils. J Immunol 1988; 140:837–9.
102. Tyler JA, Saklatavala J. Pig interleukin-1 (catabolin) induces resorption of cartilage proteoglycan and prevents synthesis of proteoglycan and collagen. Br J Rheumatol 1985; 24:(suppl)150–5.
103. Ikebe T, Hirata M, Koga T. Effect of human recombinant tumour necrosis factor-a and interleukin 1 on the synthesis of glycosaminoglycan and DNA in cultured rat costal chondrocytes. J Immunol 1988; 140:827–31.
104. Arner EC, Pratta MA. Independent effects of interleukin-1 on proteoglycan breakdown, proteoglycan synthesis and prostaglandin E_2 release from cartilage in organ culture. Arthritis Rheum 1989; 32:288–97.

105. Seow WK, Ferrante A, Si-ying L, Thong YH. Suppression of human monocyte interleukin-1 production by the plant alkaloid tetrandrine. Clin Exp Immunol 1989; 75:47–51.
106. Ferrante A, Seow WK, Rowan-Kelly B, Thong YH. Tetrandrine, a plant alkaloid, inhibits the production of tumour necrosis factor alpha (Cachectin) by human monocytes. Clin Exp Immun 1990; 80:257–62.
107. Ferrante A, Staugas REM, Rowan-Kelly B, Bresatz S, Kumaratilake LM, Rzepczyk CM, Adolf GR. Production of tumour necrosis factor alpha and beta by human mononuclear leukocytes stimulated with mitogens, bacteria and malarial paramites. Infect Immun 1990; 58:3996–4003.
108. Klebanoff SJ, Vadas MA, Harlan JM, Sparks LH, Gamble JR, Agosti JM, Watersdorph AM. Stimulation of neutrophils by tumour necrosis factor. J Immunol 1986; 136:4220–5.
109. Shalaby MR, Palladino MA Jr, Hirabayashi SE, Eessalu TE, Lewis GD, Shepard HM, Aggarwal BB. Receptor binding and activation of polymorphonuclear neutrophils by tumour necrosis factor-alpha. J Leukocyte Biol 1987; 41:196–204.
110. Gamble JR, Harlan JM, Klebanoff SJ, Vadas MA. Stimulation of the adherence of neutrophils to umbilical vein endothelium by human recombinant tumor necrosis factor. Proc Natl Acad Sci USA 1985; 82:8667–71.
111. Berger M, Wetzler EM, Wallis RS. Tumor necrosis factor is the major monocyte product that increases complement receptor expression on mature human neutrophils. Blood 1988; 71:151–8.
112. Varani J, Bendelow MJ, Sealey DE, Kunkel SL, Gannon DE, Ryan US, Ward PA. Tumour necrosis factor enhances susceptibility of vascular endothelium to neutrophil mediated killing. Lab Invest 1988; 59:292–5.
113. Humphrey DM, McManus L, Satouchi K, Hanahan DJ, Pinckard RN. Vasoactive properties of acetyl glyceryl ether phosphorylcholine and analogues. Lab Invest 1982; 46:422–7.
114. Bussolino F, Camussi G, Aglietta M, Braquet P, Bosia A, Pescarmona G, Sanavio F, D'urso N, Marchisio PC. Human endothelial cells are a target for platelet activating factor. J Immunol 1987; 139:2439–46.
115. Camussi G, Bussolino F, Salvidio G, Baglioni C. Tumour necrosis factor/cachectin stimulates peritoneal macrophages, polymorphonuclear neutrophils and vascular endothelial cells to synthesise and release platelet activating factor. J Exp Med 1987; 166:1390–404.
116. Bussolino F, Camussi G, Baglioni C. Synthesis and release of platelet activating factor by human vascular endothelial cells treated with tumour necrosis factor or interleukin-1a. J Biol Chem 1988; 263:11856–61.
117. Camussi G, Tetta C, Bussolino F, Baglioni C. Tumour necrosis factor stimulates human neutrophils to release leukotriene B_4 and platelet activating factor. Induction of phospholipase A_2 and acetyl-CoA:1-alkyl-sn-glycero-3-phosphocholine-O_2-acetyltranferase activity and inhibition of antiprotease. Eur J Biochem 1989; 182:661–6.
118. Vercellotti GM, Yin HQ, Gustafson KS, Nelson RD, Jacob HS. Platelet activating factor primes neutrophil responses to agonists: role in promoting neutrophil mediated endothelial damage. Blood 1988; 71:1110–7.
119. Paubert-Braquet M, Longchampt MO, Koltz P, Guilbaud J. Tumour necrosis factor (TNF) primes platelet activating factor (PAF) induced superoxide generation by human neutrophils (PMN): consequences in promoting PMN mediated endothelial cell (EC) damages. Prostaglandins 1988; 35(suppl):803.
120. Bussolino F, Breviario F, Tetta C, Aglietta M, Mantovani A, Dejana E. Interleukin 1 stimulates platelet activating factor production in cultured human endothelial cells. J Clin Invest 1986; 77:2027–33.
121. Breviario F, Bertocchi F, Dejana E, Bussolino F. IL-1-induced adhesion of polymorphonuclear leukocytes to cultured human endothelial cells. Role of platelet activating factor. J Immunol 1988; 141:3391–7.

122. Emeis JJ, Kluft C. PAF-Acether-induced release of tissue type plasminogen activator from vessel walls. Blood 1985; 66:86–91.
123. Campbell EJ, Senior RM, McDonald JA, Cox DL. Proteolysis by neutrophils. Relative importance of cell-substrate contact and oxidative inactivation of proteinase inhibitors *in vitro*. J Clin Invest 1982; 70:845–52.
124. Campbell EJ, Campbell MA. Pericellular proteolysis by neutrophils in the presence of proteinase inhibitors: effects of substrate opsonization. J Cell Biol 1988; 106:667–76.
125. Weiss SJ, Regiani S. Neutrophils degrade subendothelial matrices in the presence of alpha-1-proteinase inhibitor. Cooperative use of lysosomal proteinases and oxygen metabolites. J Clin Invest 1984; 73:1297–303.
126. Weiss SJ, Curnutte JT, Regiani S. Neutrophil mediated solubilization of the subendothelial matrix: oxidative and nonoxidative mechanisms of proteolysis used by normal and chronic granulomatous disease phagocytes. J Immunol 1986; 136:636–41.
127. Weitz JI, Huang AJ, Landman SL, Nicholson SC, Silverstein SC. Elastase mediated fibrinogenolysis by chemoattractant stimulated neutrophils occurs in the presence of physiologic concentrations of antiproteinases. J Exp Med 1987; 166:1836–50.
128. Kowanko IC, Ferrante A. Granulocyte-macrophage colony-stimulating factor augments neutrophil-mediated cartilage degradation and neutophil adherence. Arthritis Rheum (1991), 34:1452–1460.
129. Kowanko IC, Ferrante A. Interferon-gamma increases human neutrophil-mediated cartilage proteoglycan degradation. Clin Exp Immunol (in press).

19

Tumor Necrosis Factor Stimulation of Neutrophils for Antitumor Activity

HUNGYI SHAU and ROBERT L. ROBERTS
UCLA School of Medicine, Los Angeles, California

I. INTRODUCTION

Polymorphonuclear neutrophils (PMNs) are the first line of defense against microbial infection. However, their role in protecting hosts against tumors has not been well defined and is generally ignored by most investigators. There is some evidence that PMNs are involved in destroying tumors in vivo. Bacillus Calmette-Guerin (BCG), *Corynebacterium parvum,* and the streptococcal preparation OK-432 are reagents widely used in animal models and clinical trials to induce tumor regression. Administration of each of these reagents induces quick accumulation of PMNs at the injection site (1–3). The accumulated PMNs have been shown to have cytotoxic activity against tumor cells in vitro (1–3). Therefore, infiltrating PMNs at the tumor sites may be responsible for tumor regression caused by treatment with these microbial preparations.

When properly activated, PMNs can lyse tumor cells in vitro. Stimulators such as phorbol 12-myristate-13-acetate (PMA), Concanavalin A (Con A), BCG, *C. parvum,* or OK-432 have been shown to induce PMN production of reactive oxidants to lyse tumor cells (1–5). In addition, tumor cell destruction by activated PMNs without involvement of reactive oxygen species has also been documented. PMNs have receptors for the Fc portion of immunoglobulins and can lyse tumor target cells by interacting with the Fc portion of antibodies specific for tumor cells. This antibody-dependent cellular cytotoxicity (ADCC) can also be enhanced by stimulants or PMNs (6–11).

Tumor necrosis factor α (TNF_{α}) was originally described as a serum factor from BCG- and lipopolysaccharide (LPS)-injected animals which could induce hemorrhagic tumor necrosis in animal models (12). Monocytes treated with *C. parvum* or OK-432 in vitro or in vivo can produce large quantities of TNF (13–15). Because TNF is induced by these microbial preparations and is able to cause tumor necrosis, it is possible that TNF is a mediator for the tumor regression induced by these biological response modifiers. However, despite its antitumor efficacy in vivo, TNF when tested in vitro has no direct cytotoxic or cytostatic activity against most tumor cells, including tumor cells which are sensitive to TNF treatment in vivo (16–19). Therefore, TNF probably alters tumor growth in vivo through an indirect mechanism rather than direct toxicity to the tumor cells in most animal models.

The genes for TNF in human and mouse have been cloned, and large quantities of recombinant TNF have been produced for preclinical and clinical studies (20–24). TNF is a potent activator for PMNs, which have more surface TNF receptors than any other blood cell type (25). TNF-treated PMNs are more adherent, more phagocytic, show greater respiratory response to other stimulants, and express enhanced antibody-dependent cellular cytotoxicity (ADCC) (8,25–28). Necrotic tumors induced by BCG or TNF treatment usually involve extensive PMN infiltration (16,29). This evidence suggests that activated PMNs may constitute a significant mechanism in TNF-induced tumor regression. Therefore we undertook a series of studies to investigate the antitumor functions of TNF-activated PMNs.

II. TNF INDUCTION OF PMN CYTOSTATIC ACTIVITY

To determine the effect of TNF-activated PMNs on tumor cell growth, we cultured tumor cell lines with TNF and PMNs and then tested for the proliferative activity of the tumor cells in a 24-h assay. Incorporation of ^{3}H-thymidine in the last 4 h of the assay was measured as an indicator for proliferation. PMNs in the presence of recombinant human TNF (Cetus, Emeryville, CA) significantly inhibited proliferation of tumor cells (30,31). The cytostatic activity is dose dependent for both PMN effector cells and TNF concentration. At a TNF concentration of 50 U/ml, PMNs inhibited Raji tumor target cell proliferation at an effector cell:target ratio as low as 0.6:1. Higher PMN:Raji ratios show greater cytostatic activity. At the effector cell:target ratio of 5:1, PMNs treated with TNF at above 1 U/ml suppressed Raji proliferation. PMNs in the presence or absence of TNF do not secrete cold thymidine or incorporate tritiated thymidine.

PMN cytostatic activity is induced specifically by TNF, because it can be blocked by antibodies specific for TNF (30,31). However, TNF need not be present during the assay for the cytostatic activity. Once PMNs are activated, TNF can be washed away or blocked with anti-TNF antibodies without affecting the cytostatic activity.

PMN cytostatic activity is not restricted to one particular type of tumor cell. We have tested five different tumor cell lines, and all show sensitivity to TNF-induced PMN cytostatic activity (Table 1). These tumor cell lines include a B-cell lymphoma

Table 1 TNF Induces PMN Cytostatic Activity Against Different Tumor Cell Lines[a]

Target cells	Treatment:	Percent cytostasis ±SD PMN	TNF	PMN + TNF
Raji		11.0 ± 5.8	−10.4 ± 9.3	64.2 ± 2.3
K562		12.2 ± 5.4	10.3 ± 3.0	76.0 ± 1.5
UCLA-SO-M14		−18.4 ± 8.7	5.5 ± 5.7	57.7 ± 1.3
U937		−2.0 ± 2.7	40.7 ± 1.9	62.5 ± 3.3
SK-MES-1		9.4 ± 1.0	43.0 ± 4.8	58.6 ± 2.9

[a] Tumor target cells were treated with PMNs at the PMN:target ratio of 5:1 (except SK-MES-1, which was treated at 10:1 ratio), TNF (100 U/ml), or both in a cytostasis assay where the cell proliferation was measured by incorporation of ^{3}H-thymidine.

line Raji, an erythroleukemic cell line K562, a histiocytic cell line U937, a melanoma cell line UCLA-SO-M14, and a lung carcinoma line SK-MES-1. Among the five tumor cell lines, only two, U937 and SK-MES-1, are sensitive to TNF alone in the cytostatic assay, and TNF-activated PMNs show additive cytostatic activity over TNF against these two cell lines.

Our results indicate that PMNs can be activated by TNF to suppress tumor cell proliferation. Furthermore, this cytostatic activity can be demonstrated against different tumor cell types, including both TNF-sensitive and TNF-resistant cells.

III. INVOLVEMENT OF REACTIVE OXIDANTS IN PMN CYTOSTATIC ACTIVITY

TNF can induce an oxidative burst in adherent PMNs. Many of the reactive oxidants produced by PMNs are potentially toxic to tumor cells. It is possible that TNF induces PMN cytostatic activity by activating their production of the reactive oxidants.

Chronic granulomatous disease (CGD) is an inherited disorder in which the phagocytes are defective in generating reactive oxidants (32,33). Nonoxidative functions of CGD phagocytes, including binding of chemotactic factors, adhesion, and phagocytosis, are reported to be normal. If reactive oxidants are not involved in TNF-induced PMN cytostatic activity, we would expect PMNs from CGD patients to possess normal cytostatic function.

We have several CGD patients whose phagocytes have been characterized as totally lacking oxidative burst function (34,35). To test whether their PMNs can be activated to express cytostatic activity, we incubated Raji cells with TNF and PMNs from a CGD patient. Figure 1 shows that TNF fails to induce cytostatic activity observed even at a CGD PMN:Raji cell ratio as high as 16:1. In contrast, in the presence of TNF, PMNs from a normal control show dose-dependent cytostatic activity. The optimal cytostatic activity against Raji cells is observed at the PMN:Raji ratio of 4:1. At higher PMN:Raji ratios, normal PMNs show only suboptimal cytostatic activity. A similar lack of TNF-inducible cytostatic activity has been repeated many times with PMNs

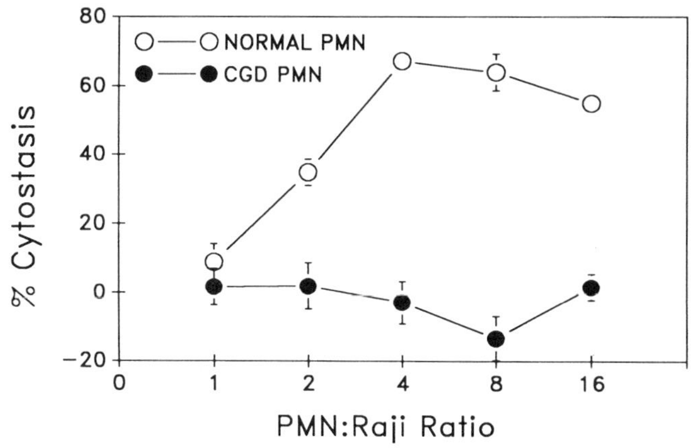

Figure 1 Induction of PMN cytostatic activity against Raji cells. Raji cells were incubated with normal or CGD PMNs in the presence of 50 U/ml of TNF. The cytostatic activity is measured as inhibition of Raji cell incorporation of ^{3}H-thymidine by the PMNs. Error bars represent SD of triplicate experiments.

from this and another CGD patient. In each experiment, PMNs from normal controls show significant cytostatic activity in the presence of TNF. The fact that TNF induces cytostatic activity only in PMNs from healthy individuals but not in PMNs from CGD patients strongly indicates that the cytostatic activity is dependent on PMN production of reactive oxidants.

To determine which reactive oxidants are involved in PMN cytostatic activity, we have tested the effect of antioxidants in the cytostasis assay of tumor cells. When catalase is added at the beginning of the co-culture of TNF, normal PMNs, and tumor cells, the PMN cytostatic activity can be totally blocked, suggesting that hydrogen peroxide (H_2O_2) is important for the cytostatic activity (30). However, catalase is effective in abrogating the cytostatic activity only when it is added within the first 2 h after the assay is initiated (31). This is consistent with the result that TNF-induced PMN H_2O_2 production reaches maximal levels in the first 2 h after TNF treatment (26,31,36).

In contrast to catalase, inhibitors for other reactive oxidants show no inhibition of PMN cytostatic activity. The reactive oxidant inhibitors which do not block PMN cytostatic activity include superoxide dismutase (SOD) for superoxide, azide for myeloperoxidase, L-methionine for myeloperoxidase products, and deferroxamine for the Haber-Weiss reaction (31). This evidence indicates that H_2O_2, but not other reactive oxidants induced by TNF, is involved in PMN cytostatic activity.

The hypothesis that TNF causes tumor regression by inducing PMN H_2O_2 production is supported by results from animal studies. Besides catalase, the glutathione redox cycle is the other major pathway by which eukaryotic cells scavenge H_2O_2 toxicity (37–39). Zimmerman et al. have shown that the content of reduced glutathione in tumor cells is inversely correlated with their sensitivity to TNF treatment in vivo (40,41). Indeed, tumor cells with a lower content of reduced glutathione are more sensitive to H_2O_2 toxicity in vitro and thus show greater response to TNF treatment in vivo. In addition, the H_2O_2 scavenger uric acid can abrogate TNF efficacy in treating Meth A-induced fibrosarcoma metastasis (40). Conversely, glutathione inhibitors increase Meth A sensitivity to TNF treatment in vivo. These data agree with the notion not only that TNF causes tumor regression by inducing PMN H_2O_2 production, but that tumor cells use the glutathione redox cycle to resist the PMN-generated H_2O_2 toxicity.

While TNF is effective in causing tumor regression in many animal models, clinical trials of cancer patients with TNF alone have yet to produce similar impressive efficacy (20–24). Part of the reason may be due to the differences between human and murine tumor cells in their sensitivity to H_2O_2. A study by O'Donnell-Tormey et al. with nine types of human cells showed that human tumor cells are more resistant to H_2O_2 toxicity than 22 types of murine cells (42). The H_2O_2 LD_{50} values of human tumor cells are 100 times higher than those of murine cells. Thus, if PMN-produced H_2O_2 is responsible for the TNF-induced tumor regression, it would not be surprising that TNF is more effective in treating tumors in the murine models than in humans, and protocols to abrogate the resistance to H_2O_2 in human tumors will be beneficial to patients receiving TNF for cancer.

IV. INVOLVEMENT OF FACTORS OTHER THAN REACTIVE OXIDANTS IN PMN CYTOSTATIC ACTIVITY

While H_2O_2 is essential for PMN cytostatic activity, there is evidence that production of H_2O_2 alone may not be sufficient to mediate the cytostatic function. We have compared the concentrations of exogenous H_2O_2 required to suppress tumor cell proliferation with the amount of H_2O_2 produced by TNF-activated PMNs (31). H_2O_2 is cytostatic to tumor cells only at concentrations above 10^{-5} M. This concentration is almost two orders of magnitude greater than the amount of H_2O_2 produced by TNF-activated PMNs at PMN concentrations sufficient to totally suppress Raji cell proliferation. In addition, culture supernatants of TNF-activated PMNs do not have any direct cytostatic activity against the tumor target cells.

One possible explanation for the discrepancy between the concentrations of H_2O_2 required to stop tumor cell proliferation and the concentrations produced by PMNs is that the tumor cells may be exposed to local high concentrations of H_2O_2 only at or near the contact area with PMNs. We and other investigators have shown that TNF-activated PMNs become more adherent to tumor cells and other surfaces (26,31,43–45). This enhanced interaction between PMNs and target cells may allow PMNs to secrete high concentrations of H_2O_2 directly on to the target cells before H_2O_2 is diluted in the culture medium. To test this hypothesis, we have cultured PMNs and tumor target cells in two different chambers of a transwell system (Costar, Cambridge, MA) where the chambers are separated by a permeable membrane. TNF induces cytostatic activity only when both PMNs and tumor target cells are placed on the same side of the permeable membrane but not when the two populations are placed on opposite sides of the membrane (Table 2). Therefore, the cytostatic activity may be mediated by local high concentrations of H_2O_2 created by enhanced adhesion of PMNs to the tumor target cells, and is not detectable when PMN-target cell contact is prevented by the permeable membrane.

Another possibility is that the low level of H_2O_2 is not directly cytostatic but acts as a cofactor to synergize with a contact-dependent cytostatic activity. PMNs contain many membrane-associated and granule-associated factors such as proteases and defensins which are potentially toxic to cells (46–49). TNF can cause moderate degranulation of PMNs and enhance their adhesion to tumor cells (26,31), thus exposing tumor target cells to these potentially toxic factors. Furthermore, H_2O_2 can synergize with proteases and defensins in cell destruction (46–50). It can also inactivate antiproteases to eliminate tumor cell defense against proteases. Under these conditions, once enough H_2O_2 is induced by TNF, the limiting factor for the cytostatic activity is probably the putative mediator, which functions only by PMN contact.

Table 2 TNF-Activated PMNs Require Contact with Tumor Target Cells to Mediate Cytostatic Activity[a]

	Percent cytostasis ±SD			
	PMN:Raji ratio			
Treatment	0.3	1	3	10
PMN (M)	2.1 ± 9.1	3.6 ± 8.6	−5.8 ± 10.7	−8.8 ± 9.1
PMN + TNF (M)	15.5 ± 7.3	32.7 ± 3.6	78.7 ± 1.1	68.4 ± 2.5
PMN (S)	−17.5 ± 6.4	−10.5 ± 6.5	−9.7 ± 9.0	17.3 ± 7.7
PMN + TNF (S)	11.6 ± 4.8	2.6 ± 4.4	10.4 ± 5.9	12.1 ± 4.4

[a] Raji cells were mixed with (M) or separated from (S) PMNs in transwells in the presence or absence of 50 U/ml of TNF.

V. TNF REGULATION OF PMN CYTOTOX ACTIVITY

Besides cytostatic activity, TNF-activated PMNs can also lyse tumor target cells. However, direct cytolytic activity is not evident in short-term assays. In a 24-h chromium release assay where cytolysis of target cells is indicated by the release of [^{51}Cr] from labeled tumor cells, we detect only marginal target cell lysis by the TNF-activated PMNs (30). The destruction of tumor target cells by TNF-treated PMNs is more significant in longer cultures. In 2-day cultures, the number of viable tumor cells is decreased to half the original number by TNF-treated PMNs (30). In contrast, the tumor cell number increases to twofold or more in control cultures. Therefore, TNF-activated PMNs are cytotoxic to tumor cells, but the cytolysis is evident only after long incubation.

VI. ANTIBODY-DEPENDENT CELLULAR CYTOTOXICITY MEDIATED BY PMN

We have shown that TNF can induce the cytotoxicity of PMNs toward tumor cell targets, and other studies revealed that agents such as granulocyte-macrophage colony-stimulating factor (GM-CSF), γ-interferon, and PMA also stimulate PMN killing of tumor cells (5,7,8,11). However, this toxicity is nonspecific, and the activated PMNs are as likely to injure host tissues such as pulmonary epithelium (51). The enhanced toxicity of PMNs by TNF must be balanced against the adverse effects on the host. This host toxicity might be decreased, however, by specifically directing the PMNs to attack only a particular target cell and decrease the adverse effects of TNF on the host. One mechanism for achieving this specificity is the use of antisera or monoclonal antibodies directed to specific antigens on the tumor cells.

Previous studies by several investigators have found that PMNs can be very effective in mediating ADCC against tumor cell targets, and that this cytotoxicity may be greatly enhanced by agents such as PMA, lectins, and various cytokines (6–11,51,52). There are few reports specifically using TNF to enhance PMN-mediated ADCC against tumor targets, although the ability of TNF to enhance various PMN functions such as oxidative metabolism and surface receptor upregulation (8,25–28,31,53,54) as well as TNF's direct antitumor activity make it a good candidate for augmenting this form of ADCC.

The cellular mechanism by which PMNs mediate ADCC is not well understood. Previous investigators have reported that oxygen intermediates such as superoxide play a role in this form of lysis, based on inhibition of lysis by superoxide scavengers and on the decreased ADCC by CGD patients whose PMNs lack the ability to make oxygen intermediates (7,55–57). However, in a recent study at UCLA, PMNs from CGD patients killed HIV-infected MOLT tumor cells as well as normal PMNs. This ADCC lysis was greatly enhanced (up to sixfold) by GM-CSF or G-CSF (11). We have also found that PMNs from CGD patients mediate ADCC as well as, or slightly better than, normal PMNs in studies in our laboratory (unpublished) using chicken erythrocyte targets. GM-CSF was also found to greatly enhance antibody-mediated lysis by both normal and CGD PMNs in those assays, and preliminary studies indicate that TNF can also enhance this cytotoxicity. It should be noted that when we use PMA instead of antibody to activate cells for killing, PMNs from CGD patients performed much less well, lysing only about a third to a fourth as many tumor cells (K562, Raji, CEM) as did normal PMNs (58). These studies indicate that oxygen intermediates may be more important in nonspecific cytotoxicity as induced by PMA but much less important in specific, antibody-mediated cytotoxicity.

Another method pursued by Fanger and associates for mediating specific killing by PMNs is the use of heteroantibodies (HAs) (59). HAs are made by covalently bonding two antibodies of different specifities together at the Fc ends of the antibodies. This results in a two-headed molecule with one Fab component directed to a target such as tumor- or virally infected cells, and the other Fab directed to the Fc receptor of a PMN or other effector cell. The linking of the target cell to the PMN by the HA activates the PMN and results in lysis of target cell. Cytokines such as TNF and GM-CSF, which increase the expression of Fc receptors on PMNs, will also enhance HA-mediated cytotoxicity. In preliminary experiments we have also found that PMNs from CGD patients mediate HA-induced cytotoxicity as well as normal PMNs and are also augmented (three- to fourfold) by GM-CSF (60).

The specificity of the HAs is such that they bind to only one particular type of Fc receptor (I, II, or III) on the PMNs. Thus the specificity of HA for both the target and effector cell has great potential for recruiting PMN to specific target cells labeled with HA. The HAs have greater avidity for the PMN Fc receptor than the Fc portion of a native IgG molecule and thus will increase binding of PMN to a particular target. It may also be possible to direct HAs to another surface receptor such as that for CD18 complex (complement C3bi receptor). TNF will also increase expression of these receptors (three- to fourfold) and thus would be expected to increase cytotoxicity (44,53).

ADCC by PMNs has been reported to be defective in PMNs from patients with lung and gastrointestinal cancer (61). Although the importance of ADCC by PMNs in combatting cancer is unknown, it may be anticipated that this form of cytotoxicity may become significant when monoclonal antibodies (or HAs) are used to treat specific malignancies. TNF could then possibly be used to bolster ADCC against cancer cells in these patients.

VII. CONCLUSION

While PMNs have only a short lifetime in vivo and in vitro, and unlike lymphocytes do not have memory response to antigenic challenges, current evidence indicates that TNF-activated PMNs can have a significant role in host antitumor defense. Once activated with TNF, PMNs are potent suppressors of tumor cell proliferation and also can eventually cause tumor cell death. This cytostatic activity is dependent on PMN production of H_2O_2 but may also require enhanced adhesion of PMNs to tumor target cells. Therefore, the effectiveness of TNF in cancer treatment may depend on the sensitivity of tumor cells to H_2O_2, and approaches to reduce tumor cell resistance to H_2O_2 may be useful in improving efficacy of TNF treatment for cancer. PMNs can mediate ADCC specifically against tumor cells in the presence of antitumor antibodies. TNF can also possibly be used to bolster ADCC against cancer cells in patients receiving tumor-specific antibody treatment.

ACKNOWLEDGMENT

This work was supported by grants from the California Institute for Cancer Research, the National Institutes of Health (HD-09800 and AI-15332), and the Pediatric AIDS

Foundation (500047). We thank Sidney H. Golub and Richard E. Stiehm for discussion, and Pornsri Lawton and Anthony Kim for excellent technical assistance.

REFERENCES

1. Lichtenstein A, Kahle J, Berek J, Zighelboim J. Successful immunotherapy with intraperitoneal *Corynebacterium parvum* in a murine ovarian cancer model is associated with the recruitment of tumor-lytic neutrophils into the peritoneal cavity. J Immunol 1984; 133:519–26.
2. Lichtenstein A. Anti-tumor effect of the streptococcal preparation OK-432 in a murine model of ovarian cancer. Cancer Immunol Immunother 1987; 24:172–7.
3. Nathan CV, Brukner LH, Silverstein SC, Cohn ZA. Extracellular cytolysis by activated macrophages and granulocytes. I. Pharmacologic triggering of effector cells and the release of hydrogen peroxide. J Exp Med 1979; 149:84–99.
4. Lichtenstein A, Seelig M, Berek J, Zighelboim J. Human neutrophil-mediated lysis of ovarian cancer cells. Blood 1989; 74:805–9.
5. Weiss SJ, Slivka A. Monocyte and granulocyte-mediated tumor cell destruction. J Clin Invest 1982; 69:255–62.
6. Shen L, Guyre PM, Fanger MW. Polymorphonuclear leukocyte function triggered through the high affinity Fc receptor for monomeric IgG. J Immunol 1987; 139:534–8.
7. Dallegri F, Patrone F, Frumento G, Sacchetti C. Antibody-dependent killing of tumor cells by polymorphonuclear leukocytes. Involvement of oxidative and non-oxidative mechanisms. J Natl Cancer Inst 1981; 73:331–9.
8. Perussia B, Kobayashi M, Rossi ME, Anegon I, Trinchieri G. Immune interferon enhances functional properties of human granulocytes: role of Fc receptors and effect of lymphotoxin, tumor ncrosis factor, and granulocyte-macrophage colony-stimulating factor. J Immunol 1987; 138:765–74.
9. Conkling P, Klassen DK, Sagone AL. Comparison of antibody-dependent cytotoxicity mediated by human polymorphonuclear cells, monocytes and alveolar macrophages. Blood 1982; 60:1290–7.
10. Spisani S, Gavioli R, Giuliani AL, Traniello S. Triggering of neutrophil cytotoxicity against an antibody-coated tumor target by TPA. Immunol Cell Biol 1989; 67:385–9.
11. Baldwin GC, Fuller ND, Roberts RL, Ho DD, Golde DW. Granulocyte- and granulocyte-macrophage colony stimulating factors enhance neutrophil cytotoxicity toward HIV-infected cells. Blood 1989; 74:1673–7.
12. Carswell EA, Old LJ, Kassel RL, Green S, Fiore N, Williamson B. An endotoxin-induced serum factor that causes necrosis of tumors. Proc Natl Acad Sci USA 1975; 73:3666–75.
13. Valone SE, Rich EA, Wallis RS, Ellner JJ. Expression of tumor necrosis factor in vitro by human mononuclear phagocytes stimulated with whole *Mycobacterium bovis* BCG and mycobacterial antigens. Infect Immun 1988; 56:3313–5.
14. Mori H, Itoh N, Tamaya T. Mechanism of induction of endogenous tumor necrosis factor in ascites of ovarian cancer patients by OK-432, a streptococcal preparation. Immunopharmacol Immunotoxicol 1989; 11:33–53.
15. Sekimoto M, Kokunai I, Shimano T, Kobayashi T, Takeda T, Haruna N, Yamaoto A, Mori T. Production of tumor necrosis factor (TNF) by monocytes from cancer patients and healthy subjects induced by OK-432 in vitro and its augmentation by human interferon-gamma. J Clin Lab Immunol 1988; 27:115–20.
16. Asher A, Mule JJ, Reichert CM, Shiloni E, Rosenberg SA. Studies on the anti-tumor efficacy of systematically administered recombinant tumor necrosis factor against several murine tumors in vivo. J Immunol 1987; 138:963–74.
17. Manda T, Shimonura K, Mukumoto S, Kobayashi K, Mizota T, Hirai O, Matsumoto S, Oku T, Nishigaki F, Mori J, Kikuchi H. Recombinant human tumor necrosis factor-alpha: evidence of an indirect mode of antitumor activity. Cancer Res 1987; 47:3707–11.

18. Palladino MA Jr, Shalaby MR, Kramer SM, Ferraiolo BL, Baughman RA, Deleo AB, Crase D, Marafino B, Aggarwal BB, Figari IS, Liggitt D, Patton JS. Characterization of the antitumor activities of human tumor necrosis factor-alpha and the comparison with other cytokines: induction of tumor-specific immunity. J Immunol 1987; 138:4023–32.
19. Shepard HM, Lewis GD. Resistance of tumor cells to tumor necrosis factor. J Clin Immunol 1988; 8:333–41.
20. Blick M, Sherwin SA, Rosenblum M, Gutterman J. Phase I study of recombinant tumor necrosis factor in cancer patients. Cancer Res 1987; 47:2986–3989.
21. Kist A, Ho AD, Rath U, Wiedenmann B, Bauer A, Schlick E, Kirchner H, Mannel DN. Decrease of natural killer cell activity and monokine production in peripheral blood of patients treated with recombinant tumor necrosis factor. Blood 1988; 72:344–8.
22. Abbruzzese JL, Levin B, Ajani JA, Faintuch JS, Saks S, Patt YZ, Edwards C, Ende K, Gutterman JU. Phase I trial of recombinant human interferon-gamma and recombinant tumor necrosis factor in patients with advanced gastrointestinal cancer. Cancer Res 1989; 49:4057–61.
23. Moritz T, Niederle N, Baumann J, May D, Kurschel E, Osieka R, Kempen J, Schlick E, Schmidt CG. Phase I study of recombinant human tumor necrosis factor alpha in advanced malignant disease. Cancer Immunol Immunother 1989; 39:144–50.
24. Demetri GD, Spriggs DR, Sherman ML, Arthur KA, Imamura K, Kufe DW. A phase I trial of recombinant human tumor necrosis factor and interferon-gamma: effects of combination cytokine administration in vivo. J Clin Oncol 1989; 7:1545-53.
25. Shalaby MR, Palladino MA Jr, Hirabayashi SE, Eessalu TE, Lewis GD, Shepard HM, Aggarwal BB. Receptor binding and activation of polymorphonuclear neutrophils by tumor necrosis factor-alpha. J Leuk Biol 1987; 41:196–204.
26. Klebanoff SJ, Vadas MA, Harlan JM, Sparks LH, Gamble JR, Agosti JM, Waltersdorph AM. Stimulation of neutrophils by tumor necrosis factor. J Immunol 1986; 136:4220–25.
27. Larrick JW, Graham D, Toy K, Lin LS, Senyk G, Fendly BM. Recombinant tumor necrosis factor causes activation of human granulocytes. Blood 1987; 69:640–4.
28. Shalaby MR, Aggarwal BB, Rinderknecht E, Svedersky LP, Findle BS, Palladino MA Jr. Activation of human polymorphonuclear neutrophil functions by interferon-gamma and tumor necrosis factor. J Immunol 1985; 135:2069–73.
29. Holmes EC, Ramming KP, Being ME, Coulson WF, Callery CD. Intralesional BCG immunotherapy of pulmonary tumors. J Thoracic Cardiovasc Surg 1979; 77:362–8.
30. Shau H. Cytostatic and tumoricidal activities of tumor necrosis factor-treated neutrophils. Immunol Lett 1988; 17:47–51.
31. Shau H. Characteristics and mechanism of neutrophil-mediated cytostasis induced by tumor necrosis factor. J Immunol 1988; 141:234–40.
32. Orkin SH. Molecular genetics of chronic granulomatous disease. Ann Rev Immunol 1989; 7:277–307.
33. Curnutte JT, Babior BM. Chronic granulomatous disease. Adv Human Genet 1987; 16:229–97.
34. Okamura N, Malawista SE, Roberts RL, Rosen HS, Ochs HD, Babior BM, Curnutte JT. Phosphorylation of the oxidase-related 48K phosphoprotein family in the unusual autosomal cytochrome-negative and X-linked cytochrome-positive types of chronic granulomatous disease. Blood 1988; 72:811–6.
35. Ohno Y, Buescher S, Roberts R, Metcalf JA, Gallin JI. Reevaluation of cytochrome b and flavin adenine dinucleotide in neutrophils from patients with chronic granulomatous disease and description of a family with probable autosomal recessive inheritance of cytochrome b deficience. Blood 1986; 67:1132–8.
36. Nathan CF. Neutrophil activation on biological surfaces. Massive secretion of hydrogen peroxide in response to products of macrophages and lymphocytes. J Clin Invest 1987; 80:1550–60.
37. Harlan JM, Levine JD, Callahan KS, Schwartz BR, Harker LA. Glutathione redox cycle

protects cultured entothelial cells against lysis by extracellularly generated hydrogen peroxide. J Clin Invest 1984; 73:706–13.
38. Nathan CF, Arrick BA, Murray HW, DeSantis NM, Cohn ZA. Tumor cell anti-oxidant defenses. Inhibition of the glutathione redox cycle enhances macrophage-mediated cytolysis. J Exp Med 1980; 153:766–82.
39. Cohen G, Hochstein P. Glutathione peroxidase: the primary agent for the elimination of hydrogen peroxide in erythrocytes. Biochemistry 1963; 2:1420–8.
40. Zimmerman RJ, Marafino BJ Jr, Chan A, Landre P, Winkelhake JL. The role of oxidant injury in tumor cell sensitivity to recombinant human tumor necrosis factor in vivo. Implications for mechanisms of action. J Immunol 1989; 142:1405–9.
41. Zimmerman RJ, Chan A, Leadon SA. Oxidative damage in murine tumor cells treated in vitro by recombinant human tumor necrosis factor. Cancer Res 1989; 49:1644–8.
42. O'Donnell-Tormey J, DeBoer CJ, Nathan CF. Resistance of human tumor cells in vitro to oxidative cytolysis. J Clin Invest 1985; 76:80–6.
43. Gamble JR, Harlan MM, Klebanoff SJ, Vadas MA. Stimulation of the adherence of neutrophils to umbilical vein endothelium by human recombinant tumor necrosis factor. Proc Natl Acad Sci USA 1985; 82:8667–71.
44. Berger M, Wetzler EM, Wallis RS. Tumor necrosis factor is the major monocyte product that increases complement receptor expression on mature human neutrophils. Blood 1988; 71:151–8.
45. Kownatzki E, Kapp A, Uhrich S. Modulation of human neutrophilic granulocyte functions by recombinant human tumor necrosis factor and recombinant human lymphotoxin. Promotion of adherence, inhibition of chemotactic migration and superoxide anion release from adherent cells. Clin Exp Immunol 1989; 74:143–8.
46. Pontremoli S, Melloni E, Michetti M, Sacco O, Sparatore B, Salamino R, Damiani G, Horecker BL. Cytolyic effects of neutrophils: role for a membrane-bound neutral proteinase. Proc Natl Acad Sci USA 1986; 83:1685–9.
47. Weiss SJ, Regiani S. Neutrophils degrade subendothelial matrices in the presence of alpha-1-proteinase inhibitor. Cooperative use of lysosomal proteinases and oxygen metabolites. J Clin Invest 1984; 73:1297–303.
48. Stroncek DF, Vercellotti GM, Huh PW, Jacob HS. Neutrophil oxidants inactivate alpha-1-protease inhibitor and promote PMN-mediated detachment of cultured endothelium. Protection by free methionine. Arteriosclerosis 1986; 6:322–40.
49. Lichtenstein AK, Ganz T, Selsted ME, Lehrer RI. Synergistic cytolysis mediated by hydrogen peroxide combined with peptide defensins. Cell Immunol 1988; 144:104–16.
50. Simon RH, Dehart PD, Todd RF III. Neutrophil-induced injury of rat pulmonary alveolar epithelia cells. J Clin Invest 1986; 78:1375–86.
51. Tsunawaki S, Oshima H, Mizuno D, Yamazaki M. Induction of polymorphonuclear leukocyte-mediated cytolysis by wheat germ agglutinin and anti-tumor antibody. Gann 1983; 74:258–64.
52. Tsunawaki W, Ikenami M, Mizuno D, Yamazaki M. Mechanisms of lectin and antibody-dependent polymorphonuclear leukocyte-mediated cytolysis. Gann 1983; 74:265–72.
53. Pichyangkul S, Schnick D, Schober W, Dixon G, Khan A. Increased expression of adhesive proteins on leukocytes. Exp Hematol 1988; 16:588–93.
54. Berkow RL, Wang D, Larrick JW, Dodson RW, Howard TH. Enhancement of neutrophil superoxide production by preincubation with recombinant human tumor necrosis factor. J Immunol 1987; 139:3783–91.
55. Clark R, Lkebanoff SJ. Studies on the mechanism of antibody-dependent polymorphonuclear leukocyte-mediated cytoxocity. J Immunol 1977; 119:1413–8.
56. Geffner JR, Giordano M, Palermo MS, Prat A, Serebrinsky GP, Isturiz MA. Neutrophil-mediated cytotoxicity triggered by immune compleses: the role of reactive oxygen metabolites. Clin Exp Immunol 1987; 69:668–75.

57. Matthews N, Neale ML, Jackson SK, Stark JM. Tumor cell killing by anaerobic conditions, free-radical scavengers and inhibitors of arachidonate metabolism. Immunology 1987; 62:153–5.
58. Roberts RL, Ank BJ, Stiehm ER. Decreased tumor cytolysis by neutrophils from patients with chronic granulomatous disease. Ped Res 1987; 21:305A.
59. Fanger MW, Shen L, Graziano RF, Guyre PM. Cytotoxicity mediated by human Fc receptors for IgG. Immunol Today 1989; 10:92–9.
60. Roberts RL, Ank BJ, Shen L, Fanger MW, Stiehm ER. Heteroantibody-dependent cytotoxicity by neutrophils from chronic granulomatous disease (CGD) patients. J Leuk Biol. 1989; 46:299.
61. Dallegri R, Ballestrero A, Ottonello L, Patrone F. Defective antibody-dependent tumor cell lysis by neutrophils from cancer patients. Clin Exp Immunol 1989; 77:58–61.

20

Interferon Activation of Eosinophils

C. De SIMONE
Università di L'Aquila, L'Aquila, Italy

S. TZANTZOGLOU, G. SANTINI, F. SORICE
Università "La Sapienza," Rome, Italy

E. JIRILLO
Università di Bari, Bari, Italy

C. RUMI
Policlinico "A. Gemelli," Rome, Italy

I. INTRODUCTION

Three major classes of interferons (IFNs)—α-IFN, β-IFN, and γ-IFN—have been identified. α-IFN is produced by B-lymphocytes, NK-cells, and macrophages; β-IFN is released by epithelial and fibroblast cells, whereas γ-IFN is secreted by T-lymphocytes. RNA and DNA viruses, microbial products, and synthetic chemicals can be considered as inducers of α/β-IFNs, while antigens and mitogens are γ-IFN inducers (Table 1) (1).

Circulating leukocytes take up IFNs, which are produced mainly in the lungs and the intestines following contact with exogenous IFN inducers, and transport them to other sites. There is conflicting evidence about whether IFNs should be internalized to act, or if the only requirement is the attachment to specific cell surface receptors (2). Two distinct IFN cell surface receptors are present in the body cells; α-IFN and β-IFN share a receptor of about 110 kDa, whereas the γ-IFN receptor has a molecular weight of approximately 54 kDa (1).

IFNs are involved in many cellular processes. It has been suggested that the antiviral activity of IFNs may be related to an exaggerated adoptive utilization (3). Some of the effects of IFNs are mediated by the ezymes 2-5A synthetase and protein kinase, whereas other functions may be elicited by still-unidentified mechanisms that are not associated with antiviral activity (1).

The current concept is that IFNs are hormonelike messengers that induce metabolic changes in distant cells. In addition, recent evidence supports a role for α-IFN as a regulatory peptide in both neuroendocrine and immune systems, possessing immunological and biological γ-endorphin and ACTH-like activities (1).

Focusing on the immune system, IFNs modulate the function of NK-cells, T-cells, B-cells, and monocytes. Low doses of these cytokines enhance and high doses suppress immunoglobulin (Ig) synthesis. On the contrary, cytotoxic and phagocytic functions of monocytes are boosted and T-suppressor functions are depressed by IFNs (Table 2).

Table 1 Human IFNs Classification

	α-IFN	β-IFN	γ-IFN
Source	B- and NK-lymphocytes; macrophages; recombinant	Fibroblasts; lymphoblasts; epithelial cells; recombinant	T-lymphocytes; recombinant
Induced by	Virus; double-stranded DNA	Virus; double-stranded DNA	Foreign antigens; mitogens
Specific activity (U/mg)	$2\text{-}4 \times 10^8$	$2\text{-}4 \times 10^8$	$> 10^8$
Number of subspecies	>15	1	1–2
Molecular weight	16,500–25,000	20,000	17,000
Functional unit	Monomer	Dimer	Trimer
pH stability	+	+	−

The activation of macrophages (M∅) and neutrophilic granulocytes (PMNs) by IFNs has been recognized for many years. Unfortunately, due to the difficulty of isolating pure eosinophilic granulocytes (EOS) from the peripheral blood of healthy donors, the effects of IFNs on EOS are little known and susceptible of bias.

II. PARTICIPATION OF EOSINOPHILS IN IMMUNOLOGICAL SYSTEMS

Almost all diseases characterized by transient or permanent eosinophilia are characterized by an "immunological momentum" during which the immune system is activated and cytokines are released (Table 3).

Table 2 Effects of IFNs on the Immune System

Effect on	In vivo	In vitro
Cell growth		−
Cell differentiation		+/−
Hematopoietic colony formation	−	−
Pinocytosis		−
DNA synthesis		−
Fc receptor expression		+
NK activity	+	+
H-2 antigen expression	+	+
HLA + β2 antigen expression		−
Antibody formation	−	−
Cytotoxicity of sensitized T-cells		+
Cytotoxicity of monocytes		+
GVHD	+/−	
Generation of allospecific suppressor T-lymphocytes		−

Table 3 Diseases Associated with Eosinophilia

Diseases	
Parasitic	Schistosomiasis, filariasis, echinococcosis, cysticercosis, coccidiosis, toxoplasmosis, trichinosis, ascariasis, teniasis, visceral larva migrans
Infectious	Mononucleosis, cat scratch diseases, chlamydia pneumonitis, chorea, brucellosis, *H. influenzae* meningitis, erythema multiforme, scarlet fever, AIDS
Allergic	Bronchial asthma, rhinitis, urticaria, angioedema, aspergillosis, drug hypersensitivity
Dermatological	Atopic dermatitis, pemphigus, herpetiform dermatitis, Well's syndrome, Kimura's disease, pustular dermatosis in AIDS
Immunitary	Eosinophilic fascitis, hyper-IgE syndrome, Churg-Strauss syndrome, GVHD, Wiskott-Aldrich syndrome, selective IgA deficiency
Hematological	Pernicious anemia, polycythemia, postsplenectomy syndrome
Respiratory	Pulmonary eosinophilia, Loffler syndrome, sarcoidosis, Wegener granulomatosis
Tumors	Hodgkin's lymphoma, sarcomas, carcinomas, leukemias

In-vitro experiments have shown that whereas freshly isolated EOS killed only 14% of antibody-coated *Schistosoma mansoni* larvae, the same EOS killed 54% of the larvae when exposed to interleukin-3 (IL-3). Moreover, EOS cultured in the presence of IL-3 and IL-5 convert from normodense to hypodense and generate two- to threefold more leukotriene C_4 (LTC_4) in response to calcium ionophore than do freshly isolated cells (4). These in-vitro changes reflect the in-vivo variations observed in hypereosinophilic subjects. Compared with normodense EOS from healthy individuals, hypodense EOS from patients with peripheral blood eosinophilia exhibit increased chemotactic responses, oxidative metabolism, and enhanced cytotoxic activity (5–9).

EOS are able to interact with IL-1 (10), IL-3 (11,12), IL-4 (13), IL-5 (14,15), IL-6 (11), colony-stimulating factors (CSFs) (11,12), and tumor necrosis factor (TNF) (16). These molecules induce a variation in the rate of EOS bone marrow production and modulate their chemotaxis, degranulation, and cytotoxicity (17).

The EOS phenotypic and functional changes induced by cytokines may be advantageous to host defense mechanisms against helminth infections and tumors but may be disadvantageous in conditions characterized by a state of chronic inflammation. A persistent and prolonged hypereosinophilia is associated with damage to the heart, lung, brain, kidney, liver, and skin (18–24), and it is likely that tissue pathology may result from the release of cytoplasmatic and/or granular products of EOS (Table 4).

III. INTERFERONS AND EOSINOPHILS

The effects of IFNs on EOS are little known. It has been shown that when EOS from the peripheral blood of individuals with parasitic diseases are preincubated in the presence of β-IFN, the number of cells expressing IgG-Fc receptors is augmented (Figure 1) (25). In addition, doses (10–500 IU) needed to induce modulation of IgG-Fc recep-

Table 4 Eosinophil-Derived Substances

Substance	Site	Activity
MBP (major basic protein)	Large granules, nucleus	Toxic against parasites, tumor cells; induces the release of histamine from basophils and mast cells; degrades airway epithelium
ECP (eosinophil cationic protein)	Large granules, matrix	Toxic against parasites; induces the release of histamine; neurotoxic
EDN/EPX (eosinophil-derived neurotoxin/eosinophil protein-X)	Large granules, matrix	Neurotoxic, toxic against parasites
EPO (eosinophil peroxidase)	Large granules, matrix	$+H_2O_2$ kills tumor cells and microorganisms; induces the release of histamine; inactivates leukotrienes
LTC_4 (leukotriene C_4)	Membrane	Bronchial spasm; mucosal edema
PAF (platelet-activating factor)	Membrane	Bronchial spasm; eosinophilotaxis; platelet activation
Arylsulfatase B	Small granules	Catabolism of proteoglycans
Acid phosphatase	Small granules	Catabolism of glycosaminoglycans

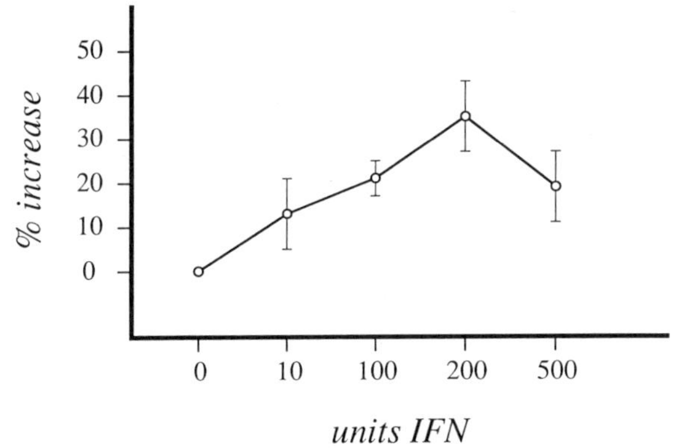

Figure 1 Effect of β-IFN on the expression of IgG-Fc receptors of eosinophilic granulocytes. To minimize some consistent subject-to-subject variations in the EA rosette-forming eosinophil percentage among the total eosinophils, the percentage among the eosinophils with IgG-Fc receptors in each subject at each time is expressed as percentage of control. The values represent the mean ±SD in 11 subjects.

tors are effective in boosting the EOS-mediated antibody-dependent cytotoxicity (Figure 2).

β-IFN has been shown to possess a protective effect in *Trypanosoma cruzi* infection (26), and has been administered alone or in combination with IL-2 to patients with advanced malignancy in therapeutic trials (27). In about 60–70% of these patients, eosinophilia follows the treatment and may be due to a hypersensitivity reaction. A recent survey of rectal cancer patients shows that the number of EOS influences the natural history of the malignancy, confirming that in neoplastic patients the number of EOS is related to a better overall survival rate (28). The possibility that the induction and/or activation of EOS is among the factors responsible for the improved survival of the β-IFN or β-IFN + IL-2-treated cancer patients is an attractive hypothesis to be confirmed.

γ-IFN is more effective as an immunomodulator than α-IFN and β-IFN and interacts more closely with other cytokines (1). Recent evidence suggests that γ-IFN and IL-4 reciprocally control Ig isotype production in T-lymphocyte-driven immune responses. In-vitro experiments have demonstrated that human alloreactive T-cell clones, producing supernatants containing IL-4, IL-5, and GM-CSF but not γ-IFN or IL-2, induce IgE synthesis by normal human peripheral blood lymphocytes (PBLs). IL-4 was shown to be necessary and sufficient for IgE synthesis; the addition of γ-IFN to supernatants resulted in inhibition of IgE production (13,29–34). IgE antibodies, although they represent a minor component of the humoral immune compartment, play a key role in allergy and parasitic diseases (35). Mast cells, basophils, EOS, mononuclear cells, and platelets express specific surface receptors for IgE at their surfaces (36). Two classes of IgE-Fc receptors (Fc R1 and Fc R2) can be distinguished; the former are present on mast cells and basophils, the latter on subpopulations of mononuclear cells, M⌀, platelets, and EOS (37). The role of IgE-Fc receptors consists of the transduction of the antigen-induced cross-linking of cytophilically bound IgE antibodies with subsequent release of pro-inflammatory and/or cytotoxic molecules.

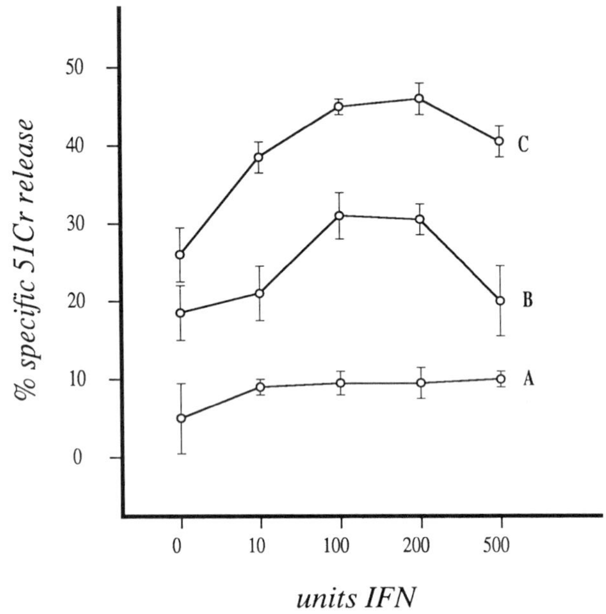

Figure 2 Dose-effect of β-IFN on eosinophil ADCC against chicken erythrocytes: A, cultures without anti-chicken erythrocyte antibodies, effector/target ratio 25:1; B, cultures with anti-chicken erythrocyte antibodies, effector/target ratio 25:1; C, effector/target ratio 50:1.

Both IL-4 and γ-IFN were able to augment significantly IgE-Fc R2/CD23 expression on a human eosinophilic cell line (EoL3) (13); a similar up-regulating activity has been shown by both cytokines on IgE-Fc R2 on normal human epithelial cells (38). The up-regulation of low-affinity IgE-Fc R2/CD23 expression by γ-IFN has been demonstrated also on the human lymphoblastoid cell line U937 (39).

The results of a study conducted by us on human EOS have shown that γ-IFN as well as IL-4 up-regulate CD23 receptor expression. Surprisingly, the simultaneous addition of γ-IFN and IL-4 to EOS resulted in a suppression of the CD23 expression (Figure 3).

These experiments suggest that the effects of γ-IFN on Fc R2 expression should be viewed in the wider context of a multicomponent network aimed at the IgE synthesis and Fc IgE receptor expression (Figure 4).

This model does not take into account the fact that γ-IFN also modulates the production of histamine by mast cells and basophils (1). Histamine up-regulates CD23 receptor expression and inhibits the synthesis of γ-IFN and IL-2 by $Leu3^+$, $Leu3^+8^+$, $Leu3^+8^-$ cell subsets via an action on both $Leu3^+18^-8^-$ and $Leu3^+18^-8^+$ cells (33,40).

γ-IFN alone or in combination with histamine also promotes the synthesis of complement components C2, C4, C3, and factor B by monocytes (41,42). IL-4 has also been shown to possess the ability to up-regulate the production of complement components by monocytes, and co-stimulation with γ-IFN results in an additive effect (42). Complement plays a major role during parasite infections, since the larvae can activate

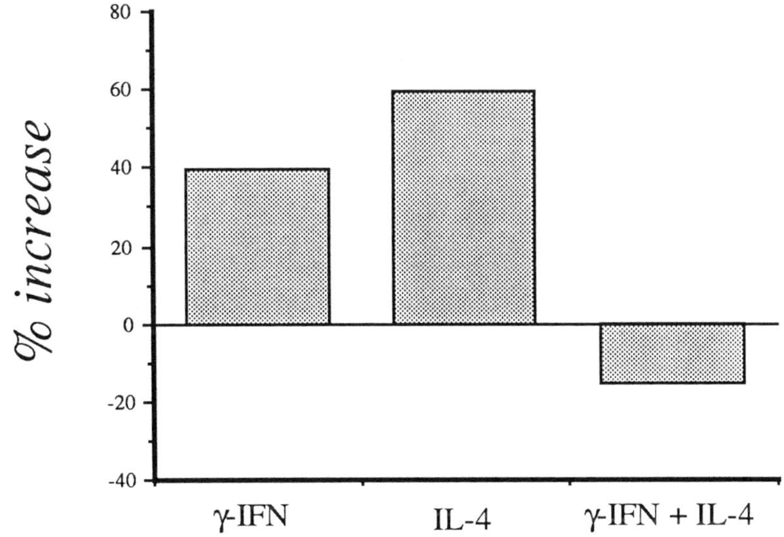

Figure 3 Effect of γ-IFN (10 IU/ml) and IL-4 (0.5 ng/ml) on the expression of CD23 on human eosinophils. A representative experiment of four performed is represented. γ-IFN and IL-4 were donated by H. Kiyono, The University of Alabama at Birmingham, Alabama.

it and bind activated complement fractions at their surfaces (43). EOS-expressing cell surface glycoproteins (CD11b; CR3; C3bi receptor) bind to the C3bi-coated parasites (44). In spite of the fact that CD11b was originally described as the receptor for C3bi, several additional ligands have recently been identified for this receptor (45). The protein gp63 of *Leishmania* binds to CD11b (46), and other ligands for CD11b are postulated to be parasite components recognized by a lectinlike or adhesion-promoting domain of the CD11b receptor with a specificity for β-glucan (47). The ability of CD11b to mediate adhesive interactions is under strict physiological control, and the stimuli which turn on the binding function of CD11b also enhance the expression of the protein on the cell surface (45). In this context, the effect of γ-IFN on CD11b expression by EOS seems to be an additional defense mechanism against the invading pathogens.

The results obtained by us in experiments where EOS were incubated with γ-IFN and evaluated for CD11b receptor expression are summarized in Figure 5.

Up-regulation of the CD11b receptor expression was observed following treatment of the cells with γ-IFN, and it is hypothesized that γ-IFN facilitates the adhesion of EOS to complement-coated microorganisms. The phenomenon could be restricted to a relatively early phase of the immune response, before the specific antibody synthesis becomes fully operating, as suggested by the observation that IL-4 and IL-4 + γ-IFN suppress the CD11b receptor expression.

It has been shown that γ-IFN enhances lymphocyte binding to endothelium and that CD4 antigens are involved in this process (48). γ-IFN is a powerful inducer of major histocompatibility complex (MHC) II antigens, and CD4 molecules may serve to increase the lymphocyte avidity toward the target cells expressing MHC II antigens

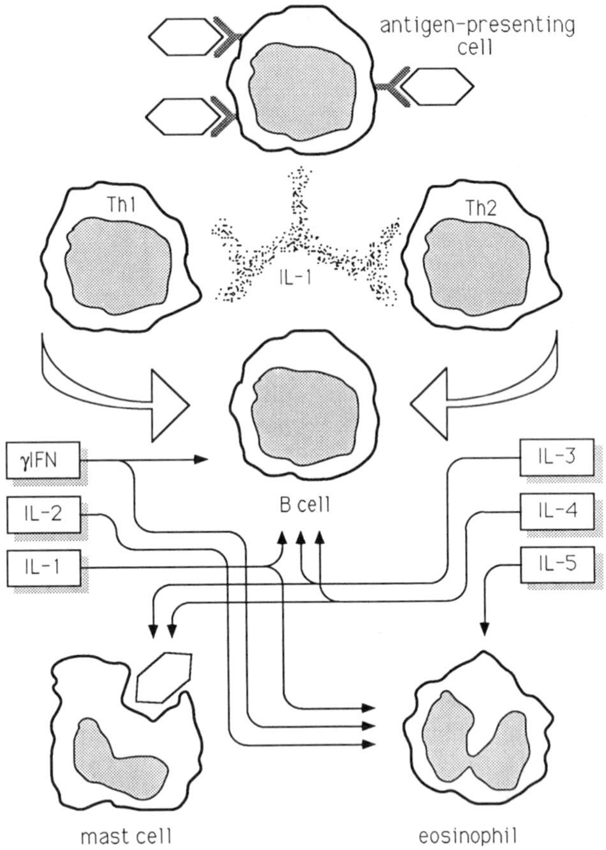

Figure 4 Schema representing the regulation of IgE synthesis and CD23 expression by immunocompetent cells and cytokines.

(49). In addition, the CD4 glycoprotein appears to form at least part of the receptor for human immunodeficiency virus (HIV) on T-cells, monocytes/macrophages, and glia cells (49). Also, human EOS express CD4 protein and bind HIV (50).

The experiments reported in Figure 6 demonstrate that γ-IFN up-regulates CD4 antigen expression on EOS from patients with AIDS. IL-4 was devoid of this property, but provided an additional stimulus for the γ-IFN-mediated CD4 up-regulation.

Blood or tissue eosinophilia is a frequent laboratory finding in AIDS patients (51,52), and serum concentrations of γ-IFN have been found to correlate positively with the gravity of the disease (53). The γ-IFN-facilitated expression of CD4 antigen on EOS could have detrimental clinical consequences if it is proven that HIV replicates inside the EOS or, alternatively, EOS represent a reservoir for the virus.

The relationship between γ-IFN, $CD4^+$ T-lymphocytes, and $CD4^+$ EOS will be the object of future research. Data available have been obtained from cryostat sections of skin biopsies of atopic individuals in which late-phase dermal reactions to allergens were induced. A strong correlation between $CD4^+$ T-cells and activated EOS, associated with indirect evidence of γ-IFN secretion, has been demonstrated. At the same

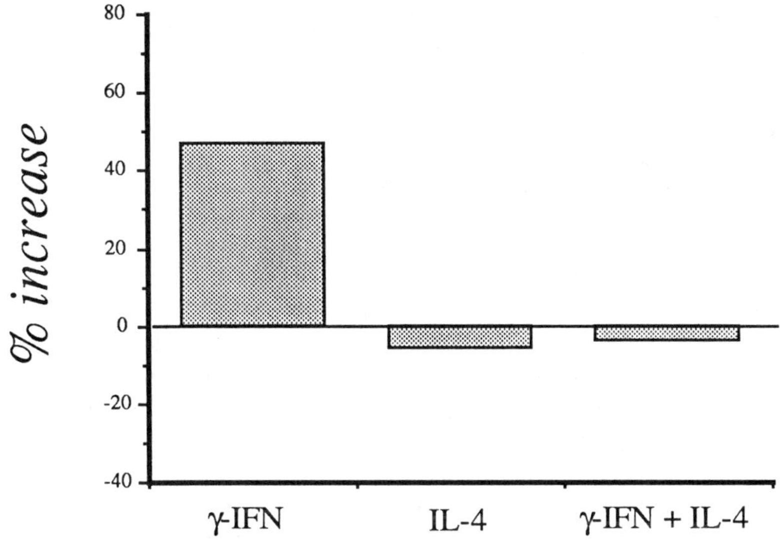

Figure 5 Effect of γ-IFN (10 IU/ml) and IL-4 (0.5 ng/ml) on the expression of CD11b on human eosinophils. A representative experiment of four performed is represented.

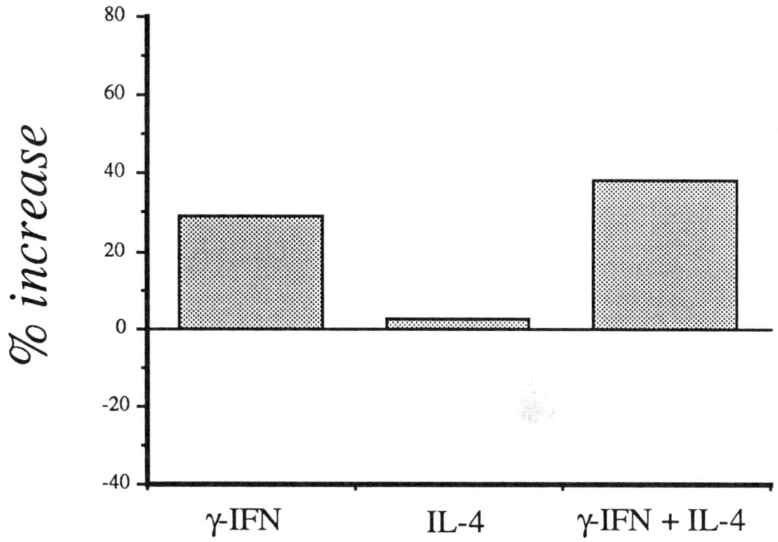

Figure 6 Effect of γ-IFN (10 IU/ml) and IL-4 (0.5 ng/ml) on the expression of CD4 on human eosinophils from an AIDS patient with Kaposi's sarcoma. Similar results were obtained employing eosinophils donated by two HIV^+ patients with opportunistic infections (*Pneumocystis carinii; Toxoplasma gondii*).

time, a few T-cells bore receptors for IL-2, and HLA-DR antigens on the endothelial cells and CD4 antigen on epidermal Langerhans cells were also present (54).

IV. CONCLUDING REMARKS

A complicated array of interactions has emerged from simple in-vitro cellular systems, and evidence is accumulating that various cytokines are involved to a different extent in the EOS-mediated immune responses (55). IL-4 has a central role in the stimulation of antibody production for EOS "arming," whereas IFNs tend to regulate many of the activities of IL-4 and the surface expression of receptors and antigens on EOS. Neither γ-IFN nor IL-4 has an effect on IgG-induced or nonspecific degranulation of EOS, whereas γ-IFN suppresses the secretory IgA-induced degranulation (17). In mice, these control interactions are supported at the T-lymphocyte level by the different properties of TH1 and TH2 cells producing lymphotoxin, IL-2, γ-IFN, and IL-4, IL-5, IL-6, respectively (56). Apparently, the presence of γ-IFN during an immune response seems to be a prerequisite for the preferential expression of helper T-lymphocytes of the TH1 phenotype. However, by employing PBLs of a patient suffering from hyper-IgE syndrome to generate phytohemagglutinin-expanded T-cell clones, it was demonstrated that several clones could secrete IL-2, IL-4, and γ-IFN. These data suggest that human T-helper cells may not occur only in the TH1 and TH2 type subsets described in the mouse (57).

Our current knowledge is provocative. Many efforts will be needed to discern the extent to which the plethora of interactions between IFNs and other peptide-regulatory factors affect the activities of EOS.

REFERENCES

1. Mannering GJ, Deloria LB. The pharmacology and toxicology of the interferons: an overview. Ann Rev Pharmacol Toxicol 1986; 26:455–515.
2. Revel M. The interferon system in man: nature of the interferon molecules and mode of action. In: Becker Y, ed. Antiviral drugs and interferon: the molecular basis of their activity. Boston, Nighoff, 1984:357–433.
3. Bocci V. Production and role of interferon in physiological conditions. Biol Rev Cambridge Physiol Soc 1981; 56:49–85.
4. Rothenberg ME, Petersen J, Stevens RL, Silberstein DS, McKenzie DT, Austen KF, Owen WF. IL-5-dependent conversion of normodense human eosinophils to the hypodense phenotype uses 3T3 fibroblasts for enhanced viability, accelerated hypodensity, and sustained antibody-dependent cytotoxicity. J Immunol 1989; 143:2311–6.
5. Kay AB, Frew AJ, Moqbel R, Walsh GM, Kurihara K, Cromwell O, Champion A, Hartnell A, Wardlaw AJ. The activated eosinophil in allergy and asthma. Biochem Acute Allergic Reactions 1989; 297:183–97.
6. Yukawa T, Kroegel C, Evans P, Fukuda T, Chung KF, Barnes PJ. Density heterogeneity of eosinophil leucocytes—induction of hypodense eosinophils by platelet-activating factor. Immunology 1989; 68:140–3.
7. Frick WE, Sedgwick JB, Busse WW. The appearance of hypodense eosinophils in antigen-dependent late phase asthma. Am Rev Respir Dis 1989; 139:1401–6.
8. Benezra J, Sheibani K, Swartz W, Stroup R, Traweek ST, Kezirian J, Rappaport H. Relationship between eosinophil density and T-cell activation markers in lymph nodes of patients with Hodgkins disease. Human Pathol 1989; 20:1181–5.

9. De Simone C, Donelli G, Meli D, Rosati F, Sorice F. Human eosinophils and parasitic diseases—II. Characterization of two cell fractions isolated at different densities. Clin Exp Immunol 1982; 48:249.
10. Whitcomb EA, Dinarello CA, Pincus SH. Differential effects of interleukin-1-alpha and interleukin-1-beta on human peripheral blood eosinophils. Blood 1989; 73:1904–8.
11. Clutterbuck EJ, Hirst EMA, Sanderson CJ. Human interleukin-5 (IL-5) regulates the production of eosinophils in human bone marrow cultures—comparison and interaction with IL-1, IL-3, IL-6, and GMCSF. Blood 1989; 73:1504–12.
12. Lopez AF, Eglinton JM, Gillis D, Park LS, Clark S, Vadas MA. Reciprocal inhibition of binding between interleukin-3 and granulocyte macrophage colony-stimulating factor to human eosinophils. Proc Natl Acad Sci USA 1989; 86:7022–6.
13. Hosoda M, Makino S, Kawabe T, Maeda Y, Satoh S, Takami M, Mayumi M, Arai K, Saitoh H, Yodoi J. Differential regulation of the low affinity Fc receptor for IgE (Fc epsilon R2/CD23) and the IL-2 receptor (Tac/p55) on eosinophilic leukemia cell line (EoL-1 and EoL-3). J Immunol 1989; 143:147–52.
14. Jabara HH, Ackerman SJ, Vercelli D, Yokota T, Arai K, Abrams J, Dvorak AM, Lavigne MC, Banchereau J, De Vries J et al. Induction of interleukin-4-dependent IgE synthesis and interleukin-5-dependent eosinophil differentiation by supernatants of a human helper T-cell clone. J Clin Immunol 1988; 8:437–46.
15. Sanderson CJ. Interleukin-5: an eosinophil growth and activation factor. Dev Biol Stand 1988; 69:23–9.
16. Whitcomb EA, Wesolek JH, Pincus SH. Modulation of human peripheral blood eosinophil function by tumor necrosis factor-alpha. Int Arch Allergy Appl Immunol 1989; 89:250–5.
17. Fujisawa T, Abughazaleh, Kita H, Sanderson CJ, Gleich GJ. Regulatory effect of cytokines on eosinophil degranulation. J Immunol 1990; 144:642–6.
18. Molina HA, Kierszenbaum F. Interaction of human eosinophils or neutrophils with *Trypanosoma cruzi* in vitro causes bystander cardiac cell damage. Immunology 1989; 66:289–95.
19. Durham SR, Loegering DA, Dunnette S, Gleich GJ, Kay AB. Blood eosinophils and eosinophil-derived proteins in allergic asthma. J Allergy Clin Immunol 1989; 84:931–6.
20. Spry CJF. The pathogenesis of endomyocardial fibrosis—the role of the eosinophil. Springer Sem Immunopathol 1989; 11:471–7.
21. Sunohara N, Furukawa S, Nishio T, Mukoyama M, Satoyoshi E. Neurotoxicity of human eosinophils toward peripheral nerves. J Neurolog Sci 1989; 92:1–7.
22. Sasano H, Virmani R, Patterson RH, Robinowitz R, Guccion JG. Eosinophilic products lead to myocardial damage. Human Pathol 1989; 20:850–7.
23. Slifman NR, Venge P, Peterson CGB, Mckean DJ, Gleich GJ. Human eosinophil-derived neurotoxin and eosinophil protein-X are likely the same protein. J Immunol 1989; 143:2317–22.
24. Ten RM, Gleich GJ, Holley KE, Perkins JD, Torres VE. Eosinophil granule major basic protein in acute renal allograft rejection. Transplantation 1989; 47:959–63.
25. De Simone C, Salvi MC, Ferrarelli G, De Santis G, Mango G, Sorice F. Human eosinophils and parasitic disease—III. β-Interferon increases eosinophil IgG-Fc receptor expression and capacity. Int J Immunopharmacol 1986; 8:479–85.
26. Kierszembaum F, Sonnenfeld G. Beta-interferon inhibits cell infection by *Trypanosoma cruzi*. J Immunol 1984; 132:905.
27. Tamura T, Sasaki Y, Shinkai T, Eguchi K, Sakurai M, Fujiwara Y, Nakagawa K, Minato K, Bungo M, Saijo N. Phase I study of combination therapy with interleukin 2 and beta-interferon in patients with advanced malignancy. Cancer Res 1989; 49:730–5.
28. Fisher ER, Paik SM, Rockette H, Jones J, Caplan R, Fisher B. Prognostic significance of eosinophils and mast cells in rectal cancer: findings from the National Surgical Adjuvant Breast and Bowel Project (protocol R-01). Human Pathol 1989; 20:159–63.

29. Galizzi JP, Cabrillat H, Rousset F, Menetrier C, de Vries JE, Banchereau J. IFN-gamma and prostaglandin E2 inhibit IL-4-induced expression of Fc epsilon R2/CD23 on B lymphocytes through different mechanisms without altering binding of IL-4 to its receptor. J Immunol 1989; 141:1982–8.
30. Heinzel FP, Sadick MD, Holaday BJ, Coffman RL, Locksley RM. Reciprocal expression of interferon gamma or interleukin 4 during the resolution or progression of murine leishmaniasis. Evidence for expansion of distinct helper T cell subsets. J Exp Med 1989; 169:59–72.
31. Jabara HH, Ackerman SJ, Vercelli D, Yokota T, Arai K, Abrams J, Dvorak AM, Lavinge MC, Banchereau J, De Vries J, et al. Induction of interleukin-4-dependent IgE synthesis and interleukin-5-dependent eosinophil differentiation by supernatants of a human helper T-cell clone. J Clin Immunol 1988; 8:437–46.
32. Gajewski TF, Joyce J, Fitch FW. Antiproliferative effect of IFN-gamma in immune regulation. III. Differential selection of TH1 and TH2 murine helper T lymphocyte clones using recombinant IL-2 and recombinant IFN-gamma. J Immunol 1989; 143:15–22.
33. Dohlsten M, Hedlund G, Fischer H, Sjogren HO, Carlsson R. Proliferation of human $CD4^{+}45R^{+}$ and $CD4^{+}45R^{-}$ T helper cells is promoted by both IL-2 and IL-4 while interferon-gamma production is restricted to IL-2 activated $CD4^{+}45^{-}$ T cells. Immunol Lett 1989; 20:29–34.
34. Tanaka M, Lee KC, Yodoi J, Saito H, Iwai Y, Kim KM, Morita M, Mayumi M, Mikawa H. Regulation of Fc epsilon receptor 2 (CD23) expression on a human eosinophilic cell line EoL3 and a human monocytic cell line U937 by transforming growth factor beta. Cell Immunol 1989; 122:96–107.
35. Vercelli D, Geha RS. The IgE system. Ann Allergy 1989; 63:4–11.
36. Capron M. Eosinophils: receptors and mediators in hypersensitivity. Clin Exp Allergy 1989; suppl 1P:3–8.
37. Ishizaka K. Basic mechanisms of IgE-mediated hypersensitivity. Curr Opinion Immunol 1989; 4:625–9.
38. Bieber T, Rieger A, Neuchrist C, Prinz JC, Rieber EP, Boltz-Nitulescu G, Scheiner O, Kraft D, Ring J, Stingl G. Induction of Fc epsilon R2/CD23 on human epidermal Langherhans cells by human recombinant interleukin-4 and gamma interferon. J Exp Med 1989; 170:309–14.
39. Mayumi M, Kawabe T, Nishioka H, Tanaka M, Kim KM, Heike T, Yodoi J, Mikawa H. Interferon and (2′5′)oligoadenylate enhance the expression of low affinity receptors for IgE (Fc epsilon R2/CD23) on the human monoblast cell line U937. Mol Immunol 1989; 26:241–7.
40. Dohlsten M, Hedlund G, Sjogren HO, Carlsson R. Inhibitory effects of histamine on interleukin-2 and gamma interferon production of different human T helper cell subsets. Scand J Immunol 1988; 28:727–33.
41. Falus A, Walcz E, Brozik M, Rokita H, Fust G, Hajnal A, Meretey K. Stimulation of histamine receptors of human monocytoid and hepatoma-derived cell lines and mouse hepatocytes modulates the production of the complement components C3, C4, factor B and C2. Scand J Immunol 1989; 30:241–8.
42. Littman BH, Dastvan FF, Carlson PL, Sanders KM. Regulation of monocyte/macrophage C2 production and HLA-DR expression by IL-4 (BSF-1) and IFN-gamma. J Immunol 1989; 142:520–25.
43. Rao UR, Chandreshekar R, Subrahmanyan D. Complement activation by eggs and microflorae of filarial parasites. Immunol Cell Biol 1987; 65:365–70.
44. Capron M, Kazatchine MD, Fisher E, et al. Functional role of a-chain of complement receptor type 3 in human eosinophil dependent antibody-mediated citotoxicity against Schistosomes. J Immunol 1987; 139:2059–65.

45. Detmers PA, Wright SD. Adhesion-promoting receptors in leucocytes. Curr Opinion Immunol 1988; 1:10–5.
46. Russel DG. The macrophage attachment glycoprotein gp63 is the predominant C3-acceptor site on *Leishmania mexicana* promastigotes. Eur J Biochem 1987; 164:213–21.
47. Wright SD, Levin SM, Jong MT, Chad Z, Kabbash LG. Cr3 (CD11b/CD18) expresses one binding site for Arg-Gly-Asp-containing peptides and a second site for bacterial lipopolysaccharide. J Exp Med 1989; 169:175–83.
48. Tornhill MH, Williams DM, Speight PM. Enhanced adhesion of autologous lymphocytes to gamma-interferon-treated human endothelial cells in vitro. Br J Exp Pathol 1989; 70:59–64.
49. McDouglas JS. Function of the CD4 molecule in normal immune responses. Curr Opinion Immunol 1988; 1:88–91.
50. Lucey DR, Dorsky DI, Nicholson-Weller A, Weller PF. Human eosinophils express CD4 protein and bind human immunodeficiency virus 1 gp120. J Exp Med 1989; 169:327–32.
51. Frentz G, Niordson AM, Thomsen K. Eosinophilic pustular dermatosis: an early skin marker of infection with human immunodeficiency virus. Br J Dermatol 1989; 121:271–4.
52. Fluery-Feith J, Van Nhieu JT, Picard C, Escudier E, Bernaudin JF. Bronchoalveolar lavage eosinophilia associated with *Pneumocystis cariniii* pneumonitis in AIDS patients. Comparative study with non-AIDS patients. Chest 1989; 95:1198–201.
53. Fuchs D, Hansen A, Reibnegger G, et al. Interferon-gamma concentrations are increased in sera from individual infected with HIV-1. J Acquired Immune Deficiency Syndromes 1989; 2:158–62.
54. Frew AJ, Kay AB. The relationship between infiltrating $CD4^+$ lymphocytes, activated eosinophils and the magnitude of the allergen-induced late phase cutaneous reaction in man. J Immunol 1988; 141:4158–64.
55. Gabrilove JL. Introduction and overview of hematopoietic growth factors. Semin Hematol 1989; 26:1–4.
56. Cambier J. Lymphocyte subsets and activation. Curr Opinion Immunol 1988; 2:220–7.
57. Quint DJ, Bolton E, McNamee LA, Solari R, Hissey PH, Champion BR, MacKenzie AR, Zanders ED. Functional and phenotypic analysis of human T-cell clones which stimulate IgE production in vitro. Immunology 1989; 67:68–74.

21

Regulation of Human Eosinophil Production and Function by Interleukin-5

ANGEL F. LOPEZ, M. FRANCES SHANNON, MON-MING CHIA
Institute of Medical and Veterinary Science, Adelaide, South Australia

LINDA PARK
Immunex Corporation, Seattle, Washington

MATHEW A. VADAS
Institute of Medical and Veterinary Science, Adelaide, South Australia

I. INTRODUCTION

Eosinophils are specialized hemopoietic cells which can be found in peripheral blood and tissues. Under normal steady-state conditions, blood eosinophils comprise only about 1–5% of circulating leukocytes; however, their absolute and relative numbers have been noted to rise in pathological conditions such as allergic reactions, parasitic infestations, and in certain neoplasias. In these cases the eosinophilia observed has two important properties. First, it is selective, in that other leukocyte numbers remain essentially unchanged. Second, it is accompanied by an increase in the state of activation of the eosinophils (1). These observations led to the notion that a regulator specific for eosinophils may exist and raised the possibility that stimulation of both eosinophil production and function was mediated by a single molecule.

In-vitro experiments strengthened this concept by the detection in spleen cell supernatants of an activity that selectively stimulated eosinophil progenitor cells as well as mature eosinophils (2,3). This eosinophil-stimulating activity was also observed in supernatants of cloned T-cells and shown to be functionally different from other growth factors with eosinophil activity such as interleukin-3 (IL-3) and granulocyte-macrophage colony-stimulating factor (GM-CSF) (4). Biochemical characterization further showed that the active factor was indeed different from IL-3 and GM-CSF (5), and because of the assay used to follow its purification it was termed eosinophil differentiation factor (EDF). Although EDF was made by mouse cells, it was active on human eosinophils, a finding that predicted the existence of the human analog (6). The selection of a mouse T-cell clone secreting only EDF facilitated the cloning of the mouse gene, and its product is now widely referred to as interleukin-5 (IL-5).

Human IL-5 has now been cloned by different groups by cross-hybridization with the mouse IL-5 probe. Expression of human IL-5 has allowed in-vitro studies confirming its high degree of specificity on the eosinophil lineage. The identification of this molecule offers much opportunity to study the regulation of eosinophils and promises to be invaluable in determining the role of the eosinophil itself. This review aims to discuss new concepts in the regulation of eosinophils by IL-5 in the light of recent findings, and seeks to identify important areas for future research.

II. STIMULATION OF EOSINOPHILS BY IL-5

A. Stimulation of Eosinophil Production

An important characteristic of IL-5 is its cross-species reactivity. In fact, the observation that mouse IL-5/EDF reacted with human cells (6) paved the way for the initial experiments examining the role of IL-5 in human eosinophil production. This is in contrast to the other two eosinophil growth factors, IL-3 and GM-CSF, which are not cross-reactive. Thus, in its ability to cross species, IL-5 mirrors granulocyte colony-stimulating factor (G-CSF), a factor that preferentially stimulates neutrophils and that cross-reacts between mouse and human (7,8).

The cloning of the mouse IL-5 gene and the subsequent cloning of the human IL-5 facilitated studies on its specificity on human cells. Unlike IL-3 and GM-CSF, IL-5 is lineage-restricted to the eosinophil lineage. Early experiments using agar cultures demonstrated that IL-5 stimulated the clonal proliferation of eosinophil progenitor cells. After 2 weeks in cultures, these colonies were composed almost exclusively of eosinophils (6). These experiments also showed that the effect of IL-5 on eosinophil progenitor cells was a direct one based on a titration of bone marrow cells and, more important, on clone transfer experiments (6). IL-5 also stimulates eosinophils selectively in liquid cultures, although these types of experiments cannot distinguish between direct effects and secondary effects by accessory cell products present in the culture system.

Although the targets for IL-5 are predominantly cells of the eosinophil lineage, it is not yet clear whether basophils can also be produced in cultures with IL-5. Some reports have noted the presence of mixed eosinophil-basophil colonies in agar (9,10), although only eosinophil numbers increase in liquid cultures stimulated by IL-5 (11,12).

As well as IL-5, human IL-3 and GM-CSF are growth factors with the ability to stimulate eosinophil production. It is not clear why three different factors exert this activity. A possible explanation may be related to the stage at which these growth factors act in the differentiation pathway of human eosinophils. This possibility is tied to the question of whether there are subpopulations of eosinophils. Thus, different subpopulations may be responding to each eosinophil-acting growth factor or, alternatively, the apparent heterogeneity in the response of progenitor cells may be explained in terms of the stage of eosinophil differentiation at which IL-5, IL-3, or GM-CSF preferentially acts. In support of the latter, IL-3 and GM-CSF have been reported to give rise to a greater number of colonies than IL-5 (11,12) (Table 1).

Morphologically, the eosinophils stimulated by IL-3 and GM-CSF are of the more immature type compared to IL-5-stimulated eosinophils (12), although these differences have not always been noted (11).

Table 1 Size of Eosinophil Clones Stimulated by IL-5

	Number of cells/clone										
Stimulus	0–10	10–20	20–30	30–40	40–50	50–60	60–70	70–80	80–90	90–100	⩾100
None	1[a]	2	1	0	0	0	0	0	0	0	0
IL-5, 3×10^{-11} M	4	7	5	1	1	0	0	0	0	0	0
IL-5, 10^{-10} M	0	2	4	10	5	1	1	3	0	0	4
IL-5, 3×10^{-10} M	0	2	3	2	2	1	3	2	1	0	14
IL-5, 10^{-9} M	0	2	1	2	1	1	0	2	0	0	19
IL-3, 10^{-9} M	0	2	1	2	0	0	3	2	1	0	36
GM-CSF, 10^{-9} M	0	1	0	1	1	2	3	0	0	2	31

[a] Number of eosinophil clones per 10^5 T-cell- and monocyte-depleted human bone marrow cells cultured in agar for 14 days at 37°C.

Using a new in-vitro system, IL-5 appears, in contrast to IL-3 and GM-CSF, incapable of initiating the proliferation of IL-5 precursors, although it was as effective as IL-3 and GM-CSF in stimulating final eosinophil differentiation in secondary cultures (13). These observations strongly indicate that while IL-3 and GM-CSF act early in the eosinophil differentiation pathway, IL-5 is important at a later stage.

While IL-5 is capable of stimulating eosinophil production by itself, it may also be able to interact with other growth factors. For example, IL-5 has been reported to have an additive effect with IL-3 and with GM-CSF in eosinophil colony formation, although it is not clear whether these factors were used at saturating concentrations. Nevertheless, these experiments point to another difference with IL-3 and GM-CSF, which clearly do not have an additive effect when added together (11). Other growth factors such as IL-1 or IL-6 do not seem to have an effect on eosinophil colony formation, either by themselves or in combination with IL-5, IL-3, or GM-CSF (11,13). On the other hand, G-CSF enhances IL-5-mediated colony formation (10), suggesting that this factor acts on an early stage of eosinophilopoiesis perhaps common to other cell lineages.

B. Stimulation of Eosinophil Function

IL-5 regulates mature eosinophils by influencing the lifespan, motility, and effector functions of these cells.

In vitro, IL-5 enhances the survival of eosinophils in the absence of other cells and growth factors (14) as well as when added to cultures containing a monolayer of fibroblasts (15). Whether IL-5 synergises with soluble fibroblast-derived products remains to be established. IL-5 from patients with eosinophilia has also been shown to exhibit this property ex vivo (16).

Crucial steps in the localization of eosinophils to the site of inflammation where they can carry out their effector functions are the egress from the circulation and their locomotion to the inflammatory foci. IL-5 has the potential to modulate these functions as it up-regulates the expression of the CD11b/CD18 antigen (6) involved in cell adhesion (17), and enhances eosinophil adherence to a variety of surfaces (18). In addition, IL-5 appears to stimulate chemotaxis of eosinophils but not of neutrophils or monocytes (19), suggesting that locally produced IL-5 may be an important determinant in the selective accumulation of eosinophils at sites of inflammation. The magnitude of the chemotactic effect of IL-5 does not seem to be as great as that of platelet-activating factor (PAF) (20); however, the main role of IL-5 may be that of priming eosinophils for an enhanced chemotactic response to PAF (21), one of the most potent inflammatory mediators.

These effects of IL-5 are accompanied by changes in the functional status of eosinophils which are important for the effector function of these cells at sites of inflammation. For example, IL-5 as well as IL-3 and GM-CSF stimulate antibody-dependent killing of tumor cells and phagocytosis of opsonized particles (6,22–25) by eosinophils. This activation is probably critical for eosinophils function as these cells—at least in vitro, and in contrast to neutrophils—display very poor or no activity in these assays and may depend on encountering these stimuli in vivo to become fully competent.

The activation of eosinophil function by IL-5 established that this factor has a dual level of activity. Like its action on progenitor cells, the activation of mature cell function is restricted predominantly to the eosinophil lineage. As illustrated in Table 2, IL-5 can enhance the function of purified blood eosinophils but not that of neutrophils or monocytes. In one case of chronic myeloid leukemia undergoing basophilic differentiation, the purified basophils responded to IL-5 by enhanced histamine release.

Table 2 Specificity of IL-5 Stimulation of Mature Cell Function

Mature cell	Function	Stimuli			
		IL-5	IL-3	GM-CSF	Medium
Eosinophils	ADCC[a]	48.6 ± 1.7	51.3 ± 3.3	48.5 ± 2.4	4.2 ± 0.3
CML basophils	Histamine release[b]	14.4 ± 0.3	21.6 ± 1.5	14.7 ± 0.9	9.2 ± 0
Monocytes	Adherence[c]	7.2 ± 1.1	48.1 ± 2.1	48.3 ± 1.8	7.0 ± 0.8
Neutrophils	O_2^- [d]	3.9 ± 1.0	3.7 ± 0.2	16.6 ± 1.8	4.0 ± 0.3

[a] Antibody-dependent cell-mediated cytotoxicity of tumor cells was performed as described (6). The values represent the mean ±SEM.

[b] Histamine released from peripheral blood basophils incubated with normal human IgE and anti-IgE antibodies expressed as percentage of calcium ionophore-stimulated release. Details of this assay have been described in detail elsewhere (74). The values represent the mean ±SEM.

[c] Percent adherence of peripheral blood monocytes after 16 h of incubation. Monocytes were purified by centrifugal elutriation and tested for their capacity to adhere to plastic as described (75). The values represent the mean ±SEM.

[d] Nanomoles of superoxide anion generated by 10^6 neutrophils after preincubation with cytokines followed by stimulation of 10^{-7} M fMLP as described (22). Mean ±SEM.

Two mechanisms probably required for eosinophil effector function and also triggered by IL-5 as well as IL-3 and GM-CSF are the respiratory burst and the release of granule contents. IL-5 as well as IL-3 and GM-CSF cause the release of superoxide anion on eosinophils directly and to a similar extent (22–25). In contrast, it seems that IL-5 is the strongest stimulus for the release of the granule-associated enzyme eosinophil-derived neurotoxin (EDN) when eosinophils are coated with secretory IgA or serum IgG (26), although it is not clear whether this difference is evident at optimal concentrations of IL-5, IL-3, and GM-CSF.

Eosinophils are end cells that are incapable of proliferation, nonetheless, they seem to retain the ability to synthesize cellular components de novo, an example of which is the biosynthesis of proteoglycans. IL-5, IL-3, and GM-CSF enhance the biosynthesis of proteoglycans and the size of the attached chondroitin sulfate chains (27). GM-CSF is probably also responsible for the increased incorporation of ^{35}S-methionine into newly synthesized eosinophil proteins (3). The IL-5, IL-3, and GM-CSF property of stimulating eosinophil protein synthesis is likely to facilitate the prolongation of eosinophil survival in vitro to weeks in culture (15). This may also represent a fundamental difference between eosinophils and neutrophils. A second contribution of IL-5, IL-3, and GM-CSF to the maintenance of eosinophil survival may be related to their ability to inhibit programmed cell death. Thus it appears that at least IL-5 is capable of inhibiting eosinophil apoptosis after a few days in culture (C. Spry, personal communication).

An interesting and typical feature of eosinophils stimulated for a few days in culture is their change in density from normodense to hypodense cells. Although the biochemical reasons for this are not clear, it is significant that this hypodense phenotype correlates with enhancement of function such as leukotriene production, helminthotoxicity, and cell survival in vitro (15). This correlation is also seen in vivo, where hypodense eosinophils from patients with hypereosinophilia were reported to exhibit enhanced leukotriene C_4 generation (28) and helminthotoxic activity. An involvement of IL-5 in this in-vivo phenomenon is further suggested by the association between the degree of hypodense eosinophils and eosinophilia (29), and more conclusively, by the ability of anti-IL-5 antibodies to inhibit the ex-vivo ability of serum of patients with the idiopathic hypereosinophilic syndrome to convert normodense eosinophils into a functionally activated hypodense phenotype (16).

The existence of three hemopoietic growth factors with the ability to stimulate eosinophil function has raised the possibility that each of them might stimulate a unique set of functions. In the few reported comparisons between IL-5, IL-3, and GM-CSF, however, these factors stimulated the same pattern of functions and the magnitude of this response was similar. In terms of potency too, IL-5, IL-3, and GM-CSF appear to stimulate 50% maximal activity at similar molar concentrations (Figure 1), although it should be noted that the patterns of glycosylation of these factors vary according to the different expression systems used to produce these factors, and this can influence their potency. These similarities may be related to the structure and the binding properties of these cytokines (see below).

Eosinophils, like other hemopoietic cells and indeed cells from other tissues, may be subjected to negative regulation. A candidate is interleukin-4, a cytokine with a similar structure and genomal organization to IL-5, IL-3, and GM-CSF (see below). IL-4 has been shown to inhibit eosinophil degranulation and eosinophil-mediated cytotoxicity of schistosomula of *Schistosoma mansoni* in the presence of IgG but not IgE (30). This

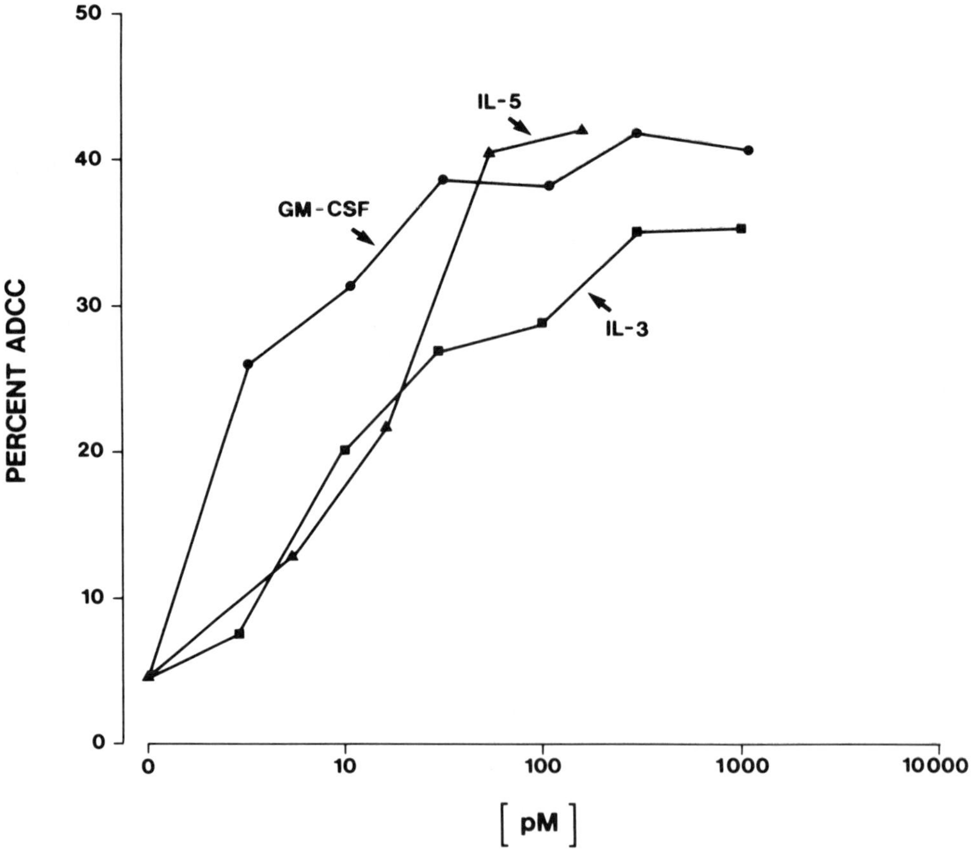

Figure 1 Comparison of human IL-5, IL-3, and GM-CSF for their ability to stimulate eosinophils to kill antibody-coated tumor cells. Each point is the mean of triplicate determinations. IL-5 was produced in yeast, IL-3 in *E. coli,* and GM-CSF in COS cells. These were specified by the suppliers to be >99% pure. The IL-5 was generously provided by Immunex Corp (Seattle, Washington), and the IL-3 and GM-CSF were kindly supplied by Genetics Institute (Cambridge, Massachusetts).

correlated with IL-4 regulation of eosinophil Fc receptors, where the IgG Fc receptor are reduced but the IgE Fc receptors remain essentially unaltered.

An important aspect of the stimulation of the eosinophil lineage by IL-5 is the relative concentrations of this factor required to stimulate the different functions. A titration of IL-5 designed to compare its relative potency on the proliferation and differentiation of eosinophil progenitors (colonies) with activation of eosinophil function (ADCC) and survival shows (Figure 2) that there is a hierarchy of eosinophil responses to IL-5. At low concentrations IL-5 preferentially maintains eosinophil numbers, followed by activation of eosinophil cytotoxicity and stimulation of eosinophil colonies at higher IL-5 concentrations. Such a pattern in vivo suggests that the amount of IL-5 produced and released into the circulation or at the inflammatory site may reflect a stepwise response, where low levels of IL-5 may be required to support eosinophil numbers, while an accelerated production of eosinophils may be needed in more demanding emergencies.

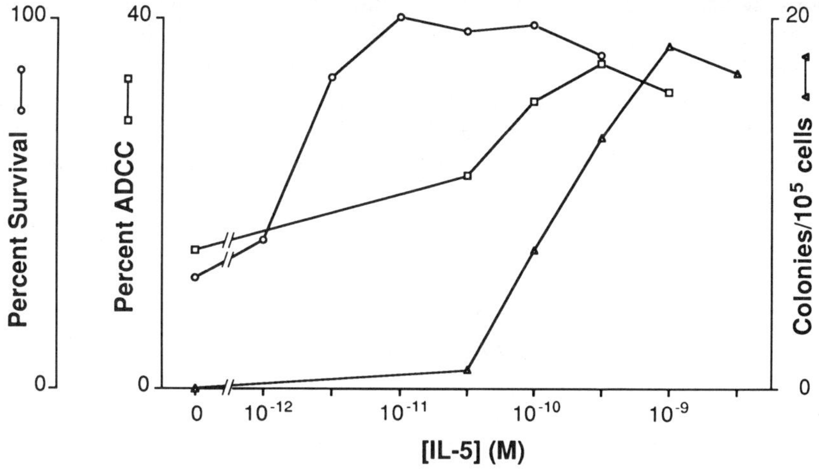

Figure 2 Relative potency of human IL-5 in stimulating eosinophil colony-forming cells (▲—▲), antibody-dependent cytotoxicity of tumor cells by eosinophils (□—□), and eosinophil survival (○—○). Each point is the mean of at least three determinations.

III. THE STRUCTURE OF HUMAN IL-5

The nucleotide sequence of human IL-5 predicts a polypeptide of 134 amino acids, which after cleavage of a signal peptide would give a processed protein of 115 amino acids with a molecular weight of about 13,000 (31). However, amino acid sequencing of native human IL-5 that can confirm this assumption has not yet been reported. Examination of the primary structure of human IL-5 reveals a high degree of homology (70%) with the mouse IL-5 protein (31). This conservation is likely to explain the biological (6,14,15,27), receptor-binding (32), and immunological (16,33) cross-reactivity of human and mouse IL-5.

Human IL-5 has two cysteines at positions 44 and 86 of the putative mature protein (Figure 3), which may form an intramolecular disulfide bridge or, by allowing disulfide bonding between two IL-5 molecules, facilitate the formation of a dimer. The latter seems to be the case, since SDS-PAGE of radiolabeled yeast-derived human IL-5 shows a molecular weight of 45,000 under nonreducing conditions, and about 22,000 under reducing conditions (32). Similarly, mouse IL-5 has been shown by gel filtration to have a molecular weight of 30,000–60,000 (5). In contrast, two cysteines of IL-3 and the four cysteines of GM-CSF form intramolecular disulfide bonds (34–36). While most studies have used IL-5 presumably in a dimer form, it is not clear whether upon reduction the IL-5 monomer exhibits typical IL-5 biological activity or is able to bind to the IL-5 receptor, behaving either as an agonist or indeed as an antagonist.

The primary structure of human IL-5 also shows two potential N-linked glycosylation sites at positions 28 and 71; however, it is not known what contribution the carbohydrate makes to the biological activity of IL-5. With other growth factors such as mouse IL-5 and human GM-CSF, the carbohydrate does not seem to be required for biological activity (37,38), and at least in the case of GM-CSF, its elimination appears to increase the specific activity of the molecule (38).

Although human IL-5 has not yet been crystallized, some physical features may be deduced by using predictive algorithms. For example, the secondary structure would have four α-helices, with the fourth α-helix containing hydrophilic amino acids (Figure 3). This hydrophilic region is the only area with significant homology to IL-3 (23) as well as GM-CSF, IL-4, and IL-6 (37), and its conservation may be important for ligand binding or for tertiary structure configuration. In fact, the fourth α-helix of IL-5 has heptad periodicities containing i/i + 3 apolar repeating sequences, suggesting long-range interactions probably with the predicted first α-helix, a feature shared with other hemopoietic growth factors (39).

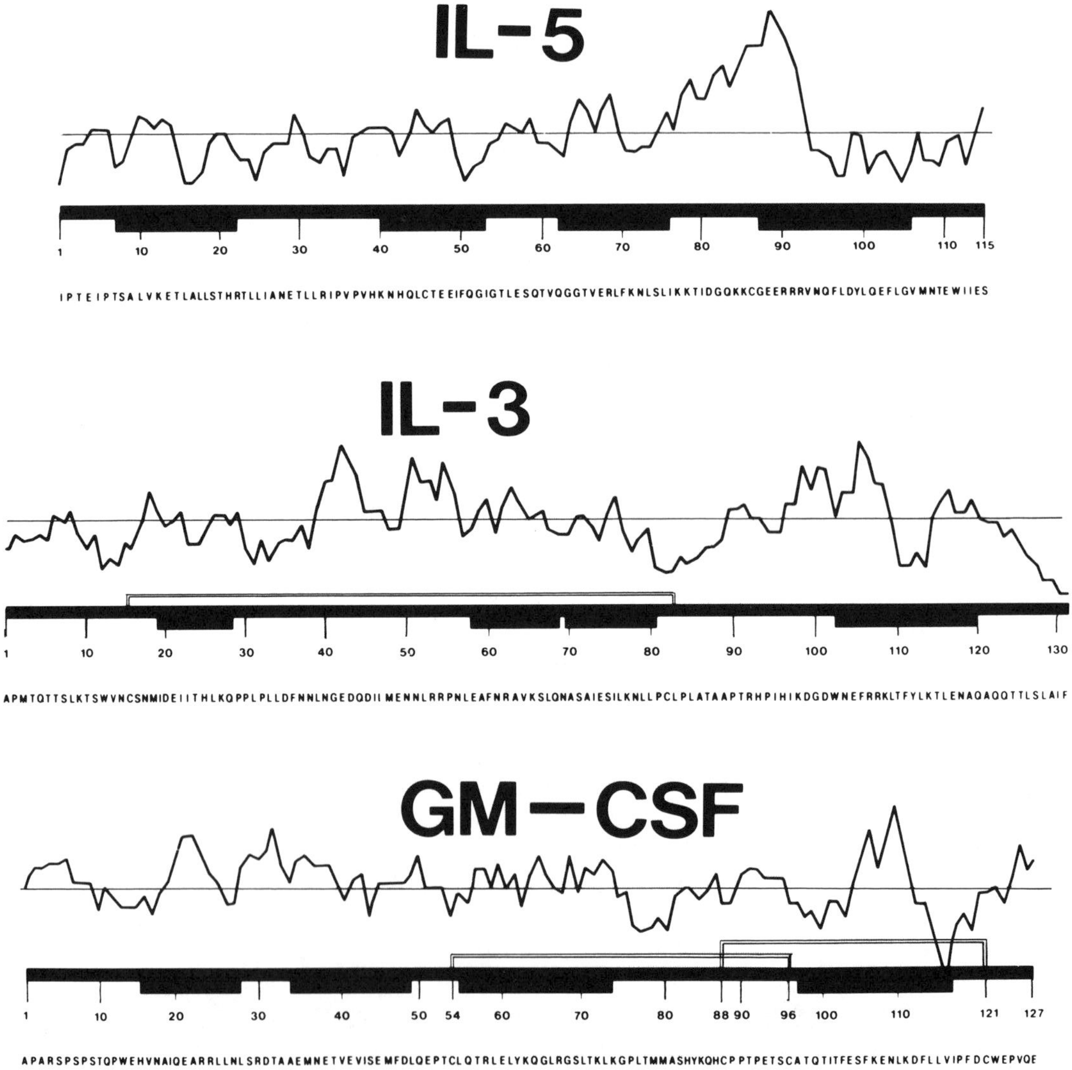

Figure 3 Comparison of the primary and predicted secondary structures of human IL-5, IL-3, and GM-CSF. The bars join the appropriate cysteine residues and represent the disulfide bonds. The predicted α-helices are represented by the solid blocks. The thin horizontal line separates the predicted hydrophilic regions (above) from the hydrophobic regions (below).

IV. BINDING OF HUMAN IL-5

Despite the multiple biological effects of human IL-5 on eosinophils, their surface receptors have only recently been described (32). Among purified primary cell types, eosinophils express IL-5 surface receptors which are low in numbers and of high affinity (Table 3). Neither neutrophils nor monocytes express detectable IL-5 receptors. Basophils from a patient with chronic myeloid leukemia also showed binding to IL-5. From a panel of human cell lines that included myeloid cells and B- as well as pre-B-cell lines (32) only HL-60 cells show detectable IL-5 receptors. This suggests that human B-cells are intrinsically different from mouse B-cells, which express receptors for mouse IL-5 (40), and it would be important to determine whether normal and activated human B-cells can bind to human IL-5.

The approximate dissociation constant (K_D) of IL-5 binding to eosinophils is of 10–100 pM (Table 3, Figure 4, and Ref. 32), a value which is consistent with the concentrations of IL-5 required to stimulate eosinophil function (see Section II.B) and similar to the K_D of IL-3 and of GM-CSF on eosinophils (41). Thus none of these three growth factors seems to have a gross advantage over the other in terms of binding affinity or relative potency.

An important consideration in studying IL-5 and indeed any ligand-receptor interaction is that of specificity. Specific binding (binding competed by the unlabeled homologous ligand but not by other ligands) of hemopoietic growth factors to some human cells has been observed; however, recent experiments demonstrated that IL-3 and GM-CSF may be different in that they inhibit the binding of each other on some cell types, including eosinophils (41–44). The competition between IL-3 and GM-CSF on eosinophils is observed both when a single concentration of radiolabeled ligand is competing with increasing concentrations of unlabeled heterologous ligand (41) and when different radioligand concentrations are competing with a 100-fold molar excess of unlabeled heterologous ligand (Figure 5). Thus IL-3 and GM-CSF receptors appear to be closely linked on the surface of eosinophils.

In the case of human IL-5, the binding to eosinophils is inhibited not only by human and mouse IL-5 but also by IL-3 and GM-CSF (Figure 6). Other growth factors with some homology in the primary and predictive tertiary structure, such as IL-4 and IL-6 (37,39), do not compete, nor does tumor necrosis factor α (TNFα), a cytokine with an unrelated structure but that is active on eosinophils (45). In addition, the cytokine leukemia-inhibitory factor (LIF)/human interleukin differentiation activity (HILDA), which has been reported to stimulate eosinophil chemotaxis and chemiluminescence (46) but is inactive in our hands at stimulating ADCC and superoxide anion generation of human eosinophils in vitro, does not compete for ^{125}I-IL-5 binding.

The ability of mouse IL-5 to fully inhibit the binding of human IL-5 is consistent with the ability of mouse IL-5 to act on human eosinophils (see above) and suggests that the binding domains of mouse and human IL-5 are in the conserved regions of these two molecules.

The inhibition of ^{125}I-IL-5 binding to eosinophils by IL-3 and GM-CSF can be readily seen when the cells are incubated for 16 h at 4°C in the presence of 0.1% sodium azide, conditions that prevent receptor trans-down-modulation. This phenomenon is observed with mouse hemopoietic growth factors and bone marrow cells at 37°C (but not at 4°C) and is characterized by the binding of one growth factor, leading to the down-modulation (internalization) of other growth factor receptors and

Table 3 Expression of Growth-Factor Receptors on Eosinophils and Other Purified Primary Myeloid Cells

	Number of receptors			K_D (M)		
Cells	IL-5	IL-3	GM-CSF	IL-5	IL-3	GM-CSF
Eosinophils	50–800	300–1000	500–900	10^{-11}–10^{-10}	5×10^{-11}–5×10^{-10}	10^{-11}–10^{-10}
Neutrophils	Absent	Absent	50–750	—	—	10^{-11}–10^{-10}
Monocytes	Absent	ha[a] = 80–600	20–500	—	10^{-11}–10^{-10}	10^{-11}–10^{-10}
		la[b] = 100–5000	100–7000		5×10^{-10}–5×10^{-9}	5×10^{-10}–5×10^{-9}
CML basophils[c]	2000	700–900	100–200	10^{-9}	10^{-11}	4×10^{-11}

[a] ha = high affinity.

[b] la = low affinity.

[c] A single case was examined.

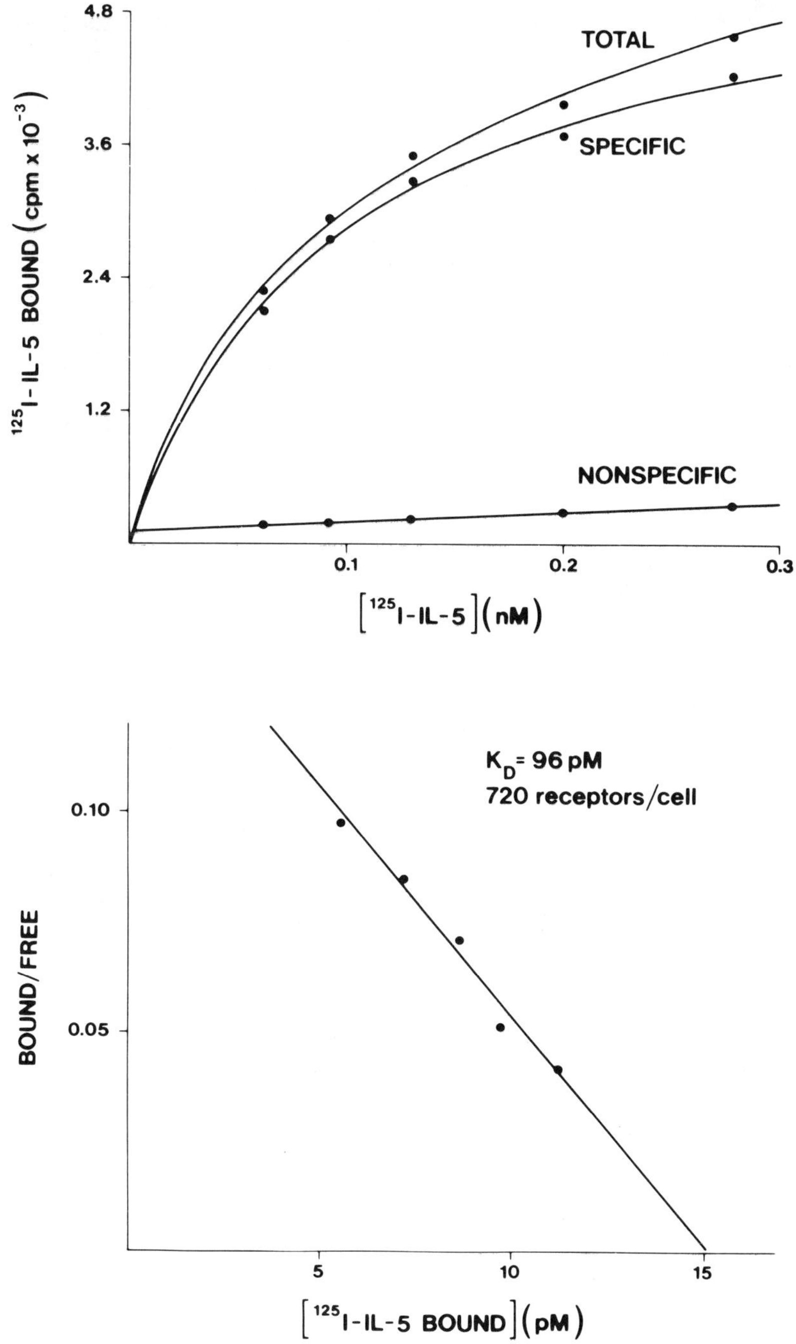

Figure 4 Equilibrium binding isotherm and Scatchard analysis of ^{125}I-IL-5 binding to human eosinophils. Each point is the mean of duplicate determinations using 2×10^6 cells each.

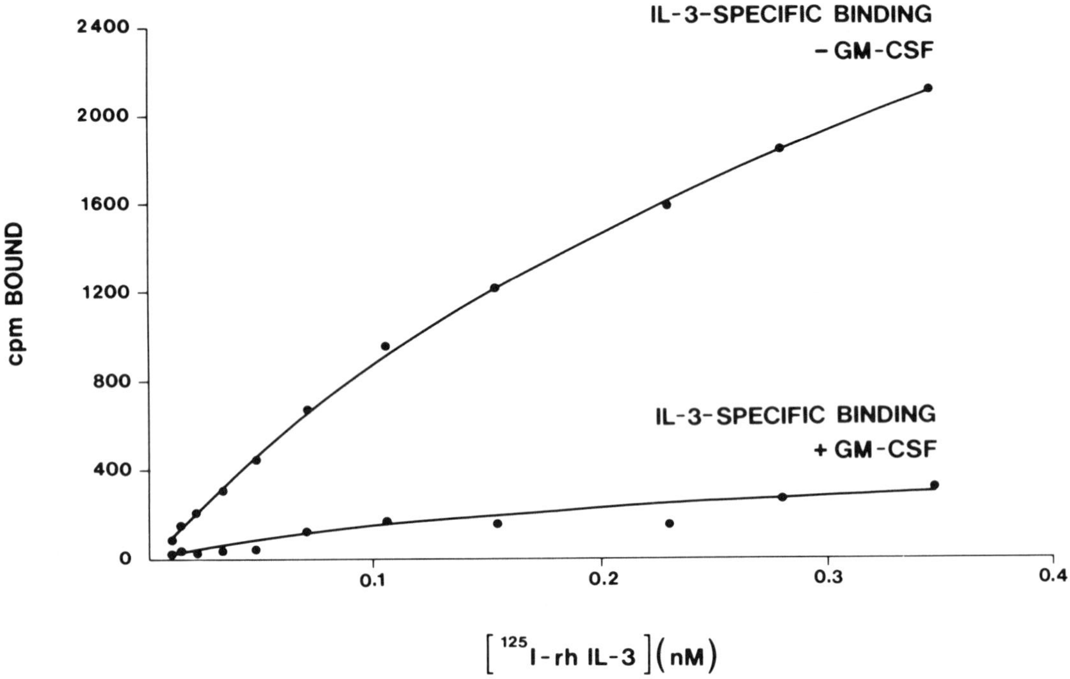

Figure 5 Competition of ^{125}I-IL-3 binding to human eosinophils by GM-CSF. Eosinophils were incubated with different concentrations of ^{125}I-IL-3 in the absence or in the presence of 100-fold molar excess GM-CSF at each point. Each point represents the mean of duplicate determinations.

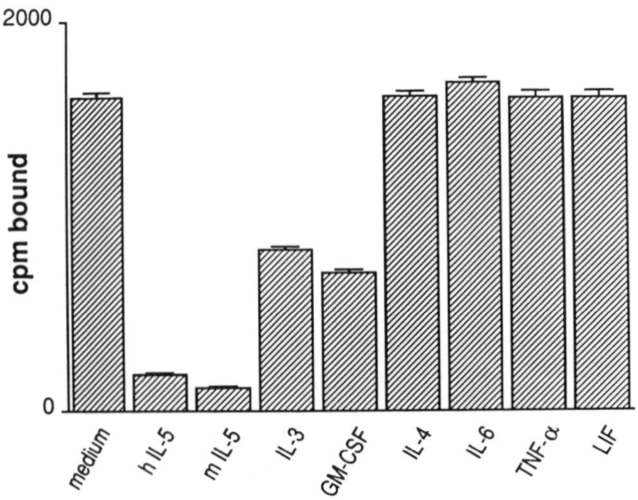

Figure 6 Competition of human ^{125}I-IL-5 (80 pM) binding to purified eosinophils by different cytokines at 100-fold molar excess.

therefore resulting in reduced binding. Evidence that human IL-5 receptor trans-down-modulation does not occur under these conditions can be obtained by acid treatment of eosinophils at the end of the incubation period, a technique that distinguishes surface-bound (acid-dissociable) from internalized ^{125}I-IL-5 (nondissociable). The fact that the majority of ^{125}I-IL-5 counts remain acid-dissociable, and that these are higher than the levels of inhibition observed (Figure 7), indicates that the competition by IL-3 and GM-CSF takes place at the level of the cell surface.

While IL-3 and GM-CSF have been consistently found to inhibit the binding of ^{125}I-IL-5 to eosinophils, IL-5 inhibits the binding of ^{125}I-IL-3 and of ^{125}I-GM-CSF to eosinophils from only some donors (Table 4; Ref. 32). The reason for this is not clear, but since the eosinophils under study are obtained from individuals with some degree of eosinophilia, the variability observed may reflect different degrees of eosinophil IL-5 receptors occupancy by IL-5 in vivo.

The competition for human ^{125}I-IL-5 binding is different from that for mouse IL-5, where mouse IL-3 and GM-CSF do not inhibit the binding of ^{125}I- or ^{35}S-labeled IL-5 to the BCL_1 mouse B-cell line (40), suggesting species differences or that each cell type expresses a unique spectrum of cross-reactivities. The latter is emphasized by analysis of the binding of IL-5, IL-3, and GM-CSF to various primary cell types, where each of these expresses a different pattern of binding and of inhibition by heterologous ligands (Table 4).

The physical nature of the relationship between IL-5, IL-3, and GM-CSF receptors on eosinophils and indeed other cell types is poorly understood. Given the apparent similarity between IL-5, IL-3, and GM-CSF in their C-termini (see above), this area may contain a polypeptide sequence that is capable of binding to a common receptor.

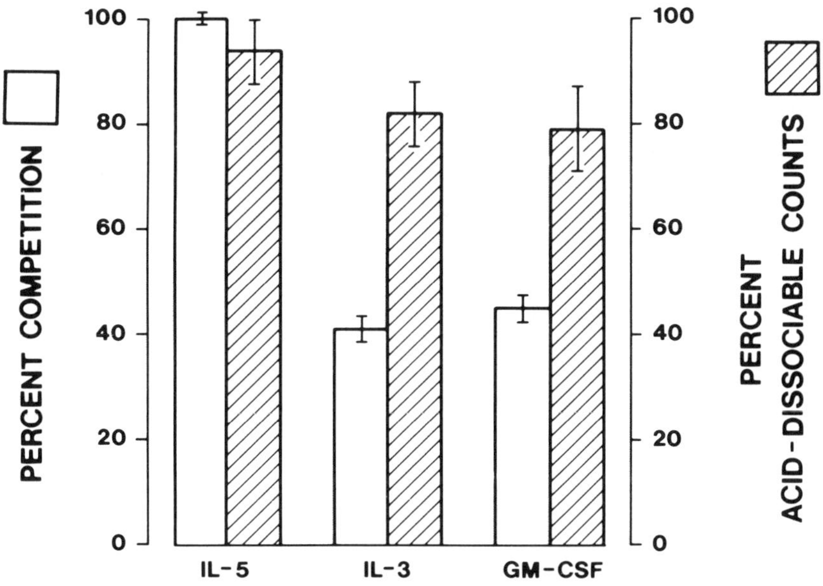

Figure 7 Comparison between the percent competition of ^{125}I-IL-5 (70 pM) binding to eosinophils by IL-3 and GM-CSF (open bars) and the percent acid-dissociable counts (hatched bars), demonstrating that the inhibition of ^{125}I-IL-5 binding occurs at the cell surface.

Table 4 Competition of ^{125}I-IL-5, ^{125}I-IL-3, and ^{125}I-GM-CSF Binding to Eosinophils and Other Myeloid Cells by Homologous and Heterologous Ligands[a]

Cells	Ligands: Competitors:	^{125}I-IL-5 IL-3	^{125}I-IL-5 GM-CSF	^{125}I-IL-3 IL-5	^{125}I-IL-3 GM-CSF	^{125}I-GM-CSF IL-5	^{125}I-GM-CSF IL-3
Eosinophils		+	+	±[a]	+	±[a]	+
Neutrophils		No binding		No binding		−	−
Monocytes		No binding		−	+	−	+
CML basophils		+	+	−	−	−	+

[a] Radioligands were used at 30–80 pM, and competition was carried out at 100-fold molar excess.

[b] ± = competition is seen in only some eosinophilic donors.

This possibility seems unlikely in view of the inability of IL-5 and IL-3 to inhibit GM-CSF binding to neutrophils and of IL-5 to compete for IL-3 or GM-CSF binding to monocytes (Table 4). This pattern rather indicates that the receptors for each of these growth factors need to be co-expressed in order for the reciprocal competition to become evident. A second possibility is therefore that IL-5, IL-3, and GM-CSF receptors become specifically associated in the cell membrane. The different ligands may then inhibit the binding of each other by steric hindrance or by sequestering a limiting polypeptide chain in a putative common receptor complex. The cloning of the IL-5 receptor will be needed before its relationship to the IL-3 and GM-CSF receptors can be fully understood.

Whatever the biochemical process involved, the competition of IL-5, IL-3, and GM-CSF for binding to peripheral blood eosinophils may provide an explanation for their similar activities on eosinophil function, in terms of the spectrum of functions stimulated, the magnitude of the response, and their relative potency as described above. In addition, the ability of these growth factors to inhibit the binding of each other may help prevent excessive eosinophil stimulation of function, with potentially deleterious effects on the host.

Whether the same relationship may be observed on eosinophil progenitor cells is not known but would appear unlikely in view of the differential effects of IL-5 on the one hand and of IL-3 and GM-CSF on the other hand (see above). It is possible that IL-5 receptors are expressed at a later stage of differentiation, with their primary role being to push the eosinophil lineage toward terminal differentiation.

V. IL-5 PRODUCTION

A. Localization of the IL-5 Gene

The similarities of human IL-5 with IL-3 and GM-CSF can be extended from their biology, structure, and binding properties to the localization and organization of their genes in the human genome.

The cDNA and genomal copies of both the human and mouse IL-5 genes have been cloned in recent years (31,47–49). The genomic structure (i.e., the intron/exon arrangement) of the human IL-5 gene is very similar to that which has been described for other hemopoietic growth factor genes, in particular for GM-CSF (50) and IL-4. The IL-3 gene is also structurally related but has a distinct feature (51). The single-copy gene for human IL-5 is located on the long arm of chromosome 5 at band q31, within 240 Kb of the human IL-4 gene (52). The genes for GM-CSF and IL-3 are also located on the same chromosomal band, separated from each other by 9 Kb (53) and probably within 500 Kb of the IL-4/IL-5 region (52). Such a clustering as well as the similarity in gene structure suggests that these genes may have arisen by duplication. Since all of these genes are expressed in T-cells, one could speculate that this region of chromosome 5 could form a DNA domain available for transcription in T-cells and allow the coordinated expression of this cluster of genes.

B. IL-5 Gene Expression

IL-5 is produced mainly by activated T-cells (4,47,54), as predicted by the seminal observations of Basten and Beeson, who, in the early 1970s, demonstrated that eosinophilia was a T-cell-dependent phenomenon (55,56). Apart from T-cells, mast cells have also been shown to express IL-5 mRNA (57), an observation that may be of relevance in allergy, where IL-5 production by both cell types may attract eosinophils to the sites of the allergic reaction.

The production of IL-5 may also be seen in cells that have undergone a malignant transformation. For instance, large-cell carcinoma of the lung has been shown to produce a factor that stimulates selective eosinophil production in vitro (58). Eosinophilia has been noted associated with lymphoid malignancies (59), and indeed IL-5 mRNA has been detected in Reed-Sternberg cells from lymph nodes of patients with Hodgkin's disease and eosinophilia (60). It will be interesting to establish whether the factor responsible for the eosinophilia seen in paraneoplastic syndromes is IL-5 itself or an IL-5-like molecule.

Although T-cells appear to be the major source of IL-5, very little is known about the stimuli that lead to IL-5 gene expression. A specific antigen seems to be one of these, as suggested by the selective production of an eosinophil colony-stimulating factor by T-cells from an eosinophilic patient with allergic bronchopulmonary eosinophilia after stimulation with aspergillus extract (61). More recently, cytokines themselves have been reported to stimulate IL-5 production. IL-2 has been shown to stimulate T-cells to produce IL-5 mRNA and protein in vitro (33), and the in-vivo administration of IL-2 leads to eosinophilia with concomitant eosinophil activation (62).

Whether there are only subsets of human T-cells that express IL-5 mRNA in an analogous situation to the mouse (63) is not known. Relevant to this point may be our observation that the human T-cell line Jurkatt does not express IL-5 mRNA under conditions where high levels of IL-3 and GM-CSF mRNA are detected (unpublished observations). Alternatively, different stimuli may operate through different second signaling pathways leading to selective gene expression. This is likely to occur by transcriptional activation of specific areas in the promoter region of these genes.

C. The IL-5 Gene Promoter

No information is available on the regions of the IL-5 gene that are involved in the regulation of its expression. However, a number of regions of the human IL-5 gene promoter have previously been shown to have some homology with the promoter regions of other T-cell expressing genes (49). Several relatively long stretches of similarity can be found between the IL-5 and IL-2 genes (Figure 8). One of these sequences (−175 to −164 in IL-5) matches an Nf-κB-like sequence in the IL-2 gene (−209 to −198). This sequence in IL-2 binds an NF-κB-like protein (64) and also other factors, one of which is AP3-like (63). This sequence can act as a T-cell-specific enhancer element (65). The function of the second similar region between IL-5 and IL-2 (Figure 8) is unknown.

A short distance upstream from the TATA box, a 15-bp sequence (−56 to −42) of the IL-5 gene is almost identical (14 of 15 bases) to a similarly positioned (−48 to −34) region of the GM-CSF gene. In the human GM-CSF gene, a DNAse 1 footprint has been observed across this region with extracts from several T-cell lines (66). We have found that bacterially expressed and purified AP1 can bind to this region of the GM-CSF promoter (−59 to −36) (unpublished data). These sequences have been shown to play an important role in GM-CSF expression in activated T-cells (66). The

```
    -300                                                   -250
TCTACCTTATACTTTGTTTTGCACACATCTTTTAAGAGGAAGTTAATTTTCTGATTTTAA
                                                       IL-2

                                               CK-1   -200
GAAATGCAAATGTGGGGCAATGATGTATTAACCCAAAGATTCTTCGTAATAGAAAATGTT

    OCT   γ-IFN

                                           -150
TTTAAAGGGGGAAACAGGGATTTTTATTATTAAAAGATAAAAGTAAATTTATTTTTTAA
             IL-2

                              -100
GATATAAGGCATTGGAAACATTTAGTTTCACGATATGCCATTATTAGGCATTCTCTATCT

                                               SRE

                     -50
GATTGTTAGAAATTATTCATTTCCTCAAAGACAGACAATAAATTGACTGGGACGCAGTC
      +1          GM-CSF

TTGTACTATGCACTTTCTTTGCCAAAGGCA
```

Figure 8 Sequence of the human IL-5 promoter region. The start of transcription (→) and the TATA box are marked. The regions of homology to other T-cells products (—) and the octamer (OCT) and serum response elements (SRE) are indicated (—).

similar sequence in the IL-5 gene may also be important in IL-5 gene expression in these cells.

The IL-5 gene also contains a 10-bp sequence (termed CK-1), which has been identified in the promoter regions of other growth-factor genes (−203 to −212, Figure 8). We have shown that this sequence from several genes binds a transcription factor, NF-GMa (67). The CK-1 sequence from G-CSF acts as a TNF_{α}- and IL-1-responsive transcription element in embryonic fibroblasts (68). Its role, if any, in the T-cell expression of GM-CSF, IL-3, and indeed IL-5, is not known. We have tested the ability of the CK-1 sequence from IL-5 to compete for binding of NF-GMa to the GM-CSF CK-1 sequence. A 40-bp fragment of DNA spanning the IL-5/CK-1 sequence can compete for binding but is fivefold less efficient than the GM-CSF or IL-3/CK-1 sequences (Figure 9). This agrees with its less than perfect match with the CK-1 consensus sequence (Figure 9). It should be noted that the IL-5/CK-1 sequence can bind NF-GMa not only from T-cells but also NF-GMa derived from a wide range of cell types (unpublished observations).

The significance of the affinity of NF-GMa being IL-3 > GM-CSF > IL-5 genes is not clear, but it is worth noting that it matches the temporal hierarchy in the stimulation of eosinophil production, where the initial stimulation of stem cell renewal and expansion of progenitor cell pools by IL-3 and GM-CSF is followed by terminal differentiation of the eosinophil lineage by IL-5. Thus the amount of NF-GMa produced may be at least one relevant factor in determining the extent of the eosinophilopoietic response.

Two other regions of the IL-5 promoter are similar to well-characterized transcriptional control elements. One is an octamer-type sequence (−254 ATGCAAAT −247; Figure 8) which is found in a wide range of genes. These sequences have been implicated in the control of many genes, including B-cell-specific expression of immunoglobulin heavy-chain genes (69). A number of octamer-binding transcription factors have recently been cloned (70). Their expression is regulated in a cell-specific manner and during embryogenesis. The possibility exists that the IL-5 octamer sequence could be involved in T-cell-specific expression, a concept reinforced by the fact that this sequence occurs in the IL-5 promoter region which has similarity to γ-interferon (64).

The IL-5 promoter also contains a serum response element (SRE) at position −80 (Figure 8). This sequence in other genes, such as the c fos protooncogene, is required for gene induction by as yet unknown factors in serum (71). The SRE is also involved in autoregulation of c fos (72) and can bind both positive and negative regulatory proteins (73). The role of these sequences in IL-5 gene expression is still obscure and awaits detailed mutational analysis of the IL-5 gene promoter.

VI. CONCLUDING REMARKS

Future research on the role of IL-5 will require a combination of cell biology and molecular biology approaches. In examining the ability of IL-5 to induce eosinophilia in vivo, the injection of IL-5 and the generation of IL-5 transgenic animals will be required. This could represent in turn a very useful model for studying the role of eosinophils in certain parasitic diseases. Ultimately, however, gene deletion experiments may prove to be the most definite way to show whether IL-5 plays a unique role in the production and function of eosinophils. These experiments may also unveil unexpected functions of IL-5 outside hemopoiesis.

a)

	-96 -87
GM-CSF	5' GAGATTCCAC 3'
	-126 -117
IL-3	5' GAGGTTCCAT 3'
	-223 -214
IL-5	5' AAGATTCTTC 3'

b)

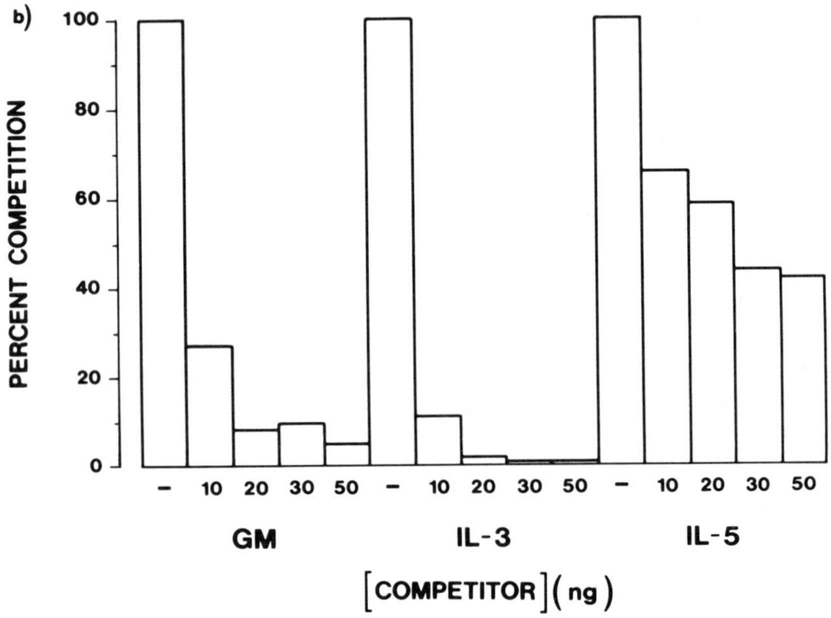

Figure 9 (a) Sequences of CK-1-like regions from GM-CSF, IL-3, and IL-5. Distances from the start of transcription of each gene are shown. Base differences between GM-CSF and the IL-3 or IL-5 sequences are underlined. (b) Binding competition experiment showing the ability of the GM-CSF, IL-3, and IL-5 sequences to compete for binding of NF-GMa to radiolabeled GM-CSF CK-1 sequence. Percent competition was estimated from densitometry of retardation gels with increasing concentrations of each competitor. Experimental design was as previously described (68).

ACKNOWLEDGMENTS

We would like to thank Genetics Institute (Cambridge, Massachusetts) and Immunex Corp. (Seattle, Washington) for gifts of reagents, and M. Walker and B. Meakins for excellent secretarial assistance. This work was supported by grants from the National Health and Medical Research Council of Australia.

REFERENCES

1. David JR, Vadas MA, Butterworth AE, de Brito PA, Carvalho EM, David RA, Bina JA, Andrade ZA. Enhanced helminthotoxic capacity of eosinophils from patients with eosinophilia. N Engl J Med 1980; 303:1147–56.
2. Metcalf D, Cutler RL, and Nicola NA. Selective stimulation by mouse spleen cell conditioned medium of human eosinophil colony formation. Blood 1983; 61:999–1005.
3. Vadas MA, Varigos G, Nicola N, Pincus S, Dessein A, Metcalf D, Battye FL. Eosinophil activation by colony-stimulating factor in man: metabolic effects and analysis by flow cytometry. Blood 1983; 61:1232.
4. Sanderson CJ, Warren DJ, Strath M. Identification of a lymphokine that stimulates eosinophil differentiation in vitro. Its relationship to interleukin 3, and functional properties of eosinophils produced in cultures. J Exp Med 1985; 162:60–74.
5. Sanderson CJ, O'Garra A, Warren DJ, Klaus GG. Eosinophil differentiation factor also has B-cell growth factor activity: proposed name interleukin 4. Proc Natl Acad Sci USA 1986; 83:437–40.
6. Lopez AF, Begley CG, Williamson DJ, Warren DJ, Vadas MA, Sanderson CJ. Murine eosinophil differentiation factor. An eosinophil-specific colony-stimulating factor with activity for human cells. J Exp Med 1986; 163:1085–99.
7. Lopez AF, Nicola NA, Burgess AW, Metcalf D, Battye FL, Sewell WA, Vadas MA. Activation of granulocyte cytotoxic function by purified mouse colony-stimulating factors. J Immunol 1983; 131:2983–8.
8. Nicola NA, Begley CG, Metcalf D. Identification of the human analogue of a regulator that induces differentiation in murine leukaemic cells. Nature 1985; 314:625–8.
9. Yokota T, Coffman RL, Hagiwara H, Rennick DM, Takebe Y, Yokota K, Gemmell L, Schrader B, Yang G, Meyerson P, Luli J, Hoy P, Pene J, Briene F, Spits H, Banchereau J, de Vries J, Lee FD, Arai N, Arai F. Isolation and characterization of lymphokine cDNA clones encoding mouse and human IgA enhancing factor and eosinophil colony-stimulating factor activities: relationship to interleukin-5. Proc Natl Acad Sci USA 1987; 84:7388–92.
10. Enokihara H, Nagashima S, Noma T, Kajitani H, Hamaguchi H, Saito K, Furusawa S, Shisido H, Honjo T. Effect of human recombinant interleukin-5 and G-CSF on eosinophil colony formation. Immunol Lett 1988; 18:73–6.
11. Clutterbuck EJ, Hirst EM, Sanderson CJ. Human interleukin-5 (IL-5) regulates the production of eosinophils in human bone marrow cultures: comparison and interaction with IL-1, IL-3, IL-6, and GMCSF. Blood 1989; 73:1504–12.
12. Sonoda Y, Arai N, Ogawa M. Humoral regulation of eosinophilopoiesis in vitro: analysis of the targets of interleukin-3, granulocyte/macrophage colony-stimulating factor (GM-CSF), and interleukin-5. Leukemia 1989; 3:14–8.
13. Clutterbuck EJ, Sanderson CJ. Regulation of human eosinophil precursor production by cytokines: a comparison of recombinant human interleukin-1 (rhIL-1), rhIL-3, rhIL-5, rhIL-6, and rh granulocyte-macrophage colony-stimulating factor. Blood 1990; 75:1774–9.
14. Begley CG, Lopez AF, Nicola NA, Wang EA, Warren DJ, Sanderson CJ, Vadas MA, Metcalf D. Purified colony-stimulating factors enhance the survival of human neutrophils and eosinophils in vitro: a rapid and sensitive microassay for colony-stimulating factors. Blood 1986; 68:162–6.
15. Rothenberg ME, Petersen J, Stevens RL, Silberstein DS, McKenzie DT, Austen KF, Owen WF Jr. IL-5-dependent conversion of normodense human eosinophils to the hypodense phenotype uses 3T3 fibroblasts for enhanced viability, accelerated hypodensity, and sustained antibody-dependent cytotoxicity. J Immunol 1989; 143:2311–6.
16. Owen WF, Rothenberg ME, Petersen J, Weller PF, Silberstein D, Sheffer AL, Stevens RL, Soberman RJ, Austen KF. Interleukin 5 and phenotypically altered eosinophils in the blood of patients with the idiopathic hypereosinophilic syndrome. J Exp Med 1989; 170:343–8.

17. Zimmerman GA, McIntyre TM. Neutrophil adherence to human endothelium in vitro occurs by CDw18 (Mol, MAC-1/LFA-1/GP 150,95) glycoprotein-dependent and -independent mechanisms. J Clin Invest 1988; 81:531–7.
18. Walsh GM, Kurihara K, Kay AB. Effect of platelet-activating factor (PAF) and interleukin (IL-5) on eosinophil adherence reactions. FASEB J 1989; 3:A1330.
19. Wang JM, Rambaldi A, Biondi A, Chen ZG, Sanderson CJ, Mantovani A. Recombinant human interleukin 5 is a selective eosinophil chemoattractant. Eur J Immunol 1989; 19:701–5.
20. Wardlaw AJ, Moqbel R, Cromwell O, Kay AB. Platelet-activating factor: a potent chemotactic and chemokinetic factor for human eosinophils. J Clin Invest 1986; 78:1701–6.
21. Numao T, Fukuda T, Akutsu I, Makino S, Enokihara H, Honjo T. Selective enhancement of eosinophil chemotaxis by recombinant human interleukin-5. J Allergy Clin Immunol 1989; 83:298.
22. Lopez AF, Williamson DJ, Gambel JR, Begley CG, Harlan JM, Klebanoff SJ, Waltersdorph A, Wong G, Clark SC, Vadas MA. Recombinant human granulocyte-macrophage colony-stimulating factor (rH GM-CSF) stimulates in vitro mature human neutrophil and eosinophil function, surface receptor expression and survival. J Clin Invest 1986; 78:1220–8.
23. Lopez AF, To LB, Yang YC, Gamble JR, Shannon MF, Burns GF, Dyson PG, Juttner CA, Clark S, Vadas MA. Stimulation of proliferation, differentiation and function of human cells by primate interleukin-3. Proc Natl Acad Sci USA 1987; 84:2761–5.
24. Lopez AF, Dyson PG, To LB, Elliott MJ, Milton SE, Russell JA, Juttner CA, Yang YC, Clark SC, Vadas MA. Recombinant human interleukin-3 stimulation of hematopoiesis in humans. Loss of responsiveness with differentiation in the neutrophilic myeloid series. Blood 1988; 72:1797–804.
25. Lopez AF, Sanderson CJ, Gamble JR, Campbell HD, Young IG, Vadas MA. Recombinant human interleukin-5 (IL-5) is a selective activator of human eosinophil function. J Exp Med 1988; 167:219–24.
26. Fujisawa T, Abu-Ghazaleh R, Kita H, Sanderson CJ, Gleich GJ. Regulatory effect of cytokines on eosinophil degranulation. J Immunol 1990; 144:642–6.
27. Rothenberg ME, Pomerantz JL, Owen WF Jr, Avraham S, Soberman RJ, Austen KF, Stevens RL. Characterization of a human eosinophil proteoglycan, and augmentation of its biosynthesis and size by interleukin 3, interleukin 5, and granulocyte/macrophage colony stimulating factor. J Biol Chem 1988; 263:13901–8.
28. Kajita T, Yui Y, Mita H, Taniguchi N, Saito H, Mishima T, Shida T. Release of leukotriene C4 from human eosinophils and its relation to the cell density. Int Arch Allergy Appl Immunol 1985; 78:406–10.
29. Fukuda T, Dunnette SL, Reed CE, Ackerman SJ, Peters MS, Gleich GJ. Increased numbers of hypodense eosinophils in the blood of patients with bronchial asthma. Am Rev Respir Dis 1985; 132:981–5.
30. Baskar P, Silberstein DS, Pincus SH. Inhibition of IgG-triggered human eosinophil function by IL-4. J Immunol 1990; 144:2321–6.
31. Campbell HD, Tucker WQJ, Hort Y, Martinson ME, Mayo G, Clutterbuck EJ, Sanderson CJ, Young IC. Molecular cloning, nucleotide sequence, and expression of the gene encoding human eosinophil differentiation factor (interleukin 5). Proc Natl Acad Sci USA 1987; 84:6627–33.
32. Lopez et al. Submitted for publication.
33. Enokihara H, Furusawa S, Nakakubo H, Kajitani H, Nagashima S, Saito K, Shishido H, Hitoshi Y, Takatsu K, Noma T, Shimizu A, Honjo T. T cells from eosinophilic patients produce interleukin-5 with interleukin-2 stimulation. Blood 1989; 73:1809–13.
34. Yang YC, Ciarletta AB, Temple PA, Chung MP, Kovacic S, Witek-Giannotti JS, Leary AC, Kriz R, Donahue RE, Wong GG, Clark SC. Human IL-3 (multi-CSF): identification

by expression cloning of a novel hematopoietic growth factor related to murine IL-3. Cell 1986; 47:3–10.

35. Clark-Lewis I, Lopez AF, To LB, Vadas MA, Schrader JW, Hood LE, Kent SB. Structure-function studies of human granulocyte-macrophage colony-stimulating factor. Identification of residues required for activity. J Immunol 1988; 141:881–9.
36. Ohgama Y, Nagase M, Nabeshima S, Fukui M, Nakazawa H. Characterization of recombinant DNA-derived human granulocyte macrophage colony stimulating factor by fast atom bombardment mass spectrometry. J Biotech 1989; 12:219–30.
37. Sanderson CJ, Campbell HD, Young IG. Molecular and cellular biology of eosinophil differentiation factor (interleukin-5) and its effects on human and mouse B cells. Immunol Rev 199; 102:29–50.
38. Kaushansky K, O'Hara PJ, Hart CE, Forstrom JW, Hagen FS. Role of carbohydrate in the function of human granulocyte-macrophage colony-stimulating factor. Biochemistry 1987; 26:4861–7.
39. Parry DA, Minasian E, Leach SJ. Conformational homologies among cytokines: interleukins and colony stimulating factors. J Mol Recog 1988; 1:107–10.
40. Mita S, Harada N, Naomi S, Hitoshi Y, Sakamoto K, Akagi M, Tominaga A, Takatsu K. Receptors for T cell-replacing factor/interleukin 5. Specificity, quantitation, and its implication. J Exp Med 1988; 168:863–78.
41. Lopez AF, Eglinton JM, Gillis D, Park LS, Clark S, Vadas MA. Reciprocal inhibition of binding between interleukin 3 and granulocyte-macrophage colony-stimulating factor to human eosinophils. Proc Natl Acad Sci USA 1989; 86:7022–6.
42. Gesner TG, Mufson RA, Norton CR, Turner KJ, Yang YC, Clark SC. Specific binding, internalization and degradation of human recombinant interleukin-3 by cells of the acute myelogenous leukemia line, KG-1. J Cell Physiol 1988; 136:493–9.
43. Park LS, Friend D, Price V, Anderson D, Singer J, Prickett KS, Urdal DL. Heterogeneity in human interleukin-3 receptors. A subclass that binds human granulocyte/macrophage colony-stimulating factor. J Biol Chem 1989; 264:5420–7.
44. Elliott MJ, Vadas MA, Eglinton JM, Park LS, To LB, Cleland LG, Clark SC, Lopez AF. Recombinant human interleukin-3 and granulocyte-macrophage colony-stimulating factor show common biological effects and binding characteristics on human monocytes. Blood 1989; 74:2349–59.
45. Silberstein DS, David JR. Tumor necrosis factor enhances eosinophil toxicity to *Schistosoma mansoni* larvae. Proc Natl Acad Sci USA 1986; 83:1055.
46. Moreau J-F, Bonneville M, Godard A, Gascan H, Gruart V, Moore M, Souilillou JP. Characterisation of a factor produced by human T cell clones exhibiting eosinophil-activating and burst-promoting activities. J Immunol 1987; 138:3844–9.
47. Azuma C, Tanabe T, Konishu M, Kinashi T, Noma T, Matsuda F, Yaoita Y, Takatsu K, Hammarstrom L, Smith CI, Severinson E, Honjo T. Cloning of cDNA for human T-cell replacing factor (interleukin-5) and comparison with the murine homologue. Nucleic Acids Res 1986; 14:9149–58.
48. Kinashi T, Harada N, Severinson E, Tanabe T, Sideras P, Konishi M, Azuma C, Tominaga A, Berstedt-Lindqvist C, Takahashi M, Matsuda F, Yaoita Y, Takatsu K, Honjo T. Cloning of complementary DNA encoding T-cell replacing factor and identity with B-cell growth factor II. Nature 1986; 324:70–3.
49. Tanabe T, Konishi M, Mizuta T, Noma T, Honjo T. Molecular cloning and structure of the human interleukin-5 gene. J Biol Chem 1987; 262:16580–4.
50. Miyatake S, Otsuka T, Yokota T, Lee F, Arai K. Structure of the chromosomal gene for granulocyte-macrophage colony stimulating factor: comparison of the mouse and human genes. EMBO J 1985; 4:2561–8.
51. Yang YC, Clark SC. In: Stamatoyannopoulos G, Nienhuis A, eds. Developmental control of globin gene expression. New York: Liss, 1987:3–11.

52. Van Leeuwen BH, Martinson ME, Webb GC, Young IG. Molecular organisation of the cytokine gene cluster, involving the human IL-4, IL-5, and GM-CSF genes, on human chromosome 5. Blood 1989; 73:1142–8.
53. Yang YC, Kovacic S, Kriz R, Wolf S, Clark SC, Wellems TE, Nienhuis A, Epstein N. The human genes for GM-CSF and IL-3 are closely linked in tandem on chromosome 5. Blood 1988; 71:958–61.
54. Tominaga A, Matsumoto M, Harada N, Takahashi T, Kikuchi Y, Takatsu K. Molecular properties and regulation of mRNA expression for murine T cell-replacing factor/IL-5. J Immunol 1988; 140:1175–81.
55. Basten A, Boyer MH, Beeson PB. Mechanisms of eosinophilia. I. Factors affecting the eosinophil response of rats to *Trichinella spiralis*. J Exp Med 1970; 131:1271–87.
56. Basten A, Beeson PB. Mechanisms of eosinophilia. II. Role of the lymphocyte. J Exp Med 1970; 131:1288–305.
57. Plaut M, Pierce JH, Watson CJ, Hanley-Hyde J, Hordan RP, Paul WE. Mast cell lines produce lymphokines in response to cross-linkage of Fc epsilon RI or to calcium ionophores. Nature 1989; 339:64–7.
58. Kodama T, Takada K, Kameya T, Shimosato Y, Tsuchiya R, Okabe T. Large cell carcinoma of the lung associated with marked eosinophilia. Cancer 1984; 54:2313–7.
59. Catovsky D, Bernasconi C, Verdonck PJ, Postma A, Hows J, van der Does-van den Berg A, Rees JKH, Castelli G, Morra E, Galton DAG. The association of eosinophilia with lymphoblastic leukaemia or lymphoma: a study of seven patients. Br J Haematol 1980; 45:523–34.
60. Samoszuk M, Nansen L. Detection of interleukin-5 messenger RNA in Reed-Sternberg cells of Hodgkin's disease with eosinophilia. Blood 1990; 75:13–6.
61. Enokihara H, Hamaguchi H, Sakamaki H, Hazama S, Saito K, Furusawa S, Shishido H. Specific production of eosinophil colony stimulating factor from sensitized T cells from a patient with allergic eosinophilia. Br J Haematol 1985; 59:85–91.
62. Silberstein DS, Schoof DD, Rodrick ML, Tai PC, Spry CJ, David JR, Eberlein TJ. Activation of eosinophils in cancer patients treated with IL-2 and IL-2-generated lymphokine-activated killer cells. J Immunol 1989; 142:2162–7.
63. Coffman RL, Seymour BW, Lebman DA, Hiraki DD, Christiansen JA, Shrader B. Cherwinski YM, Savelkoul HF, Finkelman FD, Bond MW, et al. The role of helper T cell products in mouse B cell differentiation and isotype regulation. Immunol Rev 1988; 102:5–28.
64. Lenardo MJ, Kuang A, Gifford A, Baltimore D. NF-kappa B protein purification from bovine spleen: nucleotide stimulation and binding site specificity. Proc Natl Acad Sci USA 1988; 85:8825–9.
65. Serfling E, Barthelmas R, Pfeuffer I, Schenk B, Zarius S, Swoboda R, Mercurio F, Karin M. Ubiquitous and lymphocyte-specific factors are involved in the induction of the mouse interleukin 2 gene in T lymphocytes. EMBO J 1989; 8:465–75.
66. Nimer SD, Morita EA, Martis MJ, Wachsman W, Gasson JC. Characterization of the human granulocyte-macrophage colony-stimulating factor promoter region by genetic analysis: correlation with DNase I footprinting. Mol Cell Biol 1988; 8:1979–84.
67. Shannon MF, Gamble JR, Vadas MA. Nuclear proteins interacting with the promoter region of the human granulocyte/macrophage colony-stimulating factor gene. Proc Natl Acad Sci USA 1988; 85:674–9.
68. Shannon MF, Pell LM, Lenardo MJ, Kuczek ES, Occhiodoro FS, Dunn SM, Vadas MA. A novel tumour necrosis factor-responsive transcription factor which recognises a regulatory element in hemopoietic growth factor genes. Mol Cell Biol 1990; 10:2950–9.
69. LeBowitz JH, Clerc RG, Brenowitz M, Sharp PA. The Oct-2 protein binds cooperatively to adjacent octamer sites. Genes and Develop 1989; 3:1625–38.

70. Garcia-Blanco MA, Clerc RG, Sharp PA. The DNA-binding homeo domain of the Oct-2 protein. Genes and Develop 1989; 3:739–45.
71. Prywes R, Roeder RG. Purification of the c-fos enhancer-binding protein. Mol Cell Biol 1987; 7:3482–9.
72. Schonthal A, Buscher M, Angel P, Rahsmdorf HJ, Ponta H, Hattori K, Chiu R, Karin M, Herrlich P. The Fos and Jun/AP-1 proteins are involved in the downregulation of Fos transcription. Oncogene 1989; 4:629–36.
73. Subramaniam M, Schmidt LJ, Crutchfield CE, Getz MJ. Negative regulation of serum-responsive enhancer elements. Nature 1989; 340:64–6.
74. Lopez AF, Eglinton JM, Lyons AB, Tapley PM, To LB, Park LS, Clark SC, Vadas MA. Human interleukin-3 inhibits the binding of granulocyte-macrophage factor and interleukin-5 to basophils and strongly enhances their functional activity. J Cell Physiol 1990; in press.
75. Elliott MJ, Vadas MA, Cleland LG, Gamble Jr, Lopez AF. IL-3 and GM-CSF stimulate two distinct phases of adhesion in human monocytes. J Immunol 1990; 145:167–76.

22

Cytokine Stimulation of Human Basophil Histamine Release

MARY HAAK-FRENDSCHO
Genentech, Inc., South San Francisco, California

ALLEN P. KAPLAN
State University of New York at Stony Brook, Stony Brook, New York

I. INTRODUCTION

Cytokines are products of monocytes and lymphocytes that serve as a mechanism for cell-cell interaction and modulate the immune response. These proteins can also initiate or regulate the activation or secretion of a variety of other cell types such as endothelial cells, fibroblasts, basophils, and mast cells. Cytokines that possess histamine-releasing activity represent a potentially important link between classical immediate hypersensitivity and cellular immunity. Therefore, the interactions between cytokines and secretory events in the human basophil have been the focus of investigation of the cell-cell interactions, particularly during the late phase of the allergic response.

Exposure of an allergic individual to an antigen to which the person is sensitive results in an immediate pathophysiological response that is mediated by IgE antibody. Blood basophils and tissue mast cells, which possess high-affinity IgE-Fc receptors on their plasma membranes (1), play a key role in the induction of these immediate hypersensitivity reactions (2). In the presence of specific antigen, bridging of IgE molecules occurs with resultant cell activation (3). Once activated, mast cells secrete vasoactive mediators, such as histamine, arachidonic acid metabolites, and platelet-activating factor, which facilitate migration of neutrophils, eosinophils, basophils, and mononuclear cells into a site of antigenic challenge (4,5). This is frequently followed by a late-phase reaction between 3 and 11 h after antigen challenge, particularly if the antigen dose is high (6). Evidence suggests that this late phase is associated with activation of basophils (and other cells) that are recruited from the circulation to the site of inflammation (7).

Basophils are the chief source of histamine in the circulating cells, and virtually no histamine is stored in tissues except for that found in mast cells (3). Basophils are rarely seen in tissues under normal circumstances, but they become prominent during delayed-onset human immune reactions, including the late phase of the allergic response (8). During the late phase, histamine and arachidonic acid metabolites are again released; however, there is no secondary increase in prostaglandin D_2, a product of mast cells which is not synthesized by basophils (9). Therefore, it is postulated that basophils play a major role in the late-phase mediator release, and the reaction appears to be independent of IgE antibody or the activation of complement.

The discovery of histamine-releasing factors suggests that neutrophils, platelets, and activated mononuclear cells are able to modulate basophil function, and possibly mast cell secretion, through the release of soluble mediators. Thus, it appears likely that a reciprocal interaction may occur in vivo in which the secretory products of basophils and mast cells recruit the aforementioned cells and then basophils and mast cells are activated by products of these newly arrived cells.

II. HISTAMINE-RELEASING FACTORS

The first report of basophil histamine release in response to a cytokinelike substance was by Thueson et al. (10,11), who demonstrated that supernatants from human mononuclear cells induced the release of histamine from both autologous and homologous basophils. These observations were confirmed and expanded by other investigators who found the same activity but that appeared different in terms of preliminary physicochemical characterization, from a variety of cell sources.

A. Novel Histamine-Releasing Factors (Table 1)

1. HRF-MNC

Thueson and his colleagues were first to report that cytokines, generated from antigen- or mitogen-stimulated mononuclear cells, induced both directed migration and degranulation of human basophils (11). Release of histamine from basophils by histamine-releasing factor was calcium dependent and magnesium and IgE independent (11,12). Maximal release occurred within a few minutes after exposure to the factor at 37°C (11). Size-exclusion chromatography indicated that the mononuclear cell-derived histamine-releasing factor (HRF-MNC) had an apparent molecular weight of 10,000 to 15,000 (10). Later reports largely confirmed these observations; however, it appeared that HRF-MNC is quite heterogeneous (13–17), and that histamine release is most

Table 1 Histamine-Releasing Factors

Designation	Cell source	Molecular weight	References
HRF-MNC	Peripheral blood, mononuclear cells	30, 15 kDa	15,25,36
HRA	Thoracic duct lymphocytes	50, 15, 1.3 kDa[a]	10,11
BAF-T	Peripheral blood T-cells	90, 70 kDa	30,31
HRA-N	Neutrophils	1400–2300 Da	21,39
HRF-M	Lung macrophages	18 kDa	34,36
HRF-P	Platelets	<3500 Da	35,42
HRF-NW	Nasal washings	15–30, 3.7, <3.5 kDa	35
HRF-B	RPMI 8866 cells	90, 70, 12–15 kDa	22

[a] Dependent on antigen or mitogen used to stimulate MNC.

prominent in atopic individuals (18,19). In an attempt to determine the exact cellular origin of HRF-MNC, Alam et al. (20) purified and stimulated subpopulations of peripheral blood mononuclear cells. They concluded that T-cells (both $CD4^+$ and $CD8^+$), B-cells, and monocytes each produce variable quantities of histamine-releasing factor, confirming that histamine-releasing cytokines are of multiple cellular origin. B-lymphocytes, however, appeared to be the best source.

The response of human basophils to HRF-MNC was also defined in terms of atopic status of cell donors and the role of IgE. It was found that basophils of allergic, nonallergic, or skin-test-positive but asymptomatic donors cannot be distinguished based on responsiveness to HRF-MNC (18). Although the response of basophils that have been desensitized to anti-IgE is retained when they are subsequently stimulated with HRF-MNC, one of two IgE myeloma proteins tested was capable of binding a portion of the HRF-MNC contained in concentrated supernatants, suggesting that one form of HRF may either have a relationship to previously described IgE-binding factors (18) or act by interaction with surface-bound IgE. Others have also observed a significant correlation between the ability of a single donor's basophils to response to both HRF and anti-IgE; however, there appears to be no correlation between the magnitude of response to HRF as compared to the magnitude of anti-IgE-induced histamine release (21–24).

Baeza and co-workers purified three forms of HRF-MNC with apparent molecular weights of 10 to 12 kDa, 15 to 17 kDa, and 40 to 41 kDa (25). Mouse monoclonal antibodies were prepared against the 10- to 12-kDa histamine-releasing factor (26) and were used to purify the protein in a single step by affinity chromatography. As can be seen in Figure 1, a broad band is seen at molecular weight 10,000–12,000 when a 12% gel is used. The identity of the faint band above is uncertain, but immunoblotting experiments with the monoclonal antibody confirmed reactivity with the 10,000–12,000 moeity. When this band was blotted onto a nitrocellulose membrane, divided into an upper and lower half, and subjected to amino acid sequence analysis, a striking homology was seen with connective tissue-activating peptide III (CTAP III) and neutrophil-activating peptide-2 (NAP-2). These proteins are platelet-derived factors which are formed by proteolytic cleavage of the alpha granule component, platelet basic protein. The upper half of the band had the sequence of CTAP III, while the lower half began with amino acid 16 of the CTAP III sequence. This is the same cleavage that is known to convert CTAP III to NAP-2 (28). A monoclonal antibody against 10- to 12-kDa HRF recognized CTAP III, and polyclonal antibody to CTAP III recognized HRF. Further, when CTAP III/NAP-2 was isolated directly from platelet supernatants, it was able to induce basophils histamine release, thus demonstrating the first structural, immunological, and functional relationship between a HRF and a previously described cell product. The identities of the other forms of HRF are unknown, but they do not react with the monoclonal antibody and are therefore likely to be separate gene products.

2. *HRA/BAF-T*

Earlier reports that soluble factors from antigen- or mitogen-stimulated peripheral blood lymphocytes can act directly on the basophil (11) to induce histamine release or to augment IgE-dependent histamine release (29) spurred further attempts to characterize the factor(s). The work of Sedgwick et al. (30) implicated T-lymphocytes as a main source of HRF found in stimulated mononuclear supernatants; however, production of

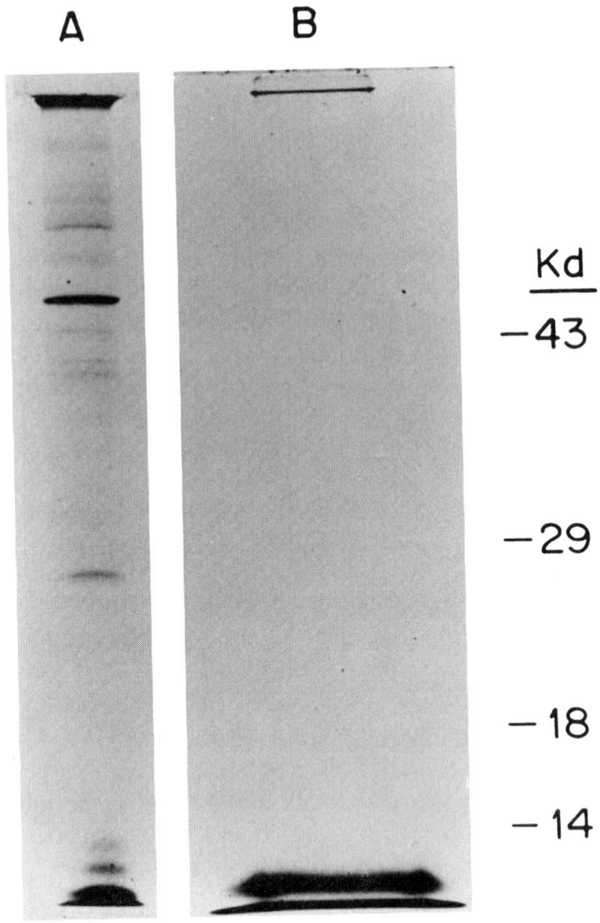

Figure 1 SDS-PAGE of HRF. Fractionated (A) or affinity-purified (B) HRF was subjected to SDS-PAGE on 12% acrylamide gels and stained with Coomassie Blue R-250.

the factor(s) appeared to be macrophage dependent. Other workers found that HRF consisted of a heterogeneous group of molecules. HRF derived from human T-cells, coined basophil-activating-factor T-cells (BAF-T), has an apparent molecular weight of 70,000 to 90,000 and is composed of two charged species with approximate pI of 4.4 and 5.2 to 5.5 (31). Lett-Brown and co-workers (32,33), using thoracic duct lymphocytes for the generation of large amounts of HRF, found that the physicochemical properties of HRF generated were dependent on the stimulant used. When lymphocytes were stimulated with streptokinase, bioactivity was associated with 10,000- to 20,000- and 1300-Da molecules (32). When thoracic duct lymphocytes were stimulated with staphylococcal enterotoxin B and the supernatants chromatographed, activity separated into two peaks at 50,000 and 15,000 molecular weight (33).

3. *HRF-M*

Macrophages are known to release monokines capable of modulating the humoral and cellular components of inflammatory reactions. Therefore it was of interest to determine whether macrophages could also produce soluble mediator(s) that activate basophils. Schulman et al. (34) reported that 24-h culture supernatants from human lung alveolar macrophages were able to induce histamine release from human basophils and, to a lesser degree, from mast cells. The basophil activation was dose, calcium, and temperature dependent. Upon chromatography, the histamine-releasing activity from the supernatants, HRF-M, migrated as a single peak with an apparent molecular weight of 18,000 (35). Further studies indicated that the ability of HRF-M to induce basophil secretion is IgE dependent, and the kinetics of HRF-M-induced histamine release are similar to that of IgE-mediated reactions (35). Evidence that this form of HRF is dependent on cell surface IgE are as follows. (a) Cells desensitized to anti-IgE failed to release histamine via IgE-dependent reactions or HRF. (b) Desensitization of cells to HRF reduced responsiveness to anti-IgE. (c) Stripping cells of their IgE eliminated responsiveness to HRF. (d) Cells from which IgE had been stripped could be rendered responsive by incubation with IgE derived from some donors [IgE(+)] but not others [IgE(−)] (36).

4. *HRA-N*

Allergic reactions consist of an immediate phase, which lasts 30 to 60 min, followed by a prolonged inflammatory reaction, the late-phase reaction (LPR) (37). Histologically, LPR are characterized by an early neutrophilic and eosinophilic infiltrate which occurs within the first 3 to 9 h, followed by a mononuclear infiltrate which peaks at 24 to 48 h (37,38). During the late-phase allergic reaction, histamine release occurs concomitant with neutrophil infiltration, and this temporal relationship suggests that neutrophils may participate in the LPR. White et al. (21,39) explored this possibility and observed that human neutrophils constitutively release a soluble factor, HRF-N, which causes the dose-related, temperature- and calcium-dependent, noncytotoxic release of histamine from basophils. HRA-N has an apparent molecular weight between 1400 and 2300 Da (39). The kinetics of HRA-N-induced histamine release was slow, with maximal release occurring at 45 to 60 min following challenge. Further study revealed that HRF-N is not only resistant to boiling, but boiling actually enhances HRA-N, suggesting the presence of a heat-labile inhibitor (40).

5. *HRF-NW*

Using an in-vivo model of intranasal antigen challenge, nasal lavage fluids obtained during the late-phase response in the nose were found to contain basophil mediators (5,41). Based on these reports, MacDonald et al. (35) examined nasal washings and found that they also contain histamine-releasing activity, HRF-NW. Upon chromatography, the majority of HRF-NW eluted at an apparent molecular weight range of 15 to 30 kDa. HRF-NW induces basophil degranulation in an IgE-dependent manner, similar to HRF as previously described from lung alveolar macrophages and platelets (34,42).

6. *HRF-P*

Previous reports suggest that platelets can be activated during allergic reactions (43). The possibility that platelets can also further stimulate basophils to enhance allergic and inflammatory reactions was therefore investigated. Supernatants from thrombin-, collagen-, or acetylglyceryl ether phosphorylcholine (PAF)-stimulated platelets have been shown to enhance both anti-IgE- and antigen-induced histamine release from human basophils (44). Orchard et al. (42) confirmed and expanded these observations, demonstrating that platelet-derived supernatants (PDS) induced histamine release from basophils.

Kinetics studies of release induced by PDS indicate that release is more rapid than that associated with IgE-dependent mechanisms. The factor responsible for this activity is nondialyzable (molecular weight greater than 3500), acid stable, and heat labile. In the future it will be of interest to determine if HRF-P is related to or a cleavage product of platelet basic protein such as CTAP-III.

7. *HRF-B*

IgE-binding factors (IgE-BF) have been shown to be capable of selectively potentiating IgE responses (46), and some observations suggest that HRF may act via interaction with cell-bound IgE. Therefore, it was of interest to determine whether IgE-BF have the ability to induce basophil histamine release. Supernatants from the human B-lymphoblastoid cell line RPMI 8866, a major source of 25,000- to 27,000-MW human IgE-binding factor (47), were screened for histamine-releasing activity. It was determined that IgE-BF, in crude supernatants and in purified form, did not cause basophil degranulation. However, RPMI 8866 cells constitutively produce histamine-releasing factors with apparent molecular weights of 90, 70, and 12–15 kDa (22). Histamine release induced by these factors had the same kinetics as that of HRF-MNC, but it was functionally and immunologically distinguishable from HRF-MNC and IgE-BF. These findings were later confirmed using purified normal human peripheral blood B-cells and sCD23 (IgE-BF) (20).

B. Cytokines and Histamine Release (Table 2)

1. *Interleukin-1*

Interleukin-1 (IL-1) is an important macrophage-derived mediator of lymphocyte activation possessing a wide range of properties, including degranulation of neutrophils (48). This, coupled with the similar physical chemical properties of IL-1 and HRF-MNC, led to the examination of the effect of IL-1 on human basophil histamine release. IL-1 was found to induce calcium-dependent release of histamine in about 30% of the donors tested (23,49). There was no relationship between responsiveness to IL-1 and anti-IgE, and their respective kinetics of histamine release were quite different. The direct histamine-releasing ability of IL-1 is, however, controversial. In the hands of others, IL-1 was only able to induce modest histamine release from a small subset of allergic donors in the presence of D_2O (19) or did not function as a secretagogue at all (50). Given the range of reported response to IL-1 [0.005 to 5 μg/ml (23)], it appears that this is too high to be physiological and that histamine release induced by IL-1 is not likely to be important.

Table 2 Cytokines with Histamine-Releasing Activity

Cytokine	Inducing	References	Potentiating	References
IL-1	+	23,49	+	19,50
IL-3	+	19,24,51	+	19,63,64,65
GM-CSF	+	19,24	+	64
IL-8	+	56	+	67
α-IFN	−		+	62
γ-IFN	−		+	63
CTAP-III	+	27	−	

2. Interleukin-3

Many cytokines have the dual capacity to stimulate progenitor cell maturation as well as activate end-stage cells. This observation, coupled with the recent availability of cloned and commercially available recombinant cytokines, provided the impetus to examine the effect of interleukin-3 (IL-3) on human basophil degranulation. Haak-Frendscho et al. (24) first reported the ability of rIL-3 to induce histamine release in the majority of donors tested. Atopic donors generally responded to a greater extent (percent responding and magnitude of response); however, nonatopics were also responsive (24,51). The kinetics of IL-3-induced histamine release were slower than that of anti-IgE-induced degranulation (24,51), and the magnitude of degranulation was enhanced by the presence of D_2O (19,24) or by increased calcium levels (51). Basophil-enrichment experiments suggest that IL-3 interacts with the basophil directly (51), and basophil receptors for IL-3 have recently been demonstrated (52).

3. Granulocyte-Macrophage Colony-Stimulating Factor

Granulocyte-macrophage colony-stimulating factor (GM-CSF) is a pluripotent growth factor for myeloid bone marrow precursors (53) that enhances the function of mature inflammatory effector cells. Based on these observations, the ability of rGM-CSF to activate human basophils was also examined. Haak-Frendscho et al. (24) reported that the majority of donor basophils tested were responsive to GM-CSF, and a dose-response release of histamine was demonstrable. When the responsiveness of atopic and nonatopic subjects was compared, atopic status did not predict responsiveness to either GM-CSF or IL-3, although atopics were generally more responsive. The rate of kinetics of histamine release was slow, similar to that of IL-3, and the response was enhanced fivefold in the presence of D_2O (19,24,45). The ability of GM-CSF to activate basophils has been confirmed (19); however, only a subset of allergic donors basophils secreted in response to GM-CSF.

4. Neutrophil Attractant/Activation Protein-1/Interleukin-8

Neutrophil attractant/activation protein-1 (NAP-1) is a monocyte-derived factor isolated from LPS-stimulated mononuclear cells supernatants (54,55). NAP-1 was first described as a neutrophil chemoattractant as well as a secretory and metabolic stimulus (55). When NAP-1 was examined for activation activity on human basophils, it was found to induce a rapid (maximal after 1 min), calcium-dependent release of histamine similar to the kinetics of IgE-mediated reactions (56). However, there was no relationship observed between the atopic status of the donors and the sensitivity of their basophils.

C. Histamine Release-Enhancing Factors

There is evidence to suggest that effector cell function is regulated by cytokine interactions. The identification of multiple cytokines possessing these related activities indicates that a complex set of molecular and cellular events may account for the pathophysiological consequences of immediate-type hypersensitivity reactions, including the acute manifestations of allergy, late-phase reactions, and shock syndromes as well as an interrelationship between cellular immunity and mast cells as described in scleroderma and rheumatoid arthritis.

1. *Histamine Release-Enhancing Activity*

Histamine release-potentiating factors have been described by several groups of investigators. Bamzai and Kretschmer (57) first reported that antigen-induced histamine release was enhanced by supernatants obtained from PHA-stimulated mononuclear cells from allergic donors. The factor(s) was capable of enhancing IgE-mediated histamine release from autologous and homologous basophils. Younger et al. (58) also demonstrated augmentation of histamine release by a 10,000- to 30,000-molecular-weight, heat-stable factor partially purified from PHA-stimulated mononuclear cells.

Ida et al. (29) reported that immune stimulation of atopic donor mononuclear cells results in the release of a soluble factor(s) that enhances IgE-mediated histamine release when incubated with leukocytes from nonatopic donor cells. A portion of the potentiating activity was acid sensitive, while the remainder was resistant to pH 2.0 treatment, suggesting that at least two mediators were released into the supernatants.

2. *Interferons*

Upper respiratory viral infections frequently precipitate asthma attacks (59,60). This observation led to investigations of the relationship between viruses and basophil degranulation. Ida et al. (61) reported enhanced histamine release to ragweed antigen E after virus-leukocyte incubation which was associated with interferon production. Busse et al. (62) then confirmed and expanded these findings. After incubation with either live or killed virus, histamine release was enhanced in response to ragweed antigen E. Incubation of the leukocyte suspension with purified α-interferon for 24 h was also associated with enhanced antigen-induced histamine release, but it did not alter calcium ionophore A23187-induced histamine release. Similarly, γ-interferon enhances anti-IgE-dependent human basophil histamine release (63).

3. *Interleukin-1*

Massey et al. (50) sought to confirm previous reports of the ability of IL-1 to induce human basophil histamine release. These investigators were unable to demonstrate IL-1α or -β as a releasing agent, even though various manipulations were employed such as increasing Ca^{2+} concentration or addition of the enhancing agents D_2O and cytochalasin B. They did, however, observe that both IL-1α and -β enhanced IgE-dependent histamine release in a dose-dependent manner. When the IgE-independent secretagogues f-Met-Leu-Phe and calcium ionophore A23187 were used, enhancement by IL-1α and β was not seen. Other investigators have also reported that IL-1 is capable of augmenting HRF- and antigen-induced histamine release (19).

4. *Interleukin-3*

Hirai et al. (64) first described the histamine release-potentiating ability of IL-3, which was observed at much lower concentrations than the amount needed to affect cell proliferation. Other workers have similarly reported that IL-3 is a direct secretagogue at high concentrations, while at low concentrations it possesses histamine release-enhancing activity (19,65). The enhancing effects are quite dramatic; thus a 10-min preexposure of cells to IL-3 at a dose insufficient to cause histamine release enhanced C5a-mediated histamine release by 40% (65). The magnitude of histamine release was enhanced, but the time course of C5a-induced release was unaltered. IL-3 potentiation is not IgE dependent, and it appears to act directly on the basophils (64). No additive effect between GM-CSF and IL-3 was observed, suggesting that they act competitively on basophils, perhaps by affecting some common process involved in histamine release (64). Moreover, these data suggest that a single basophil is responsive to both factors. Pretreatment with IL-3 also resulted in augmented secretion of arachidonate metabolites such as the sulfidoleukotrienes (SLT: LTC_4, LTD_4/LTE_4) (65). These results demonstrated that IL-3 also primes basophils to respond to secretagogue challenge with the synthesis of bioactive lipids. Other studies (63) have confirmed that, following exposure to IL-3, both IgE-dependent and peptide-mediated responses resulted in elevations in both histamine and sulfidopeptide leukotriene release. These effects were insensitive to inhibition by dexamethasone (63), thereby suggesting that IL-3 may also render human basophils unresponsive to the inhibitory effects of elevated levels of glucocorticoids.

5. *Granulocyte-Macrophage Colony-Stimulating Factor*

Hirai et al. (64) also reported that GM-CSF pretreatment of human basophils resulted in enhanced basophil histamine release. GM-CSF was equally effective in augmenting histamine release upon stimulation with IgE-dependent or IgE-independent secretagogues.

6. *Neutrophil Attractant/Activation Protein*

NAP-1 is a novel neutrophil-activating peptide which, like C5a and f-Met-Leu-Phe, activates human polymorphonuclear cells inducing chemotaxis, shape change, granule release, and respiratory burst (66). Following earlier work demonstrating that IL-3 enhances mediator release by mature basophils in response to anti-IgE, f-Met-Leu-Phe, and C5a, Dahinden et al. (67) sought to examine the effect of NAP-1 on human basophil histamine release. In their hands, both IL-3 and NAP-1 (at the concentrations utilized) failed to induce histamine release. However, when cells were exposed to IL-3 for 5 min and then stimulated with NAP-1, a marked release of histamine was observed. Kinetic studies revealed that maximum histamine release was reached within 5–10 min of stimulus addition.

III. DISCUSSION

It is clear that there are a variety of cell-derived factors that can modulate the release of histamine from human basophils and mast cells. These histamine-releasing factors include some of the known cytokines, such as interleukin-3 and interleukin-8. It has also been shown that concentrations of IL-3 and GM-CSF that are insufficient to cause histamine release can prime basophils, thereby augmenting responsiveness to other secretagogues. IL-1 causes secretion in only a small number of subjects and requires unphysiologic amounts, nevertheless, IL-1 primes cells for secretion at much lower doses. γ-Interferon also possesses this priming ability, but has not been shown to cause histamine release at any concentration. Therefore, it is likely that most, if not all, agents that can cause basophil secretion will prime cells at much lower concentrations, while there may be cytokines that can prime only. Other cytokines and colony-stimulating factors thus far tested and found to be negative for histamine-releasing ability include interleukins-2, -4, -5, -6, macrophage-CSF (CSF-1), granulocyte-CSF, tumor necrosis factors α and β, and transforming growth factor β (TGF β).

When concentrated supernatants of various cell types are fractionated and the major histamine-releasing factor(s) purified, the responsible substances do not correspond to any of the aforementioned cytokines/CSF (25). Three such substances have been isolated from concentrates derived from mononuclear cells and platelets (25,26), and one has been identified to be CTAP III and/or its derivative, NAP-2. Thus, one form of HRF that is undoubtedly a platelet-derived HRF has activity on fibroblasts (66), neutrophils (28,66), and basophils (27).

Characterization of the functional and structural properties of HRFs may best be done by assessment of each purified component. Some individual species of HRF may not share receptors, their mechanisms of signal transduction may differ, and HRF inhibitors may be specific for individual components. One form of HRF may act via surface bound IgE. This HRF, however, has not been purified to homogeneity nor characterized further. Since there is but one functional gene for IgE and reactivity of IgE-dependent HRF has been limited to some basophils [IgE(+)] but not others, the reactive portion of the IgE molecule may depend on a post-translational modification such as glycosylation. The one form of purified HRF is, based on its functional activity, the CTAP III/NAP-2 protein. This HRF does not interact with IgE, nor does responsiveness to it discriminate between allergic versus nonallergic persons. Interleukins-3 and -8 also cause histamine secretion and may synergize, but isolation of HRF directly from activated mononuclear cell supernatant does not lead to isolation of either of these cytokines. The results with GM-CSF are similar to those of IL-3 and IL-8. Thus, their role in secretion in vivo is questionable, although one can demonstrate their capacity to induce histamine release in vitro at a physiological range. Priming by certain of these factors may prove to be a more important function.

Once these series of histamine-releasing factors are purified and characterized, it will be possible to develop specific assays for each type and to assess their presence in a wide variety of disease states. The late phase of the allergic reaction as it relates to allergic rhinitis and asthma is one possible association. Others include chronic urticaria, scleroderma, and rheumatoid arthritis, in which increased numbers of cutaneous or synovial mast cells are seen in proximity to other inflammatory cell types, particularly mononuclear cells.

REFERENCES

1. Grant JA, Lett-Brown MA, Warner JA, Plaut M, Lichtenstein LM, Haak-Frendscho M, Kaplan AP. Activation of basophils. Fed Proc 1986; 42:2653–8.
2. Wasserman SI. Mediators of immediate hypersensitivity. J Allergy Clin Immunol 1983; 72:101–15.
3. Serafin WE, Austen KF. Mediators of immediate hypersensitivity reactions. N Engl J Med 1987; 317:30–4.
4. Charlesworth EN, Hood AF, Soter NA, Kagey-Sobotka A, Gillis S, Lichtenstein LM. The cutaneous late phase response to allergen: mediator release and inflammatory cell infiltration. J Clin Invest 1989; 83:1519–26.
5. Naclerio RM, Proud D, Togias A, Adkinson NF, Meyers PA, Kagey-Sobotka A, Plaut M, Norman PS, Lichtenstein LM. Inflammatory mediators in late antigen-induced rhinitis. N Engl J Med 1985; 313:65–70.
6. Dolovich J, Hargreave FE, Chalmers R, Slier KJ, Gauldie J, Bienenstock J. Late cutaneous allergic responses in isolated IgE-dependent reactions. J Allergy Clin Immunol 1973; 52:38–46.
7. Van Loveren H, Meade R, Askenase PW. An early component of delayed-type hypersensitivity mediated by T cells and mast cells. J Exp Med 1983; 157:1604–17.

8. Askenase PW. Mechanisms of hypersensitivity: cellular interactions. Basophil arrival and function in tissue hypersensitivity reactions. J Allergy Clin Immunol 1979; 64:79–89.
9. Charlesworth EN, Iliopoulos O, MacDonald SM, Kagey-Sobotka A, Lichtenstein LM. Cells and secretagogues involved in the human late-phase reponse. Int Arch Allergy Appl Immunol 1989; 88:50–3.
10. Thueson DO, Speck LS, Lett-Brown MA, Grant JA. Histamine-releasing activity (HRA): interaction with basophils and physiochemical characterization. J Immunol 1979; 123:633–9.
11. Thueson DO, Speck LS, Lett-Brown MA, Grand JA. Histamine-releasing activity (HRA): production by mitogen- or antigen-stimulated human mononuclear cells. J Immunol 1979; 123:626–32.
12. Ezeamuzie IC, Assem ESK. Histamine releasing lymphokine: preliminary evidence of membrane receptors on basophils. Agents and Actions 1985; 17:131–7.
13. Alam R, Rozniecki J, Salmaj K. A mononuclear cell derived histamine releasing factor (HRF) in asthmatic patients: histamine release from basophils in vitro. Annals of Allergy 1984; 53:66–9.
14. Dvorak AM, Lett-Brown MA, Thueson DO, Pyne K, Raghuprasad PK, Galli SJ, Grant JA. Histamine-releasing activity (HRA): HRA induces human basophil histamine release by provoking noncytotoxic granule exocytosis. Clin Immunol Immunopharm 1984; 32:142–50.
15. Kaplan AP, Haak-Frendscho M, Fauci A, Dinarello C, Halbert E. A histamine releasing factor from activated human mononuclear cells. J Immunol 1985; 135:2027–32.
16. Kaplan AP, Haak-Frendscho M, Dinarello C, Elias J, Gruber B. Mononuclear cells, mast cells and urticaria. In: Kay AB, ed. Allergy and inflammation. London: Academic Press, 1987:341–50.
17. Alam R, Rozniecki J. A mononuclear cell-derived histamine releasing factor in asthmatic patients. Allergy 1985; 40:124–9.
18. Baeza ML, Haak-Frendscho M, Satnick S, Kaplan AP. Responsiveness to human mononuclear cell-derived histamine-releasing factor. Studies of allergic status and the role of IgE. J Immunol 1988; 141:2688–92.
19. Alam R, Welter JB, Forsythe PA, Lett-Brown MA, Grant JA. Comparative effect of recombinant IL-1, -2, -3, -4, and -6, IFN-β, granulocyte-macrophage-colony-stimulating factor, tumor necrosis factor-α, and histamine-releasing factors on the secretion of histamine from basophils. J Immunol 1989; 142:3431–5.
20. Alam R, Forsythe PA, Lett-Brown MA, Grant JA. Cellular origin of histamine-releasing factor produced by peripheral blood mononuclear cells. J Immunol 1989; 142:3951–6.
21. White MV, Kaplan AP, Haak-Frendscho M, Kaliner M. Neutrophils and mast cells. Comparison of neutrophil-derived histamine-releasing activity with other histamine-releasing factors. J Immunol 1989; 1412:3575–83.
22. Haak-Frendscho M, Sarfati M, Delespesse G, Kaplan AP. Comparison of mononuclear cell and B-Lymphoblastoid histamine releasing factor and their distinction from an IgE-binding factor. Clin Immunol Immunopathol 1988; 49:72–82.
23. Haak-Frendscho M, Dinarello C, Kaplan AP. Recombinant human interleukin-1 beta causes histamine release from human basophils. J Allergy Clin Immunol 1988; 82:218–23.
24. Haak-Frendscho M, Arai N, Arai K, Baeza ML, Finn A, Kaplan AP. Human recombinant granulocyte-macrophage colony-stimulating factor and interleukin 3 cause basophil histamine release. J Clin Invest 1988; 82:17–20.
25. Baeza ML, Reddigari SR, Haak-Frendscho M, Kaplan AP. Purification and further characterization of human mononuclear cell histamine-releasing factor. J Clin Invest 1989; 1204–10.
26. Baeza ML, Reddigari SR, Kornfeld D, Gorevic PG, Kaplan AP. Further characterization of human mononuclear cell-derived histamine releasing factor (HRF) and preparation of monoclonal antibodies. J Allergy Clin Immunol 1989; 83:237.

27. Baeza ML, Reddigari SR, Kornfeld D, Ramani N, Smith EM, Hossler PA, Fischer T, Castor CN, Gorevic PG, Kaplan AP, Relationship of one form of human histamine releasing factor (HRF) to connective tissue activating peptied-III (CTAP-III). J Clin Invest 1990; 85:1516–21.
28. Walz A, Baggiolini M. Generation of the neutrophil-activating peptide NAP-2 from platelet basic protein or connective tissue-activating peptide III through monocyte proteases. J Exp Med 1989; 171:449–54.
29. Ida S, Hooks JJ, Sirganian RP, Notkins AL. Enhancement of IgE-mediated histamine release from human basophils by immune-specific lymphokines. Clin Exp Immunol 1980; 41:380–7.
30. Sedgwick JD, Holt PG, Turner KJ. Production of a histamine-releasing lymphokine by antigen- or mitogen-stimulated human peripheral T cells. Clin Exp Immunol 1981; 45:409–18.
31. Goetzl EJ, Foster DW, Payan DG. A basophil-activating factor from human T lymphocytes. Immunology 1984; 53:227–34.
32. Lett-Brown MA, Thueson DO, Plank DE, Langford MP, Grant JA. Histamine-releasing activity: Molecular heterogeneity of the activity from stimulated human thoracic duct lymphocytes. Cell Immunol 1984; 87:434–44.
33. Lett-Brown MA, Thueson DO, Plank DE, Duffy L, Grant JA. Histamine-releasing activity: Characterization and purification using high-performance liquid chromatography. Cell Immunol 1984; 87:445–51.
34. Schulman ES, Liu MC, Proud D, MacGlashan DW, Lichtenstein LM, Plaut M. Human lung macrophages induce histamine release from basophils and mast cells. Am Rev Respir Dis 1985; 131:230–5.
35. MacDonald SM, Lichtenstein LM, Proud D, Plaut M, Naclerio RM, MacGlashan DW, Kagey-Sobotka A. Studies of IgE-dependent histamine releasing factors: heterogeneity of IgE. J Immunol 1987; 139:506–12.
36. Liu MC, Proud D, Lichtenstein LM, MacGlashan DW, Schleimer RP, Adkinson NF, Kagey-Sobotka A, Schulman ES, Plaut M. Human lung macrophage-derived histamine-releasing activity is due to IgE-dependent factors. J Immunol 1986; 136:2588–95.
37. Lemanske RF, Kaliner M. Mast cell dependent late phase reactions. Clin Immunol Ref 1982; 1:547–80.
38. Allansmith MR, Baird RS, Greiner JV, Block KJ. Late phase reactions in ocular anaphylaxis in the rats. J Allergy Clin Immunol 1984; 73:49–55.
39. White MV, Kaliner MA. Neutrophils and mast cells I. Human neutrophil-derived histamine releasing activity (HRA-N). J Immunol 1987; 135:1624–30.
40. White MV, Baer H, Kubota Y, Kaliner M. Neutrophils and mast cells: characterization of cells responsive to neutrophil-derived histamine-releasing activity (HRA-N). J Allergy Clin Immunol 1989; 84:773–80.
41. Naclerio RM, Meier HL, Kagey-Sobotka A, Adkinson NF, Plaut M, Norman PS, Lichtenstein LM. Mediator release after nasal airway challenge with allergen. Ann Rev Respir Dis 1983; 128:597–602.
42. Orchard MA, Kagey-Sobotka A, Proud D, Lichtenstein LM. Basophil histamine release induced by a substance from stimulated platelets. J Immunol 1986; 136:2240–4.
43. Halomen M, Pinckard RN. Intravascular effects of IgE antibody upon basophils, neutrophils, platelets, and blood coagulation in the rabbit. J Immunol 1975; 115:519–24.
44. Knauer KA, Kagey-Sobotka A, Adkinson NF, Lichtenstein LM. Platelet augmentation of IgE-dependent histamine release from human basophils and mast cells. Int Arch Allergy Appl Immunol 1984; 74:29–35.
45. Kazimierczak W, Plaut M, Knauer KA, Meier HL, Lichtenstein LM. Deuterium-oxide-

induced histamine release from basophils of allergic subjects. Am Rev Respir Dis 1984; 129:592–6.
46. Martens CL, Huff TF, Jardieu P, Troustine ML, Coffman RF, Ishizaka K, Moore KW. cDNA clones encoding IgE-binding factors from a rat-mouse T cell hybridoma. Proc Natl Acad Sci USA 1985; 85:2460–4.
47. Sarfati M, Nakajima T, Frost H, Kilccherr E, Delespesse G. Purification and partial biochemical characterization of IgE-binding factors secreted by a human B lymphoblastoid cell line. Immunology 1987; 60:539–45.
48. Smith RJ, Bowman BJ, Speziale SC. Interleukin 1 stimulates granule exocytosis from human neutrophils. Int J Immunopharmacol 1986; 8:33–40.
49. Subramanian N, Bray MA. Interleukin 1 releases histamine from human basophils and mast cells in vitro. J Immunol 1987; 138:271–5.
50. Massey WA, Randall TC, Kagey-Sobotka A, Warner JA, MacDonald SM, Gillis S, Allison AC, Lichtenstein LM. Recombinant human IL-1α and -1β potentiate IgE-mediated histamine release from human basophils. J Immunol 1989; 143:1875–80.
51. MacDonald SM, Schleimer RP, Kagey-Sobotka A, Gillis S, Lichtenstein LM. Recombinant IL-3 induces histamine release from human basophils. J Immunol 1989; 142:3527–33.
52. Lopez AM, Lyons AB, Eglinton JM, Park LS, To LB, Clark SC, Vadas MA. Specific binding of human interleukin-3 and granulocyte-macrophage colony-stimulating factor to human basophils. J Allergy Clin Immunol 1990; 85:99–102.
53. Wodnar-Filipowicz A, Heusser CH, Moroni C. Production of the haemopoietic growth factors GM-CSF and interleukin-3 by mast cells in response to IgE receptor-mediated activation. Nature 1989; 339:150–2.
54. Yoshimura T, Matsushima K, Oppenheim JJ, Leonard EJ. Neutrophil chemotactic factor produced by lipopolysaccharide (LPS)-stimulated human blood mononuclear leukocytes: partial characterization and separation from interleukin-1 (IL-1). J Immunol 1987; 139:788–93.
55. Schroeder JM, Mrowietz U, Morita E, Christophers E. Purification and partial biochemical characterization of a human monocyte-derived, neutrophil-activating peptide that lacks interleukin 1 activity. J Immunol 1987; 139:3474-83.
56. White MV, Yoshimura T, Hook W, Kaliner MA, Leonard EJ. Neutrophil attractant/activation protein-1 (NAP-1) causes human basophil histamine release. Immunol Lett 1989; 22:151–4.
57. Bamzai AK, Kretschmer RR. Enhancement of antigen-induced leukocyte histamine release by a mononuclear cell-derived factor. J Allergy Clin Immunol 1978; 62:137–42.
58. Younger RE, Herrod HG, Lieberman PC, Valenski WR, Trony RL, Crawford LV. Characterization of mononuclear cell-derived histamine release enhancing factor. J Allergy Clin Immunol 1987; 80:547–57.
59. Horn MEC, Reed SE, Taylor P. Role of viruses and bacteria in acute wheezy bronchitis in childhood: a study of sputum. Arch Dis Child 1979; 54:587–92.
60. Minor TE, Dick EC, DeMeo AM, Ouellette JJ, Cohen M, Reed CE. Viruses as precipitants of asthmatic attacks in children. JAMA 1974; 227:292–8.
61. Ida S, Hooks JJ, Sirganian RP, Notkins AL. Enhancement of IgE-mediated histamine release from human basophils by viruses: role of interferon. J Exp Med 1977; 145:892–906.
62. Busse WW, Swenson CA, Borden EC, Treshaft MW, Dick EC. Effect of influenza: A virus on leukocyte histamine release. J Allergy Clin Immunol 1983; 71:382–8.
63. Schleimer RP, Derse CP, Friedman B, Gillis S, Plaut M, Lichtenstein LM, MacGlashan DW Jr. Regulation of human basophil mediator release by cytokines. I. Interaction with antiinflammatory steroids. J Immunol 1989; 143:1310–7.

64. Hirai K, Morita Y, Misaki Y, Ohta I, Takaishi T, Suzuki S, Motoyoshi K, Miyamoto T. Modulation of human basophil histamine release by hemopoietic growth factors. J Immunol 1988; 141:3958–64.
65. Kurimoto Y, de Weck AL, Dahinden CA. Interleukin 3-dependent mediator release in basophils triggered by C5a. J Exp Med 1989; 170:467–79.
66. Baggiolini M, Walz A, Kunkel SL. Neutrophil-activating peptide-1/interleukin 8, a novel cytokine that activates neutrophils. J Clin Invest 1989; 84:1045–9.
67. Dahinden CA, Kurimoto Y, De Weck AL, Lindley I, Dewald B, Baggiolini M. The neutrophil-activating peptide NAF/NAP-1 induces histamine release and leukotriene release by interleukin 3-primed basophils. J Exp Med 1989; 170:1787–92.

23

Hemopoietic Growth Factors Regulate Basophil Function and Viability

KOICHI HIRAI, YUTAKA MORITA, AND TERUMASA MIYAMOTO
University of Tokyo School of Medicine, Tokyo, Japan

I. INTRODUCTION

Production of white blood cells is regulated in vivo and in vitro by a variety of hormonelike mediators called by the generic names, colony-stimulating factors (CSFs) and interleukins (ILs). These factors act on hemopoietic progenitors and induce proliferation and differentiation in a sequential manner. Biological activities of these factors are believed to be exerted through their binding to specific receptors on the cell surface. In as much as such receptors developed on committed progenitors are retained by their mature progeny, hemopoietic growth factors are capable for action on end-stage cells which have lost the capacity for proliferation and differentiation. Substantial studies have documented the ability of hemopoietic growth factors to stimulate end-stage cells in a lineage-specific fashion and to enhance functional activities such as phagocytosis, cytotoxicity, motility, superoxide production, and the synthesis of biologically active molecules (1–13). In addition, hemopoietic growth factors were shown to be capable of enhancing the lifespan of mature progeny of responding hemopoietic cells (5,7,9,11–15). The action of these factors on mature cells has been well elucidated in neutrophils, eosinophils, and monocytes; however, until recently their action on human mature basophils remained obscure.

As will be discussed below, the control mechanisms of human basophilopoiesis have not been clarified in detail. Our involvement with studies of regulatory roles of hemopoietic growth factors in basophil function and viability resulted from an interest in the factors controlling human basophilopoiesis. We assumed that factors which regulate the growth of human basophils also regulate basophil function and viability. In other words, by testing the effect of hemopoietic growth factors on mature basophils, we could indirectly determine the functional receptors on basophils, and eventually conjecture the regulatory molecules for basophilopoiesis.

This review will focus on the regulatory roles of hemopoietins in basophil function and viability. We will start with a brief review of human basophilopoiesis. We will then discuss the action of hemopoietic growth factors on human basophils, including (a) enhancement of histamine release, (b) survival enhancement, and (c) chemotactic activities.

II. HUMAN BASOPHILOPOIESIS

Since the first description by Paul Ehrlich, basophils have been recognized to be unique white blood cells which stain metachromatically with a variety of chemical dyes. On their surface, they have high-affinity receptors for IgE (FcεRI), in contrast to low-affinity receptors for IgE (FcεRII) existing on many other cell types. Cross-linking of IgE molecules on the receptors by specific antigens or anti-IgE antibodies leads to the exocytosis of preformed mediators such as vasoactive amines. The activation of basophils also results in de-novo synthesis and release of lipid mediators such as leukotrienes. Through the release of preformed and newly generated mediators, basophils induce constriction of smooth muscles, alteration in vascular tone and permeability. Thus, they play an essential role in the clinical manifestation of hypersensitivity reaction in concert with mast cells.

Before discussing information on the effect of hemopoietic growth factors on basophil function and viability from our laboratory and others, it is convenient to review the current knowledge of human basophilopoiesis.

Lectin stimulation of human lymphyocytes liberates a factor which promotes the growth of human metachromatically staining cells from hemopoietic progenitors in vitro (16,17). Functional and ultrastructural studies indicated that these cultured cells belong to basophils but not to mast cells (18). Sequential fractionation of medium conditioned by lectin-stimulated human spleen cells has revealed that this molecule is a protein of a molecular weight of 23,000 Da with isoelectric points between pH 5.8 and 7.3. In addition, this human growth factor for basophils (tentatively called basophil-like cell-promoting activity) was clearly differentiated from the interleukins IL-1 and IL-2, granulocyte (G)-macrophage colony-stimulating factor (CSF), and G-CSF (19).

In 1986, a novel human hemopoietic growth factor was cloned by analysis of human genomic DNA blots with the gibbon IL-3 cDNA as probe (20). This hemopoietin possessed a multi-CSF activity and was therefore identified as a human analog to murine IL-3. In mice, IL-3 has been shown to induce the growth of mucosal-type mast cells (21) and demonstrated to be capable of propagating connective tissue-type mast cells in concert with IL-4 (22). In fact, recombinant (r) human IL-3 was able to promote the growth of metachromatically staining cells from human bone marrow or cord blood mononuclear cells (23–25), although ultrastructural and cytochemical examination revealed that these cells do belong to basophils but not to mast cells. Antibodies raised against human rIL-3 completely abolished the activity of semipurified basophil-like cell-promoting activity (25), indicating that a human lymphokine capable of inducing the proliferation of basophils is human IL-3 itself.

Because of the high degree of conservation between the gibbon and human sequence of IL-3 genes (93%), human IL-3 is able to exert biological activities on nonhuman primates. When human IL-3 was administered to nonhuman primates, Meyer et al. observed 100-fold increases in numbers of peripheral basophils (26). Thus, human IL-3 plays an essential role in proliferation and differentiation of basophils not only in vitro but also in vivo. As is true for each of the other leukocytes, not a single but several factors might potentially act on various steps of differentiation of human basophils. However, it remains obscure whether other known or unknown factors actually participate in human basophilopoiesis.

III. ENHANCEMENT OF BASOPHIL HISTAMINE RELEASE BY GM-CSF AND IL-3

The primary intent of our study was to determine the functional receptors on human basophils by testing the effects of various hemopoietic growth factors on basophil functions. The effect of factors on a basophil function was examined by using histamine release from normal human peripheral basophils. Peripheral leukocytes were incubated with various concentrations of hemopoietic growth factors for 15 min followed by stimulation with anti-IgE. Among the factors we tested, rG-CSF, M-CSF, and rIL-4 had no effect on basophil histamine release at all; however, we observed that rGM-CSF and rIL-3 enhanced IgE-mediated histamine release in a dose-dependent fashion (Figure 1). In order to determine whether both factors specifically amplify histamine release involving IgE molecules on the cell membrane, we designed similar experiments using f-Met-Leu, Pro (FMLP) and ionophore A23187, known to induce the release without

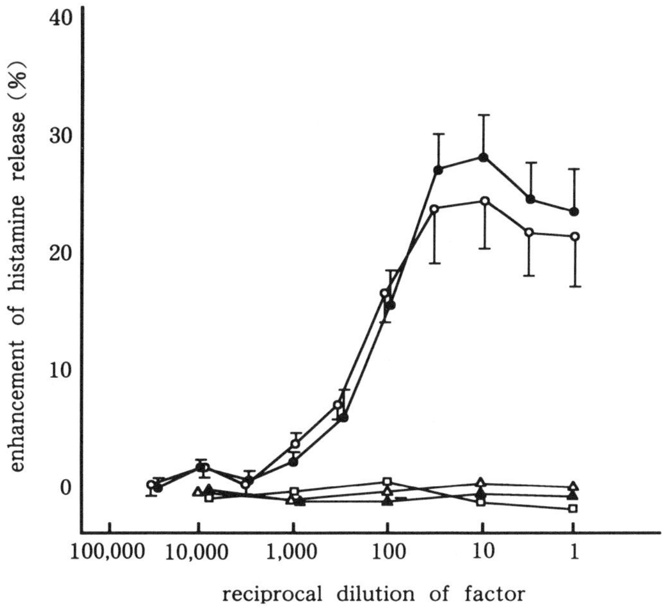

Figure 1 Effect of hemopoietins on anti-IgE-induced basophil histamine release. Leukocytes separated by dextran-glucose sedimentation were preincubated for 15 min with serially diluted hemopoietins at 37°C and then stimulated with anti-IgE. Supernatants were collected by centrifugation, and histamine was measured using an automated analizer. The enhancement of histamine release was calculated by the following formula: Enhancement = (histamine released with stimuli plus factors) − (histamine released with stimuli)/(total histamine content). Initial concentrations were 1.6 U/ml for IL-3 (●, n = 5), 600 U/ml for IL-4 (□, n = 5), 400 pM for GM-CSF (○, n = 7), 6000 U/ml for G-CSF (△, n = 5), and 6000 u/ml for M-CSF (▲, n = 5). Bars represent SEM. (Data redrawn from Ref 27.)

requiring involvement of IgE molecules, and observed that these factors augmented the histamine release evoked by both secretagogues (27) (Figures 2 and 3). Semipurified natural IL-3 (basophil-like cell-promoting activity) also augmented histamine release triggered by anti-IgE, fMLP, and ionophore A23187 in a dose-dependent fashion (28). Regardless of the stimuli employed, the enhancement occurred at similar concentrations; maximal and half-maximal enhancing activities were observed at concentrations of 20–40 pM and 2–5 pM, respectively, for GM-CSF and 0.2–0.5 U/ml and 0.02–0.05 U/ml, respectively, for IL-3. It has been shown that mature cells require lower concentrations of CSF for their activation than those required for proliferation of immature cells. The concentrations of GM-CSF and IL-3 to induce half-maximal enhancement of histamine release were 10 times lower for GM-CSF and 50 times lower for IL-3 compared with those required for half-maximal proliferation of progenitor cells. Since the enhancement was still observed using highly purified basophils (>90%) as target cells, the effect of both factors on basophils was mediated through the direct action on basophils and not through the indirect action via contaminating cells such as neutrophils, eosinophils, and lymphocytes. IL-3 and GM-CSF showed similar time kinetics, and the augmentation reached a plateau very rapidly (within 15 min). Even when factors were removed by washing after incubation, the augmentation was still observed, indicating that the presence of both factors was not essential for the enhancement of histamine release during the release process. Furthermore, the enhancement depended on temperature; preincubation at 4°C markedly decreased the augmentation of IgE-mediated release. It is of interest that the platuea levels of the enhancement achieved by both fac-

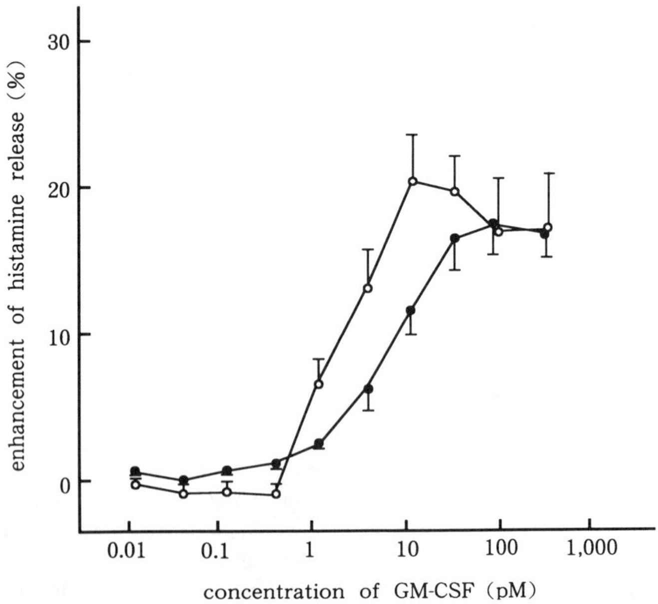

Figure 2 Effect of GM-CSF on fMLP- or A23187-induced basophil histamine release. Conditions of the experiments as described in Figure 1. Leukocytes were preincubated with different concentrations of GM-CSF and then stimulated with FMLP (●, n = 4) or ionophore A23187 (○, n = 5). Bars represent SEM. (Data redrawn from Ref 27.)

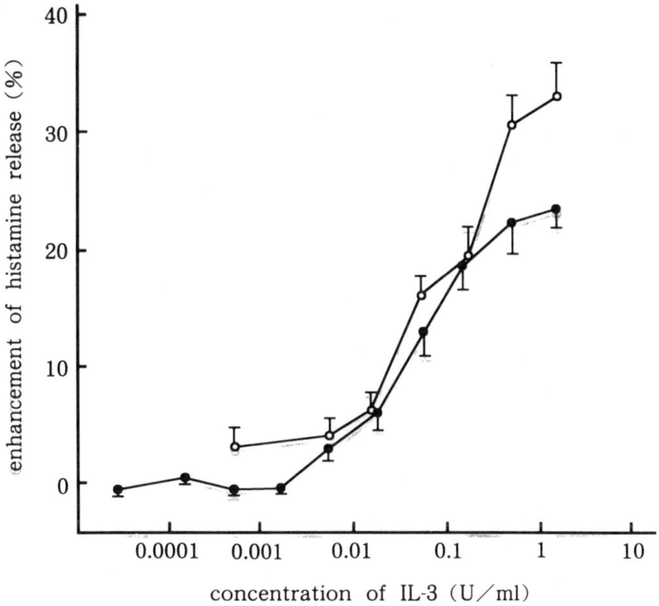

Figure 3 Effect of IL-3 on fMLP- or A23187-induced basophil histamine release. Conditions of experiments as described in Figure 1. After preincubation with IL-3, cells were stimulated with FMLP (●, n = 5) or ionophore A23187 (○, n = 5). Bars represent SEM. (Data redrawn from Ref 27.)

tors were found to be equivalent. Moreover, no additional but competitive effect on the amplification was observed between both factors (27). These results demonstrate the complete overlapping of the basophils responding to IL-3 and GM-CSF—e.g., single basophils responded to both factors—and suggest that the enhancement may be mediated either through a common receptor or through different receptors sharing a common pathway after the receptor occupancy.

Besides the enhancement of histamine release, IL-3 was shown to potentiate the production of a newly generated mediator in human basophils. Kurimoto et al. investigated the effect of IL-3 on leukotriene C_4 (LTC_4) production of human basophils. Their findings show that IL-3 markedly amplifies C5a-mediated LTC_4 production (29).

There have been no reports on the receptors for hemopoietic growth factors on normal basophils. However, two laboratories have investigated the receptors for IL-3 for GM-CSF on basophils purified from patients with chronic myelogenous leukemia. Valent et al. demonstrated the presence of a single class of high-affinity receptors for IL-3 (K_d: 160-230 pM). They failed to detect the specific binding of GM-CSF to leukemic basophils, although they observed that GM-CSF as well as IL-3 enhanced IgE-mediated histamine release from basophils separated from normal donors (30). On the other hand, Lopez et al. have recently reported that basophils expressed a single class of high-affinity receptors for both IL-3 (K_d: 26 pM) and GM-CSF (K_d: 40 pM) (31).

No report has described the mechanisms of signal transduction systems linked to receptors for IL-3 or GM-CSF in human basophils. As is observed in the other types of cells, tyrosine kinase and to a lesser extent protein kinase C might be potentially involved in human basophils. We tried to investigate second-messenger systems using a variety of inhibitors for tyrosine kinase or protein kinase C, but without success so far.

Previous reports dealing with cytokines affecting basophil histamine release are classified into two groups: (a) factors capable of inducing histamine release directly (32–41), and (b) histamine release-enhancing factors (42–46). We failed to observe any significant histamine release by GM-CSF and IL-3 in the absence of secretagogues at concentrations great enough to enhance histamine release (< 100 pM). However, there have been several reports that IL-3 itself causes basophil histamine release (47,48). The most puzzling aspect of these studies is that concentrations of IL-3 sufficient to induce histamine release were extremely different. Explaining these conflicting results might be that direct histamine release varies with the nature of the subjects and the presence of deuterium oxide. Basophils employed in our above experiments were obtained from nonatopic subjects. However, both GM-CSF and IL-3 were capable of inducing direct histamine release from basophils obtained from some atopic patients. As pointed out by Lichtenstein and co-workers, histamine releasability by IL-3 might be different between basophils in nonatopic and atopic subjects. They explained these differences on the basis of IgE heterogeneity, which they stressed exists (49).

So-called histamine-releasing factor was first described by Thueson et al. (32) and recently purified to apparent homogeneity by Baeza et al, (50). The characteristics of histamine release by "histamine-releasing factor" was found to be different from IL-3 and GM-CSF, indicating that neither IL-3 nor GM-CSF corresponds to "histamine-releasing factor" (51).

IV. ENHANCEMENT OF BASOPHIL SURVIVAL BY HEMOPOIETIC GROWTH FACTORS

It has been demonstrated that hemopoietic growth factors regulate the viability of mature end-stage cells in a lineage-specific fashion and enhance their survival in vitro. The action of hemopoietic growth factors on the survival of mature cells are well elucidated in neutrophils (5,13,14), eosinophils (5,7,9,11,12,14), and monocytes, but there is little information on the survival of normal basophils. An early report demonstrated that basophils were able to survive for 3 days in vitro without any exogenous factors (52), but the effect of hemopoietins remained obscure. Thus, we tested the effect of hemopoietic growth factors on the survival of basophils purified from normal peripheral blood. In the absence of factors, basophils started to decease rapidly; at day 7 only 10% of the cells remained in the cultures, and no viable cells were observed at day 14. Both IL-3 and GM-CSF were capable of enhancing basophil survival. The enhancing action of IL-3 on the survival was very potent—67% of cells at day 7—and even at day 14, more than 40% of the cells still survived in the cultures. GM-CSF also had an ability to enhance survival, but its action was only marginal and significantly weak compared with IL-3; 33% of the cells survived at day 7. On the other hand, G-CSF, M-CSF, and IL-4 had no enhancing activity at all. The survival was amplified by IL-3 in a dose-dependent manner; maximal and half-maximal augmentation was observed at the concentrations of 30 to 150 pM and 0.1 to 2 pM, respectively. The concentrations of IL-3 required for survival enhancement were in a range similar to those for the amplification of histamine release. Lightmicroscopic and electron microscopic examinations of cells maintained by IL-3 revealed properties of mature basophils. No findings characteristic of mast cells were observed. They contained histamine, but there was no significant difference in the content before and after culturing. Histamine release was evoked by fMLP, calcium ionophore A23187, and anti-IgE antibodies but not by compound 48/80, a secretagogue specific to mast cells. These morphological and functional characteristics documented that cultured cells maintained the properties of basophils and no phenotypic change to mast cells was observed.

It has been shown that eosinophilopoietic factors (IL-3, GM-CSF, and IL-5) regulate cellular density of eosinophils; normodense eosinophils become hypodense when exposed to these factors (7,11,12). In basophils, it has been reported that peripheral basophils are separated into two fractions with different densities (53). Functional differences were observed between two subpopulations with low and high densities (54), however, it remains unknown if IL-3 and GM-CSF regulate cellular density of basophils.

V. IL-5 REGULATES BASOPHIL FUNCTION AND VIABILITY

In contrast to mast cells, basophils exhibit a variety of myeloid-associated surface membrane antigens (55), suggesting that basophils belong to myeloid lineage. In particular, basophils share several properties with eosinophils, which are also associated with hypersensitivity reactions. First, eosinophil-specific proteins such as major basic protein (56) and lysophospholipase (57) (Charcot-Leiden crystal) are also shown to exist in basophils. Second, the major product of arachidonic acid metabolism generated by both cells is LTC_4. Third, in clonal analysis, the coexistence of eosinophils and basophils has been observed in single colonies derived from human bone marrow cells or peripheral blood mononuclear cells (58,59). Fourth, hybrid cells, which possess both eosinophilic and basophilic granules, have been found in semisolid culture systems (59), as well as in peripheral blood of patients with chronic myelogenous leukemia (60). These findings strongly indicate the close relationship between eosinophils and basophils; both cells might potentially derive from a common precursor.

The genes of GM-CSF, IL-3, and IL-5 locate very closely to each other on the long arm of chromosome 5 (61–63). All of these factors induce the proliferation and postmitotic differentiation of immature eosinophils and stimulate mature eosinophil functions. Apart from GM-CSF and IL-3, IL-5 induces selective formation of eosinophil colonies in vitro (64) and selective activation of eosinophil functions (9,10,12). Therefore, we assessed the effect of IL-5 on basophil function and viability.

Human rIL-5 amplified basophil histamine release triggered by anti-IgE, fMLP, and ionophore A23187 in a dose-dependent fashion. Maximal and half-maximal enhancement was observed at concentrations of approximately 50 pM and 5 pM, respectively. As is true for GM-CSF and IL-3, the enhancement was time and temperature dependent, and did not disappear when IL-5 was removed before stimulation. Human IL-5 shares high sequence homology with murine IL-5 (approximately 70% at the amino acid level), and murine IL-5 is shown to be capable of acting on human eosinophils (65). A similar situation has been found with basophils; murine IL-5 also amplified human basophil histamine release. IL-5 enhanced the lifespan of basophils in vitro; however, in terms of survival enhancement, the ability of IL-5 was significantly weak compared with that of IL-3.

VI. BASOPHIL CHEMOTAXIS BY IL-3 AND GM-CSF

IgE-mediated hypersensitivity reaction in the skin and in the upper and lower airways consists of an acute response followed 3-12 h later by a late-phase reaction. The late-phase reaction is characterized by the reappearance of an inflammatory reaction, which is often more severe and prolonged than the early response (66–68). Increased numbers of basophils have been observed upon histological examination in the late-phase reaction in the skin (69). In addition, symptoms of late-phase reaction coincided with a rise in histamine but were not accompanied by a rise in prostaglandin D_2, a mediator specific to mast cells (69,70). These observations suggest that basophils play a crucial role in the late-phase reaction. Accumulation of basophils at sites of inflammation indicates that mechanisms exist for the recruitment of basophils to these areas from circulating blood—implying the existence of mechanisms for basophil chemotaxis. Human stimulated lymphocytes produce a protein which is chemotactic for basophils (71,72). This lymphocyte-derived basophil chemotactic factor has not been purified, sequenced, or cloned as yet.

We tested the effects of GM-CSF and IL-3 on chemotaxis for basophils using a microchamber technique. Both factors induced migration across polycarbonate filters of purified basophils in a dose-dependent manner. Maximal and half-maximal migration was observed at concentrations of 50 pM and 5 pM, respectively, for IL-3, and 100 pM and 5 pM, respectively, for GM-CSF.

VII. SUMMARY

Table 1 summarizes the activities of hemopoietins on immature and mature basophils. IL-3, GM-CSF, and IL-5 enhanced basophil histamine release and in-vitro survival, while G-CSF, M-CSF, and IL-4 had no enhancing activities at all. In addition, IL-3 and GM-CSF induced basophil chemotaxis. Although IL-3 was proved to have proliferative and differentiation-inducing activities on basophils in vitro and in vivo, the other two factors (GM-CSF and IL-5), which are also capable of regulating basophil functions and viability, might potentially participate in proliferation or differentiation of human basophils, but this hypothesis remains without sure foundation. Studies on the roles of both factors in human basophilopoiesis need extension.

The fact that IL-3, GM-CSF, and IL-5 regulate basophil function and viability in vitro demonstrates possible mechanisms for the regulation of basophil function and viability in IgE-mediated reactions (especially in late-phase reactions) in vivo by these factors. Since these factors could be produced by antigen-stimulated T-cells or epithelial cells through the inflammatory process, these factors could participate in exacerbation and prolongation of hypersensitivity reactions by inducing the migration and enhancing functions and the lifespan of basophils.

ACKNOWLEDGMENT

We thank our colleagues Masao Yamaguchi, Toshiaki Takaishi, and Ken Ohta for their contribution to this work.

Table 1 Activities of Hemopoietins on Human Basophils

	Progenitor cells		Mature cells		
Factors	Proliferation	Differentiation	Enhancement of histamine release	Survival enhancement	Chemotactic activity
IL-3	Yes	Yes	Yes	Yes[a]	Yes
IL-4	?	?	No	No	?
IL-5	?	?	Yes	Yes[b]	?
GM-CSF	?	?	Yes	Yes[b]	Yes
G-CSF	?	?	No	No	?
M-CSF	?	?	No	No	?

[a] Potent.

[b] Marginal.

REFERENCES

1. Kurland JI, Pelus LM, Ralph P, Bockman RS, Moore MAS. Induction of prostaglandin E synthesis in normal and neoplastic macrophages: role for colony-stimulating factor(s) distinct from effects on myeloid progenitor cell proliferation. Proc Natl Acad Sci USA 1979; 76:2326–30.
2. Hamilton JA, Stanley ER, Burgess AW, Shadduck RK. Stimulation of macrophage plasminogen activator activity by colony-stimulating factors. J Cell Physiol 1980; 103:435–45.
3. Lopez AF, Nicola NA, Burgess AW, Metcalf D, Battye FL, Sewell WA, Vadas M. Activation of granulocyte cytotoxic function by purified mouse colony-stimulating factors. J Immunol 1983; 131:2983–8.
4. Weisbart RH, Golde DW, Clark SC, Wong GG, Gasson JC. Human granulocyte-macrophage colony-stimulating factor is a neutrophil activator. Nature 1985; 314:361–3.
5. Lopez AF, Williamson DJ, Gamble JR, Begley CG, Harian JM, Klebanoff SJ, Waltersdorph A, Wong G, Clark SC, Vadas MA. Recombinant human granulocyte-macrophage colony-stimulating factor stimulates in vitro mature human neutrophil and eosinophil function, surface receptor expression, and survival. J Clin Invest 1986; 78:1220–8.
6. Silberstein DS, Owen WF, Gasson JC, Dipersio JF, Golde DW, Bina JC, Soberman R, Austen KF, David JR. Enhancement of human eosinophil cytotoxicity and leukotriene synthesis by biosynthetic (recombinant) granulocyte-macrophage colony-stimulating factor. J Immunol 1986; 137:3290–4.
7. Owen WF Jr, Rothenberg ME, Silberstein DS, Gasson JC, Stevens RL, Austen KF, Soberman RJ. Regulation of human eosinophil viability, density, and function by granulocyte/macrophage colony-stimulating factor in the presence of 3T3 fibroblasts. J Exp Med 1987; 166:129–41.
8. Dahinden CA, Zingg J, Maly FE, de Weck AL. Leukotriene production in human neutrophils primed by recombinant human granulocyte/macrophage colony-stimulating factor and stimulated with the complement component C5a and FMLP as second signals. J Exp Med 1988; 167:1281–95.
9. Yamaguchi Y, Hayashi Y, Sugama Y, Miura Y, Kasahara T, Kitamura S, Torisu M, Mita S, Tominaga A, Takatsu K, Suda T. Highly purified murine interleukin 5 (IL-5) stimulates eosinophil function and prolongs in vitro survival. IL-5 as an eosinophil chemotactic factor. J Exp Med 1988; 167:1737–42.
10. Lopez AF, Sanderson CJ, Gamble JR, Campbell HD, Young IG, Vadas MA. Recombinant human interleukin 5 is a selective activator of human eosinophil function. J Exp Med 1988; 167:219–24.
11. Rothenberg ME, Owen WF Jr, Silberstein DS, Woods J, Soberman RJ, Austen KF, Stevens RL. Human eosinophils have prolonged survival, enhanced functional properties, and become hypodense when exposed to human interleukin 3. J Clin Invest 1988; 81:1986–92.
12. Rothenberg ME, Petersen J, Stevens RL, Silberstein DS, McKenzie DT, Austen KF, Owen WF Jr. IL-5-dependent conversion of normodense human eosinophils to the hypodense phenotype uses 3T3 fibroblasts for enhanced viability, accelerated hypodensity, and sustained antibody-dependent cytotoxicity. J Immunol 1989; 143:2311–6.
13. Ling CJ, Owen WF Jr, Austen KF. Human fibroblasts maintain the viability and augment the functional response of human neutrophils in culture. J Clin Invest 1990; 85:601–4.
14. Begley CG, Lopez AF, Nicola NA, Warren DJ, Vadas MA, Sanderson CJ, Metcalf D. Purified colony-stimulating factors enhance the survival of human neutrophils and eosinophils in vitro: a rapid and sensitive microassay for colony-stimulating factors. Blood 1986; 68:162–6.
15. Elliott MJ, Vadas MA, Eglinton JM, Park LS, To LB, Cleland G, Clark SC, Lopez AF. Recombinant human interleukin-3 and granulocyte-macrophage colony-stimulating factor

show common biological effects and binding characteristics on human monocytes. Blood 1989; 74:2349–59.
16. Tadokoro K, Stadler BM, de Weck AL. Factor-dependent in vitro growth of human bone marrow-derived basophil-like cells. J Exp Med 1983; 158:857–71.
17. Ogawa M, Nakahata T, Leary AG, Sterk AR, Ishizaka K, Ishizaka T. Suspension culture of human mast cells/basophils from umbilical cord blood mononuclear cells. Proc Natl Acad Sci USA 1983; 80:4494–8.
18. Ishizaka T, Dvorak AM, Conrad DH, Niebyl JR, Marquette JP, Ishizaka K. Morphologic and immunologic characterization of human basophils developed in cultures of cord blood mononuclear cells. J Immunol 1985; 134:532–40.
19. Hirai K, de Weck AL, Stadler BM. Characterization of a human basophil-like cell promoting activity. J Immunol 1988; 140:221–7.
20. Yang Y-C, Ciarletta AB, Temple PA, Chung MP, Kovacic S, Witek-Giannotti JS, Leary AC, Kriz R, Donahue RE, Wong GG, Clark SC. Human IL-3 (multi-CSF): identification by expression cloning of a novel hematopoietic growth factor related to murine IL-3. Cell 1986; 47:3–10.
21. Razin E, Ihle JN, Seldin D, Mencia-Huerta JM, Katz HR, LeBlanc PA, Hein A, Caulfield JP, Austen KF, Stevens RL. Interleukin 3: a differentiation and growth factor for the mouse mast cell that contains chondroitin sulfate E proteoglycan. J Immunol 1984; 132:1479–86.
22. Hamaguchi Y, Kanakura Y, Fujita J, Takeda S-I, Nakano T, Tarui S, Honjo T, Kitamura Y. Interleukin 4 as an essential factor for in vitro clonal growth of murine connective tissue-type mast cells. J Exp Med 1987; 165:268–73.
23. Saito H, Hatake K, Dvorak AM, Leiferman KM, Donnenberg AD, Arai N, Ishizaka K, Ishizaka T. Selective differentiation and proliferation of hematopoietic cells induced by recombinant human interleukins. Proc Natl Acad Sci USA 1988; 85:2288–92.
24. Valent P, Schmidt G, Besemer J, Mayer P, Zenke G, Liehl E, Hinterberger W, Lechner K, Maurer D, Bettelheim P. Interleukin-3 is a differentiation factor for human basophils. Blood 1989; 73:1763–9.
25. Fagg B, Hirai K, Nakajima K, Stadler BM. Human recombinant IL-3 promotes the growth of human basophils/mast cells. In: Groopman J, Evans C, Golde D, eds. Mechanisms of action and therapeutic applications of biologicals in cancer and immune deficiency disorders. UCLA Symposia on molecular and cellular biology. New York: Liss, 1988:100–4.
26. Mayer P, Valent P, Schmidt G, Liehl E, Bettelheim P. The in vivo effects of recombinant human interleukin-3: demonstration of basophil differentiation factor, histamine-producing activity, and priming of GM-CSF-responsive progenitors in nonhuman primates. Blood 1989; 74:613–21.
27. Hirai K, Morita Y, Misaki Y, Ohta K, Takaishi T, Suzuki S, Motoyoshi K, Miyamoto T. Modulation of human basophil histamine release by hemopoietic growth factors. J Immunol 1988; 141:3958–64.
28. Morita Y, Hirai K, Misaki Y, Takaishi T, Suzuki S, Ito K, Stadler BM, Miyamoto T. Enhancement of basophil histamine release by a human basophil-like cell promoting activity. Allergy 1990; 45:183–8.
29. Kurimoto Y, de Weck AL, Dahinden CA. Interleukin 3-dependent mediator release in basophils triggered by C5a. J Exp Med 1989; 179:467–79.
30. Valent P, Besemer J, Muhm M, Majdic O, Lechner K, Bettelheim P. Interleukin 3 activates human blood basophils via high-affinity binding sites. Proc Natl Acad Sci USA 1989; 86:5542–6.
31. Lopez AF, Lyons AB, Eglinton JM, Park LS, To LB, Clark SC, Vadas MA. Specific binding of human interleukin-3 and granulocyte-macrophage colony-stimulating factor to human basophils. J Allergy Clin Immunol 1990; 85:99–102.
32. Thueson DO, Speck LS, Lett-Brown MA, Grant JA. Histamine-releasing activity (HRA). I.

Production by mitogen or antigen-stimulated human mononuclear cells. J Immunol 1979; 123:626–32.

33. Thueson DO, Speck LS, Lett-Brown MA, Grant JA. Histamine-releasing activity (HRA). II. Interaction with basophils and physiocochemical characterization. J Immunol 1979; 123:633–9.
34. Sedgwick JD, Holt PG, Turner KJ. Production of a histamine-releasing lymphokine by antigen- or mitogen-stimulated human peripheral T cells. Clin Exp Immunol 1981; 45:409–18.
35. Ezeamuzie IC, Assem ESK. A study of histamine release from human basophils and lung mast cells by products of lymphocyte stimulation. Agents Actions 1983; 13:222–30.
36. Kaplan AP, Haak-Frendscho M, Fauci A, Dinarello C, Halbert E. A histamine-releasing factor from activated human mononuclear cells. J Immunol 1985; 135:2027–32.
37. Schulman ES, Liu MC, Proud D, MacGlashan DW, Lichtenstein LM, Plaut M. Human lung macrophages induce histamine release from basophils and mast cells. Am Rev Respir Dis 1985; 131:230–5.
38. Orchard MA, Kagey-Sobotka A, Proud D, Lichtenstein LM. Basophil histamine release induced by a substance from stimulated platelets. J Immunol 1986; 136:2240–4.
39. Warner JA, Pienkowski MM, Plaut M, Norman PS, Lichtenstein LM. Identification of histamine releasing factor(s) in the late phase of cutaneous IgE-mediated reactions. J Immunol 1986; 136:2583–7.
40. Subramanian N, Bray MA. Interleukin 1 releases histamine from human basophils and mast cells in vitro. J Immunol 1987; 138:271–5.
41. Haak-Frendscho M, Dinarello C, Kaplan AP. Recombinant human interleukin-1 beta causes histamine release from human basophils. J Allergy Clin Immunol 1988; 82:218–23.
42. Ida S, Hooks JJ, Siraganian RP, Notkins AL. Enhancement of IgE-mediated histamine release from human basophils by viruses: role of interferon. J Exp Med 1977; 145:892–906.
43. Goetzl EJ, Foster DW, Payan DG. A basophil activating factor from human T lymphocytes. Immunology 1984; 53:227–34.
44. Younger RE, Herrod HG, Lieberman PL, Valenski WR, Trouy RL, Crawford LV. Characterization of mononuclear cell-derived histamine release enhancing factor. J Allergy Clin Immunol 1987; 80:547–57.
45. Schleimer RP, Derse CP, Friedman B, Gillis S, Plaut M, Lichtenstein LM, MacGlashan DW Jr. Regulation of human basophil mediator release by cytokines. I. Interaction with antiinflammatory steroids. J Immunol 1989; 143:1310–7.
46. Massey WA, Randall TC, Kagey-Sobotka A, Warner JA, MacDonald SM, Gillis S, Allison AC, Lichtenstein LM. Recombinant human IL-1α and -1β potentiate IgE-mediated histamine release from human basophils. J Immunol 1989; 143:1875–80.
47. Haak-Frendscho M, Arai N, Arai K, Baeza ML, Finn A, Kaplan AP. Human recombinant granulocyte-macrophage colony-stimulating factor and interleukin 3 cause basophil histamine release. J Clin Invest 1988; 82:17–20.
48. MacDonald SM, Schleimer RP, Kagey-Sobotka A, Gillis S, Lichtenstein LM. Recombinant IL-3 induces histamine release from human basophils. J Immunol 1989; 142:3527–32.
49. MacDonald SM, Lictenstein LM, Proud D, Plaut M, Naclerio RM, MacGlashan DW Jr, Kagey-Sobotka A. Studies of IgE-dependent histamine releasing factors: heterogeneity of IgE. J Immunol 1987; 139:506–12.
50. Baeza ML, Reddigari S, Haak-Frendscho M, Kaplan AP. Purification and further characterization of human mononuclear cell histamine-releasing factor. J Clin Invest 1989; 83:1204–10.

51. Alam R, Welter JB, Forsythe PA, Lett-Brown MA, Grant JA. Comparative effect of recombinant IL-1, -2, -3, -4, and -6, IFN-γ, granulocyte-macrophage-colony-stimulating factor, tumor necrosis factor-α, and histamine-releasing factors on the secretion of histamine from basophils. J Immunol 1989; 142:3431–5.
52. Drobis JD, Siraganian RP. Histamine release from cultured human basophils: Lack of histamine resynthesis after antigenic release. J Immunol 1976; 117:1049–53.
53. Leonard EJ, Skeel A. Separation of human basophils into two fractions with different density and histamine content. J Allergy Clin Immunol 1985; 76:556–62.
54. Morita Y, Asakawa M, Hirai K, Takaishi T, Miyamoto T. Functional differences of human basophils with different densities. Int Arch Allergy Appl Immunol 1989; 88:332–336.
55. Stain C, Stockinger H, Scharf M, Jäger U, Gössinger H, Lechner K, Bettelheim P. Human blood basophils display a unique phenotype including activation linked membrane structures. Blood 1987; 70:1872–9.
56. Ackerman SJ, Kephart GM, Habermann TM, Greipp PR, Gleich GJ. Localization of eoshinophil granule major basic protein in human basophils. J Exp Med 1983; 158:946–61.
57. Ackerman SJ, Well GJ, Gleich GJ. Formation of Charcot-Leyden crystals by human basophils. J Exp Med 1982; 155:1597–609.
58. Leary AG, Ogawa M. Identification of pure and mixed basophil colonies in culture of human peripheral blood and marrow cells. Blood 1984; 64:78–83.
59. Denburg JA, Telizyn S, Messner H, Jamal BLN, Ackerman SJ, Gleich GJ, Bienenstock J. Heterogeneity of human peripheral blood eosinophil-type colonies: evidence for a common basophil-eosinophil progenitor. Blood 1985; 66:312–8.
60. Weill SC, Hrisinko MA. A hybrid eosinophilic-basophilic granulocyte in chronic granulocytic leukemia. Am J Clin Pathol 1987; 87:66–70.
61. Le Beau MM, Westbrook CA, Diaz MO, Larson RA, Rowley JD, Gasson JC, Golde DW, Sherr CJ. Evidence for the involvement of GM-CSF and FMS in the deletion (5q) in myeloid disorders. Science 1986; 231:984–7.
62. Clark SC, Kamen R. The human hematopoietic colony-stimulating factors. Science 1987; 236:1229–37.
63. Sutherland GR, Baker E, Callen DF, Campbell HD, Young IG, Sanderson CJ, Garson OM, Lopez AF, Vadas MA. Interleukin-5 is at 5q31 and is deleted in the 5q- syndrome. Blood 1988; 171:1150–2.
64. Yamaguchi Y, Suda T, Suda J, Eguchi M, Miura Y, Harada N, Tominaga A, Takatsu K. Purified interleukin 5 supports the terminal differentiation and proliferation of murine eosinophilic precursors. J Exp Med 1988; 167:43–56.
65. Lopez AF, Begley CG, Williamson DJ, Warren DJ, Vadas MA, Sanderson CJ. Murine eosinophil differentiation factor. An eosinophil-specific-colony-stimulating factor with activity for human cells. J Exp Med 1986; 163:1085–99.
66. Dolovich J, Hargreave FE, Chalmers R, Shier KJ, Gauldie J, Bienenstock J. Late cutaneous allergic responses in isolated IgE-dependent reactions. J Allergy Clin Immunol 1973; 52:38–46.
67. Gleich GJ. The late phase of the immunoglobulin E-mediated reaction: a link between anaphylaxis and common allergic disease? J Allergy Clin Immunol 1982; 70:160–9.
68. Larsen GL. Late-phase reactions: observations on pathogenesis and prevention. J Allergy Clin Immunol 1985; 76:665–9.
69. Charlesworth EN, Hood AF, Soter NA, Kagey-Sobotka A, Norman PS, Lichtenstein LM. Cutaneous late-phase response to allergen. J Clin Invest 1989; 83:1519–26.
70. Naclerio RM, Proud D, Togias AG, Adkinson MF, Meyers DA, Kagey-Sobotka A, Plaut M, Norman PS, Lichtenstein LM. Inflammatory mediators in late antigen-induced rhinitis.

N Engl J Med 1985; 313:65–70.
71. Lett-Brown MD, Boetcher B, Leonard EJ. Chemotactic responses of normal human basophils to C5a and to lymphocyte derived chemotactic factor. J Immunol 1976; 177:246–52.
72. Lett-Brown MA, Hooks JJ, Georgides JA, Thueson DO, Grant JA. Modulation of human basophil migration in vitro by a soluble factor from virus-stimulated leukocytes. Clin Immunol Immunopathol 1981; 20:179–87.

24

Effects of Hematopoietic Growth Factors on Nonhematopoietic Cells

SHOUKAT DEDHAR and CONNIE EAVES
British Columbia Cancer Agency,
Vancouver, British Columbia, Canada

I. INTRODUCTION

Growth and death are processes of major importance to tissues that are dependent on cell renewal, of which the hematopoietic system is a prime example. At the individual cell level, these processes are normally regulated at least in part by extrinsic molecular factors, generically referred to as growth factors (or inhibitors, according to their effects). Because of early, and until recently unchallenged, evidence of equisite specificity of certain growth factors for hematopoietic target cell populations, the term hematopoietic growth factors or hemopoietins gained wide acceptance, and most models of hematopoietic cell regulation assumed the existence of tissue specific molecular regulators.

Erythropoietin was the first such regulator to be recognized (1) and eventually purified (2). Early studies also showed erythropoietin to conform to the classic definition of a hormone, i.e., a molecule that is produced in one organ, in this case the kidney, and then released into the bloodstream to make its way to target cell population in another organ. For erythropoietin, the target cells are intermediate to late stages of erythroid precursors (3). Not only did these studies set a precedent for the concept of unique regulators or hematopoiesis, the apparently restricted action of erythropoietin on cells already committed to erythropoiesis suggested the likelihood of other lineage-specific regulators within the hematopoietic system.

Subsequent identification of molecules able to stimulate other subsets of hematopoietic precursors reinforced these early concepts of tissue and lineage specificity. Particularly convincing were observations derived from studies of hematopoietic colony formation by marrow cells stimulated to proliferate and differentiate in vitro. These studies showed that, according to the source of stimulatory factors incorporated into the assay medium, different types of mature blood cell colonies were generated. The concept of lineage-specific regulators became embodied in the nomenclature proposed to refer to these "colony-stimulating factors" (or CSFs), and the terms G-CSF (for granulocyte CSF), M-CSF (for macrophage CSF), GM-CSF (for granulocyte-plus-macrophage CSF) and multi-CSF (for multilineage CSF) gained wide acceptance (4). The advent of pure molecules made possible more precise examination of this general principle of lineage specificity, but because these growth factors proved extraordinarily difficult to obtain in high concentration and equally difficult to purify, progress in this regard was initially slow. Nevertheless, exceptions began to emerge almost as soon as such experiments could be undertaken (5,6).

Recombinant DNA technology and, in particular, expression cloning and methods for expressing cloned genes largely overcame these hurdles. New strategies for cloning facilitated the discovery of factors with the same apparent bioactivities, and expression systems yielded sufficient pure material for assessing defined molecules in different bioassays. As a result, in the early 1980s there was an explosion in the entire growth-factor field. From such studies, which are still ongoing, the number of factors known to be potent and direct-acting stimulators of hematopoietic cells has increased to an imponderable number. At the same time the number of different types of target cells now known to be responsive to any single factor has also increased, and responses other than growth stimulation, particularly on nondividing cells such as granulocytes, have been recognized. A list of the best-characterized cloned factors currently viewed as hemopoietins and some of their hematopoietic target populations is given in Table 1. These include not only the CSFs mentioned above but also a number of factors designated as interleukins (ILs) because they are produced by one type of leukocyte and act on another. Finally, there are other molecules whose identities were first established by recognition of other activities.

One of the interesting nonmitogenic functions of certain hemopoietins (e.g., IL-1 and GM-CSF) is to stimulate the production and release of other types of hemopoietins (reviewed in Refs. 7–9). These hematopoietic growth factors can thus be seen to operate not only as intercellular messengers but also as parts of growth-factor networks whose activation can achieve rapid localized signal amplification. Given the diversity of biological effects, both mitogenic and nonmitogenic, that these factors can have, as well as the diversity of cells on which they act, how is a given response selected in a given cell? For several of these factors, the genes encoding their specific cell surface receptors have now been cloned and shown to belong to related gene families (10,11). Although very little is as yet known about signal-transducing events associated with particular cellular responses, selectivity does not appear to be obtained through the utilization of different receptor gene products (see below).

In this review, we will briefly summarize the diversity of responses and responsive target cells now documented for some of the more intensively studied hematopoietic growth factors listed in Table 1. For organizational simplicity, effects observed on normal and transformed cells are discussed in consecutive sections. Such findings now provide strong support for the view that these factors serve as fundamental biological regulators, important to but by no means restricted to the hematopoietic system. Demonstration of responsiveness of tumor cells to factors being given therapeutically to stimulate hematopoiesis in cancer patients has raised obvious questions about potential adverse effects in such settings. Unfortunately, the experimental database in this latter area is rather limited, and there has been a certain tendency to downplay the phenomenology (12–14) rather than build on existing observations to derive new principles. Accordingly, we have also included recent new data of our own with this latter objective in mind.

II. PLEIOTROPISM OF HEMATOPOIETIC GROWTH FACTORS ON NORMAL CELLS

Examples of hematopoietic growth-factor effects on cells ontologically unrelated to the hematopoietic system have increased in number almost as rapidly as new endpoints of cellular behavior have been devised. IL-1 is a good example of this. IL-1 was initially recognized and named because it is produced by activated macrophages and itself activates T-lymphocytes. However, IL-1 was subsequently found to stimulate a variety of responses in a large number of other cell types. These include an ability to stimulate endothelial cells to increase their adhesiveness to leukocytes (15,16), to release prostaglandins (17), and to produce GM-CSF, G-CSF, and IL-6 (7,8). Some of these same responses have also been seen following IL-1 stimulation of fibroblasts (7,8,18). In addition, IL-1 stimulation of collagen type I synthesis by fibroblasts has been noted (19). IL-1 may also be involved in bone cell metabolism, since it can influence the proliferation and differentiation of osteoblasts (20,21). Even neuronal and glial cells of the central nervous system have been found to respond to IL-1 (22). IL-1 is now recognized as consisting of two very similar gene products, IL-1α and IL-1β. However, no difference has been discovered in the spectrum of activities of these two molecules, and both appear to bind to a common receptor on hematopoietic cells (23).

Other factors now recognized as having a similarly broad range of biologic functions are IL-6 (24), LIF/HILDA (25,26), and the product of the Steel gene (27). In addition to its wide range of target cells within the hematopoietic system, including pluripotent progenitors (28), granulocyte-macrophage precursors (29), megakaryocyte precursors (30), and activated B-cells (31), IL-6 leads to the release of acute-phase proteins from hepatocytes (32) and can stimulate neuronal and glial cells (22), to mention only some of its activities on nonhematopoietic cells. Both LIF/HILDA (33,34) and the product of the Steel gene (35,36) can also stimulate primitive hematopoietic cells, but the former is perhaps better known for its ability to stimulate the terminal differentiation of some leukemic cell lines (37) and to maintain embryonal carcinoma cells in vitro in an undifferentiated state (25). The latter is known to influence both germ cell and melanocyte development (27).

The extensive degree of pletotropism exhibited by these factors, in fact, calls into question the very value of their continued designation as hematopoietic growth factors. On the other hand, it may well turn out that many, even all, play a significant role in the physiological regulation of hematopoiesis in vivo, as appears to be the case for the Steel gene product. Thus far, available evidence for this comes largely from studies of in-vitro models of stromal cell-mediated support of hematopoiesis. Such studies indicate that IL-6 production by stromal cells is not an absolute requirement to sustain primitive hematopoietic cells (38), although in regular human marrow cultures, stimuli that promote stromal cell support of hematopoiesis in vitro also induce IL-6 production, and the time course of both effects do closely parallel one another (39).

In addition, other hematopoietic growth factors, for which less extensive pleiotropism has been documented, have now also been found to stimulate certain nonhematopoietic cells. For example, GM-CSF has been found to stimulate fibroblast proliferation

Table 1 Names and Activities of Cloned Hematopoietic Growth Factors (Hemopoietins) with Stimulatory Effects on Normal Hematopoietic Cells

Abbreviation	Name(s)	Some hematopoietic activities
CSF-1, M-CSF	Colony-stimulating factor-1, macrophage colony-stimulating factor	Stimulates macrophage production and activation.
G-CSF	Granulocyte colony-stimulating factor	Stimulates granulocyte production, activation, and release from bone marrow. Synergistic proliferative stimulus for early hematopoietic cells.
GM-CSF	Granulocyte-macrophage colony-stimulating factor	Stimulates granulocyte and macrophage production and activation. Proliferative stimulus for intermediate stages of erythroid, megakaryopoietic and multipotent cell development. Synergistic action on activated T-cells.
IL-1, LAF	Interleukin-1, lymphocyte-activating factor	Synergizes and stimulates proliferation of very early hematopoietic cells, B-cells, and T-cells. Activates basophils and macrophages.
IL-2, TCGF	Interleukin-2, T-cell growth factor	Stimulates T-cell proliferation. Activates NK cells.
IL-3, multi-CSF	Interleukin-3, multipotential colony-stimulating factor.	Alone or in combination with other factors, stimulates proliferation and differentiation of early and late hematopoietic (myeloid) cells of all lineages. Activates basophils and eosinophils.
IL-4, BSF-1	Interleukin-4, B-cell stimulating factor-1	Co-stimulates proliferation of many hematopoietic cell types as well as B- and T-cells. Promotes secretion by activated B-cells of IgG and IgE.
IL-5, BCGF-2, EDF	Interleukin-5, B-cell growth factor-2, T-cell replacing factor, eosinophil differentiation factor	Stimulates production of eosinophils. Promotes B-cell differentiation.

IL-6, BSF-2, β_2-IFN	Interleukin-6, B-cell stimulating factor-2, β_2-interferon	Stimulates granulocyte production (murine only). Synergizes to stimulative primitive hematopoietic cells. Stimulates activated B-cell proliferation and Ig secretion.
IL-7	Interleukin-7	Stimulates proliferation of pre B-cells, T-cells and megakaryocyte precursors.
IL-8, NAP-1, LAI[a]	Interleukin-8, neutrophil-activating protein-1, leukocyte-adhesion inhibitor	Stimulates neutrophil and T-cell chemotaxis
IL-9, P40	Interleukin-9, T-cell growth factor P40	Stimulates proliferation of mast cells, erythroid cells, and a subset of helper T-cells.
IL-10, B-TCGF, CSIF	Interleukin-10, B-cell-derived T-cell growth factor, cytokine synthesis-inhibitory factor	Co-stimulates proliferation of mature and immature T-cells and mast cells. Inhibits T-cell production of γ-IFN and TNF.
IL-11	Interleukin-11	Stimulates proliferation of activated B-cells and early multipotential hematopoietic cells. Co-stimulates production of megakaryocytes.
LIF, HILDA, DIA	Leukemia-inhibitory factor, differentiation-inhibiting activity, human interleukin for DA cells	Co-stimulates proliferation of primitive multipotential cells.
SCF, MGF, c-kit ligand	Stem-cell factor, mast-cell growth factor, c-kit ligand, Steel factor	Co-stimulates early hematopoietic cells, including multipotential cells, pre B-cells, early erythroid cells, and early granulopoietic cells.

[a] This is the only factor on this list that as yet has no known ability to stimulate the proliferation of a hematopoietic cell.

(40), and erythropoietin and G-CSF as well as GM-CSF were able to stimulate endothelial cell proliferation and migration (41,42). Interestingly, endothelial cell migration was not affected by exposure of these cells to IL-1, in spite of the ability of IL-1 to profoundly affect other responses by these cells (42).

Another approach to inferring hematopoietic growth-factor responsiveness by candidate target cells relies not on the demonstration of a biological response but on the detection of specific receptors for the factor of interest. Such studies have shown that receptors for G-CSF, GM-CSF, and M-CSF may be found on human placenta and trophoblastic cells (43–45), and receptors for IL-4 have been demonstrated on a variety of neuroblastic, mesodermal, and epithelial cell types (46). Whether or not factor binding in all of these cases also mediates a change in cell behavior is not yet established; however, a role for M-CSF in the development of the placenta seems likely, since *op/op* mice that carry a defective M-CSF gene are fertile but have difficulties in bringing their litters to term (47,48).

III. HEMATOPOIETIC GROWTH FACTOR EFFECTS ON TRANSFORMED NONHEMATOPOIETIC CELLS

Given the widely distributed effects of many hematopoietic growth factors on normal cells of nonhematopoietic origin, it is no longer surprising to learn that these factors can also stimulate a variety of nonhematopoietic tumor cells or cell lines. Recent data from a number of laboratories have revealed both stimulatory and inhibitory effects of these molecules on transformed cell growth.

Ruff et al. (49) were the first to document such a phenomenon in their description of the ability of GM-CSF to modulate the expression of certain surface antigens and to inhibit the growth of several human small-cell lung carcinoma (SCLC) cell lines. A subsequent study with another SCLC cell line confirmed these initial findings (50), but they did not prove to be a consistent observation (51,52) and, in the report by Baldwin et al. (52), GM-CSF enhanced the proliferation of the particular SCLC cell line used in their study. These different responses cannot be correlated with differences in receptor affinity, since high-affinity receptors were found on cells that were inhibited and stimulated (50,52). Similar heterogeneity in effects of GM-CSF on the growth in vitro of primary lung tumor cells has also been reported. Most samples showed no response, but some were inhibited and, in occasional samples (~10%), evidence of GM-CSF enhancement of proliferation was noted (13,14). Responses of primary lung tumor cells to other hematopoietic growth factors have not yet been as well studied, although in one of the surveys just referred to, one of 11 SCLC lines was shown to express receptors for, and to be stimulated to proliferate by, IL-3 (51).

Our own group was the first to document a growth-stimulatory effect of GM-CSF on a nonhematopoietic tumor cell. The responsive cells identified in this initial study (40) were an osteosarcoma cell line and two breast carcinoma cell lines (see also Figure 1). Berdel et al. (53) reported that the proliferation of some colon carcinoma cell lines could also be stimulated by GM-CSF and extended these observations to IL-3 and G-CSF. In the two surveys of primary human tumor cell responses to GM-CSF recently reported (13,14), positive examples were rare and growth inhibition was as common as growth simulation. Tumor types most commonly found to show a response to GM-CSF were breast, colon, ovary, and, as mentioned above, lung.

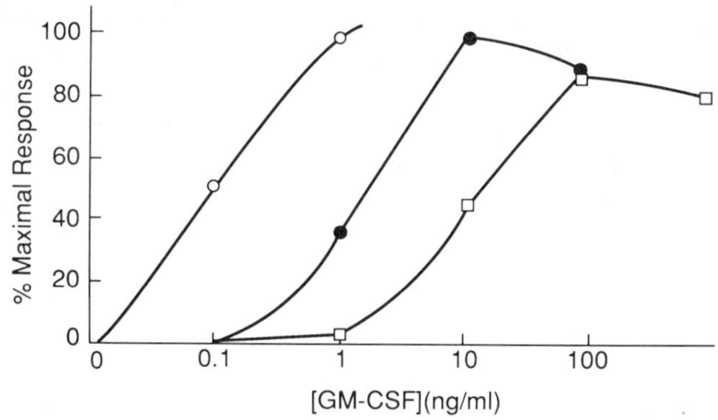

Figure 1 Proliferative response of granulocyte-macrophage colony-forming cells (CFU-GM) and two human tumor cell lines to GM-CSF. The proliferative response of CFU-GM (-○-) to GM-CSF was determined in assays of 5×10^4 nonadherent human marrow cells cultured in standard methylcellulose cultures as described in Ref. 40. The proliferative response of the two human tumor cell lines, MG-63 osteosarcoma (-●-), and MCF-7 breast carcinoma (-□-) was determined by measuring ^{3}H-thymidine incorporation under defined, serum-free conditions (DMEM/Hams F12 medium containing insulin/transferrin/selenium). For details, see Ref. 40.

IL-6 has been shown to stimulate primary lymphoma cells (14) and EBV-transformed human B-cells (54) but inhibited the proliferation of a number of breast carcinoma cell lines (55). It is interesting that IL-1 has also been found to inhibit the proliferation of some tumor cell lines (21). IL-1 is a potent inducer of IL-6 (7,8,24). Thus the inhibitory effect of IL-1 might be indirectly mediated by IL-6. IL-6 has also been found to decrease the intercellular adhesion of breast carcinoma cells to one another and to increase their motility (56). Such effects might alter the invasiveness of such cells, with important implications for therapy, although this is difficult to predict as in-vivo studies have not yet been reported.

It can be seen that a variety of human tumor cells, including cells in fresh biopsy samples, have the molecular apparatus to respond to some hematopoietic growth factors. Such factors have only recently become readily available in pure form, and this type of testing has thus been carried out only on a limited scale. Nevertheless, it is noteworthy that initial studies with the first factors introduced into clinical trials, primarily on cancer patients, have already revealed their variable potential for enhancement of transformed cell growth and more recently of invasiveness in some model situations. Such findings have not, however, triggered significant alarms sufficient to result in discontinuation of their clinical evaluation for a number of reasons. First, significant relapses or stimulation of nonhematopoietic tumor growth in treated patients has not occurred. Second, in most tissue culture studies, effective concentrations of factor have been several-fold higher than those able to stimulate hematopoietic progenitors (e.g., see Figure 1). Thus it has been argued that clinical regiments designed to stimulate hematopoiesis in vivo might not pose a significant hazard to most patients with nonhematopoietic malignancies even if the latter were factor responsive (12). Finally, in some instances stimulatory responses have been detected in the absence of other potential stimulators, including those present in serum (40). Although it may be biologically relevant and even important to define the factor response potential of different tumor cells, what matters clinically is whether and how a given hematopoietic growth factor might additionally modify the growth or metastasis of a tumor in the milieu in which it finds itself in vivo. Suitable strategies for addressing such questions in experimental models are extremely difficult to devise and test, and in the end the most fruitful approach may be to rely on clinical experience from carefully implemented trials (57,58).

IV. FURTHER IN-VITRO STUDIES

The findings summarized above suggest that the potential of human tumor cells to respond to hematopoietic growth factors may be much more extensive than previously anticipated. To understand this biology better, we have begun experiments to extend the range of factors evaluated using the same target cells and exposure conditions. In addition, we have begun to test the effects of specific growth factor combinations.

MG-63 (osteosarcoma) and MCF-7 (breast carcinoma) are cell lines we had previously shown to be stimulated by GM-CSF to proliferate under serum-free conditions (40). As shown in Figures 2 and 3, we have now established that MG-63 cells can also respond to G-CSF, IL-4, and IL-3, and that MCF-7 cells can also respond to IL-3. G-CSF and IL-4 are stimulators of MG-63 proliferation but are less potent in this regard than GM-CSF (Figure 2). In contrast, the effect of IL-3 on both MG-63 and MCF-7 cells is inhibitory. To our knowledge, these are the first examples of opposing effects of these two factors on the same responsive cell. On some human cells, GM-CSF and IL-3 cross-compete for binding, suggesting a common signal-transducing mechanism (59). The MG-63 and MCF-7 cell lines may therefore be of interest for further dissection of how GM-CSF and IL-3 may activate different intracellular events in different target cell populations.

We have previously shown that the proliferation of MG-63 cells is also inhibited by IL-1β (21). To determine whether IL-β had any influence on the stimulatory action of GM-CSF on these cells, MG-63 cells were preincubated with IL-1β for 5 h. As shown

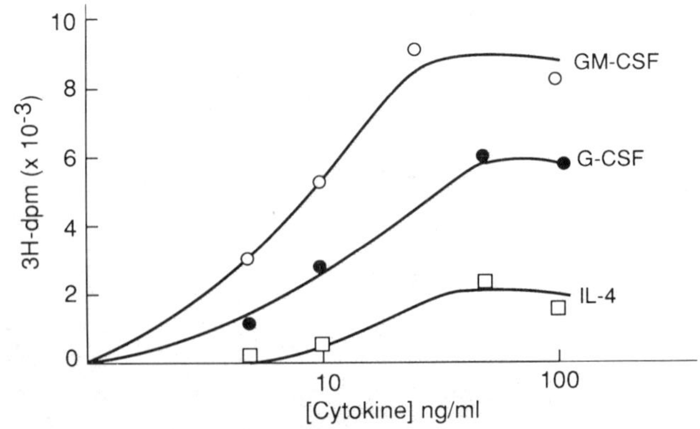

Figure 2 Comparative effects of GM-CSF and IL-4 on the proliferation of MG-63 cells. The effect of human recombinant GM-CSF, G-CSF, and IL-4 on the proliferation of MG-63 cells was determined by measurement of ^{3}H-thymidine incorporation under defined, serum-free conditions as described previously (40). -○-, GM-CSF; -●-, G-CSF; -□-, IL-4.

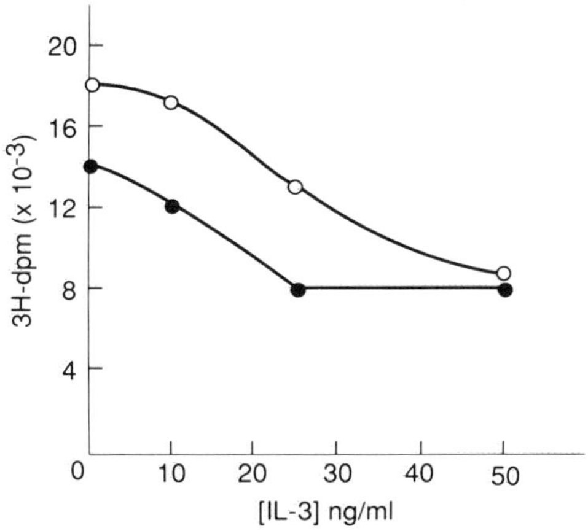

Figure 3 Effect of IL-3 on the proliferation of MCF-7 and MG-63 cells. Human MCF-7 breast carcinoma cells (-●-) and human MG-63 osteosarcoma cells (-○-) were treated with IL-3 under defined, serum-free conditions and proliferation determined by measurement of ^{3}H-thymidine incorporation as described previously (40).

in Figure 4, this eliminated the subsequent ability of MG-63 cells to respond to GM-CSF. Pretreatment with TGF-β partially reduced their subsequent responsiveness to GM-CSF. MG-63 cells can also be induced to proliferate by PDGF, and pretreatment with IL-1β blocks this mitogenic action of PDGF (data not shown). Recent studies have shown that the ability of IL-1β to inhibit the MG-63 cell response to PDGF is correlated with an IL-1β-induced down-regulation of PDGF receptor expression on the cell surface. Whether GM-CSF receptors are similarly affected has not yet been tested.

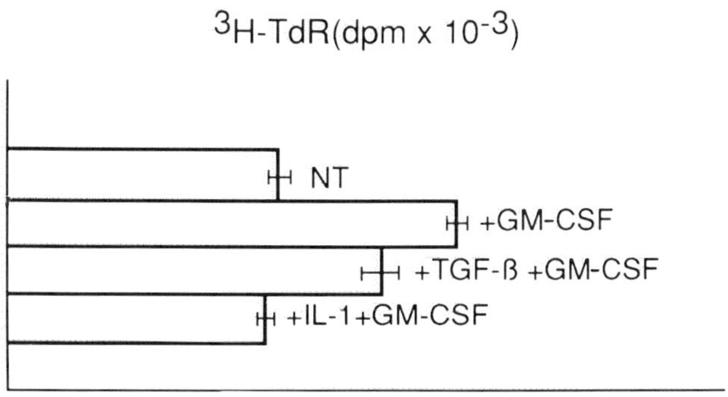

Figure 4 Modulatory effects of IL-1 and TGF-β on the growth stimulatory effect of GM-CSF on MG-63. MG-63 human osteosarcoma cells were placed under serum-free conditions (40) for 5 h at 37°C in 5% CO_2 in the presence or absence of either IL-1β (10 pM) or human TGF-β (1 nM). The medium was then removed, and the cells were washed extensively and overlayed with medium containing human recombinant GM-CSF (80 ng/ml) (Biogen). ^{3}H-thymidine (1 μCi; 2 G/mMol) was then added. ^{3}H-thymidine incorporation was measured after 20 h at 37°C. NT, no treatment.

V. CONCLUSION

Advances in biomedical and recombinant DNA technology have introduced a new era of molecular isolation and characterization that has allowed the rapid identification and production of a multitude of new growth factors that interact with specific receptors on the cell surface. More than a dozen such factors have been well characterized with respect to their ability to stimulate the proliferation of various stages of hematopoietic cell development. Because these factors are also potent stimulators of hematopoiesis in vivo, they offer great promise as therapeutic agents in patients whose conditions are severely limited by hematologic insufficiency. However, coincident with the initiation of clinical trials to evaluate such possibilities has emerged unanticipated but irrefutable evidence that perhaps none of these factors has the hematopoietic tissue specificity suggested by earlier studies.

It is now clear that many of the so-called hematopoietic growth factors are effective stimulators of a variety of nonhematopoietic cell types including certain transformed cells, and the spectrum of responses elicited is as broad as the spectrum of responsive target cells. Nevertheless, particular cells respond to certain factors and not others, and the response elicited by a given cell is also not necessarily the same (see Table 2). Such findings highlight the need to proceed cautiously in any future clinical trial of hematopoietic growth-factor therapy and the need for more information about the role and actions of these factors in vivo. Such findings also reinforce the same molecules being used in a variety of cellular settings to achieve different effects, with specificity being attained by selectivity in intracellular pathway activation. The genes encoding the cell surface receptors for many of these factors have recently been cloned, and their analysis and manipulation should provide new clues about the molecular mechanisms activated in different responsive cell types. Elucidation of the physiological significance of hematopoietic growth factor action on nonhematopoietic cells is thus likely to provide information of general biological significance, and may even open up new possibilities for the treatment of nonhematopoietic tumors.

ACKNOWLEDGEMENTS

This work was supported by operating grants from the National Cancer Institute of Canada. C. J. Eaves is a Terry Fox Cancer Research Scientist of the National Cancer Institute of Canada.

Table 2 Summary of Various Hematopoietic Growth-Factor Effects on Human Osteosarcoma and Breast Carcinoma Cell Lines

Growth factor	Cell line	Concentration for maximal effect	Stimulator
GM-CSF	MCF-7	8 ng/ml	Stimulator
GM-CSF	MG-63	80 ng/ml	Stimulator
G-CSF	MG-63	80 ng/ml	Stimulator
IL-4	MG-63	80 ng/ml	Stimulator
IL-3	MG-63	50 ng/ml	Inhibitor
IL-3	MCF-7	25 ng/ml	Inhibitor
IL-1	MG-63	10^{-11} M	Inhibitor

REFERENCES

1. Erslev AJ, Caro J. Pathophysiology of erythropoietin. In: Dunn CDR, ed. Current concepts in erythropoiesis. New York: Wiley, 1983:1–19.
2. Miyake T, Kung CKH, Goldwasser E. Purification of human erythropoietin. J Biol Chem 1977; 252:5558–64.
3. Eaves CJ, Eaves AC, Erythropoiesis. In: Golde DW, Takaku F, eds. Hematopoietic stem cells. New York: Marcel Dekker, 1985:19–43.
4. Metcalf D. The granulocyte-macrophage colony-stimulating factors. Science 1985; 229:16–22.
5. Metcalf D, Johnson GR, Burgess AW. Direct stimulation by purified GM-CSF of the proliferation of multipotential and erythroid precursor cells. Blood 1980; 55:138–47.
6. Metcalf D, Nicola NA. Proliferative effects of purified granulocyte colony-stimulating factor (G-CSF) on normal mouse hemopoietic cells. J Cell Physiol 1983; 116:198–206.
7. Clark SC, Kamen R. The human hematopoietic colony-stimulating factors. Science 1987; 236:1229–37.
8. Oster W, Lindemann A, Mertelsmann R, Herrmann F. Regulation of gene expression of M-, G-, GM-, and multi-CSF in normal and malignant hematopoietic cells. Blood Cells 1988; 14:443–62.
9. Gimble JM. The function of adipocytes in the bone marrow stroma. New Biologist 1990; 2:304–12.
10. Bazan JF. Structural design and molecular evolution of a cytokine receptor superfamily. Proc Natl Acad Sci USA 1990; 87:6934–8.
11. Krystal G, Alai M, Cutler RL, Dickeson H, Mui ALF, Wognum AW. Hematopoietic growth factor receptors. Hematol Pathol 1991; 5:141-162.
12. Onetto N. Extra hematopoietic effect of colony-stimulating factors. Blood 1989; 74:1446–7.
13. Foulke RS, Marshall MH, Trotta PP, Von Hoff DD. In vitro assessment of the effects of granulocyte-macrophage colony-stimulating factor on primary human tumors and derived lines. Cancer Res 1990; 50:6264–7.
14. Salmon SE, Liu R. Effects of granulocyte-macrophage colony-stimulating factor on in vitro growth of human solid tumors. J Clin Oncol 1989; 7:1346–50.
15. Bevilacqua MP, Pober JS, Wheeler ME, Cotran RS, Gimbrone MA Jr. Interleukin 1 acts on cultured human vascular endothelium to increase the adhesion of polymorphonuclear leukocytes, monocytes, and related leukocyte cell lines. J Immunol 1985; 76:2003–11.
16. Caverder DE, Haskard DO, Joseph B, Ziff M. Interleukin 1 increases the binding of human B and T lymphocytes to endothelial cell monolayers. J Immunol 1986; 136:203–7.
17. Rossi V, Breviario F, Ghezzi P, Dejani PF, Mantovani A. Prostacyclin synthesis induced in vascular cells by Interleukin 1. Science 1985; 229:174–6.
18. Mizel SB, Dayer JM, Krane SM, Mergenhagen SE. Stimulation of rheumatoid synovial cell collagenase and prostaglandin production by partially purified lymphocyte-activating factors (interleukin 1). Proc Natl Acad Sci USA 1981; 78:2474–7.
19. Postlethwaite AE, Raghour R, Stricklin GP, Poppleton H, Seyer JM, Kang AH. Modulation of fibroblast function by interleukin 1: increased steady state accumulation of type 1 procollagen messenger RNAs and stimulation of other functions but not chemotaxis by human recombinant interleukin 1 α and β. J Cell Biol 1988; 106:311–8.
20. Cowen M, Wood DD, Russell GG. Stimulation of the proliferation of human bone cells in vitro by human monocyte products with interleukin 1 activity. J Clin Invest 1985; 75:1223–9.
21. Dedhar S. Regulation of expression of the cell adhesion receptors, integrins, by recombinant human interleukin 1-β in human osteosarcoma cells: inhibition of cell proliferation and stimulation of alkaline phosphatase activity. J Cell Physiol 1989; 138:291–9.

22. Merril JE, Macroglia: Neural cells responsive to lymphokines and growth factors. Immunol Today 1987; 8:146–50.
23. Dower SK, Kronheim SR, Hopp TP, et al. The cell surface receptors for interleukin-1α and interleukin-1β are identical. Nature 1986; 324:266–8.
24. Sehgal PB, May LT, Tamm I, Vilcek J. Human β_2 interferon and B-cell differentiation factor BSF-2 are identical. Science 1987; 235:731–2.
25. Smith AG, Heath JK, Donaldson DD, et al. Inhibition of pluripotential embryonic stem cell differentiation by purified polypeptides. Nature 1988; 336:688–90.
26. Yamamori T, Fukada K, Aebersold R, Korsching S, Fann M-J, Patterson PH. The cholinergic neuronal differentiation factor from heart cells is identical to leukemia inhibitory factor. Science 1989; 246:1412–6.
27. Matsui Y, Zsebo KM, Hogan BLM. Embryonic expression of a haematopoietic growth factor encoded by the S1 locus and the ligand for c-kit. Nature 1990; 347:667–9.
28. Ogawa M, Ikebuchi K, Leary AG. Humoral regulation of stem cell proliferation. Ann NY Acad Sci 1989; 554:185–91.
29. Wong GG, Witek-Giannotti JS, Temple PA, et al. Stimulation of murine hemopoietic colony formation by human IL-6. J Immunol 1988; 140:3040–4.
30. Ishibashi T, Kimura H, Uchida T, Kariyone S, Friese P, Burstein SA. Human interleukin 6 is a direct promoter of maturation of megakaryocytes in vitro. Proc Natl Acad Sci USA 1989; 86:5953–7.
31. Hirano T, Yasukawa K, Harada H, et al. Complementary DNA for a novel human interleukin (BSF-2) that induces B lymphocytes to produce immunoglobulin. Nature 1986; 324:73–6.
32. Gauldie J, Richards C, Harnish D, Lansdorp P, Baumann H. Interferon βb2/B-cell stimulatory factor type 2 shares identity with monocyte-derived hepatocyte-stimulating factor and regulates the major acute phase protein response in liver cells. Proc Natl Acad Sci USA 1987; 84:7251–5.
33. Leary AG, Wong GG, Clark SC, Smith AG, Ogawa M. Leukemia inhibitory factor differentiation-inhibiting activity/human interleukin for DA cells augments proliferation of human hematopoietic stem cells. Blood 1990; 75:1960–4.
34. Verfaillie C, McGlave P. Leukemia inhibitory factor/human interleukin for DA cells: a growth factor that stimulates the in vitro development of multipotential human hematopoietic progenitors. Blood 1991; 77:263–70.
35. Martin FH, Suggs SV, Langley KE, et al. Primary structure and functional expression of rat and human stem cell factor DNAs. Cell 1990; 63:203–11.
36. Anderson DM, Lyman SD, Baird A, et al. Molecular cloning of mast cell growth factor, a hematopoietin that is active in both membrane bound and soluble forms. Cell 1990; 63:235–43.
37. Gearing DP, Gough NM, King JA, et al. Molecular cloning and expression of cDNA encoding a murine myeloid leukaemia inhibitory factor (LIF). EMBO J 1987; 6:3995–4002.
38. Sutherland HJ, Eaves CJ, Lansdorp PM, Thacker JD, Hogge DE. Differential regulation of sequential stages of human hematopoiesis in long-term cultures of highly purified hematopoietic stem cells maintained on genetically engineered murine stromal cells. Blood 1991; 78:666–672.
39. Eaves CJ, Cashman JD, Kay RJ, et al. Mechanisms that regulate the cell cycle status of very primitive hematopoietic cells in long-term human marrow cultures. II. Analysis of positive and negative regulators produced by stromal cells within the adherent layer. Blood 1991; 78:110–117.
40. Dedhar S, Gaboury L, Galloway P, Eaves C. Human granulocyte-macrophage colony-

stimulating factor is a growth factor active on a variety of cell types of nonhemopoietic origin. Proc Natl Acad Sci USA 1988; 85:9253–7.
41. Anagnostou A, Lee ES, Kessimian N, Levinson R, Steiner M. Erythropoietin has a mitogenic and positive chemotactic effect on endothelial cells. Proc Natl Acad Sci USA 1990; 87:5978–82.
42. Bussolino F, Wang JM, Defilippi P, et al. Granulocyte- and granulocyte-macrophage-colony stimulating factors induce human endothelial cells to migrate and proliferate. Nature 1989; 337:471–3.
43. Uzumaki H, Okabe T, Sasaki N, et al. Identification and characterization of receptors for granulocyte colony-stimulating factor on human placenta and trophoblastic cells. Proc Natl Acad Sci USA 1989; 86:9323–6.
44. Gearing DP, King JA, Gough NM, Nicola NA. Expression cloning of a receptor for human granulocyte-macrophage colony-stimulating factor. EMBO J 1989; 8:3667–76.
45. Rettenmier CW, Sacca R, Furman WL, et al. Expression of the human c-fms proto-oncogene product (colony-stimulating factor-1 receptor) on peripheral blood mononuclear cells and choriocarcinoma cell lines. J Clin Invest 1986; 77:1740–6.
46. Lowenthal JW, Castle BE, Christiansen J, et al. Expression of high affinity receptors for murine interleukin 4 (BSF-1) on hemopoietic and nonhemopoietic cells. J Immunol 1988; 140:456–64.
47. Wiktor-Jedrzejczak W, Bartocci A, Ferrante AW Jr, et al. Total absence of colony-stimulating factor 1 in the macrophage-deficient osteopetrotic (op/op) mouse. Proc Natl Acad Sci USA 1990; 87:4828–32.
48. Yoshida H, Hayashi S-I, Kunisada T, et al. The murine mutation osteopetrosis is in the coding region of the macrophage colony stimulating factor gene. Nature 1990; 345:442–3.
49. Ruff MR, Farrar WL, Pert CB. Interferon γ and granulocyte/macrophage colony-stimulating factor inhibit growth and induce antigens characteristic of myeloid differentiation in small-cell lung cancer cell lines. Proc Natl Acad Sci USA 1986; 83:6613–7.
50. Yamashita Y, Nara N, Aoki N. Antiproliferative and differentiative effect of granulocyte-macrophage colony-stimulating factor on a variant human small cell lung cancer cell line. Cancer Res 1989; 49:5334–8.
51. Vellenga E, Biesma B, Meyer C, Wagteveld L, Esselink M, de Vries EGE. The effects of five hematopoietic growth factors on human small cell lung carcinoma cell lines: interleukin 3 enhances the proliferation in one of the eleven cell lines. Cancer Res 1991; 51:73–6.
52. Baldwin GC, Gasson JC, Kaufman SE, et al. Nonhematopoietic tumour cells express functional GM-CSF receptors. Blood 1989; 73:1033–7.
53. Berdel WE, Danhauser-Riedl S, Steinhauser G, Winton EF. Various human hematopoietic growth factors (interleukin-3, GM-CSF, G-CSF) stimulate clonal growth of nonhematopoietic tumor cells. Blood 1989; 73:80–3.
54. Tosabo G, Seamon KB, Goldman ND, et al. Identification of a monocyte-derived human B cell growth factors as interferon-β2 (BSF-2, IL-6). Science 1988; 239:502–4.
55. Chen L, Mony Y, Zilberstein A, Revel M. Growth inhibition of human breast carcinoma and leukemia/lymphoma cell lines by recombinant interferon-β2. Proc Natl Acad Sci USA 1988; 85:8037–41.
56. Tamm I, Cardinale I, Krueger J, Murphy JS, May LT, Sehgal PB. Interleukin 6 decreases cell-cell association and increases motility of ductal breast carcinoma cells. J Exp Med 1989; 170:1649–69.
57. Antman KS, Griffin JD, Elias A, et al. Effect of recombinant human granulocyte-macrophage colony-stimulating factor on chemotherapy-induced myelosuppression. N Engl J Med 1988; 319:593–8.

58. Mitsuyasu RT, Golde DW. Clinical role of granulocyte-macrophage colony-stimulating factor. In: Golde DW, ed. Hematology/oncology/clinics of North America, vol. 3. Philadelphia: WB Saunders, 1989:411–21.
59. Elliott MJ, Vadas MA, Eglinton JM, et al. Recombinant human interleukin-3 and granulocyte-macrophage colony-stimulating factor show common biological effects and binding characteristics on human monocytes. Blood 1989; 74:2349–59.

25

Effects of Cytokines on the Expression of Adhesion Molecules in Allergic Diseases

EDUARDO CALDERON
James A. Haley V.A. Hospital and University of South Florida, Tampa, Florida

I. INTRODUCTION

The binding of a specific allergen, by an IgE-dependent mechanism, to mast cells or basophils results in degranulation, vesicular transport, and release of inflammatory mediators. This reaction induces the early-phase allergic response, leading to smooth-muscle contraction, increased mucus production, and tissue swelling. Four to eight hours after the early phase, the late-phase response begins. It is characterized by the presence of an inflammatory cellular infiltrate. A variety of cells are involved in this hypersensitivity type I reaction, such as epithelial cells, granulocytes (neutrophils, basophils, eosinophils, and mast cells), mononuclear cells (lymphocytes, monocytes, and antigen-presenting cells), and platelets. In addition to chemical mediators, the orchestration of the allergic response depends on communication between interacting cells by a variety of cytokines. Although they have transient and local actions, the production and effects of cytokines are key events for the inflammatory reaction.

Adhesion molecules are cell surface antigens which are essential for the adhesion, activation, and tissue transmigration of circulating blood cells. Adhesion molecules can be constitutively expressed on the surface of human cells or can be induced by inflammatory mediators or cytokines released by cells involved in allergic diseases. Inflammatory mediators which increase or promote expression of adhesion molecules include: histamine, leukotrienes B_4, C_4, and D_4, platelet-activating factor (PAF), hydrogen peroxide, substance P, and neuropeptide Y. Cytokines which cause expression of adhesion molecules include: interleukin (IL)-1, IL-2, IL-3, IL-4, IL-5, IL-6, IL-7, IL-8, tumor necrosis factor (TNF), granulocyte-macrophage colony-stimulating factor (GM-CSF), and immune interferon (γ-IFN). Therefore, interactions among cytokines and adhesion molecules may represent a novel regulatory mechanism of cellular interactions in the pathogenesis of allergic diseases.

II. FUNCTION AND CLASSIFICATION: BASIC ASPECTS

Adhesion molecules are essential for (1–3): (a) adhesion of cells to cells and to the extracellular tissue matrix, (b) leukocyte activation and transmigration from vessels into the tissues, (c) cell growth and proliferation, (d) promotion of antigen-specific recognition and co-stimulatory signals for T-lymphocytes, and (e) leukocyte cytotoxicity and phagocytosis. These membrane antigens have been grouped into three structurally related families (1,4–6) (Table 1).

A. Immunoglobulin Supergene Family

The large immunoglobulin supergene family of glycoproteins shows diversity in function and tissue distribution. It has been named "immunoglobulin" because its members share one or more immunoglobulin domains. This family includes the following 10 members: (a) lymphocyte function-associated antigen (LFA)-2 (CD2), which has a cytoplasmic domain which may be a binding domain for a cytoplasmic enzyme or a cytoskeletal element which facilitates migration of T-cells; (b) T-cell receptor (TCR or

Table 1 Classification of Adhesion Molecules and Their Ligands

A.	*Immunoglobulin supergene family*	*Ligand*
	LFA-2 (CD2)	LFA-3
	T-cell receptor (TCR or CD3)	
	LFA-3 (CD58)	CD2
	ICAM-1 (CD54)	LFA-1
	ICAM-2	LFA-1
	VCAM-1	VLA-4
	MHC class I	CD8
	MCH class II	CD4
B.	*Integrin family*	
	1. Very late activation antigens or β_1 (CD29) group:	
	VLA-1	Laminin, collagen
	VLA-2	Laminin, collagen
	VLA-3	Laminin, collagen, fibronectin
	VLA-4	VCAM-1, fibronectin
	VLA-5	Fibronectin
	VLA-6	Laminin
	2. Leu-CAMs or β_2 (CD18) group:	
	LFA-1 (CD11a/CD18)	ICAM-1, ICAM-2 and an unknown antigen
	Mac-1 (CD11b/CD18)	ICAM-1, iC3b, fibrinogen
	p150,95 (CD11c/CD18)	ICAM-1, iC3b
	3. Cytoadhesins or β_3 group:	
	VNR	Fibrinogen, vWf, fibronectin, vitronectin
	Platelet glyc IIb/IIIa	Vitronectin, vWf, fibrinogen
C.	*Selectin family*	
	ELAM-1	Sialyl-Lewis X determinant
	LAM-1	Unknown
	GMP-140 (CD62)	CD15 (lacto-N-fucopentose III)

CD3), which is expressed by T-cells; (c) LFA-3 (CD58), which is the cell surface adhesive ligand for CD2 and has a broad tissue distribution; (d) intercellular adhesion molecule (ICAM)-1 (CD54), expressed at low levels on most leukocytes, is the ligand for integrins LFA-1, Mac-1, and p150,95. ICAM-1 is expressed close to the high-affinity IL-2 receptor (R) and due to their close proximity and possibly to their functions, the two are named "ICAM-1-IL-2R complex" (7); (e) ICAM-2, which is homologous to ICAM-1, consists of two immunoglobulin domains and is constitutively present on endothelial cells; (f) vascular cell adhesion molecule (VCAM)-1, which is expressed by cytokine-stimulated vascular endothelial cells. It allows eosinophils, lymphocytes, and/or monocytes to adhere through their integrin ligand, VLA-4; (g) CD8, present on cytotoxic and suppressor lymphocytes; and (h) CD4, present on T-helper cells and eosinophils, the reciprocal or counter-receptors for (i,j) major hystocompatibility complex (MHC) classes I and II, respectively. Of great significance, Corrigan and Kay showed an increased expression of MHC class II on $CD4^+$ lymphocytes of acute severe asthmatic patients (8).

B. Integrin Family

Integrins, expressed by almost all human cells, are heterodimers composed of an α and a β chain (9). Integrins have been classified in seven groups because seven β chains have been identified. The name "integrin" is due to the ability of these antigens to link or "integrate" the extracellular space with the cytoskeleton. Integrins play a role in platelet aggregation, tissue repair, and tumor invasion, but their outstanding functions are for cell-matrix adhesion and leukocyte transmigration to inflammatory sites. Integrins facilitate the movement of immunological cells into an inflammatory site and promote their physical attachment to their targets at the site of an ongoing immune response. Integrins mediate the adhesion of cells to fibronectin, laminin, or collagens by recognizing specific peptide sequences. The first tripeptide to be identified as an adhesive recognition sequence for β_1, β_3, and β_5 integrins was L-arginine-L-glycyl-L-aspartyl (RGD) (5). The three first groups of integrins are well known:

(a) The "very late activation" (because the first two members appear after prolonged lymphocyte stimulation) or β_1 group includes six members with the common denomination VLA. In this regard, $CD4^+$ lymphocytes of patients with acute severe asthma showed an increased expression of VLA-1 as compared with those from healthy control individuals (8).

(b) The LeuCAM (β_2 or CD18) group has three members: LFA-1, Mac-1, and p150,95. LFA-1, present only on leukocytes, is the receptor for ICAM-1 and ICAM-2. There is evidence for the existence of a third ligand for LFA-1 which has a strength of interaction between that of ICAM-1 and ICAM-2 (10). The interaction of LFA-1 and ICAM-1 is a potent co-stimulus for TCR-mediated lymphocyte activation, suggesting that LFA-1/ICAM-1 is of major physiological importance as a co-stimulatory signal (11). Mac-1 is present on neutrophils, monocytes, macrophages, large granular lymphocytes, and some B-cells. p150,95 is found on the membranes of macrophages, monocytes, and granulocytes. Leukocyte adhesion deficiency (LAD) is a disease caused by genetic mutations of the gene of the CD18 chain (12). Leukocytes of LAD patients cannot migrate from the intravascular to the extravascular space, resulting in recurrent life-threatening bacterial infections, progressive periodontitis, lack of pus formation, and leukocytosis.

(c) The cytoadhesins or β_3 group includes the vitronectin receptor (VNR) and the platelet glycoprotein IIb/IIIa (gpIIb/IIIa) complex, which bind to vitronectin, fibrinogen, and von Willebrandt factor (9). Cytoadhesins are expressed on platelets, endothelial cells, fibroblasts, and smooth muscle cells. Patients with Glanzmann's thrombasthenia have a genetic deficiency of gpIIb/IIIa. In consequence, platelets are not able to bind vitronectin, fibrinogen, and von Willebrandt factor.

C. Selectin Family

Selectins, or LECCAMs, are membrane antigens with a lectin domain in the N-terminus, suggesting that members of this family bind to sugars. The name "selectin" was suggested to indicate the ability to select cells trafficking across the vascular endothelium. Selectins are expressed on activated lymphocytes, neutrophils, endothelial cells, and platelets. Members of this family include LAM-1, ELAM-1, and GMP-140. Leukocyte adhesion molecule (LAM)-1, the human homolog to murine MEL-14, participates in neutrophil extravasation under conditions of flow at inflamed tissues (13). Endothelial cell adhesion molecule (ELAM)-1 is not constitutively present on endothelium in vitro or in vivo but it is expressed by cytokine-stimulated endothelial cells. ELAM-1 is involved mainly in neutrophil adhesion to endothelium (14). Granule membrane protein (GMP)-140 (CD62) can be mobilized in 5 min from Palade-Weibel bodies to the surface of thrombin- or histamine-stimulated endothelial cells and platelets (15). Its glycoprotein receptor, containing sialic acid, is constitutively expressed on neutrophils (16).

1. Low-Affinity IgE Receptor

The low-affinity IgE receptor ($Fc_{\epsilon}RII$) contains the tripeptide RGD and has homology with the selectin family. Therefore, it may function, in part, as a member of the adhesion molecule system for two reasons:

(a) The extracellular C-terminus of $Fc_{\epsilon}RII$ contains RGD (17). The immunoprecipitation of some molecules of $Fc_{\epsilon}RII$ by polyclonal anti-RGDS (L-arginine-L-glycyl-L-aspartyl-L-serine) antibody, and the inhibition of the binding of monoclonal antibody (MAb) BB10 (anti-eosinophil $Fc_{\epsilon}RII$) to eosinophils and a B-lymphocyte line using the polypeptide RGDS, indicate the presence of RGD on both eosinophil and B-cell $Fc_{\epsilon}RII$. Additionally, a cross-reactivity reaction between monoclonal antibodies BB10 and gp63 (anti-*Leishmania*), which contains RGD, suggests that both of them share the RGD sequence. The significant inhibition of the IgE-dependent cytotoxicity against leishmania by preincubation of eosinophils with MAb BB10, gp63, and MAb 135 (anti-CD23), or polyclonal anti-RGDS antibody or RGDS, suggests that the tripeptide RGD is necessary for $Fc_{\epsilon}RII$ function. Therefore $Fc_{\epsilon}RII$ may play a role in eosinophil and B-cell adhesion to integrins located on endothelial cells (i.e., vitronectin receptors) and on activated leukocytes (i.e., VLA group).

(b) The extracellular C-terminus of $Fc_{\epsilon}RII$ also possesses a marked homology with human lectins (18), and lectin is the important domain in the N-terminus of the selectin family. These adhesion molecules bind sugars through the lectin domain. The binding region of $Fc_{\epsilon}RII$ to IgE, the most heavily glycosylated of the immunoglobulins, corresponds to those amino acids homologous to the carbohydrate-binding domain of lectins. $Fc_{\epsilon}RII$ shares other basic structures with selectins (19). Structural homology includes four conserved cysteines and several amino acid sequences. Therefore, it is possible that besides binding IgE, $Fc_\epsilon RII$ has additional functions where carbohydrate binding is critical. For instance, it has been shown that IgE-coated particles are phagocytosed by $Fc_\epsilon RII$-bearing macrophages, $Fc_\epsilon RII$ acts synergistically with Mac-1 and both are required for lysis of parasites, and $Fc_\epsilon RII$ promotes release of inflammatory mediators by monocytes, eosinophils, and platelets (20–22).

III. CYTOKINES INVOLVED IN ALLERGIC DISEASES ENHANCE THE EXPRESSION OF ADHESION MOLECULES

Cytokines with a regulatory role in leukocyte participation in the early- and late-phase allergic responses induce and/or increase the expression of some adhesion molecules (Table 2).

A. IL-1 and Tumor Necrosis Factor

The abilities of (a) eosinophils to produce IL-1 and IL-1α mRNA, (b) human circulating monocytes to secrete IL-1β and TNF_α, (c) lung cells to release TNF-$_\alpha$, and (d) mast cells to produce IL-1 and TNF_α, in an IgE-dependent fashion suggest that IL-1 and TNF play a role in the allergic response (23–26). Since these cytokines can induce the expression of adhesion molecules by inflammatory cells, IL-1 and TNF can also induce the expression of adhesion molecules on cells involved in the pathogenesis of the allergic diseases.

1. Recombinant (r) rIL-1β-activated endothelium facilitates PMNL adhesion and transmigration, which requires the coordinated and sequential expression of ELAM-1 and ICAM-1 (27). After 4 h of incubation with rIL-1β, leukocyte adhesion and transmigration were increased three- to fourfold at a time when ELAM-1 expression had peaked and ICAM-1 was modestly increased. PMNL transmigration was blocked by >90% using monoclonal antibodies anti-ELAM-1 or anti-ICAM-1. After 24 to 48 h, ELAM-1 expression decreased and ICAM-1 expression peaked. This was coincident with PMNL adhesion, while transmigration had returned to basal levels. Monoclonal antibodies anti-LFA-1, Mac-1, or CD18 (counter-receptor of ICAM-1) also blocked PMNL transmigration. This study suggests that IL-1β promotes PMNL transmigration by inducing the coordinate and sequential expression of ELAM-1 and ICAM-1.

2. TNF_α stimulates neutrophil adhesion to fibrinogen-coated surfaces, which is mediated by CD11c/CD18. p150,95 is a receptor that recognizes the sequence L-glycine-L-proline-L-arginine (Gly-Pro-Arg) in the N-terminal domain of the Aα-chain of fibrinogen (28). Monoclonal antibodies of LeuM5 and 3.9 (anti-α-subunit of p150,95) inhibit adhesion of TNF-stimulated neutrophils to surfaces coated with fibrinogen. Therefore, in vivo, TNF_α-stimulated neutrophils can also show increased adhesion to fibrinogen present in basement membranes.

3. Human circulating neutrophils adhere to IL-1-stimulated human umbilical vein endothelial cell (HUVEC) monolayers in vitro by the expression of the lectin adhesion molecule-1 (LAM-1) (13). Under conditions of flow, MAb DREG-56 (anti-LAM-1) reduces adhesion of neutrophils by >50%, indicating that LAM-1 on the surface of neutrophils plays a basic role in the adhesion of circulating neutrophil to endothelium. LAM-1 is necessary to bind unstimulated neutrophils in the circulation to IL-1-stimulated endothelial cells.

Table 2 Adhesion Molecules Expressed by Granulocytes After Cytokine Stimulation over a Given Time Period

Granulocyte	Adhesion molecule expressed/activated	Cytokine inducer	Time	Ref.
Neutrophil	Sialyl-Lewis X determinant[a,b]			
	LAM-1	IL-1	3–10 min	13
	CD18	TNF_{α}	5–30 min	69
	Mac-1	GM-CSF	60 min	62
	LNR	TNF	60 min	67
Eosinophil	VLA-4[a,c]			
	Mac-1	IL-5, IL-3, and GM-CSF	60 min	44
	p150,95	IL-5, IL-3 and GM-CSF	60 min	44
Basophil	ICAM-1[a]			
	VLA-4[a]			
	CD11b	IL-3	1h	81
	CD11c	IL-3	1h	81
Mast cell	Laminin receptor[a]	IL-3 (enhances)		85
	Fibronectin receptor[a]			
	ICAM-1	IL-4	4 days	42

[a] Constitutively expressed.

[b] ELAM-1, the ligand for Sialyl-Lewis X determinant, can be expressed on epithelial cells within 6 h after cytokine stimulation.

[c] VCAM-1, the ligand for VLA-4, can be expressed by epithelial cells after 4 to 6 h by cytokine stimulation.

4. Either IL-1 or TNF_α induces the expression of VCAM-1 on endothelial cells in vitro after 4 to 6 h of stimulation, and VCAM-1 remains at high levels for at least 72 h (29). VCAM-1 mRNA is present on endothelial cells after 2 h of stimulation, and the lymphocyte binding to endothelium parallels the mRNA induction. These findings are consistent with an active role for IL-1 and TNF_α inducing, on endothelial cells, expression of VCAM-1 to recruit inflammatory cells to sites of aseptic inflammation or infection (i.e., eosinophils). The induction kinetics suggest that VCAM-1 may act in both acute and chronic inflammation.

5. Either rIL-1β or rTNF_α induces the expression of ELAM-1 on human endothelial cells in vitro (14). ELAM-1 expression peaked at 4 to 6 h and was decaying at 24 h. Cell surface ELAM-1 expression paralleled that of its mRNA. Since the early induction and high turnover rates of ELAM-1 mRNA and ELAM-1 are consistent with the rapid neutrophil migration at sites of acute inflammation, this study suggests that IL-1β and TNF_α, by inducing ELAM-1, promote neutrophil adhesion to endothelium. A complementary study showed that ELAM-1 expression by endothelial cells in vivo occurred concurrently with the inflammatory cell infiltrate by 4 h after an intradermal skin test using specific allergens in allergic patients (30). In vitro, anti-TNF_α and anti-IL-1 antibodies blocked the expression of ELAM-1, suggesting that ELAM-1 expression by endothelial cells may have a role in leukocyte transmigration into allergic skin reactions.

6. Either IL-1β or TNF_α enhances ICAM-1 expression by monkey bronchial epithelial and endothelial cells in vitro (31). The distribution of ICAM-1 is topographically correlated with areas containing inflammatory cells. Therefore, the expression of several adhesion molecules on both endothelial cells and granulocytes is evoked by either IL-1β or TNF_α cytokines.

B. IL-2

IL-2 may play a role in the pathogenesis of allergic diseases because IL-2 increases the production of several cytokines by lymphocytes. IL-2 production in vitro by T-lymphocytes from children with asthma, but not from controls, has been observed after stimulation with *Dermatophagoides farinae* antigens (32). IL-2 stimulates circulating eosinophils to increase absolute counts and to become hypodense (33). Human eosinophils express IL-2R, and its binding leads to eosinophil activation and migration (34). IL-2 was 1000-fold more potent on a molar basis than PAF or C5a.

IL-2 increases the expression of ICAM-1 by memory T-cells after 24-48 h of incubation (35). MAb RR1/1 (anti-ICAM-1) blocks ICAM-1 expression and T-cell proliferation as well, suggesting a role for ICAM-1 in the immune response. This study demonstrated the autocrine capacity of activated T-cells to express ICAM-1 because they have the ability to produce IL-2. Using an immunoperoxidase technique, an in-vivo study of patients on IL-2 therapy for metastatic cancer showed that IL-2 induced the expression of ELAM-1 and ICAM-1 (36). Although the mechanism to produce these adhesion molecules is not clear (because IL-2 is able to induce the production of other cytokines, which can also induce ELAM-1 and ICAM-1), the study showed that IL-2 stimulated the expression of ELAM-1 by postcapillary venular endothelium and ICAM-1 by stromal cells and mononuclear cells.

C. IL-3

IL-3 increases eosinophil survival and histamine release by basophils which possess IL-3 high-affinity receptors. Indirect immunofluorescence and flow cytometric analysis revealed that rIL-3 treatment led to rapid and sustained increases in basophil surface expression of CD11 (37). Monoclonal anti-CD11 and anti-CD18 decreased the basophil adherence induced by rIL-3, suggesting important roles for the α and β chains of the integrin family. Additionally, human (h)rIL-3 stimulated human monocyte adhesion to endothelium (38). Monocyte adhesion was, in part, inhibited by MAb 60.3 (anti-CD18) but not by MAb 60.1 (anti-CD11b). The stimulation had biphasic kinetics: an early phase detectable by 10 min, and a late phase seen after 9 h of incubation. The early phase did not result from protein synthesis, but the late phase was totally dependent on de novo protein synthesis. These results suggest that the CD18 chain of the integrins but not the α chain of Mac-1 is important for monocyte adhesion to endothelial cells.

D. IL-4

IL-4, produced by mast cells and T-lymphocytes, induces mast cell differentiation and IgE synthesis and thus exacerbates allergic diseases. IL-4 induces the expression of VCAM-1 by endothelial cells, increases the expression of ICAM-1 by mast cells and macrophages, but decreases the expression of ICAM-1 and ELAM-1 by endothelial cells. IL-4 decreases ICAM-1 expression on endothelial cells (39). In addition, IL-4 inhibits, at least in part, ICAM-1 expression of cytokine-stimulated endothelial cells which was induced by IL-1, TNF, and γ-IFN. Furthermore, ELAM-1 expression is induced by IL-1 and TNF. The inhibitory effect of IL-4 on the expression of ICAM-1 and ELAM-1, antigens related to PMNL adhesion to endothelial cells, suggests that IL-4 does not allow PMNL attachment to endothelium. However, IL-4 augments adhesiveness of endothelial cells for T-cells (40). IL-4 induces the adhesion of lymphocytes to microvascular endothelial cells, and IL-1β enhances this action (41). This suggests that IL-4 enhances binding by increasing the expression or accessibility of endothelial cell surface receptors for lymphocytes. MAb anti-LFA-1 did not diminish the increased adhesion resulting from IL-4 stimulation. It was concluded that the adhesion molecule induced by IL-4 is unknown. MAb 6G10 (anti-VCAM-1) blocks the lymphocyte adhesion to these microvascular endothelial cells, suggesting that VCAM-1 is the adhesion molecule which mediates lymphocyte binding to microvascular endothelium. IL-4 promotes expression of ICAM-1 and ICAM-1 mRNA by human mast cells and macrophages (42). Therefore, there are several mechanisms by which IL-4 exerts its pro-inflammatory effects in allergic diseases.

E. IL-5

IL-5, produced by lymphocytes, mast cells, and eosinophils, promotes terminal differentiation of eosinophil precursors, enhances the effector capacity of mature eosinophils, and prolongs the survival of eosinophils in vitro. Furthermore, IL-5 mRNA is present in the bronchial mucosa of asthmatics (43). The presence of IL-5 explains, in part, the eosinophilic infiltration present in asthma and in other allergies. IL-5 enhances the in-vitro eosinophil adherence to human vascular endothelial cells which is dependent on the CD11/18 expression (44). The enhancement attachment is not observed for neutrophils. Therefore, IL-5 (and to a lesser extent IL-3) is a potent and selective stimulant for eosinophil but not neutrophil adhesion to endothelial cells.

F. IL-6

Epithelial cells and leukocytes involved in allergic diseases, such as T-cells, mast cells, and activated macrophages, produce IL-6 (45). IL-6 probably has adverse actions on allergies, since it potentiates IL-4-dependent IgE synthesis and also promotes the in-vitro survival of eosinophils (45,46). Recombinant hIL-6 induces on cultured U937 cells (human promonocytic cells) the expression of ICAM-1 as well as the integrins CD18, CD11b, and CD11c (47). IL-6 induces both a dose-dependent growth inhibition and expression of those adhesion molecules. A specific anti-rhIL-6 antiserum completely inhibits IL-6 effects.

G. IL-7

Roles for IL-7 in allergic diseases have not been established yet. However, IL-7 may play a role, since it has lymphopoietic properties and since lymphocytes have critical function due to their immunoregulatory functions. IL-7 is an important growth factor for human lymphocyte progenitors and for mature T-cells and is also a potent stimulus for proliferation (48,49). IL-7 gives a weak costimulatory signal that promotes T-cell proliferation triggered by MAb anti-CD3; however, after 2 h of stimulation, it did not influence the expression of ICAM-1 (49). Additionally, IL-7 increased the IL-2-induced proliferation by MAb 64.1 (anti-CD3) or T-cells compared to IL-2 or IL-7 alone. IL-2, IL-6, or IL-7 alone or in combination did not increase ICAM-1 expression in T-cells stimulated with lesser concentrations of MAb 64.1. Stimulation of CD3 augmented ICAM-1 expression by more than 85%. However, another study showed an opposite effect in that IL-7 induced a high degree of expression of ICAM-1 on lymphokine-activated killer cells (48). This paralleled the enhanced expression of IL-2R. No effect was observed for LFA-1 and LFA-3.

H. IL-8

IL-8 induces the expression of Mac-1 and p150,95 on PLMNLs and decreases the expression of ELAM-1 by endothelial cells. IL-1 and TNF stimulate the production of IL-8 by bronchial epithelial and endothelial cells, alveolar macrophages, monocytes, and T-lymphocytes. IL-8 is a cytokine chemotactic for human basophils and neutrophils, stimulates the histamine release by basophils from normal and allergic individuals, and induces neutrophils to produce leukotriene B_4 (LTB_4) (50–52).

A leukocyte adhesion inhibitor is secreted by endothelial cells. It is apparently identical to IL-8 and acts on neutrophils to inhibit binding to ELAM-1 (53). This suggests that IL-8 may act to limit the extent of leukocyte-vessel wall adhesion. However, IL-8 increases in PMNLs the expression of Mac-1 and p150,95, in 15 min, promoting adherence to endothelial cells (54).

I. γ-Interferon

Viral infections stimulate inflammatory cells to increase the production of γ-IFN. This helps to explain the bronchial hyperresponsiveness observed in viral infections in allergic asthmatic patients. Several effects of γ-IFN on endothelial cell expression of adhesion molecules have been observed. γ-IFN augmented and prolonged the expression of ELAM-1 by human endothelial cells (55). ELAM-1 is not constitutively expressed by endothelial cells, but its expression was induced by IL-1 or TNF. Whereas γ-IFN, per se, did not induce expression of ELAM-1, it enhanced and prolonged the expression of ELAM-1. γ-IFN increased the expression of ICAM-1. γ-IFN plus TNF, but not plus IL-1, synergistically increased ICAM-1, ELAM-1, and MHC class I expression. It is necessary to note that treatment of HUVEC with either TNF or IL-1 caused transient induction of ELAM-1 and sustained expression of ICAM-1 (56). TNF but not IL-1 also increased the expression of MHC class I. γ-IFN stimulated lymphocyte adhesion and migration through endothelial cell monolayers (57). γ-IFN, which is more potent than IL-1β and TNF_{α}, enhanced ICAM-1 expression by cultured monkey bronchial epithelial cells in a concentration-dependent fashion (31). ICAM-1 contributed to the eosinophil in-vivo infiltration and increase in airway responsiveness. Finally, on cultured human keratinocytes, γ-IFN induced the expression of ICAM-1 (58). Using indirect immunofluorescence, it was observed that ICAM-1 was strongly expressed in a diffuse cytoplasmic pattern with an intense cell surface expression. The induced expression of ICAM-1 provides evidence for a modulatory function of keratinocytes in epidermal leukocyte trafficking.

J. Granulocyte-macrophage Colony-stimulating Factor

GM-CSF, produced by T-cells, endothelial cells, epithelial cells, neutrophils, and eosinophils, induces eosinophilopoiesis and activates mature eosinophils and increases eosinophil survival in vitro (59,60). In addition, GM-CSF mRNA is present in allergen-induced late-phase cutaneous reactions in allergic individuals (61). Therefore, GM-CSF may have a negative effect in the pathogenesis of the allergic diseases.

GM-CSF induces the expression of CD11b and decreases the expression of LAM-1 on the surface of neutrophils (62). The exposure of neutrophils, monocytes, and their precursors to GM-CSF induced the rapid and complete loss of LAM-1 from the cell surface but did not have an effect on LAM-1 expressed on lymphocytes. hrGM-CSF enhanced the adhesion of human monocytes to HUVEC and to plastic surfaces (38). MAb 60.3 (anti-CD18) inhibited this adhesion by 50% and MAb 60.1 (anti-Mac-1) did not inhibit it. This study suggested that CD18 may have an essential function for monocyte adhesion. GM-CSF induced the rapid expression of CD11b on human granulocytes in vivo (63). GM-CSF was administered as a continuous infusion at a dose of 32 or 64 μg/kg/day to nine adult patients with sarcoma. A transient leukopenia developed within 15 min of the initiation of the treatment, which was associated with a significant increase in the expression of CD11b by granulocytes compared to basal levels. The increase in CD11b was seen within 30 min of administration of GM-CSF in two of three patients and was present even 24 h later in all patients.

IV. RELATIONSHIPS BETWEEN CYTOKINES AND ADHESION MOLECULES EXPRESSED BY GRANULOCYTES INVOLVED IN THE PATHOGENESIS OF THE ALLERGIC DISEASES.

A. Neutrophils (Figure 1)

Histologic analysis indicates that cutaneous leukocyte infiltration occurs after IgE stimulation and mast cell degranulation. The infiltration is TNF_{α} dependent. Neutrophils represent more than 90% of the leukocyte infiltrate, reaching the highest levels by 6 to 12 h and diminishing by 24 h (64). In addition, neutrophil chemotactic activity appears in serum of asthmatic patients undergoing a provocative challenge by allergen

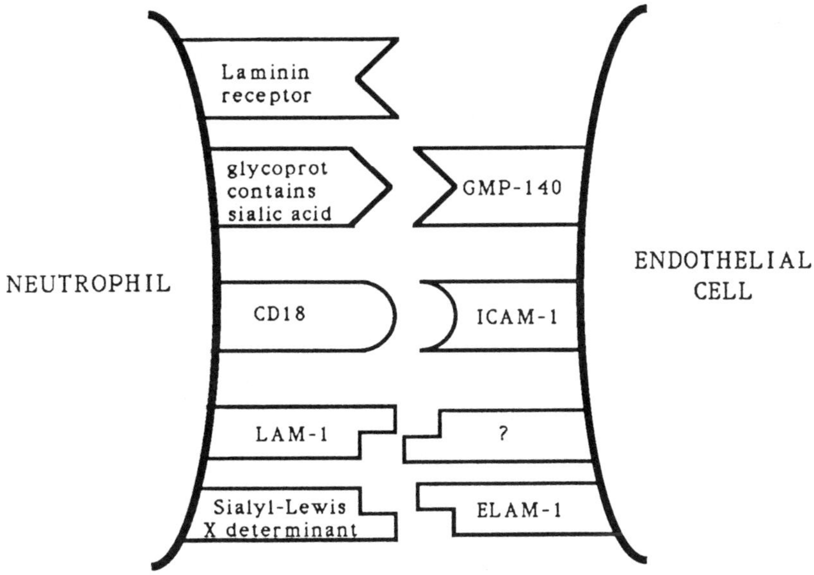

Figure 1 Schematic representation of neutrophil adhesion molecules and their ligands expressed by vascular endothelial cells.

or exercise, during the early and late phases of the asthmatic response (65). Both studies support the concept that neutrophils accumulate and participate in challenged tissues for IgE-dependent allergic responses.

PMNL granules containing CD11b, CD18, LNR, FNR, and VNR have been named adhesomes (66). rTNF stimulation induces fusion of adhesomes with the plasma membrane and expression of both CD18 and LNR. Therefore, through the fused adhesomes, PMNLs may express several extracellular matrix receptors. Human neutrophils express integrins of the CD18 group in an inactive form. After stimulation, these integrins convert to an active status. Mac-1 participates in both neutrophil adhesion and communication between the plasma membrane and the cytoskeleton during ingestion (67). Chemotactic peptides and lipid mediators enhance human neutrophil adherence in vitro to endothelial cells in a dose-dependent manner with a rapid time course (68). Stimulated neutrophil adherence to human endothelial cells is dependent on cell surface expression of the LFA-1, Mac-1, and p150,95 molecules. In addition, $hTNF_{\alpha}$ increases neutrophil adhesion for endothelial cells in 5 to 30 min, and MAb 60.3 (anti-CD18) blocks that adhesion (69). IL-1 stimulated HUVEC increases adhesion of PMNLs, and MAb DREG56 (anti-LAM-1) reduces the adhesion by 30% (70). MAb TS1/18 (anti-CD18) inhibits the adhesion by 57%, and both monoclonal antibodies increase the inhibition by 76%. This study suggests that the LAM-1 and CD18 are both required for maximum PMNL adhesion.

Stimulation of endothelial cells by IL-1 and TNF_{α}, after 6 h of incubation, causes endothelial cell binding to inactivated PMNLs. This process is mediated by ELAM-1 expression. However, there is a more rapid mechanism which is stimulated by PAF, histamine, or thrombin in 5 min, inducing the expression of CD11/CD18 or GMP-140 by endothelial cells. There is a complementary mechanism, which is mediated by the expression of GMP-140 on oxygen radical-stimulated endothelial cells between 1 and 4 h of incubation (71). ELAM-1, expressed by cytokine-stimulated endothelial cells, participates in PMNL adhesion through the expression of the ligand sialyl-Lewis X determinant. Soluble ELAM-1 serves as a conventional neutrophil chemoattractant (72). After binding its neutrophil ligand, ELAM-1 recruits the participation of additional adhesion molecules by triggering activation of LFA-1 and Mac-1 on the surface of neutrophils, all of which participate in diapedesis. Therefore ELAM-1 has the ability to generate responses in cells that bear it.

B. Eosinophils (Figure 2)

ICAM-1, which is upregulated on inflamed monkey bronchial epithelial and endothelial cells in vivo, mediates eosinophil adhesion to endothelial cells in vitro (31). Monoclonal antibodies RR1/1 or R15.7 (anti-ICAM-1) inhibit eosinophil adhesion to cultured airway epithelial cells. Treatment of monkeys intravenously with MAb R6.5 (anti-ICAM-1) diminishes the eosinophil infiltration and bronchial hyperresponsivenss. Bronchial eosinophilic infiltrate, which is characteristic of asthmatic inflammation, is blocked by intravenous MAb R6.5. Therefore, ICAM-1, expressed by inflamed airway epithelium, contributes to eosinophil adhesion and may also participate in eosinophil migration into the bronchi. IL-1 or TNF, through the expression of both ELAM-1 and ICAM-1, induce adhesion of eosinophils and neutrophils to endothelial cells (73). The kinetics and dose responses of adhesions of both granulocytes to IL-1- and TNF-stimulated endothelial cells appear similar. However, this study shows that the eosinophil adhesion peaks later and persists longer than the neutrophil adhesion.

In addition to cytokine (i.e., IL-3, IL-5, and GM-CSF) induction of eosinophil adhesion, inflammatory mediators may augment the eosinophil-selective adhesion mechan-

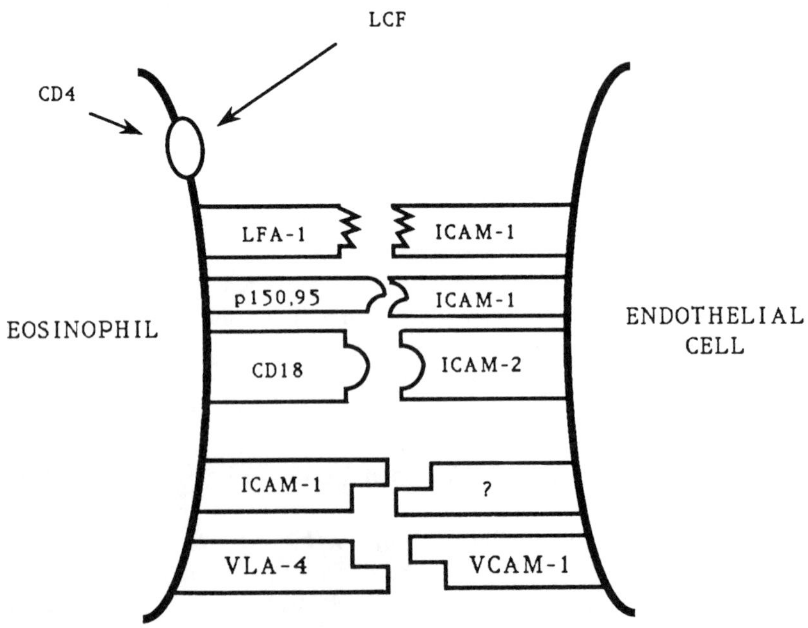

Figure 2 Schematic representation of adhesion molecules expressed by eosinophils and their reciprocal receptors on endothelial cells.

ism and the accumulation of eosinophils in asthmatic airway, providing a greater capacity as compared with neutrophils to survive in the bronchial tissue. Expression of LFA-1, p150,95, and ICAM-1 by human eosinophils in vitro is greater than that observed in peripheral eosinophils from atopic individuals (74). Another study showed that human eosinophils express CD18, and its expression is significantly reduced on hypodense eosinophils (75), which may signify that these activated eosinophils do not transmigrate. CD18 also is expressed by endothelial cells after 4 h of stimulation with IL-1 and TNF, thus increasing their adhesiveness to eosinophils. IL-1, $rTNF_{\alpha}$, and LPS stimulate the adhesion of endothelial cells to eosinophils in time and dose-dependent reactions. Moreover, PAF but not lyso-PAF increases eosinophil adhesion to endothelial cells twofold (76). MAb 60.3 (anti-CD18) inhibits eosinophilic binding to endothelial cells, demonstrating that CD18 adhesion molecules are involved in the induced adherence. This study suggests that the initiation of the tissue eosinophilic infiltration may result from both eosinophil and endothelium activation. However, it may be the result of the endothelial cell activation alone.

Human eosinophils constitutively express VLA-4, which mediates specific adhesion to endothelial cells (77). After 6 h of incubation with IL-1 or TNF, endothelial cells express VCAM-1, the VLA-4 ligand, which increases eosinophil but not neutrophil binding. MAb anti-VLA-4 almost completely inhibited the eosinophil adhesion. The common expression by human eosinophils and lymphocytes of VLA-4 and its role in mediating their adhesion to VCAM-1, expressed by endothelial cells, may facilitate the eosinophil and lymphocyte infiltration present in allergic diseases (78). In this regard, IL-4, a key cytokine in allergic diseases, has particular functions increasing expression of VCAM-1 and decreasing expression of ICAM-1 and ELAM-1 on endothelial cells. All of the above contribute to eosinophil and lymphocyte infiltration rather than neutrophil infiltration. Eosinophil adherence and transmigration to nonstimulated endothelial cells are physiological characteristics of blood eosinophils and require Ca^{2+} and Mg^{2+} (79). Stimulated eosinophils adhere to endothelial cells by the expression of CD11/CD18, while resting eosinophils adhere to stimulated endothelium by the expression of VCAM-1. This suggests that VCAM-1 and the endothelial ligand for CD11/CD18, probably ICAM-1, mediate the endothelial adhesion of eosinophils. Finally, binding of eosinophilic CD4 for the lymphocyte chemoattractant factor (LCF) allows eosinophils to migrate on nitrocellulose membranes (80). rLCF does not influence other eosinophilic functions, such as degranulation, superoxide production, leukotriene C_4 production, in-vitro survival, and expression of CD11 or IL-2R. Therefore, at sites of inflammatory responses, where activated T-cells are present, CD4 can also mediate eosinophil migration into the tissues.

C. Basophils (Figure 3)

Human anti-IgE-mediated basophil degranulation is associated with a rapid and sustained increase in the surface expression of CD11b and CD11c and decreases in LAM-1 (81). The CD11 expression was more sensitive and rapid than histamine release. This study suggests that anti-IgE basophil degranulation in vivo may be accompanied or preceded by CD11b and CD11c expression, which in turn may activate some cellular functions. Human basophils express ICAM-1 to a greater extent than lung mast cells. This suggests that mast cells, compared to basophils, express a lower number of ICAM-1 molecules and/or that mast cells may express distinct epitopes of the ICAM-1 (82).

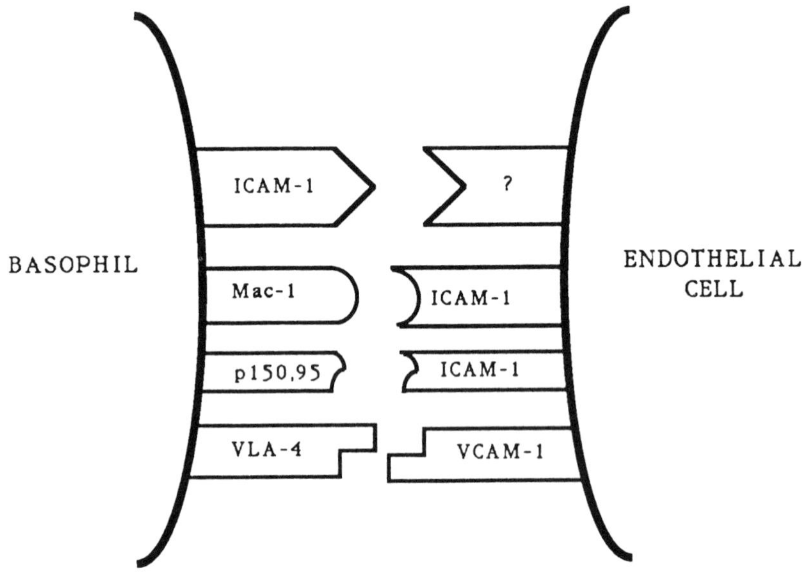

Figure 3 Adhesion molecules expressed on basophils and their counter-receptors on the surface of endothelial cells.

Basophils also express VLA-4α, and endothelial cells express the counter-receptor, VCAM-1 (83). IL-1-stimulated endothelial cells, within 4 h, demonstrate four- to eightfold increased adhesion to basophils. Treatment with anti-VCAM-1 inhibits adhesion. Basophils, eosinophils, lymphocytes, and monocytes, but not neutrophils, bind via VLA-4 to VCAM-1 expressed by endothelial cells. This represents a novel mechanism for endothelium facilitating adhesion of these leukocytes.

D. Lung and Dermal Mast Cells (Figure 4)

Mast cells bind to fibronectin and laminin, which are ubiquitous adhesion proteins of the extracellular matrix (84,85). The adherence appears to be mediated by an integrin on mast cells and the tripeptide RGD in both proteins. In addition, when mast cells adhere to laminin, they exhibit adhesion spreading and redistribution of histamine-containing granules on a laminin substratum (85). Mast cell adhesion to laminin is enhanced by IL-3 and inhibited by both monoclonal antibodies to laminin and to laminin receptors. The expression of receptors for fibronectin and laminin by mast cells explains the tissue distribution and accumulation at sites of epithelial injury where these proteins are present. Exposure of fibronectin and laminin by shedding epithelium facilitates mast cell adhesion and explains the accumulation of mast cells seen in the allergic inflammation.

Endothelial cells lining microvessels express ELAM-1 2 h after degranulation of human mast cells in vitro (86). This induction is also dependent of the endogenous release of TNF_{α}. This study shows that anti-IgE-mediated degranulation causes rapid and cytokine-dependent induction of ELAM-1 by mast cells in the adjacent microvessels. ELAM-1 expression, by endothelial cells, was blocked by anti-TNF_{α}. A complementary study shows that human dermal mast cell degranulation in vivo and in vitro causes release of preformed TNF_{α}, which in turn induces ELAM-1 expression by der-

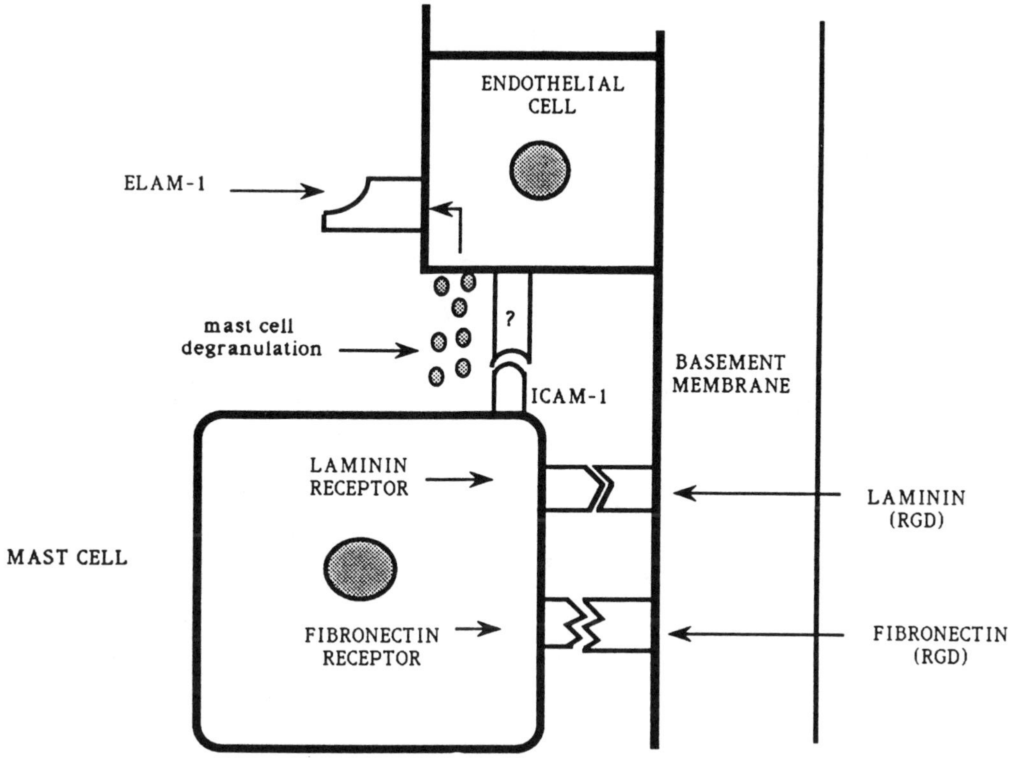

Figure 4 Schematic representation of adhesion molecules expressed by mast cells. Mast cell degranulation induces the expression of ELAM-1 by endothelial cells.

mal endothelium (87). Both studies provide evidence for human mast cells as regulatory cells for dermal endothelium in ELAM-1 production. In addition, mast cell mediators more than vasoactive amines may regulate endothelium during the allergic inflammation. Finally, substance P (SP), by inducing dermal mast cell degranulation, stimulates expression of ELAM-1 on adjacent human postcapillary microvascular endothelium (88). This study, by suggesting that SP is a potential determinant of endothelium-leukocyte adhesion, provides evidence for additional functions in the pathogenesis of allergic diseases.

To summarize, mast cell adhesion to airway epithelium may be essential for mast cell-epithelial cell interactions, and thus, in allergies respiratory and airway function can be injured by intraluminal mast cells more than is currently appreciated.

V. ADHESION MOLECULES AS A COMPONENT IN THE INFLAMMATORY NETWORK OF THE ALLERGIC LATE-PHASE RESPONSE

Leukocyte transmigration is a physiological process, contributing to immune surveillance (Figure 5). However, in pathologic conditions, this process causes tissue damage and disease in the host. Neutrophils are initially the predominant type of leukocyte at inflammatory sites, with the peak of adhesion and transmigration occurring within the first hours after the onset of an allergic response. However, after 8 to 12 h eosinophils

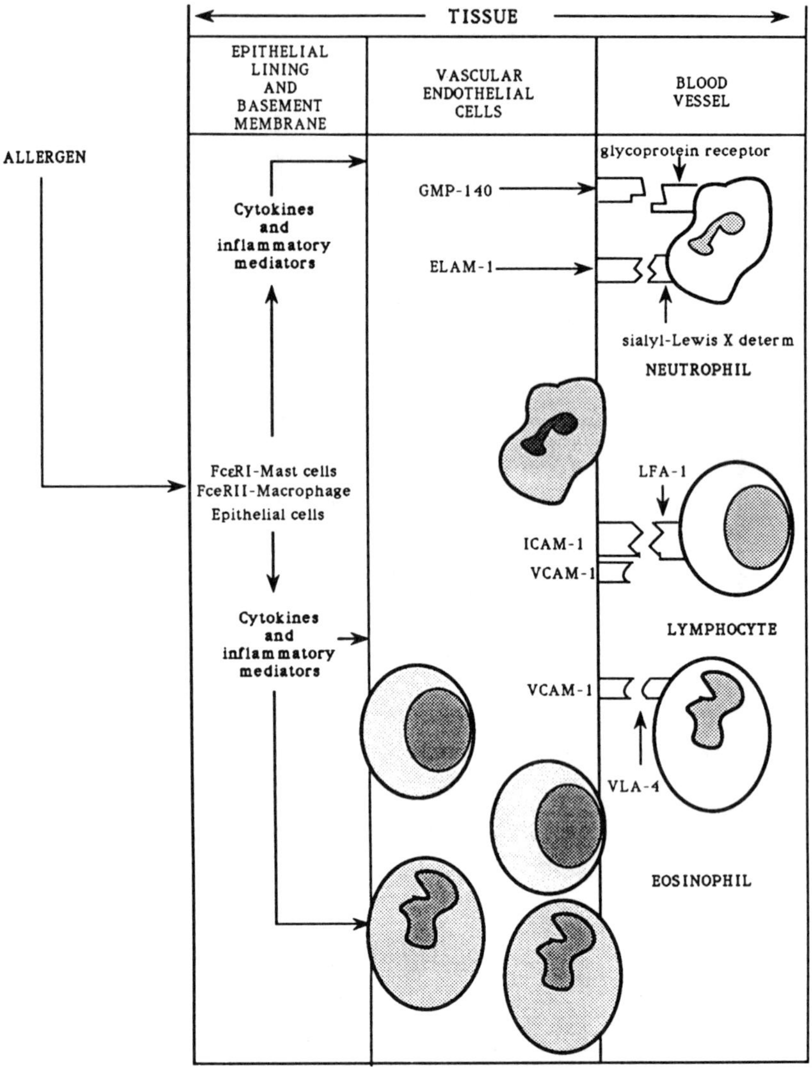

Figure 5 After contact with allergens, tissular cells bearing IgE release chemical mediators and cytokines. They induce the expression of a variety of adhesion molecules by endothelial cells over a given time period. GMP-140, expressed in less than 5 min, binds to its glycoprotein receptor, which is constitutively expressed by neutrophils. Within the following 4 to 6 h, endothelial cells express ELAM-1, which binds to its reciprocal receptor on neutrophils. Adherent neutrophils are activated and express other adhesion molecules after stimulation by chemical mediators and cytokines present in the endothelium. Then, neutrophils can transmigrate into the tissue. Endothelial cells also express ICAM-1 and VCAM-1 in 4 to 6 h, allowing lymphocytes and eosinophils to adhere. A sequence of activation and transmigration allows these cells to infiltrate the tissue.

and lymphocytes increase their presence in the IgE-dependent inflamed tissue. The different kinetics for neutrophil, eosinophil, and lymphocyte adhesion to vascular endothelium may be explained by differences in expression of adhesion molecules on vascular endothelial cells and/or by each type of leukocyte.

Following the cross-linking of IgE on the surface, mast cells and basophils release chemical mediators and cytokines which, after contact with vascular endothelial cells, induce the synthesis and expression of adhesion molecules. A variety of them can be expressed at different times. In-vitro studies suggest that activated vascular endothelial cells rapidly increase the expression of adhesion molecules such as GMP-140, ELAM-1, and ICAM-1. These molecules have the ability to bind neutrophils, which constitutively express the reciprocal receptors (CD15, sialyl-Lewis X determinant, and LFA-1, respectively). Then, endothelial cells can decrease the expression of ELAM-1 (probably induced by IL-4), thereby inhibiting the neutrophil binding. Concurrently, activated endothelial cells increase the expression of different adhesion molecules, such as ICAM-1 and VCAM-1, which allow adherence to lymphocytes and eosinophils. These molecules bind ligands constitutively expressed by eosinophils and lymphocytes (LFA-1 and VLA-4, respectively). Therefore, inflammatory mediators and cytokines released by IgE-stimulated epithelium, which characterize allergic asthma and rhinitis, induce resting circulating leukocytes to attach to activated vascular endothelial cells. In addition, it is possible that activated leukocytes, through a systemic stimulation (i.e., atopic dermatitis), increase or induce the expression of their adhesion molecules, which bind ligands, constitutively expressed on vascular endothelial cells. Finally, both circulating eosinophils and vascular endothelial cells can be activated, facilitating the adhesive process even more.

Adherent leukocytes can be activated either by contact with inflammatory mediators and cytokines present in the endothelium or by intracellular mechanisms which communicate surface antigens to metabolic pathways (i.e., the protein kinase C system). This process includes both the expression of adhesion molecules that allow leukocytes to transmigrate (i.e., CD18, ICAM-1, and ELAM-1) and the cytoskeleton activation which enables the cells to become fluid and capable of penetrating into the tissue. In addition to adhesion, transmigration requires the de-adhesion mechanism which is regulated by phosphorylation of the cytoplasmic domain of the β_2 subunit of the integrins (89). Leukocytes such as mast cells, eosinophils, and lymphocytes that express VLA integrins can migrate more easily through basement membranes which have high concentrations of laminin, fibronectin, and collagens containing the adherent sequence RGD.

Chemoattractant mediators such as PAF, LTB_4, and IL-2 can facilitate leukocyte motility into the tissue. This infiltrative process, combined with the effects of GM-CSF, increases the leukocyte tissular survival. Finally, activated and transmigrated leukocytes with a longer survival time release enzymes and catabolic mediators that cause tissue inflammation which is the characteristic feature of the allergic late phase.

VI. SUMMARY AND PERSPECTIVES

The importance of chemical mediators, cytokines and cell adhesion molecules in the pathogenesis of inflammatory diseases now appears to be established. Soluble mediators and adhesion molecules may also play an essential role in the pathogenesis of the allergic diseases. After IgE challenge, in sensitized individuals, granulocytes bearing high-affinity IgE receptors (FcεRI) and low-affinity IgE receptors (FcεRII) migrate into epithelial tissues and release inflammatory mediators and cytokines which stimulate the adjacent vascular endothelium to express adhesion molecules. Owing to these vascular cell adhesion molecules which act as receptors, resting circulating leukocytes find points of attachment, because leukocytes also constitutively express adhesion molecule which act as reciprocal or counter receptors. Adhered leukocytes, stimulated by cytokines and inflammatory mediators within the tissue, are activated to express other adhesion molecules. As a consequence, leukocytes undergo activation of the cytoskeleton and become capable of penetrating into the tissue. Finally, activated and transmigrated leukocytes cause tissue inflammation, a characteristic feature of the late phase allergic response. In addition to these properties, adhesion molecules are important for leukocyte functions such as cytotoxicity, phagocytosis, growth and proliferation. Antiadhesion molecule therapy, using nonspecific antiinflammatory drugs or specific monoclonal antibodies to directly block adhesion molecules, may constitute a novel approach to the treatment of allergic diseases.

Future studies will provide additional information about functions of adhesion molecules which have already been identified and for those not yet identified. After activation by allergens, adhesion molecules expressed by bronchial and dermal endothelium participate in localization to the epithelium of granulocytes and mononuclear cells. The identification of a physiological anti-adhesion molecule system which might regulate cellular mechanisms triggered by adhesion molecules will facilitate the unveiling of additional pathways involved in the pathophysiology of allergies. Several genes have already been identified which encode DNA for adhesion molecules. It is possible that such genes may, in atopic individuals, be easily activated under physiologic conditions, or by mild stimulation, to produce adhesion molecules with high affinity for their reciprocal receptors. It seems reasonable to correlate fluctuations of serum levels of soluble fragments of adhesion molecules during exacerbation and remission periods of chronic allergic symptoms to predict possible usefulness of specific antiadhesion therapy. One such study, already in progress, is evaluating the therapeutic potential of monoclonal antibody to ICAM-1 in monkeys. The direct blocking of adhesion molecules by either specific antibodies or with nonspecific anti-inflammatory drugs may constitute a novel method of controlling the symptoms of allergic diseases.

REFERENCES

1. Springer TA. Adhesion receptors of the immune system. Nature 1990; 346:425–34.
2. Carlos TM, Harlan JM. Membrane proteins involved in phagocyte adherence to endothelium. Immunol Rev 1990; 114:5–22.
3. Wardlaw A. Leukocyte adhesion to endothelium. Clin Exp Med 1990; 20:619–26.
4. Osborn L. Leukocyte adhesion to endothelium in inflammation. Cell 1990; 62:3–6.
5. Yamada KM. Adhesive recognition sequences. J Biol Chem 1991; 266:12809–12.
6. Patarroyo M, Makgoba MW. Leukocyte adhesion to cells in immune and inflammatory responses. Lancet 1989(II):1139–41.
7. Burton J, Goldman CK, Rao P, et al. Association of intercellular adhesion molecule 1 with the multichain high-affinity interleukin 2 receptor. Proc Natl Acad Sci USA 1990; 87:7329–33.

8. Corrigan CJ, Kay AB. CD4 T-lymphocyte activation in acute severe asthma. Am Rev Respir Dis 1990; 141:970–7.
9. Hynes RO. Integrins, a family of cell surface receptors. Cell 1987; 48:549–55.
10. de Fourgerolles AR, Stacker SA, Schwarting RS, Springer TA. Characterization of ICAM-2 and evidence for a third counter-receptor for LFA-1. J Exp Med 1991; 174:253–67.
11. Van Seventer GA, Shimizu Y, Horgan KJ, Shaw S. The LFA-1 ligand ICAM-1 provides an important costimulatory signal for T cell receptor-mediated activation of resting cells. J Immunol 1990; 144:4579–86.
12. Kishimoto TK, Hollander N, Roberts TM, et al. Heterogeneous mutations in the β subunit common to the LFA-1, Mac-1, and p150,95 glycoproteins cause leukocyte adhesion deficiency. Cell 1987; 50:193–202.
13. Smith CW, Kishimoto TK, Abbassi O, et al. Chemotactic factors regulate lectin adhesion molecules 1 (LECAM-1)-dependent neutrophil adhesion to cytokine-stimulated endothelial cells *in vitro*. J Clin Invest 1991; 87:609–18.
14. Bevilacqua MP, Stengelin S, Gimbrone MA, Seed B. Endothelial leukocyte adhesion molecules 1: An inducible receptor for neutrophils related to complement regulatory proteins and lectins. Science 1989; 243:1160–5.
15. McEver RP, Beckstead JH, Moore KL, et al. GMP-140, a platelet α-granule membrane protein, is also synthesized by vascular endothelial cells and is localized in Weibel-Palade bodies. J Clin Invest 1989; 84:92–9.
16. Moore KL, Varki A, McEver RP. GMP-140 binds to a glycoprotein receptor on human neutrophils: evidence for a lectin-like interaction. J Cell Biol 1991; 112:491–9.
17. Grangette C, Gruart V, Ouaissi MA, et al. IgE receptor on human eosinophils (FcϵRII). Comparison with B cell CD23 and association with an adhesion molecule. J Immunol 1989; 143:3580–8.
18. Kikutani H, Inui S, Sato R, et al. Molecular structure of human lymphocyte receptor for immunoglobulin E. Cell 1986; 47:657–65.
19. Conrad DH. Fc_ϵRII/CD23: the low affinity receptor for IgE. Ann Rev Immunol 1990; 8:623–45.
20. Boltz-Nitulescu G, Wiltschke C, Langer K, et al. Augmentation of IgE receptor expression and IgE receptor-mediated phagocytosis of rat bone marrow-derived macrophages by murine interferons. Immunology 1988; 63:529–35.
21. Capron M, Kazatchkine MD, Fischer E, et al. Functional role of the α chain of complement receptor type 3 in human eosinophil-dependent antibody-mediated cytotoxicity against schistosomes. J Immunol 1987; 139:2059–65.
22. Delespesse G, Sarfati M, Hofstetter H. Human IgE-binding factors. Immunol Today 1989; 10:159–64.
23. Del pozo V, de Andres B, Martin E, et al. Murine eosinophils and IL-1: αIL-1 mRNA detection by *in situ* hybridization. J Immunol 1990; 144:3117–22.
24. Borish L, Mascali JJ, Rosenwasser LJ. IgE-dependent cytokine production by human peripheral blood mononuclear phagocytes. J Immunol 1991; 146:63–7.
25. Ohno I, Ohkawara Y, Yamauchi K, et al. Production of tumor necrosis factor with IgE receptor triggering from sensitized lung tissue. Am J Respir Cell Mol Biol 1990; 3:285–9.
26. Gordon JR, Galli SJ. Release of both preformed and newly synthesized tumor necrosis factor α (TNF α)/cachectin by mouse mast cells stimulated via the FcϵRI. A mechanism for the sustained action of mast cell-derived TNF α during IgE-dependent biological responses. J Exp Med 1991; 174:103–7.
27. Luscinskas FW, Cybulsky MI, Kiely JM, et al. Cytokine-activated human endothelial monolayers support enhanced neutrophil transmigration via a mechanism involving both endothelial-leukocyte adhesion molecule-1 and intercellular adhesion molecule-1. J Immunol 1991; 146:1617–25.
28. Loike JD, Sodeik B, Cao L, et al. CD11c/CD18 on neutrophils recognizes a domain at the N terminus of the Aα chain of fibrinogen. Proc Natl Acad Sci USA 1991; 88:1044–8.

29. Osborn L, Hession C, Tizard R, et al. Direct expression cloning of vascular cell adhesion molecule 1, a cytokine-induced endothelial protein that binds to lymphocytes. Cell 1989; 59:1203–11.
30. Leung DYM, Pober JS, Cotran RS. Expression of endothelial-leukocyte adhesion molecule-1 in elicited late phase allergic reactions. J Clin Invest 1991; 87:1805–9.
31. Wegner CD, Gundell RH, Reilly P, et al. Intercellular adhesion molecule-1 (ICAM-1) in the pathogenesis of asthma. Science 1990; 247:456–9.
32. Yoshizawa I, Noma T, Kawano Y, Yata J. Allergen-specific induction of IL-2 responsiveness in lymphocytes from children with asthma. J Allergy Clin Immunol 1989; 84:246–55.
33. Sedgwick JB, Frick WE, Sondel PM, et al. The appearance of hypodense eosinophils during interleukin-2 treatment. J Allergy Clin Immunol 1990; 85:557–66.
34. Rand TH, Silberstein DS, Kornfeld H, Weller PF. Human eosinophils express functional interleukin 2 receptors. J Clin Invest 1991; 88:825–32.
35. Buckle AM, Hogg N. Human memory T cells express intercellular adhesion molecule-1 which can be increased by interleukin 2 and interferon-γ. Eur J Immunol 1990; 20:337–41.
36. Cotran RS, Pober JS, Gimbrone MA, et al. Endothelial activation during interleukin 2 immunotherapy. A possible mechanism for the vascular leak syndrome. J Immunol 1987; 139:1883–8.
37. Bochner BS, McKelvey AA, Sterbinsky SA, et al. IL-3 augments adhesiveness for endothelium and CD11b expression in human basophils but not for neutrophils. J Immunol 1990; 145:1832–7.
38. Elliott MJ, Vadas MA, Cleland LG, et al. IL-3 and granulocyte-macrophage colony-stimulating factor stimulate two distinct phases of adhesion in human monocytes. J Immunol 1990; 145:167–76.
39. Thornhill MH, Haskard DO. IL-4 regulates endothelial cell activation by IL-1, tumor necrosis factor, or IFNγ. J Immunol 1990; 145:865–72.
40. Thornhill MH, Kyan-Aung U, Haskard DO. IL-4 increases human endothelial adhesiveness for T cells but not for neutrophils. J Immunol 1990; 144:3060–5.
41. Masinovsky B, Urdal D, Gallatin M. IL-4 acts synergistically with IL-1β to promote lymphocyte adhesion to microvascular endothelium by induction of vascular cell adhesion molecule-1. J Immunol 1990; 145:2886–95.
42. Valent P, Bevec D, Maurer D, et al. Interleukin 4 promotes expression of mast cell ICAM-1 antigen. Proc Natl Acad Sci USA 1991; 88:3339–42.
43. Hamid Q, Azzawi M, Ying S, et al. Expression of mRNA for interleukin-5 in mucosal bronchial biopsies from asthma. J Clin Invest 1991; 87:1541–6.
44. Walsh GM, Hartnell A, Wardlaw AJ, et al. IL-5 enhances the *in vitro* adhesion of human eosinophils, but not neutrophils, in a leukocyte integrin (CD11/18)-dependent manner. Immunology 1990; 71:258–65.
45. Lu L, Lin ZH, Shen RN, et al. Influence of interleukins 3, 5 and 6 on the growth of eosinophil progenitors in highly enriched human bone marrow in the absence of serum. Exp Hematol 1990; 18:1180–6.
46. Maggi E, Del Prete GF, Parronchi P, et al. Role for T cells, IL-2 and IL-6 in the IL-4-dependent *in vitro* human IgE synthesis. Immunology 1989; 68:300–6.
47. Duits AJ, Jainandunsing SM, Van de Winkel GJ, Capel PJA. Selective enhancement of Leu-Cam expression by interleukin 6 during differentiation of human promonocytic U937 cells. Scand J Immunol 1991; 33:151–9.
48. Stötter H, Custer MC, Bolton ES, et al. IL-7 induces human lymphokine-activated killer cell activity and is regulated by IL-4. J Immunol 1991; 146:150–5.
49. Barth C, O'Connell P, Zanker B, Strom TB. Interleukin-7 (IL-7) and its effect on the expression of the intercellular adhesion molecule (ICAM-1) in T cells. Transplant Proc 1991; 23:824–5.
50. Matsushima K, Oppenheim JJ. Interleukin 8 and MCAF: novel inflammatory cytokines inducible by IL 1 and TNF. Cytokine 1989; 1:2–13.

51. Standiford TJ, Kunkel SL, Basha MA, et al. Interleukin-8 gene expression by a pulmonary epithelial cell line. A model for cytokine networks in the lung. J Clin Invest 1990; 86:1945–53.
52. Schröder JM. The monocyte-derived neutrophil activating peptide (NAP/interleukin 8) stimulates human neutrophil arachidonate-5-lipoxygenase, but not the release of cellular arachidonate. J Exp Med 1989; 170:847–63.
53. Gimbrone MA, Obin MS, Brock AF, et al. Endothelial interleukin-8: a novel inhibitor of leukocyte-endothelial interactions. Science 1989; 246:1601–3.
54. Detmers PA. Neutrophil-activating protein 1/interleukin 8 stimulates the binding activity of the leukocyte adhesion receptor CD11b/CD18 on human neutrophils. J Exp Med 1990; 171:1155–62.
55. Leeuwenberg JF, von Asmuth EJ, Jeunhomme TM, Buurman WA. IFN-gamma regulates the expression of the adhesion molecule ELAM-1 and IL-6 production by human endothelial cells *in vitro*. J Immunol 1990; 145:2110–4.
56. Doukas J, Pober JS. IFN-γ enhances endothelial activation induced by tumor necrosis factor but not IL-1. J Immunol 1990; 145:1727–33.
57. Issekutz TB. Effects of six different cytokines on lymphocyte adherence to microvascular endothelium and *in vivo* lymphocyte migration in the rat. J Immunol 1990; 144:2140–6.
58. Griffiths CE, Voorhees JJ, Nickoloff BJ. Gamma interferon induces different keratinocyte cellular patterns of expression of HLA-DR and DQ and intercellular adhesion molecule-1 (ICAM-1). Br J Dermatol 1989; 120:1–8.
59. Moqbel R, Hamid Q, Ying S, et al. Expression of mRNA and immunoreactivity for the granulocyte/macrophage colony-stimulating factor in activated human eosinophils. J Exp Med 1991; 174:749–52.
60. Kita H, Ohnishi T, Okubo Y, et al. Granulocyte/macrophage colony-stimulating factor and interleukin 3 release from human peripheral blood eosinophils and neutrophils. J Exp Med 1991; 174:745–8.
61. Kay AB, Ying S, Varney V, et al. Messenger RNA expression of the cytokine gene cluster, interleukin 3 (IL-3), IL-4, IL-5, and granulocyte/macrophage colony-stimulating factor, in allergen-induced late-phase cutaneous reactions in atopic subjects. J Exp Med 1991; 173:775–8.
62. Griffin JD, Spertini O, Ernst TJ, et al. Granulocyte-macrophage colony-stimulating factor and other cytokines regulate surface expression of the leukocyte adhesion molecule-1 on human neutrophils, monocytes, and their precursors. J Immunol 1990; 145:576–84.
63. Socinski MSA, Cannistra R, Sullivan A, et al. Granulocyte-macrophage colony stimulating factor induces the expression of the CD11b surface adhesion molecule on human granulocytes *in vivo*. Blood 1988; 72:691–7.
64. Wershil BK, Wang ZS, Gordon JR, Galli SJ. Recruitment of neutrophils during IgE-dependent cutaneous late phase reactions in the mouse is mast cell-dependent. J Clin Invest 1991; 87:446–53.
65. Virant FS, Bierman CW. The role of the neutrophil in the late-phase asthmatic reaction and airway hyperresponsiveness. Immunol Allergy Clin North Am 1990; 10:283–93.
66. Singer II, Scott S, Kawka DW, Kazazis DM. Adhesomes: specific granules containing receptors for laminin, C3bi/fibrinogen, fibronectin and vitronectin in human polymorphonuclear leukocytes and monocytes. J Cell Biol 1989; 109:3169–82.
67. Graham IL, Brown EJ. Extracellular calcium results in a conformational change in Mac-1 (CD11b/CD18) on neutrophils. J Immunol 1991; 146:685–91.
68. Tonnesen MG, Anderson DC, Springer TA, et al. Adherence of neutrophils to cultured human microvascular endothelial cells. J Clin Invest 1989; 83:637–46.
69. Zimmerman GA, McIntyre TM. Neutrophil adherence to human endothelium in vitro occurs by CDw18 (Mol, MAC-1/LFA-1/GP 150,95). J Clin Invest 1988; 81:531–7.
70. Hallmann R, Jutila MA, Smith CW, et al. The peripheral lymph node homing receptor, LECAM-1, is involved in CD18-independent adhesion of human neutrophils to endothelium. Biochem Biophys Res Commun 1991; 174:236–43.

71. Patel KD, Zimmerman GA, Prescott, et al. Oxygen radicals induce human endothelial cells to express GMP-140 and bind neutrophils. J Cell Biol 1991; 112:749–59.
72. Lo S, Lee S, Ramos RA, et al. Endothelial-leukocyte adhesion molecule 1 activates the adhesive activity of leukocyte integrin CR3 (CD11b/CD18, Mac-1, $\alpha_m\beta_2$) on human neutrophils. J Exp Med 1991; 173:1493–500.
73. Kyan-Aung U, Haskard DO, Poston RN, et al. Endothelial leukocyte adhesion molecule-1 and intercellular adhesion molecule-1 mediate the adhesion of eosinophils to endothelial cells *in vitro* and are expressed by endothelium in allergic cutaneous inflammation *in vivo*. J Immunol 1991; 146:521–8.
74. Walsh GM, Hartnell A, Moqbel R, et al. Receptor expression and functional status of cultured human eosinophils derived from umbilical cord blood mononuclear cells. Blood 1990; 76:105–11.
75. Hartnell A, Moqbel R, Walsh GM, et al. Fcγ and CD11/CD18 receptor expression on normal density and low density human eosinophils. Immunology 1990; 69:264–70.
76. Lamas AM, Mulroney CM, Scheleimer RP. Studies of the adhesive interaction between purified human eosinophils and cultured vascular endothelial cells. J Immunol 1988; 140:1500–5.
77. Walsh GM, Mermod JJ, Hartnell A, et al. Human eosinophil, but not neutrophil, adherence to IL-1 stimulated human umbilical vascular endothelial cells is $\alpha_4\beta_1$ (very late antigen-4) dependent. J Immunol 1991; 146:3419–23.
78. Weller PF, Rand TH, Goelz SE, et al. Human eosinophil adherence to vascular endothelium mediated by binding to vascular cell adhesion molecule 1 and endothelial leukocyte adhesion molecule 1. Proc Natl Acad Sci USA 1991; 88:7430–3.
79. Dobrina A, Menegazzi R, Carlos TM, et al. Mechanisms of eosinophil adherence to cultured vascular endothelial cells. J Clin Invest 1991; 88:20–6.
80. Rand TH, Cruikshank WW, Center DW, Weller PF. CD4-mediated stimulation of human eosinophils: lymphocyte chemoattractant factor and other CD4-binding ligands elicit eosinophil migration. J Exp Med 1991; 173:1521–8.
81. Bochner BS, Sterbinsky SA. Altered surface expression of CD11 and Leu 8 during human basophil degranulation. J Immunol 1991; 146:2367–73.
82. Valent P, Majdic O, Maurer D, et al. Further characterization of surface membrane structures expressed on human basophils and mast cells. Int Arch Allergy Appl Immunol 1990; 91:198–203.
83. Bochner BS, Luscinskas FW, Gimbrone MA, et al. Adhesion of human basophils, eosinophils, and neutrophils to interleukin 1-activated human vascular endothelial cells: contributions of endothelial cell adhesion molecules. J Exp Med 1991; 173:1553–6.
84. Castych J, Costa JJ, Thompson HL, Metcalfe DD. Mast cell adhesion to fibronectin. Immunology 1991; 73:478–84.
85. Thompson HL, Burbelo PD, Segui-Real B, et al. Laminin promotes mast cell attachment. J Immunol 1989; 143:2323–7.
86. Klein LM, Lavker RM, Matis WL, Murphy GF. Degranulation of human mast cells induces an endothelial antigen central to leukocyte adhesion. Proc Natl Acad Sci USA 1989; 86:8972–6.
87. Walsh LJ, Trinchieri G, Waldorf HA, et al. Human dermal mast cells contain and release tumor necrosis factor α, which induces endothelial leukocyte adhesion molecule 1. Proc Natl Acad Sci USA 1991; 88:4220–4.
88. Matis WL, Lavker RM, Murphy GF. Substance P induces the expression of an endothelial-leukocyte adhesion molecule by microvascular endothelium. J Invest Dermatol 1990; 94:492–5.
89. Hibbs ML, Xu H, Stacker SA, Springer TA. Regulation of adhesion to ICAM-1 by the cytoplasmic domain of LFA-1 integrin β subunit. Science 1991; 251:1611–3.

C

Effects of Cytokines: Clinical Research

26

Granulocyte Colony-Stimulating Factors as Therapeutic Agents

ROBERT E. DONAHUE
National Heart, Lung, and Blood Institute, Bethesda, Maryland

STEVEN C. CLARK
Genetics Institute, Inc., Cambridge, Massachusetts

I. INTRODUCTION

With the development of in-vitro assays for hematopoietic progenitors (1,2), it became clear that there are factors in a variety of cell-derived conditioned media that allow hematopoietic progenitors to survive, proliferate, and terminally differentiate. Over the past two decades these culture systems have been modified significantly to allow the identification and enrichment of lineage-specific and multilineage progenitors. These progenitors, residing mostly in the bone marrow, give rise to the large numbers of circulating red cells, neutrophils, basophils, eosinophils, monocytes, platelets, and lymphocytes. As many of these blood elements are short-lived, they must be continually replenished.

A number of hematopoietic colony-stimulating factors have been identified that play a role in granulocyte and red blood cell production. These have been identified based on their in-vitro activities. Factors can be relatively lineage specific; e.g., colonies grown in the presence of erythropoietin (EPO) consist largely of nucleated red blood cells, colonies grown in the presence of granulocyte-CSF (G-CSF) consist largely of neutrophils, and colonies grown in the presence of macrophage-CSF (M-CSF, also known as CSF-1) consist largely of macrophages (phagocytic cells derived from circulating monocytes) (3). Still other CSFs, e.g. IL-3 (also known as multipotential CSF), and granulocyte/macrophage-CSF (GM-CSF), are capable of acting on multilineage hematopoietic progenitors. In addition, there is another group of cytokines that alone have little if any colony-stimulating activity, but, when combined with other hematopoietic growth factors, are capable of enhancing colony formation. IL-7, IL-6, and the newly described cytokines IL-11 (93) and the ligand for the C-kit protoncogene (also known as stem cell factor (SCF), mast cell growth factor (MCGF), and kit ligand (KL) (94–95) fall within this category. These in-vitro results define a hierarchy of progenitor cells capable of responding to the CSFs. G-CSF, M-CSF, and EPO support the growth

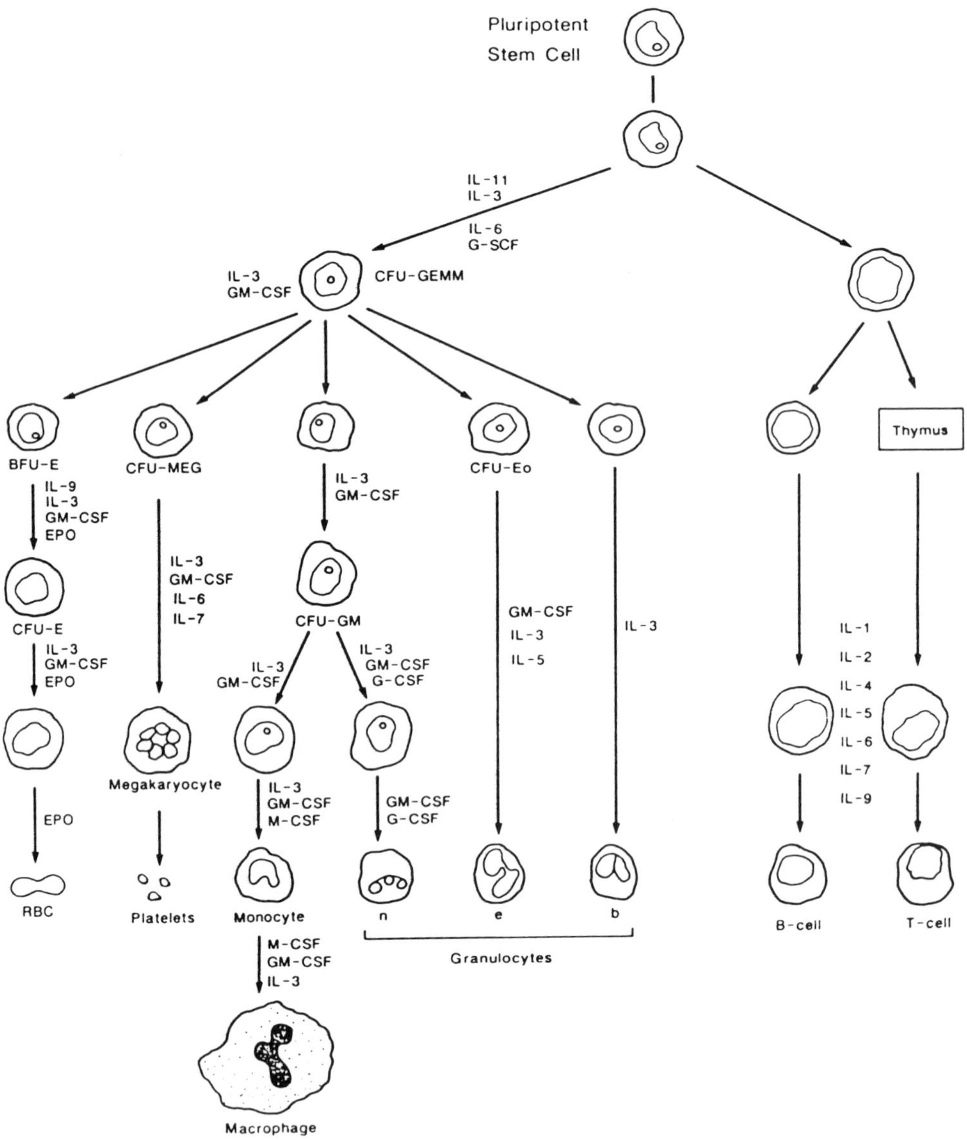

Figure 1 Interactions of the CSFs with hematopoietic cells (3).

and proliferation of relatively late progenitors, while GM-CSF interacts, in addition, with earlier progenitors, and IL-3 interacts with even earlier progenitors (Figure 1).

Recombinant DNA technology has recently been employed to isolate cDNA clones encoding these hematopoietic growth factors. These advances have facilitated the large-scale production of these important regulatory molecules, thereby making it possible to study the biological effects of these factors in-vitro and in-vivo. Murine hematopoietic growth factor genes that have been molecularly cloned include the genes for IL-3 (4), GM-CSF (5), G-CSF (6), M-CSF (7), and EPO (8). Similarly, in the human system, the genes encoding GM-CSF (9), G-CSF (10,11), EPO (12,13), and IL-3 or multi-CSF (14) have also been cloned. Interestingly, two different cDNAs encoding different forms of human M-CSF have been molecularly cloned and expressed (15,16). Numerous preclinical and clinical studies have been initiated using these hematopoietic growth factors. The results clearly demonstrate that these cytokines are functionally active in vivo. The responses elicited reflect the in-vitro activities of the proteins.

II. INFECTIOUS DISEASES AND INFLAMMATION

Many in-vitro activities have been ascribed to the colony-stimulating factors. Some of these have been reviewed previously (17). Over the past several years a literature has accumulated describing the effects of GM-CSF and its ability to enhance the responsiveness of granulocytes to various microbial and parasitic agents. For example, it has been shown that GM-CSF can inhibit neutrophil migration (18) as well as act as a chemotactic agent (19).

The ability of the cytokine GM-CSF to stimulate neutrophil oxidative metabolism and chemotaxis to the bacterial chemoattractant f-Met-Leu-Phe and other major physiological chemoattractants, such as C5a and leukotriene B_4, has been studied extensively in vitro (20–23). The effect of GM-CSF on augmenting granulocyte oxidative metabolism and f-Met-Leu-Phe-induced chemotaxis appears to be associated with changes in f-Met-Leu-Phe receptor number and affinity (24). Several investigators have also shown that GM-CSF can enhance neutrophil and eosinophil phagocytosis of serum-opsonized baker's yeast (20,22,25), neutrophil phagocytosis of the opsonized bacterium *Staphylococcus aureus* (26), eosinophil cytotoxicity for opsonized *Schistosoma mansoni* larvae (27), and intracellular killing of *Leishmani donovani* by human monocyte-derived macrophages (28) and *Trypanosoma cruzi* by murine macrophages (29). M-CSF has also been found to enhance killing of *Candida albicans* by murine macrophages, possibly by augmenting expression of mannose receptors (30). As has been discussed in the past (31), these results imply that GM-CSF and potentially other hematopoietic growth factors could assist in the recovery of patients with either local or systemic infections by enhancing the activity of preexisting leukocytes and/or by increasing the number of leukocytes important in eliminating infections.

Direct evidence in vivo suggesting that cytokines may play a role in activating leukocytes and subsequently limiting infections, however, continues to be meager. Data is now beginning to accumulate in some studies suggesting that granulocytes isolated from primates (32–35) and humans (36,37) receiving GM-CSF or G-CSF parenterally have enhanced oxidative metabolism and increased bactericidal activity. In a study where neutrophils were isolated from AIDS patients treated with GM-CSF, the neutrophils appeared to have increased oxidative metabolism, phagocytosis, and antibody-dependent cellular cytotoxicity (36). Increases in superoxide anion release from granulocytes were also observed in patients with sarcomas after a 12–24 h of constant intravenous infusion of rhGM-CSF (37). The primed granulocytes may prove beneficial in limiting infections and promoting wound healing. Patients with transitional-cell carcinomas of the urothelium receiving rhG-CSF were found to have a reduced incidence and severity of mucositis associated with chemotherapy (38).

Similar evidence for granulocyte priming by parenterally administered GM-CSF has been demonstrated in primates (32–35). In one study, granulocytes isolated from primates infused with GM-CSF have had augmented oxidative metabolism when stimulated with PMA or f-Met-Leu-Phe, and increased bactericidal activity against *Escherichia coli* (33). In another primate study (34), the use of fluorescence-activated flow cytometry and luminol-enhanced chemiluminescence showed a significant priming effect of rhGM-CSF on the response of granulocytes to stimuli for membrane depolarization and respiratory burst activity. These granulocytes following in-vivo priming with rhGM-CSF had increased random migration and migration to f-Met-Leu-Phe and platelet-activating factor (35).

These observations, however, contrast with other studies involving the administration of GM-CSF to patients transplanted with autologous bone marrow (39) or diagnosed as having a myelodysplastic syndrome (40,41). In the study of cancer patients receiving autologous bone marrow transplants, the ability of granulocytes to phagocytize *Cryptococcus neoformans* and release hydrogen peroxide were similar both before and during GM-CSF infusion and similar to granulocytes isolated from patients treated with the same high-dose chemotherapy and autologous bone marrow support but not receiving growth factor (39). These cancer patients also demonstrated diminished neutrophil migration to a sterile inflammatory site during the rhGM-CSF infusion. This observation can potentially be explained by the earlier observation that rhGM-CSF can inhibit neutrophil migration (18) in the absence of a secondary stimulus. In another study (40,41), patients receiving rhGM-CSF and having a myelodysplastic syndrome had no alteration in neutrophil function, as measured by oxidative metabolism and chemotaxis to f-Met-Leu-Phe. Further work is required to resolve these findings from those previously mentioned.

It remains unclear what the role of colony-stimulating factors may be in disease states that involve an inflammatory and/or an autoimmune response. With the development of radioimmunoassay and immunoenzyme assays, local and systemic levels of the cytokines may now begin to be determined in a variety of pathologic conditions. A wide variety of cell lineages involved in the inflammatory response (fibroblasts, endothelial cells, T-lymphocytes, and macrophages) can be induced to produce CSFs. Murine peritoneal macrophages, for example, have been shown to synthesize mRNA and release GM-CSF in response to phagocytosis, adherence to fibronectin, M-CSF, and a variety of other inflammatory stimuli (42). This local production of CSFs can then prime granulocytes to become activated.

The potential role of the hematopoietic growth factors in inflammation is furthered supported by the in-vitro observation that rhGM-CSF increased the surface expression of CD11b(Mol) and CD11c (p150,95), two members of a family of leukocyte adhesion molecules, on mature granulocytes (43). Subsequent in-vivo studies confirmed this initial observation. Patients with sarcomas receiving rhGM-CSF had increased expression of CD11b on their granulocytes (44). In studying the migration patterns of granulocytes of patients receiving rhGM-CSF, it was also noticed that there is a rapid but transient leukopenia associated with the administration of rhGM-CSF (45). This leukopenia was due to the rapid margination of granulocytes to the endothelium of the lung, at least in part due to the increased expression of adhesion-promoting glycoproteins (46). The demargination of the granulocytes from the lung endothelium, however, appears to depend on factors other than down-regulation of CD11b.

Coinciding with the initial neutropenia associated with GM-CSF administration due to neutrophil margination is a secretion by the neutrophils of their secondary granules (47). This results in an elevation in circulating plasma levels of lactoferrin and transcobalamin 1 and 3, potentially leading to the appearance of hypofunctional neutrophils in the circulation. Such results support the contention that hematopoietic growth factors may play a role in regulating an inflammatory response. If the colony-stimulating factors are important in the regulation and recruitment of cells involved in inflammation or autoimmunity, then factors that will inhibit the activities of these CSFs locally may limit the tissue damage that occurs with these responses.

III. INDUCED CYTOPENIAS AND CANCER

Patients undergoing intensive chemotherapy or radiation therapy for cancer frequently develop leukopenia and thrombocytopenia. This leukopenia is associated with an increased susceptibility to infection-related morbidity and mortality. To reduce the chance of infection and hemorrhage, one would like to have not only adequate supportive care, but also a therapy capable of accelerating neutrophil and platelet recovery. Administration of the hematopoietic growth factors either singly or in combinations may prove useful in accelerating leukocyte and platelet recovery.

We (48–50), as well as others (33), have demonstrated in a primate model that rhGM-CSF administration alone or in combination with IL-3 (50) elicits increased levels of circulating leukocytes in primates. The degree of leukocytosis is dose dependent and rapidly resolves once the protein administration is discontinued. Similar results have been made in studies with G-CSF in primates (32). To evaluate whether GM-CSF (51–53) and G-CSF (54) treatment could accelerate leukocyte recovery following autologous bone marrow transplantation, several primate models have been employed. In these studies, an acceleration in granulocyte recovery was observed in all instances when compared to the control group. Pretreatment with either G-CSF or GM-CSF did not prevent the leukocyte nadir associated with the total body irradiation. An accelerated recovery of platelet count was observed in primates treated with GM-CSF but not G-CSF. Along with the observation that GM-CSF could accelerate neutrophil recovery following autologous bone marrow transplantation, GM-CSF was also found to increase neutrophil and platelet counts in two primates experiencing poor bone marrow engraftment (51) and in primates exposed to partial body irradiation (52). These experiments have demonstrated that the colony-stimulating factors should prove useful in accelerating leukocyte recovery following bone marrow transplantation. This was shown in autologous bone marrow transplant studies in human patients having melanoma (55), breast cancer (55), Hodgkin's disease (56), or acute lymphoblastic leukemia (ALL) (57) following intensive preparative therapy employing high-dose chemotherapy, and, for the ALL patients, marrow purging. Enhanced granulocyte but not platelet recovery was observed in the patients receiving GM-CSF. Accelerated neutrophil recovery was also observed in another study using G-CSF where single patients (with hematological malignancies) received a syngeneic, allogeneic, or autologous bone marrow transplant (58).

Colony-stimulating factors have also been found to accelerate the rate of recovery of leukocytes and platelets following chemotherapy alone. Encouraging results were initially observed in two primates who received G-CSF following two doses of the alkylating agent cyclophosphamide (60 mg/kg/day) (32). Several studies have now been reported evaluating the effects of G-CSF (38,59–60) and GM-CSF (61,62) on neutropenias induced by cytotoxic chemotherapy in patients with a variety of malignancies. In these instances, enhanced recoveries of neutrophil counts were observed. The use of CSFs in treating leukemia patients, however, must be carefully evaluated because of the responsiveness of many primary leukemic cells to the different hematopoietic growth factors (63,64). It is possible, however, that responsiveness might be exploited. In-vitro (65) and preliminary in-vivo (66) evidence suggests that rhGM-CSF will enhance the cytotoxic effects of the S-phase-specific agent cytosine arabinoside on myeloblasts in acute myeloblastic leukemia and in the myeloid blast crisis phase of chronic myeloid leukemia.

In addition to their use in treating the side effects of cancer therapy, the colony-stimulating factors may prove useful directly in treating malignant disease. The observation that systemic administration of autologous lymphokine-activated killer (LAK) cells and recombinant IL-2 (67) can, in some cases, prove beneficial to patients with metastatic disease at least suggests the possibility that the different CSFs might also be used in vivo or ex vivo to expand different populations of effector cells. Both GM-CSF and G-CSF have been shown to enhance tumoricidal activity of effector cells in vitro, either alone or in combination with tumor-specific monoclonal antibodies (68–73). These observations have opened the door for many exciting new approaches to cancer therapy.

IV. BLOOD REPLACEMENT

Blood transfusion therapy is common practice in modern medicine and surgery. Hazards associated with transfusion therapy include immediate and hemolytic transfusion reactions, graft-versus-host disease, allergic reactions, and transmission of bacterial, parasitic, and viral agents to the recipient. With the development of new technologies, leukocyte transfusions have also become available. Granulocyte transfusions have been shown to be efficacious in combination with antibiotics in the treatment of granulocytopenic patients that are septicemic. A problem with leukocyte transfusion, however, is that granulocyte storage life is short. Colony-stimulating factors may prove beneficial here. For example, GM-CSF has been shown to enhance the survival and function of purified human blood neutrophils and eosinophils (74). This suggests that GM-CSF could aid in extending the granulocyte storage life and enhance the activity of granulocyte transfusions.

Still another potential for hematopoietic growth factors is to expand either ex vivo or in vivo a population of cells that could subsequently be purified and transfused into a patient. For example, erythropoietin could be used to increase red blood cell numbers, G-CSF to increase neutrophil count, or GM-CSF to increase the number of circulating granulocytes and monocytes. These cells could then be transfused into another patient or autotransfused into the donor following surgery or myelosuppressive therapy, enhancing host defense and/or minimize transmission of infectious agents such as cytomegalovirus and HIV.

Similarly, one may wish to expand the progenitor pool of a donor with CSFs prior to the harvest of bone marrow or peripheral blood leukocytes for transplant. rhGM-CSF has been shown in humans to expand both circulating (75) and bone marrow-derived (76,77) hematopoietic progenitor compartments in vivo. Initial studies in humans suggest that circulating stem cells mobilized using GM-CSF and subsequently harvested by apheresis will prove effective in accelerating hemopoietic recovery following myeloablative therapy in cancer patients when reinfused alone (78) or in combination with bone marrow (79). Preliminary studies further suggest that IL-3 (80,81) and G-CSF (82) may also prove effective in expanding the circulating pool of progenitors.

The use of such regimens could potentially eliminate the leukocyte nadirs associated with myeloablative therapies and increase the therapeutic index of chemotherapeutic agents used in treating cancer. These leukocytes can also be used as potential targets for gene therapy.

V. NATURALLY OCCURRING CYTOPENIAS

Bone marrow failure syndromes are associated with a decreased output of either one or multiple mature hematopoietic cell types into the circulation. The pathophysiology and etiology of many of these syndromes remain unclear. They can result from defects at the level of the stem cell or the microenvironment. For example, cytopenias can be due to functional defects and/or reduced numbers of stem or progenitor cells; stromal or microvascular defects; cellular or humoral inhibitory mechanisms; or a deficiency in a cellular or humoral element important in the proliferation and maturation of hematopoietic progenitors (83).

In certain cases, hematopoietic growth factors may prove useful in expanding the stem or progenitor cell pool and/or stimulate the maturation of preexisting progenitors. The effectiveness of a hematopoietic growth factor in a bone marrow failure syndrome was demonstrated initially with GM-CSF in the treatment of a pancytopenic primate naturally infected with a type D retrovirus having an acquired immunodeficiency syndrome (48). In this case a dramatic leukocytosis and reticulocytosis was elicited upon treatment with GM-CSF. Phase I trials of GM-CSF in leukopenic patients having the acquired immunodeficiency syndrome (84) or patients with myelodysplastic syndromes (85–89) have now been completed. In all instances GM-CSF was capable of elevating white blood cell counts, but the effects on the other cell lineages were variable. Phase I trials of GM-CSF in patients with aplastic anemia have also been attempted. As this disorder is quite heterogeneous in nature (83), it is not too surprising that the responses of the patients to GM-CSF were also quite variable (90–92). Lack of responsiveness may correlate with either the absence of responsive progenitors or the presence of inhibitors.

With a better understanding of the pathogenesis of naturally occurring cytopenias, additional uses for the hematopoietic growth factors will certainly emerge. We expect that combinations of hematopoietic factors will soon be used in various clinical situations and, if the clinical results are as promising as the results from primate studies, they should provide powerful new therapies for the clinician.

REFERENCES

1. Pluznik DH, Sachs L. The colony of normal "mast" cells in tissue culture. J Cell Comp Physiol 1965; 66:319–24.
2. Bradley TR, Metcalf D. The growth of mouse bone marrow cells in vitro. Aust J Exp Biol Med Sci 1966; 44:287–300.
3. Clark SC, Kamen R. The human hematopoietic colony-stimulating factors. Science 1987; 236:1229–37.
4. Fung MC, Hapel AJ, Ymer S, Cohen DR, Johnson RM, Campbell HD, Young IG. Molecular cloning of cDNA for murine interleukin-3. Nature 1984; 307:233–7.
5. Gough NM, Gough J, Metcalf D, Kelso A, Grail D, Nicola NA, Burgess AS, Dunn AR. Molecular cloning of cDNA encoding a murine hematopoietic growth regulatory granulocyte-macrophage colony-stimulating factor. Nature 1984; 309:763–6.

6. Tsuchiya M, Asano S, Kaziro Y, Nagata S. Isolation and characterization of the cDNA for murine granulocyte colony-stimulating factor. Proc Natl Acad Sci USA 1986; 83:7633–7.
7. Rajavashisth TB, Eng R, Shadduck RK, Waheed A, Ben-Avram CM, Shively JE, Lusis AJ. Cloning and tissue-specific expression of mouse macrophage colony-stimulating factor mRNA. Proc Natl Acad Sci USA 1987; 84:1157–61.
8. Shoemaker CB, Mitsock LD. Murine erythropoietin gene: cloning, expression, and human gene homology. Mol Cell Biol 1986; 6:849–58.
9. Wong GG, Witek JS, Temple PA, Wilkens KM, Leary AC, Luxenberg DP, Jones SS, Brown EL, Kay RM, Orr EC, Shoemaker C, Golde DW, Kaufman RJ, Hewick RM, Wang EA, Clark SC. Human GM-CSF: molecular cloning of the complementary DNA and purification of the natural and recombinant proteins. Science 1985; 228:810–5.
10. Nagata S, Tsuchiya M, Asano S, Kaziro Y, Yamazaki T, Yamamoto O, Hirata Y, Kubota N, Oheda M, Nomura H, Ono M. Molecular cloning and expression of cDNA for human granulocyte colony-stimulating factor. Nature 1986; 319:415–8.
11. Souza LM, Boone TC, Grabilove J, Lai PH, Zsebo KM, Murdock DC, Chazin VR, Bruszewski J, Lu H, Chen KK, Barendt J, Platzer E, Moore MAS, Mertelsmann R, Welte K. Recombinant human granulocyte colony-stimulating factor: effects on normal and leukemic myeloid cells. Science 1986; 232:61–5.
12. Jacobs K, Shoemaker C, Rudersdorf R, Neill SD, Kaufman RJ, Mufson A, Seehra J, Jones SS, Hewick R, Fritsch EF, Kawakita M, Shimizu T, Miyake T. Isolation and characterization of genomic cDNA clones of human erythropoietin. Nature 1985; 313:806–10.
13. Lin FK, Suggs S, Lin CH, Browne JK, Smalling R, Egrie JC, Chen KK, Fox GM, Martin F, Stabinsky Z, Badrawi SM, Lai PH, Goldwasser E. Cloning and expression of the human erythropoietin gene. Proc Natl Acad Sci USA 1985; 82:7580–4.
14. Yang YC, Ciarletta AB, Temple PA, Chung MP, Kovacic S, Witek-Giannotti JS, Leary AC, Kriz R, Donahue RE, Wong GG, Clark SC. Human IL-3 (multi-CSF): identification by expression cloning of a novel hematopoietic growth factor related to murine IL-3. Cell 1986; 47:3–10.
15. Kawasaki ES, Ladner MB, Wang AM, Arsdell JV, Warren MK, Coyne MY, Schweickart VL, Lee MT, Wilson KJ, Boosman A, Stanley ER, Ralph P, Mark DF. Molecular cloning of a complementary DNA encoding human macrophage-specific colony-stimulating factor (CSF-1). Science 1985; 230:291–6.
16. Wong GG, Temple PA, Leary AC, Witek-Giannotti JS, Yang YC, Ciarletta AB, Chung M, Murtha P, Kriz R, Kaufman RJ, Ferenz CR, Sibley BS, Turner KJ, Hewick RM, Clark SC, Yanai N, Yokota H, Yamada M, Saito M, Motoyoshi K, Takaku S. Human CSF-1: molecular cloning and expression of a 4kb cDNA encoding the human urinary protein. Science 1987; 235:1504–8.
17. Metcalf D. The hemopoietic colony stimulating factors. Amsterdam: Elsevier, 1984.
18. Gasson JC, Weisbart RH, Kaufman SE, Clark SC, Hewick RM, Wong GG, Golde DW. Purified human granulocyte-macrophage colony-stimulating factor: direct action on neutrophils. Science 1984; 226:1339–42.
19. Wang JM, Colella S, Allavena P, Mantovani A. Chemotactic activity of human recombinant granulocyte-macrophage colony-stimulating factor. Immunology 1987; 60:439–44.
20. Lopez AF, Williamson J, Gamble JR, Begley CG, Harlan JM, Klebanoff SJ, Waltersdorph A, Wong G, Clark SC, Vadas MA. Recombinant human granulocyte-macrophage colony-stimulating factor stimulates in vitro mature human neutrophil and eosinophil function, surface receptor expression, and survival. J Clin Invest 1986; 78:1220–8.
21. Weisbart RH, Golde DW, Clark SC, Wong GG, Gasson JC. Human granulocyte-macrophage colony-stimulating factor is a neutrophil activator. Nature 1985; 314:361–3.
22. Burgess AW, Begley CG, Johnson GR, Lopez AF, Williamson DJ, Mermod JJ, Simpson RJ, Schmitz A, DeLamarter JF. Purification and properties of bacterially synthesized human granulocyte-macrophage colony stimulating factor. Blood 1987; 69:43–51.

23. Weisbart RH, Kwan L, Golde DW, Gasson JC. Human GM-CSF primes neutrophils for enhanced oxidative metabolism in response to the major physiological chemoattractants. Blood 1987; 69:18–21.
24. Weisbart RH, Golde DW, Gasson JC. Biosynthetic human GM-CSF modulates the number and affinity of neutrophil f-Met-Leu-Phe receptors. J Immunol 1986; 137:3584–7.
25. Metcalf D, Begley CG, Johnson GR, Nicola NA, Vadas MA, Lopez AF, Williamson DJ, Wong GG, Clark SC, Wang EA. Biologic properties in vitro of a recombinant human-granulocyte-macrophage colony-stimulating factor. Blood 1986; 67:37–45.
26. Fleischmann J, Golde DW, Weisbart RH, Gasson JC. Granulocyte-macrophage colony-stimulating factor enhances phagocytosis of bacteria by human neutrophils. Blood 1986; 68:708–11.
27. Silberstein DS, Owen WF, Gasson JC, DiPersio JF, Golde DW, Bina JC, Soberman R, Austen KF, David JR. Enhancement of human eosinophil cytotoxicity and leukotriene synthesis by biosynthetic (recombinant) granulocyte-macrophage colony-stimulating factor. J Immunol 1986; 137:3290–4.
28. Weiser WY, Niel AV, Clark SC, David JR, Remold HG. Recombinant human granulocyte/macrophage colony-stimulating factor activates intracellular killing of *Leishmani donovani* by human-derived macrophages. J Exp Med 1987; 166:1436–46.
29. Reed SG, Nathan CF, Phil DL, Rodricks P, Shanebeck K, Conlon PJ, Grabstein KH. Recombinant granulocyte/macrophage colony-stimulating factor activates macrophages to inhibit *Trypanosoma cruzi* and release hydrogen peroxide. J Exp Med 1987; 166:1734–46.
30. Karbassi A, Becker JM, Foster JS, Moore RN. Enhanced killing of *Candida albicans* by murine macrophages treated with macrophage colony-stimulating factor: evidence for augmented expression of mannose receptors. J Immunol 1987; 139:417–21.
31. Metcalf D. The molecular biology and functions of the granulocyte-macrophage colony-stimulating factors. Blood 1986; 67:257–67.
32. Welte K, Bonilla M, Gillio AP, Boone TC, Potter GK, Gabrilove JL, Moore MAS, O'Reilly RJ, Souza LM. Recombinant human G-CSF: effects on hematopoiesis in normal and cyclophosphamide treated primates. J Exp Med 1987; 165:941–8.
33. Mayer P, Lam C, Obenaus H, Liehl E, Besemer J. Recombinant human GM-CSF induces leukocytosis and activates peripheral blood polymorphonuclear neutrophils (PMNs) in nonhuman primates. Blood 1987; 70:206–13.
34. MacVittie TJ, D'Alesandro MM, Monroy RL. Kaffenberger W, Patchen ML, Clark SC, Donahue RE. Recombinant human granulocyte-macrophage colony-stimulating factor (rh GM-CSF): effects of *in vivo* infusion into monkeys on hemopoiesis and priming of circulating neutrophils. (Submitted.)
35. Linnekin DM, Monroy RL, Donahue RE, MacVittie TJ. Priming effects of recombinant human granulocyte-macrophage colony-stimulating factor on nonhuman primate polymorphonuclear neutrophil motility. (Submitted.)
36. Baldwin GC, Gasson JC, Quan SC, Fleischmann J, Weisbart R, Oette D, Mitsuyasu RT, Golde DW. Granulocyte-macrophage colony-stimulating factor enhances neutrophil function in acquired immunodeficiency syndrome patients. Proc Natl Acad Sci USA 1988; 85:2763–6.
37. Sullivan R, Fredette JP, Socinski M, Elias A, Antman K, Schnipper L, Griffin JD. Enhancement of superoxide anion release by granulocytes harvested from patients receiving granulocyte-macrophage colony-stimulating factor. Br J Haematol 1989; 71:475–9.
38. Gabrilove JL, Jakubowski A, Scher H, Sternberg C, Wong G, Grous J, Yagoda A, Fain K, Moore MAS, Clarkson B, Oettgen HF, Alton K, Welte K, Souza L. Effect of granulocyte colony-stimulating factor on neutropenia and associated morbidity due to chemotherapy for transitional-cell carcinoma of the urothelium. New Engl J Med 1988; 318:1414–42.
39. Peters WP, Stuart A, Affronti ML, Kim CS, Coleman E. Neutrophil migration is defective during recombinant human granulocyte-macrophage colony stimulating factor (rHuGM-

CSF) infusion after autologous bone marrow transplantation in humans. Blood 1988; 72:1310–5.
40. Vadhan-Raj S, Hittelman WW, Ventura C, Bueshcher S, Keating MJ, Gutterman JU. Granulocyte-macrophage colony-stimulating factor and myelodysplastic syndromes. New Engl J Med 1988; 319:51–3.
41. Buescher ES, McIlheran SM, Vadhan-Raj S. Effects of *in vivo* administration of recombinant human granulocyte-macrophage colony-stimulating factor on human neutrophil chemotaxis and oxygen metabolism. J Infect Dis 1988; 158:1140–2.
42. Thorens B, Moermod J, Vassalli P. Phagocytosis and inflamatory stimuli induce GM-CSF mRNA in macrophages through post-transcriptional regulation. Cell 1987; 48:671–9.
43. Arnaout MA, Wang EA, Clark SC, Sieff C. Human recombinant granulocyte-macrophage colony-stimulating factor increases cell-to-cell adhesion and surface expression of adhesion-promoting surface glycoproteins on mature granulocytes. J Clin Invest 1986; 78:597–601.
44. Socinski MA, Cannistra SA, Sullivan R, Elias A, Antman K, Schnipper L, Griffin JD. Granulocyte-macrophage colony-stimulating factor induces the expression of the CD11b surface adhesion molecule on granulocytes *in vivo*. Blood 1988; 72:691–7.
45. Devereux S, Linch DC, Campos-Costa D, Spittle MF, Jelliffe AM. Transcient leucopenia induced by granulocyte-macrophage colony-stimulating factor. Lancet 1987; ii:1523–4.
46. Devereux S, Bull HA, Campos-Costa D, Saib R, Linch DC. Granulocyte macrophage colony-stimulating factor induced changes in cellular adhesion molecule expression and adhesion to endothelium: *in vitro* and *in vivo* studies in man. Br J Haematol 1989; 71:323–30.
47. Devereux S, Porter JB, Hoyes KP, Abeysinghe RD, Said R, Linch DC. Secretion of neutrophil secondary granules occurs during granulocyte-macrophage colony stimulating factor induced margination. Br J Haematol 1990; 74:17–23.
48. Donahue RE, Wang EA, Stone DK, Kamen R, Wong GG, Sehgal PK, Nathan DG, Clark SC. Stimulation of hematopoiesis in primates by continuous infusion of recombinant human GM-CSF. Nature 1986; 321:872–5.
49. Donahue RE, Wang EA, Kaufman RJ, Foutch L, Leary AC, Witek-Giannotti JS, Metzger M, Hewick RM, Steinbrink DR, Shaw G, Kamen R, CLark SC. Effects of N-linked carbohydrate on the *in vivo* properties of human GM-CSF. Cold Spring Harbor Symp Quant Biol 1986; 51:685–92.
50. Donahue RE, Seehra J, Metzger M. Lefebvre D, Rock B, Carbone S, Nathan DG, Garnick M, Sehgal PK, Laston D, LaVallie E, McCoy J, Schendel PF, Norton C, Turner K, Yang YC, Clark SC. Human IL-3 and GM-CSF act synergistically in stimulating hematopoiesis in primates. Science 1988; 241:1820–3.
51. Nienhuis AW, Donahue RE, Karlsson S, Clark SC, Agricola B, Antinoff N, Pierce JE, Turner P, Anderson WF, Nathan DG. Recombinant human granulocyte-macrophage colony stimulating factor (GM-CSF) shortens the period of neutropenia following autologous bone marrow transplantation in a primate model. J Clin Invest 1987; 80:573–7.
52. Monroy RL, Skelly RR, MacVittie TJ, Davis TA, Sauber JJ, Clark SC, Donahue RE. The effect of recombinant GM-CSF on the recovery of monkeys transplanted with autologous bone marrow. Blood 1987; 70:1696–9.
53. Monroy RL, Skelly RR, Taylor P, Dubois A, Donahue RE, MacVittie TJ. Recovery from severe hematopoietic suppression using recombinant human granulocyte-macrophage colony stimulating factor. Exp Hematol 1988; 16:344–8.
54. Gillio AP, Bonilla MA, Potter GK, Gabrilove JL, O'Reilly RJ, Souza LM, Welte K. Effects of recombinant human granulocyte-colony stimulating factor on hematopoietic reconstitution after autologous bone marrow transplantation in primates. Transplant Proc 1987; 19:153–6.
55. Brandt SJ, Peters WP, Atwater SK, Kurtzberg J, Borowitz MJ, Jones RB, Shpall EJ, Bast

RC, Gilbert CJ, Oette DH. Effect of recombinant human granulocyte-macrophage colony-stimulating factor on hematopoietic reconstitution after high-dose chemotherapy and autologous bone marrow transplantation. New Engl J Med 1988; 318:869–76.

56. Devereaux S, Linch DC, Gribben JG, McMillan A, Patterson K, Goldstone AH. GM-CSF accelerates neutrophil recovery after autologous bone marrow transplantation for Hodgkin's disease. Bone Marrow Transplant 1989; 4:49–54.

57. Blazer BR, Kersey JH, McGlave PB, Vallera DA, Lasky LC, Haake RJ, Bostrom B, Weisdorf R, Epstein C, Ramsay NKC. *In vivo* administration of recombinant human granulocyte/macrophage colony stimulating factor in acute lymphoblastic leukemia patients receiving purged autografts. Blood 1989; 73:849–57.

58. Kodo H, Tajika K, Takahashi S, Ozawa K, Asano S, Fumimaro T. Acceleration of neutrophilic granulocyte recovery after bone-marrow transplantation by administration of recombinant human granulocyte colony-stimulating factor. Lancet 1988; ii:38–9.

59. Morstyn G, Souza LM, Keech J, Sheridan W, Campbell L, Alton NK, Green M, Metcalf D. Effect of granulocyte colony stimulating factor on neutropenia induced by cytotoxic chemotherapy. Lancet 1988; ii:667–72.

60. Bronchud MH, Scarffe JH, Thatcher N, Crowther D, Souza LM, Alton NK, Testa NG, Dexter TM. Phase I/II study of recombinant human granulocyte colony-stimulating factor in patients receiving intensive chemotherapy for small cell lung cancer. Br J Cancer 1987; 56:809–13.

61. Antman KS, Griffin JD, Elias A, Socinski MA, Ryan L, Cannistra SA, Oette D, Whitley M, Frei E, Schnipper LE. Effect of recombinant human granulocyte-macrophage colony-stimulating factor on chemotherapy-induced myelosuppression. N Engl J Med 1988; 319:593–8.

62. Gattringer C, Thaler J, Drach J, Micksche M, Huber H. GM-CSF treatment in aplasia after cytotoxic therapy. Onkologie 1989; 12:16–18.

63. Griffin JD, Lowenberg B. Review: clonogenic cells in acute myeloblastic leukemia. Blood 1986; 68:1185–95.

64. Young DC, Wagner K, Griffin JD. Constitutive expression of the granulocyte-macrophage colony-stimulating factor gene in acute myeloblastic leukemia. J Clin Invest 1987; 79:100–6.

65. Cannistra SA, Groshek P, Griffin JD. Granulocyte-macrophage colony-stimulating factor enhances the cytotoxic effects of cytosine arabinoside in acute myeloblastic leukemia and in the myeloid blast crisis phase of chronic myeloid leukemia. Leukemia 1989; 3:382–34.

66. Ganser A, Ottmann OG, Schulz G, Ohelzer D. Recombinant human granulocyte-macrophage colony-stimulating factor and low-dose cytosine arabinoside in patients with myelodysplastic syndrome: a pilot study. Onkologie, 1989; 12:13–5.

67. Rosenberg SA, Lotze MT, Muhl LM, Leitman S, Chang AE, Ettinghausen SE, Matory YL, Skibber JM, Shiloni E, Vetto JT, Seipp CA, Simpson C, Reichert CN. Observations on the systemic administration of autologous lymphokine-activated killer cells and recombinant interleukin-2 to patients with metastatic cancer. N Engl J Med 1985; 313:1485–92.

68. Grabstein KH, Urdal DL, Tushinski RJ, Mochizuki DY, Price VL, Cantrel MA, Gillis S, Conlon PJ. Induction of macrophage tumoricidal activity by granulocyte-macrophage colony-stimulating factor. Science 1986; 232:506–8.

69. Fabian I, Baldwin GC, Golde DW. Biosynthetic granulocyte-macrophage colony-stimulating factor enhances neutrophil cytotoxicity toward human leukemia cells. Leukemia 1987; 1:613–7.

70. Matsuda A, Shirafuji N, Kodo H, Ieki R, Uemura N, Watari K, Nagata S, Sekiguchi M, Asano S. Enhancement of antibody-dependent neutrophil-mediated cytoxicity against human melanoma cells by human granulocyte colony-stimulating factor (hG-CSF). Exp Hematol 1987; 15:525.

71. Mufson RA, Aghajanian J, Wong G, Woodhouse C, Morgan AC. Macrophage colony-

stimulating factor enhances monocyte and macrophage antibody-dependent cell-medicated cytotoxicity. Cell Immunol 1989; 119:182–92.
72. Kushner H, Cheung NKV. GM-CSF enhances 3F8 monoclonal antibody-dependent cellular cytotoxicity against human melanoma and neuroblastoma. Blood 1989; 73:1936–41.
73. Munn DH, Cheung NKV. Antibody-dependent antitumor cytotoxicity by human monocytes cultured with recombinant macrophage colony-stimulating factor. J Exp Med 1989; 170:511–26.
74. Begley CG, Lopez AF, Nicola NA, Warren DJ, Vadas MA, Sanderson CJ, Metcalf D. Purified colony-stimulating factors enhance the survival of human neutrophils and eosinophils in vitro: a rapid and sensitive microassay for colony-stimulating factors. Blood 1986; 68:162–6.
75. Socinski MA, Cannistra SA, Elias A, Antman KH, Schnipper L, Griffin JD. Granulocyte-macrophage colony stimulating factor expands the circulating haemopoietic progenitor cell compartment in man. Lancet 1988; ii:1194–8.
76. Broxmeyer H, et al. Kinetics of human hemopoietic cells after *in vivo* administration of granulocyte-macrophage colony-stimulating factor. J Clin Invest 1989; 83:551–7.
77. Aglietta M, et al. Kinetics of human hemopoietic cells after *in vivo* administration of granulocyte-macrophage colony-stimulating factor. J Clin Invest 1989; 83:551–7.
78. Haas R, Ho AD, Bredthauer U, Cayeux S, Egerer G, Knauf W, Hunstein W. Successful autologous transplantation of blood stem cells mobilized with recombinant human granulocyte-macrophage colony-stimulating factor. Exp Hematol 1990; 18:94–8.
79. Gianni AM, Siena S, Bregni M, Tarella C, Stern AC, Pileri A, Bonadonna G. Granulocyte-macrophage colony-stimulating factor to harvest circulating haemopoietic stem cells for autotransplantation. Lancet 1989; ii:580–5.
80. Monroy RL, Davis TA, Donahue RE, MacVittie TJ. Collection of enriched peripheral blood stem cells from primates treated with IL-1 and IL-3 in vivo. Blood 1989; 74 (suppl):75a.
81. Geissler K, Valent P, Mayer P, Liehl E, Hinterberger W, Lechner K, Bettelheim P. RhIL-3 expands the pool of circulating hemopoietic stem cells in primates—synergism with rhGM-CSF. Blood 1989; 74(suppl):151a.
82. Kurtzberg J, Kirkpatrick G, Atwater S, Peters W. Differential effects of continuous in vivo administration of G-CSF vs GM-CSF on bone marrow progenitor cell growth. Blood 1989; 74(suppl):17a.
83. Alter BP, Rappeport JM, Parkman SC (1981). The bone marrow failure syndromes. In: Nathan DG, Oski FA, eds. Hematology of infancy and childhood. Philadelphia: WB Saunders, 1981:168–249.
84. Groopman JE, Mitsuyasu RT, DeLeo MJ, Oette DH, Golde DW. Effect of recombinant human granulocyte-macrophage colony-stimulating factor on myelopoiesis in the acquired immunodeficiency syndrome. New Engl J Med 1987; 317:593–8.
85. Vadhan-Raj S, Buescher S, LeMaistre A, Keating M, Walters R, Ventura C, Hittelman W, Broxmeyer HE, Gutterman JU. Stimulation of hematopoiesis in patients with bone marrow failure and in patients with malignancy by recombinant human granulocyte-macrophage colony-stimulating factor. Blood 1988; 72:134–41.
86. Vadhan-Raj S, Keating M, LeMaistre A, Hittelman WN, McCredie K, Trujillo JM, Broxmeyer HE, Henney C, Gutterman JU. Effects of recombinant human granulocyte-macrophage colony-stimulating factor in patients with myelodysplastic syndromes. New Engl J Med 1987; 317:1545–52.
87. Ganser A, Volkers B, Greher J, Ottmann OG, Walther F, Becher R, Bergmann L, Schulz G, Hoelzer D. Recombinant human granulocyte-macrophage colony-stimulating factor in patients with myelodysplastic syndromes—a Phase-I/II trial. Blood 1989; 73:31–7.

88. Herrmann F, Lindemann A, Klein H, Lubbert M, Schulz G, Mertelsmann R. Effect of recombinant human granulocyte-macrophage colony-stimulating factor in patients with myelodysplastic syndrome with excess blasts. Leukemia 1989; 3:335–8.
89. Thompson JA, Lee DJ, Kidd P, Rubin E, Kaufmann J, Bonnem EM, Fefer A. Subcutaneous granulocyte-macrophage colony-stimulating factor in patients with myelodysplastic syndrome: toxicity, pharmacokinetics, and hematological effects. J Clin Oncol 1989; 7:629–37.
90. Nissen C., et al. Failure of recombinant human granulocyte-macrophage colony-stimulating factor therapy in aplastic anemia patients with very severe neutropenia. Blood 1988; 72:2045–7.
91. Vadhan-Raj S, et al. Stimulation of myelopoiesis in patients with aplastic anemia by recombinant human granulocyte-macrophage colony-stimulating factor. N Engl J Med 1988; 319:1628–34.
92. Champlin RE, Nimer SD, Ireland P, Oette DH, Golde DW. Treatment of refractory aplastic anemia with recombinant human granulocyte-macrophage colony-stimulating factor. Blood 1989; 73:694–9.
93. Paul SR, Bennett F, Calvetti JA, Kelleher K, Wood CR, O'Hara RM, Leary AC, Sibley B, Clark SC, Williams DA, Yang YC. Molecular cloning of a cDNA encoding interleukin 11, a novel stromal cell dervied lymphopoietic and hematopoietic cytokine. Proc Natl Acad Sci, USA 1990:7512–7516.
94. Zsebo KM, Wypych J, McNiell IK, Lu HS, Smith KA, Karkare SB, Sachdev RK, Yuschenkoff VN, Birnett NC, Williams LR, Satyagal VN, Tung W, Bosselman RA, Mendiaz EA, Langley KE. Identification, purification, and biological characterization of hematopoietic stem cell factor from buffalo rat liver-conditioned medium. Cell 1990; 63:195–201.
95. Anderson DM, Lyman SD, Baird A, Wignall JM, Eisenman J, Rauch C, March CJ, Boswell HS, Gimpel SD, Cosman D, Williams DE. Molecular cloning of mast cell growth factor, a hematopoietin that is active in both membrane bound and soluble forms. Cell 1990; 63:235–243.

27

G-CSF and M-CSF: Preclinical and Clinical Results

F. HERRMANN, A. LINDEMANN and R. MERTELSMANN
University of Freiburg, Freiburg, Germany

I. INTRODUCTION

Our knowledge of the colony-stimulating factors (CSFs) has increased dramatically over the past several years. Today, cDNAs for all human CSFs have been isolated, molecularly cloned, and expressed in large quantities for experimentation and clinical application. In this chapter, the molecular biology, biochemistry, physiology, pathobiology, and clinical promise of two CSFs [granulocyte (G)-CSF and macrophage (M)-CSF] will be briefly reviewed.

II. MOLECULAR BIOLOGY AND BIOCHEMISTRY OF G-CSF

G-CSF was the first of the human CSFs to be cloned based on amino acid sequence analysis and use of oligonucleotide probes to isolate the respective cDNA clones (1,2). The sources of protein and mRNA were the bladder carcinoma cell line 5637 and the squamous carcinoma cell line (CHU-2) (3,4). The G-CSF protein has 204 amino acids (AA), including a 30-AA signal sequence. The natural protein has a molecular weight (MW) of 19.6 kDa and contains a small amount of O-linked carbohydrate sites (1). The gene for human G-CSF has also been cloned (5). Five exons and four introns span the gene. A region of about 300 bp upstream of the transcription initiation site controls G-CSF gene expression. Within the G-CSF mRNA an elimination of three AA after position 35 results from an alternative splicing (5). The protein which lacks the three AA was shown to have much greater biological activity than the protein containing the insert (2,5). No homology of G-CSF with any other CSF exists, but several positions of identity and similarities in the gene structure are shared with human interleukin (IL)-6 (6). The human G-CSF gene maps to chromosome 17q 11–21 (7). G-CSF, expressed in *Escherichia coli* (1) and mammalian cells (2), is currently being explored in clinical trials (see below). There is no obvious difference in the biological activity of the molecule with or without glycosylation. In vitro, G-CSF is produced by mesenchymal cells such as vascular endothelial cells and fibroblasts, and by monocytes/macrophages and granulocytes (8–12) upon appropriate stimulation. These stimuli can be provided by second-messenger agonists (see Ref. 13 for review) of the three major signal transduction pathways (i.e., diacylglycerol-, cAMP-, and Ca^{2+}-activated pathways) or inflammation-associated mediators such as bacterial products and cytokines including IL-1, IL-4, IL-6, and tumor necrosis factor (TNF) (see Ref. 14 for review; 15). Interestingly, other CSFs including GM-CSF and multi-CSF (IL-3) may also stimulate expression of the G-CSF gene (11). The regulation of expression of the G-CSF gene can occur at the level of transcription as well as at the level of mRNA stabilization, although primarily post-transcriptional means are used (16,17). The presence of an AU-rich sequence in the 3′ noncoding region of the G-CSF mRNA may be a critical site for regulation of mRNA stability (18), which may serve as a recognition site for destabilizers of G-CSF mRNA (17). Ongoing research includes more precise definition of the sequences responsible for the control of G-CSF gene expression and the mechanisms involved.

III. PHYSIOLOGY AND PATHOBIOLOGY OF G-CSF

In vitro, natural and recombinant human (rh) G-CSF have been shown to stimulate proliferation and differentiation of progenitor cells committed to the granulocyte lineage (1,3,19). Analysis of the colonies formed in the presence of G-CSF indicated growth of predominantly neutrophil granulocytes (>90%) and of few monocytes. In addition, G-CSF has been shown to exert an in-vitro effect on the functional activity of mature neutrophils. In this regard, an enhancement of antibody-dependent cellular cytotoxicity (ADCC) (20), of surface expression of the chemotactic peptide receptor for fMLP (21), and of adhesion molecules of the LFA family has been demonstrated (22). G-CSF is also a weak inducer of secretion of arachidonic acid metabolites by neutrophils (23). Evidence for induction of differentiation of myeloid leukemia blasts by G-CSF came from studies utilizing the murine myelomonocytic leukemia line WEHI-3B, which in its D+ subline could be induced to develop a mature phenotype associated with loss of self-renewing potential (1). In contrast, the D− subline was incapable of differentiation upon exposure to G-CSF. Comparable results have been obtained with the human promyelocytic leukemia line HL60 and the human monoblast line U937, which can be induced to differentiate by G-CSF (24,25). Recently, other cytokines have been identified that may accelerate the process of differentiation induced by G-CSF, including rh leukemia-inhibitory factor (26) and rh IL-6 (unpublished observations). Cells obtained from fresh acute myelogenous leukemia (AML) samples have also been shown to be responsive for G-CSF. In short-term agar cultures, G-CSF promoted primarily proliferation of leukemic colony-forming cells (L-CFCs) (27); whereas in long-term cultures of AML cells, spontaneous differentiation was not augmented by exogenous G-CSF (28). In contrast to normal cells, which require prior stimulation to express G-CSF, leukemic blasts from 30–50% of AML patients were shown to constitutively synthesize various CSFs including G-CSF. Moreover, leukemia in-vitro growth of some of these patients was due to endogenous CSF in an autocrine fashion (29,30). There is also evidence to assume that AML cells use paracrine mechanisms to supply growth-promoting molecules and thus to escape growth restrictions, involving secretion of mediators such as IL-1 and TNF by leukemia cells that stimulate release of CSFs (e.g., G-CSF) by neighboring bone marrow stroma cells (31,32). It has also been shown that cells of stable-phase chronic myelogenous leukemia (CML) patients express G-CSF and use this factor to stimulate terminal divisions in maturing leukemic cells in vitro (33). Thus, unregulated expression of G-CSF may be part of the process of expansion of the myeloid compartment in CML. The reason for constitutive growth factor expression in acute and chronic myelogenous leukemia is presently unknown. There are, however, some indications to assume that activation of certain c-onc genes may contribute to growth-factor expression (34).

IV. PRECLINICAL ANIMAL STUDIES WITH rh G-CSF

In the preclinical setting, several animal models have been instrumental in predicting the in-vivo response to exogenous G-CSF. In mice, injection of G-CSF into the intraperitoneal cavity induced a neutrophilia and hastened neutrophil recovery following total body irradiation (TBI) and 5-fluorouracil treatment (35,36) due to stimulation of granulopoiesis. Similarly, continuous infusion of rh G-CSF to hamsters increased selectively the peripheral blood neutrophil count (NC) and reduced the duration of 5-fluorouracil-induced myelosuppression (37). Subcutaneous administration of rh G-CSF to cynomolgus monkeys also resulted in a selective and dose-dependent increase of the absolute NC. In all monkeys, the NC returned to baseline 3 to 7 days after cessation of G-CSF (38). The effects of rh G-CSF on cyclophosphamide-induced myelosuppression and on reconstitution of myelopoiesis after marrow-ablative TBI followed by autologous bone marrow transplantation (ABMT) was also examined. The results demonstrated that rh G-CSF could abbreviate the period of cyclophosphamide-induced neutropenia significantly (38) and could also stimulate the reconstitution of myelopoiesis following TBI/ABMT, but had no detectable effect on thrombopoiesis and erythropoiesis (39).

V. CLINICAL STUDIES WITH rh G-CSF

Since preclinical studies suggested that G-CSF would be an effective agent for reducing the infection-associated morbidity and mortality of severe neutropenia, rh G-CSF was introduced in clinical studies. Early clinical trials showed that rh G-CSF was active in humans. G-CSF induced a dose-dependent granulocytosis when administered by constant intravenous (i.v.) infusion (40), by short intravenous infusion (41), and by subcutaneous (s.c.) injection (22,42). Doses of G-CSF in the range 1–60 μg/kg/day by either i.v. or s.c. administration proved to be well tolerated. Some patients experienced bone discomfort, which was controlled by acetaminophen. Related to the increased granulocytosis and increased cell turnover, increased serum levels of lactate dehydrogenase and uric acid were recorded. Increases of the levels of leukocyte alkaline phosphatase, serum elastase, and lysozyme were attributed to an increase of the functional activity of phagocytes. The only reported adverse event related to G-CSF administration that required discontinuation of G-CSF was the induction of acute neutrophilic dermatosis (Sweet syndrome) in a patient with preexisting cutaneous vasculitis (43).

Based on these early Phase I clinical studies, rh G-CSF was evaluated in various nonneoplastic disease states associated with absolute neutropenia, such as severe congenital neutropenia (SCN; also referred to as Kostman's syndrome) (44,45), cyclic neutropenia (46), and idiopathic neutropenia (47), as well as in disease states associated with neutropenia due to neoplastic bone marrow infiltration including myelodysplastic syndrome (MDS) (48,49) and hairy cell leukemia (43). In addition, several studies were reported of G-CSF in combination with chemotherapy and associated myelosuppression without (40,41,50–52) or with autologous bone marrow support (53–55). Welte et al. (45) have administered rh G-CSF to 15 patients with SCN for 240 to 600 days at a dose of 3–60 μg/kg/day subcutaneously. Thirteen of the patients responded with an elevation of the NC above 1000μ/L, and this level of NC could be maintained during the entire treatment period. In three patients the increase in NC was associated with an improvement of severe bacterial infections resistant to antibiotic treatment. In another study (44), five SCN patients were treated with rh G-CSF. G-CSF led to an increase in the numbers of functional neutrophils in all patients. Hammond and co-workers undertook a study of the effects of rh G-CSF in six patients with cyclic neutropenia (46). Administration of G-CSF to cyclic neutropenic patients dramatically reduced cycle length and frequency of infective episodes but failed to eliminate the recurrent cycle count fluctuation. The effects of rh G-CSF in idiopathic neutropenia were investigated by Jakubowski et al. (47). A patient who was severely neutropenic responded to the administration of rh G-CSF with normalization of NC as long as the factor was given (160 days). The patient had no infections during the treatment period, and preexisting ulcers of the gingiva and hard palate showed healing within 10 weeks after initiation of G-CSF therapy. Studies using rh G-CSF in MDS patients were reported by Negrin et al. (49) and Kobayashi et al. (48). Negrin et al. observed in 10 of 12 patients a 5- to 40-fold increase of NC over the 8-week treatment period. Increased reticulocyte counts occurred in five patients, and were associated with decreased transfusion requirements. Platelet counts were stable or slightly increased. Kobayashi et al. reported similar results in five of five MDS patients treated. G-CSF administration after chemotherapy for small-cell lung cancer (40) and bladder cancer (50,51) resulted in shortening of the neutropenic period, independent of whether the factor was given in the first or the second cycle of chemotherapy. The neutrophil nadir occurred earlier in the cycle when rh G-CSF was given. Prechemotherapy G-CSF was shown to be unnecessary for the period of neutropenia to be reduced. Studies of Morstyn et al. (41) have investigated the optimal scheduling of G-CSF following chemotherapy. It was shown that s.c. administration was more effective than short i.v. infusions. It was unnecessary to elevate the levels of NC with G-CSF to supranormal levels before the time of the expected neutrophil nadir. It was also unnecessary to administer G-CSF following neutrophil recovery.

Studies which have directly compared cycles of chemotherapy with and without G-CSF showed a reduction in febrile days (50,52), fewer infections (40), fewer days on i.v. antibiotics (50,52), shortening of the duration of hospitalization (52), and reduction of the degree of mucositis (50). Some studies have also observed a favorable effect on platelet counts (50), most likely due to lower frequency of the use of platelet-toxic antibiotics, whereas others observed a fall in platelet levels when high doses (30–60 μg/kg/day) of G-CSF were used, which was most likely related to an enhanced consumption of platelets (22). In this study a transient decrease of neutrophil and monocyte counts in the first 30 min after G-CSF injection was reported. A modulation of surface adhesion structures was shown to result in aggregation and adhesion of these cells to the vessel endothelium and transient depletion of neutrophils and monocytes from the circulation.

G-CSF has also been used in three studies so far reported (53–55) in conjunction with ABMT. Sheridan et al. (53) treated a total of 16 patients with high-risk acute lymphoblastic leukemia (ALL), non-Hodgkin's lymphoma (NHL), Hodgkin's disease, and germ cell tumors in partial or complete remission with busulphan and cyclophosphamide as a preparative regimen followed by AMBT. G-CSF was started the following day at a dose of 60 μg/kg/day as a continuous subcutaneous infusion until a NC of ≥1500/μL was reached for 3 consecutive days and was stepwise reduced thereafter. Mean time to recovery to a NC of 500/μL was 11 days and to a NC of 1000/μL was 13 days, significantly less than in the matched historical control group, where the respective numbers were 20 and 29 days. No influence on the onset of fever and/or proven infection could be seen when the growth factor was given compared to the historical control group. However, patients receiving G-CSF had a statistically significant reduced requirement for parenteral antibiotics. Also reduced was the length of hospitalization and days of isolation. The M. D. Anderson transplant group (54) reported similar results on 18 patients with relapsed/refractory Hodgkin's disease treated with cyclophosphamide, carmustine, and etoposide as myeloablative protocol followed by AMBT on day 0. G-CSF was started on day 1 at a dose of 60 μg/kg/day as a 30-min i.v. infusion for a maximum of 28 days. The dose was reduced stepwise according to the NC in a manner similar to the study of Sheridan et al., once an adequate granulocyte count was obtained. Again, patients were compared to a matched historical control group including similar areas of previous irradiation and an identical number of previous cycles of chemotherapy. Also, identical numbers of nucleated cells were reinfused in the two groups. Whereas a NC of 0.1×10^9/L was reached after a median of 9 days in the group receiving G-CSF, the historical control group achieved this level not earlier than after 13 days. The number of days to recovery to a NC of 500/μL was 13 versus 22 and 16 versus 30, respectively.

A third study was performed by Peters et al. (55). This group explored different doses of G-CSF in a total of 24 patients with either advanced breast cancer or advanced melanoma. A preparative regime with cisplatinum, carmustine, and cyclophosphamide was given followed by ABMT and G-CSF 3 days later. The patients received G-CSF at doses of 16, 32, and 64 μg/kg/day as a 14-day continuous i.v. infusion. The time to the first appearance of neutrophils in the peripheral blood was 9 days and was not changed by application of G-CSF. However, the neurophil recovery was hastened by administration of G-CSF in the immediate phase thereafter, leading to a mean leucocyte count at day 14 of 6400/μL in the G-CSF-treated patient group compared to 900/μL in patients receiving no growth factor. In this study, administration of growth factors led to a decrease of the incidence of bacteremias from 35% in the historical control group to 18%.

Further studies are required to assess the safety and efficacy of long-term administration of G-CSF. In particular, more data are required from multiple courses of G-CSF in the chemotherapy setting. Dose-intensification studies of antineoplastic agents need to be performed to assess the clinical benefit to cancer patients in terms of improvement in survival rates. The possibility that G-CSF may promote tumor growth in patients with cancer or leukemia must also be considered.

VI. MOLECULAR BIOLOGY AND BIOCHEMISTRY OF M-CSF

The molecular biology of M-CSF is by far the most complex of all CSFs. The M-CSF gene contains 10 exons and 9 introns (56). Resulting from alternate splicing within exon 6, three forms of M-CSF RNA appear in the cytoplasma. All three RNAs are translated into different proteins, termed M-CSF-alpha, -beta, and -gamma (57). They share a common signal sequence of 32 AA, followed by 149 AA which represent the biologically active part of the molecule, share a transmembrane domaine of 23 AA and a 36-AA cytoplasmic domain. Genomic and cDNA clones of the three different M-CSFs have been cloned (58–60). M-CSF-alpha is 256 AA long, M-CSF-beta has 298 AA inserted after AA 181, and M-CSF-gamma has 182 AA inserted at the same position. The first 182 AA of this insertion are common to M-CSF-beta and -gamma (57). In the common 149-AA N-terminal domain are two N-linked glycosylation sites and seven cysteine residues. The M-CSF-alpha-soluble protein is a disulfide-bonded homodimer with a MW of 44–56 kDa (57). The M-CSF-beta and -gamma-secreted proteins are disulfide-bonded homodimers of 88 kDa. The presence of a transmembrane hydrophobic region of M-CSF has led to the speculation that M-CSF might be synthesized as a membrane-bound precursor that would be proteolytically cleaved to release the soluble form. This hypothesis has been substantiated by demonstrating that removal of the transmembrane and cytoplasmic domains by deletion mutagenesis abolished M-CSF surface expression and favored a more sufficient secretion of the protein (61). In contrast to other CSFs, the M-CSF gene lacks the long AU-rich sequences (59). Nevertheless, primarily post-transcriptional mechanisms control M-CSF gene expression (17,62). Several short AU-rich streches (58,59) may, however, contribute to the instability of the M-CSF mRNA. The cellular sources and mechanisms of induction of M-CSF correspond to those of G-CSF (17,62–69). Interestingly, M-CSF expression in monocytes is also subjected to autocrine regulation (70). Monocytes which are a major source of M-CSF also express high-affinity M-CSF receptors (70). The M-CSF receptor and the product of the c-fms proto-oncogene have been shown to be identical molecules (72).

VII. PHYSIOLOGY AND PATHOBIOLOGY OF M-CSF

M-CSF acts autocrinously as a circulating regulator of the mononuclear phagocyte system (73). It spurs proliferation and differentiation of monocytic bone marrow progenitor cells into mature monocytes, in synergy with granulocyte-macrophage (GM)-CSF (74,75). M-CSF stimulation also leads to differentiation of monocytes into macrophages (76). Mature macrophages are dependent on M-CSF for the maintenance of protein synthesis (77) and other functions, including stimulation of killing of *Candida albicans* (78), protection of macrophages from viral infection (79), stimulation of macrophage tumoricidal activity (80), and induction of secretion of secondary cytokines (64,65,70), prostaglandins (80), and plasminogen activator (82). These effects of M-CSF are mediated by binding to the high-affinity M-CSF receptor encoded by c-fms (72). The c-fms gene is the normal cellular homolog of the v-fms oncogene from the McDonough strain of the feline sarcoma virus (83). Furthermore, the c-fms gene product is expressed by monocytes and macrophages (71,84) and displays tyrosine kinase activity (84). C-fms gene expression during monocytic differentiation is regulated through post-transcriptional stabilization by a labile protein activated through the protein kinase C pathway (85). Clearance of M-CSF by M-CSF receptor-mediated endocytosis and intracellular destruction by Kupfer cells of the liver and spleen macrophages (73) appears to be the negative feedback control for monocyte/macrophage production. There are also indications from experiments in mice to assume that M-CSF produced by the gravid uterus plays a role in placental development (86). Synthesis of M-CSF secretion by uterine decidual cells appears to be controlled by chorionic gonadotropin (87).

There is also experimental evidence to suggest that M-CSF and its receptor can contribute to the development of neoplasia. A variety of epithelial neoplasms (uterus, ovary, breast, lung) and myeloid leukemias have been shown to express M-CSF and/or its receptor (30,88–90). Interestingly, in ovarian cancer, elevation of M-CSF serum levels was correlated with cancer activity (88). In addition, one integration site for the Friend murine leukemia virus is utilized in about 20% of in-vivo primary myeloid leukemias is the 5′ end of c-fms (91). Proviral integration at this side results in high levels of c-fms transcripts in multipotent bone marrow stem cells and could thus contribute to the development of leukemia. It has also been shown that infection of M-CSF-dependent cells with v-fms results in factor independence and tumorigenicity (92). Similarly, co-transfection of c-fms and M-CSF into 3T3 fibroblasts led to cellular transformation (93).

VIII. PRECLINICAL ANIMAL STUDIES WITH rh M-CSF

Single daily intravenous administration of rh M-CSF to mice (94) for a period of 4 days caused a dose-dependent increase in circulating monocyte counts that was 10-fold at the highest dose tested (20,000 U/day). M-CSF treatment also resulted in an increase of the macrophage content of the liver and peritoneal cavity (94) and a significant hematopoietic progenitor cell cycling rate (95). Multiple daily injections (>2 injections) of rh M-CSF to mice, however, suppressed progenitor cell cycling and failed to increase bone marrow, spleen, or blood cellularity (95).

IX. CLINICAL STUDIES WITH M-CSF

Recently the first preliminary results from clinical application of rh M-CSF in six patients have been obtained (96). At a dose of 30 μg/kg/day given as a continuous infusion, a doubling of the number of circulating monocytes with no obvious change of bone marrow cellularity was observed. Also, no adverse effects were recorded. More experience exists with the clinical use of purified urinary human M-CSF. Motoyoshi and Takaku (97) reported on results of Phase I/II studies of the Japanese M-CSF study group. In healthy volunteers, urinary M-CSF given once daily (8×10^6 U total dose) for 7 days (2-h infusion) caused a significant increase of the number of circulating monocytes. Urinary M-CSF given at the same dose after chemotherapy for urogenital cancer significantly increased the nadir of circulating leukocytes as compared to an identical preceding chemotherapy course without M-CSF, but had no effect on the duration of severe neutropenia. In a randomized controlled study of patients with gynecologic malignancies, 46 individuals received urinary M-CSF (8×10^6 U) for 7 days (2-h infusion). Interestingly, the average period of neutropenia (<500/μL) was significantly shortened and the average nadir of platelets significantly increased in chemotherapy courses with M-CSF compared to identical chemotherapy cycles in the same patient performed in the absence of exogenous M-CSF. A Phase II clinical study of urinary M-CSF was also performed after ABMT (98). In these studies the average number of days needed to recover to 1000/μL leukocytes in a control group (not receiving M-CSF) was 22.6 ±6.0 days. Recovery to 1000/μL leukocytes was, however, 16.7 ±5.7 days in patients who had received M-CSF.

X. CONCLUSION

Recombinant DNA technology has been central in answering questions in the research of regulation of development and function of hematopoietic cells. As a result of these studies, hematopoietic growth factors are now part of therapeutic thinking in hematology/oncology. Although clinical studies with M-CSF are still preliminary, Phase I and Phase II studies with recombinant human G-CSF have shown convincingly that this factor is able to correct various forms of impaired neutropoiesis. Factor-induced augmentation of neutrophil number and function, however, lasts only as long as the factor is continued. More data are required to show whether factor-associated elevation of neutrophils does indeed protect patients from or improve recovery from infections. There are also several rationales to use the above CSFs after high-dose anticancer chemotherapy. Acceleration of neutrophil recovery by exogenous CSF could contribute to reducing morbidity or mortality at current chemotherapy doses, or to increasing the dose intensity, and to allow administration of more repeated cycles of chemotherapy. The future will show whether this approach will live up to expectations and result in therapeutic benefit to cancer patients.

REFERENCES

1. Souza LM, Boone TC, Gabrilove J, et al. Science 1986; 232:61.
2. Nagata S, Tsuchiya M, Asano S, et al. Nature 1986; 319:415.
3. Welte K, Platzer E, Lu L, et al. Proc Natl Acad Sci USA 1985; 82:1526.
4. Nomura H, Imazeki I, Oheda M, et al. EMBO J 1986; 5:87.
5. Nagata S, Tsuchiya M, Asamo S, et al. EMBO J 1986; 5:575.
6. Hirano T, Yasukawa K, Harada H, et al. Nature 1986; 324:73.
7. Simmers RN, Weber CM, Shannon MF, et al. Blood 1987; 70:330.
8. Zsebo KM, Yuschenkoff VN, Schiffer S, et al. Blood 1988; 71:99.
9. Koeffler HP, Gasson J, Ranyard J, et al. Blood 1987; 70:55.
10. Vellenga E, Rambaldi A, Ernst TH, et al. Blood 1988; 71:1529.
11. Oster W, Lindemann A, Mertelsmann R, Herrmann F. Blood 1989; 73:64.
12. Lindemann A, Riedel D, Oster W, et al. J Clin Invest 1989; 83:1308.
13. Akashi M, Yamamoto K, Koeffler HP. In: (Mertelsmann R, Herrmann F, eds.) Hematopoietic growth factors in clinical application. New York: Marcel Dekker, 1990, 41.
14. Herrmann F, Mertelsmann R. Blut 1989; 58:117.
15. Wieser M, Bonifer R, Oster W, et al. Blood 1989; 73:1105.
16. Koeffler HP, Gasson J, Tobler A. Mol Cell Biol 1988; 8:3423.
17. Ernst TJ, Ritchie AR, Demetri GD, Griffin JD. J Biol Chem 1989; 264:5700.
18. Caput D, Beutler B, Hartog K, et al. Proc Natl Acad Sci USA 1986; 83:1670.
19. Strife A, Lambek C, Wisniewski D, et al. Blood 1987; 69:1508.
20. Platzer E, Welte K, Gabrilove J, et al. J Exp Med 1985; 162:1788.
21. Platzer E, Oez S, Welte K, et al. Immunobiology 1987; 172:185.
22. Lindemann A, Herrmann F, Oster W, et al. Blood 1989; 74:2644.
23. Herrmann F, Gauss J, Lindemann A, Mertelsmann R. Eur J Immunol 1990; 20:2513.
24. Elias L, Epps DEV. Leukemia 1988; 2:763.
25. Geissler K, Harrington M, Srivastava C, et al. J Immunol 1989; 143:140.
26. Maekawa T, Metcalf D. Leukemia 1989; 3:270.
27. Miyauchi J, Kelleher CA, Yang YC, et al. Blood 1987; 69:657.
28. Vellenga E, Ostapovicz D, O'Rourke B, Griffin JD. Leukemia 1987; 1:584.
29. Young DC, Demetri GD, Ernst TJ, et al. Exp Hematol 1988; 16:378.
30. Oster W, Lindemann A, Mertelsmann R, Herrmann F. Blood Cells 1988; 14:443.

31. Griffin JD, Rambaldi A, Vellenga E, et al. Blood 1987; 70:1218.
32. Oster W, Cicco NA, Klein H, et al. J Clin Invest 1989; 84:451.
33. Klein H, Becher R, Lübbert M, et al. J Exp Med 1990; 171:1785.
34. Graf T, v. Weizsäcker FV, Grieser S, et al. Proc Natl Acad Sci USA 1986; 83:2484.
35. Kobayaski Y, Okabe T, Urabe A, et al. Jpn J Cancer Res 1987; 78:763.
36. Shimamura M, Kobayaski Y, Yuo A, et al. Blood 1987; 69:353.
37. Cohen AM, Zsebo KM, Inoue H, et al. Proc Natl Acad Sci USA 1987; 84:2884.
38. Welte K, Bonilla MA, Potter GK, et al. J Exp Med 1987; 165:941.
39. Gillio AP, Bonilla MA, Potter GK, et al. Transplant Proc 1987; 19:153.
40. Bronchud MH, Scarffe JH, Thatcher N, et al. Br J Cancer 1987; 56:809.
41. Morstyn G, Campbell L, Souza LM, et al. Lancet 1988; 1:667.
42. Asamo S, Shirafuji N, Watari K, et al. Behring Inst Mitt 1988; 83:222.
43. Glaspy JA, Baldwin GC, Robertson PA, et al. Ann Intern Med 1988; 109:789.
44. Bonilla MA, Gillio AP, Ruggeiro M, et al. N Engl J Med 1989 320:1574.
45. Welte K, Zeidler C, Reiter A, et al. Blood 1990; 75:1056.
46. Hammond WP, Price TH, Souza LM, Dale DC. N Engl J Med 1989; 320:1306.
47. Jakubowski AA, Souza L, Kelly F, et al. N Engl J Med 1989; 320:38.
48. Kobayashi Y, Okabe T, Ozawa K, et al. Am J Med 1989; 86:178.
49. Negrin RS, Haeuber DH, Naglar A, et al. Ann Int Med 1989; 110:976.
50. Gabrilove JL, Jakubowski AA, Scher H, et al. N Engl J Med 1988; 312:1414.
51. Gabrilove JL, Jakubowski AA, Fain K, et al. J Clin Invest 1988; 82:1454.
52. Neidhart J, Mangalik A, Kohler W, et al. J Clin Oncol 1989; 7:1685.
53. Sheridan W, Wolf M, Lusk J, et al. Lancet 1989; 2:891.
54. Taylor K, Jagannath S, Spitzer G, et al. J Clin Oncol 1990; 8:1607.
55. Peters WP. Semin Hematol 1989; 26 (suppl 2):18.
56. Ladner MB, Martin GA, Noble JA, et al. EMBO J 1987; 6:2693.
57. Cosman D, Wignal J, Anderson D, et al. Behring Inst Mitt 1988; 83:15.
58. Kawasaki ES, Ladner MB, Wang AM, et al. Science 1986; 230:291.
59. Wong GG, Temple PA, Leary AC, et al. Science 1987; 235:1504.
60. Ceretti DP, Wignall J, Anderson D, et al. Mol Immunol 1988; 25:761.
61. Heard JM, Roussel MF, Rettenmier CW, Sherr CJ. Oncogene Res 1987; 1:423.
62. Horiguchi J, Sariban E, Kufe D. Mol Cell Biol 1988; 8:3951.
63. Oster W, Lindemann A, Horn S, et al. Blood 1987; 70:1700.
64. Rambaldi A, Young DC, Griffin JD. Blood 1987; 69:1409.
65. Horiguchi J, Warren MK, Kufe D. Blood 1987; 69:1259.
66. Seelentag WK, Mermod JJ, Montesano R, Vasalli P. EMBO J 1987; 6:2261.
67. Akaski M, Saito M, Koeffler HP. Blood 1989; 74:2383.
68. Mantovani L, Henschler R, Brach M, et al. FEBS Lett 1991; 280:97.
69. Oster W, Lindemann A, Mertelsmann R, Herrmann F. Eur J Immunol 1989; 19:543.
70. Warren MK, Ralph P. J Immunol 1986; 137:2281.
71. Nienhuis AW, Bunn HF, Turner PH, et al. Cell 1985; 42:421.
72. Sherr CJ, Rettenmier CW, Sacca R, et al. Cell 1985; 41:665.
73. Bartocci A, Mastrogiannis DS, Migliovati G, et al. Proc Natl Acad Sci USA 1987; 84:6179.
74. Stanley ER, Guilbert LJ, Tushinski RJ, Barelmez SH. J Cell Biochem 1983; 21:151.
75. Caracciolo D, Shirsat N, Wong GG, et al. J Exp Med 1987; 166:1851.
76. Becker S, Warren MK, Haskill S. J Immunol 1987; 139:3703.
77. Tushinski RJ, Stanley ER. J Cell Physiol 1983; 116:67.
78. Karbassi A, Becker JM, Foster JS, Moore RN. J Immunol 1987; 139:417.
79. Lee MT, Warren MK. J Immunol 1987; 139:3019.
80. Ralph P, Nakoinz I. Cell Immunol 1987; 105:270.
81. Herrmann F, Gauss J, Lindemann A, Mertelsmann R. Blood 1992; in press.

82. Hamilton JA, Stanley ER, Burgess AW, Shadduck RK. J Cell Physiol 1980; 103:435.
83. Donner L, Fedele LA, Garon CF, et al. J Virol 1982; 41:489.
84. Woolford J, Rothwell V, Rohrschneider L. Mol Cell Biol 1985; 5:3458.
85. Weber B, Horiguchi J, Luebbers R, et al. Mol Cell Biol 1989; 9:769.
86. Pollard JW, Bartocci A, Arceci R, et al. Nature 1987; 330:484.
87. Baccarimi M, Stanley ER. In: Habenicht A, ed. Growth factors, differentiation factors and cytokines. Berlin: Springer Verlag, 1989: 188.
88. Kacinski BM, Bloodgood RE, Carter D, et al. Int J Radiat Oncol Biol Phys 1988 (suppl 1):140.
89. Herrmann F, Oster W, Cicco NA, et al. In: Habenicht A, ed. Growth factors, differentiation factors, and cytokines. Berlin: Springer Verlag, 1989:292.
90. Rambaldi A, Wahamiya N, Vellenga E, et al. J Clin Invest 1988; 81:1030.
91. Gisselbrecht S, Fichelson S, Sola B, et al. Nature 1987; 329:259.
92. Wheeler EF, Rettenmier CW, Look AT, et al. Nature 1986; 324:377.
93. Roussel MF, Dull TJ, Rettenmier CW, et al. Nature 1986; 325:549.
94. Hume DA, Pavli P, Donahue RE, Fidler IJ. J Immunol 1988; 141:3405.
95. Chikkapa G, Broxmeyer HE, Cooper S, et al. Cancer Res 1989; 49:3558.
96. Jakubowski A, Cody B, Chapman P, et al. Blood 1989; 74 (suppl 1):1222 (abstr).
97. Motoyoshi K, Takaku F. (1990). In: Mertelsmann R, Herrmann F, eds. Hematopoietic growth factors in clinical application. New York: Marcel Dekker, 1990: 161.
98. Masaoka T, Motoyoshi K, Takaku F, et al. Bone Marrow Transplant 1988; 3:121.

28

Clinical Trials of Granulocyte-Macrophage Colony-Stimulating Factor for the Treatment of Aplastic Anemia

SAROJ VADHAN-RAJ
University of Texas, M. D. Anderson Cancer Center, Houston, Texas

I. INTRODUCTION

Aplastic anemia is a group of heterogenous disorders characterized by pancytopenia and a hypocellular bone marrow (1,2). Various mechanisms have been implicated in the pathogenesis of the disease. These include loss of hemopoietic cells, dysfunctional stem cells, defects in bone marrow microenvironment, and cellular- or humoral-mediated suppression of hematopoiesis (1–3). Aplastic anemia may be congenital or acquired. Although initiation of acquired aplastic anemia has been associated with exposure to drugs, toxic agents, radiation, viral infections, or other diseases, in the majority of patients the exact cause is unknown.

The severity of the hematopoietic insufficiency is classified using criteria defined by the International Aplastic Anemia Study Group. Patients with severe disease (as defined by a presence of any two of the three findings in peripheral blood—neutrophil counts $< 500/mm^3$, platelets $< 20{,}000/mm^3$, and a corrected reticulocyte count $< 1\%$, and a severe or moderate hypocellularity of the bone marrow), if untreated, have a median survival of 3 to 6 months, and 80% mortality within 1 year (4).

Bone marrow transplantation from a histocompatible donor is currently the treatment of choice for patients under the age of 40 years (5–7). However, this option is not available to a majority of the patients because of their older age or lack of an HLA-matched donor. Patients not suitable for bone marrow transplantation are generally treated with immunosuppressive agents such as antithymocyte globulin (ATG) (8–10). However, about half of the patients fail to respond to ATG or have only a temporary benefit from such treatment. Patients with severe aplastic anemia who cannot undergo marrow transplantation and who fail standard therapy have a high mortality from complications related to cytopenias (9,11,12). Consequently, supportive therapy with transfusion of blood products and antibiotics to combat infections remains the mainstay of treatment in a significant number of patients.

II. HEMATOPOIETIC GROWTH FACTORS

Most mature blood cells are short-lived and must be continually replenished (13–15). Production of mature blood cells is a multistep process that involves interactions of hematopoietic progenitor cells, cytokines, and accessory cell populations. Hematopoietic growth factors are a group of polypeptide hormones that stimulate the growth and differentiation of hematopoietic progenitor cells along multiple pathways. In both murine and human systems, several of these growth factors have been identified based on their ability to support the growth of colonies of progenitor cells in semisolid media, and classified depending on the type of cells seen in these colonies. Granulocyte colony-stimulating factor (G-CSF) and macrophage CSF (M-CSF) appear to be lineage specific, stimulating predominantly the growth of granulocytes and monocytes, respectively. Granulocyte-macrophage CSF (GM-CSF) and interleukin-3 (IL-3), on the other hand, have broader effects and stimulate proliferation of several cell lineages.

In addition to stimulating proliferation of hematopoietic progenitor cells, these hormones also augment select functions of mature cells (16–20). For instance, GM-CSF enhances superoxide production and lysozyme secretion in response to bacterial chemoattractant N-formyl-methionyl-leucyl-phenylalanine (fMLP), and phagocytosis of yeast by neutrophils. GM-CSF also stimulates antibody-dependent killing of tumor cells by neutrophils and eosinophils, and tumoricidal activity of monocytes.

The recent cloning of human genes encoding these proteins, and the availability of recombinant hematopoietic growth factors in sufficient quantities for clinical trials provides a possibility of a novel therapeutic approach to stimulate bone marrow function in patients with bone marrow failure states (21).

III. CLINICAL STUDIES OF GM-CSF IN APLASTIC ANEMIA

Based on its ability to stimulate the production and functions of granulocytes and monocytes, the potential role of GM-CSF has been evaluated in patients with aplastic anemia by several investigators. In the initial Phase I study of GM-CSF in patients with bone marrow failure, we observed a marked stimulation of myelopoiesis (Figures 1 and 2) in a patient with severe aplastic anemia who had relapsed after an initial temporary response to ATG (22). Based on this favorable experience, we evaluated the biological effects of GM-CSF in a total of 10 patients with aplastic anemia (23). Seven patients had a severe disease, and three had a moderate disease. Nine patients had acquired disease, while one patient had a familial type of congenital hypoplastic anemia. Nine of these 10 patients were not suitable for bone marrow transplantation, and many of these patients had received prior therapies with ATG (4 pts), steroids (8 pts), androgens (4 pts), and splenectomy (1 pt). All patients had pancytopenia and hypocellular or acellular bone marrow (cellularity $\leqslant$ 10% in nine patients). Seven patients were receiving red cell transfusions, and four patients were requiring periodic platelet transfusions. Baseline median neutrophil counts were 599/mm^3 (range, 99 to 1560/mm^3).

GM-CSF (60–500 μg/m^2/day) was administered by continuous intravenous infusion daily for 14 days. The 2-week treatment cycles alternated with 2-week rest periods. The treatment resulted in increases in white blood cell counts (1.6- to 10-fold) in all patients and neutrophils (1.5- to 20-fold). Nine of the 10 patients had $>$1500/mm^3 neutrophils during GM-CSF treatment. Significant increases were also seen in eosinophils (12- to $>$70-fold) and monocytes (2- to 32-fold). The counts returned to baseline levels

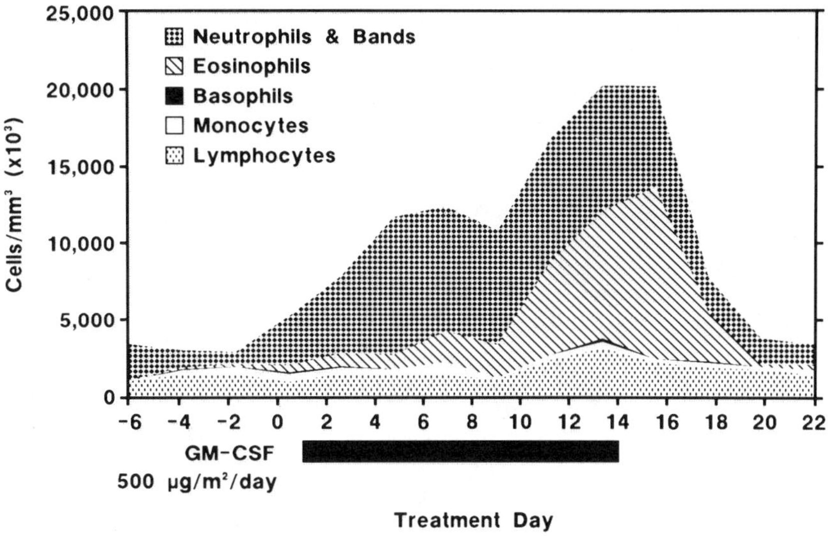

Figure 1 Effects of GM-CSF treatment on peripheral blood white cell counts and differential cells in a patient with aplastic anemia.

when GM-CSF infusion was discontinued, indicating that continuous administration of hormone was necessary to maintain the hematologic effect. However, white cells increased with repeated cycles of treatment.

While no increases in the concentration of bone marrow myeloid and erythroid colony-forming cells were seen, the responses in white blood cell counts were accompanied by increases in bone marrow cellularity [from baseline median 3% (range, 1% to 20%) to 42% (5 to 70%)], myeloid precursor cells (from baseline mean level of 20.5% to maximal mean level of 52.4%), and myeloid:erythroid cell ratios (from baseline mean of 2.2 to maximal mean of 12.5). These findings indicated that the responses in white blood cell counts were related to the proliferative effect of GM-CSF on myeloid compartment. The magnitude of myeloid response was dependent on the severity of the disease, indicating that the preserved level of hematopoiesis may be a critical factor for predicting the response to the growth factor.

Granulocytes derived after GM-CSF treatment were examined for locomotion and hydrogen peroxide production. Chemotaxis in response to formyl peptide (fMLP) was depressed prior to treatment and was not significantly affected by GM-CSF treatment. However, the rates of hydrogen peroxide production were significantly enhanced after GM-CSF treatment (152% of control values). Despite the increases in numbers of granulocytes and oxidative metabolism of phagocytic cells, four patients had episodes of sepsis during the study. This finding might be related to the need for central venous catheter for continuous infusion, intermittent schedule-dependent rise and fall in granulocyte counts, or persistence of impaired chemotaxis. Alteration of route (i.e., s.c. injections) and schedule (i.e., uninterrupted cycles) might overcome some of these problems.

In order to determine whether the pathophysiologic process of aplastic anemia is related to inappropriate levels of circulating growth-stimulatory or -inhibitory factors, serum samples were examined for the presence of various cytokines (Table 1). While

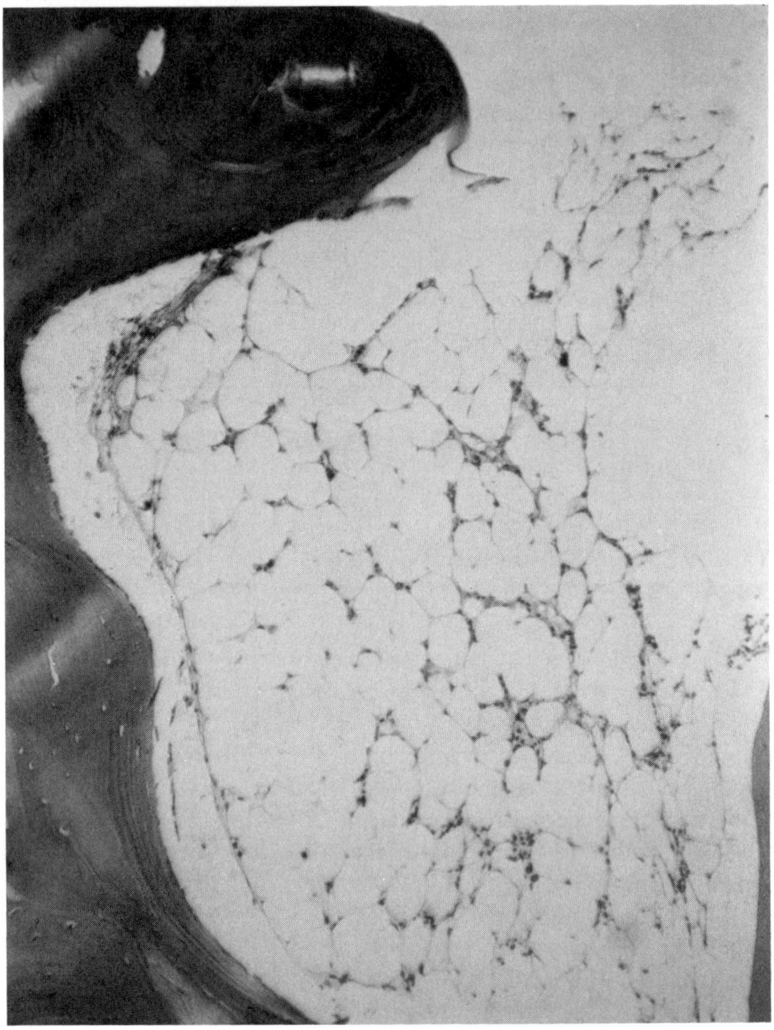

(a)

Figure 2 Bone marrow biopsy sections prior to (a) and after (b) GM-CSF treatment in the patient with aplastic anemia.

we did not detect any myeloid growth-factor activity in the serum from these patients, their serum erythropoietin levels were markedly elevated. Despite the presence of high levels of endogenous erythropoietin, erythropoietic responses were not seen in most of these patients. One possible explanation for the lack of erythropoietic response may be persistence of hematopoietic suppressors. While we did not detect any γ-interferon in patients' serum, circulating levels of interleukin-2 were detected in serum from eight patients. Thus it is possible that IL-2 may be one of the mediators involved in suppression of hematopoiesis.

Antin et al. treated seven patients with severe aplastic anemia with GM-CSF (24). All patients required red cell transfusions, and six required platelet transfusions. All

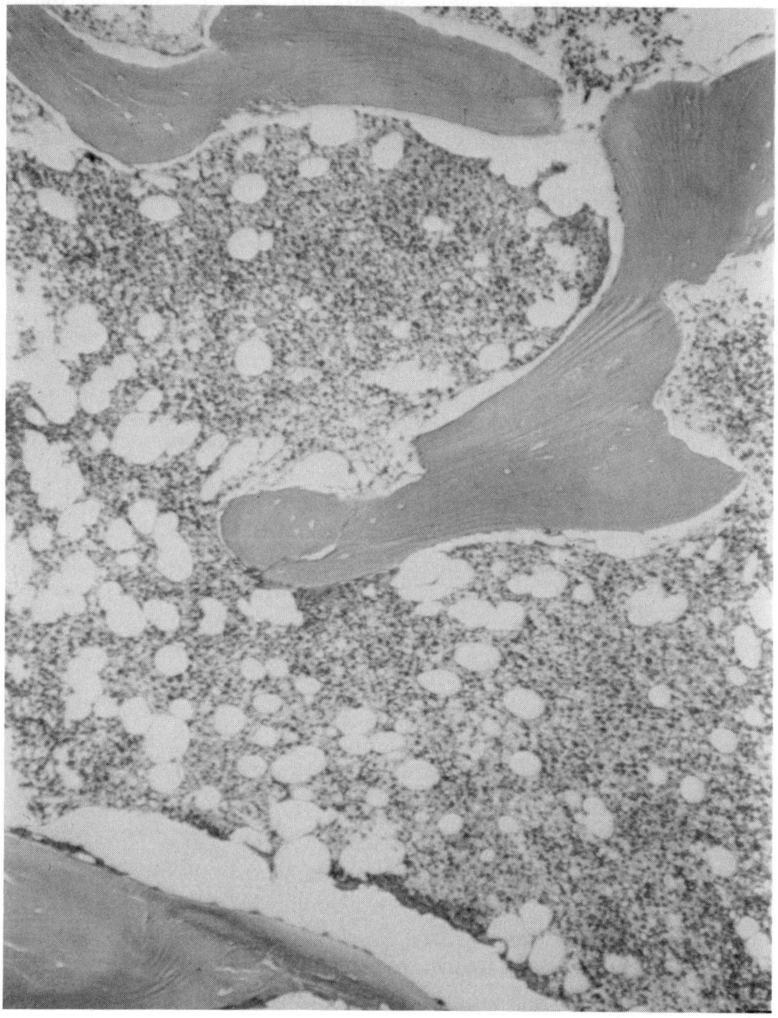

(b)

patients had granulocytopenia (median 192, range, 0–925/mm^3). Prior therapies included ATG (4 pts), androgen (3 pts), thymosin (1 pt), prednisone (2 pts), and cyclophosphamide and hydroxyurea (1 pt). GM-CSF (15 to 480 μg/m^2/day) was administered by 1- or 4-h infusion for 7 days or 12-h infusion for 14 days. Patients were treated at progressively higher dose levels if there was no observed toxicity.

Increases in granulocytes and monocytes were seen at the lowest doses used, whereas increases in reticulocytes were generally observed at the higher dose levels. At least a 100% increase was seen in granulocytes in 13 of 22 courses, in monocytes in 14 of 22 courses, and in reticulocytes in 13 of 16 courses. No increases were seen in eosinophils, immature myeloid cells, or platelets. Despite increases in reticulocytes, no amelioration of red-cell transfusion requirements were seen. The increases in granuocytes, monocytes, and reticulocytes were often seen 7 to 14 days after the discontinuation of infusion, suggesting an effect on early progenitors.

Table 1 Circulating Levels of Endogenous Serum Cytokines in Patients with Aplastic Anemia

Patient no.	Erythropoietin (mμ/mL)	Hemopoietic growth factors[a]	Il-2[b] (U/mL)	Il-1 (pg/ml)	γ-IFN (U/ml)
1	234	N[c]	15	N	<0.01
2	445	N	7	240	<0.01
3	>175	N	4	N	<0.01
4	81	N	2	N	<0.01
5	650	N	6	N	<0.01
6	126	N	3	N	<0.01
7	1200	N	8	N	<0.01
8	620	N	ND	N	<0.01
9	>175	N	9	N	<0.01
10	250	N	N	N	<0.01
Normal levels	4–26	N	N	N	<0.01
(Number of controls)	(25)	(20)	(5)	(5)	(10)

[a] Serum samples were tested for hemopoietic growth-factor by human bone marrow proliferation assay (G-CSF, GM-CSF, interleukin-3, or IL-5), 32D cell line proliferation assay (G-CSF), and CESS cell line immunoglobulin production assay (IL-6).

[b] Interleukin-2 assay was also negative in serum samples from five patients with cancer.

[c] N denotes negative. ND denotes not done.

Nissen et al. treated four patients with very severe aplastic anemia refractory to ATG (25). All patients had severe neutropenia ($\leqslant$ 30/mm^3) and were red cell and platelet transfusion dependant. GM-CSF (4–32 μg/kg/day) was administered by continuous i.v. infusion daily for 14 days or subcutaneously in twice-daily doses. One patient with evidence of residual marrow myelopoiesis responded to GM-CSF with increases in neutrophil counts, and recovered from septicemia and bilateral pneumonia that had been resistant to conventional therapy. In contrast, three patients with no evidence of residual myelopoiesis (neutrophil counts 0–10/mm^3) did not respond to GM-CSF. These results again support the observation that the level of residual hematopoiesis is an important determinant for response to GM-CSF.

Champlin et al. treated 13 patients with refractory aplastic anemia who had either failed to respond to ATG (10 patients) or relapsed after an initial response (3 pts) (26). Two of these three patients then failed on repeat treatment with ATG. Nine of these 13 patients had severe disease, and four had moderate disease. All patients required red cell transfusions, and 11 required platelet transfusions. All patients had granulocytopenia (median, 340; range, 30 to 770/mm^3) and monocytopenia (median, 70; range, 20 to 150/mm^3). GM-CSF (4 to 64 μg/kg/day) was administered by continuous i.v. infusion daily for 14–28 days.

Of the 11 evaluable patients, 10 had significant increments in neutrophils, eosinophils and monocytes. Seven had complete normalization of granulocyte counts, and three had partial responses (>500mm^3). Patients with pretreatment granulocyte counts >300/mm^3 had more increases in circulating myeloid cells than those with more severe granulocytopenia. Eight patients had normalization of their monocyte counts, and two had partial responses. Substantial increases were also seen in eosinophils.

White blood cell counts returned to baseline upon discontinuation of GM-CSF. The response in white blood cells was associated with significant increases in bone marrow cellularity [from baseline median 3% (range, 2% to 15%) to 36% (10% to 55%)] and myeloid hyperplasia. Of interest, one patient had increases in hemoglobin (from 7 to 11 gm/dL) and platelets (from 20 to 45 × $10^3/mm^3$). The transfusion requirements were unaffected in the remaining patients.

Guinan et al. have investigated the tolerance and efficacy of GM-CSF in nine pediatric patients with aplastic anemia (27). Seven patients had received treatment with ATG; four patients had relapsed after an initial response and two had received more than one course of treatment. Eight patients were red-cell transfusion dependent, and seven patients were platelet transfusion dependent. Bone marrow cellularity was less than 5% in eight patients and 10 to 15% in one patient. GM-CSF was administered by continuous intravenous infusion for 28 days. The dose of GM-CSF was doubled after 14 days in patients who failed to have a complete hematologic response. Patients with a partial or complete response were continued on study for two additional months.

All eight evaluable patients had increases in white blood cell counts, and six of these eight patients had partial responses in granulocytes ($> 500/mm^3$). The median neutrophil counts increased fourfold in responding patients (range, 2.5- to 31-fold). The majority of patients also had increases in monocytes and eosinophils. Five of the six patients who were eligible for maintenance therapy completed two further months of planned therapy with persistent or improved neutrophil responses.

Upon disontinuation of GM-CSF, neutrophils returned to baseline levels in three patients. However, in one patient the response was maintained for 2 months after drug discontinuation and the other had a trilinileage response, characterized by increases in neutrophils, hemoglobulin, and platelets, which has lasted for greater than 1 year despite the discontinuation of GM-CSF. While three additional patients had increases in reticulocyte counts, no effects were seen on RBC or platelet transfusion requirements.

Despite the need for central venous catheter, no infectious episodes were seen in this study. Of interest, all four patients who completed maintenance treatment or received extended GM-CSF treatment were alive at the time of their report. This was in contrast to patients who received more abbreviated treatment.

More recently, a multicenter, randomized controlled trial of GM-CSF in aplastic anemia has been initiated (28). Patients were randomized to receive GM-CSF (3 μg/kg) daily s.c. over a 90-day period, or observation. Patients on observation arm were allowed to cross over to GM-CSF after 90 days, if at least one major infection occurred during observation period. All patients had neutropenia ($<1500/mm^3$). Baseline neutrophil counts in GM-CSF and observation arms were 330 and $242/mm^3$, respectively.

At the time of their preliminary report, 41 patients were evaluable for efficacy. The median granulocyte counts of patients on GM-CSF increased to 1077, 2622, and 1452/mm^3 after 1, 2, and 3 months of treatment, whereas the control group had neutrophil counts of 185, 723, and $924/mm^3$, respectively. GM-CSF-treated patients experienced fewer major infections (30% versus 61%, $p = 0.05$). No significant differences in platelets, hemogloblin levels, or transfusion requirements were seen.

A. Side Effects of GM-CSF

GM-CSF was generally well tolerated in these trials. The side effects were relatively mild and included constitutional symptoms such as myalgias, bone pain, headache, fatigue, fever, anorexia/nausea, rash, and occasional thrombocytopenia. At higher doses ($\geqslant$16 μg/kg/day), thrombophlebitis, pulmonary infiltrates, and serositis have been observed (26). However, generally such high doses of GM-CSF are not necessary to achieve white cells in the physiological range. Thus, it might be prudent to titrate the dose of GM-CSF according to the biological endpoint to avoid the potential toxicity of higher doses.

IV. DISCUSSION

The results of the reported clinical trials demonstrate that GM-CSF is effective in stimulating myelopoiesis in most patients with aplastic anemia. The response in myeloid elements was characterized by significant increases in neutrophils, eosinophils, and monocytes, and accompanied by increases in bone marrow cellularity and myeloid hyperplasia. This latter finding suggests that the rise in white count was not due merely to mobilization of mature cells but also to the proliferative effect of GM-CSF on the myeloid compartment.

These findings have several potential clinical ramifications. For instance, short-term treatment with GM-CSF might be useful to expedite myelopoietic recovery following bone marrow transplantation. Second, GM-CSF might enhance hematopoietic recovery following ATG treatment. In patients refractory to standard therapies, GM-CSF may be useful in correcting granulocytopenia and monocytopenia, and in reducing infectious morbidity. The preliminary results of the multiinstitutional trial have shown a reduction in the incidence of major infections in patients treated with GM-CSF. However, data from larger studies with long-term followup are necessary to firmly establish whether increasing the number and function of white blood cells by GM-CSF translates into ultimate clinical benefit.

The vast majority of patients treated in these initial trials had refractory or long-standing disease. The magnitude of white cell response in these patients was inversely related to the severity of the disease, and some failures were seen in patients with very severe disease. This finding suggests that the response to hematopoietic growth factors is dependent on the size of the progenitor cell pool. Furthermore, in occasional patients, an initial response to GM-CSF has been followed by a subsequent reduction in response. It is unclear whether this finding represents the development of refractoriness to CSFs by receptor modulation or other mechanisms, stem cell depletion, or the natural history of the disease.

While GM-CSF may be useful to overcome some of the problems associated with myeloid leukopenia, two observations suggest that treatment with GM-CSF alone may not be enough to influence the underlying disease process. First, continuous treatment is necessary to maintain the hematopoietic effects. Second, no consistent stimulatory effects have been seen on red cells and platelets. Interestingly, in occasional patients with aplastic anemia and in a few patients with myelodysplasia who have exhibited trilinileage responses, the hematopoietic response was maintained despite the discontinuation of GM-CSF, indicating that the treatment expanded the progenitor cell pool in these patients. This observation suggests that the combination of GM-CSF with hematopoietic growth factors acting at the primitive progenitor cell level (such as GM-CSF plus IL-1, IL-3, or IL-6) might augment multilineage responses in these disorders. Synergistic effects between various growth factors and cytokines have already been demonstrated in vitro as well as in preclinical studies (29,30). Recent advances in the understanding of the biological effects of hematopoietic growth factors promise future clinical applications of these agents in bone marrow failure states.

V. REFERENCES

1. Boggs DR, Boggs SS. The pathogenesis of aplastic anemia: a defective pluripotent hematopoietic stem cell with inappropriate balance of differentiation and self-replication. Blood 1976; 48:71–6.
2. Gale RP, Champlin RE, Feig SA, Fitchen JH. Aplastic anemia: biology and treatment. Ann Intern Med 1981; 95:477–94.
3. Ascensao J, Pahwa R, Kagan W, Malcolm M, Hansen J, Good R. Aplastic anemia: evidence for an immunological mechanism. Lancet 1976; 1:669–71.
4. Camitta BM, Thomas ED, Nathan DG, et al. Severe aplastic anemia: a prospective study of the effect of early marrow tranplantation on acute mortality. Blood 1976; 48:63.
5. Gluckman E. Current status of bone marrow transplantation for severe aplastic anemia: a preliminary report from the International Bone Marrow Transplant Registry. Transplant Proc 1987; 19:259709.
6. Storb R, Thomas ED, Buckner CD, et al. Marrow transplantation for aplastic anemia. Semin Hematol 1984; 21:27–35.
7. Thomas EE, Storb R, Clift RA, et al. Bone-marrow transplantation. N Engl J Med 1975; 292:832–43.
8. Gluckman E, Devergie A, Poros A, Degoulet R. Results of immunosuppression in 170 cases of severe aplastic anaemia: report of the European Group of Bone Marrow Transplant (EGBMT). Br J Haematol 1982; 51:541–50.
9. Champlin R, Ho W, Gale RP. Antithymocyte globulin treatment in patients with aplastic anemia: a prospective randomized trial. N Engl J Med 1983; 308:113–8.
10. Hunter RF, Huang AT. Antithymocyte globulin: a realistic approach to therapy for sever aplastic anemia. South Med J 1986; 79:1121–5.
11. Camitta B, O'Reilly RJ, Sensenbrenner L, et al. Antithoracic duct lymphocyte globulin therapy of sever aplastic anemia. Blood 1983; 62:883–3.
12. Marsh JC, Hows JM, Bryett KA, Al-Hashimi S, Fairhead SM, Gordon-Smith EC. Survival after antilymphocyte globulin therapy for aplastic anemia depends on disease severity. Blood 19XX; 70:1046–52.
13. Metcalf D. The granulocyte-macrophage colony-stimulating factor. Science 1985; 229 (4708):16–22.
14. Clark SC, Kamen R. The human hematopoietic colony stimulating factors. Science 1987; 236 (4806):1229–37.
15. Broxmeyer HE, Williams DE. The production of myeloid blood cells and their regulation during health and disease. CRC Crit Rev Oncol Hematol 1988; 8(3):173–226.
16. Weisbart RH, Golde DW, Clark SC, Wong GG, Gasson JC. Human granulocyte-macrophage colony-stimulating factor is a neutrophil activator. Nature 1985; 315:361.
17. Metcalf D, Begley CG, Johnson GR, Nicola NA, Vadas MA, Lopez AF, Williamson DJ, Wong GG, Clark SC, Wang EA. Biologic properties in vitro of a recombinant human granulocyte-macrophage colony-stimulating factor. Blood 1986; 1:37.
18. Burgess AW, Begley G, Johnson GR, Lopez AF, Williamson DJ, Mermod JJ, Simpson RJ, Schmitz A, DeLamarter JF. Purification and properties of bacterially synthesized human granulocyte-macrophage colony-stimulating factor. Blood 1987; 69:43.
19. Vadas MA, Nicola NA, Metcalf D. Activation of antibody dependent cell mediated cytotoxicity of human neutrophils and eosinophils by separate colony-stimulating factors. J Immunol 1983; 130:795.
20. Grabstein KH, Urdal DL, Tushinski RJ, Mochizuki DY, Price VL, Cantrell MA, Gillis S, Conlon PJ. Induction of macrophage tumoricidal activity by granulocyte-macrophage colony-stimulating factor. Science 1988; 232:506.
21. Broxmeyer HE, Vadhan-Raj S. Preclinical and clinical studies with the hematopoietic colony stimulating factors and related interleukins. Immunol Res 1989; 8:185–201.

22. Vadhan-Raj S, Buescher S, LeMaistre A, Keating M, Walters R, Ventura C, Hittelman W, Broxmeyer HE, Gutterman JU. Stimulation of hematopoiesis in patients with bone marrow failure and in patients with malignancy by recombinant human granulocyte-macrophage colony-stimulating factor. Blood 1988; 72(1):134–41.
23. Vadhan-Raj S, Buescher S, Broxmeyer HE, LeMaistre A, Lepe-Zuniga JL, Ventura G, Jeha S, Horwitz LJ, Trujillo JM, Gillis S, Hittelman WN, Gutterman JU. Stimulation of myelopoiesis in patients with aplastic anemia by recombinant human granulocyte-macrophage colony-stimulating factor. N Engl J Med 1988; 319:1628–34.
24. Antin JH, Smith BR, Holmes W, Rosenthal DS. Phase I/II study of recombinant human granulocyte-macrophage colony-stimulating factor in aplastic anemia and myelodysplastic syndrome. Blood 1988; 72(2):705–13.
25. Nissen C, Tichelli A, Gratwohl A, Speck B, Milne A, Gordon-Smith EC, Schaedelin J. Failure of recombinant human granulocyte-macrophage colony-stimulating factor therapy in aplastic anemia patients with very severe neutropenia. Blood 1988; 72(6):2445–7.
26. Champlin RE, Nimer SD, Ireland P, Oette DH, Golde DW. Treatment of refractory aplastic anemia with recombinant human granulocyte-macrophage colony-stimulating factor. Blood 1989; 73(3):694–9.
27. Guinan EC, Sieff CA, Oette DH, Nathan DG. A phase I/II trial of recombinant granulocyte-macrophage colony-stimulating factor for children with aplastic anemia. Blood 1990; 76(6):1077–82.
28. Schuster MW, Liu ET, Solberg LA, Stadtmauer E, Bennett JM, Israel RJ. Granulocyte-macrophage colony-stimulating factor for aplastic anemia: preliminary results of a multicenter randomized controlled trial. Blood 1990; 76:10(177):47a.
29. Broxmeyer HE, Williams DE, Hangoc G, et al. Synergistic myelopoietic action in vivo of combinations of purified natural murine colony stimulating factor-1, recombinant murine interleukin-3, and recombinant murine granulocyte-macrophage colony-stimulating factor administered to mice. Proc Natl Acad Sci USA 1987; 84:3871.
30. Donahue RE, Seehra J, Metzgar M, et al. Human IL-3 and GM-CSF act synergistically in stimulating hematopoiesis in primates. Science 1988; 241(4874):1820–3.

29

Clinical Trials of Granulocyte Colony-Stimulating Factors for Treatment of Bone Marrow Depression Associated with Cancer Chemotherapy

GRAHAM J. LIESCHKE and GEORGE MORSTYN
Ludwig Institute for Cancer Research,
The Royal Melbourne Hospital, Victoria, Australia

I. INTRODUCTION

Myelosuppression is a common effect of many chemotherapeutic drugs. A recent tabulation attributes "moderate" or "marked" myelosuppression to 40 of 58 common schedules (69%) of administration of 36 frequently used single chemotherapeutic agents (1). Except in the treatment of hematological malignancies such as acute leukemia, where myelotoxic therapy is required to treat the underlying disease, myelosuppression is presumed to be an unnecessary effect of chemotherapy which exposes the patient to risks of significant morbidity and mortality related to sepsis. The correlation between increasing severity and duration of neutropenia and an increasing risk of infection was documented in 1966 (2). Improvements to antibiotic therapy since then have improved the management of septic neutropenic patients (3), but prior to the clinical availability of the hemopoietic growth factors there was no generally applicable therapy that addressed the underlying vulnerability to infection that a persistently neutropenic state conferred.

Following the cloning of the cDNAs for human granulocyte colony-stimulating factor (G-CSF) and granulocyte-macrophage colony-stimulating factor (GM-CSF), sufficient amounts of recombinant colony-stimulating factors (CSFs) became available for preclinical and clinical studies to commence. Initial studies showed not only that the CSFs elevated neutrophil levels in mice (4,5) and nonhuman primates (6–8) but also that the CSFs were effective at accelerating neutrophil recovery in models of chemotherapeutically induced myelosuppression. G-CSF, which is active in different species, accelerated neutophil recovery after aplasia-inducing doses of cyclophosphamide in monkeys (6), and G-CSF treatment protected cyclophosphamide-treated mice from death from infective challenges (9). Studies with GM-CSF were restricted by the lack of cross-species activity of human GM-CSF. GM-CSF accelerated hemopoietic recovery in monkeys following irradiation and autologous marrow transplantation

(10,11). Recombinant murine GM-CSF improved survival of mice from melphalan-induced neutropenia (12).

This review considers the data from clinical studies in humans that address the role of the CSFs in the therapy of patients with malignancy. To understand the interactions between chemotherapeutic and CSF therapies when administered together, it is first necessary to examine the effects of CSF administration in the absence of chemotherapy.

II. G-CSF

A. Effects of G-CSF Alone

The initial Phase I studies of G-CSF in patients with cancer were reported in 1987 (13), 1988 (14,15), and 1989 (16,17). In these patients, intravenous G-CSF administration alone resulted in a dose-dependent neutrophilia which was sustained for periods of daily G-CSF administration of up to 14 days. Three groups observed a monocytosis and increase in circulating lymphocytes during this period (14–16). The neutrophilia resolved over 2–4 days upon cessation of G-CSF administration. Immediately after each dose of G-CSF there was a transient marked reduction in the number of circulating neutrophils before the onset of the G-CSF-driven elevation in neutrophil levels (14,16), and one group observed a transient monocytopenia as well (16). These changes also occurred after subcutaneously administered G-CSF (17). Patients previously treated with chemotherapy or radiotherapy appeared to have a lesser response to exogenous G-CSF than previously untreated patients (14,15,17).

During G-CSF therapy, the peripheral blood showed a marked left shift, with the appearance of circulating myelocytes and promyelocytes after 4-5 days of G-CSF administration (14). Neutrophils contained Dohle bodies and toxic granules (14–16,18), and in addition large polylobulated "macropolycytes" were sometimes seen (14), some of which are tetraploid and may therefore represent skipped cell divisions (L. Campbell, personal communication). Not only did the peripheral blood contain morphologically immature neutrophil precursors, but G-CSF therapy alone resulted in a marked increase in the number and frequency of circulating hemopoietic progenitor cells, not only of the granulocyte-macrophage lineage (15,19), but also of erythroid, megakaryocytic, and multipotential lineages (19).

Marrow examination during G-CSF therapy revealed an increase in the myeloid-to-erythroid ratio in most patients (15), associated with an increase in cellularity (14,15). The most marked change was an increase in the number of promyelocytes (14,15). The frequency of marrow hemopoietic progenitor cells were generally unaltered during G-CSF therapy (15,19). However, if the observed increase in marrow cellularity upon marrow biopsy was indicative of changes in the entire marrow compartment, it could be extrapolated that there was an increase in the total number of marrow progenitor cells.

Kinetic studies of tritiated thymidine-labeled marrow cells from a G-CSF-treated patient showed increased proliferation at all stages of granulopoiesis, particularly at myeloblast production. The time for labeled cells to enter the circulation was decreased from 4–5 days to 1 day. The calculated minimum half-life of labeled granulocytes was comparable to the normal range of 7–8 h, and the calculated increase in amplification divisions necessary to maintain the G-CSF-driven neutrophilia was 3.2 additional divisions (20).

Generally, no effect of G-CSF on platelet levels during short courses of administration has been noted (13–15,17), but Lindemann et al. (16) observed a reduction in circulating platelet levels of up to 40% on the tenth day of a 14-day treatment period for patients who received 30–60 μg/kg/day of G-CSF. Following cessation of G-CSF, there was a modest rebound in platelet levels correcting this change.

G-CSF therapy was associated with few adverse effects. Some patients experienced bone pain, which was most frequently described as a retrosternal discomfort, or as aching in the lower back (13–17). Analgesic therapy with acetaminophen was sometimes required. Subcutaneous administration by continuous infusion has not been associated with significant local inflammation (17). G-CSF therapy was associated with elevated serum urate, lactate dehydrogenase, elastase, lysozyme, and alkaline phosphatase levels (14–17). Other monitored parameters have not been affected, including circulating levels of tumor necrosis factor alpha and interleukin-1β (16). Splenomegaly, which has been noted in patients with cyclic neutropenia treated with G-CSF (21), and acute febrile neutrophilic dermatosis (the Sweet syndrome), which has been noted in a patient with hairy-cell leukemia treated with G-CSF (22), have not been observed in patients with malignancy. The Phase I studies did not define a maximal tolerated dose on the basis of clinical toxicity, but daily doses above 30–60 μg/kg/day resulted in marked neutrophilia, exceeding 50×10^9/L in some patients (14–17). Further dose escalation was not undertaken because excessive leukocytosis may be associated with risks of leukostasis.

B. Effects of G-CSF After Chemotherapy

The published studies combining G-CSF with chemotherapy are listed in Table 1 (13,14,23–25). Initially, the effects of G-CSF administration after conventional chemotherapy doses were studied.

Bronchud et al. (13) studied patients with small-cell lung cancer receiving chemotherapy with adriamycin, ifosfamide, and etoposide. Intravenous administration of G-CSF for 14 days commenced 1 day after the last dose of antineoplastic drug. This regimen of G-CSF reduced both the degree and duration of neutropenia during the chemotherapy cycle, and in G-CSF-supplemented cycles there were significantly fewer infective episodes than in other cycles.

Gabrilove et al. (23) examined the effect of G-CSF in patients with transitional cell bladder tumors receiving "M-VAC" combination chemotherapy with methotrexate, doxorubicin, vincristine, and cisplatin. In the first cycle of chemotherapy, intravenous G-CSF was administered for 8 days following the first component of M-VAC chemotherapy. Not only did G-CSF therapy reduce the duration of neutropenia, but these patients required fewer days of antibiotic therapy, were eligible to receive scheduled mid-cycle chemotherapy more often, and experienced a reduced incidence of mucositis. Patients who had undergone previous pelvic radiotherapy were less protected against neutropenia by G-CSF therapy than were nonirradiated patients. By studying some patients in whom the chemotherapy was supplemented by G-CSF in the second rather than the first cycle, the effect of G-CSF was shown to be cycle independent.

Morstyn et al. (14) initially examined the effect of G-CSF after a single intravenous dose of melphalan (25 mg/m^2). In previously untreated patients, 8 days of intravenous G-CSF therapy at doses of 3 μg/kg/day or more reduced the duration of leukopenia from 8 days to 3 days or less. The neutrophil nadir occurred earlier at efficacious G-

Table 1 Clinical Studies Combining Chemotherapy and Colony-Stimulating Factor Administration[a]

Reference	Type of cancer	Type of chemotherapy	Type of CSF	CSF schedule: Dose range (μg/kg/day)	CSF schedule: Route	CSF schedule: Duration (days)
13	Small-cell lung	DOX, IFOS, VP-16	G-CSF	1–40	i.v. cont	14
14,17	Various advanced malignancies	Melphalan	G-CSF	1–60	i.v. bol s.c. bol s.c. cont	8 8 8–16
23	Bladder	M-VAC	G-CSF	1–60	i.v. bol	7
24	Various refractory malignancies	CTX, VP-16, DDP	G-CSF	20–60	i.v.	20
25	Breast and ovary	DOX	G-CSF	10	i.v. bol	11
35,36	Sarcoma	DOX, IFOS, DTIC	GM-CSF	4–64	i.v. cont	10
45	Small-cell lung	CBDCA, VP-16	GM-CSF	15	s.c. bol	7–21
46	Breast, lymphoma	CTX	GM-CSF	5.5	i.v. cont	7–14
47	Various advanced malignancies	Various	GM-CSF	250 μg/m^2/day	s.c. bol	10
48	Acute myeloid leukemia	ARA-C	GM-CSF	120 μg/m^2/day	i.v. cont	11–40

[a] Abbreviations: CSF = colony-stimulating factor; G = granulocyte; GM = granulocyte-macrophage; DOX = doxorubicin; IFOS = ifosfamide; VP-16 = etoposide; M-VAC = methotrexate, vinblastine, doxorubicin, cisplatinum; CTX = cyclophosphamide; DDP = cisplatinum; DTIC = dacarbazine; CBDCA = carboplatin; ARA-C = cytosine arabinside; i.v. = intravenous; s.c. = subcutaneous; cont = continuous infusion; bol = bolus.

Source: Adapted from Ref. 50.

CSF doses, and followed an initial phase in which leukocyte levels were elevated above normal by G-CSF therapy.

More detailed studies to determine the optimal schedule of G-CSF extended these observations considerably (17). Subcutaneous administration of G-CSF was shown to be at least equally as effective as intravenous administration. The period of G-CSF therapy before chemotherapy that had been part of the initial Phase I/II studies of G-CSF was shown to be unnecessary for the beneficial effect of G-CSF on neutrophil levels. By varying the schedule of G-CSF administration following chemotherapy, it was shown that even when G-CSF was started 8 days after this dose of melphalan, the period of neutropenia could be abrogated, and that 7 days of G-CSF therapy was sufficient. The minimal schedule of G-CSF administration following a standard dose of a chemotherapeutic drug, therefore, did not require continuous G-CSF therapy during the chemotherapy cycle for the optimal effect on neutrophil levels. This observation supports the hypothesis that G-CSF may not need to be administered continuously and prophylactically to all patients receiving standard-dose chemotherapy for the optimal clinical benefit to accrue. Phase III studies that explore the role of both prophylactic and minimal G-CSF schedules are warranted to address these issues.

G-CSF therapy has not been associated with consistent modulations of the course of thrombocyopenia following chemotherapy (13,14,17,23–25), although it may be expected that if the detrimental effect of sepsis on platelet survival was removed by a reduction in the rate of sepsis, there may be an indirect beneficial effect. This issue can be addressed only by Phase III studies.

In all of these studies, the combination of G-CSF with chemotherapy was well tolerated by the patients. Bone pain has also occurred when G-CSF was given after chemotherapy, although after high-dose chemotherapy followed by marrow transplantation supplemented with G-CSF, 15 patients on a Phase II study did not experience bone pain (26). It is possible that chemotherapeutic agents may modify the cellular mechanisms mediating the generation of bone pain during G-CSF therapy, and that this effect may not be as frequent when G-CSF is given after high doses of chemotherapy.

III. GM-CSF

A. Effects of GM-CSF Alone

Although there were reports of the effects of GM-CSF in patients with aquired immunodeficiency syndrome (27), primary marrow disorders such as the myelodysplastic syndromes and aplastic anemia (28,29), and in patients after marrow transplantation (30), an assessment of in-vivo effects of GM-CSF in these patients was complicated by the possibility that the underlying disease state may have influenced the response to GM-CSF, therefore making the observations not truly representative of the response of the normal or nondiseased but infiltrated marrows of cancer patients. Studies that have assessed the effect of GM-CSF administration alone in cancer patients have used nonglycosylated GM-CSF synthesized by *E. coli* (31–33) and glycosylated GM-CSF synthesized in yeast expression systems (34–38) or a mammalian cell expression system (39).

Antman et al. (35,36) administered GM-CSF by continuous intravenous infusion to patients with inoperable or metastatic sarcomas without marrow involvement for up to 7 days at doses of 4–32 μg/kg/day. These patients developed leukocytosis with both neutrophilia and eosinophilia. Marrow biopsies taken after GM-CSF therapy showed increased cellularity and increased myeloid-to-erythroid ratios. There was an increase in circulating granulocyte-macrophage and erythroid progenitor cells, which was not reflected by an alteration in the frequency of marrow progenitor cells. However, as the median marrow cellularity increased during GM-CSF therapy, it is possible that the total marrow progenitor pool was expanded.

Lieschke et al. (31) reported observations from a Phase I study in patients with malignancy treated with subcutaneously administered GM-CSF for 10 consecutive days. In addition to observing a dose-related neutrophilia and eosinophilia during GM-CSF therapy, a dose-related monocytosis was observed. Some patients also developed a lymphocytosis. When these patients were retreated with the same dose of GM-CSF after 10 days without GM-CSF, there was an accentuated response, suggesting that even after 10 days without exogenous GM-CSF exposure, the marrow remained primed for a heightened response to the resumption of GM-CSF therapy. Furthermore, alternate-day therapy at higher doses also maintained an elevated leukocyte count. This group also conducted a study of intravenously administered GM-CSF by bolus injection or short intravenous infusion (32). The similar design of the two studies and the use of the same form of GM-CSF permitted a comparison of the relative efficacy of subcutaneously and intravenously administered GM-CSF. For a given dose, subcutaneously administered GM-CSF had a greater biological effect, as assessed by the effect on peripheral blood parameters. Using a sensitive immunoassay developed by Cebon et al. (40), it was shown that serum levels above that achieving maximal in-vitro stimulation of marrow progenitor cells were maintained for long periods by subcutaneous dosing, suggesting that favorable pharmacokinetics contributed to the greater effect of subcutaneous dosing.

GM-CSF was also noted to cause a transient leukopenia immediately following the administration of a dose (31–34,38,41,42), due to the transient disappearance of not only neutrophils, but also monocytes and eosinophils from the circulating pool (31,32,38). As the circulating pool of neutrophils was replenished over 2–4 h, there was an early increase in the proportion of immature forms, indicating an early redistribution of leukocytes (32). GM-CSF therapy induced expression of surface adhesion molecules CD 11b (Mo-1), with variable effects on CD 11a (LFA-1) and CD 11c (Leu M5) (34,42). The effect on CD 11a was evident within 60 min of in-vivo exposure to GM-CSF (42). The fate of redistributed leukocytes is unknown, although there is some evidence to suggest that there may be accumulation of leukocytes in the lungs during the transient leukopenia (41,43). These observations provide evidence for immediate biological effects of exogenous GM-CSF on the functions of cells expressing GM-CSF receptors. Furthermore, these effects have been observed even at the lowest doses of GM-CSF administered, which have no detectable proliferative effect evidenced by peripheral blood leukocyte levels (31,32), suggesting that GM-CSF has biological actions at doses below those affecting circulating leukocyte levels.

The effects of GM-CSF therapy on platelet levels have been variable. Shorter courses (35) and higher doses (38) of therapy have been reported to be associated with decreases in platelet levels, and other studies have described a transient decrease (32,34). A history of idiopathic thrombocytopenic purpura (ITP) would appear to contraindicate GM-CSF therapy, because one patient with a low-grade lymphoma and history of ITP in remission appeared to have immediate reactivation of platelet destruction after GM-CSF (31). No consistent effect on erythrocyte parameters has been observed.

A variety of adverse effects have been observed during GM-CSF therapy, which have led to the definition of the maximal tolerated dose. Significant toxicities observed in Phase I studies at high GM-CSF doses have been thrombotic events, pleural and pericardial effusions and inflammation, and edema (31–35). These effects have been observed at doses of 30 μg/kg/day and above. The dose-response curve to GM-CSF is not clearly linear as assessed by fold-neutrophil increase over baseline (31–33), and doses in the range of 3–15 μg/kg/day are recommended for further studies. Even at lower doses of GM-CSF, other adverse effects are observed: generalized skin rash (sometimes with pruritus), myalgia and arthralgia, malaise and lethargy, anorexia and nausea, and fever. Subcutaneous administration can be associated with local inflammation at injection sites (31). The first dose of GM-CSF in a treatment cycle can be followed by a significant reaction characterized by flushing, tachycardia, hypotension, musculoskeletal pain, and dyspnea, during which there is significant arterial oxygen desaturation (31,32,44). This first-dose reaction is more common after short intravenous administrations of GM-CSF, and has usually not been observed after second or subsequent consecutive daily GM-CSF doses (44). It has frequently been observed in patients with lung cancer receiving GM-CSF (44), including patients with small-cell lung cancer treated with carboplatin and etoposide followed by GM-CSF. Particularly severe reactions were seen in a patient with the Eaton-Lambert myasthenic syndrome (44,45).

The initial studies combining CSFs with chemotherapy regimes were designed to temporally separate the administration of CSF and chemotherapeutic agents because of concern that the myelotoxicity of the antineoplastic agent may be accentuated if hemopoietic progenitor cells were pushed into cell cycle by G-CSF or GM-CSF. The validity of this concern was suggested by the observation of Welte et al. (6) that nonhuman primates that received G-CSF concurrently with cyclophosphamide appeared to have a more severe degree of transient neutropenia than animals that received G-CSF only after cyclophosphamide treatment. Cell kinetic studies during GM-CSF therapy of solid tumor patients with normal marrows have shown that not only did GM-CSF administration result in increased numbers of circulating hemopoietic progenitor cells, but during GM-CSF therapy, there were increased proportions of marrow myeloblasts, promyelocytes, myelocytes, granulocyte-macrophage colony-forming units (CFU-GM), and erythroid burst-forming units (BFU-E) in S-phase (39). Kinetic studies showed that the birth rate of marrow cycling cells was doubled during GM-CSF administration, the duration of S-phase was decreased by 40%, and the cell cycle time was reduced to one-third of baseline. Following cessation of GM-CSF administration, the proportion of cycling marrow cells reduced to levels below baseline. The clinical importance of this effect has not yet been tested, but the observation has favorable implications for the myelotoxic effect of cell cycle-specific chemotherapeutic agents in cycles subsequent to the first if the marrow is left in a relatively refractory state upon cessation of supportive postchemotherapy GM-CSF, because of a post-GM-CSF reduction in the proportion of cycling marrow cells.

B. Effects of GM-CSF After Chemotherapy

The published studies combining GM-CSF with chemotherapy are listed in Table 1 (35,36,45–48). Initially, patients receiving conventional chemotherapy doses have been studied.

Antman et al. (35,36) reported a study in which combination chemotherapy for sarcoma (doxorubicin, ifosfamide, dacarbazine) was supplemented during the first cycle with GM-CSF (4–64 μg/kg/day) in a dose-finding study. To derive comparative data, observations made during the second cycle of chemotherapy were collated. This approach has been criticized (47,49,50) because the control second cycle may have been unfairly disadvantaged by the possibility of cumulative myelosuppression from the first cycle. However, this study suggested a beneficial effect of GM-CSF administration, as the GM-CSF-supplemented first cycle was characterized by neutropenia of shorter duration and less severe degree. The platelet nadir in the first cycle was also less severe than in the second cycle, but this may also have reflected the differences between that first and second cycle of chemotherapy rather than a specific effect of GM-CSF.

Hermann et al. (47) reported observations made in a group of patients with lymphoma and solid tumors in whom the second chemotherapy cycle was supplemented with GM-CSF (250 $\mu g/m^2$/day for 10 days). In this study, the GM-CSF-supplemented second cycle was characterized by a shorter duration and less severe neutropenia. No difference in red cell or platelet parameters was observed in this study. The GM-CSF-supplemented cycle was characterized by fewer days with fever above 38.5°C, and fewer days on parenteral antibiotics. This observation is important, because it demonstrates clinical advantage from GM-CSF on clinical parameters of sepsis, of which fever is the most common clinical sign, even though Phase I studies demonstrated that GM-CSF administration alone can be associated with fever.

Morstyn et al. (45) have conducted studies in patients with small-cell lung cancer undergoing treatment with carboplatin (100 mg/m^2/day, 3 days) and etoposide (120 mg/m^2/day, 3 days). Initial observations indicated a reduction in degree of neutropenia in the first cycle compared with historical controls for patients receiving this chemotherapy regimen supplemented by subcutaneously administered GM-CSF (15 $\mu g/kg$/day). Systematic studies to optimize both the dose and schedule of GM-CSF administration in this chemotherapy context have shown that GM-CSF does not have to start immediately following the chemotherapy to abrogate the chemotherapy-induced neutropenia, and that if GM-CSF therapy is continued for too long, an excessive leukocytosis is induced after the leukocyte nadir. There was also a trend for worsening thrombocytopenia (Morstyn et al., unpublished observations).

Standard-dose chemotherapy treatment did not appear to significantly influence the spectrum of adverse effects of GM-CSF. Skin rash, bone pain, abdominal cramps, fever, and the first-dose reaction have all been reported with GM-CSF therapy after chemotherapy (35,36,44–48). The dose of bacterially synthesized nonglycosylated GM-CSF recommended for further studies was 5–15 $\mu g/kg$/day. Many studies now use the lower dose of 5 $\mu g/kg$/day, at which there is still an observable leukopoietic response, but at which the adverse effects may be less. Some of the adverse effects may be due to the release of other cytokines such as tumor necrosis factor-alpha or interleukin-1β by GM-CSF-activated monocytes (51). It is possible that after high-dose chemotherapy, effector cells may be obliterated or their function impaired, and some of these adverse effects may not be seen.

IV. EFFECTS OF IN-VIVO CSF ADMINISTRATION ON EFFECTOR CELL FUNCTIONS

A variety of neutrophil functions have been shown to be influenced by in-vitro exposure of neutrophils to G-CSF, and similarly monocyte and neutrophil functions are influenced by in-vitro exposure to GM-CSF. In particular, GM-CSF-activated macrophages were shown to inhibit tumor cell growth by a tumor necrosis factor-alpha-dependent mechanism (52,53). Other neutrophil functions which are believed to be important for the antimicrobial activities of neutrophils are augmented by in vitro by GM-CSF (54,55). Encouragingly, neutrophils from patients treated with both G-CSF and GM-CSF show enhanced activity in these functional assays in some reports (Table 2) (15,16,22,56–63). One difference between G-CSF and GM-CSF is their effect on neutrophil mobility. In-vivo administration of G-CSF does not alter the normal response of neutrophils to chemotactic factors (15,57,58), but neutrophils from patients receiving GM-CSF show an impaired chemotactic response (60,61). Whether or not this difference is of clinical relevance is unknown. Another difference is the apparently greater activation of monocytes and macrophages by GM-CSF. Whether or not it is activated monocytes that contribute to the broader spectrum of adverse effects of GM-CSF is unknown, but some of the adverse effects may be mediated by products of activated monocytes such as tumor necrosis factor-alpha or interleukin 1β (51). These modulations of effector cell function may be of clinical importance for cancer patients.

In vitro, effector cell function is modified at significantly lower doses than those required for the maximal proliferative effect on hemopoietic progenitor cells (64), sug-

Table 2 Effects of in-Vivo Colony-Stimulating Factor Administration on in-Vitro Assays of Leukocyte Functional Activities[a]

Functional activity	Response[b] of cells exposed in vivo to CSF (references)	
	G-CSF	GM-CSF
Neutrophil functions		
Superoxide/peroxide production[c]		
fMLP stimulated	+ (16)	+ (59,60)
PMA stimulated	+ (56)	N (61) and + (59,60)
Phagocytosis	N (57) and + (22)[d]	N (61) and N+ (62)[e]
Mobility/chemotactic response	N (15,57,58)	D (60,61)
Intracellular bacterial killing	+ (22)[d]	N+ (62)[e]
Antibody-dependent cell-mediated cytotoxicity	+ (22)[d]	+ (62)[e]
Monocyte functions		
Antibody-dependent cell-mediated cytotoxicity	—	+ (63)
Tumor necrosis factor-alpha production	—	+ (63)
Interferon production	—	+ (63)

[a] Abbreviations: CSF = colony-stimulating factor; G = granulocyte; GM = granulocyte/macrophage; fMLP = f-Met-Leu-Phe; PMA = phorbol myristate acetate.

[b] + = augmented response; N = response unchanged from normal; N+ = impaired baseline response normalized; D = decreased response

[c] Measured by nitroblue tetrazolium reduction (56), cytochrome C reduction (59,60), hydrogen peroxide production (61), or chemiluminescence (16).

[d] Neutrophils tested from G-CSF-treated patients with hairy-cell leukemia.

[e] Neutrophils tested from GM-CSF-treated patients with acquired immunodeficiency syndrome.

gesting that lower GM-CSF doses that are free of the dose-related adverse effects may still confer clinical benefit. The occurrence of a transient leukopenia following low GM-CSF doses that do not induce a leukocytosis with repeated daily dosing is evidence for the in-vivo biological activity of low GM-CSF doses. Much more work is therefore required on the in-vivo effects of G-CSF and GM-CSF on neutrophil and monocyte function.

Circulating cells from CSF-treated patients show a marked left shift, and in-vitro studies on populations of cells harvested from CSF-treated patients may show functional differences which reflect the immaturity of the cell population studied, rather than a change in the functional state of the mature effector cells. It is also possible that the functional changes observed in populations of circulating cells do not reflect the changes that occur in cells that have already entered the tissues. The functional state of tissue-localized effector cells is probably more important than that of circulating cells in preventing infection or exhibiting anticancer activity.

V. CLINICAL BENEFITS OF SUPPLEMENTING CHEMOTHERAPY WITH CSF ADMINISTRATION

The Phase II studies of G-CSF and GM-CSF described above demonstrated potential clinical advantages for patients which are summarized in Table 3 (13,14,17,23–25,33,35,46,47,65,66). Although the quantitative relationship between neutrophil levels and the risk of infection has long been accepted (2), it does not immediately follow that a CSF-driven accelerated neutrophil recovery will confer clinical advantage to the patients. This must be demonstrated in well-designed, prospective, randomized clinical studies.

Preclinical data indicate that considerable protection from infection can be conferred by both G-CSF and GM-CSF. G-CSF was administered for 4 days to cyclophosphamide-treated mice, who were then challenged with an infective inoculum. G-CSF treatment almost completely protected these mice from inoculums of *Pseudomonas aeruginosa, Escherichia coli, Serratia marcescens, Staphylococcus aureus,* and *Candida albicans* which were lethal to non-G-CSF-treated control mice (9). The ability of GM-CSF to protect against infection was tested in lethally irradiated mice transplanted with syngeneic marrow cells followed by intraperitoneal GM-CSF therapy. Control mice were treated with saline alone. On day 9 after marrow transplantation, mice were challenged with an inoculum of *Salmonella typhimurium* which led to death within 14 days for all non-GM-CSF-treated control mice, but 35% of GM-CSF treated mice survived for 30 days (67).

In the clinical setting, CSF therapy may be administered in two ways to improve the outcome for patients at risk of infection. The CSF may be administered prophylactically to all patients at risk, aiming to reduce the overall risk of fever or sepsis for all patients. While this may decrease the morbidity and mortality due to fever and sepsis for the whole group, with standard doses of chemotherapy many patients would be unnecessarily treated with CSF. It is possible that an equivalent improvement in mortality with reduced morbidity may be conferred on such groups of patients if only those patients who develop a febrile or septic episode are treated with CSF. In this circumstance, CSF therapy may shorten the period for which antibiotic therapy is required, and may accelerate neutrophil recovery sufficiently to reduce the mortality associated with febrile neutropenic episodes. Both these approaches are being exam-

Table 3 Clinical and Hematological Benefits Suggested from Studies Combining Colony-Stimulating Factor Administration with Chemotherapy in Cancer Patients[a]

Reported clinical benefit	References	
	G-CSF	GM-CSF
Hematologic effects		
Shorter duration of neutropenia	13,14,17,23,24,25,65	35,46,47
Less severe degree of neutropenia	—	35,46,47
Eosinophila	—	35
Accelerated monocyte recovery	23,24	—
Reduced thrombocytopenia	—	35,46
No effect on thrombocytopenia	13,14,17,23,24,25	47
Effects on parameters of sepsis		
Fewer febrile days	23	47
Fewer infections	13,65	—
Fewer days on antibiotics	23,65	47
Effects on delivery of chemotherapy		
Eligible for scheduled chemotherapy	23	46
Higher chemotherapy dose delivered	25	—
Other effects		
Fewer days of hospitalization	65	—
Reduced mucositis	23	47
Possible CSF antitumor effect	66	33

[a] Abbreviations: CSF = colony-stimulating factor; G = granulocyte; GM = granulocyte-macrophage.
Source: Adapted from Ref. 50.

ined. Interim analysis of a randomized study of G-CSF for the chemotherapy of lung cancer showed a G-CSF-related reduction in the duration of neutropenia by 50%, a reduced incidence of febrile neutropenia by approximately 40%, and a reduction in the number of days of hospitalization and days on antibiotics by 40–50% (65). Morstyn et al. are examining the use of G-CSF as an adjunctive therapy to standard antibiotics in the management of chemotherapy-related febrile neutropenic episodes in a prospective, randomized, double-blind Phase III study (data not yet available).

A further clinical advantage to patients might be that GM-CSF-stimulated in-vitro tumoricidal activity of monocytes (52,53) translates into a clinically relevant antitumor effect. Only one tumor response was reported from Phase I GM-CSF studies, which occurred in a patient with a sarcoma (33). It is important to monitor tumor responses, because in-vitro data show not only that some nonhemopoietic tumor cell lines express CSF receptors (68), but that their growth may be either inhibited (69), unaffected (70), or stimulated (68,71) by in-vitro exposure to CSFs. The role of these receptors on solid tumor cell lines is unknown, and the in-vitro stimulatory effects are small, and so it seems unlikely that CSF administration will compromise tumor responses. Trials are now commencing in which antitumor antibodies are being administered with GM-CSF to examine if GM-CSF-augmented antibody-dependent cell-mediated anticancer effects can be elicited.

VI. CSFs AND HIGH-DOSE CHEMOTHERAPY

In addition to the potential benefits to patients of the clinical use of the hemopoietic growth factors to modulate myelosuppression and its clinical consequences, a potentially more significant benefit is the possibility that higher or more intense chemotherapy doses may perhaps be safely administered. For some antineoplastic agents, there is a dose-related antitumor effect, but the delivery of maximal doses of antineoplastic drug has been limited by clinical toxicity, often myelosuppression. If CSF-supplemented chemotherapy with increased antineoplastic dose intensity were to translate into increased antitumor effect and concomitant increased patient cure or survival, this would represent a significant improvement in anticancer therapy. The evidence for a favorable result from increased dose intensity has been recently reviewed (72). There are three possible ways that the dose intensity (that is, the amount of antineoplastic drug delivered per unit time) could be increased:

1. Increased individual doses of antineoplastic drug. If individual doses are increased, it may be possible to deliver an adequate total dose in a shorter time; or, alternatively, a larger total dose may be safely delivered over a significantly shortened time. The total dose of antineoplastic drug delivered, however, may be an independent outcome-determining factor unrelated to the intensity with which that total dose is delivered, and therefore should be considered separately. Supplementary CSF therapy may permit the safe administration of individual doses of antineoplastic drugs for which the maximal individual dose is limited by the degree of myelosuppression.
2. The dosage interval could be decreased. It is often the need to wait for recovery from myelosuppression that dictates whether or not the next scheduled dose can be delivered. CSFs, by accelerating recovery from myelosuppression, may permit shorter dosage intervals.
3. Combinations of antineoplastic agents with overlapping myelotoxicity but independent antineoplastic actions may be possible with favorable myeloproliferative effects from supplementary CSF administration.

In designing studies that address this issue, it is important that it is clear which of the determinants of dose intensity is being addressed, and that the regimen of CSF usage has been optimized for the circumstances.

There are two reported studies that examine the possibility of increased dose intensity in the context of CSF administration. Bronchud et al. (25) examined the possibilities of escalating the individual dose of doxorubicin and shortening the dosage interval in the context of supplementary G-CSF therapy in a Phase II study. For patients with advanced breast or ovarian cancer, it was possible to deliver doxorubicin at doses of 75–150 mg/m^2 every 14 days for three cycles with supplementary G-CSF administration by continuous infusion (10 μg/kg/day, 7 days; followed by 5 μg/kg/day, 4 days). In four control patients treated with doxorubicin (75 mg/m^2), neutrophil levels of 2.5 $\times$ 10^9/L were achieved only after 19–21 days. Tumor response rates were encouraging. However, one of the limitations of this approach was also demonstrated. At the higher and most intensely delivered doxorubicin dose, patients experienced significant epithelial and mucosal toxicity, including blistering and desquamation of the palms and soles. This demonstrates that although CSF therapy may reduce myelotoxicity and therefore permit dose escalation, by doing so other toxicities may be unmasked which may become dose limiting.

Gianni et al. (46) studied the effect of GM-CSF on the delivery of high doses of cyclophosphamide (7 g/m^2) that are associated with significant myelosuppression but compatible with spontaneous marrow reconstitution, but were below the myeloablative doses requiring marrow transplantation support. After this dose of cyclophosphamide, a schedule finding study showed that GM-CSF (250 $\mu g/m^2$/day, glycosylated mammalian-cell synthesized) was most effective at minimizing the duration of neutropenia when started the day after cyclophosphamide, rather than 5 days later, and when continued for 14 days, rather than ceased earlier. GM-CSF therapy following cyclophosphamide reduced the duration of neutropenia, accelerated the rate of platelet recovery and reduced the need for platelet transfusions, and moved forward the day on which patients would be eligible for additional chemotherapy (on the basis of recovery from myelosuppression) from day 20 to day 14. Most studies have not shown any benefit in platelet recovery (Table 3). There were fewer documented infections in the GM-CSF treated group, but this did not attain statistical significance.

These studies document the potential utility of both G-CSF and GM-CSF for ameliorating the myelosuppressive effects of increased doses of antineoplastic agents, thereby supporting dose-intensifying regimens.

VII. USE OF CSFs IN THE TREATMENT OF MYELOID MALIGNANCIES

The potential interactions between myeloid malignancies, their treatment with chemotherapeutic agents, and the CSFs are complex. Human leukemic promyelocytes are able to bind G-CSF, and some proliferate in vitro under this stimulus (73). Some myeloid malignancies can utilize GM-CSF as a proliferative stimulus in vitro (74,75). These observations raise the possibility that in-vivo administration of G-CSF or GM-CSF to patients with myeloid malignancies may lead to stimulated proliferation of the leukemic clone. Indeed, in a proportion of patients with myelodysplastic syndromes, particularly those with more than 15% blast cells in the marrow, stimulation of proliferation of the abnormal blast cells has been observed (76). However, there are also observations that indicate that, for some leukemic clones, the CSFs alone can inhibit proliferation. For example, C3H/He mice with myeloid leukemia, or inoculated with the myeloid leukemic cell line C2M, have improved survival when treated with daily G-CSF or GM-CSF (77,78). Improved survival was also seen when the C2M leukemic cells were preincubated with G-CSF or GM-CSF before inoculation, which was shown in vitro to inhibit the proliferation of the leukemic stem cells. However, for patients it is not presently possible to correlate the in-vitro effects of the CSFs on leukemic stem cells with the outcome of in-vivo CSF therapy.

A potentially favorable interaction between CSFs and chemotherapeutic agents can be envisaged even for patients with CSF-responsive leukemic stem cells. If an increased percentage of CSF-responsive leukemic stem cells were pushed into cell cycle by CSF administration, increased kill of leukemic stem cells might be anticipated with the administration of cycle-specific antineoplastic agents. This phenomenon has been demonstrated in vitro with cytosine arabinoside and hydroxyurea after G-CSF and GM-CSF treatment of acute myeloid leukemic stem cells (79,80). A drawback of this approach is that normal myeloid progenitor cells would also be expected to be pushed into cell cycle, also increasing their susceptibility to antiproliferative effects of cycle-specific chemotherapy drugs. A differential effect on normal and leukemic cells could be achieved if there was differential uptake of the antineoplastic agent. Alternatively, myeloablative doses of antineoplastic drugs and CSF could be given, followed by infusion of autologous remission or allogeneic marrow to achieve hemopoietic reconstitution.

A few small studies have been reported exploring the effect of CSF in patients with myeloid leukemia. Buechner et al. (81) administered GM-CSF to six patients with acute leukemia rendered aplastic by chemotherapy. Early neutrophil recovery was seen in some patients, without evidence for stimulated leukemic regrowth in four patients with acute myeloid leukemia. In a larger study (82), the same group studied 29 patients, 23 of whom had acute myeloid leukemia. Significant acceleration of neutrophil recovery by postaplasia GM-CSF administration was demonstrated compared to historical controls. Following chemotherapeutically induced aplasia, myeloid leukemic regrowth was seen in three patients while on GM-CSF; the regrowth in one of them disappeared upon cessation of GM-CSF. Estey et al. (48) also gave postchemotherapy GM-CSF to patients with poor-prognosis acute myeloid leukemia, and observed no significant differences in their clinical course from historical controls. Teshima et al. (66) reported 13 patients with acute or chronic myeloid leukemia who were treated empirically with G-CSF. In only one patient with chronic myeloid leukemia did G-CSF appear to stimulate leukemic regrowth, and this patient subsequently received G-CSF and antineoplastic therapy concurrently, following which both neutrophils and leukemic blasts were reduced. A second patient in this group was interesting in that G-CSF appeared to suppress the leukemic clone. This patient had an elevated blast level and profound sepsis 1 month after combination antileukemic chemotherapy. G-CSF was commenced to supplement antibiotic therapy for septicemia and pneumonia. While on G-CSF, the blast level decreased and normal neutrophil level increased. This possible favorable effect of G-CSF may have reflected its ability to induce differentiation of some myeloid leukemic cells in vitro (83). In a recently reported randomized study of GM-CSF in myelodysplastic syndromes, there was equal progression to leukemia in the control group observed for 12 weeks after randomization as in the group treated with GM-CSF for 12 weeks after randomization. Interestingly, the occurrence of infection was reduced by GM-CSF treatment, and lower doses of GM-CSF were necessary in this setting (84).

Overall, it is concluded that in this clinical setting the risk of CSF-induced leukemic growth in vivo seems low, and further studies are required.

VIII. EFFECTS OF CSFs AFTER MYELOABLATIVE CHEMOTHERAPY WITH MARROW TRANSPLANTATION

High-dose chemotherapy given with myeloablative intent requires that hematopoietic reconstitution be achieved with hemopoietic progenitor cells infused after the chemotherapy is given. The sources of these stem cells that have been used are autologous marrow, harvested in the remission phase of leukemia or from a noninvolved marrow in the case of solid tumors, allogeneic marrow suitable donors, or stem cells harvested by leukopheresis from the peripheral blood. The clinical use of CSFs has been investigated in this setting.

A. G-CSF After Marrow Transplantation

Two studies show favorable effects of G-CSF in autologous bone marrow transplantation (AtBMT). Sheridan et al. (26) administered G-CSF (20 μg/kg/day, adjusted to neutrophil level, by subcutaneous continuous infusion) to 15 patients treated with busulphan and cyclophosphamide followed by AtBMT. Compared to similarly treated historical controls, the mean time to a neutrophil level exceeding 1×10^9/L was reduced from 20 to 11 days. The acceleration in neutrophil repopulation appeared to translate into clinical benefit for the patients, who had fewer days on parenteral antibiotics, fewer days in reverse barrier nursing, and fewer days of parenteral nutrition. There was no discernable effect on red cell or platelet reconstitution. Taylor et al. (85) administered G-CSF (60 μg/kg/day, adjusted to neutrophil level, short daily intravenous infusion) to 18 patients with relapsed or refractory Hodgkin's disease treated with cyclophosphamide, carmustine, and etoposide, and observed a reduction in the median time to a neutrophil level exceeding 1×10^9/L from 30 days in an historical control series to 16 days in G-CSF-treated patients.

Masaoka et al. (86) reported that results of G-CSF therapy in allogeneic bone marrow transplantation (AlBMT). G-CSF was commenced 3–5 days after marrow infusion (200–800 μg/m^2/day, short intravenous infusion). Compared with historical controls, there was accelerated neutrophil recovery, which was accentuated in the subset of patients not given methotrexate for graft-versus-host prophylaxis, and there was no difference in the incidence of graft-versus-host disease.

During G-CSF administration alone, there is a marked increase in the number and frequency of circulating hemopoietic progenitor cells. Collected circulating hemopoietic progenitor cells shorten the time for neutrophil recovery when reinfused after marrow transplantation (87). The repopulating ability and long-term durability of neutrophil recovery from peripheral blood stem cell reinfusion is not known, but G-CSF administration provides an opportunity for collection of blood enriched for circulating stem cells with relatively few leukopheresis attendances. It is potentially a superior method for in-vivo enrichment than collection during the rebound phase after cyclophosphamide administration, and given the minimal toxicity of G-CSF, may also be applicable to normal allogeneic donors. Preliminary data have been reported from a study in which, after high-dose chemotherapy, both autologous circulating progenitor cells harvested during G-CSF therapy and autologous marrow were reinfused and patients received G-CSF during the period of progenitor cell engraftment. There was a small change in the time for neutrophil recovery compared to comparable patients who had received only autologous marrow and post-transplantation G-CSF from 11 to 9 days, but a marked reduction in the time to platelet recovery with platelet levels of 20×10^9/L attained by day 14 (88).

B. GM-CSF After Marrow Transplantation

The initial studies of GM-CSF after myeloablative conditioning and AtBMT are difficult to assess because they were also dose-finding studies using wide dose ranges of GM-CSF (30,89–91), and in one study purged marrows with low numbers of remaining granulocyte-macrophage progenitor cells were also used (91). Compared to historical controls, it appeared that GM-CSF accelerated neutrophil recovery, particularly at higher GM-CSF doses, but in the studies where GM-CSF was stopped after 14 days (30,90), there were decreases in neutrophil levels, suggesting that the neutrophil recovery was still dependent on exogenous GM-CSF at that stage. Possible GM-CSF related toxicity was seen, particularly at higher doses (30,91), but in the clinical context of AtBMT it was difficult to distil the effects of GM-CSF from the usual course of AtBMT patients.

Devereaux et al. (89) reported observations from 10 evaluable patients with resistant Hodgkin's disease, all of whom received 3–21 days of GM-CSF (100 $\mu g/m^2$/day, continuous intravenous infusion). Compared to a series of predominantly historical controls, there was accelerated neutrophil recovery, with the mean time to a neutrophil level exceeding 0.5×10^9/L being reduced from 25 to 18 days. Platelet recovery was comparable to the control group, and there were similar rates of infection, febrile days, and similar durations of hospital stay in the two groups.

Gianni et al. (92) reported an interesting study of complex design that demonstrated GM-CSF administration after cyclophosphamide facilitated stem cell collection from the peripheral blood, and also the marrow. Following irradiation and melphalan, collected stem cells from both sources were reinfused, and some patients received further GM-CSF. GM-CSF administration at the time of cell collection significantly accelerated both neutrophil and platelet recovery compared to a matched control group, but GM-CSF administration after stem cell reinfusion did not further shorten the time to attain a neutrophil level exceeding 0.5×10^9/L. The only clinical benefit reported was a reduction in neutropenia. Nemunaitis et al. (93) reported preliminary results from a randomized placebo controlled study of GM-CSF (250 $\mu g/m^2$/day, 20 days) in AtBMT. Patients who received GM-CSF had significantly fewer transfusions of platelet and red cells, and had fewer days of fever, antibiotic therapy, nausea, and parenteral nutrition, even though the day of attainment of a neutrophil count exceeding 1×10^9/L was not significantly different between the two groups at the time of this interim analysis. It remains important to demonstrate that accelerated neutrophil recovery translates into clinical benefit in Phase III studies such as this study and the ongoing European study in AlBMT recipients (94).

Preliminary data from studies of GM-CSF in AlBMT have been reported, and also suggest more rapid neutrophil recovery without effects on acute graft-versus-host disease (94,95).

IX. CONCLUSION

There is now abundant evidence from Phase II data to suggest a clinical role for both G-CSF and GM-CSF in cancer patients receiving chemotherapy. The clinical advantage of these hematologic effects and validity of Phase II observations now needs to be demonstrated by Phase III studies in the contexts considered above. Furthermore, clinical advantage resulting from modified chemotherapy-induced myelosuppression may permit new approaches to the clinical application of antineoplastic agents, such as those described above, and lead to a better antitumor outcome with improved response rates and patient survival.

REFERENCES

1. Chabner BA, Myers CE. Clinical pharmacology of cancer chemotherapy. In: DeVita VT Jr, Hellman S, Rosenberg SA, eds. Cancer: principles and practice of oncology, 3rd ed. Philadelphia: JB Lippincott, 1989:349–95.
2. Bodey GP, Buckley M, Sathe YS, Freireich EJ. Quantitative relationship between circulating leukocytes and infection in patients with acute leukemia. Ann Intern Med 1966; 64:328–40.

3. Lieschke GJ, Bell D, Rawlinson W, Green MD, Sheridan W, Morstyn G, Stuart-Harris R, Kefford RF, Levi J, Sorrell T. Empiric single agent or combination antibiotic therapy for febrile episodes in neutropenic patients: an overview. Eur J Cancer Clin Oncol 1989; 25 (suppl 2):S37–42.
4. Fujisawa M, Kobayashi Y, Okabe T, Takaku F, Komatsu T, Itoh S. Recombinant human granulocyte colony-stimulating factor induces granulocytosis in vivo. Jpn J Cancer Res 1987; 77:866–9.
5. Metcalf D, Begley CG, Williamson DJ, Nice EC, DeLamarter J, Mermod JJ, Thatcher D, Schmidt A. Hemopoietic responses in mice injected with purified recombinant murine GM-CSF. Exp Hematol 1987; 15:1–9.
6. Welte K, Bonilla MA, Gillio AP, Boone TC, Potter GK, Gabrilove JL, Moore MAS, O'Reilly RJ, Souza LM. Recombinant human granulocyte colony-stimulating factor: effects on hematopoiesis in normal and cyclophosphamide-treated primates. J Exp Med 1987; 165:941–8.
7. Donahue RE, Wang EA, Stone DK, Kamen R, Wong GG, Sehgal PK, Nathan DG, Clark SC. Stimulation of hematopoiesis in primates by continuous infusion of human GM-CSF. Nature 1986; 321:872–5.
8. Mayer P, Lam C, Obenaus H, Liehl E, Besemer J. Recombinant human GM-CSF induced leukocytosis and activates peripheral blood polymorphonuclear neutrophils in nonhuman primates. Blood 1987; 70:206–13.
9. Ono M, Matsumoto M, Matsubara S, Tomiko S, Asano S. Protective effect of human granulocyte colony-stimulating factor on bacterial and fungal infection in neutropenic mice. Behring Inst Mitt 1988; 83:216–21.
10. Nienhuis AW, Donahue RE, Karlsson S, Clark SC, Agricola B, Antinoff N, Pierce JE, Turner P, Anderson WF, Nathan DG. Recombinant human granulocyte-macrophage colony stimulating factor (GM-CSF) shortens the period of neutropenia after autologous marrow transplantation in a primate model. J Clin Invest 1987; 80:573–7.
11. Monroy RL, Skelly RR, MacVittie TJ, Davis TA, Sauber JJ, Clark SC, Donahue RE. The effect of recombinant GM-CSF on the recovery of monkeys transplanted with autologous bone marrow. Blood 1987; 170:1696–9.
12. Douer D, Sagi O, Shaked N, Witz IP, Ramot B. Response to recombinant murine GM-CSF in melphalan treated mice. Blood 1987; 70 (suppl 1):133a. (abstr).
13. Bronchud MH, Scarffe JH, Thatcher N, Crowther D, Souza LM, Alton NK, Testa NG, Dexter TM. Phase I/II study of recombinant human granulocyte colony-stimulating factor in patients receiving intensive chemotherapy for small cell lung cancer. Br J Cancer 1987; 56:809–13.
14. Morstyn G, Campbell L, Souza LM, Alton NK, Keech J, Green M, Sheridan W, Metcalf D, Fox R. Effect of granulocyte colony-stimulating factor on neutropenia induced by cytotoxic chemotherapy. Lancet 1988; i:667–72.
15. Gabrilove JL, Jakubowski A, Fain K, Grous J, Scher H, Sternberg C, Yagoda A, Clarkson B, Bonilla MA, Oettgen HF. Phase I study of granulocyte colony-stimulating factor in patients with transitional cell carcinoma of the urothelium. J Clin Invest 1988; 82:1454–61.
16. Lindemann A, Hermann F, Oster W, Haffner G, Meyenburg W, Souza LM, Mertelsmann R. Hematologic effects of recombinant human granulocyte colony-stimulating factor in patients with malignancy. Blood 1989; 74:2644–51.
17. Morstyn G, Campbell L, Lieschke G, Layton JE, Maher D, O'Connor M, Green M, Sheridan W, Vincent M, Alton K. Treatment of chemotherapy-induced neutropenia by subcutaneously administered granulocyte colony-stimulating factor with optimization of dose and duration of therapy. J Clin Oncol 1989; 7:1554–62.
18. Kerrigan DP, Castillo A, Foucar K, Townsend K, Niedhart J. Peripheral blood morphologic changes after high-dose antineoplastic chemotherapy and recombinant human granulocyte colony-stimulating factor. Am J Clin Pathol 1989; 92:280–5.

19. Duhrsen U, Villeval J-L, Boyd J, Kannourakis G, Morstyn G, Metcalf D. Effects of recombinant human granulocyte colony-stimulating factor on hematopoietic progenitor cells in cancer patients. Blood 1988; 72:2074–81.
20. Lord BI, Bronchud MH, Owens S, Chang J, Howell A, Souza L, Dexter TM. The kinetics of human granulopoiesis following treatment with granulocyte colony-stimulating factor in vivo. Proc Natl Acad Sci USA 1989; 86:9499–9503.
21. Hammond WP IV, Price TH, Souza LM, Dale DC. Treatment of cyclic neutropenia with granulocyte colony-stimulating factor. N Engl J Med 1989; 320:1306–11.
22. Glaspy JA, Baldwin GC, Robertson PA, Souza L, Vincent M, Ambersley J, Golde DW. Therapy for neutropenia in hairy cell leukemia with recombinant human granulocyte colony-stimulating factor. Ann Intern Med 1988; 109:789–95.
23. Gabrilove JL, Jakubowski A, Scher H, Sternberg C, Wong G, Grous J, Yagoda A, Fain K, Moore MA, Clarkson B. Effect of granulocyte colony-stimulating factor on neutropenia and associated morbidity due to chemotherapy for transitional cell carcinoma of the urothelium. N Engl J Med 1988; 318:1414–22.
24. Niedhart J, Kohler B, Castillo A, Mangalik A, Saiki J, Duncan P, Sousa L, Downing M. Recombinant human granulocyte colony stimulating factor (G-CSF) shortens duration of granulocytopenia and thrombocytopenia following intensive chemotherapy dosing. Proc Am Assoc Cancer Res 1988; 29:356a (abstr 1415).
25. Bronchud MH, Howell A, Crowther D, Hopwood P, Souza L, Dexter TM. The use of granulocyte colony-stimulating factor to increase the intensity of treatment with doxorubicin in patients with advanced breast and ovarian cancer. Br J Cancer 1989; 60:121–5.
26. Sheridan WP, Morstyn G, Wolf M, Dodds A, Lusk J, Maher D, Layton JE, Green MD, Souza L, Fox RM. Granulocyte colony-stimulating factor and neutrophil recovery after high-dose chemotherapy and autologous bone marrow transplantation. Lancet 1989; ii:891–5.
27. Groopman J, Mitsuyasu RT, DeLeo MJ, Oette D, Golde DW. Effect of recombinant human granulocyte-macrophage colony stimulating factor on myelopoiesis in the acquired immunodeficiency syndrome. N Engl J Med 1987; 317:593–8.
28. Vadhan-Raj S, Keating M, LeMaistre A, Hittelman WN, McCredie K, Trujillo JM, Broxmeyer HE, Henney C, Gutterman JU. Effects of human granulocyte-macrophage colony-stimulating factor in patients with myelodysplastic syndromes. N Engl J Med 1987; 317:1545–52.
29. Vadhan-Raj S, Buescher S, LeMaistre A, Keating M, Walters R, Ventura C, Hittelman W, Broxmeyer HE, Gutterman JU. Stimulation of hematopoiesis in patients with bone marrow failure and in patients with malignancy by recombinant human granulocyte-macrophage colony-stimulating factor. Blood 1988; 72:134–41.
30. Brandt SJ, Peters WP, Atwater SK, Kurtzberg J, Borowitz MJ, Jones RB, Shpall EJ, Bast RC Jr, Gilbert CJ, Oette DH. Effect of recombinant human granulocyte-macrophage colony-stimulating factor on hematopoietic reconstitution after high-dose chemotherapy and autologous marrow transplantation. N Engl J Med 1988; 318:869–76.
31. Lieschke GJ, Maher D, Cebon J, O'Connor M, Green M, Sheridan W, Boyd A, Rallings M, Bonnem E, Metcalf D. Effects of bacterially synthesized recombinant human granulocyte-macrophage colony stimulating factor in patients with advanced malignancy. Ann Intern Med 1989; 110:357–64.
32. Lieschke GJ, Maher D, Cebon J, O'Connor M, Green M, Sheridan W, Rallings M, Bonnem E, Burgess AW, McGrath K, Fox RM, Morstyn G. Phase I study of intravenously administered bacterially synthesized granulocyte-macrophage colony-stimulating factor and comparison with subcutaneous administration. Cancer Res 1990; 50:606–14.
33. Steward WP, Scarffe JH, Austin R, Bonnen E, Thatcher N, Morgenstern G, Crowther D. Recombinant human granulocyte-macrophage colony stimulating factor (rhGM-CSF) given as daily short infusions—a phase I dose-toxicity study. Br J Cancer 1989; 59:142–5.

34. Hermann F, Schulz G, Lindemann A, Meyenburg W, Oster W, Krumwieh D, Mertelsmann R. Hematopoietic responses in patients with advanced malignancy treated with recombinant human granulocyte-macrophage colony-stimulating factor. J Clin Oncol 1989; 7:159–67.
35. Antman KS, Griffin JD, Socinski MA, Ryan L, Cannistra SA, Oette D, Whitley M, Frei E 3rd, Schnipper LE. Effect of recombinant human granulocyte-macrophage colony stimulating factor on chemotherapy-induced myelosuppression. N Engl J Med 1988; 319:593–8.
36. Socinski MA, Cannistra SA, Elias A, Antman KH, Schnipper L, Griffin JD. Granulocyte-macrophage colony stimulating factor expands the circulating haemopoietic progenitor cell compartment in man. Lancet 1988; i:1194–8.
37. Rifkin RM, Hersh EM, Salmon SE. A phase I study of therapy with recombinant human granulocyte-macrophage colony stimulating factor (rhGM-CSF) administered by IV bolus or continuous infusion. Behring Inst Mitt 1988; 83:125–33.
38. Phillips N, Jacobs S, Stoller R, Earle E, Przepiorka D, Shadduck RK. Effect of recombinant human granulocyte-macrophage colony-stimulating factor on myelopoiesis in patients with refractory metastatic carcinoma. Blood 1989; 74:26–34.
39. Aglietta M, Piacibello W, Sanavio F, Stacchini A, Apria F, Schena M, Mossetti C, Carnino F, Caligaris-Cappio F, Gavosto F. Kinetics of human hemopoietic cells after in vivo administration of granulocyte-macrophage colony-stimulating factor. J Clin Invest 1989; 83:551–7.
40. Cebon J, Dempsey P, Fox R, Kannourakis G, Bonnem E, Burgess AW, Morstyn G. Pharmacokinetics of human granulocyte-macrophage colony-stimulating factor using a sensitive immunoassay. Blood 1988; 72:1340–7.
41. Devereux S, Linch DC, Campos-Costa D, Spittle MF, Jelliffe AM. Transient leukopenia induced by granulocyte-macrophage colony stimulating factor. Lancet 1987; ii:1523.
42. Socinski MA, Cannistra SA, Sullivan R, Elias A, Antman K, Schnipper L, Griffin JD. Granulocyte-macrophage colony stimulating factor induces the expression of the CD11b surface adhesion molecule on human granulocytes in vivo. Blood 1988; 72:691–7.
43. Devereux S, Bull HA, Campos-Costa D, Saib R, Linch DC. Granulocyte macrophage colony stimulating factor induced changes in cellular adhesion molecule expression and adhesion to endothelium: in-vitro and in-vivo studies in man. Br J Haematol 1989; 71:323–30.
44. Lieschke GJ, Cebon J, Morstyn G. Characterization of the clinical effects after the first dose of bacterially synthesized recombinant human granulocyte-macrophage colony-stimulating factor. Blood 1989; 74:2634–43.
45. Morstyn G, Stuart-Harris R, Bishop J, Raghavan D, Kefford R, Lieschke G, Bonnem E, Olver I, Green M, Rallings M, Fox R. Optimal scheduling of granulocyte-macrophage colony-stimulating factor for the abrogation of chemotherapy induced neutropenia in small cell lung cancer. Proc Am Soc Clin Oncol 1989; 8:218a (abstr 850).
46. Gianni AM, Bregni M, Siena S, Orani A, Stern AC, Gandola L, Bonadonna G. Recombinant human granulocyte-macrophage colony-stimulating factor reduces hematologic toxicity and widens clinical applicability of high-dose cyclophosphamide treatment in breast cancer and non-Hodgkin's lymphoma. J Clin Oncol 1990; 8:768–78.
47. Hermann F, Schulz G, Wieser M, Kolbe K, Nicolay U, Noack M, Lindemann A, Mertelsmann R. Effects of granulocyte-macrophage colony-stimulating factor on neutropenia and related morbidity induced by myelotoxic chemotherapy. Am J Med 1990; 88:619–24.
48. Estey EH, Dixon D, Kantarjian HM, Keating M, McCredie K, Bodey GP, Kurzrock R, Talpaz M, Freireich EJ, Deisseroth AB, Gutterman JU. Treatment of poor-prognosis, newly diagnosed acute myeloid leukemia with ara-C and recombinant human granulocyte-macrophage colony stimulating factor. Blood 1990; 75:1766–9.
49. Brennan LV. Recombinant GM-CSF in myelosuppression of chemotherapy (letter). N Engl J Med 1989; 320:253.

50. Lieschke GJ, Morstyn G. Role of G-CSF and GM-CSF in the prevention of chemotherapy-induced neutropenia. In: Mertelsmann R, Hermann F, eds. Hematological growth factors in clinical applications. New York: Marcel Dekker 1990:191–223.
51. Hart PH, Whitty GA, Piccoli DS, Hamilton JA. Synergistic activation of human monocytes by granulocyte-macrophage colony stimulating factor and IFN-gamma: increased TNF-alpha but not IL-1 activity. J Immunol 1988; 141:1516–21.
52. Grabstein KH, Urdal DL, Tushinski RJ, Mochizuki DY, Price VL, Cantrell MA, Gillis S, Conlon PJ. Induction of macrophage tumoricidal activity by granulocyte-macrophage colony-stimulating factor. Science 1986; 232:506–8.
53. Cannistra SA, Vellenga E, Groshek P, Rambaldi A, Griffin JD. Human granulocyte-macrophage colony stimulating factor and interleukin 3 stimulate monocyte cytotoxicity through a tumor necrosis factor dependent mechanism. Blood 1988; 71:672–6.
54. Wiesbart RH, Golde DW, Clark SC, Wong GC, Gasson JC. Human granulocyte macrophage colony-stimulating factor is a neutrophil activator. Nature 1985; 314:361–3.
55. Lopez AF, Williamson J, Gamble JR, Begley CG, Harlan JM, Klebanoff SJ, Waltersdorph A, Wong G, Clark SC, Vadas MA. Recombinant human granulocyte-macrophage colony stimulating factor stimulates in vitro mature human neutrophil and eosinophil function, surface receptor expression and survival. J Clin Invest 1986; 78:1220–8.
56. Jakubowski AA, Souza L, Kelly F, Fain K, Budman D, Clarkson B, Bonilla MA, Moore MA, Gabrilove J. Effects of human granulocyte colony-stimulating factor in a patient with idiopathic neutropenia. N Engl J Med 1989; 320:38–42.
57. Bronchud MH, Potter MR, Morgenstern, Blasco MJ, Scarffe JH, Thatcher N, Crowther D, Souza LM, Alton NK, Testa NG, Dexter TM. In vitro and in vivo analysis of the effects of recombinant human granulocyte colony-stimulating factor in patients. Br J Cancer 1988; 58:64–9.
58. Toner GC, Jakubowski AA, Crown JPL, Meisenberg B, Sheridan C, Gabrilove JL. Colony-stimulating factors and neutrophil migration (letter). Ann Intern Med 1989; 110:846–7.
59. Sullivan R, Fredette JP, Socinski M, Elias A, Antman K, Schnipper L, Griffin JD. Enhancement of superoxide anion release by granulocytes harvested from patients receiving granulocyte-macrophage colony stimulating factor. Br J Haematol 1989; 71:475–9.
60. Kaplan SS, Basford RE, Wing EJ, Shadduck RK. The effect of recombinant human granulocyte macrophage colony stimulating factor on neutrophil activation in patients with refractory carcinoma. Blood 1989; 73:636–8.
61. Peters WP, Stuart A, Affronti ML, Kim CS, Coleman RE. Neutrophil migration is defective during recombinant human granulocyte-macrophage colony-stimulating factor infusion after autologous bone marrow transplantation in humans. Blood 1988; 72:1310–5.
62. Baldwin GC, Gasson JC, Quan SG, Fleischmann J, Weisbart R, Oette D, Mitsuyasu RT, Golde DW. Granulocyte-macrophage colony-stimulating factor enhances neutrophil function in acquired immunodeficiency syndrome patients. Proc Natl Acad Sci USA 1988; 85:2763–6.
63. Wing EJ, Magee DM, Whiteside TL, Kaplan SS, Shadduck RK. Recombinant human granulocyte/macrophage colony-stimulating factor enhances monocyte cytotoxicity and secretion of tumor necrosis factor α and interferon in cancer patients. Blood 1989; 734:643–6.
64. Burgess AW, Begley CG, Johnson GR, Lopez AF, Williamson DJ, Mermod JJ, Simpson RJ, Schmitz A, DeLamarter JF. Purification and properties of bacterially synthesized human granulocyte-macrophage colony stimulating factor. Blood 1987; 69:43–51.
65. Crawford J, Ozer H, Johnson D, and the G-CSF study group. Granulocyte colony stimulating factor: prevention of chemotherapy induced febrile neutropenia (FN) in patients with

small cell lung cancer (SCLC). A randomized double blind placebo controlled trial. Proc Am Soc Clin Oncol 1990; 9:229 (abstr).

66. Teshima H, Ishikawa J, Kitayama H, Yamagami T, Hiraoka A, Nakamura H, Shibata H, Masaoka T, Takaku F. Clinical effects of recombinant human granulocyte colony-stimulating factor in leukemia patients: a phase I/II study. Exp Hematol 1989; 17:853–8.
67. Bleiberg I, Riklis I, Fabian I. Enhanced resistance of bone marrow transplanted mice to bacterial infection induced by recombinant granulocyte-macrophage colony-stimulating factor. Blood 1990; 75:1262–6.
68. Baldwin CG, Gasson JC, Kaufmann SE, Quan SG, Williams RE, Avalos BR, Gazdar AF, Golde DW, DiPerso JF. Nonhematopoietic tumor cells express functional GM-CSF receptors. Blood 1989; 73:1033–7.
69. Ruff MR, Farrar WL, Pert CB. Interferon γ and granulocyte/macrophage colony-stimulating factor inhibit growth and induce antigens characteristic of myeloid differentiation in small-cell lung cancer cell lines. Proc Natl Acad Sci USA 1986; 83:6613–7.
70. Wilson W, Rubin M, Mechinaud F, Mertins S, Walsh T, Magrath I, Longo D, Pizzo PA. The effect of recombinant human (rh) GM-CSF on the proliferation of human B cell lymphomas. Blood 1987; 70:145a (abstr).
71. Berdel WE, Danhauser-Reidl S, Steinhauser G, Winton EF. Various human hematopoietic growth factors (interleukin-3, GM-CSF, G-CSF) stimulate clonal growth of nonhematopoietic tumor cells. Blood 1989; 73:80–3.
72. Dodwell DJ, Gurney H, Thatcher N. Dose intensity in cancer chemotherapy. Br J Cancer 1990; 61:789–94.
73. Begley CG, Metcalf D, Nicola NA. Binding characteristics and proliferative action of purified granulocyte colony-stimulating factor on normal and leukemic human promyelocytes. Exp Hematol 1988; 16:71–9.
74. Vellenga E, Young DC, Wagner K, Wiper D, Ostapovicz D, Griffin JD. The effects of GM-CSF and G-CSF in promoting growth of clonogenic cells in acute myeloblastic leukemia. Blood 1987; 69:1771–6.
75. Motoji T, Takanashi M, Masuda M, Oshimi K, Mizoguchi H. Effect of recombinant GM-CSF and recombinant G-CSF on colony formation of blast progenitors in acute myeloblastic leukemia. Exp Hematol 1989; 17:56–60.
76. Ganser A, Volkers B, Greher J, Ottmann OG, Walther F, Becher R, Bergmann L, Schulz G, Hoelzer D. Recombinant human granulocyte-macrophage colony-stimulating factor in patients with myelodysplastic syndromes—a phase I/II trial. Blood 1989; 73:31–7.
77. Bessho M, Jinnai I, Hirashima K. Suppressive effect of G-CSF, GM-CSF and [71SER]IL-1beta (OCT-43) on development of murine myeloid leukemia. Exp Hematol 1990; 18:604 (abstr).
78. Bessho M, Susaki K, Hirashima K, Tamura M, Ono M. Prolonged survival of mice injected with myeloid leukemia by subcutaneous injection of recombinant human G-CSF. Leuk Res 1989; 13:1001–7.
79. Cannistra SA, Groshek P, Griffin JD. Granulocyte-macrophage colony-stimulating factor enhances the cytotoxic effects of cytosine arabinoside in acute myeloblastic leukemia and in the myeloid blast crisis phase of chronic myeloid leukemia. Leukemia 1989; 3:328–34.
80. Hiddemann W, Kiehl M, Schleyer E, Worman B, Zuhlsdorf M, Buchner T. Stimulatory effect of GM-CSF and IL3 on the metabolism and cytotoxic activity of cytosine arabinoside (ara-C) in leukemic blasts from patients with acute myeloid leukemia. Blood 1989; 74:230a (abstr).
81. Buechner T, Hiddemann W, Zuhlsdorf M, Koenigsmann M, Bochmann A, Vandeloo J, Schulz G. Human recombinant granulocyte macrophage colony stimulating factor (GM-

CSF) treatment of patients with acute leukemia in aplasia and at high risk of early death. Behring Inst Mitt 1988; 83:308–12.

82. Buechner T, Hiddemann W, Koenigsmann M, Zuehlsdorf M, Woermann B, Boeckmann A, Aguion-Freire E, Innig G, Maschmeyer G, Ludwig W-D, Heinecke A, Schulz G. Hematologic and therapeutic effects of recombinant human GM-CSF following chemotherapy (CT) in patients with acute leukemias at higher age or after relapse. Blood 1989; 74:271a (abstr 1021).
83. Metcalf D. Actions and interactions of G-CSF, LIF and IL-6 on normal and leukemic murine cells. Leukemia 1989; 3:349–55.
84. Schuster MW, Larson RA, Thompson JA, Coiffier B, Bennett JM, Israel RJ, for the Schering-Plough/Sandoz MDS Study Group. Granulocyte-macrophage colony-stimulating factor (GM-CSF) for myelodysplastic syndrome (MDS): Results of a multi-center randomized controlled trial. Blood 1990; 76 (suppl 1):318 (abstr 1261).
85. Taylor K McD, Jagannath S, Spitzer G, Spinolo JA, Tucker SL, Fogel B, Cabanillas RB, Hagemeister FB, Souza LM. Recombinant human granulocyte colony-stimulating factor hastens granulocyte recovery after high-dose chemotherapy and autologous bone marrow transplantation in Hodgkin's disease. J Clin Oncol 1989; 12:1791–9.
86. Masaoka T, Takaku F, Kato S, Moriyama Y, Kodera Y, Kanamura A, Shimosaka A, Shibata H, Nakamura H. Recombinant human granulocyte colony-stimulating factor in allogeneic bone marrow transplantation. Exp Hematol 1989; 17:1047–50.
87. To LB, Dyson PG, Bradford A, Russell JA, Haylock DN, Ho JQK, Kimber RJ, Juttner CA. Peripheral blood stem cells collected in very early remission produce rapid and sustained autologous hematopoietic reconstitution in acute non-lymphoblastic leukemia. Bone Marrow Transplant 1987; 2:103–8.
88. Sheridan WP, Juttner C, Szer J, Begley G, De Luca E, McGrath K, Vincent M, Souza L, Morstyn G, Rox RM. Granulocyte colony-stimulating factor (G-CSF) in peripheral blood stem cell (PBSC) and bone marrow (BM) transplantation. Blood 1990; 76 (supp 1):565 (abstr 2251).
89. Devereaux S, Linch DC, Gribben JG, McMillan A, Patterson K, Goldstone AH. GM-CSF accelerates neutrophil recovery after autologous bone marrow transplantation for Hodgkin's disease. Bone Marrow Transplant 1989; 4:49–54.
90. Nemunaitis J, Singer JW, Buckner CD, Hill R, Storb R, Thomas ED, Appelbaum FR. Use of recombinant human granulocyte-macrophage colony-stimulating factor in autologous marrow transplantation for lymphoid malignancies. Blood 1988; 72:834–6.
91. Blazar BR, Kersey JH, McGlave PB, Vallera DA, Lasky LC, Haake RJ, Bostrom B, Weisdorf DR, Epstein C, Ramsey NK. In vivo administration of recombinant human granulocyte/macrophage colony-stimulating factor in acute lymphoblastic leukemia patients receiving purged autografts. Blood 1989; 73:849–57.
92. Gianni AM, Siena S, Bregni M, Tarella C, Stern AC, Peleri A, Bonadonna G. Granulocyte-macrophage colony-stimulating factor to harvest circulating haemopoietic stem cells for autotransplantation. Lancet 1989; ii:580–5.
93. Nemunaitis J, Singer JW, Buckner CD, Epstein C, Hansen J, Hill R, Storb R, Thomas ED, Appelbaum FR. Preliminary analysis of a randomized, placebo-controlled trial of rhGM-CSF in autologous bone marrow transplantation (ABMT). Proc Am Soc Clin Oncol 1990; 9:10 (abstr 34).
94. De Witte T, Gratwohl A, Van der Lely N, Muus P, Stern A, Speck B, Nissen C, Marmont A, Bacigalupo A, Gluckman E, Zwaan F. A multicenter double blind randomized trial of recombinant human granulocyte-macrophage colony stimulating factor (rhGM-CSF) in recipients of allogeneic T-cell depleted bone marrow. Blood 1989; 74:84a (abstr 311).

95. Nemunaitis J, Anasetti C, Appelbaum FR, Buckner CD, Epstein CD, Hansen J, Oldham F, Storb R, Thomas ED, Singer JW. Phase I/II trial of RHGM-CSF after allogeneic bone marrow transplantation (BMT). Blood 1989; 74:123a (abstr 457).

Abbreviations

AA	arachidonic acid
ABMT (AtBMT)	autologous bone marrow transplantation
ACTH	adrenocorticotropic hormone
ADCC	antibody dependent cell cytotoxicity
ALL	acute lymphoblastic leukemia
alpha-1 PI	alpha-1 proteinase inhibitor
AML	acute myelogenous leukemia
ANAP	anionic neutrophil-activating peptide
AND	anaphylactic degranulation
ARDS	adult respiratory distress syndrome
ATG	antithymocyte globulin
B-TCGF	B-cell derived TCGF
BAF	basophil activating factor (HRA,HRF)
BCG	Bacillus Calmette-Guerin
BCGF	B-cell growth factor
BCGFII	IL-5
BFU	burst forming unit
BPI	bactericidal/permeability increasing protein
BSF	B-cell stimulating factor
BSF-1	IL-4
c-kit ligand	SCF
C. parvum	*Corynebacterium parvum*
cAMP	adenosine 3′,5′-cyclic monophosphate
CD	cluster of differentiation (cell surface antigen)
CD11a/CD18	LFA-1
CD2	LFA-2
CD3	T-cell receptor, TCR
CD54	ICAM-1
CD58	LFA-3

CFU	colony forming unit
CGD	chronic granulomatous disease
cGMP	guanosine 3′,5′-cyclic monophosphate
CML	chronic myelogenous leukemia
CR	complement receptor
CR1	complement receptor type 1 (C3B-R)
CR3	complement receptor type 3 (C3Bi-R; CD11b)
CR4	complement receptor type 4 (gp95,150)
CSF	colony-stimulating factor
CSF-1	M-CSF
CSF-alpha	GM-CSF
CSF-beta	G-CSF
CSIF	cytokine synthesis inhibitory factor
CT	cholera toxin
CTAP	connective tissue activating peptide
Cyt.b558	cytochrome b558, b-245, X-CGD protein
DAG	diacylglycerol
DFP	diisopropyl phosphofluoridate
EC	endothelial cell
ECP	eosinophil cationic proteins
EDF	eosinophil differentiation factor
EDN	eosinophil-derived neurotoxin
ELAM	endothelial leukocyte adhesion molecule
ENAP	endothelial cell-derived neutrophil activating peptide
EPA	erythroid potentiating factor
EPO	erythropoietin
EPO	eosinophil peroxidase
ETAF	epidermal cell-derived thymocyte-activating factor (IL-1)
Fc-R	Fc (of immunoglobulin) receptor
FINAP	fibroblast-derived neutrophil activating peptide
FLAP	5-lipoxygenase activating protein
FMLP	N-formyl-methionyl-leucyl-phenylalanine
G	granulocyte
G-CSF	granulocyte colony-stimulating factor
G-protein	guanine nucleotide binding regulatory protein
GCP	granulocyte chemotactic peptide (IL-8)
GM-CSF	granulocyte-macrophage colony-stimulating factor
GMP-140	granule membrane protein (CD62)
gro	growth stimulating gene product (MGSA)
H-7	1-(5-isoquinolinylsulfonyl)-2-methylpiperazine
HETE	hydroxyeicosatetraenoic acid
HILDA	human interleukin for DA cells
HPETE	hydroperoxyeicosatetraenoic acid
HRA	histamine releasing activity (HRF)
HRF	histamine releasing factor
HRIF	histamine release-inhibiting factor
HUVEC	human umbilical vein endothelial cells
ICAM	intercellular adhesion molecule
IFN	interferon
IFN_{γ}	interferon type II, immune IFN
Ig	immunoglobulin
IL	interleukin

IL-1	hemopoietin-1, lymphocyte activating factor
IL-2	T-cell growth factor
IL-3	multi-CSF
IL-4	BSF-1
IL-5	BCGF-2, EDF
IL-6	BSF-2; IFN-beta 2
IL-8	MONAP, LYNAP, MDNCF, NAF, GCP, NAP-1
IL-9	p40
IL-10	B-TCGF, CSIF
IP3	inositol-1,4,5-trisphosphate
ITP	idiopathic thrombocytic purpurea
LAD	leukocyte adhesion deficiency
LAF	lymphocyte activating factor (IL-1)
LAM	leukocyte adhesion molecule
LCF	lymphocyte chemotactic factor (IL-8)
LDCF	lymphocyte derived chemotactic factor (IL-8)
Leu M5	P150,95
LF	lactoferrin
LFA-1	leukocyte functional antigen-1 (CD11a/CD18)
LIF	leukocyte inhibitory factor (chapter 12)
LIF (HILDA)	leukemia inhibitory factor
LPS	lipopolysaccharide (endotoxin)
LT	leukotriene
LYNAP	lymphocyte/neutrophil activating protein (IL-8)
M	monocyte
M-CSF	macrophage colony-stimulating factor (CSF-1)
Mac-1	CD11b/CD18
MBP	major basic protein (eosinophil)
MCAF	monocyte chemotactic and activating factor
MCF	monocyte chemotactic factor
MDNCF	monocyte derived neutrophil chemotactic factor (IL-8)
MDS	myelodysplastic syndrome
MGF	mast-cell growth factor
MGSA	melanoma growth stimulating activity (gro oncogene)
MIF	migration inhibitory factor
MIP	macrophage inflammatory protein
MONAP	monocyte-derived neutrophil activating factor (IL-8)
MPO	myeloperoxidase
multi-CSF	IL-3
NAF	neutrophil activating factor
NAP-1	neutrophil activating protein (IL-8)
NCF	neutrophil chemotactic factor (IL-8)
NHL	non-Hodgkin's lymphoma
NK	natural killer cell
O_2^-	superoxide
OH	hydroxyl radical
p150,95	CD11c/CD18
p40	IL-9
PA	phosphatidic acid
PAF	platelet activating factor
PBP	platelet basic protein
PDGF	platelet-derived growth factor

PF-4	platelet factor 4
PG	prostaglandin
PHA	phytohemagglutinin
PI	phosphatidyl inositol
PIP_2	phosphatidylinositol 4,5-bisphosphate
PKA	cyclic AMP-dependent protein kinase
PKC	protein kinase C
PMA	phorbol 12-myristate 13-acetate
PMD	peicemeal degranulation
PMN	polymorphonuclear leucocyte (neutrophil)
PMSF	phenylmethyl sulfonylfluoride
PT	pertussis toxin
PWM	pokeweed mitogen
RBC	red blood cell
RBL	rat basophilic leukocyte
RGD	arg-gly-asp, an integrin recognition sequence
SBTI	soybean trypsin inhibitor
SCF	stem-cell factor, MGF, lc-kit ligand, Steel factor
SCLC	small-cell lung carcinoma
SCN	severe congenital neutropenia
SDS	sodium dodecylsulfate
Steel factor	SCF
TBI	total body irradiation
TCF	T-cell chemotactic factor (IL-8)
TCGF	T-cell growth factor (IL-2)
TGF	transforming growth factor
TH	helper T-cell
TNF_α	tumor necrosis factor (cachectin)
TNF_β	lymphotoxin
TRF	T-cell replacing factor (IL-5, IL-8)
VCAM	vascular cell adhesion molecule
VIP	vasoactive intestinal polypeptide
VLA	very late activation antigen
VNR	vitronectin receptor
W-7	N-(6-aminohexyl)-5-chloro-1-naphthalenesulfonamide

Index

3-deaza-SIBA, mast cell inhibition, 311
3-isobutyl-1-methylxanthine (IBMX)
basophil histamine release, inhibition of, 304
5-HETE, basophils and mast cells, production of, 274–275
A23187 calcium ionophore
basophil degranulation, 188,237–240,282,285,289
leukotriene formation, 89,94
mast cell cAMP, effects on, 307–308
NADPH oxidase, activation of, 52,55
neutrophil activation, 314–316
neutrophil activation, GM-CSF augmention of, 467–468
AA release, neutrophil, GM-CSF enhancement of, 458–470,490
ABMT
G-CSF administration, 654–655,685
GM-CSF administration, 685–686
ABMT following bone marrow suppression, M-CSF administration, 657
Acetylcholine, neutrophil responses to, 319
Acid phosphatase, eosinophil, glycosaminoglycan degradation, 538
Acidic isoferritin (AIF), hemopoiesis, effect on, 340,347
ACTH
mast cell cAMP, 307
release by IL-1, 363
Actin polymerization, role of PIP_2, 117–124
Activin, hemopoiesis, effect on, 340, 346
Acute intersitial nephritis, eosinophilia in, 143
Acute myeloid leukemia, GM-CSF in therapy, 674
Acute-phase reactant, alpha-MSH, inhibition by, 362
ADCC by monocytes, GM-CSF in vivo, effects on, 679
ADCC by neutrophils
G-CSF enhancement of, 652
G-CSF, GM-CSF in vivo, effects on, 679
GM-CSF, augmentation of, 486
increased by TNF, 420
potentiation by LIF, 382
ADCC of RBC by eosinophils, IFN-β enhancement of, 540
ADCC of tumor cells by neutrophils, 523–524
TNF enhancement of, 529,628–629

ADCC of tumor cells by neutrophils, GM-CSF enhancement of, 458–459
Adenine, mast cell cAMP, 307
Adenocarcinoma, basophil degranulation in, 178,215–217
Adenoma, renal mast cell degranulation in, 215
Adenosine
endothelial cell metabolism, 26
histamine release, inhibition of, 304–307
neutrophil cAMP, stimulation of, 108,117
neutrophils, effects on, 314–318
Adenosine triphosphate (ATP), source of hypoxanthine, 25
Adenylate cyclase
GM-CSF, effect on, 459
mechanism of activation, 302
stimulation of, 108–111
Adenylate cyclase, neutrophil, GM-CSF decrease of, 492
Adherence of neutrophils to endothelial cells, 17–18,352–364
Adherence of neutrophils
effect of cytokines on, 125
IL-1 and IL-2 decrease of, 418–419
IL-8, stimulation of, 397
LTB_4, stimulation of, 96
TNF augmentation of, 418–419
Adherence of monocytes, IL-3, GM-CSF stimulation of, 552
Adhesion molecules, leukocytes, GM-CSF in vivo, stimulation of, 676
Adhesion of neutrophil
GM-CSF, augmentation of, 486
LIF stimulation of, 379–381
tumor cytotoxicity, role in, 527–529
Adhesion to tumor cells, TNF enhancement of, 527
ADP-ribosylation, of G proteins, 109–114
Adrenergic receptor activation
atopic disease, abnormality, 322
mast cell cAMP, 307
Adult respiratory distress syndrome (ARDS), neutrophil, role in, 17–19
Affective illness, cAMP, reduced activation in, 323
Aggregation of neutrophils
effect of cytokines on, 125,379
LIF stimulation of, 379–381
LTB4, stimulation of, 95–97
Aging, cAMP, cGMP abnormalities in, 324
AIDS
eosinophil, role in, 143
GM-CSF therapy for, 639,643,675
Allergic conjunctivitis, basophil infiltration in, 178
Allergic contact dermatitis, basophil degranulation in, 213–215
Allergic disease, adhesion molecules, role in, 615–636
Allergic response, late phase, basophil role in, 573–577
Allergy
basophil infiltration, 176–178
basophils and mast cells role in, 273
eosinophil, role in, 141–142
Allograft rejection, mast cell degranulation in, 203–215
Allopurinol, in protection from neutrophils, 24
Alopecia areata, basophil infiltration in, 176–178
α1-antiproteinase, PAF synthesis, regulation of, 514
α1-proteinase inhibitor, suppression by neutrophil HOC1, 503
α-mannosidase, neutrophil primary granule component, 6
α-MSH, neutrophil emigration, inhibition of, 362–363
Amphitropic proteins, roles in NADPH oxidase, 60
Anaphylactic degranulation (AND) of basophils, mast cells, 169–247
Anaphylaxis of basophils, mast cells, 176
Anemias induced by irradiation
G-CSF therapy, 641
GM-CSF therapy, 641
IL-3 therapy, 641
Angioedema, episodic, role of eosinophil, 143
Anionic neutrophil-activating peptide (ANAP), IL-8, relation to, 388

Anti-DNP in mast cell degranulation, ultrastructure, 188
Anti-IgE
degranulation, ultrastructure, 188
mast cell activation, 308–311
Anti-IgE, basophil, adhesion molecule expression, influence on, 627
Anti-microbial activity, neutrophil, GM-CSF enhancement of, 458–459
Antibody–antigen complex, neutrophil emigration, 352
Antigen
degranulation, ultrastructure, 188–198,230
mast cell cGMP, activation of, 307,308
Antithymocyte globulin (ATG) in immunosuppression, hemopoiesis, 661–667
Aplastic anemia, GM-CSF in therapy for, 661–670
Arachidonic acid
as second messenger, 120–125
granule fusion, role in, 16
in PL-A_2 activation, 52
lipoxygenase substrate, 77–81,87–89
metabolism in basophils, mast cells, 274
Arthus reaction, neutrophil emigration, 351
Arylsulfatase B, eosinophil, proteoglycan degradation, 538
Ascorbic acid, neutrophil cAMP, effects on, 314
Asthma
adhesion molecules, role in, 615–636
eosinophil, role in, 141–142
neutrophil cAMP abnormalities in, 321
Athero-embolic renal disease, eosinophil, role in, 143
Atopic, dermatitis, eosinophil, role in, 142
Atopic disease, neutrophil cAMP abnormalities in, 321
ATP
activation of NADPH oxidase, 54
decrease by H_2O_2, 503
regulation of lipoxygenases, 78–83
ATPase, inhibition by MBP, 138

Bacteria
cytotoxicity by neutrophils, 316
cytotoxicity mechanisms, 8–10
Bacteria killing by neutrophil, IFN-γ, enhancement of, 447–448
Bactericidal action of neutrophils G-CSF, GM-CSF in vivo, effects on, 679
effect of cytokines on, 125
BAF, cells sources and degranulation actions, 574
Band cell in neutrophil differentiation, 3
Basophil
activation mechanisms, 273–299
adhesion and inflammation, role in, 620–628
mechanism of release reaction, 273–291
regulation by cyclic nucleotides, 302–305
Basophil histamine release, cytokine stimulation of, 573–586
Basophil-activating factor (BAF), basophil degranulation, 236
Basophilia, cytokine dependence, 176,228
Basophilic leukemia, mast cell degranulation, 203
Basophilopoiesis, 588–595
Basophils, piecemeal degranulation, 169–271
BCG, neutrophil infiltration, 523
Behcet's syndrome, basophil infiltration in, 176–178
β-adrenergic receptor stimulation of neutrophil cAMP, 108–111, 117
β-adrenergic responses, cAMP mechanisms, abnormalities of, 302,322
β-galactosidase in neutrophil primary granules, 5–6
β-glucuronidase abnormality in atopy, 323
β-glucuronidase in neutrophil primary granules, 5–6
β-glucuronidase release by IL-8, 395–400
β-thromboglobulin, IL-8, similarity to, 391–393

BFU-E, hemopoiesis, role in, 343
Bladder cancer, G-CSF in therapy of, 674
Bone marrow, neutrophils, release from, 356-361
Bone marrow depression after cancer chemotherapy, G-CSF and GM-CSF in therapy of, 671–686
Bone marrow transplantation, G-CSF and GM-CSF administration after, 684–686
Botulinum toxin, effects on neutrophil functions, 115
Bradykinin, skin mast cell release, activation of, 276
Breast and ovary cancers, G-CSF in therapy, 674
Breast, lymphoma cancers, GM-CSF in therapy, 674
Bullous pemphigoid, basophil, mast cell degranulation in, 178,203,215
Butyrate, mast cell maturation, 233

c-fos mRNA, neutrophil, GM-CSF, augmentation of, 491
C-I, NADPH oxidase, inhibition of, 57
C-reactive protein, neutrophil cAMP, 314
C. parvum, neutrophil infiltration, 523
C3a
  basophil histamine release, activation of, 276
  neutrophil emigration, 352
C3b, NADPH oxidase, activation of, 52–53
C3b, expression, stimulation by LTB4, 97
C3bi receptor, in neutrophil secondary granule, bactericidal, 6–9
C5a
  basophil degranulation, 187–190,237–240,276,580
  eosinophil chemotaxis, 147
  histamine release, induction of, 276,286
  neutrophil activation, regulation by cyclic nucleotides, 316
  neutrophil chemoattractant, 9–17,52
  neutrophil emigration, 352
  neutrophil, stimulation of IL-1 production, 352–364
  neutrophils, activation of, 387–401
Calcium
  5-lipoxygenase requirement, 89–95
  basophil secretion, 282–289
  basophil, IgE induced increase, 279–280
  granule fusion, role in, 14–15
  lipoxygenases, regulation of, 81–83
  mast cell cGMP, 307
  NADPH oxidase, activation of, 53–55
  neutrophil activation, role in, 111–120,125
Calcium channel, basophil, 280
Calcium oscillations, basophil, 282–283
Calcium, basophil, histamine release, dependence on, 577–579
Calcium, neutrophil
  GM-CSF and PAF, augmentation of, 489–493
  IL-8, response to, 399–400
  LIF and FMLP, stimulation of, 374–375
Calmodulin
  histamine release, role in, 284
  NADPH oxidase, stimulation of, 56
Calmodulin, neutrophil, TNF activation, role in, 431
cAMP
  granulocyte functions, regulation of, 301–325
  histamine release, inhibition of, 285,289–290
  inhibition of neutrophil activation, 108–117
cAMP-dependent protein kinase, NADPH oxidase, effect on, 49,56
Cancer, basophil, mast cell degranulation in, 203
Cancer chemotherapy and bone marrow suppression
  G-CSF administration, 654–655
  M-CSF administration, 657
Cancer, chemotherapy-induced leukopenia
  G-CSF therapy for, 653–655,671–686
  CM-CSF therapy for, 671–686
Cancer, radiation-induced leukopenia
  G-CSF therapy for, 639–642
  GM-CSF therapy for, 640,671–686
Cancer, urogenital and gynecological, M-CSF in therapy for, 657

Cancer, neutrophils, role in cytotoxicity of, 527–529, *see also* tumor
Candida, neutrophil cytotoxicity, regulation by cyclic nucleotides, 316
Carbamylcholine neutrophil chemotaxis, effect on, 319
Carcinoma, IL-8, source of, 406
Carcinoma of breast (MCF7) and colon, G-CSF, GM-CSF, IL-3 stimulation of growth, 606–610
Catalase
  antioxidant, 17–18
  neutrophil microbicidal activity, inhibition by, 448
Cathepsin in host defense; tissue injury, 5–20
Cationic proteins of rat mast cells, 309
Cationic proteins, defensins in neutrophil primary granule, bactericidal, 8,27
CD11/CD18 integrins, expression increased by IL-8, 398
CD11b
  GM-CSF, augmentation of, 486
  induction by GM-CSF, 640
CD11b, eosinophil, IFN-γ, IL4 effects on expression of, 541–543
CD11b/CD18, eosinophil, up regulation by IL-5, 552
CD14, adhesion molecules, ligand for, 616,631
CD18, neutrophil, increased expression by IFN-γ, 440,451
CD2, adhesion molecule, ligand for, 616
CD20, homology to IgE receptor, 279
CD3 (T-cell receptor, TCR), adhesion molecule, 616
CD35 expression, neutrophil, GM-CSF, stimulation of, 459
CD4
  adhesion molecule, ligand for, 616,627–628
  T-cell migration, 359
CD4 expression, eosinophil, IFN-γ, up regulation by, 542–543
CD8, adhesion molecule, ligand for, 616
CD45
  hemopoiesis, role in, 342
  NADPH oxidase, regulation of, 58
Cell-mediated immunity, basophils, mast cells in, 197
Ceruloplasmin, antioxidant, 11–12
CFU-Eo, hemopoiesis, role in, 343
CFU-G, hemopoiesis, role in, 343
CFU-GM, hemopoiesis, role in, 343
CFU-M, hemopoiesis, role in, 343
CFU-mast, hemopoiesis, role in, 343
CFU-Meg, hemopoiesis, role in, 343
CFU-Mix, hemopoiesis, role in, 343
CGD neutrophils
  IFN-γ restoration of O_2^- production, 444–447
  mechanism of cytotoxicity, 503–514
  O_2^-, cytostasis defects, 525–528
  respiratory burst defect, 48
cGMP
  influence on granulocyte functions, 301–325
  role in neutrophil functions, 118,125
cGMP, neutrophils, regulation of LIF, 374
Charcot-Leyden crystals, basophil ultrastructure, 177,182–183,212
Chediak-Higashi Syndrome, cyclic nucleotide abnormalities in, 323
Chemiluminescence, neutrophil, IL-8, response to, 399–400
Chemoattractants in neutrophil activation, 107
Chemotaxins
  basophils, mast cells, 223–228
  effect of cytokines on, 125
  eosinophil, 147
  GM-CSF enhancement of, 459
  neutrophil, 17–18,109–155,351–364
  neutrophil cAMP, cGMP effects on, 314,316
  T-cells, stimulation by IL-8, 389
Chemotaxis of eosinophils, IL-5 stimulation, 552
Chemotaxis of neutrophils
  IL-8 and MCAF, stimulation of, 344,399–400
  lack of effect by IL-1, IL-2, 420
  LIF potentiation, 377
  TNF, regulation of, 419–430
  LTB_4 stimulation, 95,97

Cholera toxin
granulocyte cAMP, 302,307,314
Gs ADP-ribosylation, 109–111
Cholinergic receptor, augmentation of neutrophil functions, 109
Cholinergic receptor activation of neutrophil cGMP, 314
Chondrocytes, IL-8, source of, 406
Chrohn's disease, mast cell degranulation in, 176–178,203,215–216
Chronic glomerulonephritis
mast cell degranulation, 215
respiratory burst defect, 48
CK-1 sequence in growth promoter genes, 565–566
Colchicine, neutrophil cAMP, effects on, 313–314
Collagen, adhesion molecule, ligand for, 616
Collagen sponges, in assay of neutrophil emigration, 356–363
Collagenase
in neutrophil secondary granule, 6–8
tissue injury, 6–20
Collagenase, neutrophil, HOC1 activation of, 508
Colony-forming unit (CFU), hemopoiesis, 341–342
Complement, C3b, C5a receptors on eosinophil, 139
Complement receptors
effects of cytokines on, 125
eosinophil adherence, 139
Compound 48/80
degranulation, ultrastructure, 188
mast cell cGMP, activation of, 307–308
Concanavalin A basophil degranulation 196,209,231
mast cell cAMP, activation, 307–308
neutrophil O_2^-, cAMP, effect on, 316
Connective tissue activating peptide (CTAP) III, IL-8, similarity to, 392,405–407
Corticosteroids, IL-1 synthesis, inhibition of, 351,361
Cortisone, effect on basophil numbers, 175
CR1
NADPH oxidase activation, effect on, 53
CR1, neutrophils
expression increased by LIF, 379–380
induction of expression, 354,360
NADPH oxidase activation, effect on, 53
CR3, neutrophils
emigration, induction of and role in, 358–361
IFN-γ, increased expression of, 440,451
LIF, stimulation of expression, 379–380
LTB4, stimulation of expression of, 96
Crohn's disease, basophil infiltration, degranulation, 176–178,203,215
CSF-1, bone marrow hemopoiesis, 604
CTAP III, histamine releasing activity, 578–581
CTAP III, platelets, homology to HRF, 575–582
Cutaneous basophil hypersensitivity (CBH), basophil infiltration in, 179,199,218–222
Cutaneous necrotizing angiitis, basophil infiltration in, 178
Cyclophosphamide induced neutropenia, GM-CSF correction for, 677–686
Cystic fibrosis, leukocyte cAMP abnormality in, 323
Cytoadhesins (β3 group), adhesion molecules, 16
Cytochalasin B,
neutrophil enzyme release, 108
neutrophil respiratory burst, role in, 428–430
Cytochrome b558 (B-245)
component of respiratory burst, 47–49
in neutrophil secondary granules, 6
neutrophil expression enhanced by IFN-γ, 444–451
Cytostasis, MCAF, stimulation of, 345
Cytotoxicity, by eosinophil granule proteins, 137–145
Cytotoxicity by neutrophils, 22
GM-CSF, augmentation of, 486
cAMP regulation of, 316

D_2O, basophil, potentiation of histamine release, 579,592
DAG lipase in neutrophil activation, 121
DAG, neutrophil, GM-CSF, effects on, 489–490
Darier's disease, basophil infiltration in, 179
Defensins, neutrophil, anti-microbial effects, 6–8, 505–508
Deferoxamine, iron binding, inhibition of cytotoxicity, 23
Degranulation
  basophils, mast cells, 169–247
  effect of cytokines on, 125
  eosinophils, 146
Degranulation of neutrophil
  effect of cytokines on, 354,360
  GM-CSF enhancement of, 459
  LIF, stimulation of, 378
  regulation by cAMP, cGMP, 316
  TNF, IL-1 and IL-2, effects on, 426–427
Delayed hypersensitivity, basophil infiltration, 176–178,198,215
Dermatitis
  basophil infiltration, 176–178,203
  eosinophil, role in, 142
Dermatitis herpetiformis, basophil infiltration in, 178
Dermatomyositis, basophil infiltration in, 179
Desensitization of IgE-mediated histamine release, 286–288
Desensitization, neutrophils, effect of cytokines on, 123
DFP inactivation of LIF, 374
Diacylglycerol (DAG)
  basophils, 280,288
  in neutrophil activation, 13,111–123
  NADPH oxidase, activation of, 52–55
Diapedesis of neutrophil, 17–18
Diazoxide, mast cell cAMP, 307
Differentiation
  basophils, mast cells, 228–235
  eosinophil, 144
  hemopoiesis, role in, 339–347
Differentiation, leukemic cells, G-CSF induction of, 652
Dimethylthiourea, inhibition of cytotoxicity, 23
Dipeptidase, LTD_4 metabolism, 88
Disodium cromoglycate, mast cell cAMP, cGMP, effects on, 307
DNA breaks caused by H_2O_2, $OH^{\bullet}$, 503
Dopamine, neutrophil O_2^-, effect on, 318
Doxorubicin, G-CSF co-administration, 682

Early response genes, fos, myc, TIS-8, GM-CSF stimulation of, 459
ECP, eosinophil, parasite cytotoxicity of, 538
Eczema, basophil infiltration in, 176–178
EGTA inhibition of LIF activity, 375
Ehrlich, Paul
  eosinophil variability, description of, 140
  first description of basophils and mast cells, 169
ELAM-1
  adhesion molecule, 616–631
  tissue injury, role in, 17,19
Elastase
  host defense; tissue injury, 5–20
  in neutrophil primary granules, 5–6
  release by IL-8, 395–400
Elastase release, neutrophil, cartilage degradation, 504,514
Emigration/margination of neutrophils, 351–364
Emphysema, neutrophil, role in, 20
Endocytosis by basophils, 209–211
Endothelial cell growth factor, enhanced by heparin, 274
Endothelial cell-leukocyte adhesion molecule (ELAM), neutrophil adherence and emigration, role in, 352–358
Endothelial cells
  adhesion and inflammation, role in, 616–632
  basophil, mast cell interaction, 245
  effect of LIF on, 380–381
  hemopoiesis, role in, 344–345
  neutrophil adhesion to, 352–360,398

[Endothelial cells]
response to LTB_4, 96–97
tissue injury target, 18–29
Endotoxin
induction of IL-8, 344
neutrophil emigration, effects on, 352
Enkephalin, neutrophil cAMP, cGMP, 314,324
Eosinophil
activation, functions, 137–168
activation by LIF, 382
adhesion and inflammation, role in, 620–627
basophil, mast cell interaction, 222, 245
IL-5 in regulation of, 549–572
Eosinophil cationic proteins (ECP)
eosinophil specific granules, 137
cytotoxicity of parasites, 141
Eosinophil peroxidase (EPO)
in eosinophil specific granules, 137–146
tumor cytotoxicity, 538
Eosinophil-derived neurotoxin (EDN)
in eosinophil specific granules, 137–138
parasite, nerve cytotoxicity, 538
release, stimulation by IL-5, 553
Eosinophilia
allergy, asthma, parasitic infestation, role in, 537
conditions associated with, 141–144
diseases associated with, 537
GM-CSF stimulation of, 675–676
Eosinophilia-myalgia syndrome, eosinophil and tryptophan, role in, 142
Eosiniphilic pustular folliculitis, eosinophil, role in, 142
Epithelial cells, source of IL-1, 354
Epithelium, basophil, mast cell interaction, 245
EPO in hemopoiesis, 638
Erythema multiforme, basophil infiltration in, 178
Erythroid potentiating activity (EPA), hemopoiesis, role in, 346
Erythropoietin (EPO)
hemopoiesis, erythroid cells, 601
hemopoiesis, role in, 340,343
Eserine inactivation of LIF, 374
Esterase activity of LIF, 374
Esthesioneuroblastoma, basophil infiltration in, 178
Estrogens, effect on basophil numbers, 176
Ethanol, neutrophil cAMP, 314,324

F-actin polymerization, GM-CSF, stimulation of, 459–472
Familial polyposis, basophil infiltration in, 178
Fc_γ receptor, neutrophil
effect on cytokines on, 125
increased expression by IFN-γ, 438,451
in neutrophil activation, 108,116
NADPH oxidase activation, 53
mediation of phagocytosis; LIF augmentation of, 381
Fc I, III receptors, neutrophils, expression, effect of IFN-γ, 354
Fc receptor, eosinophil, 139–140
Fc_ε receptor, basophil degranulation, 187
Fc_γ II-receptor, basophil histamine release, 275
Fenton reaction, hydroxyl ion formation, 9
Fes protooncogene, hemopoiesis, role in, 342
Fever, GM-CSF, side effect, 678–686
Fibrinogen, adhesion molecule, ligand for, 616–619
Fibroblasts
hemopoiesis, role in, 344–345
IL-8, source of, 354,406–409
Fibronectin, adhesion molecule, ligand for, 616–629
Fibrosarcoma, virus-induced, basophil degranulation in, 215
Fibrosis, basophil infiltration in, 178–179
FLAP
5-lipoxygenase, translocation of, 82
structure and function, 88–93

Fluoride, neutrophil cAMP, 314
FMLP
basophil degranulation, 187–188,211–215,237–240,275–281
effects on pH, 491
eosinophil chemotaxis, 147
LT synthesis stimulation, 94
neutrophil activation, 6–12,109–124,423–432
neutrophil activation and cAMP inhibition of, 315–318
neutrophil calcium, chemotaxis, stimulation of, 375–380
neutrophil chemoattractant, activation, 9,12,22,52,358–361,387–401,442
FMLP activation of neutrophils, GM-CSF augmentation of, 467–468
FMLP receptor expression, neutrophil,
G-CSF enhancement of, 652
GM-CSF stimulation of, 459,486–489
Follicle stimulating hormone (FSH), hemopoiesis, role in, 346
Forskolin
basophil histamine release, inhibition of, 304
mast cell, neutrophil cAMP, 307,314
Forssman glycolipid, fibroblast, mast cell interaction, 245
Fungi killing by neutrophils, IFN-γ, enhanced by, 447–448
Fura-2, inhibition of LIF activity, 375

G-CSF
clinical use, 637–649,653–658,671–676
effect on neutrophil functions, 125
hemopoiesis, role in, 4,340–345,638,651
neutrophil emigration, stimulation of, 354–361
preclinical studies, 653
side effects and toxicities, 673–675
structure, molecular biology, 651
synthesis by AML cells, 652–653
G-CSF, bone marrow hemopoiesis, 604
G-CSF, osteosarcoma growth, stimulation of, 608–610
G-CSF, primates, enhanced neutrophil activities, 639–640
G-protein
basophil activation, mediation of, 279–290
link to LTB_4 receptor, 95
respiratory burst, component of, 47
role in neutrophil activation, 13–14,107–127
G-protein, neutrophil
GM-CSF, stimulation of, 459,466–472,291
mechanism of IL-8 activation, 399–400
Gamma-glutamyl transferase in LTD_4 synthesis, 88
Gelatinase
in neutrophil tertiary granule, 6–8
tissue injury, role in
Glomerulonephritis, neutrophil role in, 508
Glucagon, neutrophil cAMP, 314
Glucocorticoids
effect on cAMP, 307,313
histamine release, inhibition of, 285,290
Glutathione peroxidase, antioxidant, 11–12
Glutathione, tumor, TNF and H_2O_2, sensitivity to, 526
GM-CSF
adhesion molecules, promotion of expression, 615,620–624
cellular sources, 457–458
clinical uses, 637–649,661–670,671–686
effects on neutrophil functions, 109,122–125
eosinophil survival and functions, stimulation of, 144,149
G-CSF production, stimulation of, 652
hemopoiesis, role in, 340–345, 485–486,638
histamine releasing activity, 237–244,578–581
leukopenia induction, 640
mast cell secretion, stimulation of, 243
NADPH oxidase, priming for activation of, 52–54
neutrophil activation, mechanism, 457–498,500

[GM-CSF]
neutrophil cAMP, cGMP, effects on, 314,321
neutrophil differentiation, 4
neutrophil emigration, stimulation of, 354–361
priming of neutrophils, 94,486–487
side effects and toxicities, 471–472,667–668,677
GM-CSF receptor binding, eosinophil, neutrophil, basophil, monocyte, 557–562
GM-CSF receptors in neutrophils, regulation of, 458
GM-CSF, bone marrow hemopoiesis, 604
GM-CSF, eosinophil hemopoiesis, 550–551
GM-CSF, fibroblast proliferation, 603
GM-CSF, neutrophil
activation, synergism with TNF, 427
damage to cartilage increased by, 511
GM-CSF, neutrophil and eosinophil, activation for phagocytosis, cytotoxicity, 639
GM-CSF, primates, enhanced neutrophil activities, 639–640
GM-CSF, tumor cell growth, stimulation of, 606–610
GMP-140 (CD62), adhesion molecule, 616–630
Golgi, mast cell granule synthesis, 195–198,225
Gordon phenomenon, caused by EDN, 138
gp91-phox, respiratory burst, component of, 48
GppNHp
G-protein binding, 110
neutrophil cAMP, 314
Graft rejection, eosinophil, role in, 143
Granules, morphology of basophils, mast cells, 177–186
Granulocyte chemotactic peptide (GCP), IL-8, identity to, 389
Granulocytopenia, GM-CSF in therapy for, 661–668
Granulocytosis
G-CSF stimulation of, 653
[Granulocytosis]
IL-8, response to, 401
Growth stimulating gene product (gro, an oncogene), IL-8, similarity to, 394
GTP
effect on LTB_4 synthesis, 95
G-protein binding, 110,114
NADPH oxidase activation, 52
GTPase
G-protein function, 110–112
in neutrophil activation, 14
LTB_4, stimulation of, 96
GTPγS, mast cell activation, 309
NADPH oxidase, stimulation of, 55
Guanylate cyclase
basophils, mast cells, 302,312
neutrophils, GM-CSF stimulation of, 459

H_2O_2
adhesion molecules, promotion of expression, 615
tumor cytostasis, 525–526
H_2O_2 production, neutrophils, 47
effect of cytokines on, 125
GM-CSF in vivo, stimulation of, 663
IFN-γ, enhanced by, 441
H_2O_2, neutrophil tissue injury and inflammation, role in, 7–29,501–511
Haber Weiss reaction, hydroxyl ion formation, 9
Helminths, cytotoxicity by eosinophils, 138,145
Hemopoiesis (hematopoiesis)
cytokines, effects on, 4,339–340,485,638
effect of cyclic nucleotides on, 321
neutrophil, 2–4
Hemopoietic progenitor cells in blood, G-CSF stimulation of, 672
Heparin
basophils and mast cells, release from, 274
mast cell morphology, 234–245
Hepatocytes, secretion of IL-8, 404–406
Herpes, basophil infiltration in, 179
HETE
as neutrophil second messenger, 111,121–122

[HETE]
basophils and mast cells, production of, 274–275
effects on neutrophils, 98
neutrophil cGMP, 314
HETEs, eosinophil chemotaxis, 147
Histamine
adhesion molecules, promotion of expression, 615
eosinophil chemotaxis, 147
histamine release, inhibition of, 304–308
neutrophil cAMP, 314
Histamine release
basophil, mast cell release, 169–237
effect of cAMP, cGMP on, 301–312
from basophils and mast cells, 274–290
Histamine release, basophil, cytokine stimulation of, 573–586
Histamine release, basophil, IL-3, IL-5, GM-CSF stimulation of, 552
Histamine releasing factors (HRF, HRA, BAF)
cell sources and actions, 574–582,592
leukocyte sources, 226–239
several cell sources, 276
Histamine release, IL-8, stimulation of, 400
Histone, tissue injury, role in, 27–29
HL-60 cells, GM-CSF receptor regulation of, 458
HOC1, product of respiratory burst, 47
HOC1, neutrophil, tissue injury and inflammation, role in, 501–514
Hodgkin's disease
basophil infiltration, 177–178
eosinophil infiltration, 142
GM-CSF in therapy for, 686
HPETE
neutrophil cGMP, 314
product of, and regulation of lipoxygenases, 81–82
Human umbilical vein endothelial cells (HUVEC)
adhesion of neutrophils to, 619
IL-8, source of, 403
Hyaluronic acid, degradation by OH•, HOC1, 502
Hydroxyl radical in host defense; tissue injury, 10–19
Hypodense eosinophils
IL-3 and IL-5 enhancement of change to, 537,553
in eosinophilia, allergy, asthma, 140–142,149
Hypoxanthine, endothelial cell metabolism, 26

ICAM-1 (CD54)
adhesion molecule, 616–631
neutrophil adherence and emigration, role in, 352–361
tissue injury, role in, 17,29
upregulation of expression by LIF, 381
ICAM-2, adhesion molecule, 616
Idiopathic hypereosinophil syndrome
eosinophil, role in, 143
Idiopathic thrombocytic purpurea (ITP), GM-CSF, contraindicated for, 676
IFN
eosinophil activation, role in, 535–547
sources, inducers, 536
IFN production, monocytes, GM-CSF in vivo, effects on, 679
IFN receptors, leukocytes, 535
IFN-α
effects on neutrophil functions, 125
hemopoiesis, role in, 346
histamine releasing activity, 578–580
IFN-α, IFN-β
IL-1 production, stimulation of, 353
IFN-β, hemopoiesis, role in, 346
IFN-β, eosinophil IgG Fc receptors, 537–539
IFN-γ
adhesion molecules, promotion of expression, 615,623
basophil secretion, 239–244,290
IFN-γ
binding of lymphocytes to endothelium increased by, 541–543
effects on neutrophil functions, 125–126
hemopoiesis, role in, 340,346
histamine releasing activity, 578–580

inhibition of eosinophil degranulation, 149
mast cell secretion, stimulation of, 243
MHC-II, induction of, 541–543
neutrophil emigration, stimulation of, 358,361
neutrophil functions, effects on, 437–456,500
no effect on LT biosynthesis, 94
priming neutrophils for respiratory burst, 54
IFN-γ receptors, neutrophils, 449
lack of effect on calcium, PL-C activation, 443
mechanism of activation, 449–452IFN-
IFN-γ, monocytes
complement components increased by, 540
Ig supergene family, adhesion molecules, 616
IgA, association with asthma, eosinophils, degranulation, 146–148
IgA Fc receptor expression, GM-CSF, stimulation of, 459,461
IgA receptor, neutrophil, GM-CSF, augmentation of, 486,489
IgE
basophil release, activation of, 273–289
basophil, mast cell degranulation, 187,229–244
inflammation re adhesion molecules, 615–631
stimulation of EPO release, 146
IgE binding factors, histamine release, role in, 578
IgE Fc-RI, basophils, 588
IgE, Fc_{ε}-RII,
adhesion molecule, homology to, 618–619
eosinophils, platelets, macrophages, 540
IgE production, IFN-γ, IL-4, effects on, 539
IgE receptors, basophil, mast cell degranulation, 169
IgE, basophil, histamine release by cytokines, dependence on, 573–580
IgE receptor structure, 278–279
IgG
basophil release, activation of, 275
NADPH oxidase activation, 52
neutrophil cGMP, 315–316
opsonized RBC, 381
IL-1
adhesion molecules, promotion of expression of, 615,620–621
basophil degranulation, effect on, 238–244
contaminant of IL-8 preparations, 396
eosinophil and mast cell sources, 619
eosinophil enzyme release, 147–148
G-CSF production, stimulation of, 652
hemopoiesis, role in, 340–345,638
IL-8 production, stimulation of, 388–404
mast cell secretion, effect on, 243
neutrophil activation, effects on, 125–126,417–436,500
neutrophil adherence, stimulation of, 381
neutrophil chemotaxis and emigration, effects on, 351–358
neutrophil production, GM-CSF stimulation of, 459
no effect on LT biosynthesis, 94
not chemotactic for neutrophils, 388–420
priming neutrophil for activation of respiratory burst, 54
production by neutrophils, 509
tissue injury, role in, 17,29
IL-1 receptor antagonist, regulation of IL-1 responses, 362
IL-1, basophil, histamine releasing activity, 290,578–580
IL-1, bone marrow, hemopoiesis, 604
IL-1, fibroblasts, stimulation, 603
IL-1, neutrophil, IFN-γ receptors, effect on, 449
IL-1, tumor cells, growth, inhibition of, 607–610
IL-2
adhesion molecules, promotion of expression, 615,621
allergic disease, role in, 621
blood levels in aplastic anemia, 664–666

cancer therapy, with LAK cells, 642
eosinophil, hypodense, conversion to, 621
hemopoiesis, role in, 638,340–345
induction of eosinophilia, 148
neutrophil activation, effects on, 417–436,500
no effect on LT biosynthesis, 94
IL-3
adhesion molecules, promotion of expression, 615,620–628
basophil histamine releasing activity, 286–290,578–580,589–595
basophilopoiesis, 588–589,595
G-CSF production, stimulation of, 652
hemopoiesis, role in, 340,343,638
mast cell secretion, effect on, 243
IL-3, neutrophil differentiation, 4
IL-3 infusion, basophil degranulation, 175,205–245
IL-3 receptor binding, eosinophil, neutrophil, basophil, monocyte, 557–562
IL-3, bone marrow, hemopoiesis, 604
IL-3, eosinophil
change to hypodense form, effects on, 537
degranulation and survival, stimulation of, 147
hemopoiesis, promotion of, 144,148,550–551
killing of *Shistosoma mansoni* enhanced by, 537
survival, histamine release, 622
IL-3, osteosarcoma and breast carcinoma growth, inhibition of, 608–610
IL-4
adhesion molecules, promotion of expression, 615,621–631
G-CSF production, stimulation of, 652
hemopoiesis, role in, 340–345,604, 638
mast cell secretion, effect on, 241–244
neutrophil functions, effects on, 500
IL-4, eosinophil
degranulation and cytotoxicity, inhibition by, 553
[IL-4, eosinophil]
IgG Fc-R, reduction of, 554
IL-4, osteosarcoma growth, stimulation of, 608–610
IL-5
adhesion molecules, promotion of expression, 615,620–626
basophil secretion, effect on, 229,239–244
cell sources, 563
gene expression, 562–565
hemopoiesis, role in, 340,343,638
mast cell secretion, stimulation of, 243
IL-5 receptor binding, eosinophil, neutrophil, basophil, monocyte, 557–562
IL-5, eosinophil
change to hypodense form, effects on, 537
chemotaxis, activation, 146
degranulation and survival, stimulation of, 148–149
regulation of function by, 551–556
regulation of hemopoiesis by, 549–555,604
IL-6
adhesion molecules, promotion of expression, 615,623
G-CSF production, stimulation of, 652
hemopoiesis, role in, 340,345,605,638
hepatocytes, acute phase proteins, 603
mast cell secretion, effect on, 241–243
neutrophil differentiation, 4
neutrophil functions, effects on, 500
tumor cell growth, stimulation and inhibition of, 607
IL-7
adhesion molecules, promotion of expression, 615,623
hemopoiesis, role in, 340,605,638
IL-8 (NAP-1)
adhesion molecules, promotion of expression, 615, 623
basophil histamine releasing activity, 578–581
cellular origin, 402–406
hemopoiesis, role in, 340,344
inflammation, role in, 17

neutrophil chemotaxis and emigration, effects on, 352–361
neutrophil functions, effects on, 386–416,500
neutrophils, T-cells, effect on chemotaxis of, 605
nomenclature, 389
purification and structure, 388–394
stimulation of LT biosynthesis, 94
IL-8 receptors, neutrophil, GM-CSF, effect on, 461
IL-9, hemopoiesis, role in, 340,605,638
IL-10, hemopoiesis, 605
IL-8, similarity to, 393
IL-10, T-cells, inhibition of TNF, IFN-γ production, 605
IL-11, hemopoiesis, 605
Immunosuppresion, bone marrow, ATG, steroids, cyclophosphamide, 661–670
Indoleamine 2,3-dioxygenase, neutrophil, stimulation by IFN-γ, 450–451
Indomethacin
basophil histamine release, effect on, 304
IgE-induced histamine release, regulation of, 277–278
neutrophilia, effect on, 358
Infection, G-CSF therapy for, 639
Infection, bone marrow suppressed cancer patients, G-CSF, GM-CSF, protection from, 680–683
Inflammation
adhesion molecules, role in, 615–636
basophils, mast cells, role in, 169,176
eosinophil role in, 552
GM-CSF role, 638–641
GM-CSF, side effects of therapy, 677
IL-8, role in, 386–408
neutrophil emigration, role in, 17,351–364,499–521
Inhibin, hemopoiesis, effect on, 340,346
Inosine, endothelial cell metabolism, 26
Inositol phosphates, neutrophil, GM-CSF, effects on, 489–490
Insulinoma, basophil infiltration in, 179
Integrins
adhesion molecules, 616–628
expression enhanced by LTB4, 96–97
Interstitial cystitis, basophil infiltration in, 179
Ionomycin, NADPH oxidase, activation of, 52–55
IP_3
basophil activation, role in, 279,281,287
neutrophil activation, role in, 13
neutrophil second messenger, 113–119,125
stimulation of NADPH oxidase, 55
IP_3 kinase regulation in neutrophil, 119
IP_3, mast cell, cAMP, effect on, 309
IP_4 formation in neutrophils, 119–120
Iron
in hydroxyl radical formation, 8–10,23–26
lipoxygenase, 78–79

JE, mast cell secretion, effect on, 243–244
Jones, T.W., first description of eosinophils, 137

K562 cells in assay for neutrophil ADCC, 382,524–525
Kallikrein, mast cells, release by cGMP, 312
Keratinocytes, IL-8, source of, 388–408
Kinetics of lipoxygenase, 79–81

Lactoferrin
hemopoiesis, effect on, 340,347
Lactoferrin, neutrophil
iron-binding, secondary granule, 4–11
OH• production, enhanced by, 501
release stimulated by IL-8, 395–400
release stimulated by LIF, 378
LAD, leukocyte adhesion, migration defect, 617
LAM-1 adhesion molecule, 616–619,624
LAM-1 receptors, neutrophils, GM-CSF effect on, 461
Laminin
adhesion molecule, ligand for, 616–629
in neutrophil tertiary granules, 6
Late phase of allergic reaction, neutrophil role in, 577

Late phase, asthma and allergy, adhesion molecules, role in, 615
Latex, neutrophil cAMP, 315
Legionnaire's disease, basophil infiltration in, 177–178
Leu M5 (P150,95) expression, GM-CSF augmentation of, 489
LeuCAM (β2 or CD18), adhesion molecule, 616
Leukemia
  basophilia, 176
  hemopoiesis, 347
Leukocyte adhesion inhibitor (LAI), IL-8, similarity to, 398
Leukocytosis
  GM-CSF stimulation of, 675–676
  in bacterial infections, 1
Leukokinin, activation by cathepsins, 5
Leukopenia, transient, GM-CSF stimulation of, 676–678
Leukotriene B_4 (LTB_4), chemotactic stimulus for granulocytes, 14
Leukotrienes, formation and actions, 87–89
Levamisole, neutrophil cAMP, cGMP, 314
LFA-1
  adhesion molecule, 616–627
  adhesion molecule, ligand for, 616–631
  G-CSF enhancement of, 652
  neutrophil adhesion, role in, 17
  neutrophil emigration, role in, 357,361
LFA-2, LFA-3, adhesion molecules, 616
Lichen planus bullosus, basophil infiltration in, 179
LIF, effects on neutrophil functions, 373–385
  hemopoiesis, effect on, 340,347
  neutrophil cGMP, 314,321
LIF (HILDA)
  eosinophil chemotaxis and chemiluminescence, stimulation by, 557
  hemopoiesis, 605
  leukemic cell differentiation, 603
Lipoxin synthesis, neutrophil, GM-CSF, stimulation of, 458–466
Lipoxins, actions on LTB_4 receptor, 99
Lipoxygenase
  basophil histamine release, augmentation of, 304
  neutrophil activation, role in, 111
  neutrophil, GM-CSF activation of, 468
  regulation of activities, 77–86
Lipoxygenases, mechanisms of activation, 87–106
Lithium, regulation of IP hydrolysis, 119
Lodoxamide in protection from neutrophils, 24
LPS
  IL-8 production, stimulation of, 388–406
  neutrophil emigration, stimulation of, 360–362
  neutrophil O_2^- activation, cAMP effect on, 316
  priming neutrophils for respiratory burst, 54
LTB_4
  adhesion molecules, promotion of expression, 615
  eosinophil chemotaxis, 147
  NADPH oxidase, activation of, 62–63
  by neutrophil activation, 107–121
  IL-8 effects on, 387–401
  neutrophil adhesion, role in, 17
  neutrophil aggregation, stimulation of, 380
  neutrophil cAMP, effects on, 314–316
  neutrophil chemotaxis, emigration, 358
  release from mast cells, 274–275
LTB_4 receptor, roles in neutrophil activation, 94–96,99
  GM-CSF, effect on, 459,461,468–469
LTB_4 synthesis, neutrophil,
  GM-CSF, stimulation of, 458–459,490
LTC_4
  adhesion molecules, promotion of expression, 615,627
  basophils and mast cells, release from, 187,213,237,274–275,285–290
LTC_4 production by eosinophil, 538
LTC_4, basophil, IL-2 augmentation of secretion, 581
LTC_4 , LTD_4 , LTE_4, cAMP inhibition of release, 306

LTD_4, adhesion molecules,
  promotion of expression, 615
Lupus erythematosus, basophil infiltration in, 176–178
LY83583, neutrophil activation, inhibition of, 321
Lymphocyte, adhesion molecule expression, 630–631
Lymphocyte-T, basophil, mast cell interactions, 238–239,245
Lymphoma, gastric, basophil infiltration, 178,203,215
Lymphotoxin (TNF-β)
  hemopoiesis, role in, 340
  neutrophil chemotaxis, emigration, 354,358
Lysophosphatidylcholine, tissue injury, role in, 27–29
Lysosomal enzyme release, LTB_4 stimulation in neutrophils, 95–97
Lysozyme (muramidase)
  neutrophil secondary granule component, bactericidal, 5–8
  neutrophil release stimulated by LIF, 378

M-CSF
  clinical use, 657
  hemopoiesis, role in, 4,340–345,638
  structure, molecular biology, 655–656
M-CSF receptor (c-fms proto-oncogene product), regulation of, 656
M-CSF, macrophage
  activation for cytotoxicity, 639
  activation for cytotoxicity, cytokine production, 656
Mac-1, adhesion molecule, 616–628
Macrophage inflammatory protein-1 (MIP-1)
  IL-8, similarity to, 393–394
  mast cell secretion, stimulation of, 241–244
Macrophage inflammatory protein 2 (MIP-2), IL-8, similarity to, 394,408
Macrophages
  basophil, mast cell interaction, 245
  source of IL-1, TNFα, 354
Major basic protein (MBP), in eosinophil specific granules, 137–144
Mannitol
  basophil degranulation, 187–188
  inhibition of cytotoxicity, 23
MARCKS, substrate for PKC, 54
Mast cells
  activation mechanisms, 273–299
  adhesion and inflammation, role in, 620–630
  degranulation, 169–271
  regulation by cyclic nucleotides, 305–312
Mastocytosis, 176
MBP, eosinophil, tumor and parasite killing, role in, 538
MCAF, hemopoiesis, role in, 340,344
MDP, neutrophil, cAMP, cGMP, effects on, 314
Melanoma, mast cell degranulation, 203,215
Melanoma growth-stimulating activity (MGSA), IL-8, similarity to, 360,394,407
Metamyelocyte, neutrophil differentiation, 3
MHC class I expression, GM-CSF, stimulation of, 459
MHC-I, MHC-II, adhesion molecule, 616
Microbicidal activity, neutrophil
  GM-CSF, augmentation of, 486
  IFN-γ, enhanced by, 447–448
Migration-inhibiting factor (MIF), mast cell migration inhibition, 226
MIP-1, MIP-2, in hemopoiesis, inflammation, 340,345
MIP-2, IL-8, similarity to, 360
MK-886, inhibition of FLAP translocation, 90
MO-1, neutrophil adhesion, role in, 17
Mo-1 expression, neutrophil, GM-CSF, stimulation of, 459,489
Mobility, chemotaxis, neutrophil, G-CSF, GM-CSF in vivo, effects on, 679
Monensin, IL-8 receptors, inhibition of, 364
Monocyte, IL-1 source of, 351–354
Monocyte chemotactic activating protein (MCAF, MCP-1)
  IL-8, similarity to, 394

Monocyte tumoricidal activity in vivo, GM-CSF stimulation, 681
Monocyte-derived neutrophil activating peptide (MONAP), IL-8, identity to, 389–390
Monocytes
- hemopoiesis, 344–345
- IL-8, source of, 388–409
- NADPH oxidase defect in CGD, 444–447

Monocytopenia, GM-CSF in therapy for, 661–668
Monocytosis, GM-CSF stimulation of, 676
Morphine, skin mast cell release, activation of, 276
MPO, neutrophil, tissue injury, role in, 502–509
Myeloblasts
- G-CSF stimulation of, 672
- neutrophil differentiation, 2–3

Myelocytes
- basophil hemopoiesis, 177–180
- neutrophil differentiation, 3

Myelodysplastic syndrome
- G-CSF stimulation of, 653
- GM-CSF therapy for, 468,640

Myeloid leukemia, G-CSF, GM-CSF, effects on differentiation and growth of, 683–684
Myeloperoxidase (MPO)
- neutrophil primary granule component, 6–10
- neutrophil release by IL-8, 395–400
- tissue injury, role in, 6–10

Myelopoiesis, GM-CSF actions on, 662
Myelosuppression due to chemotherapy, G-CSF stimulation of, 653
Myxedema, increase in basophil numbers, 176

Na^+/H^+ antiport, neutrophil
- effect of cytokines on, 125
- GM-CSF, augmentation of, 460,487

NADPH oxidase, neutrophil
- IFN-γ, enhanced by, 444–452
- IL-8, response to, 396

[NADPH oxidase, neutrophil]
- respiratory burst (O_2^-), 9–10,47–56,111–127

NaF, NADPH oxidase, stimulation of, 52
NAP-1, IL-8, identity to, 387–409
NAP-2, IL-8 (NAP-1), similarity to, 405–407
NAP-2, platelets, homology to HRF, 575–582
NAP-3 (MGSA/GRO), IL-8 (NAP-1), similarity to, 405
NECA, neutrophil functions, inhibition of, 315,318
Nematode, basophil infiltration, 179
Neuropeptide Y, adhesion molecules, promotion of expression, 615
Neutropenia, GM-CSF in therapy for, 661–670
Neutropenia associated with cancer chemotherapy, G-CSF, GM-CSF, effects on, 673–686
Neutrophil
- adhesion and inflammation, role in, 616–626
- basophil, mast cell interactions, 239,245
- emigration, 351–372
- G-proteins, 107–127
- IL-8 activation of, 386–416
- in respiratory burst, 47–56
- leukotriene synthesis and actions, 87–89
- physiological roles, 1–46
- regulation by cyclic nucleotides, 312–325

Neutrophil activating factor (NAF), IL-8, identity to, 389
Neutrophilia
- G-CSF stimulation of, 672
- GM-CSF stimulation of, 675–676

Neutrophilic dermatosis, G-CSF stimulation of, 653
Nippostrongylus brasiliensis, basophil infiltration in, 229
Nitric oxide, neutrophil cGMP stimulation of, 314
Nucleus, distinctive in neutrophils, 1–2

O_2^- production, neutrophil, 47,95
GM-CSF, stimulation of, 458–459,486
tissue injury and inflammation, role in, 501
tumor cytotoxicity, role in, 528
OH˙, neutrophil, tissue injury and inflammation, role in, 501
Oncostatin M, hemopoiesis, cytostasis, effects on, 340,346
Osteosarcoma (MG-63), GM-CSF stimulation of growth, 606–610
Ovulation, decrease in basophil numbers, 176
Oxidative burst, G-CSF, GM-CSF in vivo, effects on, 679
Oxypurinol, protection from neutrophils, 24

P-cells, relation to mast cells, 233–244
p150,95, adhesion molecule, 616–628
neutrophil adhesion, role in, 17
p22-phox, respiratory burst, component of, 48
p47-phox, role in NADPH oxidase, 48–49,58
p67-phox, role in NADPH oxidase, 48–49
PA release, neutrophil, GM-CSF enhancement of, 460,473
PAF
adhesion molecules, promotion of expression, 615,627,631
decrease of proteoglycan synthesis, 510
eosinophil chemotaxis, 147,552
eosinophil degranulation, LTC4, calcium, 149
hypodense eosinophil, stimulation of conversion to, 149
neutrophil chemoattractant, 14,22,357
neutrophils, activation of, 387,432
product of phospholipase action, 53
receptor on eosinophils, 140
release from mast cells, 275
PAF production by eosinophil, 538
PAF release, neutrophil, regulation by cAMP, cGMP, 316
PAF synthesis, neutrophil, GM-CSF, stimulation of, 458–471
PAF, neutrophil, tissue damage enhanced by, 512
Pain, mediation by LTB_4, 98
Pain, bone, G-CSF and GM-CSF, effects on, 673–675,677–678
Parasite killing by eosinophils, 537–539
Parasites
basophil, mast cell maturation, effects on, 230
eosinophils in defense against, 141–145
PDGF, osteosarcoma, growth stimulation of, 609
Pemphigus, basophil infiltration in, 176–178
Pentose phosphate pathway, regulation by cAMP, cGMP, 316
Permeability increasing protein, in neutrophil primary granules, 6
Permeabilization, in neutrophil studies, 14–15
Peroxides, activation of 5-lipoxygenase, 82
Pertussis toxin
histamine release, effect on, 279,285
inhibition of 5-lipoxygenase activation, 82
inhibition of G-protein, neutrophil activation, 13–14
inhibition of Gi, 109
Pertussis toxin, neutrophil
GM-CSF effects, inhibition of, 472–473,491–492
TNF activation, lack of effect on, 430
PGD_2
basophil, mast cell interactions in synthesis of, 245
mast cell cAMP, effects on, 307
mast cells, synthesis and release from, 275
PGE
histamine release, inhibition of, 304–308
neutrophil cAMP, 314
PGE_1, PGE_2,
hemopoiesis, effects on, 347
PGE_2
IL-8 production, inhibition of, 357–361
neutrophils, chemotaxis of (with IL-8), 401–402

PGE_2, neutrophils, GM-CSF
increase of, 466
$PGF_{2\alpha}$, mast cell cAMP,
neutrophil cGMP, effects on,
307,314
PGI_2
basophil histamine release, inhibition
of, 304
neutrophil cAMP, 314
vasodilation, 357
pH changes, neutrophil
GM-CSF effects on, 459,474,491
second messenger role, 116,122
Phagocytosis by neutrophils
bactericidal function, 7
G-CSF, GM-CSF in vivo, effects on,
679
GM-CSF enhancement of, 459
LIF stimulation, 379–381
neutrophil, G protein role, 108,115,125
neutrophils, effect on cAMP, 319
Phosphatidic acid (PA)
formation in neutrophil, 116–121
product of phospholipase, 53
Phosphatidylcholine (PC)
inhibition of 15-lipoxygenase, 83
source of arachidonic acid, 121
Phosphatidylethanolamine (PE), source of
arachidonic acid, 121
Phosphatidylinositol (PI), formation in
neutrophils, 113,120–121
Phosphatidylserine, inhibition of 15-
lipoxygenase, 83
Phosphodiesterase (PDE)
basophil histamine release, regulation
of, 314
cyclic nucleotide regulation, 307,314
effect on enzyme release, 114,117
Phospholipase A_2 (PL-A_2)
histamine release from basophil, mast
cell, role in, 279–281
leukotriene biosynthesis, 89,92
neutrophil activation, 16,111–121
neutrophil, GM-CSF activation of,
466,493
NADPH oxidase activation, role in, 52
regulation by cAMP, 319
Phospholipase C (PL-C)
histamine release from basophil, mast
cell, role in, 279–281
neutrophil activation, 13–14,109–121
neutrophil, FMLP activation of, 488
NADPH oxidase activation, role in, 52
regulation by cAMP, 319
Phospholipase D (PL-D)
histamine release from basophil, mast
cell, role in, 279–281
NADPH oxidase activation, role in, 52
neutrophil activation, 111,114
neutrophil activation, GM-CSF
augmentation of, 460,473,490
Phosphorylation of IgE receptors,
basophil desensitization, 287
Phytohemagglutinin (PHA), basophil,
mast cell maturation, 230,236
PI turnover, inhibition by cAMP, 316
Piecemeal degranulation (PMD), ba-
sophils, mast cells, 169–247
PIP_2
as neutrophil second messenger, 118
formation in neutrophil, 111–124
neutrophil activation, role in, 13–14
PKC
basophil secretion, controversial role
in, 280–289,302
NADPH oxidase, role in activation of,
57
neutrophil activation, role in,
13–14,111–122,316
PKC, HL-60 cells, GM-CSF stimulation
of, 492–493
PKC, neutrophil
FMLP, role in activation by, 488
GM-CSF, no effect on, 467,492–493
in mechanism of IL-8 activation,
399–400
TNF activation, lack of effect on, 431
PLAP, TNF activation of, 470
Plasminogen activator, in neutrophil
secondary granules, 6
Plasminogen activator, neutrophil, in
cartilage degradation, 504–505
Platelet activating factor (PAF) formation
in neutrophil, 107–112
mast cell production and release,
275–279

Platelet basic protein (PBP), IL-8, similarity to, 392,405
Platelet factor 4 (PF-4), IL-8, similarity to, 360,391–393
Platelet glycoprotein IIb/IIIa, adhesion molecule, 616
Platelet synthesis of PAF, LTB_4, cooperation with neutrophils, 470–471
Platelets
basophil, mast cell interaction, 239,245
G-CSF, effects on, 673
Pluripotential stem cell, neutrophil differentiation in, 3
PMA
activation of NADPH oxidase, 52–55
basophil activation, 281–289
inflammation, mast cells, 246
mast cell activation, 308
neutrophil activation, 14–22,314–319
PKC activator, 122
PMA, neutrophil
in endothelial cell killing, 506
in proteoglycan degradation, 505–507
pH, effects on, 491
tumor cytotoxicity, role of O_2^- in, 528–529
PMSF
inactivation of LIF, 374
LIF inactivation, cGMP protection, 321
Pneumocystis carinii, bronchoalveolar eosinophilia in, 143
Polyanthole sulfonate, inhibition of tissue injury, 27
Polycythemia vera, increase in basophil numbers, 176
Polymyxin B, basophil degranulation, effect on, 188
Porphyria, basophil infiltration, 179
Pregnancy, onset of labor, MBP elevated in serum, 144
Primary (azurophilic) granule, neutrophil structure, 2–8
Priming of neutrophils
GM-CSF enhancement of, 459–468
PAF, LTB_4, LPS, FMLP, 460
Progenitor cells
hemopoiesis, 341,342
neutrophil differentiation, 2–4
Progesterones, decrease in basophil numbers, 176
Promyelocytes
G-CSF stimulation of, 672
neutrophil differentiation, 3
Prostaglandin, regulation of neutrophil functions, 108–121
Proteases, tissue injury, role in, 6,20–22
Protein synthesis, neutrophil, IFN-γ stimulation of, 450–451
Proteoglycan, immature mast cells, 234
Proteoglycan synthesis, degradation, TNF-activated neutrophils, effects on, 509–512
Proteoglycan synthesis, inhibition by H_2O_2, 502,504
Proteoglycan synthesis, eosinophil, IL-3, IL-5, GM-CSF stimulation of, 553
Protozoa killing by neutrophils, IFN-γ enhancement of, 447–448
Psoriasis
basophil infiltration, 176–178
IL-8 and neutrophils, roles in, 386–388
Psoriatic scales, IL-8, source of, 388

Raf kinase, neutrophils, GM-CSF enhancement of, 466,474–475
Raji tumor cells, cytostasis by neutrophils, 524–527
Random migration, neutrophils, GM-CSF, effect on, 459–461
Rap-1 protoncogene,
NADPH oxidase, role in, 48–49
neutrophil G-protein, 115
Ras protoncogene, neutrophil G-protein, 115
Rat basophilic leukemia cells (RBL), histamine release, 276–290
Renal disease, eosinophil, role in, 143
Respiratory burst (O_2^-), eosinophil, IL-3, IL-5, GM-CSF stimulation of, 553
Respiratory burst, neutrophil
IFN-γ enhancement of, 441
IL-8, response to, 396–400
potentiation by LIF, 378,383

tissue injury and inflammation, role in, 501–514
TNF, effects on, 423–432
RGD, integrin recognition sequence, 617–618,628–629
Rheumatoid arthritis, neutrophils, H_2O_2, HOC1, roles in, 19,502
Rheumatoid synovitis, source of mast cell growth factor, 235
Rhinitis, basophil infiltration, 177–178
Rho, neutrophil G-protein, 115
R020-1724, PDE inhibition, 309,315,318
Rolipram, PDE inhibition, 309,315

Sarcoidosis, basophil infiltration, 179
Sarcoma, GM-CSF in therapy, 674
Scabies, basophil infiltration in, 179
SCF, bone marrow, hemopoiesis, 605
Schistosoma mansoni, cytotoxicity by eosinophils, 139,141,145
Schistosomiasis, basophil infiltration in, 179
SDS, NADPH oxidase, stimulation of, 55
Secondary (specific) granules, neutrophil structure, 2–8
Secondary granules, eosinophil specific granules, 137
Secretion, mast cells, basophils in disease, 207–216
Selectins, adhesion molecules, 616–631
Sertoli cells, hemopoiesis, role in, 346
Serum, neutrophil activation, synergism with TNF, 428
Sezary's syndrome, basophil degranulation in, 203,215
Sialyl-Lewis X determinant, adhesion molecules, 616,625,630
Side effects and toxicities
G-CSF, 673–675
GM-CSF, 667–668,677
SK-MES-1, cytostasis by neutrophils, 524–525
Small granules, eosinophil, 139
Small-cell lung cancer
G-CSF and GM-CSF in therapy, 674
GM-CSF stimulation of growth, 606
SOD, neutrophil, microbicidal activity, inhibition of, 448
Sodium azide, no effect on neutrophil cytotoxicity, 23
Somatostatin
mast cell cAMP, effects on, 307
skin mast cell release, effect on, 276
Sonication, neutrophil hormonal responses, effects on, 313
Soybean trypsin inhibitor, no effect on neutrophil cytotoxicity, 23
Specific granule, source of cytochrome b558, 49
SQ22536, adenylate cyclase inhibition, 318
Staurosporine
histamine release inhibition, 281,285
inhibition of IL-8 effects, 399–400
Steel gene product, hemopoiesis, 603
Stem cells, hemopoiesis, role in, 341,343
Substance P
augmentation of neutrophil responses, 109,124
skin mast cell release, activation of, 276
Substance P, mast cells, adhesion molecules, promotion of expression, 615,629
Superoxide (O_2^-)
host defense; tissue injury, 9–22
MCAF, stimulation of, 345
product of respiratory burst, 47
stimulation by LTB_4, 95,97
Superoxide dismutase (SOD), in oxidative burst, tissue injury, 11–23
Superoxide production
effect of cytokines on, 125,458,486
inhibition by cAMP, 117,316–319
Survivial of eosinophil prolonged by IL-5, GM-CSF, 551–555
Survival of neutrophils, GM-CSF, stimulation of, 459
Synexin, role in neutrophil granule fusion, 16
Synovial cells, IL-8, source of 406–408

T-cells, IL-5 production stimulated by, 563
T-cells, NK cells, activation, 604
T-lymphocytes, hemopoiesis, role in, 344–345

T-lymphocytes, IL-8 and TNF-β source of, 354
TCA3, secretion by mast cells, 243–244
Terfenadine, mast cell cAMP, effects on, 307
Tertiary granule, neutrophil structure, 2
TGF-β
  hemopoiesis, effect on, 340,346
  IL-1, inhibition of, 353–361
  osteosarcoma growth, inhibition of, 609
TH1, TH2 lymphocytes, sources of cytokines regulating eosinophils, 542–543
Thrombocytopenia, G-CSF and GM-CSF effects on, 675–686
Thyrotoxicosis, decrease in basophil numbers, 176
Thyrotropic hormone, decrease in basophil numbers, 175–176
Thyroxine, effect on basophil numbers, 175
Tinea circinata, basophil infiltration, 179
Tissue damage by neutrophils, cytokines, effects on, 499–521
TMB-8, inhibition of LIF activity, 375
TNF
  adhesion molecules, promotion of expression, 615–628
  G-CSF production, stimulation of, 652
  IL-8 production, stimulation of, 403
  neutrophil activation, 417–436
TNF-α
  eosinophil cytotoxicity of parasites, enhancement of, 144
  hemopoiesis, effect on, 340–345
  LTB_4 synthesis, enhancement of, 94
  NADPH oxidase, priming for activation of, 52–54
  neutrophil chemotaxis and emigration, stimulation of, 351–364
  neutrophil functions, effects on, 500
  production by mast cells, 241–244,619
  production by neutrophils, 509
  tissue injury, role in, 4,17,29
TNF-α production, effect of cytokines on, 125
TNF-α production, monocytes, GM-CSF in vivo, effects on, 679
TNF-α,β, neutrophil, proteoglycan degradation enhanced by, 509
TNF-β, neutrophil functions, effects on, 500
TNF-β, neutrophil, proteoglycan synthesis, effect on, 509
TNF receptors, regulation in neutrophils, 418
TNF, neutrophil
  chemiluminescence enhanced by, 513
  IFN-γ receptors, effect on, 449
  increased antimicrobial activity, 420–423
  increased cytotoxicity, 420–423
  priming for respiratory burst, 423–432
  antitumor activity, stimulation of, 523–533
Transferrin (TF)
  hemopoiesis, effect on, 340,347
  iron binding, 11
Transferrin receptor, effect of cytokines on expression of, 125
Transmigration, leukocytes, allergy and inflammation, role in, 617,630–631
Trichinella spiralis, basophil infiltration, 229
Tryptase, mast cells, 274–275
Tuftsin, neutrophil cAMP and cGMP, effects on, 314,321
Tumor cell growth, GM-CSF, effects on, 681
Tumor cells
  G-CSF, GM-CSF stimulation of, 601–614,683–684
Tumor cytostasis by neutrophils, TNF stimulation of, 523–533
Tumor cytotoxicity by mast cells, 244
Tumor cytotoxicity by neutrophils, regulation by cAMP, 316
Tyrosine kinase, NADPH oxidase, regulation of, 58
Tyrosine kinase, neutrophil, GM-CSF, augmentation of, 459,466,474,492–493
Tyrosine phosphatase, NADPH oxidase, regulation of, 58

U937 tumor cells, cytostasis by neutrophils, 524–525
UCLA-SO-M14 melanoma, cytostasis by neutrophils, 524–525

Ulcerative colitis, basophil infiltration, degranulation, 176–178,203,215
Urate crystals, IL-1 production, stimulation of, 353
Uromodulin, IL-1, inhibition of, 361
Uropod, basophil morphology, 228
Urticaria, basophil infiltration, 176–178
UV irradiation, IL-1 production, stimulation of, 353

Vaccinia, basophil infiltration, 179
Vascular permeability mediated by LTB_4, 98
Vasoactive intestinal polypeptide (VIP), skin mast cell release, activation of, 276
VCAM, tissue injury, role in, 29
VCAM-1
  adhesion molecule, 616–628
  ligand for adhesion molecules, 616–628
Viruses, IL-1 production, stimulation of, 353
Vitamin B12 binding protein
  in neutrophil secondary granules, 6
    release by IL-8, 395–400
Vitamin C, antioxidant, 11
Vitamin E, antioxidant, 11
VLA-1, VLA-6, adhesion molecules, 616
VLA-4, adhesion molecule, 616,625
VNR, adhesion molecule, 616,625

W-7, inhibition of NADPH oxidase, 56
WEHI-3 growth factor, identity to IL-3, 234
Whipple's disease, mast cell degranulation in, 203,215

Xanthine, endothelial cell metabolism, 26
Xanthine oxidase, endothelial cell, 24

Zymosan
  neutrophil activation, 22
  neutrophil aggregation, stimulation of, 388
  neutrophil cAMP and cGMP, effects on, 314–316